CU00920300

DIAGNOSTIC IMAGING
SPINE

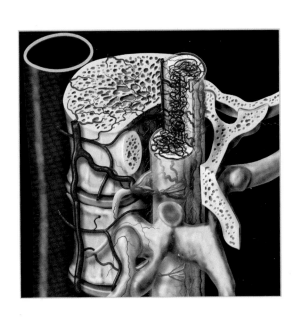

DIAGNOSTIC IMAGING
SPINE

Jeffrey S. Ross, MD

Staff Neuroradiologist
Head, Radiology Research
Cleveland Clinic Foundation

Michael Brant-Zawadzki, MD, FACR

Medical Director
Department of Radiology
Hoag Memorial Hospital
Newport Beach, CA

Stanford University
Volunteer Professor of Radiology
Stanford, CA

Kevin R. Moore, MD

Adjunct Assistant Professor of Radiology
Section of Neuroradiology
University of Utah, School of Medicine

Pediatric Neuroradiologist
Primary Children's Medical Center
Salt Lake City, UT

Julia Crim, MD

Chief of Musculoskeletal Radiology
Associate Professor of Radiology
University of Utah, School of Medicine
Salt Lake City, UT

Mark Z. Chen, MD

Department of Radiology
Hoag Memorial Hospital
Newport Beach, CA

Assistant Clinical Professor
Department of Radiology
UCSF School of Medicine

Gregory L. Katzman, MD

Associate Professor, Neuroradiology
Adjunct Associate Professor, Medical Informatics
University of Utah, School of Medicine
Chief, Radiology VA Hospital
Salt Lake City, UT

AMIRSYS®
Names you know, content you trust®

AMIRSYS®

Names you know, content you trust®

First Edition

Text - Copyright Jeffrey S. Ross, MD 2004

Drawings - Copyright Amirsys Inc 2004

Compilation - Copyright Amirsys Inc 2004

Composition by Amirsys Inc, Salt Lake City, Utah

Printed by Friesens, Altona, Manitoba, Canada

ISBN: 0-7216-2880-X
ISBN: 0-8089-2315-3 (International English Edition)

Notice and Disclaimer

Library of Congress Cataloging-in-Publication Data

Diagnostic imaging. Spine / Jeffrey S. Ross ... [et al.].— 1st ed.
    p. cm.
  Includes index.
  ISBN 0-7216-2880-X
  1. Spine—Imaging. I. Title: Spine. II. Ross, Jeffrey S. (Jeffrey Stuart)

  RD768.D535 2005
  616.7'30754—dc22
                          2004057457

With love to Peg, Whitney, Tyler and Jamie
The ladies in my life

The fear of the Lord is the beginning of knowledge, but fools despise wisdom and discipline.
Proverbs 1:7

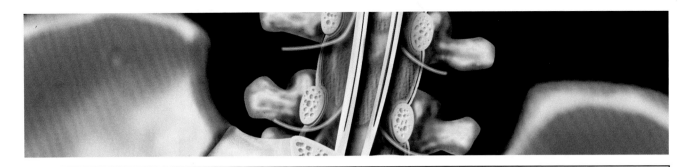

DIAGNOSTIC IMAGING: SPINE

We at Amirsys and Elsevier are proud to present <u>Diagnostic Imaging: Spine</u>, the fourth volume in our acclaimed *Diagnostic Imaging* series. This precedent-setting, image- and graphic-packed series began with David Stoller's <u>DI: Orthopaedics</u>. The next two volumes, <u>DI: Brain</u> and <u>DI: Head and Neck</u> are now joined by Jeff Ross and Michael Brant-Zawadzki's <u>DI: Spine</u>. The current practice of neuroradiology demands expertise in all three core areas. <u>Spine</u>, the last in the neuroradiology "triumvirate," covers the major (and most important minor) diagnoses that affect the axial skeleton, intradural space, spinal cord and peripheral nerves.

Again, the unique bulleted format of the *Diagnostic Imaging* series allows our authors to present approximately twice the information and four times the images per diagnosis compared to the old-fashioned traditional prose textbook. All the *DI* books follow the same format, which means the same information is in the same place: Every time! In every organ system. The innovative visual differential diagnosis "thumbnail" that provides an at-a-glance look at entities that can mimic the diagnosis in question has been highly popular. "Key Facts" boxes provide a succinct summary for quick, easy review.

In summary, *Diagnostic Imaging* is a product designed with you, the reader, in mind. Today's typical practice settings demand efficiency in both image interpretation and learning. We think you'll find the new *Spine* volume a highly efficient and wonderfully rich resource that will complete your core neuroradiology reference books. Enjoy!

Anne G. Osborn, MD
Executive Vice President and Editor-in-Chief, Amirsys Inc.

H. Ric Harnsberger, MD
CEO, Amirsys Inc.

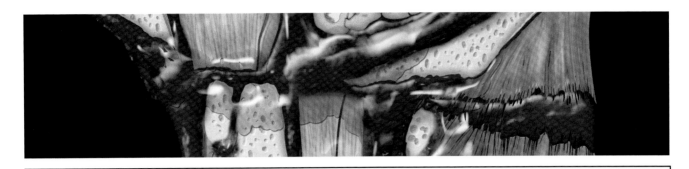

FOREWORD

Signs and symptoms referable to the spine are among the most common reasons for seeking medical attention and stimulus for imaging. While most symptoms are related to self-limiting disorders, they occur across a backdrop of morphologic changes that range from subtle to extraordinarily complex in terms of appearances and differentials. Sorting these considerations out requires more than deciding between normal and abnormal, but also normal and unusual, abnormal but not relevant, abnormal and not much we can do and abnormal and not a moment to lose. Where and when to go next requires one to sort through differential considerations and subsequent options, whether imaging, intervention or tincture of time. The imager in this environment requires a blend of experience and expertise in interpretation, technical knowledge, judgment and common sense. While noble and sought after qualities we all wish to possess in some abundance, in today's world of rapidly evolving technology and new knowledge, we all need quick, accurate and easy to acquire supplemental intelligence. Hence the need for a usable, compact up to date reference that will enable our decision-making. Such a reference companion becomes invaluable in our efforts to move from observation to wisdom.

What lies within is the result of selection, common sense and thoughtful labor. The review of the literature is current and the layout is practical and logical. Not only are the primary disease considerations well illustrated, but the differential considerations as well. A format extremely helpful in the decision making process. This is not a text in the traditional sense and the verbiage has been trimmed to the absolute minimum. As one who as always been drawn to dense prose, the format was at first unsettling. If the absence of punctuation and complete sentence is offensive, this text is not for you. If you are fond of word smithing in your medical texts, this format is not for you. If, however, you want data nuggets in lieu of word streams and real life illustrations in lieu of descriptions, you are home free. Succinct bullets, copious illustrations and images are the format. One need not wade through paragraphs to extract information about the disease, differentials, genetics, imaging findings and technical considerations. These are conveyed more succinctly and efficiently than one could possibly expect.

While this is not the text you will curl up with next to a fire on a cold winter night, it is the text you will always keep within arms reach in the reading room.

Michael T. Modic, MD
Chairman, Division of Radiology
Cleveland Clinic Foundation

Chairman and Professor
Department of Radiology
Cleveland Clinic Lerner College of Medicine

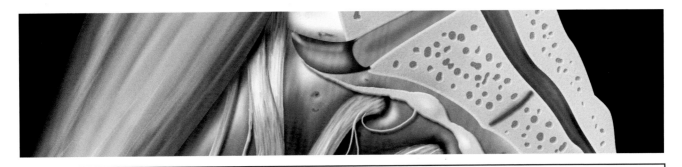

PREFACE

It's about time! Hard to comprehend that 10 years have gone by since I last was co-author on a major spine imaging text. Bifocals, gray hair and innumerable MRI's of degenerated disc disease have occurred, and have been read in the interim. Hanging of film hardcopies has become a rare and rather quaint experience. Voice recognition is now a dictation mainstay. "Hanging chad" is now a part of my vocabulary.

Spine MR imaging has also undergone a gentler evolution typical of a mature technology and sits squarely at the forefront of spinal diagnosis. CT is enjoying another resurgence given multi-detector technology and ease of use of 3D workstations and PACS systems.

With the publication of DI spine, my distinguished co-authors and I are pleased to be part of an evolution in educational textbooks. Gone is the prose, replaced by a tight outline format allowing not only a dense amount of information for each diagnosis, but also the ability to rapidly scan the material for areas of particular interest by well-defined subheadings. There is the highest priority on images, with space for multiple examples of a given pathologic diagnosis.

Diagnoses have been divided into sections, with easy color coding and numbering for quick reference. Differential considerations are highlighted by smaller thumbnail images. Really stressed for time? Try the key facts box for each diagnosis. Integral to the book are the over 130 illustrations, superbly rendered by James Cooper.

Each diagnosis is meant to stand by itself, yet maintain a close integration within the section. The number of unique diagnoses is exhaustive giving the reader an in depth coverage of all the essential diagnoses in a given area of the spine. With this highly structured approach to spine information, the production of a second edition is possible in a much shorter time interval than seen with my previous spine textbook.

I am indebted to my co-authors and to the entire Amirsys team for their dedication and diligence in producing this work. I hope you find this book not only visually pleasing but of real and timely use in your practice.

Jeffrey S. Ross, MD

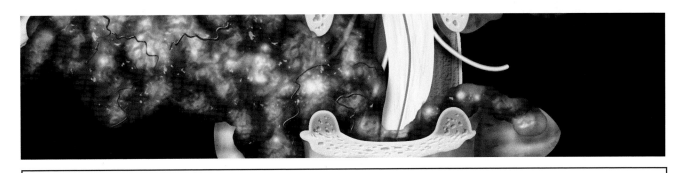

ACKNOWLEDGMENTS

Illustrations

James A. Cooper, MD

Art Direction and Design

Lane R. Bennion, MS
Richard Coombs, MS

Image/Text Editing

Angie D. Mascarenaz
Kaerli Main

Medical Text Editing

Anne G. Osborn, MD
Karen L. Salzman, MD
Richard H. Wiggins III, MD
Akshay Gupta, MD

Case Management

Cassie L. Dearth
David Harnsberger
Roth LaFleur

Production Lead

Melissa A. Morris

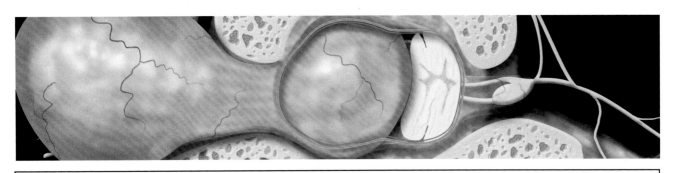

SECTIONS

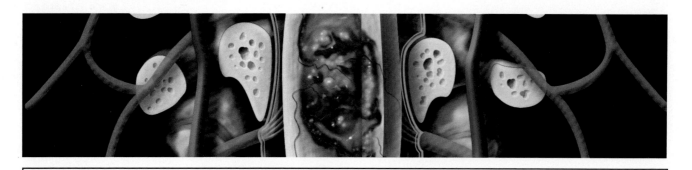

TABLE OF CONTENTS

PART II
Trauma, Degeneration, and Inflammatory Arthritides

SECTION 1
Trauma

Introduction and Overview

Vertebral Column, Discs, and Paraspinal Muscle

SECTION 2
Degenerative Disease and Inflammatory Arthritides

Introduction and Overview

Degenerative Diseases

Inflammatory Arthritides

PART III
Infection and Inflammatory Disorders

SECTION 1
Infections

Introduction and Overview

Infections

SECTION 2
Inflammatory & Autoimmune

PART IV
Neoplasms, Cysts, and Other Masses

SECTION 1
Neoplasms

Introduction and Overview

Extradural

Intradural Extramedullary

SECTION 2
Non-Neoplastic Cysts and Tumor Mimics

PART V
Vascular and Systemic Disorders

SECTION 1
Vascular Lesions

SECTION 2
Spinal Manifestations of Systemic Diseases

PART VIII
Potpourri

SECTION 1
Gamuts

DIAGNOSTIC IMAGING
SPINE

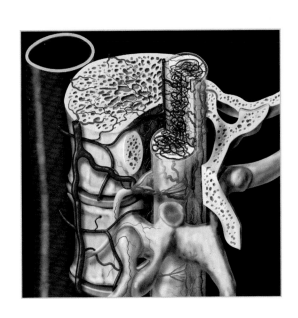

I

1

PART I
Congenital

Congenital and Developmental Disorders 1

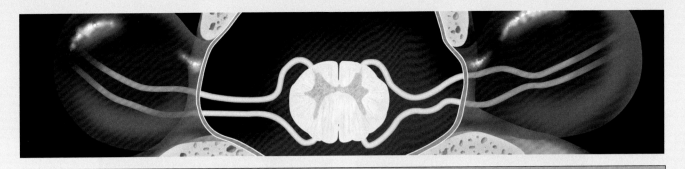

SECTION 1: Congenital and Developmental Disorders

SPINE EMBRYOLOGY

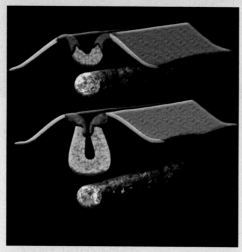

3D graphic shows normal formation of neural plate (top) and neural groove (bottom). Cutaneous epithelium (orange), neural crest (red), neural ectoderm (green), and notochord (gray).

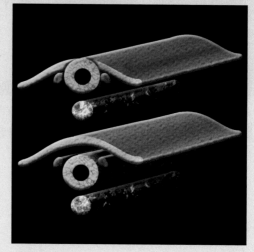

3D graphic shows normal neural tube closure (top) and dysjunction (bottom). Cutaneous epithelium (orange), neural crest (red), neural ectoderm (green), and notochord (gray).

TERMINOLOGY

Definitions
- Canalization and retrogressive differentiation: Development of caudal cell mass into distal spinal cord, filum terminalis
- Canal of Kovalevsky (neurenteric canal): Transient communication of amnion to yolk sac through notochordal canal
- Caudal cell mass: Undifferentiated pluripotential cells that form distal spinal cord/filum
- Closed neural tube defect (closed spinal dysraphism, CSD): Neural elements covered by skin or other cutaneous appendage
  ○ Meningocele, lipomyelomeningocele, myelocystocele, spinal lipoma, dorsal dermal sinus
- Dysjunction - separation of neural tube from overlying ectoderm during neural tube closure
- Neural crest: Origin of peripheral nervous system (PNS)
  ○ Specialized neuroectodermal cells arising between neural tube, cutaneous ectoderm
  ○ Differentiate into sensory neurons of dorsal root ganglia (DRG) and sympathetic/parasympathetic motor neurons of autonomic ganglia
- Neural tube: Origin of central nervous system (CNS)
  ○ Fuses first in cervical region, then irregularly in cephalic and caudal directions
    ▪ Proximal 2/3 → future brain
    ▪ Caudal 1/3 → future spinal cord
- Neurulation: Process of spinal cord formation (cervical → midlumbar segments)
- Notochord
  ○ Cellular rod that defines embryonic primitive axis, provides rigidity to developing embryo
  ○ Induces neuroectoderm → neural tube, neural crest
  ○ Actuates induction of mesodermal germ layer → to spinal axis mesenchymal elements

- Open neural tube defect (open spinal dysraphism, OSD): Neural elements not covered by skin or other cutaneous appendage
  ○ Myelocele, myelomeningocele
- Somites: Paired blocks of solid mesoderm around neural tube
  ○ Dorsolateral somite (dermatomyotome) → skeletal muscles, dermis
  ○ Ventromedial somite → vertebral column cartilage, bone, ligaments
- Spina bifida: Incomplete closure of dorsal osseous spinal elements (spinous processes, lamina)

IMAGING ANATOMY

Anatomic Relationships
- Spine formation includes spinal cord and spinal column development
  ○ Occur simultaneously rather than as separate events
  ○ Begins in future occipital region, subsequently commences at multiple other sites simultaneously
    ▪ Sites progress at different rates, will be at different developmental stages at any given point in time
  ○ Cephalic spinal cord forms via process of neurulation
  ○ Caudal spinal cord forms via canalization and retrogressive differentiation
- End of 2nd gestational week: Bilaminar embryo forms "primitive knot" (Hensen node), adjacent primitive streak
- Beginning of 3rd week: Cardinal event is neural plate appearance during process of gastrulation (transformation of 2 germ cell layer embryo → 3 germ layers)
- Day 16-17: Primitive streak regresses, cells at rostral lip of primitive knot migrate to form notochordal process
  ○ Notochordal process elongates, canalizes → notochord

SPINE EMBRYOLOGY

DIFFERENTIAL DIAGNOSIS

Notochord anomalies
- Split notochord syndromes; dorsal enteric cyst/sinus/fistula/diverticulum, neurenteric cyst
- Diastematomyelia

Premature dysjunction anomalies
- Intradural spinal lipoma (rostral to filum)
- Lipomyelocele
- Lipomyelomeningocele
- Terminal lipoma

Nondysjunction anomalies
- Myelocele
- Myelomeningocele
- Dorsal dermal sinus
- Cervical myelocystocele

Caudal cell mass anomalies
- Caudal regression syndrome
- Filum fibrolipoma
- Tight filum terminale (tethered cord syndrome)
- Terminal myelocystocele
- Anterior sacral meningocele
- Sacrococcygeal teratoma

Vertebral formation and segmentation anomalies
- Hemivertebra, butterfly vertebra, block vertebra, "Klippel-Feil syndrome"

Malformations of unconfirmed mechanism
- Simple (dorsal) meningocele
- Lateral meningocele

- o Transient communication of amnion through notochordal canal to yolk sac (canal of Kovalevsky - neurenteric canal)
- End of 3rd week: Neural fold/groove formation (neurulation)
  - o Neural folds elongate, fuse in midline → neural tube
    - ■ Fusion occurs at multiple sites simultaneously
  - o Temporary openings at cranial and caudal ends (neuropores)
    - ■ Normally close day 25 → 27, signaling completion of neurulation
  - o Notochord induces surrounding paraxial mesoderm derived from primitive streak → paired somite blocks (myotomes, sclerotomes)
    - ■ Myotomes → paraspinal muscles, skin cover
    - ■ Medial sclerotomes → vertebral body, intervertebral disc, meninges, spinal ligaments
    - ■ Lateral sclerotomes → posterior spinal elements
  - o Neuroepithelial cells (neuroblasts) around central tube form mantle layer → spinal cord gray matter
    - ■ Dorsal neuroblasts → sensory neurons
    - ■ Ventral neuroblasts → motor neurons
    - ■ Intermediate horn neuroblasts → sympathetic autonomic nervous system neurons
  - o Outermost spinal cord layer forms marginal layer, myelinates → spinal cord white matter
  - o Central neuroepithelial cells differentiate into ependymal cells along central canal
  - o Neural crest cells appear along each side of neural groove → spinal sensory ganglia (DRG), autonomic ganglia, Schwann cells, meninges (pia, arachnoid), pigment cells, adrenal medulla
- Day 24: Sclerotomal resegmentation begins, continues through 5th week
  - o Caudal half of superior vertebra combines with rostral half of inferior vertebra after split at sclerotomal cleft → "new" vertebral body
    - ■ Intersegmental arteries trapped in center of new vertebral body
  - o Notochord within vertebral body degenerates; intervertebral notochordal remnant → vertebral disc nucleus pulposus

- Day 30: Neural tube development below caudal neuropore commences within undifferentiated caudal cell mass (of primitive streak)
  - o Less precise process than neurulation
  - o Cysts develop in caudal cell mass, coalesce into ependymal lined tubular structure, unite with rostral neural tube
  - o Transient ventriculus terminalis appears (day 43 to 48)
  - o Retrogressive differentiation → caudal conus medullaris, filum terminale
- Days 40-60: Vertebra undergo chondrification (within specific centers)
- About 3rd gestational month, spinal cord extends nearly entire length of developing spinal column
  - o During further development, vertebral column and dura elongate faster than spinal cord, producing apparent shift of terminal cord to higher level
    - ■ Conus near adult level by infancy
  - o Lower spinal nerves (cauda equina) descend obliquely to exit through corresponding vertebral foramen
- After chondrification, vertebral ossification commences (4 distinct centers in vertebral body, vertebral arches), continues through birth into young adulthood

CLINICAL IMPLICATIONS

Clinical Importance
- Abnormal neurenteric canal ⇒ persistent enteric-spinal canal connection (canal of Kovalevsky)
  - o Dorsal-enteric anomalies (neurenteric cyst) spectrum
- Failure of correct neural groove closure 2° teratogen or faulty notochordal induction ⇒ neural tube defect disorders
  - o Myelocele, myelomeningocele
  - o Lower extremity paralysis, associated brain anomalies (callosal dysgenesis, Chiari 2 malformation)
- Failure of vertebral formation, segmentation ⇒ segmentation and fusion anomalies (SFAs)

SPINE EMBRYOLOGY

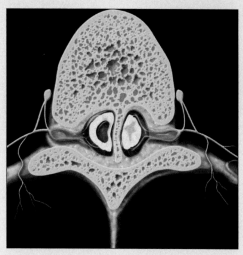

Axial graphic demonstrates type 1 diastematomyelia with large osseous spur connecting vertebral body to posterior elements. Spinal cord is divided into two hemicords, each within a separate dural tube (right hemicord has syrinx).

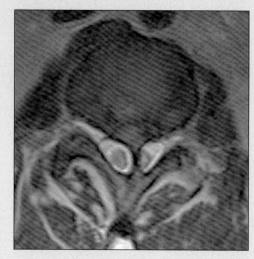

Axial T2WI MR depicts classic type 1 diastematomyelia, with ossified spur dividing dural sac, spinal cord (note syringomyelic left hemicord).

- ○ Butterfly vertebra, hemivertebra, block vertebra
- ○ Scoliosis, respiratory compromise, "Klippel-Feil syndrome"
- • Incomplete primitive streak regression may leave caudal remnant ⇒ sacrococcygeal teratoma
- • Notochordal remnant within posterior vertebral body, clivus, or sacrum may undergo malignant degeneration ⇒ chordoma

- • Vertebral formation and segmentation disorders
  - ○ Hemivertebra, butterfly vertebra, block vertebra
- • Malformations of unconfirmed mechanism
  - ○ Simple (dorsal) meningocele
  - ○ Lateral meningocele

CUSTOM DIFFERENTIAL DIAGNOSIS

Pertinent differential diagnosis

- • Notochordal anomalies
  - ○ Neural plate incompletely splits from notochord
    - ▪ Split notochord syndrome (dorsal enteric cyst/sinus/fistula/diverticulum)
    - ▪ Diastematomyelia
- • Neurulation anomalies
  - ○ Premature dysjunction
    - ▪ Dysjunction prior to neural tube closure permits perineural mesenchyme access to neural groove and ependymal lining → differentiation into fat, incomplete neural tube closure
    - ▪ Intradural spinal lipoma (rostral to filum), lipomyelo(meningo)cele
  - ○ Nondysjuction
    - ▪ Produces focal ectodermal/neuroectodermal tract and prevents mesenchymal migration → focal or widespread dysraphism
    - ▪ Myelo(meningo)cele, dorsal dermal sinus, cervical myelocystocele
- • Caudal cell mass anomalies
  - ○ Faulty caudal cell mass canalization and retrogressive differentiation
  - ○ Insult occurs prior to 4th gestational week
  - ○ Filum fibrolipoma, tight filum terminale (tethered cord syndrome), caudal regression syndrome, terminal myelocystocele, anterior sacral meningocele

SELECTED REFERENCES

1. Larsen WJ: Human embryology. 3rd ed. New York: Churchill-Livingstone. 47-59, 2001
2. Jinkins JR: Atlas of neuroradiologic embryology, anatomy, and variants. Philadelphia. Lippincott Williams & Wilkins. 1-38, 2000
3. Barkovich A: Pediatric Neuroimaging. 3rd ed. Philadelphia: Lippincott-Raven 621-665, 2000
4. Tortori-Donati P et al: Spinal dysraphism: a review of neuroradiological features with embryological correlations and proposal for a new classification. Neuroradiology. 42(7):471-91, 2000
5. Moore K et al: The developing human; clinically oriented embryology. Philadelphia: W.B.Saunders Co. 53-63, 1993
6. Pang D: Sacral agenesis and caudal spinal cord malformations. Neurosurgery. 32(5): 755-78, discussion 778-9, 1993
7. DeLaPaz RL: Congenital anomalies of the lumbosacral spine. Neuroimaging Clinics of North America. 3(3):439-40, 1993
8. Pang D et al: Split cord malformation: Part I: A unified theory of embryogenesis for double spinal cord malformations. Neurosurgery. 31(3):451-80, 1992
9. Sadler TW: Langman's medical embryology. 5th ed. Baltimore: WIlliams and Wilkins, 1985
10. Naidich TP et al: Diastematomyelia: hemicord and meningeal sheaths; single and double arachnoid and dural tubes. AJNR Am J Neuroradiol. 4(3):633-6, 1983

IMAGE GALLERY

Typical

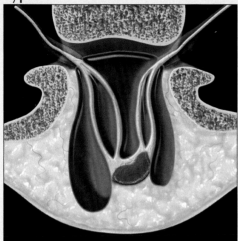 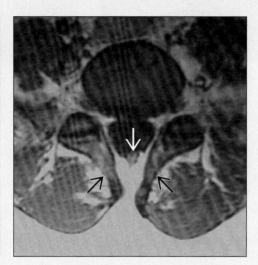

(Left) Axial graphic shows lipomyelomeningocele (premature dysjunction). Neural placode (red) attaches to overlying (skin-covered) fat. Note posterior dysraphism from incomplete neural tube closure. *(Right)* Axial T1WI MR shows wide posterior dysraphism (black arrows), insertion of rotated neural placode (white arrow) into a dorsal lipomatous mass.

Typical

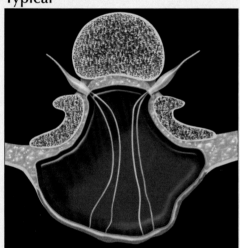 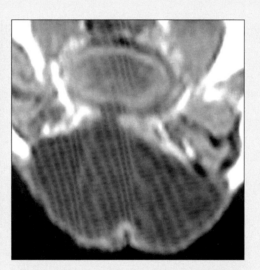

(Left) Axial graphic reveals myelomeningocele, with elongated nerve roots inserting into the exposed dorsal neural placode. Dilated CSF sac is characteristic, and lacks skin covering. *(Right)* Axial T1WI MR reveals unrepaired lumbar myelomeningocele. Neural elements lack skin covering and are in direct contact with environment (Courtesy S. Blaser, MD).

Typical

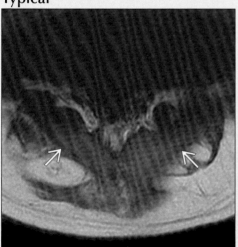 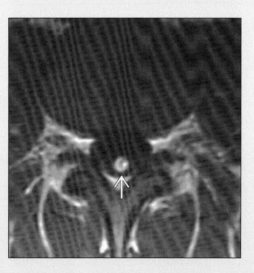

(Left) Axial T2WI MR demonstrates severe caudal regression syndrome, with absence of sacrum and small, dysplastic iliac wings (arrows). *(Right)* Axial T1WI MR reveals filum fibrolipoma (arrow) producing clinical tethered cord symptoms.

CHIARI II MALFORMATION

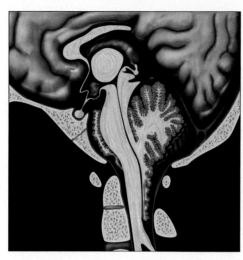
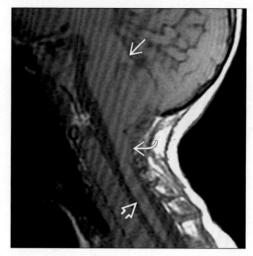

Sagittal graphic shows characteristic findings of Chiari II malformation, including callosal dysgenesis, tectal beaking, small posterior fossa, vermian ectopia, and medullary kinking.

Sagittal T1WI MR depicts classic small posterior fossa with beaked tectum (arrow), vermian ectopia (curved arrow), and a small syrinx (open arrow).

TERMINOLOGY

Abbreviations and Synonyms
- Synonyms: CM 2, Arnold-Chiari malformation type 2 (AC2), Chiari type II

Definitions
- Complex hindbrain malformation
  - Virtually 100% associated with neural tube closure defect (NTD), usually lumbar myelomeningocele (MMC)
    - Rare reports in closed spinal dysraphism; most probably misinterpreted Chiari I

IMAGING FINDINGS

General Features
- Best diagnostic clue: Cerebellar herniation with concurrent myelomeningocele
- Location: Posterior fossa, upper cervical spine; syrinx may involve entire cord
- Size: Posterior fossa smaller than normal
- Morphology: Cerebellum "wraps" around medulla and "towers" through incisura, with beaked tectum and heart-shaped midbrain

Radiographic Findings
- Radiography: Lateral skull ⇒ low torcular herophili +/- "lacunar" skull (universal at birth, largely resolves by 2nd year)

CT Findings
- NECT: Crowded posterior fossa, widened tentorial incisura, tectal beaking, and inferior vermian displacement
- Bone CT
  - Small posterior fossa (PF)
    - Low lying tentorium/torcular inserts near foramen magnum
    - Large, funnel-shaped foramen magnum with "notched" opisthion
    - "Scalloped" posterior petrous pyramids, clivus
  - Posterior C1 arch anomalies (66%), enlarged cervical canal

MR Findings
- T1WI
  - "Cascade" or "waterfall" of cerebellum/brainstem downwards
    - Uvula/nodulus/pyramid of vermis ⇒ sclerotic "peg"
    - Medulla "heaps up" over cord tethered by dentate ligaments ⇒ cervicomedullary "kink" (70%)

DDx: Chiari II Malformation

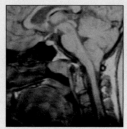
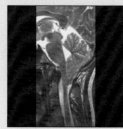
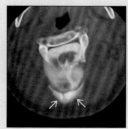
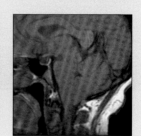

Chiari 1 Malformation

Chiari 1 Malformation

Chiari III Malformation

CSF Hypotension

CHIARI II MALFORMATION

Key Facts

Terminology
- Synonyms: CM 2, Arnold-Chiari malformation type 2 (AC2), Chiari type II
- Virtually 100% associated with neural tube closure defect (NTD), usually lumbar myelomeningocele (MMC)

Imaging Findings
- Small posterior fossa (PF)
- "Cascade" or "waterfall" of cerebellum/brainstem downwards
- Medulla "heaps up" over cord tethered by dentate ligaments ⇒ cervicomedullary "kink" (70%)

Top Differential Diagnoses
- Chiari I malformation
- Chiari III malformation

- Intracranial CSF hypotension
- Severe, chronic shunted hydrocephalus (congenital)

Pathology
- Secondary to sequelae of CSF leakage through open spinal dysraphism during gestation (4th fetal week)

Clinical Issues
- Usually presents within context of known MMC
- Chiari II malformation most common cause of death in MMC

Diagnostic Checklist
- Low torcular herophili indicates small posterior fossa
- CT or MR showing towering cerebellum, downward vermian displacement, +/- brainstem compression diagnostic of Chiari II

- "Towering" cerebellum ⇒ compresses midbrain, causes "beaked" tectum
- 4th ventricle elongated with no posterior point (fastigium)
- ○ Open dysraphism, MMC ≈ 100% (lumbar > > cervical)
- ○ Hydrosyringomyelia (20-90%)
- T2WI
  - ○ Similar to T1WI + hyperintense gliotic brain tissue
  - ○ +/- 4th ventricular lesions (rare)
    - Roof of IV ventricle adjacent/within choroid plexus
    - Glial or arachnoidal cysts, glial or choroidal nodules, subependymoma
- Other MR findings
  - ○ Phase contrast cine MR ⇒ restricted CSF flow through foramen magnum, decreased conus movement

Ultrasonographic Findings
- Real Time
  - ○ Fetal obstetrical ultrasound (US) pivotal for early diagnosis
    - MMC may be identified as early as 10 weeks
    - Characteristic brain findings ("lemon" and "banana" signs) seen as early as 12 weeks

Imaging Recommendations
- Initial screening using MR imaging (brain and spine)
- Follow-up CT or MRI to assess hydrocephalus status; MRI for progressive brainstem or spinal symptoms

DIFFERENTIAL DIAGNOSIS

Chiari I malformation
- No association with myelomeningocele
- Tonsillar herniation (not vermis)

Chiari III malformation
- Chiari II malformation + cervical dysraphism, cephalocele

Intracranial CSF hypotension
- Symptomatic expression of low CSF pressure; distinguishable by clinical onset and symptoms
- Slumping posterior fossa with pons compressed against clivus, dural thickening/enhancement

Severe, chronic shunted hydrocephalus (congenital)
- May cause collapsed brain, upwardly herniated cerebellum

PATHOLOGY

General Features
- General path comments: Hydrocephalus and severity of brain malformation relate to size of PF, degree of caudal hindbrain descent
- Genetics
  - ○ Methylene-Tetra-Hydrofolate-Reductase (MTHFR) mutations associated with abnormal folate metabolism
    - MTHFR mutations PLUS folate deficiency ⇒ ↑ risk NTD ⇒ Chiari II
    - 4-8% recurrence risk if one affected child
- Etiology
  - ○ Secondary to sequelae of CSF leakage through open spinal dysraphism during gestation (4th fetal week)
    - Abnormal neurulation ⇒ CSF escapes through NTD ⇒ failure to maintain 4th ventricular distention ⇒ hypoplastic PF chondrocranium ⇒ displaced/distorted PF contents
    - Exceedingly rare cases of closed spinal dysraphism with Chiari II malformation may contradict this theory
  - ○ Alternative theory proposes association between Chiari II malformation and myelomeningocele is due to rostral and caudal neural tube dysgenesis
- Epidemiology: Incidence: 0.44 per 1,000 births, ↓ with folate replacement therapy
- Associated abnormalities
  - ○ Spine

CHIARI II MALFORMATION

- Open dysraphism (MMC) ≈ 100% (lumbar > > cervical)
  - Posterior arch C1 anomalies (66%)
  - Hydrosyringomyelia (20-90%)
  - Diastematomyelia (5%)
  - Klippel-Feil syndrome
  - Cervical myelocystocele
  - Brain/skull
    - Corpus callosum (CC) dysgenesis (90%), aqueductal stenosis, rhombencephalosynapsis, gray matter malformations, absent septum pellucidum, fused forniceal columns
    - Lacunar skull (lückenschädel)

Gross Pathologic & Surgical Features

- Small PF ⇒ contents shift down into cervical spinal canal
  - Cerebellar hemispheres/tonsils "wrap" around medulla
  - Pons/cranial nerve roots often elongated
  - Compressed/elongated/low IV ventricle ⇒ pouch in cervical canal
  - +/- Hydrosyringomyelia

Microscopic Features

- Purkinje cell loss, sclerosis within herniated tissues

CLINICAL ISSUES

Presentation

- Most common signs/symptoms
  - Neonate: MMC, enlarging head circumference +/- hydrocephalus symptoms
  - Older child/adult: Clinical hydrocephalus, symptoms referable to tethered cord (MMC repair),
  - All age groups: Varying degrees of lower extremity paralysis/sphincter dysfunction/bulbar signs
- Clinical profile
  - Usually presents within context of known MMC
    - Infants: Enlarging head circumference
    - Child/adult: Known Chiari II malformation, signs of hydrocephalus/shunt failure +/- bulbar symptoms
- Laboratory
  - Fetal screening: ↑ α-feto protein

Demographics

- Age: Usually presents at birth with MMC +/- hydrocephalus
- Gender: M = F

Natural History & Prognosis

- Chiari II malformation most common cause of death in MMC
  - Brainstem compression/hydrocephalus, intrinsic brainstem "wiring" defects
- Progression of spinal neurological deficits is rare; suspect hydrocephalus, associated undiagnosed spinal deformity (diastematomyelia), tethered cord

Treatment

- Folate supplement for pregnant mothers (pre-conception ⇒ 6 weeks post conception) significantly decreases MMC risk

- Surgical management
  - Chiari decompression with resection of posterior foramen magnum, C1 ring
  - CSF diversion/shunting
  - Fetal MMC repair in selected patients may ameliorate Chiari II severity

DIAGNOSTIC CHECKLIST

Consider

- Brain/spinal axis MR to detect presence of Chiari II, assess severity, look for complications

Image Interpretation Pearls

- Low torcular herophili indicates small posterior fossa
- CT or MR showing towering cerebellum, downward vermian displacement, +/- brainstem compression diagnostic of Chiari II

SELECTED REFERENCES

1. McLone DG et al: The Chiari II malformation: cause and impact. Childs Nerv Syst. 19(7-8):540-50, 2003
2. Tubbs RS et al: Chiari II malformation and occult spinal dysraphism. Case reports and a review of the literature. Pediatr Neurosurg. 39(2):104-7, 2003
3. Sener RN et al: Rhombencephalosynapsis and a Chiari II malformation. J Comput Assist Tomogr. 27(2):257-9, 2003
4. McDonnell GV et al: Prevalence of the Chiari/hydrosyringomyelia complex in adults with spina bifida: preliminary results. Eur J Pediatr Surg. 10 Suppl 1:18-9, 2000
5. Ojemann JG et al: Prepontine lesions with chiari II malformation. Report of two cases. Pediatr Neurosurg. 33(3):113-7, 2000
6. Northrup H et al: Spina bifida & other neural tube defects. Curr Probl Pediatr 30:313-32, 2000
7. McLone DG: Hydromyelia in a child with chiari II. Pediatr Neurosurg. 32(6):328, 2000
8. Tulipan N: Intrauterine MMC repair reverses hindbrain herniation. Pediatr Neurosurg 31(3):137-42, 1999
9. Piatt JH Jr et al: The Chiari II malformation: lesions discovered within the fourth ventricle. Pediatr Neurosurg. 30(2):79-85, 1999
10. Nishino A et al: Cervical myelocystocele with Chiari II malformation: magnetic resonance imaging and surgical treatment. Surg Neurol. 49(3):269-73, 1998
11. La Marca F et al: Presentation and management of hydromyelia in children with Chiari type-II malformation. Pediatr Neurosurg. 26(2):57-67, 1997
12. Cama A et al: Chiari complex in children--neuroradiological diagnosis, neurosurgical treatment and proposal of a new classification (312 cases). Eur J Pediatr Surg. 5 Suppl 1:35-8, 1995
13. Shuman RM: The Chiari malformations: a constellation of anomalies. Semin Pediatr Neurol. 2(3):220-6, 1995
14. Ruge JR et al: Anatomical progression of the Chiari II malformation. Childs Nerv Syst. 8(2):86-91, 1992
15. Nishimura T et al: Brain stem auditory-evoked potentials in meningomyelocele. Natural history of Chiari II malformations. Childs Nerv Syst. 7(6):316-26, 1991
16. Peach B: Arnold-Chiari malformation with normal spine. Arch Neurol. 10:497-501, 1964

IMAGE GALLERY

Typical

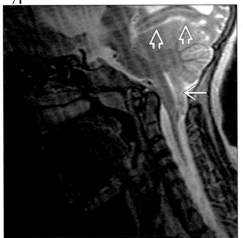 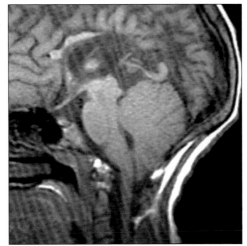

(Left) Sagittal T2WI MR demonstrates typical small posterior fossa with towering cerebellum (open arrows), vermian ectopia (arrow), and enlarged upper cervical canal. (Right) Sagittal T2WI MR reveals relatively mild Chiari II findings including small posterior fossa, minor tectal beaking and vermian ectopia, and callosal dysgenesis.

Typical

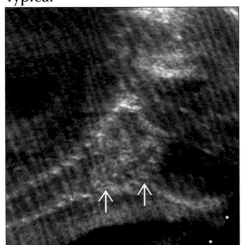 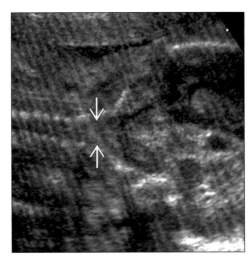

(Left) Sagittal ultrasound real time demonstrates characteristic cerebellar vermis descent into the upper cervical canal (arrows). (Right) Coronal ultrasound real time shows descent of cerebellar vermis (arrows) into the upper cervical canal.

Variant

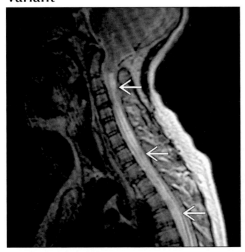 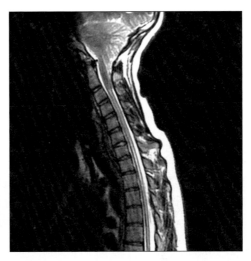

(Left) Sagittal T2WI MR shows relatively mild posterior fossa changes in conjunction with long segment (holocord) syringomyelia (arrows). (Right) Sagittal T2WI MR reveals characteristic Chiari II posterior fossa findings in conjunction with long segment syringomyelia.

MYELOMENINGOCELE

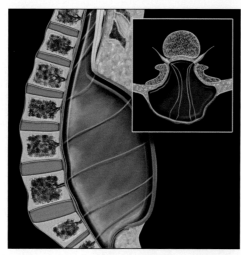

Sagittal graphic shows a patulous dural sac without skin covering protruding through a dysraphic defect. Inset shows wide open dysraphism, with nerve roots dangling from ventral placode.

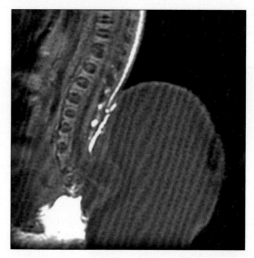

Sagittal T1WI MR depicts a large unrepaired lumbar myelomeningocele, with neural elements protruding into the sac (Courtesy R. Boyer, MD).

TERMINOLOGY

Abbreviations and Synonyms

- Synonyms: MMC, meningomyelocele, open spinal dysraphism (OSD), spina bifida aperta, spina bifida cystica

Definitions

- Posterior spinal defect lacking skin covering ⇒ neural tissue, CSF, and meninges exposed to air

IMAGING FINDINGS

General Features

- Best diagnostic clue: Wide osseous dysraphism, low-lying cord/roots, post-operative skin closure changes
- Location: Lumbosacral (44%) > thoracolumbar (32%) > lumbar (22%) > thoracic (2%)
- Size: Small ⇒ large, depending on extent of neural tube defect
- Morphology: Exposed CSF sac + neural elements protrude through wide dorsal dysraphism

Radiographic Findings

- Radiography
  - Posterior spina bifida with wide eversion of lamina

- Most rostral normal lamina = superior margin of myeloschisis defect
- Myelography: +/- CSF loculations, absence of CSF between placode and dura, low-lying cord

CT Findings

- NECT
  - Wide posterior osseous dysraphism, skin covered CSF sac (post-operative)
  - Associated anomalies, post-operative complications
    - Spine CT: Diastematomyelia spur, dural constriction, or cord ischemia sequelae (abrupt cord termination)
    - Head CT: Hydrocephalus from VP shunt failure

MR Findings

- T1WI
  - Wide spinal dysraphism, flared laminae, low-lying cord/roots; skin covered CSF sac (post-operative)
  - Loss of normal posterior epidural fat segmentation at anomaly level (sagittal imaging)
    - Epidural fat contiguous on two or more adjacent levels ⇒ suspicious for dysraphism
- T2WI: Nerve roots originate from ventral placode surface; ventral roots exit medial to dorsal roots

Ultrasonographic Findings

- Real Time
  - Obstetrical ultrasound ⇒ antenatal diagnosis

DDx: Myelomeningocele

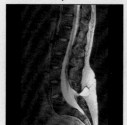

Dorsal Meningocele

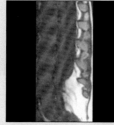

Lipomyelomeningocele

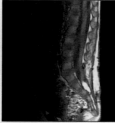

Terminal Lipoma

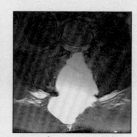

Pseudomeningocele

MYELOMENINGOCELE

Key Facts

Terminology
- Synonyms: MMC, meningomyelocele, open spinal dysraphism (OSD), spina bifida aperta, spina bifida cystica
- Posterior spinal defect lacking skin covering ⇒ neural tissue, CSF, and meninges exposed to air

Imaging Findings
- Best diagnostic clue: Wide osseous dysraphism, low-lying cord/roots, post-operative skin closure changes

Top Differential Diagnoses
- Dorsal meningocele
- Closed (occult) spinal dysraphism
- Post-operative pseudomeningocele

Pathology
- Red, exposed neural placode leaking CSF protrudes through osseous midline defect

Clinical Issues
- Stable post-operative deficit expected → best possible outcome

Diagnostic Checklist
- Imaging untreated MMC rarely indicated
- MMC patients frequently have other CNS abnormalities; neurological deterioration requires assessment of entire craniospinal axis
- Low-lying cord on MR imaging does not always equate to clinical tethering

---

- Open neural arch, flared laminae, protruding myelomeningocele sac, and Chiari II brain findings ("lemon" sign, "banana" sign, hydrocephalus)

Other Modality Findings
- Sagittal cine phase contrast MR ⇒ diminished conus pulsation may indicate tethering

Imaging Recommendations
- Best imaging tool: MR imaging
- Protocol advice
  - Obstetrical ultrasound: Initial MMC diagnosis, delivery planning (Caesarian section), triaging for possible fetal surgery
  - Head CT: Hydrocephalus evaluation
  - MRI: Sagittal and axial T1WI and T2WI; must include entire sacrum

DIFFERENTIAL DIAGNOSIS

Dorsal meningocele
- Meninges protrude through dorsal dysraphism into subcutaneous fat
- Skin covered, usually does not contain neural elements

Closed (occult) spinal dysraphism
- Dorsal osseous dysraphism; cord may be low-lying
- Skin or other cutaneous derivative (e.g., lipoma) covers neural elements

Post-operative pseudomeningocele
- History, clinical exam permit distinction
- Look for surgical laminectomy defect, absence of spina bifida osseous changes

PATHOLOGY

General Features
- General path comments

  - Dysjunction = normal neural tube separation from overlying ectoderm during neural tube closure
  - Open neural tube defects (NTD) arise from dysjunction failure ⇒ neural placode
    - Anterior placode surface ⇒ external pia mater cord surface
    - Posterior placode surface ⇒ internal neural tube ependyma
  - Placode may be segmental or terminal
    - Segmental (lumbar, thoracolumbar, thoracic) ⇒ spinal cord continues distally
    - Terminal (lumbosacral, sacral) ⇒ placode at end of spinal cord
- Genetics
  - Pax 3 paired box gene derangements
  - Methylene-tetra-hydrofolate-reductase (MTHFR) mutations associated with abnormal folate metabolism
    - MTHFR mutations + folate deficiency ⇒ increased risk of NTD
  - Trisomy 13, 18 (14% of NTD fetuses)
- Etiology
  - Lack of complex carbohydrate molecule expression on neuroectodermal cell surface ⇒ failed neural tube closure
  - NTD deficits worsened by chronic mechanical injury, amniotic fluid chemical trauma
- Epidemiology
  - Incidence 0.44-0.6/1,000 live births
  - Maternal folate deficiency, obesity, anti-epileptic therapy (lowers folate bioavailability)
- Associated abnormalities
  - Kyphoscoliosis: Neuromuscular imbalance +/- vertebral segmentation anomalies
    - Developmental (65%): Neuromuscular imbalance, anterior displacement of spinal extensor muscles
    - Congenital (30%): Congenital osseous anomalies (hemivertebrae, bony bar)
  - Diastematomyelia, dermal sinus (31-46%)
    - Cord split above (31%), below (25%), or at (22%) MMC level
    - Hemimyelocele variant (10%) → asymmetric deficits

MYELOMENINGOCELE

- ○ Syrinx (30-75%)
- ○ Chiari II malformation (≈ 100%), hydrocephalus requiring shunting (80%)
- ○ Orthopedic abnormalities (80%); 2° to muscular imbalance

Gross Pathologic & Surgical Features
- Red, exposed neural placode leaking CSF protrudes through osseous midline defect
- Spinal cord always physically tethered; +/- clinical neurologic deterioration

Microscopic Features
- Purkinje cell loss, sclerosis of herniated posterior fossa tissues related to Chiari II malformation

CLINICAL ISSUES

Presentation
- Most common signs/symptoms
  - ○ Stable neurological deficits expected following closure
    - Neurological deterioration ⇒ imaging evaluation for tethered cord, dural ring constriction, cord ischemia, or syringohydromyelia
- Clinical profile
  - ○ Newborn with midline raw, red, exposed neural placode
    - Lesion level determines severity of neurological deficits
    - Hydrocephalus 2° to Chiari II malformation
  - ○ Post-operative: Fixed paraparesis and sensory deficits concomitant with defect level, large heads (hydrocephalus), neurologically induced orthopedic disorders, neurogenic bladder (90%), +/- kyphoscoliosis
- Laboratory findings: Elevated maternal serum alpha fetoprotein (AFP)

Demographics
- Age: Always present at birth
- Gender: M < F (1:3)
- Ethnicity: ↑ Frequency in Irish/Welsh populations (4-8x), families with other affected children (7-15x)

Natural History & Prognosis
- Stable post-operative deficit expected → best possible outcome
  - ○ Hydrocephalus, tethered cord determine prognosis for deterioration
  - ○ Neurological deterioration suggests complication
    - Tethering by scar or second (unrecognized) malformation → most common
    - Constricting post-operative dural ring
    - Cord compression by epidermoid/dermoid tumor or arachnoid cyst
    - Cord ischemia
    - Syringohydromyelia (29-77%)
- Chiari II malformation is the most common cause of death in MMC patients

Treatment
- Folate supplementation to pregnant/conceiving women

- MMC closure < 48 hours to stabilize neural deficits, prevent infection
  - ○ Some tertiary centers perform in-utero surgical repair; may lessen Chiari II, neurological deficit severity
- Subsequent management revolves around treating post-operative complications
  - ○ Cord untethering, hydrocephalus management, treatment of kyphoscoliosis

DIAGNOSTIC CHECKLIST

Consider
- Imaging untreated MMC rarely indicated
- MMC patients frequently have other CNS abnormalities; neurological deterioration requires assessment of entire craniospinal axis
- Cord re-tethering = most common spinal cause of delayed deterioration

Image Interpretation Pearls
- Low-lying cord on MR imaging does not always equate to clinical tethering

SELECTED REFERENCES
1. Johnson MP et al: Fetal myelomeningocele repair: short-term clinical outcomes. Am J Obstet Gynecol. 189(2):482-7, 2003
2. Hirose S et al: Fetal surgery for myelomeningocele: panacea or peril? World J Surg. 27(1):87-94, 2003
3. Rintoul NE et al: A new look at myelomeningoceles: functional level, vertebral level, shunting, and the implications for fetal intervention. Pediatrics. 109(3):409-13, 2002
4. Ertl-Wagner B et al: Fetal magnetic resonance imaging: indications, technique, anatomical considerations and a review of fetal abnormalities. Eur Radiol. 12(8):1931-40, 2002
5. Trivedi J et al: Clinical and radiographic predictors of scoliosis in patients with myelomeningocele. J Bone Joint Surg Am. 84-A(8):1389-94, 2002
6. Bowman RM et al: Spina bifida outcome: a 25-year prospective. Pediatr Neurosurg. 34(3):114-20, 2001
7. Tortori-Donati P et al: Magnetic resonance imaging of spinal dysraphism. Top Magn Reson Imaging. 12(6):375-409, 2001
8. Unsinn KM et al: US of the spinal cord in newborns: spectrum of normal findings, variants, congenital anomalies, and acquired diseases. Radiographics. 20(4):923-38, 2000
9. Tortori-Donati P et al: Spinal dysraphism: a review of neuroradiological features with embryological correlations and proposal for a new classification. Neuroradiology. 42(7):471-91, 2000
10. Barkovich A: Pediatric Neuroimaging. 3rd ed. Philadelphia: Lippincott-Raven, 627-34, 2000
11. Shurtleff DB et al: Epidemiology of tethered cord with meningomyelocele. Eur J Pediatr Surg 7 suppl 1: 7-11, 1997
12. Shaw GM et al: Risk of neural tube defect-affected pregnancies among obese women. JAMA. 275(14):1093-6, 1996
13. McLone DG et al: Complications of myelomeningocele closure. Pediatr Neurosurg. 17(5):267-73, 1991-92

IMAGE GALLERY

Typical

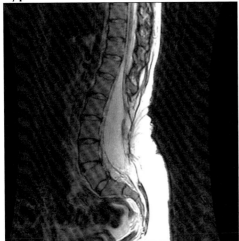
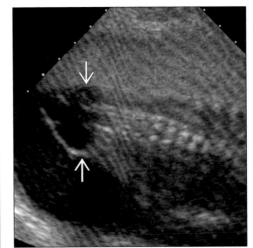

(Left) Sagittal T2WI MR displays the typical post-operative appearance following MMC closure, with patulous sac, tethered cord, and skin covering. *(Right)* Coronal ultrasound real time in utero shows dorsal open dysraphism with complex cystic myelomeningocele (arrows) (Courtesy A. Kennedy, MD).

Variant

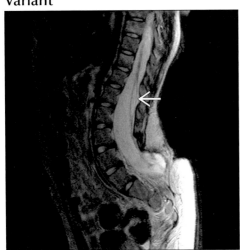
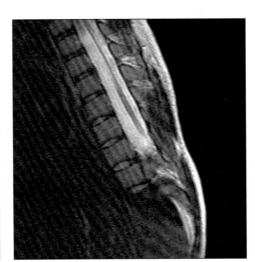

(Left) Sagittal T2WI MR depicts a variant post-operative appearance following MMC closure. Atrophic distal cord is low-lying with terminal syrinx (arrow) (Courtesy G. Hedlund, DO). *(Right)* Sagittal T2WI MR in a patient with repaired lumbosacral myelomeningocele reveals severe caudal regression in conjunction with atrophic tethered cord (Courtesy G. Hedlund, DO).

Variant

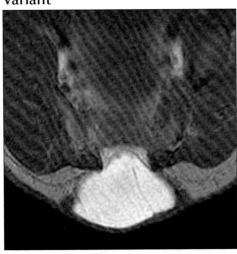
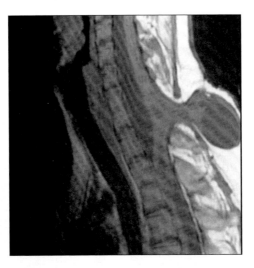

(Left) Sagittal T2WI MR shows a sacral myelomeningocele herniating through a wide dysraphic defect. Sac is not skin covered (Courtesy R. Boyer, MD). *(Right)* Sagittal T1WI MR reveals a thoracic myelomeningocele with dysmorphic cord and syrinx covered by skin (following operative closure).

LIPOMYELOMENINGOCELE

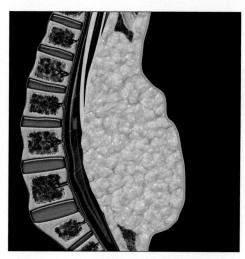

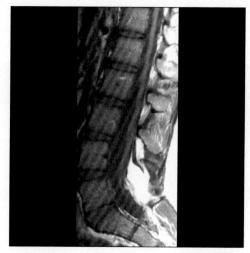

Sagittal graphic shows a low-lying conus with syrinx terminating in a large dorsal lipomyelomeningocele.

Sagittal T1WI MR displays typical features of LMMC, with tethered spinal cord terminating in a large lipoma contiguous with subcutaneous fat through a large dysraphic defect.

TERMINOLOGY

Abbreviations and Synonyms
- Synonyms: LMMC, lipomyelocele (LMC), lipomyeloschisis

Definitions
- Lipomyelocele = neural placode-lipoma complex contiguous with subcutaneous fat through dysraphic defect, attaching to and tethering spinal cord
- Lipomyelomeningocele = lipomyelocele + meningocele, enlargement of subarachnoid space, displacement of neural placode outside of spinal canal

IMAGING FINDINGS

General Features
- Best diagnostic clue: Subcutaneous fatty mass contiguous with neural placode/lipoma through posterior dysraphism
- Location: Lumbosacral
- Size: Skin mass varies from nearly imperceptible ⇒ large
- Morphology: Tethered low-lying spinal cord inserts into lipoma through dysraphic defect

Radiographic Findings
- Radiography: Multilevel dorsal spinal dysraphism +/- hypodense soft tissue mass
- Myelography: Dorsal dysraphism + dilated dural sac; low-lying conus inserts into hypodense lipoma

CT Findings
- NECT
  - Ventral neural placode/tethered cord +/- terminal hydromyelia, cord myeloschisis
  - Hypodense dorsal lipoma is contiguous with subcutaneous fat through posterior spina bifida
- Bone CT
  - Multilevel dysraphism, enlarged canal at placode level

MR Findings
- T1WI
  - Hyperintense lipoma contiguous with subcutaneous fat, tethered cord/placode
    - Herniation of placode-lipoma complex immediately inferior to last intact lamina above dorsal defect
    - Lipoma may be rotated (40%)
    - +/- Intramedullary, intradural, or extradural lipoma - actually occult extension from LMMC rather than discrete second lesion

DDx: Lipomyelomeningocele

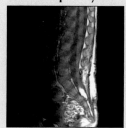

Terminal Lipoma

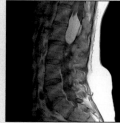

Intradural Lipoma

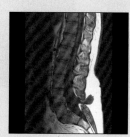

Dorsal Meningocele

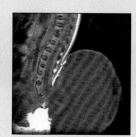

Myelomeningocele

Key Facts

Terminology
- Synonyms: LMMC, lipomyelocele (LMC), lipomyeloschisis

Imaging Findings
- Best diagnostic clue: Subcutaneous fatty mass contiguous with neural placode/lipoma through posterior dysraphism
- Ventral neural placode/tethered cord +/- terminal hydromyelia, cord myeloschisis

Top Differential Diagnoses
- Terminal lipoma
- Intradural (juxtamedullary) lipoma
- Dorsal meningocele
- Myelocele/myelomeningocele

Pathology
- Cord always tethered
- Lipoma may be asymmetric (40%), rotating placode and elongating roots on one side, shortening on other

Clinical Issues
- Soft midline or paramedian skin covered mass above buttocks
- Cutaneous stigmata (50%); hemangioma, dimple, dermal sinus, skin tag, hairy patch

Diagnostic Checklist
- Determination of re-tethering following surgery primarily clinical diagnosis; use imaging to search for complications

---

- ○ Cord tethering +/- myeloschisis, terminal hydromyelia
- T2WI: Hyperintense lipoma; neural elements isointense on background of hyperintense CSF
- STIR: Lipoma → hypointense, confirming fat composition

Ultrasonographic Findings
- Real Time: Echogenic intradural spinal mass contiguous with tethered cord through dorsal dysraphism

Imaging Recommendations
- Best imaging tool: MR imaging
- STIR or chemical fat-saturated techniques confirm fat composition

DIFFERENTIAL DIAGNOSIS

Terminal lipoma
- Lipoma tethers low-lying conus, stretching cord; merges through sacral spina bifida to join subcutaneous fat
- No spinal canal enlargement
- Rotation of lipoma, vertebral segmentation and fusion anomalies (SFA) rare

Intradural (juxtamedullary) lipoma
- Enclosed by intact dura; cutaneous manifestations unusual
- Cervical, thoracic spine most common

Dorsal meningocele
- Skin covered, no lipomatous elements
- More limited dysraphic defect

Myelocele/myelomeningocele
- Clinically obvious open dysraphism; no skin or subcutaneous fat covering, no lipoma

PATHOLOGY

General Features
- General path comments
  - ○ LMC and LMMC are analogous to myelocele and myelomeningocele respectively except that a lipoma is attached to dorsal placode surface and intact skin overlies lesion
  - ○ Cord always tethered
- Etiology
  - ○ Neural tube normally forms by infolding and closure of neural ectoderm as it separates from cutaneous ectoderm during 3rd and 4th week ⇒ neurulation and disjunction
    - In LMMC, premature disjunction of neural ectoderm from cutaneous ectoderm ⇒ mesenchymal tissue direct access to incompletely closed neural tube
    - Mesenchyme is incorporated between neural folds
    - Neural folds remain open, forming neural placode at site of premature disjunction
    - Ependymal lining of primitive neural tube induces mesenchyme to form fat ⇒ lipoma
- Epidemiology
  - ○ 20-56% of occult spinal dysraphism; 20% of skin covered lumbosacral masses
  - ○ Incidence not impacted by folate supplementation to pregnant women (unlike MMC)
- Associated abnormalities
  - ○ +/- Intramedullary, intradural, or extradural lipoma → occult extension of LMMC
  - ○ Butterfly vertebrae, hemivertebrae, fused vertebrae (≤ 43%)
  - ○ Sacral abnormalities (≤ 50%); confluent foramina and partial sacral dysgenesis
  - ○ Anorectal and GU abnormalities (5-10%); if concurrent sacral anomalies → 90%
  - ○ Terminal diastematomyelia (≤ 10%)
  - ○ (Epi)dermoid tumor, dermal sinus, angioma, arachnoid cyst (rare)
  - ○ Arteriovenous malformation (very rare)

LIPOMYELOMENINGOCELE

Gross Pathologic & Surgical Features
- Canal enlarged at placode, spina bifida level
- Lipoma may envelop both dorsal and ventral nerve roots, dorsal nerve roots only, or filum terminale/conus
- Dura deficient at spina bifida zone → does not close neural tube
  - Attached laterally to neural placode, posterior to dorsal nerve roots as they emerge from cord
- Lipoma may be asymmetric (40%), rotating placode and elongating roots on one side, shortening on other
  - Predisposes to operative injury, incomplete tether release

Microscopic Features
- Dorsal placode surface adjacent to lipoma has no ependymal lining; covered by connective tissue mixed with islands of glial cells, smooth muscle fibers

CLINICAL ISSUES

Presentation
- Most common signs/symptoms: Back/leg pain, scoliosis, lower extremity paraparesis, sacral sensory loss, limb atrophy, orthopedic foot deformity, bladder/bowel dysfunction
- Clinical profile
  - Soft midline or paramedian skin covered mass above buttocks
    - Lumbosacral mass: Clinical attention within 6 months
    - No mass: Present when neurological deficits manifest (5 years ⇒ adulthood)
  - Cutaneous stigmata (50%); hemangioma, dimple, dermal sinus, skin tag, hairy patch

Demographics
- Age: Infancy (most common) ⇒ adulthood
- Gender: F > M

Natural History & Prognosis
- Potentially irreversible progressive neurological impairment (cord tethering, enlarging lipoma)
  - Lipoma grows with infant
  - Bladder dysfunction usually persists if not operated early
- ≤ 45% of children neurologically normal at diagnosis
  - 16-88% develop neurological symptoms if left untreated
  - Most symptomatic patients progress if untreated
- Neurologically intact patients at surgery usually remain intact on long term follow-up
- Post-operative exam should not deteriorate with longitudinal growth; neurological decline raises suspicion of re-tethering, warrants repeat imaging
- Symptomatic re-tethering common; weeks to years after initial surgery
  - Median time between initial procedure and reoperation for re-tethering ⇒ 52 months

Treatment
- Early prophylactic surgery (< 1 year of age) to untether cord, resect lipoma, and reconstruct dura

DIAGNOSTIC CHECKLIST

Consider
- Presence/absence of placode rotation important pre-operative information for surgeon

Image Interpretation Pearls
- Determination of re-tethering following surgery primarily clinical diagnosis; use imaging to search for complications

SELECTED REFERENCES
1. McNeely PD et al: Ineffectiveness of dietary folic acid supplementation on the incidence of lipomyelomeningocele: pathogenetic implications. J Neurosurg. 100(2):98-100, 2004
2. Schoenmakers MA et al: Long-term outcome of neurosurgical untethering on neurosegmental motor and ambulation levels. Dev Med Child Neurol. 45(8):551-5, 2003
3. Tortori-Donati P et al: Magnetic resonance imaging of spinal dysraphism. Top Magn Reson Imaging. 12(6):375-409, 2001
4. Bulsara KR et al: Clinical outcome differences for lipomyelomeningoceles, intraspinal lipomas, and lipomas of the filum terminale. Neurosurg Rev. 24(4):192-4, 2001
5. Lee JH et al: Combined anomaly of intramedullary arteriovenous malformation and lipomyelomeningocele. AJNR Am J Neuroradiol. 21(3):595-600, 2000
6. Barkovich AJ: Pediatric Neuroimaging. 3rd ed. Philadelphia, Lippincott, Williams, and Wilkins. 641-646, 2000
7. Kim SY et al: Prenatal diagnosis of lipomyelomeningocele. J Ultrasound Med. 19(11):801-5, 2000
8. Cochrane DD et al: The patterns of late deterioration in patients with transitional lipomyelomeningocele. Eur J Pediatr Surg. 10 Suppl 1:13-7, 2000
9. Iskandar BJ et al: Congenital tethered spinal cord syndrome in adults. J Neurosurg. 88(6):958-61, 1998
10. Wu HY et al: Long-term benefits of early neurosurgery for lipomyelomeningocele. J Urol. 160(2):511-4, 1998
11. Colak A et al: Recurrent tethering: a common long-term problem after lipomyelomeningocele repair. Pediatr Neurosurg. 29(4):184-90, 1998
12. Ball W: Pediatric Neuroradiology. Philadelphia, Lippincott-Raven, 724-725, 1997
13. Chreston J et al: Sonographic detection of lipomyelomeningocele: a retrospective documentation. J Clin Ultrasound. 25(1):50-1, 1997
14. Sutton LN: Lipomyelomeningocele. Neurosurgery Clinics of North America 6:325-38, 1995
15. Kanev PM et al: Reflections on the natural history of lipomyelomeningocele. Pediatr Neurosurg. 22(3):137-40, 1995
16. Herman JM et al: Analysis of 153 patients with myelomeningocele or spinal lipoma reoperated upon for a tethered cord. Presentation, management and outcome. Pediatr Neurosurg. 19(5):243-9, 1993
17. Kanev PM et al: Management and long-term follow-up review of children with lipomyelomeningocele, 1952-1987. J Neurosurg. 73(1):48-52, 1990

LIPOMYELOMENINGOCELE

IMAGE GALLERY

Typical

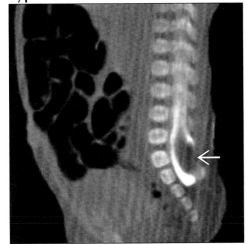
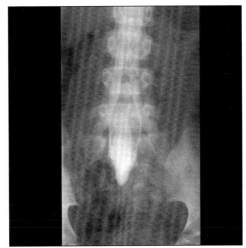

(Left) Sagittal NECT following myelography shows a dilated dural sac and low-lying cord terminating in a large hypodense lipoma (arrow). Subcutaneous fat is contiguous with lipoma through spina bifida. *(Right)* Anteroposterior myelography depicts splitting ("myeloschisis") of a low-lying spinal cord within the dilated distal dural sac.

Typical

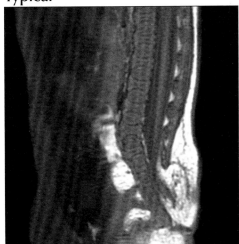
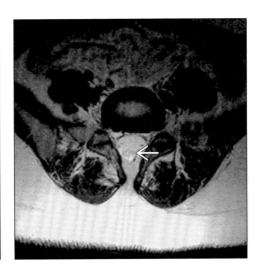

(Left) Sagittal T1WI MR shows a lipomyelocele with tethered cord terminating in a large lipoma contiguous with subcutaneous fat (Courtesy R. Boyer, MD). *(Right)* Axial T2WI MR in LMMC reveals dilation of the distal dural sac, with low-lying cord (arrow) terminating in lipoma contiguous with subcutaneous fat through dorsal dysraphism.

Variant

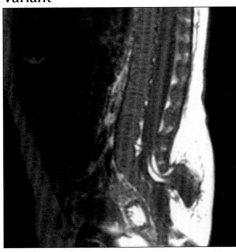
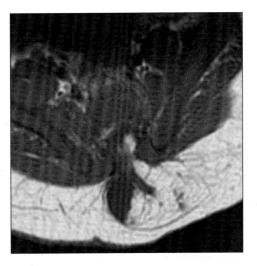

(Left) Sagittal T1WI MR shows a tethered cord terminating in a lipomyelomeningocele. Dural sac protrudes through dysraphic defect with lipoma to merge into subcutaneous fat (Courtesy G. Hedlund, DO). *(Right)* Axial T1WI MR depicts a lipomyelomeningocele with rotated neural placode, dural sac, and lipoma protruding through dorsal defect into subcutaneous tissues (Courtesy G. Hedlund, DO).

SPINAL LIPOMA

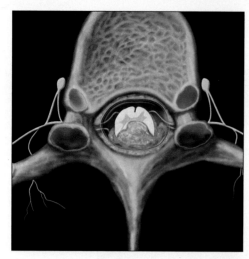

Axial graphic shows incomplete closure of the dorsal spinal cord around a dorsal juxtamedullary conus lipoma, encompassing the dorsal roots.

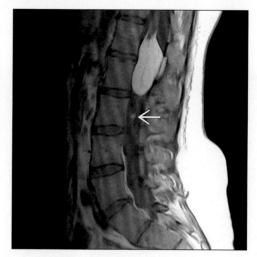

Sagittal T1WI MR shows a fatty intradural mass encircling the conus, producing focal canal enlargement. A small amount of fat is also present within the filum terminale (arrow).

TERMINOLOGY

Abbreviations and Synonyms
- Intradural (juxtamedullary, subpial) or terminal lipoma

Definitions
- Spinal lipoma intimately associated with spinal cord (intradural) or distal cord/filum insertion (terminal)

IMAGING FINDINGS

General Features
- Best diagnostic clue: Hyperintense (T1WI) intradural mass
- Location
  - Intradural
    - Thoracic (30%) > cervicothoracic (24%) > cervical (12%) > lumbosacral spine
    - Dorsal (73%) > lateral/anterolateral (25%) > anterior (2%)
  - Terminal
    - Lumbosacral
- Size: Range: Tiny → huge

- Morphology: Lipoma invaginates into cord substance (intradural lipoma) or tether cord with extension through dorsal dysraphism into subcutaneous fat (terminal lipoma)

Radiographic Findings
- Radiography
  - Intradural lipoma
    - Hypodense mass +/- dysraphism; posterior elements generally intact but show focal canal widening 2° to bony erosion
  - Terminal lipoma
    - Hypodense mass +/- posterior dysraphism
- Myelography
  - Intradural or terminal hypodense mass partially surrounded by hyperdense contrast
  - Large tumors may produce spinal block

CT Findings
- NECT
  - Intradural lipoma: Focal lobulated hypodense intradural mass +/- central canal, neural foraminal widening at lipoma level
  - Terminal lipoma: Elongated hypodense mass at filum termination; may extend into subcutaneous fat through dysraphic defect

MR Findings
- T1WI

DDx: Spinal Lipoma

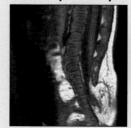

Lipomyelocele

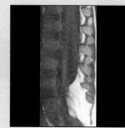

Lipomyelomeningocele

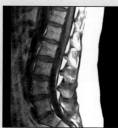

Filum Fibrolipoma

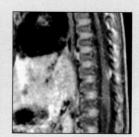

Dermoid Tumor

SPINAL LIPOMA

Key Facts

Terminology
- Spinal lipoma intimately associated with spinal cord (intradural) or distal cord/filum insertion (terminal)

Imaging Findings
- Best diagnostic clue: Hyperintense (T1WI) intradural mass
- Real Time: Echogenic intraspinal mass +/- reduced conus motion

Top Differential Diagnoses
- Lipomyelocele/lipomyelomeningocele
- Filum fibrolipoma
- Dermoid cyst

Pathology
- Composed of normal fat

- Arise from premature separation (dysjunction) of cutaneous ectoderm from neuroectoderm during neurulation

Clinical Issues
- Intradural lipoma: Patient complains of weakness and sensory anomalies referable to lesion level
- Terminal lipoma: Patient presents with clinical appearance of "Tethered cord syndrome" and (frequently) cutaneous stigmata

Diagnostic Checklist
- Profound hypodensity on CT myelography and T1WI hyperintensity distinctively characteristic of lipoma
- Use chemical fat-saturation or inversion recovery MR technique to confirm fat content

---

- Intradural lipoma
  - Lobulated ovoid/rounded intradural hyperintense mass intimately associated with cord
  - +/- Canal widening, local dysraphism
  - ↓ Signal intensity on fat saturation sequences
- Terminal lipoma
  - Hyperintense mass attached to distal cord/filum; extends through lumbosacral dysraphism ⇒ subcutaneous fat
  - Thin, "stretched" cord usually tethered +/- syrinx
- T2WI
  - Similar signal intensity, imaging appearance to T1WI
  - +/- Spinal cord compression (intradural) ⇒ hyperintense cord signal
- STIR: ↓ Signal intensity confirms fat
- T1 C+: No lipoma enhancement

Ultrasonographic Findings
- Real Time: Echogenic intraspinal mass +/- reduced conus motion

Other Modality Findings
- Sagittal PC MRI: Decreased conus motion ⇒ tethered cord

Imaging Recommendations
- Best imaging tool: MR imaging
- Protocol advice
  - Ultrasound in infants for screening; confirm with MRI if positive
  - Sagittal, axial T1WI to define lipoma(s) extent and relationship to neural placode, adjacent tissues
    - Image through tip of thecal sac to avoid missing fibrolipoma or terminal lipoma

DIFFERENTIAL DIAGNOSIS

Lipomyelocele/lipomyelomeningocele
- Skin covered (closed) neural placode-lipoma complex contiguous with subcutaneous fat through dysraphic defect
- Mass often palpable +/- cutaneous stigmata

Filum fibrolipoma
- Common; 4-6% population, mostly asymptomatic but symptomatic patients present with "tethered cord"
- Hyperintense/hypodense mass in filum +/- tethering, low-lying conus

Dermoid cyst
- Mixed density/signal intensity mass; lack of homogeneous hyperintensity +/- dermal sinus help to distinguish

PATHOLOGY

General Features
- General path comments
  - Three main types of spinal lipomas: Intradural, lipomyelo(meningo)cele/terminal lipoma, and filum lipoma
  - Composed of normal fat
    - Fat cells ↑ in size considerably during infancy; tiny lipomas in neonates may grow substantially during infancy
    - Conversely, lipomas ↓ in size if patient loses weight
- Etiology
  - Arise from premature separation (dysjunction) of cutaneous ectoderm from neuroectoderm during neurulation
    - Surrounding mesenchyme enters ependyma-lined central spinal canal, impeding closure of neural folds ⇒ open placode
    - Mesenchyme differentiates into fat
    - Similar mechanism ⇒ dermal sinus tract; explains their frequent association
- Epidemiology
  - Intradural lipoma (4%)
    - < 1% of primary intraspinal tumors
  - Lipomyelo(meningo)cele (includes terminal lipoma) (84%)
  - Filum lipoma (12%)
- Associated abnormalities

SPINAL LIPOMA

- ○ Intradural lipoma: +/- Localized dysraphism at lipoma level; segmentation anomalies rare
- ○ Terminal lipoma: Sacral hypogenesis, anorectal malformations, genitourinary (GU) malformations (5-10%), terminal diastematomyelia, epidermoid, dermal sinus, angioma, arachnoid cyst
  - ▪ Sacral anomalies much more likely if GU, anorectal malformations present (≥ 90%)

Gross Pathologic & Surgical Features

- Intradural lipoma
  - ○ Partially encapsulated sessile (55%) or exophytic (45%) juxtamedullary fatty mass entirely enclosed within dural sac
  - ○ Midline spinal cord "open"; subpial lipoma nestled between open lips
- Terminal lipoma
  - ○ Delicately encapsulated fatty mass attached to cord/filum; frequently contiguous with subcutaneous fat through dorsal lumbosacral dysraphism
    - ▪ Rotation uncommon (unlike LMMC)
  - ○ Cord almost always tethered; stretched and thinned +/- hydrosyringomyelia (20%)

Microscopic Features

- Homogeneous mass of mature fat separated into globules by strands of fibrous tissue
  - ○ +/- Calcification, ossification, muscle fibers, nerves, glial tissue, arachnoid, ependyma

CLINICAL ISSUES

Presentation

- Most common signs/symptoms
  - ○ Cervical, thoracic intradural lipoma: Slow ascending mono- or paraparesis, spasticity, cutaneous sensory loss, deep sensory loss
  - ○ Lumbosacral intradural lipoma: Flaccid lower extremity paralysis, sphincter dysfunction
  - ○ Terminal lipoma: Bowel/bladder dysfunction, lower extremity weakness/sensory abnormality, foot deformity, scoliosis
  - ○ Symptoms may be exacerbated by pregnancy
- Clinical profile
  - ○ Intradural lipoma: Patient complains of weakness and sensory anomalies referable to lesion level
    - ▪ Overlying skin usually looks normal; no cutaneous stigmata
  - ○ Terminal lipoma: Patient presents with clinical appearance of "Tethered cord syndrome" and (frequently) cutaneous stigmata

Demographics

- Age
  - ○ 3 age peaks for presentation
    - ▪ < 5 years (24%)
    - ▪ 2nd → 3rd decades (55%)
    - ▪ 5th decade (16%)
- Gender
  - ○ Intradural: M ≤ F
  - ○ Terminal: M < F

Natural History & Prognosis

- Small lipomas may grow dramatically during infancy
- Symptomatic patients unlikely to improve spontaneously without intervention
  - ○ Caveat: Lipomas may shrink if patient loses weight

Treatment

- Surgical resection, untethering of cord (if applicable)
- Weight loss may be conservative management method to avoid surgery in highly selected obese patients

DIAGNOSTIC CHECKLIST

Consider

- Follow-up even small lipomas in neonates; they may grow significantly!

Image Interpretation Pearls

- Profound hypodensity on CT myelography and T1WI hyperintensity distinctively characteristic of lipoma
- Use chemical fat-saturation or inversion recovery MR technique to confirm fat content

SELECTED REFERENCES

1. Bulsara KR et al: Clinical outcome differences for lipomyelomeningoceles, intraspinal lipomas, and lipomas of the filum terminale. Neurosurg Rev. 24(4):192-4, 2001
2. Tortori-Donati P et al: Magnetic resonance imaging of spinal dysraphism. Top Magn Reson Imaging. 12(6):375-409, 2001
3. Arai H et al: Surgical experience of 120 patients with lumbosacral lipomas. Acta Neurochir (Wien). 143(9):857-64, 2001
4. van Leeuwen R et al: Surgery in adults with tethered cord syndrome: outcome study with independent clinical review. J Neurosurg. 94(2 Suppl):205-9, 2001
5. Barkovich A: Pediatric neuroimaging. 3rd ed. Philadelphia, Lippincott-Raven. 636-640, 2000
6. Unsinn KM et al: US of the spinal cord in newborns: spectrum of normal findings, variants, congenital anomalies, and acquired diseases. Radiographics. 20(4):923-38, 2000
7. Iskandar BJ et al: Congenital tethered spinal cord syndrome in adults. J Neurosurg. 88(6):958-61, 1998
8. Endoh M et al: Spontaneous shrinkage of lumbosacral lipoma in conjunction with a general decrease in body fat: case report. Neurosurgery. 43(1):150-1; discussion 151-2, 1998
9. Ball W: Pediatric Neuroradiology. Philadelphia, Lippincott-Raven, 723-724, 1997
10. Byrne RW et al: Operative resection of 100 spinal lipomas in infants less than 1 year of age. Pediatr Neurosurg. 23(4):182-6; discussion 186-7, 1995
11. Fujiwara F et al: Intradural spinal lipomas not associated with spinal dysraphism: a report of four cases. Neurosurgery. 37(6):1212-5, 1995
12. Aoki N: Rapid growth of intraspinal lipoma demonstrated by magnetic resonance imaging. Surg Neurol. 34(2):107-10, 1990

SPINAL LIPOMA

IMAGE GALLERY

Typical

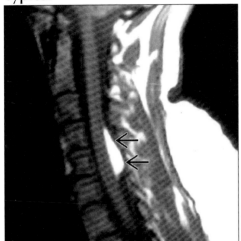
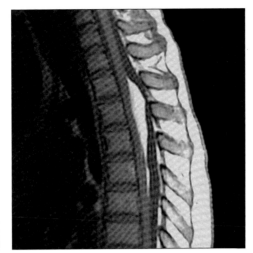

(Left) Sagittal T1WI MR shows an intradural lipoma (arrows) adherent to the dorsal cervical spinal cord (Courtesy G. Hedlund, DO). *(Right)* Sagittal T1WI MR depicts a large intradural thoracic lipoma which invaginates into the dorsal cord surface and remodels the central spinal canal (Courtesy R. Boyer, MD).

Typical

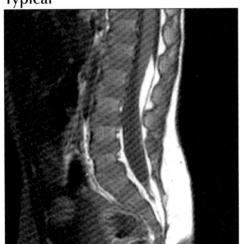
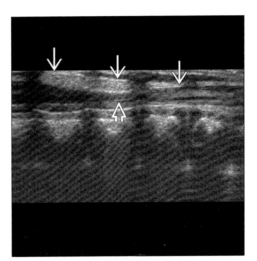

(Left) Sagittal T1WI MR demonstrates a large intradural juxtamedullary conus lipoma with low-lying conus at the L3 level (Courtesy G. Hedlund, DO). *(Right)* Lateral ultrasound real time shows an echogenic dorsal mass (arrows) representing a juxtamedullary lipoma tethering the conus tip (open arrow) at L3 (Courtesy G. Hedlund, DO).

Typical

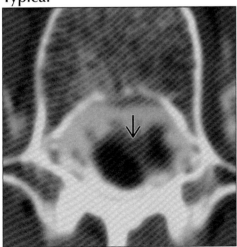
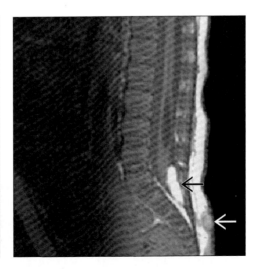

(Left) Axial NECT following myelography reveals a dorsal hypodense subpial lipoma that encircles and distorts the conus (arrow). *(Right)* Sagittal T1WI MR shows a terminal lipoma (black arrow) tethering a low-lying syringomyelic cord. White arrow indicates Vitamin E capsule at skin opening of dermal sinus (Courtesy R. Boyer, MD).

POSTERIOR ELEMENT INCOMPLETE FUSION

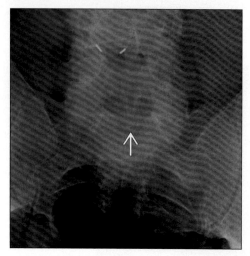

Anteroposterior radiography shows incomplete fusion of the S1 posterior ring. A small ossicle resides within the osseous defect (arrow).

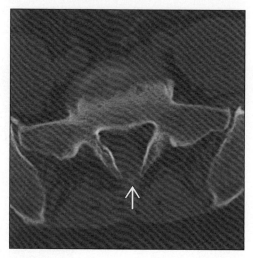

Axial bone CT depicts incomplete fusion of the S1 posterior elements. Ossicle (arrow) within defect is an occasionally noted variant.

TERMINOLOGY

Abbreviations and Synonyms
- Synonym: "Spina bifida occulta"

Definitions
- Spinous process/lamina fusion failure without underlying neural or dural abnormality

IMAGING FINDINGS

General Features
- Best diagnostic clue: Incomplete lumbosacral posterior element fusion
- Location: Lumbosacral junction (L5 > S1) > > cervical (C1 > C7 > T1), thoracic
- Size: Defect usually small
- Morphology: Posterior elements do not fuse in midline; margins are rounded, well-corticated, and may overlap

Radiographic Findings
- Radiography: Unfused spinous process/lamina approximate at midline

CT Findings
- NECT: No abnormal neural, dural, or lipomatous tissue within posterior osseous defect

MR Findings
- T1WI
  - Normal dural sac, conus position, and filum thickness
  - No abnormal neural, dural, or lipomatous tissue within posterior osseous defect
- T2WI: Same as T1WI

Ultrasonographic Findings
- Real Time: Posterior element defect; normal conus level and periodic motion

Imaging Recommendations
- Best imaging tool
  - Plain films most economical screening tool
  - MR best for definitive exclusion of significant underlying abnormality
- Protocol advice
  - Ultrasound for infants with sacral dimples or other cutaneous stigmata
  - Sagittal and axial T1WI, T2WI best screen for tethered cord, neural anomalies

DDx: Posterior Element Incomplete Fusion

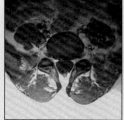

Lipomyelomeningocele

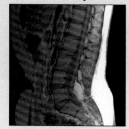

Lipomyelomeningocele

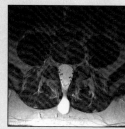

Dorsal Meningocele

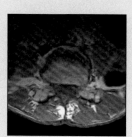

Laminectomy Defect

POSTERIOR ELEMENT INCOMPLETE FUSION

Key Facts

Terminology
- Synonym: "Spina bifida occulta"
- Spinous process/lamina fusion failure without underlying neural or dural abnormality

Imaging Findings
- Best diagnostic clue: Incomplete lumbosacral posterior element fusion

- Location: Lumbosacral junction (L5 > S1) > > cervical (C1 > C7 > T1), thoracic
- Normal dural sac, conus position, and filum thickness
- No abnormal neural, dural, or lipomatous tissue within posterior osseous defect

Top Differential Diagnoses
- Closed spinal dysraphism (CSD)
- Surgical laminectomy defect
- Normal progression of ossification

DIFFERENTIAL DIAGNOSIS

Closed spinal dysraphism (CSD)
- Lipoma, tethered cord, lipomyelomeningocele, dorsal meningocele, dorsal dermal sinus
- Search for clinical cord tethering symptoms, cutaneous stigmata

Surgical laminectomy defect
- Surgical history present; look for incision scar, denervation of paraspinal muscles, laminectomy defect

Normal progression of ossification
- Normal L5 laminae may remain unfused until 5-6 years of age

PATHOLOGY

General Features
- Etiology: Unknown; probably not linked to neurulation process aberrations
- Epidemiology: Up to 30% of US population

Gross Pathologic & Surgical Features
- Non-fused spinous processes and lamina overlie normal dural sac

Microscopic Features
- Histologically normal corticated bone

CLINICAL ISSUES

Presentation
- Most common signs/symptoms
  - Usually asymptomatic if no cutaneous stigmata
  - Occasionally skin dimple on back
    - Dimples within gluteal cleft almost always pilonidal sinuses; need no further evaluation
    - Dimples above gluteal cleft have higher incidence of associated abnormalities; merit further evaluation with MRI
- Clinical profile: Patient presents with low back or leg pain; finding is incidentally noted during imaging

Demographics
- Age: All ages; more common < 40 years of age
- Gender: F > M

Natural History & Prognosis
- Usually incidental finding of no clinical significance

Treatment
- Conservative

DIAGNOSTIC CHECKLIST

Consider
- Incomplete posterior fusion is an incidental finding that is very rarely of neurological significance
  - Plain films economical screening tool, but positive finding rarely significant
  - MR best for definitive exclusion of significant underlying abnormality, but yield is exceedingly low in absence of cutaneous stigmata or neurological deficits

SELECTED REFERENCES

1. Frymoyer et al: The Adult Spine. Vol 2. 2nd ed. Philadelphia, Lippincott-Raven. 1923-1926, 1997
2. Avrahami E et al: Spina bifida occulta of S1 is not an innocent finding. Spine. 19(1):12-5, 1994
3. Boone D et al: Spina bifida occulta: lesion or anomaly? Clin Radiol. 36(2):159-61, 1985

IMAGE GALLERY

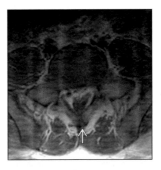 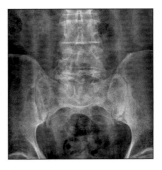

(Left) Axial T1WI MR reveals incidental incomplete posterior fusion (arrow). Osseous margins are rounded and well-corticated. *(Right)* Anteroposterior radiography depicts incomplete fusion of the S1 laminae. This variation demonstrates rotation and overlap of the posterior elements.

DORSAL DERMAL SINUS

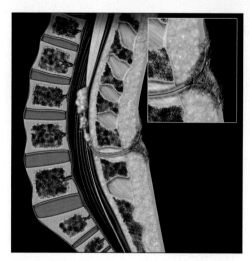

Sagittal graphic shows a dermal sinus extending from skin surface into spinal canal to terminate in an epidermoid. A skin dimple with capillary angioma and hairy tuft marks sinus opening.

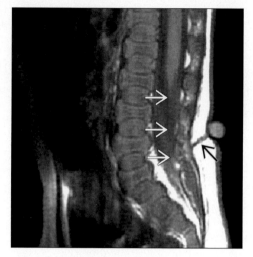

Sagittal T1WI MR shows a typical dermal sinus (black arrow) entering at L4/5 and coursing cranially (white arrows), terminating at the conus. A Vitamin E capsule marks the skin opening.

TERMINOLOGY

Abbreviations and Synonyms
- Synonyms: DST, dermal sinus tract

Definitions
- Midline/paramedian stratified squamous epithelial-lined sinus tract extending inward from skin surface for a variable distance

IMAGING FINDINGS

General Features
- Best diagnostic clue: Hypointense sinus tract superimposed on hyperintense subcutaneous fat
- Location: Lumbosacral (60%) > occipital (25%) > thoracic (10%) > cervical (1%)
- Size: Tract is thin (several mm); length variable
- Morphology
  - Subcutaneous tract +/- dysraphism
  - Length of tract varies short → long; may end in subcutaneous tissue or extend to terminus
    - Terminus usually conus medullaris (lumbosacral lesions) or central spinal canal (cervical, thoracic lesions)

Radiographic Findings
- Radiography: +/- Dysraphism, laminar defect

- Myelography: Dorsal dural tenting +/- (epi)dermoid, nerve root clumping

CT Findings
- CECT: +/- (Epi)dermoid, +/- ring-enhancement (abscess, arachnoiditis), or nerve root clumping (adhesive arachnoiditis; prior infection, (epi)dermoid rupture)
- Bone CT
  - Osseous findings range from normal → groove in lamina/spinous process → multilevel dysraphism

MR Findings
- T1WI
  - Sinus tract hypointense to subcutaneous fat
    - Extraspinal tract passes inferiorly and ventrally to lumbodorsal fascia, turns upward to ascend within spinal canal
  - Dorsal dural tenting indicates → dural penetration
    - Intradural sinus course nearly impossible to follow; indistinguishable from cauda equina, filum
  - +/- (Epi)dermoid cyst
    - Dermoid: Hypo- → hyperintense (fat)
    - Epidermoid: Hypointense
    - Extradural lesions may be subtle; look for nerve root or cord displacement
    - Ruptured (epi)dermoid difficult to detect; look for nerve clumping, CSF "smudging"

DDx: Dorsal Dermal Sinus

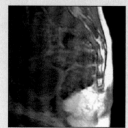

Low Dimple/Tract

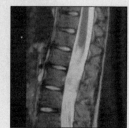

Epidermoid Cyst

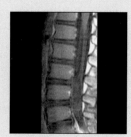

Epidermoid Cyst

DORSAL DERMAL SINUS

Key Facts

Terminology
- Synonyms: DST, dermal sinus tract

Imaging Findings
- Best diagnostic clue: Hypointense sinus tract superimposed on hyperintense subcutaneous fat
- Osseous findings range from normal → groove in lamina/spinous process → multilevel dysraphism
- Dorsal dural tenting indicates → dural penetration
- Lumbosacral sinus ⇒ tethered cord, low-lying conus
- Thoracic, cervical sinuses ⇒ normal conus position

Top Differential Diagnoses
- Low sacrococcygeal midline dimple
- Pilonidal sinus
- (Epi)dermoid tumor without dermal sinus

Pathology
- Focal incorporation of cutaneous ectoderm into neural ectoderm during disjunction at a circumscribed point only ⇒ focal segmental adhesion

Clinical Issues
- Progressive neurological deterioration from cord tethering, (epi)dermoid enlargement, mass effect on spinal cord or cauda equina, sequelae of meningitis/abscess

Diagnostic Checklist
- Dorsal dermal sinus must be differentiated from simple sacral dimple or pilonidal sinus
- Maintain a high index of suspicion for all dimples above intergluteal fold

---

- +/- Tethered cord
  - Lumbosacral sinus ⇒ tethered cord, low-lying conus
  - Thoracic, cervical sinuses ⇒ normal conus position
- T2WI
  - Sinus tract hypointense to subcutaneous fat
  - +/- Hyperintense (epi)dermoid cyst
  - +/- Nerve root clumping (adhesive arachnoiditis)
- DWI: +/- Hyperintense epidermoid cyst
- T1 C+: +/- Intra/extramedullary abscess, infectious or chemical arachnoiditis

Ultrasonographic Findings
- Real Time
  - Shows entire length of tract from skin to spinal cord
    - Subcutaneous tract slightly hypoechoic, hard to detect
    - Echogenic subarachnoid tract clearly demonstrated within anechoic CSF
  - +/- Low-lying conus, thick filum, ↓ nerve mobility, intrathecal mass

Other Modality Findings
- Sagittal phase contrast cine MRI
  - Loss of normal conus pulsation
  - Increased contrast between free-flowing CSF, solid epidermoid tumor

Imaging Recommendations
- Best imaging tool: MR imaging
- Protocol advice
  - Sagittal and axial T1WI, T2WI
    - Adjust window/level to best delineate subcutaneous tract
  - Ultrasound supplements MR in infants < 1 year; use MR to confirm positive ultrasound study

DIFFERENTIAL DIAGNOSIS

Low sacrococcygeal midline dimple
- 2-4% of infants

- Small (< 5 mm), low (< 2.5 cm from anus), extend inferiorly or horizontally toward coccyx
- Usually no associated masses, other cutaneous stigmata

Pilonidal sinus
- Common; nearly always incidental
- Low ostium, do not enter spinal canal

(Epi)dermoid tumor without dermal sinus
- No skin stigmata or sinus tract

PATHOLOGY

General Features
- General path comments
  - Three clinically important types of sinus tracts
    - Low sacral or coccygeal dermal sinuses form embryologically differently; always terminate in sacral or coccygeal fascia and never extend into subarachnoid space
    - Pilonidal sinus: Low ostium, do not enter spinal canal
    - Congenital dorsal dermal sinus + atypical dimple (large (> 5 mm), remote from anus (> 2.5 cm), combined with other lesions)
  - Midline dimple/pit is one of most common referrals to pediatric neurosurgeons
    - Regardless of depth, dimples below top of intergluteal crease end blindly and never extend intraspinally
    - Sinus opening dermatomal level correlates with metameric cord level of attachment
- Etiology
  - Focal incorporation of cutaneous ectoderm into neural ectoderm during disjunction at a circumscribed point only ⇒ focal segmental adhesion
    - Spinal cord ascends relative to spinal canal, stretches adhesion into a long, tubular tract
- Epidemiology
  - Low sacrococcygeal dimple: 2-4% of all infants

DORSAL DERMAL SINUS

- ○ Pilonidal sinus: Common
- ○ DST: Uncommon, midline > paramedian ostium
- • Associated abnormalities
  - ○ (Epi)dermoid tumor (30-50%)
    - ▪ Midline sinus ostia ⇒ usually dermoid
    - ▪ Paramedian ostia ⇒ epidermoid more common
    - ▪ May be multiple; most common at conus
  - ○ Epidural/subdural abscess, meningitis, or intramedullary abscess 2° to staphylococcal or coliform bacteria
  - ○ Lipoma (15-20%)
  - ○ Cutaneous stigmata; angioma, pigment abnormalities, hypertrichosis, lipoma, skin tag, or (rarely) supranumerary sinus tracts

Gross Pathologic & Surgical Features

- • Sinus tract course varies short → long; may terminate extraspinal
- • Intraspinal extension of sinus tract ≥ 50%
  - ○ May terminate in subarachnoid space, conus medullaris, filum terminale, nerve root, fibrous nodule on cord surface, or (epi)dermoid cyst
- • Palpable sinus tract
- • (Epi)dermoid tumor
  - ○ +/- Cheesy, oily material (dermoid) or discrete pearly white (epidermoid) tumor
  - ○ Capsule often adherent to surrounding neural structures

Microscopic Features

- • Sinus tract lined by stratified squamous epithelium
- • Epidermoid: Desquamated epithelium
- • Dermoid: Skin adnexa

CLINICAL ISSUES

Presentation

- • Most common signs/symptoms
  - ○ Asymptomatic; incidentally noted skin dimple
  - ○ Neurological deficits below level of tract secondary to tethering or cord compression
  - ○ Other signs/symptoms
    - ▪ Meningitis, intraspinal abscess (retrograde passage of pathogens)
- • Clinical profile: Atypical sacral dimple with pinpoint ostium, cutaneous stigmata

Demographics

- • Age: Infancy ⇒ 3rd decade
- • Gender: M = F

Natural History & Prognosis

- • Progressive neurological deterioration from cord tethering, (epi)dermoid enlargement, mass effect on spinal cord or cauda equina, sequelae of meningitis/abscess
  - ○ Early surgical intervention ⇒ normal neurological development possible
- • Most important factor influencing outcome is total excision of sinus before development of infection, neural compression

Treatment

- • Surgical excision of sinus tract, tethered cord release, and treatment of complications
- • Long term antibiotics (if infected)

DIAGNOSTIC CHECKLIST

Consider

- • Dorsal dermal sinus must be differentiated from simple sacral dimple or pilonidal sinus
- • Regardless of depth, dimples below top of intergluteal crease end blindly and never extend intraspinally
- • Maintain a high index of suspicion for all dimples above intergluteal fold

Image Interpretation Pearls

- • Critical to identify dermal sinus course and termination for surgical planning
- • Up to 50% of dermal sinuses associated with (epi)dermoid tumor
- • Dural "nipple" on sagittal image indicates dural penetration

SELECTED REFERENCES

1. Tubbs RS et al: Isolated flat capillary midline lumbosacral hemangiomas as indicators of occult spinal dysraphism. J Neurosurg. 100(2):86-9, 2004
2. Ackerman LL et al: Cervical and thoracic dermal sinus tracts. A case series and review of the literature. Pediatr Neurosurg. 37(3):137-47, 2002
3. Lee JK et al: Cervical dermal sinus associated with dermoid cyst. Childs Nerv Syst. 17(8):491-3, 2001
4. Aydin K et al: Thoracocervical dorsal dermal sinus associated with multiple vertebral body anomalies. Neuroradiology. 43(12):1084-6, 2001
5. Shen WC et al: Dermal sinus with dermoid cyst in the upper cervical spine: case note. Neuroradiology. 42(1):51-3, 2000
6. Unsinn KM et al: US of the spinal cord in newborns: spectrum of normal findings, variants, congenital anomalies, and acquired diseases. Radiographics. 20(4):923-38, 2000
7. Chen CY et al: Dermoid cyst with dermal sinus tract complicated with spinal subdural abscess. Pediatr Neurol. 2:157-60, 1999
8. Tindall et al: The Practice of Neurosurgery. Baltimore, Williams and Wilkins, 2760-2764, 1996
9. Gibson PJ et al: Lumbosacral skin markers and identification of occult spinal dysraphism in neonates. Acta Paediatr. 84(2):208-9, 1995
10. Kanev PM et al: Dermoids and dermal sinus tracts of the spine. Neurosurg Clin N Am. 6(2):359-66, 1995
11. Avrahami E et al: Spina bifida occulta of S1 is not an innocent finding. Spine. 19(1):12-5, 1994
12. Herman TE et al: Intergluteal dorsal dermal sinuses. The role of neonatal spinal sonography. Clin Pediatr (Phila). 32(10):627-8, 1993
13. Barkovich AJ et al: MR evaluation of spinal dermal sinus tracts in children. AJNR 12:123-9, 1990
14. HAWORTH JC et al: Congenital dermal sinuses in children; their relation to pilonidal sinuses. Lancet. 269(6879):10-4, 1955

IMAGE GALLERY

Typical

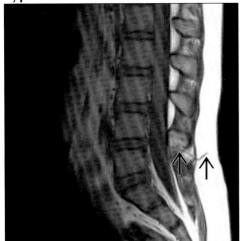
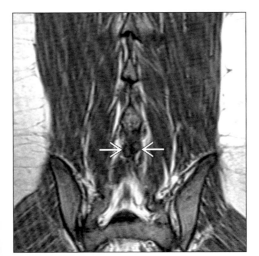

(Left) Sagittal T1WI MR shows a sinus tract (arrows) passing through a bifid L5 spinous process, and tethered cord with low-lying conus at L3/4 (Courtesy R. Boyer, MD). *(Right)* Coronal T1WI MR demonstrates a bifid L5 spinous process (arrows), the point of spinal entry for a dorsal dermal sinus (Courtesy R. Boyer, MD).

Variant

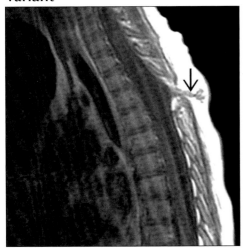
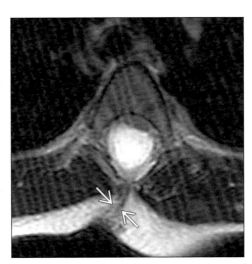

(Left) Sagittal T1WI MR demonstrates a thoracic dermal sinus tract (arrow) terminating in an intradural dermoid tumor. The dura is tented outward at point of sinus tract entry. *(Right)* Axial T2WI MR reveals a double "tram track" sinus tract (arrows) terminating in a hyperintense intradural dermoid tumor. The sinus tract enters the dural sac through a dysraphic defect.

Variant

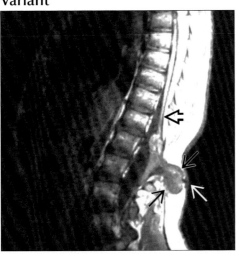
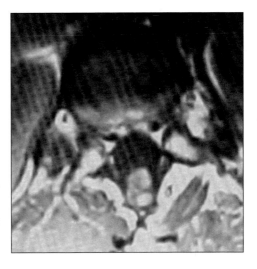

(Left) Sagittal T1WI MR depicts a dermoid tumor (black arrows) within the spinal canal, filling the sinus tract nearly to the cutaneous opening (white arrow) and tethering the low-lying conus (open arrow). *(Right)* Axial T1WI MR reveals a heterogeneous intraspinal dermoid tumor associated with dermal sinus tract. Hyperintense tumor elements reflect fat content.

DERMOID AND EPIDERMOID TUMORS

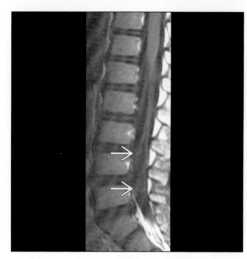

Sagittal T1WI MR shows a hypointense intradural epidermoid within the cauda equina that displaces nerve roots. Arrows demarcate rostral and caudal extent.

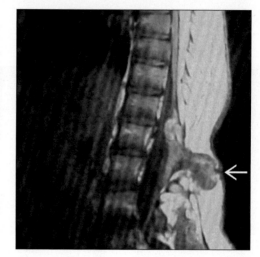

Sagittal T1WI MR shows a mixed signal intensity intra-extradural dermoid that tethers the spinal cord and expands outward into a dermal sinus (skin opening indicated by arrow).

TERMINOLOGY

Abbreviations and Synonyms
- Synonym: (Epi)dermoid cyst

Definitions
- Benign spinal tumor composed of cells that embryologically comprise skin and its appendages (hair follicles, sweat glands, and sebaceous glands)

IMAGING FINDINGS

General Features
- Best diagnostic clue: Lumbosacral or cauda equina CSF isointense/isodense mass
- Location
  - 40% intramedullary, 60% extramedullary; extradural rare
    - Dermoid: Lumbosacral (60%), cauda equina (20%), infrequent in the cervical and thoracic spine
    - Epidermoid: Upper thoracic (17%), lower thoracic (26%), lumbosacral (22%), and cauda equina (35%)
  - Acquired epidermoid cysts almost uniformly occur at cauda equina
- Size: Range: Tiny subpial masses → huge growths

- Morphology: Uni- or multilobular round/ovoid mass

Radiographic Findings
- Radiography: Focal vertebral osseous erosion, spinal canal widening, and flattening of pedicles and laminae
- Myelography
  - CSF or fat density mass adjacent to bright CSF; most useful in conjunction with CT
  - Frequently myelographic block if symptomatic
  - Largely replaced by FLAIR, DWI MRI

CT Findings
- CECT
  - Dermoid: Well-demarcated isodense mass +/- regions of fat hypodensity, calcification
    - +/- Minimal enhancement
  - Epidermoid: Well-circumscribed hypodense mass with attenuation similar to CSF +/- calcification (rare)
    - Rarely hyperdense on nonenhanced images reflecting high protein content, hemorrhage, or cellular debris
    - Minimal to no enhancement unless infected
- Bone CT
  - Focal osseous erosion, spinal canal widening, flattening of pedicles and laminae at spinal level of mass

DDx: Dermoid and Epidermoid Tumors

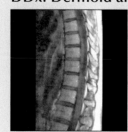

Arachnoid Cyst

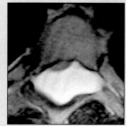

Arachnoid Cyst

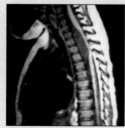

Neurenteric Cyst

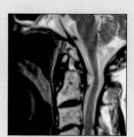

Neurenteric Cyst

DERMOID AND EPIDERMOID TUMORS

Key Facts

Terminology
- Synonym: (Epi)dermoid cyst

Imaging Findings
- 40% intramedullary, 60% extramedullary; extradural rare
- Dermoid: Well-demarcated isodense mass +/- regions of fat hypodensity, calcification
- Epidermoid: Well-circumscribed hypodense mass with attenuation similar to CSF +/- calcification (rare)
- Dermoid: T1 hypo- to hyperintense signal intensity mass
- Epidermoid: Usually T1 isointense to CSF, occasionally mildly hyperintense
- DWI: Distinguishes epidermoid (hyperintense) from arachnoid cyst (isointense to CSF)

Top Differential Diagnoses
- Arachnoid cyst
- Neurenteric cyst

Pathology
- Congenital (100% dermoid, 60% epidermoid)
- Acquired (40% epidermoid)

Clinical Issues
- Slowly progressive compressive radiculopathy/myelopathy

Diagnostic Checklist
- Diagnosis requires high index of suspicion; look for mass effect on regional structures
- FLAIR and DWI may distinguish epidermoid from CSF, arachnoid cyst

MR Findings
- T1WI
  - Dermoid: T1 hypo- to hyperintense signal intensity mass
    - Hypointensity may reflect increased water content from sweat gland secretions
    - Fat hyperintensity is most specific for dermoid but least common appearance; intrinsic T1 shortening permits differentiation of dermoid from epidermoid
  - Epidermoid: Usually T1 isointense to CSF, occasionally mildly hyperintense
- T2WI: Both show high T2 signal intensity
- FLAIR: Mild hyperintensity to CSF may help detect occult epidermoid tumor, differentiate from arachnoid cyst
- DWI: Distinguishes epidermoid (hyperintense) from arachnoid cyst (isointense to CSF)
- T1 C+: +/- Mild ring-enhancement; more avid contrast-enhancement if infected

Ultrasonographic Findings
- Real Time: Hypoechoic mass lesion with internal echoes, focal areas of hyperechogenicity (if fat present → dermoid)

Imaging Recommendations
- Best imaging tool: MRI; reserve CT myelography for patients with MR contraindications, inconclusive MR studies
- Protocol advice: Sagittal and axial T1WI and T2WI MRI to include entire conus and cauda equina to coccyx

DIFFERENTIAL DIAGNOSIS

Arachnoid cyst
- Follows CSF signal intensity/density on all sequences
- DWI MR useful to distinguish arachnoid cyst (isointense to CSF) from epidermoid (hyperintense)

Neurenteric cyst
- Intradural cyst; usually ventral to cord but may be dorsal or intramedullary
- +/- Vertebral anomalies, hyperdense/hyperintense proteinaceous content
- Definitive diagnosis is pathological

PATHOLOGY

General Features
- General path comments: Benign tumor arising from cells that produce skin and its appendages (hair follicles, sweat glands, sebaceous glands)
- Etiology
  - Congenital (100% dermoid, 60% epidermoid)
    - Arise from dermal/epidermal rests or focal expansion of a dermal sinus
  - Acquired (40% epidermoid)
    - Iatrogenic lesion resulting from implantation of viable dermal and epidermal elements following lumbar puncture (non-trocar spinal needle) or following surgery (myelomeningocele closure)
    - Cells slowly grow until large enough to cause symptoms
    - Link between lumbar puncture and subsequent epidermoid tumor is particularly strong in neonatal period
- Epidemiology
  - (Epi)dermoid comprise 1-2% of all spinal cord tumors, up to 10% of spinal cord tumors under age 15 years
  - Dermoid and epidermoid occur roughly equally in spine; ≈ 40% single epidermoid, 35% single dermoid, and 5% multiple dermoid or epidermoid
- Associated abnormalities
  - Dermal sinus (20%)
  - Vertebral abnormalities (diastematomyelia, hemivertebra, scoliosis)
  - Closed dysraphism (anterior sacral meningocele, "spina bifida occulta") - rare

DERMOID AND EPIDERMOID TUMORS

Gross Pathologic & Surgical Features

- Epidermoid
  - Striking white pearly sheen capsule; may be smooth, lobulated, or nodular
  - Cyst filled with creamy, waxy, pearly material
  - Either easy to shell out or firmly affixed to regional structures (result of local inflammation)
- Dermoid
  - Well-demarcated smooth mass; wall may be thickened by skin appendages or calcifications
  - Cyst filled with thick cheesy, buttery, yellowish material

Microscopic Features

- Epidermoid
  - Outer connective tissue capsule lined with stratified squamous epithelium; calcification rare
  - Centrally contains desquamated epithelial keratin, cholesterol crystals; positive staining with antibodies to EMA and cytokeratin
- Dermoid
  - Uni- or multilocular; outer connective tissue capsule lined with stratified squamous epithelium containing hair follicles, sebaceous glands, and sweat glands
  - +/- Inflammation (if ruptured)
  - Centrally contains desquamated epithelial keratin, lipid material

CLINICAL ISSUES

Presentation

- Most common signs/symptoms
  - Asymptomatic
  - Slowly progressive compressive radiculopathy/myelopathy
  - Other signs/symptoms
    - Cauda equina syndrome
    - Acute chemical meningitis secondary to rupture and discharge of inflammatory cholesterol crystals into CSF
    - Meningitis; most common in association with dermal sinus

Demographics

- Age
  - Dermoids usually cause symptoms before 20 years of age
  - Epidermoids are slower growing; symptoms usually arise in early adult hood (3rd to 5th decade)
- Gender
  - Dermoids M = F
  - Epidermoids M > F

Natural History & Prognosis

- Symptoms slowly progress if untreated
- Complete surgical resection offers best opportunity for good neurologic outcome
  - Incomplete resection frequently recurs; malignant transformation very rare

Treatment

- Standard treatment is complete surgical excision

- Radiotherapy not established for the treatment of epidermoid cysts
  - May be an alternative to palliative operation or for patients who cannot undergo surgery

DIAGNOSTIC CHECKLIST

Consider

- Dermoid is a congenital lesion and presents during childhood/adolescence
- Epidermoid may be congenital or acquired, and usually arises later during 3rd to 5th decade

Image Interpretation Pearls

- Epidermoids/dermoids are frequently difficult to diagnosis on CT and MRI
  - Diagnosis requires high index of suspicion; look for mass effect on regional structures
  - FLAIR and DWI may distinguish epidermoid from CSF, arachnoid cyst

SELECTED REFERENCES

1. Ziv ET et al: Iatrogenic intraspinal epidermoid tumor: two cases and a review of the literature. Spine. 29(1):E15-8, 2004
2. Bretz A et al: Intraspinal epidermoid cyst successfully treated with radiotherapy: case report. Neurosurgery. 53(6):1429-31; discussion 1431-2, 2003
3. Ferrara P et al: Intramedullary epidermoid cyst presenting with abnormal urological manifestations. Spinal Cord. 41(11):645-8, 2003
4. Amato VG et al: Intramedullary epidermoid cyst: preoperative diagnosis and surgical management after MRI introduction. Case report and updating of the literature. J Neurosurg Sci. 46(3-4):122-6, 2002
5. Graham D et al: Greenfield's Neuropathology. 7th ed. London, Arnold. 964-966, 2002
6. Scarrow AM et al: Epidermoid cyst of the thoracic spine: case history. Clin Neurol Neurosurg. 103(4):220-2, 2001
7. Barkovich A: Pediatric neuroimaging. 3rd ed. Philadelphia, Lippincott-Raven. 669-70, 2000
8. Kikuchi K et al: The utility of diffusion-weighted imaging with navigator-echo technique for the diagnosis of spinal epidermoid cysts. AJNR Am J Neuroradiol. 21(6):1164-6, 2000
9. Potgieter S et al: Epidermoid tumours associated with lumbar punctures performed in early neonatal life. Dev Med Child Neurol. 40(4):266-9, 1998
10. Machida T et al: Acquired epidermoid tumour in the thoracic spinal canal. Neuroradiology. 35(4):316-8, 1993
11. Toro VE et al: MRI of iatrogenic spinal epidermoid tumor. J Comput Assist Tomogr. 17(6):970-2, 1993
12. Lunardi P et al: Long-term results of the surgical treatment of spinal dermoid and epidermoid tumors. Neurosurgery. 25(6):860-4, 1989
13. Shikata J et al: Intraspinal epidermoid and dermoid cysts. Surgical results of seven cases. Arch Orthop Trauma Surg. 107(2):105-9, 1988
14. Phillips J et al: Magnetic resonance imaging of intraspinal epidermoid cyst: a case report. J Comput Tomogr. 11(2):181-3, 1987

IMAGE GALLERY

Typical

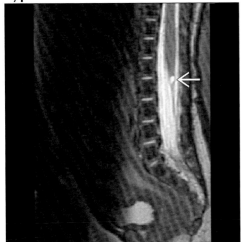 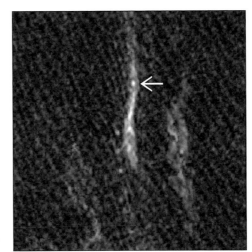

(Left) Sagittal T2WI MR demonstrates a small intradural epidermoid cyst (arrow) at the conus tip (Courtesy R. Boyer, MD). *(Right)* Sagittal DWI MR shows hyperintense diffusion restriction within an intradural cyst (arrow), confirming the diagnosis of epidermoid tumor (Courtesy R. Boyer, MD).

Typical

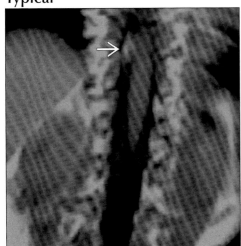 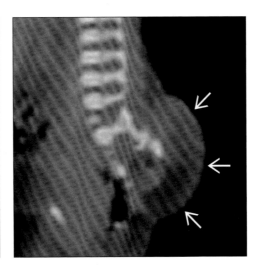

(Left) Coronal T1WI MR depicts a small intradural dermoid tumor with intrinsic hyperintense signal from fat (arrow). *(Right)* Sagittal NECT shows a mixed intradural/extradural dermoid tumor with osseous remodeling producing a large palpable sacral mass (arrows) in a patient with Currarino triad (Courtesy G. Hedlund, DO).

Variant

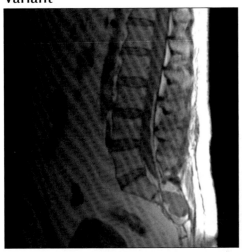 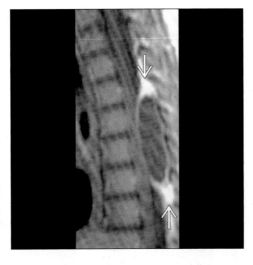

(Left) Sagittal T1WI MR shows a low-lying tethered cord with filum lipoma, ending in a large sacral dermoid tumor. The dermoid displays mixed isointense and hyperintense (fat) signal intensity. *(Right)* Sagittal T1WI MR reveals a large hypointense extradural epidermoid tumor. Fat capping at the poles (arrows) confirms epidural location (Courtesy M. Huckman, MD).

CAUDAL REGRESSION SYNDROME

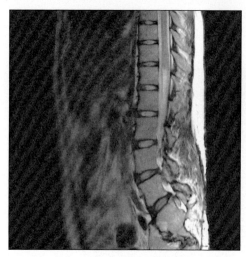

Sagittal T2WI MR shows wedge-shaped conus termination and sacral hypogenesis, characteristic of group 1 CRS patients.

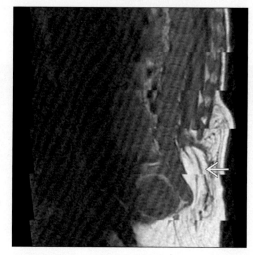

Sagittal T1WI MR demonstrates a low-lying conus terminating in a large lipoma (arrow). These findings in conjunction with sacral hypogenesis are typical of group 2 CRS patients.

TERMINOLOGY

Abbreviations and Synonyms
- Synonyms: CRS, sacral agenesis, lumbosacral dysgenesis

Definitions
- Constellation of caudal developmental growth abnormalities with associated regional soft tissue anomalies

IMAGING FINDINGS

General Features
- Best diagnostic clue: Lumbosacral dysgenesis with abnormal distal spinal cord
- Location: Lumbosacral spine
- Size: Variable diminution of caudal spine
- Morphology
  - Spectrum ranging in severity from absent coccyx to lumbosacral agenesis
    - Partial or total unilateral dysgenesis with oblique lumbosacral joint
    - Bilateral total lumbosacral dysgenesis; vertebral column terminates in thoracic spine
  - Caudal vertebral bodies often fused
  - Severe canal narrowing rostral to last intact vertebra

- Osseous vertebral excrescences, fibrous bands connecting bifid spinous processes, or severe distal dural tube stenosis

Radiographic Findings
- Radiography: Lumbosacral osseous hypogenesis
- Myelography: Caudal hypogenesis +/- dural stenosis; most useful in conjunction with CT

CT Findings
- CECT
  - Lumbosacral dysgenesis with distal spinal stenosis
  - May see prominent nerve/DRG enhancement

MR Findings
- T1WI
  - Vertebral body dysgenesis/hypogenesis
  - Group 1: Distal spinal cord hypoplasia ("wedge-shaped" cord termination), severe sacral osseous anomalies
    - +/- Dilated central canal, conus CSF cyst
  - Group 2: Tapered, low-lying, distal cord elongation with tethering, less severe sacral anomalies
- T2WI: Same findings as T1WI; best for depicting dural stenosis
- T1 C+: Hypertrophied DRG/nerve roots may enhance

Ultrasonographic Findings
- Real Time

DDx: Caudal Regression Syndrome

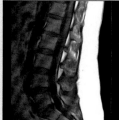

Tethered Cord

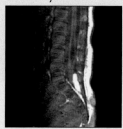

Terminal Lipoma

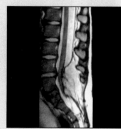

Lipomyelomeningocele

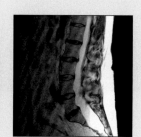

Occult Meningocele

CAUDAL REGRESSION SYNDROME

Key Facts

Terminology
- Synonyms: CRS, sacral agenesis, lumbosacral dysgenesis

Imaging Findings
- Best diagnostic clue: Lumbosacral dysgenesis with abnormal distal spinal cord
- Spectrum ranging in severity from absent coccyx to lumbosacral agenesis
- Group 1: Blunt spinal cord termination above L1; central canal may be prominent
- Group 2: Elongated conus with thick filum +/- intraspinal lipoma

Top Differential Diagnoses
- Tethered spinal cord
- Closed spinal dysraphism

- Occult intrasacral meningocele (OIM)

Pathology
- Most severe cases ⇒ sirenomelia ("mermaid")
- Most cases sporadic
- 1/7,500 births (milder forms > severe forms)
- 15-20% are infants of diabetic mothers; 1% of offspring from diabetic mothers affected
- Genitourinary abnormalities (24%)

Diagnostic Checklist
- MR imaging most useful imaging tool for characterizing abnormalities and surgical planning
- Caudal spine anomalies should be sought out in patients with genitourinary or anorectal anomalies and vice versa

---

- ○ Group 1: Blunt spinal cord termination above L1; central canal may be prominent
- ○ Group 2: Elongated conus with thick filum +/- intraspinal lipoma

Imaging Recommendations
- Consider ultrasound for infant screening
- MR imaging to confirm ultrasound findings, treatment planning
  - ○ Sagittal MRI to demonstrate extent of lumbosacral deficiency, distal spinal cord morphology, and presence/absence of tethering
  - ○ Axial MRI to detect osseous spinal narrowing, hydromyelia, other associated lesions

DIFFERENTIAL DIAGNOSIS

Tethered spinal cord
- Low-lying spinal cord +/- thickened or fatty filum, no caudal dysgenesis
- Difficult to clinically discern from mild sacral dysgenesis
  - ○ +/- Associated imaging abnormalities may help distinguish

Closed spinal dysraphism
- Dorsal dysraphism without severe vertebral column agenesis
- Ex: Lipomyelomeningocele (lipomyeloschisis)

Occult intrasacral meningocele (OIM)
- Sacrum thinned and remodelled, sometimes imitating caudal regression

PATHOLOGY

General Features
- General path comments
  - ○ Sequela of caudal cell mass dysplasia with spectrum of severity

- ○ Lower extremity deformities, lumbosacral agenesis, anorectal abnormalities, renal/pulmonary hypoplasia characteristic
  - ■ Most severe cases ⇒ sirenomelia ("mermaid")
  - ■ 20% ⇒ tethering subcutaneous lesions (group 2)
- Genetics
  - ○ Most cases sporadic
  - ○ Dominantly inherited form recently described; defect in the HLBX9 homeobox gene (chromosome 7)
    - ■ HLBX9 also expressed in pancreas ⇒ possible association between diabetes hyperglycemia and caudal regression
- Etiology
  - ○ Normal caudal spine development ⇒ canalization and retrogressive differentiation
    - ■ Anorectal and genitourinary structures form contemporaneously in close anatomic proximity
  - ○ Insult prior to fourth gestational week ⇒ caudal cell mass developmental abnormalities
    - ■ Hyperglycemia, infectious, toxic, or ischemic insult postulated to impair spinal cord, vertebral formation
    - ■ Signaling defects by retinoic acid and sonic hedgehog during blastogenesis and gastrulation
    - ■ Abnormal neural tube, notochord development ⇒ impaired migration of neurons and mesodermal cells
- Epidemiology
  - ○ 1/7,500 births (milder forms > severe forms)
  - ○ 15-20% are infants of diabetic mothers; 1% of offspring from diabetic mothers affected
  - ○ Association with VACTERL (10%), omphalocele, exstrophy bladder, imperforate anus, spinal anomaluies (10%), and Currarino triad syndromic complexes
- Associated abnormalities
  - ○ Tethered cord
    - ■ ≈ 100% of CRS patients with conus terminating below L1
    - ■ Thickened filum (65%) +/- dermoid or lipoma
  - ○ Other spinal anomalies

CAUDAL REGRESSION SYNDROME

- Vertebral anomalies (22%), diastematomyelia, terminal hydromyelia (10%), myelomeningocele (35-50%), lipomyelomeningocele (10-20%), terminal myelocystocele (15%), anterior sacral meningocele
  - ○ Congential cardiac defects (24%), pulmonary hypoplasia
  - ○ Genitourinary abnormalities (24%)
    - Renal agenesis/ectopia, hydronephrosis, Müllerian duct malformations, urinary bladder malformation
  - ○ Anorectal anomalies (particularly anal atresia)
    - Higher level of anal atresia ⇒ more severe lumbosacral dysgenesis, genitourinary anomalies
  - ○ Orthopedic abnormalities; extreme cases ⇒ lower extremity fusion (sirenomelia)

Gross Pathologic & Surgical Features
- Severity of vertebral dysgenesis, presence/absence of tethering, and osseous canal diameter impact surgical planning

Microscopic Features
- Findings typical for tissue content

Staging, Grading or Classification Criteria
- Group 1: More severe caudal dysgenesis with high-lying, club-shaped cord terminus (decreased number of anterior horn cells)
  - ○ Distal cord hypoplasia with wedging seen in all patients with partial or complete dysgenesis and termination of spinal cord above L1
  - ○ Termination of the conus above L1 highly correlated with sacral malformations ending at S1 or above
- Group 2: Less severe dysgenesis with low-lying, tapered, distal cord tethered by tight filum, lipoma, lipomyelomeningocele, or terminal myelocystocele
  - ○ Conus termination below L1 highly correlated with sacral malformations ending at S2 or below
  - ○ Tethering is thus more common in milder sacral dysgenesis

CLINICAL ISSUES

Presentation
- Most common signs/symptoms
  - ○ Neurogenic urinary bladder dysfunction (nearly all patients)
  - ○ Sensorimotor paresis (group 2 > group 1)
    - Severity of motor deficit > sensory
    - Sacral sensory sparing common, even in severe cases
  - ○ Neurologically asymptomatic (group 1 > group 2)
- Clinical profile
  - ○ Broad spectrum ranging from neurologically normal ⇒ complete lumbosacral agenesis and fusion of lower extremities (sirenomelia)
    - Always accompanied by narrow hips, hypoplastic gluteal muscles, and shallow intergluteal cleft
  - ○ Symptomatic patient presentation ranges from mild foot disorders ⇒ complete lower extremity paralysis and distal leg atrophy
    - Motor level usually higher than sensory level

- Level of vertebral aplasia correlates with motor but not sensory level

Demographics
- Age
  - ○ Severe cases identified in utero (obstetrical ultrasound) or at birth
  - ○ Mild cases may not be identified until adulthood
- Gender: M = F

Natural History & Prognosis
- Variable depending on severity

Treatment
- Surgical untethering if clinically symptomatic
- Surgical release/duraplasty may improve neurological function in patients with distal spinal canal stenosis
- Orthopedic procedures to improve lower extremity functionality

DIAGNOSTIC CHECKLIST

Consider
- MR imaging most useful imaging tool for characterizing abnormalities and surgical planning

Image Interpretation Pearls
- Caudal spine anomalies should be sought out in patients with genitourinary or anorectal anomalies and vice versa

SELECTED REFERENCES

1. Nievelstein RA et al: Magnetic resonance imaging in children with anorectal malformations: embryologic implications. J Pediatr Surg. 37(8):1138-45, 2002
2. Barkovich A: Pediatric neuroimaging. 3rd ed. Philadelphia, Lippincott-Raven, 650-53, 2000
3. Tortori-Donati P et al: Spinal dysraphism: a review of neuroradiological features with embryological correlations and proposal for a new classification. Neuroradiology 42(7): 471-91, 2000
4. Catala M: Embryogenesis. Why do we need a new explanation for the emergence of spina bifida with lipoma? Childs Nerv Syst. 13(6):336-40, 1997
5. Ball W: Pediatric Neuroradiology. Philadelphia, Lippincott-Raven, 735-36, 1997
6. Heij HA et al: Abnormal anatomy of the lumbosacral region imaged by magnetic resonance in children with anorectal malformations. Arch Dis Child. 74(5):441-4, 1996
7. Long FR et al: Tethered cord and associated vertebral anomalies in children and infants with imperforate anus: evaluation with MR imaging and plain radiography. Radiology. 200(2):377-82, 1996
8. Nievelstein RA et al: MR of the caudal regression syndrome: embryologic implications. AJNR Am J Neuroradiol. 15(6):1021-9, 1994
9. Pang D: Sacral agenesis and caudal spinal cord malformations. Neurosurgery 32(5): 755-78, discussion 778-9, 1993
10. Barkovich AJ et al: The wedge-shaped cord terminus: a radiographic sign of caudal regression. AJNR Am J Neuroradiol. 10(6):1223-31, 1989

CAUDAL REGRESSION SYNDROME

IMAGE GALLERY

Typical

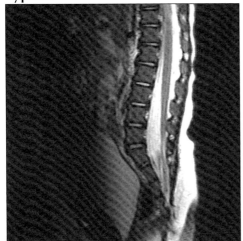
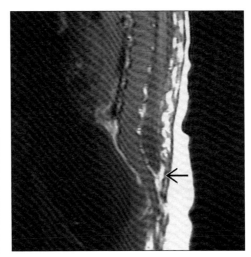

(Left) Sagittal T2WI MR shows a low-lying, tethered conus and mild sacral hypogenesis (four sacral vertebrae). Findings are diagnostic of mild group 2 CRS (Courtesy R. Boyer, MD). *(Right)* Sagittal T1WI MR demonstrates a small lipoma at the filum terminus (arrow), in conjunction with low-lying tethered conus and mild sacral hypogenesis (four sacral vertebrae).

Variant

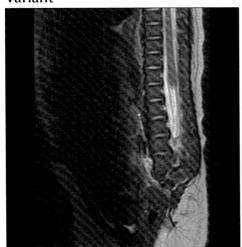
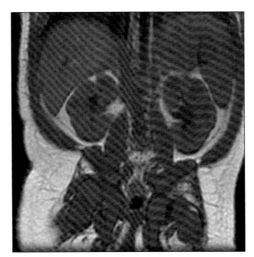

(Left) Sagittal T2WI MR in a CRS patient following myelomeningocele repair shows wedge-shaped conus (group 1) and severe sacral dysgenesis. *(Right)* Coronal T1WI MR depicts marked pelvic hypogenesis (group 1 CRS).

Variant

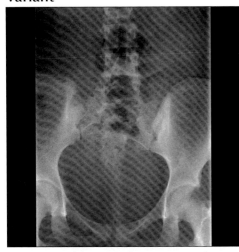
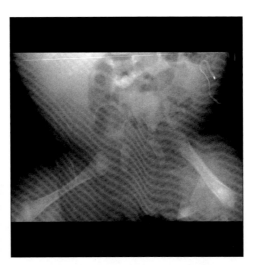

(Left) Anteroposterior radiography shows left hemisacral caudal dysgenesis (Courtesy R. Boyer, MD). *(Right)* Anteroposterior radiography depicts marked pelvic hypogenesis and pubic deficiency correlating with clinical bladder exstrophy and lower extremity under-development (Courtesy G. Hedlund, DO).

TETHERED SPINAL CORD

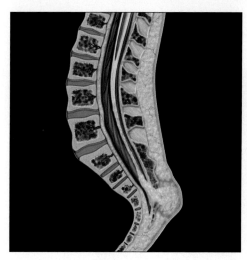

Sagittal graphic shows a low-lying hydromyelic tethered cord with fibrolipoma inserting into a terminal lipoma. Lipoma is contiguous with subcutaneous fat through dorsal dysraphism.

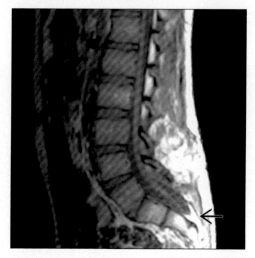

Sagittal T1WI MR shows an elongated, attenuated spinal cord terminating directly into a small terminal lipoma (arrow). No distinguishable filum is detected.

TERMINOLOGY

Abbreviations and Synonyms
- Synonyms: "Tethered cord syndrome (TCS)", "tight filum terminale syndrome"

Definitions
- Symptoms and imaging findings referable to low-lying conus medullaris tethered by a short, thick filum terminale

IMAGING FINDINGS

General Features
- Best diagnostic clue: Conus ends below L2 inferior endplate; tethered by thickened filum +/- fibrolipoma, terminal lipoma
- Location: Thoracolumbar junction → sacrum
- Size: Filum thickened (> 2 mm at L5-S1, axial MRI)
- Morphology: Attenuated conus terminates lower than normal

Radiographic Findings
- Radiography
  ○ May be normal, but nearly always shows localized dysraphism or incomplete posterior fusion
  ○ +/- Scoliosis (20%)

CT Findings
- NECT: Stretched, thinned cord with low-lying conus, thickened filum +/- fibrolipoma, dysraphism, vertebral segmentation and fusion anomalies

MR Findings
- T1WI
  ○ Thickened filum +/- hyperintense lipoma
  ○ Filum > 2 mm (L5-S1, axial MRI)
  ○ +/- Low-lying conus; may be difficult to distinguish from thickened filum
  ○ Dorsal positioning of conus medullaris, filum terminale in thecal sac
    ■ Noted even in prone position; normally cord falls into anterior 2/3 of canal when prone
- T2WI
  ○ Findings similar to T1WI
  ○ +/- Hyperintense dilatation of conus central canal 2° to hydromyelia or myelomalacia (25%)
  ○ Fatty filum ⇒ chemical shift artifact
  ○ Dural sac widened; dorsal dura tense, tented posteriorly by thickened filum

Ultrasonographic Findings
- Real Time: +/- Low-lying conus, thickened filum terminale, reduced or absent spinal cord movement

DDx: Tethered Cord Syndrome

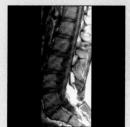

Lipomyelomeningocele

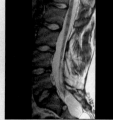

Occult Meningocele

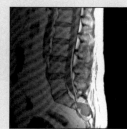

Filum lipoma/Dermoid

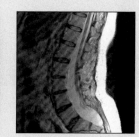

Post-op TCS Release

TETHERED SPINAL CORD

Key Facts

Terminology

- Synonyms: "Tethered cord syndrome (TCS)", "tight filum terminale syndrome"
- Symptoms and imaging findings referable to low-lying conus medullaris tethered by a short, thick filum terminale

Imaging Findings

- Best diagnostic clue: Conus ends below L2 inferior endplate; tethered by thickened filum +/- fibrolipoma, terminal lipoma
- Size: Filum thickened (> 2 mm at L5-S1, axial MRI)

Top Differential Diagnoses

- Normal variant low-lying conus
- Open or closed spinal dysraphism
- Post-surgical low-lying conus

Pathology

- Widened dural sac; thickened filum closely applied to or indistinguishable from dural sac

Clinical Issues

- Low back and leg pain; worst in morning, exacerbated by exertion
- Urinary bladder dysfunction

Diagnostic Checklist

- Tethered cord syndrome is a clinical diagnosis; imaging role is detection of low-lying conus/thick filum, associated anatomic abnormalities for surgical decision making
- Measure filum thickness at L5/S1; stretching at more rostral levels may erroneously thin filum into "normal" size range

Other Modality Findings

- Phase contrast MRI
  - ↓ Spinal cord motion
  - ≤ 1/3 show return of normal cord motion after untethering, even if symptoms resolve

Imaging Recommendations

- Best imaging tool: MRI
- Protocol advice
  - Ultrasound < 1 year old; confirm positive study with MRI
  - Thin-section sagittal, axial T1WI and T2WI, phase contrast MRI; extend axial slices to thecal sac termination

DIFFERENTIAL DIAGNOSIS

Normal variant low-lying conus

- Asymptomatic patient with normal filum thickness

Open or closed spinal dysraphism

- Spinal lipoma, myelomeningocele, meningocele, (epi)dermoid, diastematomyelia, dermal sinus tract

Post-surgical low-lying conus

- Imaging shows low-lying conus irrespective of symptoms; cannot exclude re-tethering by imaging alone
  - Ultrasound, PC MRI helpful to evaluate conus motion
  - Diagnosis of re-tethering must be made on clinical grounds

PATHOLOGY

General Features

- General path comments
  - Incomplete retrogressive differentiation with failure of terminal cord involution or failure of filum terminale to lengthen

- Conus normally terminates at or above inferior L2 in ≥ 98% of normal population
  - Conus should be at normal position by birth → 2 months old
  - Conus terminating below L2/3 is always abnormal at any post-natal age
  - May not be distinct filum; spinal cord sometimes elongated, ends directly in small terminal lipoma
- Etiology: Tethering stretches nerve fibers, arterioles, and venules ⇒ impairs oxidative metabolism of conus and nerve roots ⇒ syringohydromyelia/myelomalacia
- Epidemiology: Prevalence unknown; probably more common than appreciated
- Associated abnormalities
  - Lumbosacral hypogenesis, VACTERL syndrome
  - Open or closed spinal dysraphism, incomplete posterior fusion (up to 100%)
    - Diastematomyelia, spinal lipoma, intrasacral or dorsal meningocele, lipomyelomeningocele, myelomeningocele
  - Cutaneous stigmata (50%)
  - Hydromyelia/myelomalacia (25%)
  - Scoliosis (functional adaption to ↓ length of spinal cord course, ↓ intramedullary tension)

Gross Pathologic & Surgical Features

- Widened dural sac; thickened filum closely applied to or indistinguishable from dural sac
- Thickened fibrotic filum (55%), small fibrolipoma within thickened filum (23%), or filar cyst (3%)

Microscopic Features

- Tethered filum histologically abnormal, even if conus terminates at normal level
  - Normal filum ⇒ mainly collagen fibers
  - TCS filum ⇒ more connective tissue with dense collagen fibers, hyalinization and dilated capillaries

CLINICAL ISSUES

Presentation

- Most common signs/symptoms

TETHERED SPINAL CORD

- ○ Low back and leg pain; worst in morning, exacerbated by exertion
- ○ Gait spasticity, weakness, muscular atrophy
- ○ ↓ Sensation, abnormal lower extremity reflexes
- ○ Urinary bladder dysfunction
- ○ Orthopedic foot abnormalities (usually clubfoot)
- ○ Cutaneous stigmata (≤ 50%); simple dimple, hairy tuft, or hemangioma
- • Clinical profile
  - ○ Adults and children present differently
    - ▪ Adults: Pain first (2° degenerative changes), followed later by weakness +/- incontinence
    - ▪ Children: Incontinence, scoliosis, weakness

Demographics
- • Age: Symptomatic presentation most common during rapid somatic growth (adolescent growth spurt, school age 4 to 8 years), or in elderly 2° kyphosis
- • Gender: M = F

Natural History & Prognosis
- • Progressive, irreversible neurological impairment
  - ○ Majority of patients show improvement or stabilization of neurological deficits following surgical untethering; motor weakness (12-60%), sensory dysfunction (40-60%), pain (50-88%), bladder dysfunction (19-67%)
  - ○ Better outcome if symptom duration shorter or conus moves to more normal level following surgery
- • Post-operative symptom recurrence rare; prompts consideration for re-tethering

Treatment
- • Symptomatic patients: Early prophylactic surgery
  - ○ Resect tethering mass, release cord, and repair dura
- • Asymptomatic patients with radiographic tethering: Management controversial
  - ○ Some advocate prophylactic surgery ⇒ low morbidity, prognosis for asymptomatic patients better than symptomatic
  - ○ Others advocate prophylactic surgery only for asymptomatic adults who lead physically active lifestyles

DIAGNOSTIC CHECKLIST

Consider
- • Clinical tethering may occur despite normal conus level
  - ○ Tethered cord syndrome is a clinical diagnosis; imaging role is detection of low-lying conus/thick filum, associated anatomic abnormalities for surgical decision making
- • Distinguish cord tethering 2° tight/thickened filum terminale from tethering due to other lesions

Image Interpretation Pearls
- • Measure filum thickness at L5/S1; stretching at more rostral levels may erroneously thin filum into "normal" size range
- • Determine conus level using axial images; cauda equina may obscure conus tip on sagittal images ⇒ imitate elongated conus

SELECTED REFERENCES

1. Yamada et al: Neurosurg Focus 16(2), 2004
2. Haro H et al: Long-term outcomes of surgical treatment for tethered cord syndrome. J Spinal Disord Tech. 17(1):16-20, 2004
3. Selcuki M et al: Is a filum terminale with a normal appearance really normal? Childs Nerv Syst. 19(1):3-10, 2003
4. Unsinn KM et al: US of the spinal cord in newborns: spectrum of normal findings, variants, congenital anomalies, and acquired diseases. Radiographics. 20(4):923-38, 2000
5. Barkovich A: Pediatric neuroimaging. 3rd ed. Philadelphia, Lippincott-Raven. 648-650, 2000
6. Yamada S et al: Adult tethered cord syndrome. J Spinal Disord. 13(4):319-23, 2000
7. Selcuki M et al: Management of tight filum terminale syndrome with special emphasis on normal level conus medullaris (NLCM). Surg Neurol. 50(4):318-22; discussion 322, 1998
8. Souweidane MM et al: Retethering of sectioned fibrolipomatous filum terminales: report of two cases. Neurosurgery. 42(6):1390-3, 1998
9. Iskandar BJ et al: Congenital tethered spinal cord syndrome in adults. J Neurosurg. 88(6):958-61, 1998
10. Sharif S et al: "Tethered cord syndrome"--recent clinical experience. Br J Neurosurg. 11(1):49-51, 1997
11. Yundt KD et al: Normal diameter of filum terminale in children: in vivo measurement. Pediatr Neurosurg. 27(5):257-9, 1997
12. Beek FJ et al: Sonographic determination of the position of the conus medullaris in premature and term infants. Neuroradiology. 38 Suppl 1:S174-7, 1996
13. Gilmore RL et al: The clinical neurophysiology of tethered cord syndrome and other dysraphic syndromes, in Yamada S (ed): Tethered Cord Syndrome. Park Ridge, IL: AANS, 167–182, 1996
14. Beek FJ et al: Sonographic determination of the position of the conus medullaris in premature and term infants. Neuroradiology. 38 Suppl 1:S174-7, 1996
15. Brunelle F et al: Lumbar spinal cord motion measurement with phase-contrast MR imaging in normal children and in children with spinal lipomas. Pediatr Radiol. 26(4):265-70, 1996
16. Yamada S et al: Pathophysiology of tethered cord syndrome. Neurosurg Clin N Am. 6(2):311-23, 1995
17. Warder DE et al: Tethered cord syndrome: the low-lying and normally positioned conus. Neurosurgery. 34(4):597-600; discussion 600, 1994
18. Warder DE et al: Tethered cord syndrome and the conus in a normal position. Neurosurgery. 33(3):374-8, 1993
19. Chestnut R et al: The Vater association and spinal dysraphia. Pediatr Neurosurg. 18(3):144-8, 1992
20. Raghavan N et al: MR imaging in the tethered spinal cord syndrome. AJR Am J Roentgenol. 152(4):843-52, 1989
21. Wilson DA et al: John Caffey award. MR imaging determination of the location of the normal conus medullaris throughout childhood. AJR Am J Roentgenol. 152(5):1029-32, 1989
22. Kang JK et al: Effects of tethering on regional spinal cord blood flow and sensory-evoked potentials in growing cats. Childs Nerv Syst. 3(1):35-9, 1987
23. Pang D et al: Tethered cord syndrome in adults. J Neurosurg. 57(1):32-47, 1982

IMAGE GALLERY

Typical

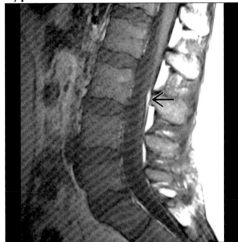
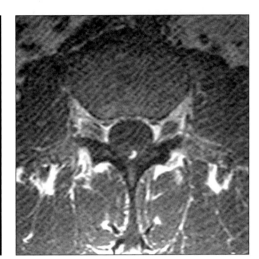

(Left) Sagittal T1WI MR depicts a low-lying, tethered conus with thickened fatty filum (arrow). *(Right)* Axial T1WI MR shows a small filum lipoma in conjunction with filum thickening in a symptomatic TCS patient.

Typical

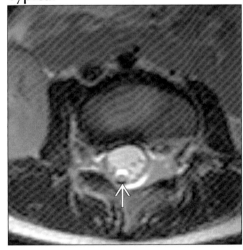
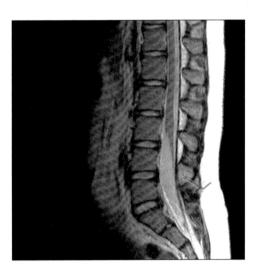

(Left) Axial T2WI MR of TCS patient demonstrates chemical shift artifact (arrow) confirming fat content in thickened filum. *(Right)* Sagittal T2WI MR shows a low-lying conus at L3 with thickened filum and dorsal positioning of tethered cord related to dermal sinus tract (Courtesy G. Hedlund, DO).

Typical

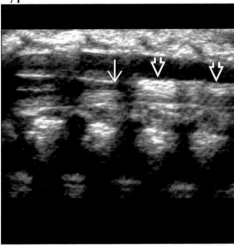
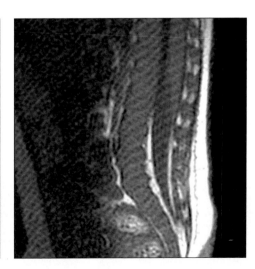

(Left) Sagittal ultrasound real time depicts a low-lying conus (arrow) with echogenic thickening of the filum (open arrows) corresponding to filum lipoma. Conus movement was reduced (Courtesy R. Boyer, MD). *(Right)* Sagittal T1WI MR reveals a low-lying conus at L3, with thickened fatty filum. The cord/conus is displaced dorsally (Courtesy R. Boyer, MD).

TERMINAL MYELOCYSTOCELE

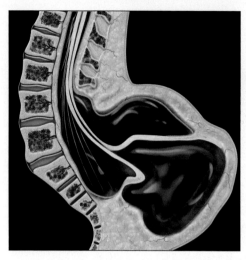

Sagittal graphic displays a low-lying, hydromyelic spinal cord piercing an expanded subarachnoid space (meningocele), to terminate in a myelocystocele.

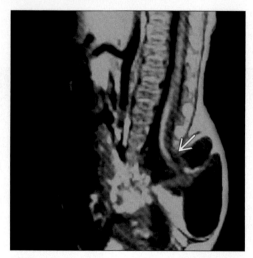

Sagittal T1WI MR depicts a low-lying hydromyelic cord traversing meningocele, expanding into a large terminal cyst. Arrow marks dorsal fibrous band (Courtesy R. Boyer, MD).

TERMINOLOGY

Abbreviations and Synonyms
- Synonym: Terminal syringocele

Definitions
- Complex spinal malformation → hydromyelic low-lying tethered spinal cord traversing a meningocele to terminate in myelocystocele

IMAGING FINDINGS

General Features
- Best diagnostic clue: Hydromyelic tethered cord traversing dorsal meningocele to terminate in a dilated terminal ventricle cyst
- Location: Sacrum/coccyx
- Size: Mass varies from small → huge (> 10 cm diameter)
- Morphology: Closed spinal dysraphism, large skin covered mass, terminal cord cyst traversing meningocele

Radiographic Findings
- Radiography
  - Lumbosacral dysraphism +/- soft tissue mass
  - +/- Pubic diastasis (usually + bladder exstrophy)
- Myelography

  - Hydromyelic cord passes through meningocele, terminates in separate sac caudal to contrast filled meningocele
  - Delayed imaging → +/- contrast imbibition into hydromyelic cord/terminal cyst

CT Findings
- NECT
  - Lumbosacral dysraphism
  - Hydromyelic cord penetrates meningocele sac, ends in caudal terminal cystic sac

MR Findings
- T1WI
  - Hypointense cephalic dorsal meningocele ⇒ back mass
  - Tethered distal cord shows "trumpet-like flaring" into hypointense caudal terminal cyst
- T2WI
  - Hypointense dorsal fibrous band at cephalic margin of meningocele constrains cord
  - Fibrolipomatous tissue surrounds both sacs

Ultrasonographic Findings
- Real Time
  - Sagittal plane: Spinal cord passes through hypoechoic, dilated subarachnoid space (meningocele), terminates in cord cyst

DDx: Terminal Myelocystocele

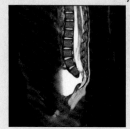
Ant. Meningocele

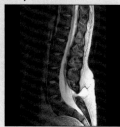
Dorsal Meningocele

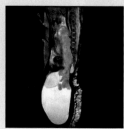
Sacrococc. Teratoma

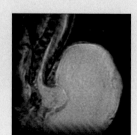
Myelomeningocele

TERMINAL MYELOCYSTOCELE

Key Facts

Terminology
- Synonym: Terminal syringocele
- Complex spinal malformation → hydromyelic low-lying tethered spinal cord traversing a meningocele to terminate in myelocystocele

Imaging Findings
- Best diagnostic clue: Hydromyelic tethered cord traversing dorsal meningocele to terminate in a dilated terminal ventricle cyst
- Lumbosacral dysraphism

Top Differential Diagnoses
- Anterior sacral meningocele
- Simple dorsal meningocele
- Sacrococcygeal teratoma
- Myelomeningocele

Pathology
- Skin covered lumbosacral dysraphism
- Arachnoid lined meningocele directly contiguous with spinal subarachnoid space
- Low-lying hydromyelic cord traverses meningocele, expands into large contiguous ependymal-lined terminal cyst

Clinical Issues
- Presents at birth with large skin-covered back mass
- Majority neurologically intact at diagnosis

Diagnostic Checklist
- Early diagnosis and surgery → best chance for normal neurological outcome
- Non-neurological prognosis largely linked to severity of associated anomalies

---

- o Axial plane: Bifid hydromyelic dorsal spinal cord within meningocele

Imaging Recommendations
- Best imaging tool: MRI
- Protocol advice
  - o Sagittal MR imaging for diagnosis and estimating length of hydromyelia, sizing cysts, and identifying associated abnormalities
  - o Axial MR imaging to clarify extent of rachischisis, evaluate associated anomalies

DIFFERENTIAL DIAGNOSIS

Anterior sacral meningocele
- Anterior meningocele protrudes thorough an enlarged sacral neural foramen into pelvis

Simple dorsal meningocele
- Dorsal meningocele protrudes thorough focal dysraphism
- Cord rarely tethered or hydromyelic

Sacrococcygeal teratoma
- Similar clinical appearance of skin mass
- Distinguish by presence of solid tumor elements within cysts, calcifications

Myelomeningocele
- Open spinal dysraphism; no skin covering, clinically obvious

PATHOLOGY

General Features
- General path comments
  - o Classic pathological triad
    - Skin covered lumbosacral dysraphism
    - Arachnoid lined meningocele directly contiguous with spinal subarachnoid space

- Low-lying hydromyelic cord traverses meningocele, expands into large contiguous ependymal-lined terminal cyst
  - o Terminal cyst does not communicate directly with subarachnoid space
  - o Some speculate → most severe manifestation of persistent terminal ventricle (ventriculus terminalis) spectrum
- Etiology
  - o Postulated to result from deranged secondary neurulation of caudal cell mass; typically associated with other caudal tail-fold malformations
    - CSF unable to normally exit from early neural tube ⇒ terminal ventricle balloons into cyst ⇒ disrupts overlying dorsal mesenchyme but not superficial ectoderm
    - Posterior elements do not form normally ⇒ spina bifida with intact skin
    - Terminal ventricle dilatation ⇒ distends arachnoid cord lining ⇒ meningocele
    - Cyst bulk prevents cord ascent ⇒ tethered cord
    - After arachnoid formation, progressive distention of distal cord causes caudal bulge below end of meningocele into extra-arachnoid space and cephalically to expand distal cord, producing flaring of distal spinal cord
    - Disruption of caudal motor segments ⇒ progressive symptoms present at birth or that appear later
- Epidemiology
  - o Rare: 1-5% of skin covered lumbosacral masses
    - Much more common in cloacal exstrophy patients
  - o Sporadic; no familial incidence
  - o Postulated associations with teratogens retinoic acid, hydantoin, ioperamid hydrochloride
  - o No known association with diabetes mellitus (unlike caudal regression syndrome)
- Associated abnormalities
  - o Cloacal exstrophy, imperforate anus, omphalocele, pelvic deformities, equinovarus, ambiguous hypoplastic genitalia, and renal abnormalities
  - o Syndromal associations
    - Caudal regression syndrome

TERMINAL MYELOCYSTOCELE

- OEIS syndrome constellation (omphalocele, exstrophy of the bladder, imperforate anus, and spinal anomalies)
  - Chiari I and II malformations, hydrocephalus, and vertebral segmentation anomalies (rare)

Gross Pathologic & Surgical Features
- Lumbosacral dysraphism with hypoplastic, widely everted laminae
- Proximal (smaller, rostral) sac resembles typical meningocele, with inner surface lined by arachnoid and thick fibrous layer
- Distal spinal cord herniates under fibrous band between medial ends of most cephalic widely bifid lamina, traverses meningocele → terminal cyst (larger, caudal)
  - Cord narrowed by fibrous band where it exits spinal canal, then widens distally due to concurrent hydromyelia
  - Distal spinal nerve roots arise from ventral surface of intra-arachnoid segment of spinal cord, traverse meningocele, and re-enter spinal canal before exiting at their root sleeves or via bony clefts

Microscopic Features
- Meningocele lined by arachnoid, thick fibrous layer
- Terminal cyst lined by ependyma, dysplastic glia; directly contiguous with central cord canal
- Outer cord surface pia, arachnoid continuous with meningocele

CLINICAL ISSUES

Presentation
- Most common signs/symptoms
  - Presents at birth with large skin-covered back mass
    - Skin appears normal or exhibits hemangioma, nevus, or hypertrichosis
    - Rare patients without back mass present later with progressive neurological deficits
  - Majority neurologically intact at diagnosis
  - Later presentation or untreated lesion may develop progressive lower extremity paresis
- Clinical profile
  - Usually neurologically intact at birth but may present with lower extremity sensorimotor deficits
  - Large mass obliterates intergluteal cleft, extends upward from perineum for a variable distance
  - +/- Concurrent midline cecal and paramedian bladder exstrophy, other visible anomalies

Demographics
- Age: Infancy
- Gender: F > M

Natural History & Prognosis
- Normal intellectual potential
- Mass size and deficits tend to progress with time, may be partially or totally reversible with prompt surgical repair
  - Main goals of neurosurgical intervention are to reduce mass size and un-tether cord

- Operation soon after diagnosis is indicated to prevent progression of neurological abnormalities, cyst growth
- Persistent neurological deficits usually permanent
- Overall prognosis is mainly related to other associated anomalies (OEIS constellation)

Treatment
- Early diagnosis and surgical repair maximizes probability of a normal neurological outcome
- Delayed recognition and operation increase odds of onset, progression of lower extremity paresis

DIAGNOSTIC CHECKLIST

Consider
- Early diagnosis and surgery → best chance for normal neurological outcome
- Non-neurological prognosis largely linked to severity of associated anomalies

Image Interpretation Pearls
- Tethered hydromyelic cord traversing meningocele to terminate in a separate caudal cyst is unique imaging finding diagnostic of terminal myelocystocele

SELECTED REFERENCES

1. Lemire RJ et al: Tumors and malformations of the caudal spinal axis. Pediatr Neurosurg. 38(4):174-80, 2003
2. Kumar R et al: Terminal myelocystocele. Indian J Pediatr. 69(12):1083-6, 2002
3. Midrio P et al: Prenatal diagnosis of terminal myelocystocele in the fetal surgery era: case report. Neurosurgery. 50(5):1152-4; discussion 1154-5, 2002
4. Unsinn KM et al: US of the spinal cord in newborns: spectrum of normal findings, variants, congenital anomalies, and acquired diseases. Radiographics. 20(4):923-38, 2000
5. Cartmill M et al: Terminal Myelocystocele: an unusual presentation. Pediatr Neurosurg. 32(2):83-5, 2000
6. Barkovich A: Pediatric neuroimaging. 3rd ed. Philadelphia, Lippincott-Raven, 653-654, 2000
7. Tortori-Donati P et al: Spinal dysraphism: a review of neuroradiological features with embryological correlations and proposal for a new classification. Neuroradiology 42(7): 471-91, 2000
8. Choi S et al: Long-term outcome of terminal myelocystocele patients. Pediatr Neurosurg. 32(2):86-91, 2000
9. Meyer SH et al: Terminal myelocystocele: important differential diagnosis in the prenatal assessment of spina bifida. J Ultrasound Med. 17(3):193-7, 1998
10. Byrd SE et al: Imaging of terminal myelocystoceles. J Natl Med Assoc. 88(8):510-6, 1996
11. Byrd SE et al: MR of terminal myelocystoceles. Eur J Radiol. 20(3):215-20, 1995
12. Peacock WJ et al: Magnetic resonance imaging in myelocystoceles. Report of two cases. J Neurosurg. 70(5):804-7, 1989
13. McLone DG et al: Terminal myelocystocele. Neurosurgery. 16(1):36-43, 1985
14. Lemire RJ et al: Skin-covered sacrococcygeal masses in infants and children. J Pediatr. 79(6):948-54, 1971

IMAGE GALLERY

Typical

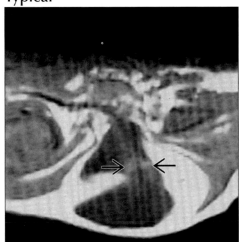

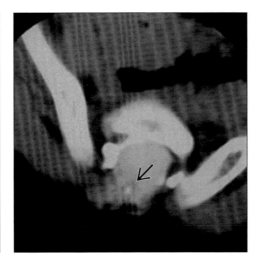

(Left) Axial T1WI MR depicts passage of bifid hydromyelic, low-lying cord (arrows) through the arachnoid-lined meningocele (Courtesy G. Hedlund, DO). *(Right)* Axial NECT following myelography shows a hydromyelic low-lying spinal cord (arrow) traversing the meningocele sac. Wide dorsal dysraphism is present (Courtesy R. Boyer, MD).

Variant

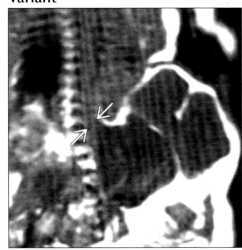

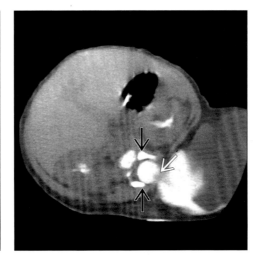

(Left) Coronal T1WI MR shows a low-lying spinal cord (arrows) traversing a large dorsolateral meningocele that atypically extends into the left flank (Courtesy R. Boyer, MD). *(Right)* Axial CECT following myelography shows wide posterior dysraphism (black arrows). The spinal cord (white arrow) traverses a large eccentric dorsolateral meningocele (Courtesy R. Boyer, MD).

Variant

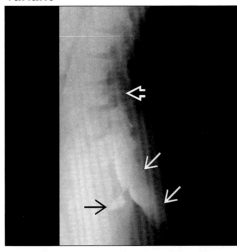

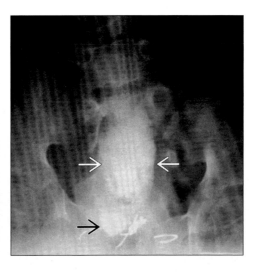

(Left) Lateral myelography demonstrates the hydromyelic low-lying cord (open arrow) passing through the dorsal meningocele (white arrows) to terminate in a small caudal terminal cyst (black arrow). *(Right)* Anteroposterior myelography shows the meningocele's (white arrows) relationship to wide dysraphism and terminal cyst (black arrow). Surgical wires indicate prior bladder exstrophy repair.

ANTERIOR SACRAL MENINGOCELE

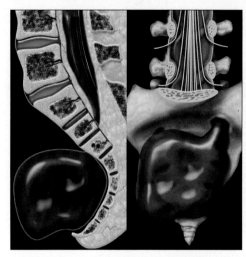
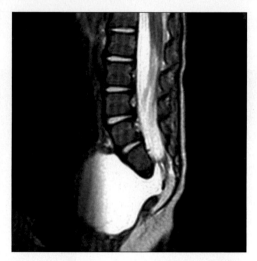

Sagittal graphic (left) depicts characteristic anterior sacral "scimitar" remodeling by large anterior cyst. Coronal graphic (right) shows cyst origin through an enlarged neural foramen.

Sagittal T2WI MR shows a large anterior sacral cyst, contiguous with the meninges, extending through an enlarged neural foramen (Courtesy G. Hedlund, DO).

TERMINOLOGY

Abbreviations and Synonyms
- Anterior sacral meningocele (ASM)

Definitions
- Sacral meninges herniate anteriorly into the pelvis through focal erosion or hypogenesis of sacral +/- coccygeal vertebral segments

IMAGING FINDINGS

General Features
- Best diagnostic clue: Presacral cyst, contiguous with thecal sac, protruding through an anterior osseous defect
- Location: Sacrum/coccyx
- Size: Variable
- Morphology
  - Uni- or multi-loculated cyst; usually devoid of neural tissue but may have traversing nerve roots
  - Sacral defect is 2° to neural foraminal widening
    - May be unilateral or bilateral, symmetrical or asymmetrical, and single or multiple level

Radiographic Findings
- Radiography
  - Widened sacral canal and neural foramina

- Scalloping of anterior sacrum wall
    - Curved "scimitar" sacrum on lateral projection
  - +/- Scoliosis
- Myelography
  - Thecal sac continuity with cyst
    - Most useful in conjunction with NECT (CT myelography)
  - Rarely used unless MR contraindicated or non-diagnostic

CT Findings
- CECT
  - Deficient sacrum with variably sized anterior cyst
    - +/- Nerve roots traversing sacral defect
  - +/- Lipoma/dermoid (hypodense)
  - Enhancement absent

MR Findings
- T1WI
  - Deficient sacrum with variably sized presacral cyst
    - Sagittal images confirm cyst/thecal sac continuity
  - +/- Cord tethering
  - +/- Lipoma/dermoid (hyperintense)
- T2WI
  - Homogeneous hyperintense CSF signal intensity cyst (similar to thecal sac)
  - Best sequence to identify nerve roots traversing sacral defect
- T2* GRE

DDx: Anterior Sacral Meningocele

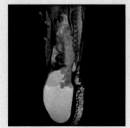
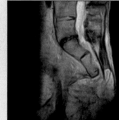
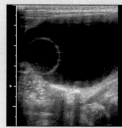
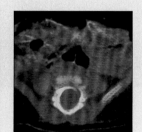

| *Sacrococc. Teratoma* | *Chordoma* | *Ovarian Cyst* | *Neurenteric Cyst* |

ANTERIOR SACRAL MENINGOCELE

Key Facts

Terminology
- Anterior sacral meningocele (ASM)
- Sacral meninges herniate anteriorly into the pelvis through focal erosion or hypogenesis of sacral +/- coccygeal vertebral segments

Imaging Findings
- Best diagnostic clue: Presacral cyst, contiguous with thecal sac, protruding through an anterior osseous defect
- Widened sacral canal and neural foramina
- Curved "scimitar" sacrum on lateral projection

Top Differential Diagnoses
- Sacrococcygeal teratoma (SGT)
- Sacral chordoma
- Ovarian cyst

- Neurenteric cyst
- Cystic neuroblastoma

Pathology
- 5% of retrorectal tumors
- Associated abnormalities: Anorectal anomalies, epidermoid/dermoid tumor or other tethering lesion, Currarino triad

Diagnostic Checklist
- MR imaging to identify and characterize cyst location and contents, confirm abnormal ultrasound findings
- Continuity of cyst with thecal sac necessary to ensure diagnosis
- Soft tissue mass or calcification implies tumor
- Presence/absence of neural tissue within cyst important for surgical planning

---

  - No hypointensity (calcification) within cyst wall
    - Distinguishes from sacrococcygeal teratoma
- DWI: Hypointense signal confirms CSF composition, excludes epidermoid cyst (hyperintense)
- T1 C+: Enhancement absent

Ultrasonographic Findings
- Real Time
  - Cystic hypoechoic pelvic mass anterior to sacrum
  - Complex internal echoes if prior/concurrent inflammation or infection

Imaging Recommendations
- Best imaging tool
  - MR imaging confirms cyst contiguity with thecal sac
    - T1WI also shows +/- epidermoid, lipoma/dermoid
    - T2WI demonstrates +/- entrapped neural tissue
  - CT imaging best depicts osseous defect, absence of rim calcification (that would imply SGT)
- Protocol advice
  - Ultrasound for initial screening during infancy
  - Sagittal and axial MR imaging to confirm positive ultrasound studies, pre-operative planning, and post-operative surveillance

DIFFERENTIAL DIAGNOSIS

Sacrococcygeal teratoma (SGT)
- Cystic SGT may be difficult to distinguish from ASM
  - Look for soft tissue mass, enhancement, calcification

Sacral chordoma
- Mixed solid/cystic destructive sacral mass
  - Bone CT shows destructive margins
  - Rare in children; peak incidence 5th → 6th decade

Ovarian cyst
- Ultrasound may reveal surrounding ovarian tissue that clinches diagnosis

Neurenteric cyst
- Cyst usually within spinal canal +/- rachischisis, vertebral formation anomalies

Cystic neuroblastoma
- Search for calcifications, metastatic lesions

PATHOLOGY

General Features
- General path comments
  - First described in 1837
  - 5% of retrorectal tumors
  - Osseous sacral remodeling in large meningoceles ⇒ classic "scimitar" shape
- Genetics
  - Sporadic (most patients)
  - Minority show inherited predisposition
    - Currarino triad: Autosomal dominant with variable penetration (HLXB 9 gene, chromosome 7q36)
    - Conditions where dural ectasia is prominent (NF1, Marfan, Homocystinuria)
- Etiology
  - Embryogenesis not definitively known; classified within caudal mass anomalies spectrum
    - Erosion or dysgenesis of sacral/coccygeal segments permits herniation of meningeal sac into anterior pelvis
  - Possible associations
    - Simple form: Marfan, NF1
    - Complicated form: Familial, partial sacral agenesis, imperforate anus or anal stenosis, and tethered cord
- Epidemiology: Rare; less common than dorsal meningoceles
- Associated abnormalities: Anorectal anomalies, epidermoid/dermoid tumor or other tethering lesion, Currarino triad

Gross Pathologic & Surgical Features
- Widened sacral dural sac communicates with pelvic cyst through a narrow neck within sacral defect
- +/- Neural tissue within cyst sac

ANTERIOR SACRAL MENINGOCELE

Microscopic Features
• Characteristic features of dural sac tissue; may reveal signs of prior inflammation

CLINICAL ISSUES

Presentation
• Most common signs/symptoms
  ○ Constipation, urinary frequency, incontinence, dysmenorrhea, dyspareunia, low back/pelvic pain
    ▪ 2° to pressure on pelvic viscera
  ○ Other signs/symptoms
    ▪ Sciatica, diminished rectal/detrusor tone, numbness/paresthesias in lower sacral dermatomes (nerve root pressure)
    ▪ Intermittent positional high or low pressure headaches due to fluid shifts between ASM and spinal subarachnoid space
    ▪ Superinfection +/- meningitis (uncommon)
• Clinical profile
  ○ Most present with urinary or bowel complaints; ASM is discovered during imaging evaluation
  ○ Rare finding in headache patient

Demographics
• Age: Onset of symptoms in 2nd to 3rd decade
• Gender
  ○ M = F (children)
  ○ M < F (adults)

Natural History & Prognosis
• Good prognosis following successful repair

Treatment
• Open posterior trans-sacral approach, patching of meningocele - dural sac connection
  ○ Easier if cyst does not contain neural elements, permitting simple ligation of cyst neck
• Endoscopic approach ⇒ lower morbidity

DIAGNOSTIC CHECKLIST

Consider
• Ultrasound for infant screening
• MR imaging to identify and characterize cyst location and contents, confirm abnormal ultrasound findings
• Bone CT to demonstrate characteristic osseous findings that permit a specific diagnosis

Image Interpretation Pearls
• Continuity of cyst with thecal sac necessary to ensure diagnosis
• Soft tissue mass or calcification implies tumor
• Presence/absence of neural tissue within cyst important for surgical planning

SELECTED REFERENCES

1. Rigante D et al: Anterior sacral meningocele in a patient with Marfan syndrome. Clin Neuropathol. 20(2):70-2, 2001
2. Barkovich A: Pediatric neuroimaging. 3rd ed. Philadelphia, Lippincott-Raven, 654-55, 2000
3. Clatterbuck RE, Jackman SV, Kavoussi LR, Long DM. Laparoscopic treatment of an anterior sacral meningocele. J Neurosurg (Spine). 92: 246, 2000
4. Shamoto H et al: Anterior sacral meningocele completely occupied by an epidermoid tumor. Childs Nerv Syst. 15(4):209-11, 1999
5. Fitzpatrick MO, Taylor WAS. Anterior sacral meningocele associated with a rectal fistula. Case report and review of the literature. J Neurosurg (Spine). 91: 124-127, 1999
6. Voyvodic F et al: Anterior sacral meningocele as a pelvic complication of Marfan syndrome. Aust N Z J Obstet Gynaecol. 39(2):262-5, 1999
7. Ball W: Pediatric Neuroradiology. Philadelphia, Lippincott-Raven, 737, 1997
8. Lee SC et al: Currarino triad: anorectal malformation, sacral bony abnormality, and presacral mass--a review of 11 cases. J Pediatr Surg. 32(1):58-61, 1997
9. Gaskill SJ et al: The Currarino triad: its importance in pediatric neurosurgery. Pediatr Neurosurg. 25(3):143-6, 1996
10. Kochling J et al: The Currarino syndrome--hereditary transmitted syndrome of anorectal, sacral and presacral anomalies. Case report and review of the literature. Eur J Pediatr Surg. 6(2):114-9, 1996
11. Funayama CA et al: Recurrent meningitis in a case of congenital anterior sacral meningocele and agenesis of sacral and coccygeal vertebrae. Arq Neuropsiquiatr. 53(4):799-801, 1995
12. Raftopoulos C et al: Anterior sacral meningocele and Marfan syndrome: a review. Acta Chir Belg. 93(1):1-7, 1993
13. Chamaa MT et al: Anterior-sacral meningocele; value of magnetic resonance imaging and abdominal sonography. A case report. Acta Neurochir (Wien). 109(3-4):154-7, 1991
14. North RB et al: Occult, bilateral anterior sacral and intrasacral meningeal and perineurial cysts: case report and review of the literature. Neurosurgery. 27(6):981-6, 1990
15. McGuire RA Jr et al: Anterior sacral meningocele. Case report and review of the literature. Spine. 15(6):612-4, 1990
16. Brem H et al: Neonatal diagnosis of a presacral mass in the presence of congenital anal stenosis and partial sacral agenesis. J Pediatr Surg. 24(10):1076-8, 1989
17. Lee KS et al: The role of MR imaging in the diagnosis and treatment of anterior sacral meningocele. Report of two cases. J Neurosurg. 69(4):628-31, 1988
18. Martin B et al: MR imaging of anterior sacral meningocele. J Comput Assist Tomogr. 12(1):166-7, 1988
19. Dyck P et al: Anterior sacral meningocele. Case report. J Neurosurg. 53(4):548-52, 1980
20. Sherman et al. Anterior Sacral Meningocele. Am J Surg 79:743-747, 1950
21. Bryant T. Case of deficiency of the anterior part of the sacrum with a thecal sac in the pelvis, similar to the tumor of spina bifida. Lancet. 1: 258-360, 1937
22. Fiumara F et al: Purulent meningitis due to spontaneous anterior sacral meningocele perforation. Case report

OCCULT INTRASACRAL MENINGOCELE

Key Facts

Terminology
- Synonyms: Occult intrasacral meningocele (OIM), sacral meningeal cyst, type 1B meningeal cyst

Imaging Findings
- Best diagnostic clue: Smooth, cystic enlargement of central sacral canal
- Cyst follows CSF signal intensity
- No neural elements within cyst

Top Differential Diagnoses
- Tarlov cyst
- Dorsal meningocele
- Dural dysplasia

Pathology
- Extradural arachnoid cyst

- No herniation of meninges, hence not a true meningocele
- Cyst is connected to thecal sac by a pedicle that permits contiguous CSF flow
- CSF pulsation +/- raised intraspinal pressure (across stenotic pedicle) pressure erodes and remodels sacral canal

Clinical Issues
- Most patients are asymptomatic and need no specific treatment
- Symptomatic patients or very large cysts may require surgery

Diagnostic Checklist
- MRI best modality for diagnosis of sacral cyst, pre-operative planning

Imaging Recommendations
- Best imaging tool
  - Magnetic resonance imaging best modality for initial diagnosis
  - CT myelography may help reveal connection between cyst and subarachnoid space
- Protocol advice: Sagittal and axial T1WI and T2WI to identify cyst, clarify relationship to adjacent structures

DIFFERENTIAL DIAGNOSIS

Tarlov cyst
- Etiologically similar to OIM; congenital dilatation of nerve root meningeal sleeves
- Large cysts may remodel sacrum, but will be eccentrically centered over neural foramen
- Frequently multiple

Dorsal meningocele
- True meningocele; protrudes through dorsal dysraphism into subcutaneous tissues

Dural dysplasia
- Vertebral scalloping usually present in lumbar spine as well as sacrum, +/- lateral meningocele
- Search for characteristic imaging and clinical stigmata of etiological disorder

PATHOLOGY

General Features
- General path comments
  - Extradural arachnoid cyst
    - No herniation of meninges, hence not a true meningocele
    - No neuronal elements within cyst
  - Cyst is connected to thecal sac by a pedicle that permits contiguous CSF flow
  - CSF pulsation +/- raised intraspinal pressure (across stenotic pedicle) pressure erodes and remodels sacral canal

- Etiology: Diverticulum of sacral subarachnoid space ⇒ expands into sacral cyst 2° to valve-like mechanism ⇒ secondary remodeling of sacral canal
- Epidemiology
  - Spinal meningeal cysts are uncommon
    - Comprise 1 to 3% of all spinal tumors
  - Prevalence of occult sacral meningocele unknown, but < prevalence of Tarlov cyst
- Associated abnormalities
  - Tarlov cyst(s)
  - Posterior spinal dysraphism
  - Tethered cord syndrome

Gross Pathologic & Surgical Features
- Sacral laminectomy ⇒ thinned sacral vertebral laminae
  - Cyst may be attached to distal thecal sac by a narrow pedicle that permits one-way (mostly) CSF flow into cyst
  - Symptomatic cysts less likely to communicate with subarachnoid space than asymptomatic cysts

Microscopic Features
- Cyst is lined by fibrous connective tissue +/- single inner layer of arachnoid membrane

Staging, Grading or Classification Criteria
- Nabors classification: Type IB meningeal cyst

CLINICAL ISSUES

Presentation
- Most common signs/symptoms
  - Asymptomatic; incidental discovery on MRI
  - Symptomatic: Chronic low back pain, sciatica, perineal paresthesias, and bladder dysfunction
  - Less common signs/symptoms
    - Intermittent, severe lower back pain
    - Atypical bowel symptoms, severe constipation, and stool incontinence
    - Tethered cord syndrome
- Clinical profile

- ○ Specific symptoms are referable to sacral root compression
- ○ May be exacerbated by positional change or Valsalva maneuver

Demographics
- Age
  - ○ Teen → elderly
  - ○ Rarely diagnosed in children
- Gender: Some series report M > F, others M < F

Natural History & Prognosis
- Most patients are asymptomatic and need no specific treatment
  - ○ Asymptomatic cysts are most commonly identified and referred to specialists following incidental discovery on MRI
- Symptomatic patients or very large cysts may require surgery
  - ○ Indications for operative intervention include increased cyst size on serial exams, or onset of symptoms referable to cyst
  - ○ Good prognosis for recovery following surgery

Treatment
- Conservative approach recommended for asymptomatic cysts, especially when small
- Symptomatic cysts may require treatment
  - ○ Percutaneous cyst aspiration may relieve symptoms temporarily
    - ■ May be used as diagnostic test prior to definitive therapy
    - ■ Percutaneous cyst aspiration with fibrin glue therapy may produce definitive long-lasting symptom reduction
  - ○ Operative therapy ⇒ sacral laminectomy to expose, resect cyst
    - ■ May not be necessary to completely resect entire cyst
    - ■ Primary goal is to close dural defect ⇒ eradicate one-way valve communication, prevent cyst recurrence
    - ■ If adhesions prevent full excision, may partially resect posterior wall or marsupialize cyst to subarachnoid space

DIAGNOSTIC CHECKLIST

Consider
- MRI best modality for diagnosis of sacral cyst, pre-operative planning
- Definitive cyst characterization based on operative inspection, histological examination

Image Interpretation Pearls
- Classic appearance is an intrasacral cyst producing smooth sacral canal expansion with outward displacement of nerve roots
- OIM centered in midline; center over neural foramen implies Tarlov cyst

SELECTED REFERENCES

1. Nishio Y et al: A case of occult intrasacral meningocele presented with atypical bowel symptoms. Childs Nerv Syst. 20(1):65-7, 2004
2. Sato et al: Spinal Extradural Meningeal Cyst: Correct Radiological and Histopathological Diagnosis. Neurosurg Focus 13(4), 2002
3. Diel J et al: The sacrum: pathologic spectrum, multimodality imaging, and subspecialty approach. Radiographics. 21(1):83-104, 2001
4. Patel MR et al: Percutaneous fibrin glue therapy of meningeal cysts of the sacral spine. AJR Am J Roentgenol. 168(2):367-70, 1997
5. Okada T et al: Occult intrasacral meningocele associated with spina bifida: a case report. Surg Neurol. 46(2):147-9, 1996
6. Tindall et al: The Practice of Neurosurgery. Baltimore, Williams and Wilkins, Pages A-B, 1996
7. Doi H et al: Occult intrasacral meningocele with tethered cord--case report. Neurol Med Chir (Tokyo). 35(5):321-4, 1995
8. Tatagiba M et al: Management of occult intrasacral meningocele associated with lumbar disc prolapse. Neurosurg Rev. 17(4):313-5, 1994
9. Davis SW et al: Sacral meningeal cysts: evaluation with MR imaging. Radiology. 187(2):445-8, 1993
10. Bayar MA et al: Management problems in cases with a combination of asymptomatic occult intrasacral meningocele and disc prolapse. Acta Neurochir (Wien). 108(1-2):67-9, 1991
11. Doty JR et al: Occult intrasacral meningocele: clinical and radiographic diagnosis. Neurosurgery. 24(4):616-25, 1989
12. Nabors MW et al: Updated assessment and current classification of spinal meningeal cysts. J Neurosurg. 68(3):366-77, 1988
13. Goyal RN, Russell NA, Benoit BG, et al: Intraspinal cysts: a classification and literature review. Spine 12:209-213, 1987
14. Genest AS: Occult intrasacral meningocele. Spine. 9(1):101-3, 1984
15. Grivegnee A et al: Comparative aspects of occult intrasacral meningocele with conventional X-ray, myelography and CT. Neuroradiology. 22(1):33-7, 1981
16. Fortuna A et al: Arachnoid diverticula: a unitary approach to spinal cysts communicating with the subarachnoid space. Acta Neurochir 39:259-268, 1977
17. Lamas E et al: Occult intrasacral meningocele. Surg Neurol. 8(3):181-4, 1977
18. Lombardi G et al: Congenital cysts of the spinal membranes and roots. Br J Radiol 36:197-205, 1963

OCCULT INTRASACRAL MENINGOCELE

IMAGE GALLERY

Typical

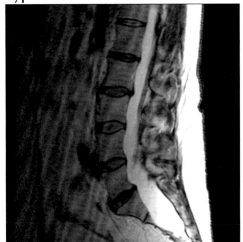 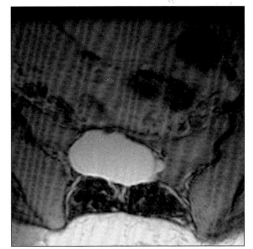

(Left) Sagittal T2WI MR demonstrates large sacral meningocele with extensive remodeling of sacral canal. *(Right)* Axial T2WI MR shows marked enlargement and remodeling of sacrum by a large intrasacral meningocele. No neural elements reside within the extradural cyst, and posterior elements are intact.

Typical

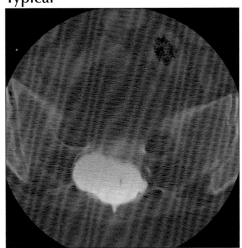 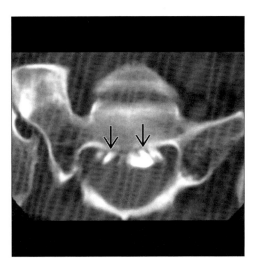

(Left) Axial bone CT following myelography shows a large intrasacral meningocele with contrast opacification indicating contiguity with thecal sac. Posterior elements are intact but markedly thinned. *(Right)* Axial NECT following myelography shows a large extradural cyst with sacral remodeling that anteriorly displaces nerve root sleeves (arrows). Mild contrast uptake indicates contiguity with thecal sac.

Variant

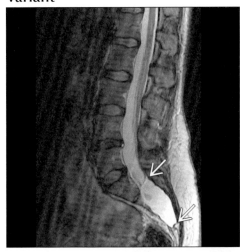 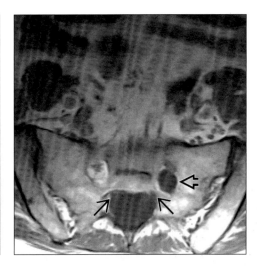

(Left) Sagittal T2WI MR shows a large intrasacral meningocele in conjunction with low-lying tethered cord and syringomyelia. Arrows mark rostral and caudal cyst margins. *(Right)* Axial T1WI MR reveals an intrasacral meningocele that anteriorly displaces the bilateral sacral nerve roots (black arrows). Also noted is a left S1 Tarlov cyst (open arrow).

SACROCOCCYGEAL TERATOMA

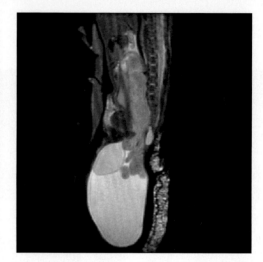

Sagittal graphic depicts a typical large, heterogeneous, partially cystic sacrococcygeal teratoma located anterior to the sacrum, without osseous invasion.

Sagittal T2WI MR shows a large (AAP type II) mixed cystic/solid tumor, with mostly solid internal portion and mostly cystic external portion (Courtesy R. Boyer, MD).

TERMINOLOGY

Abbreviations and Synonyms
- Synonyms: SGT, germ cell tumor of coccyx

Definitions
- Congenital sacral tumor containing elements of all three germ layers

IMAGING FINDINGS

General Features
- Best diagnostic clue: Large heterogeneous sacral mass in an infant
- Location: Sacrum/coccyx
- Size
  - Usually large at diagnosis
    - Mature teratomas ≈ 7.5 cm
    - Immature teratomas ≈ 11.6 cm
- Morphology: Heterogeneous mass containing calcifications, mixed solid and cystic components, fat-debris levels, bone, hair, teeth, or cartilage

Radiographic Findings
- Radiography: Soft tissue mass, calcifications (≤ 60%)

CT Findings
- CECT

- Complex mixed attenuation cystic/solid pelvic mass with enhancement of solid portions
  - Calcifications (≤ 60%); small punctate foci → well formed teeth, bones
  - Calcium (hyperdense), fluid (hypodense), and fat (markedly hypodense)

MR Findings
- T1WI: Heterogeneous mixed signal intensity; fat (hyperintense), soft tissue (isointense), cyst fluid (hypointense), and calcium (markedly hypointense)
- T2WI: Heterogeneous signal intensity; fat (hyperintense), soft tissue (isointense), cyst fluid (hyperintense), and calcium (markedly hypointense)
- STIR: Depicts lobulated, sharply demarcated tumor margins against dark marrow background
- T2* GRE: Shows calcifications best; hemorrhage presents similar imaging appearance
- T1 C+: Heterogeneous enhancement of solid portions

Ultrasonographic Findings
- Real Time
  - Complex mixed hypo-/hyperechoic sacral mass
    - Obstetrical: In-utero diagnosis ⇒ cesarian section, possible fetal surgery or radiofrequency ablation (RFA)
    - Post-natal: Visualization hampered by fat/calcium shadowing, posterior bone elements, large size

DDx: Sacrococcygeal Teratoma

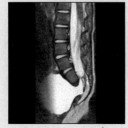
Ant. Meningocele

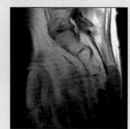
Chordoma

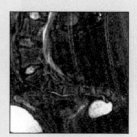
Dermoid

SACROCOCCYGEAL TERATOMA

Key Facts

Terminology
- Synonyms: SGT, germ cell tumor of coccyx

Imaging Findings
- Complex mixed attenuation cystic/solid pelvic mass with enhancement of solid portions
- Calcifications (≤ 60%); small punctate foci → well formed teeth, bones

Top Differential Diagnoses
- Anterior sacral meningocele (ASM)
- Chordoma
- Dermoid tumor
- Exophytic rhabdomyosarcoma

Pathology
- Most common newborn tumor

- Malignant risk ↑ with age at diagnosis, higher surgical subtype, male gender, presence of necrosis or hemorrhage
- Epidemiology: 1:35,000 to 40,000 births

Clinical Issues
- Most common: Neonate with large benign sacral tumor noted prenatally or at delivery
- Less common: Newborn with buttock asymmetry or delayed presentation at > 1 month with presacral tumor

Diagnostic Checklist
- AAP type influences prognosis, treatment approach
- Heterogeneous sacral tumor +/- calcification, cysts, hemorrhage suggests diagnosis

Imaging Recommendations
- Best imaging tool
  - Prenatal: Obstetrical ultrasound +/- fetal MRI
  - Post-natal: MRI
- Protocol advice
  - MRI +/- CT to determine full extent of mass, treatment planning
    - Sagittal and axial MR imaging for surgical planning
    - CT with oral/IV contrast to delineate extent of bone destruction, calcification

DIFFERENTIAL DIAGNOSIS

Anterior sacral meningocele (ASM)
- Cystic mass; no solid component or enhancement
- Enlarges with Valsalva maneuver

Chordoma
- Mixed solid/cystic destructive sacral mass
- Rare in children; peak incidence 5th → 6th decade
- T2WI → markedly hyperintense
- Bone CT → destructive margins

Dermoid tumor
- Isointense/hyperintense (T1WI) → hyperintense (T2WI)
- Smaller, more homogeneous than SGT

Exophytic rhabdomyosarcoma
- Aggressive appearing tumor without calcium, bone, or hair

PATHOLOGY

General Features
- General path comments
  - Most common newborn tumor
    - 80% mature, 20% immature; immature teratomas have greater risk of malignancy

  - Malignancy risk 10% at term; ↑ to 65-90% if diagnosed > 2 months
    - Malignant risk ↑ with age at diagnosis, higher surgical subtype, male gender, presence of necrosis or hemorrhage
- Genetics
  - Most cases are sporadic; some syndromic associations (Currarino triad)
  - Scattered reports of familial parent-child associations (autosomal dominant)
    - Congenital sacral deformities, anorectal stenosis, vesicoureteral reflux, retrorectal abscess, and skin dimple
- Etiology
  - Originate from totipotential cell rests at caudal spine/notochord (Hensen node)
    - Degree of totipotential cell differentiation ⇒ tumor type
    - Undifferentiated cells ⇒ more malignant tumors
  - Alternative hypothesis: "Twinning" accident ⇒ incomplete separation during embryogenesis
- Epidemiology: 1:35,000 to 40,000 births
- Associated abnormalities: Currarino triad, anorectal or genitourinary abnormalities (10%)

Gross Pathologic & Surgical Features
- Benign teratomas (83%)
  - Heterogeneous noninvasive, partially cystic, calcified soft tissue mass; rarely invade spinal canal
  - Multiple tissue types show varying stages of differentiation, maturation
- Malignant teratomas (17%)
  - More likely intrasacral, aggressive local behavior
  - Malignancy postulated to arise from differentiated cell lines within teratoma ⇒ neuroblastoma, adenocarcinoma, or rhabdomyosarcoma, embryonal cell carcinoma, or anaplastic carcinoma

Microscopic Features
- Elements derived from all three germ layers (endoderm, mesoderm, and ectoderm)

Staging, Grading or Classification Criteria
- Four surgical subtypes (Altman/AAP classification)

SACROCOCCYGEAL TERATOMA

○ Type I: Primarily external (47%) ⇒ best prognosis
○ Type II: Dumbbell shape, equal external/internal portions (34%)
○ Type III: Primarily internal within abdomen/pelvis (9%)
○ Type IV: Entirely internal; no visible external component (10%) ⇒ worst prognosis

CLINICAL ISSUES

Presentation
• Most common signs/symptoms
  ○ Back/pelvic mass in a newborn
    ▪ Exophytic masses easily diagnosed, but internal (type III, IV) occult ⇒ delayed diagnosis
  ○ In-utero presentation
    ▪ Polyhydramnios, high output cardiac failure with hydrops, hepatomegaly, placentomegaly
  ○ Urinary retention, constipation (larger tumors)
• Clinical profile
  ○ Most common: Neonate with large benign sacral tumor noted prenatally or at delivery
  ○ Less common: Newborn with buttock asymmetry or delayed presentation at > 1 month with presacral tumor
• Laboratory: Serum α- fetoprotein (AFP), β-human chorionic gonadotropin (HCG) levels post-operative tumor markers

Demographics
• Age: 50-70% diagnosed in-utero or during first days of life, 80% by 6 months, and fewer than 10% beyond 2 years
• Gender: M < F 4:1

Natural History & Prognosis
• Prognosis excellent in benign tumors
  ○ Mature or mostly cystic ⇒ good prognosis
  ○ Immature teratomas ⇒ greater risk of malignancy if not totally resected
• Malignant tumors have variable prognosis; later diagnosis (> 1st birthday), internal location ⇒ worse prognosis
• Fetal mortality rate 20-65% (2° to polyhydramnios, tumor hemorrhage, high-output cardiac failure)
  ○ Hydrops fetalis portends grim prognosis; > 30 weeks gestation ⇒ 25% mortality, < 30 weeks gestation ⇒ 93% mortality
• Postpartum morbidity attributable to associated congenital anomalies, tumor mass effects, recurrence, and intra-operative/post-operative complications

Treatment
• Surgery alone curative if entire benign tumor and coccyx removed; recurs if coccyx not resected
• Cytoreduction surgery + radiation, chemotherapy may be palliative for malignant tumors; early diagnosis, resection best chance for cure
• Fetal surgery, (RFA) offered at some specialized centers; good outcome requires careful patient selection

DIAGNOSTIC CHECKLIST

Consider
• Imaging goals: Imperative to confirm diagnosis, determine intra/extrapelvic extent and size, relationship to adjacent structures, and presence/absence of metastatic disease
• AAP type influences prognosis, treatment approach

Image Interpretation Pearls
• Heterogeneous sacral tumor +/- calcification, cysts, hemorrhage suggests diagnosis

SELECTED REFERENCES

1. Hirose S et al: Fetal surgery for sacrococcygeal teratoma. Clin Perinatol. 30(3):493-506, 2003
2. Graf JL et al: Fetal sacrococcygeal teratoma. World J Surg. 27(1):84-6, 2003
3. Axt-Fliedner R et al: Prenatal diagnosis of sacrococcygeal teratoma: a review of cases between 1993 and 2000. Clin Exp Obstet Gynecol. 29(1):15-8, 2002
4. Perrelli L et al: Sacrococcygeal teratoma. Outcome and management. An analysis of 17 cases. J Perinat Med. 30(2):179-84, 2002
5. Avni FE et al: MR imaging of fetal sacrococcygeal teratoma: diagnosis and assessment. AJR Am J Roentgenol. 178(1):179-83, 2002
6. Monteiro M et al: Case report: sacrococcygeal teratoma with malignant transformation in an adult female: CT and MRI findings. Br J Radiol. 75(895):620-3, 2002
7. Paek BW et al: Radiofrequency ablation of human fetal sacrococcygeal teratoma. Am J Obstet Gynecol. 184(3):503-7, 2001
8. Barkovich A: Pediatric neuroimaging. 3rd ed. Philadelphia, Lippincott-Raven, 655, 2000
9. Holterman AX et al: The natural history of sacrococcygeal teratomas diagnosed through routine obstetric sonogram: a single institution experience. J Pediatr Surg. 33(6):899-903, 1998
10. Ball W: Pediatric Neuroradiology. Philadelphia, Lippincott-Raven, 736-37, 1997
11. Schropp KP et al: Sacrococcygeal teratoma: the experience of four decades. J Pediatr Surg. 27(8):1075-8; discussion 1078-9, 1992
12. Wells RG et al: Imaging of sacrococcygeal germ cell tumors. Radiographics. 10(4):701-13, 1990
13. Noseworthy J et al: Sacrococcygeal germ cell tumors in childhood: an updated experience with 118 patients. J Pediatr Surg. 16(3):358-64, 1981
14. Schey WL et al: Clinical and radiographic considerations of sacrococcygeal teratomas: an analysis of 26 new cases and review of the literature. Radiology. 125(1):189-95, 1977
15. Altman RP et al: Sacrococcygeal teratoma: American Academy of Pediatrics Surgical Section Survey-1973. J Pediatr Surg. 9(3):389-98, 1974
16. Huddart SN et al: Sacrococcygeal teratomas: the UK Children's Cancer Study Group's experience. I. Neonatal.

IMAGE GALLERY

Typical

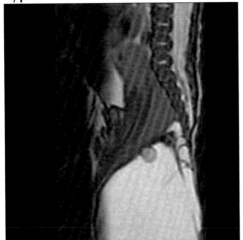 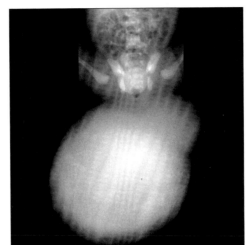

(Left) Sagittal T2WI MR shows a predominately cystic external (AAP I) teratoma that displaces the pelvic viscera rostrally (Courtesy G. Hedlund, DO). *(Right)* Anteroposterior radiography shows a large external sacral teratoma (AAP type 1) (Courtesy R. Boyer, MD).

Typical

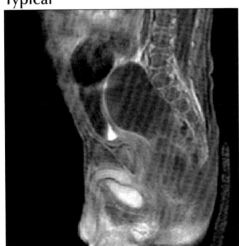 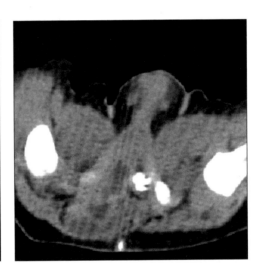

(Left) Sagittal T1 C+ MR reveals a predominately internal (AAP III) heterogeneous enhancing partially cystic tumor (Courtesy G. Hedlund, DO). *(Right)* Axial CECT reveals a mixed solid/cystic enhancing tumor extending into perineum, with several large well-formed internal calcifications (Courtesy G. Hedlund, DO).

Typical

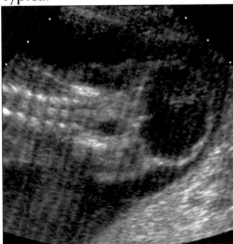 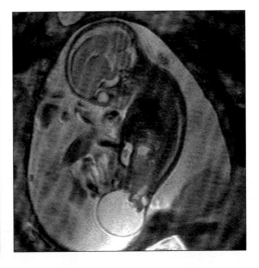

(Left) Coronal ultrasound real time of a fetus reveals a mixed echogenicity solid/cystic sacral mass (Courtesy A. Kennedy, MD). *(Right)* Sagittal T2WI MR fetal MR depicts a heterogeneous solid/cystic sacral mass (AAP type II) with concurrent polyhydramnios (Courtesy A. Kennedy, MD).

DIASTEMATOMYELIA

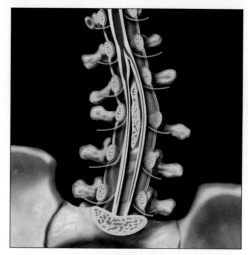
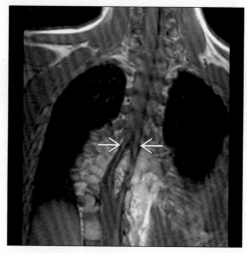

Coronal graphic demonstrates type I SCM with large osseous marrow-filled spur dividing syringomyelic tethered spinal cord into two hemicords contiguous with thoracic syrinx.

Coronal T1WI MR (Type I SCM) demonstrates an ossified septum dividing the two hemicords (arrows). Scoliosis and fusion of the posterior elements is also apparent.

TERMINOLOGY

Abbreviations and Synonyms
- Synonyms: SCM, split cord malformation, "diastem"

Definitions
- Sagittal division of spinal cord into two hemicords, each with one central canal, dorsal horn, and ventral horn

IMAGING FINDINGS

General Features
- Best diagnostic clue
  - Fibrous or osseous spur splits spinal cord into two hemicords
    - Split cord and spur often occur in conjunction with intersegmental fusion
- Location: Thoracolumbar cleft (85% between T9 and S1) > > upper thoracic, cervical clefts
- Size: Range focal ⇒ extensive
- Morphology
  - Hemicords usually reunite above and below cleft
  - +/- Spur (fibrous, osteocartilaginous, or osseous), thickened filum, cord tethering

Radiographic Findings
- Radiography

  - Quantify kyphoscoliosis, "count" level of vertebral segmentation anomalies
  - Detects spur < 50% of cases
- Myelography
  - Split cord; one or two dural tubes
  - Excellent delineation of spur location and meningocele manqué (if present); most useful in conjunction with CT

CT Findings
- NECT
  - Osseous spur often visible; fibrous spurs are frequently occult
  - Vertebral segmentation anomalies

MR Findings
- T1WI
  - Two hemicords +/- syringohydromyelia (50%)
  - +/- Isointense (fibrous) or hyperintense (osseous - contains marrow) spur
- T2WI
  - Two hemicords +/- syringohydromyelia (50%) in one or both cords, surrounded by bright CSF
  - Hypointense (fibrous or osseous) spur; fibrous spur best seen in axial or coronal plane
- T2* GRE: Myelographic effect produces bright CSF adjacent to dark bones, highlights hypointense spur

DDx: More Examples of Diastematomyelia

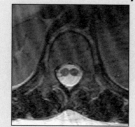
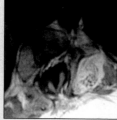
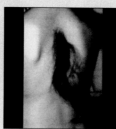
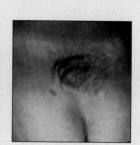

Type II Diastem. *Meningocele Manqué* *High Hair Patch* *Low Hair Patch*

DIASTEMATOMYELIA

Key Facts

Terminology
- Synonyms: SCM, split cord malformation, "diastem"
- Sagittal division of spinal cord into two hemicords, each with one central canal, dorsal horn, and ventral horn

Imaging Findings
- Location: Thoracolumbar cleft (85% between T9 and S1) > > upper thoracic, cervical clefts
- Hemicords usually reunite above and below cleft
- Split cord; one or two dural tubes
- Osseous spur often visible; fibrous spurs are frequently occult
- Vertebral segmentation anomalies

Top Differential Diagnoses
- Duplicated spinal cord (diplomyelia)

Pathology
- "Split notochord syndrome" spectrum
- Epidemiology: 5% of congenital scoliosis
- Congenital spinal deformities (85%)
- Nerve roots may become adherent to dura and tether cord ⇒ "meningocele manqué"

Clinical Issues
- Cutaneous stigmata high on back indicates diastematomyelia level (> 50%); "fawn's tail" hair patch most common

Diagnostic Checklist
- Search for DSM in patients with cutaneous stigmata, intersegmental fusion of posterior elements, clinical tethered cord

Ultrasonographic Findings
- Real Time
  - Obstetrical ultrasound → "extra" posterior echogenic focus, splaying of fetal posterior spinal elements
  - Post-natal imaging → spur, tethered cord

Imaging Recommendations
- Best imaging tool: MR imaging
- Protocol advice
  - Consider ultrasound to screen infants with skin dimple or cutaneous marker
  - MR imaging most definitive
    - Coronal, axial images best demonstrate hemicords, spur
    - T1WI to evaluate for filum lesions (e.g., fibrolipoma), vertebral anomalies
    - T2WI to determine number of dural sacs, +/- syringohydromyelia
    - T2* GRE to detect spur
- Supplement with bone CT +/- myelography to optimally define spur anatomy for surgical planning
  - Sagittal, coronal reformats excellent for depicting osseous anatomy, extent of spur

DIFFERENTIAL DIAGNOSIS

Duplicated spinal cord (diplomyelia)
- Two complete spinal cords, each with two anterior and two posterior horns and roots
- Exceedingly rare, seen only in presence of spinal canal duplication; many authors dispute its true existence, believe it represents a severe form of diastematomyelia

PATHOLOGY

General Features
- General path comments
  - Septum inhibits normal spinal cord movement during activity ⇒ symptom progression
  - Spinal cord damage occurs via direct pressure and by traction ⇒ cord ischemia

- Cleft splits cord, with single cord above and below split
  - Most (91%) hemicords reunite caudally to terminate in a single filum terminale
- Roots may adhere to dura ⇒ "meningocele manqué"
- Genetics: Sporadic; rare familial cases described
- Etiology
  - "Split notochord syndrome" spectrum
    - Congenital splitting of notochord ⇒ "split notochord syndrome" spectrum; diastematomyelia, dorsal enteric fistula/sinus, and dorsal enteric cysts/diverticula
  - Notochord directly influences vertebral body formation ⇒ segmentation anomalies
    - Lateral notch produces hemivertebra
    - Cleft produces butterfly vertebra
- Epidemiology: 5% of congenital scoliosis
- Associated abnormalities
  - Other split notochord syndromes (20%)
  - Congenital spinal deformities (85%)
    - Segmentation and fusion anomalies (SFA)
    - Intersegmental laminar fusion (60%); virtually pathognomonic for diastematomyelia
    - Spinal dysraphism (myelocele/myelomeningocele 15-25%, hemimyelocele 15-20%)
    - Tethered spinal cord (75%); thickened filum terminale (40-90%)
    - Syringohydromyelia (50%) one or both hemicords, usually above diastematomyelia
    - Congenital scoliosis (79%)
    - 15-20% of Chiari II malformations

Gross Pathologic & Surgical Features
- Sagittal spinal cord split into symmetric or asymmetric hemicords, residing in either one or two dural tubes
  - Symmetric: Each hemicord contains one central canal, dorsal horn/root, and one ventral horn/root surrounded by pial layer
  - Asymmetric: Division of anterior or posterior hemicord - "partial diastematomyelia"
- Two dural tubes, each with own pial, arachnoid, and dural sheaths for several spinal segments (50%)

DIASTEMATOMYELIA

○ Bony or cartilaginous spur at inferior cleft, originating from lamina or vertebral body
○ Vertebral anomalies more severe (block or butterfly vertebrae, hemivertebrae, and posterior spina bifida)
○ Hydromyelia common
• Single dural tube, subarachnoid space (50%)
○ No bony spur; nearly always have a fibrous band coursing thru inferior cleft inserting into dura → tethers cord
○ Vertebral anomalies less severe (usually butterfly vertebrae)
○ Nerve roots may become adherent to dura and tether cord ⇒ "meningocele manqué"

Microscopic Features
• Single ependymal lined central canal, ventral horn/root, and dorsal horn/root per hemicord

Staging, Grading or Classification Criteria
• Pang type I SCM
○ Separate dural sac, arachnoid space surrounds each hemicord
○ Osseous/fibrous spur
○ More commonly symptomatic than type II
• Pang type II SCM
○ Single dural sac, arachnoid space
○ No osseous spur; +/- adherent fibrous bands tether cord
○ Rarely present with symptoms unless hydromyelia, tethering

CLINICAL ISSUES

Presentation
• Most common signs/symptoms
○ Clinically indistinguishable from other causes of tethered cord
○ Cutaneous stigmata high on back indicates diastematomyelia level (> 50%); "fawn's tail" hair patch most common
○ Other signs/symptoms
  ▪ Progressive kyphoscoliosis in older children, adults
  ▪ Orthopedic foot problems (50%); especially clubfoot
  ▪ Urologic dysfunction
• Clinical profile
○ Mild cases normal +/- cutaneous stigmata
○ Severe cases → kyphoscoliosis, neurological and musculoskeletal abnormalities

Demographics
• Age: Diagnosis in childhood; adult presentation uncommon
• Gender
○ Pediatric: F > > M (80-94%)
○ Adult: M < F 1:3.4

Natural History & Prognosis
• Stable or progressive disability if untreated
○ Late onset or previously stable patients may become symptomatic following relatively minor back injury or surgery requiring spinal manipulation

• ≥ 90% of patients stabilize or improve following surgery
○ Caveat: Scoliosis rarely affected by surgical untethering

Treatment
• Surgical tethered cord release, spur resection, and dural repair for progressive symptoms, prophylactic precursor to scoliosis surgery

DIAGNOSTIC CHECKLIST

Consider
• Scrutinize images for presence of spur; type I DSM generally has more severe symptoms and anomalies, worse prognosis
• Search for DSM in patients with cutaneous stigmata, intersegmental fusion of posterior elements, clinical tethered cord

Image Interpretation Pearls
• Segmentation anomalies with intersegmental laminar fusion virtually pathognomonic for diastematomyelia

SELECTED REFERENCES

1. Balci S et al: Cervical diastematomyelia in cervico-oculo-acoustic (Wildervanck) syndrome: MRI findings. Clin Dysmorphol. 11(2):125-8, 2002
2. Tortori-Donati P et al: Magnetic resonance imaging of spinal dysraphism. Top Magn Reson Imaging. 12(6):375-409, 2001
3. Barkovich A: Pediatric neuroimaging. 3rd ed, Philadelphia, Lippincott-Raven, 655-65, 2000
4. Balci S et al: Diastematomyelia in two sisters. Am J Med Genet. 86(2):180-2, 1999
5. Ersahin Y et al: Split spinal cord malformations in children. J Neurosurg. 88(1):57-65, 1998
6. Frymoyer et al: The Adult Spine. Vol 2. 2nd ed. Philadelphia, Lippincott-Raven. 1923-1926, 1997
7. Miller A et al: Evaluation and treatment of diastematomyelia. J Bone Joint Surg Am. 75(9):1308-17, 1993
8. Pang D et al: Split cord malformation: Part I: A unified theory of embryogenesis for double spinal cord malformations. Neurosurgery. 31(3):451-80, 1992
9. Pang D et al: Split cord malformation: Part II: Clinical syndrome. Neurosurgery 31(3): 481-500, 1992
10. Kaffenberger DA et al: Meningocele manque: radiologic findings with clinical correlation. AJNR Am J Neuroradiol. 13(4):1083-8, 1992
11. Naidich TP et al: Diastematomyelia: hemicord and meningeal sheaths; single and double arachnoid and dural tubes. AJNR Am J Neuroradiol. 4(3):633-6, 1983
12. Harwood-Nash DC et al: Diastematomyelia in 172 children: the impact of modern neuroradiology. Pediatr Neurosurg. 16(4-5):247-51, 1990-91
13. Russell NA et al: Diastematomyelia in adults. A review. Pediatr Neurosurg. 16(4-5):252-7, 1990-91

DIASTEMATOMYELIA

I

1

59

IMAGE GALLERY

Typical

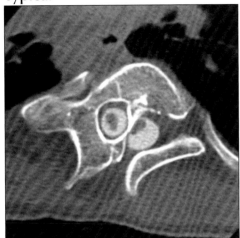
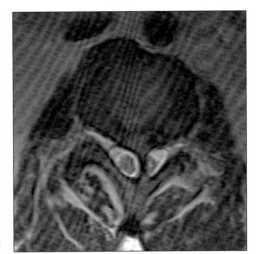

(Left) Axial bone CT following myelography shows dural tube division by an osseous septum (type 1 SCM). The left lamina is dysraphic. (Right) Axial T2WI MR shows two hemicords within individual dural tubes, separated by an osseous spur (type I SCM). The left hemicord demonstrates syringomyelia.

Variant

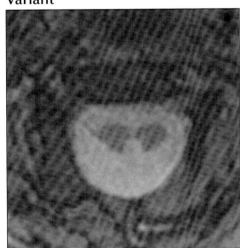
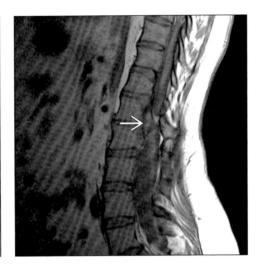

(Left) Axial T2 GRE MR shows a rare cervical type II SCM. The two hemicords share a single dural tube. (Right) Sagittal T1WI MR (type 1 SCM) depicts an osseous spur (arrow) at L1 vertebral level that splits, tethers cord. The conus resides at L3 level.*

Variant

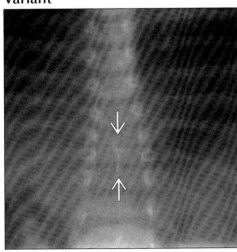
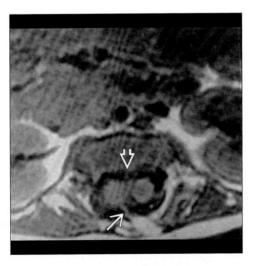

(Left) Anteroposterior radiography (type I SCM) depicts widening of the spinal canal, with a midline osseous spur (arrows) (Courtesy of R. Boyer, MD). (Right) Axial T1WI MR depicts a thin fibrous septum (open arrow) dividing two hemicords (type II SCM). A dorsal nerve root (arrow) affixes right hemicord to the dorsal dural sac (meningocele manqué).

NEURENTERIC CYST

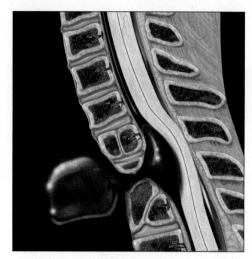

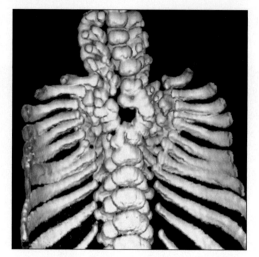

Sagittal graphic shows a large mediastinal enteric cyst extending into the ventral spinal canal through a patent canal of Kovalevsky to produce cord compression.

Coronal bone CT (3D reformat) shows extensive vertebral segmentation anomalies, multiple abnormal fused ribs, and a large patent canal of Kovalevsky (Courtesy S. Blaser, MD).

TERMINOLOGY

Abbreviations and Synonyms
- Synonyms: Spinal enterogenous cyst, spinal enteric cyst, spinal dorsal-enteric cyst

Definitions
- Intraspinal cyst lined by enteric mucosa

IMAGING FINDINGS

General Features
- Best diagnostic clue: Intraspinal cyst + vertebral abnormalities (persistent canal of Kovalevsky, segmentation and fusion anomalies)
- Location: Thoracic (42%) > cervical (32%) > > lumbar spine, intracranial/basilar cisterns (rare)
- Size: Range small → large
- Morphology: Intraspinal or "dumbbell" shaped abdominal or mediastinal enteric/spinal cyst; ventral > dorsal, extramedullary (80-85%) > intramedullary (10-15%), midline > paramedian

Radiographic Findings
- Radiography
  - Enlarged spinal canal, widening of interpedicular distance

  - +/- Vertebral segmentation/fusion anomalies, midline circular vertebral defect (canal of Kovalevsky)
- Myelography
  - Focal spinal canal enlargement, contrast filling defect
    - Invaginating cyst mimics intramedullary lesion

CT Findings
- CECT: Hypodense intraspinal cyst with minimal to no enhancement
- Bone CT
  - Focal osseous canal enlargement, widening of interpedicular distance
  - Vertebral anomalies (≤ 50%, usually pediatric patient); vertebral clefts, butterfly vertebra, segmentation anomalies

MR Findings
- T1WI
  - Well-circumscribed fluid-intensity lesion +/- vertebral anomalies
    - Iso- → hyperintense (to CSF) depending on protein/mucin content
- T2WI
  - Well-circumscribed fluid-intensity cystic lesion
    - Hypo- → isointense (to CSF) depending on protein/mucin content
  - +/- Cord myeloschisis, focal cord atrophy

DDx: Neurenteric Cyst

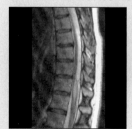

Arachnoid Cyst

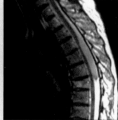

Arachnoid Cyst

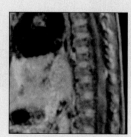

Dermoid

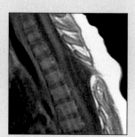

Dermoid/Dermal Sinus

NEURENTERIC CYST

Key Facts

Terminology
- Synonyms: Spinal enterogenous cyst, spinal enteric cyst, spinal dorsal-enteric cyst

Imaging Findings
- Best diagnostic clue: Intraspinal cyst + vertebral abnormalities (persistent canal of Kovalevsky, segmentation and fusion anomalies)
- Location: Thoracic (42%) > cervical (32%) > > lumbar spine, intracranial/basilar cisterns (rare)
- Focal osseous canal enlargement, widening of interpedicular distance

Top Differential Diagnoses
- Arachnoid cyst
- (Epi)dermoid cyst
- Anterior thoracic meningocele

Pathology
- Single smooth unilocular (rarely multilocular) cyst containing clear or proteinaceous fluid (milky, cream-colored, yellowish, xanthochromic)
- Demonstrable cyst connection with spinal cord, vertebrae, or both; dorsal spinal-enteric tract traverses cartilage-lined canal of Kovalevsky through small dysplastic vertebra

Clinical Issues
- Back/radicular pain
- Progressive paraparesis/paresthesias

Diagnostic Checklist
- Degree of cord compression, size of cyst, and severity of associated anomalies determine disease course and prognosis

---

- T1 C+: Mild to no rim-enhancement

Ultrasonographic Findings
- Real Time: Hypoechoic intraspinal cyst

Nuclear Medicine Findings
- Technetium Tc-99m cyst uptake (gastric mucosa) confirms diagnosis

Imaging Recommendations
- Multiplanar T1WI, T2WI to assess for vertebral anomalies, cord compression, and cyst relationship to adjacent structures
- Bone CT/3D CT to characterize osseous anomalies, surgical planning

DIFFERENTIAL DIAGNOSIS

Arachnoid cyst
- CSF density/intensity on all pulse sequences
- Generally located within dorsal spinal canal
- Vertebral anomalies uncommon

(Epi)dermoid cyst
- Most common at conus/cauda equina level
- +/- Sinus tract, cord tethering, skin dimple

Anterior thoracic meningocele
- Anterior dumbbell shape, contiguous with dural sac

PATHOLOGY

General Features
- General path comments
  - Enteric cysts not limited to spinal column; may be found within brain, mediastinum, abdomen, pelvis, subcutaneous tissues
  - Neurenteric cyst is a subgroup of split notochord syndrome spectrum
    - Dorsal enteric diverticulum: Diverticulum from dorsal mesenteric border of bowel
    - Dorsal enteric enterogenous cyst: Prevertebral, intraspinal, postvertebral, mediastinal, or mesenteric location
    - Dorsal enteric sinus: Blind ending tract with opening on dorsal skin surface
    - Dorsal enteric fistula (most severe): Connects intestinal cavity with dorsal skin surface, traversing through soft tissues and spine
- Etiology
  - Putative derivation from abnormal connection between primitive endoderm and ectoderm during 3rd embryonic week
    - Notochord normally separates dorsal ectoderm (skin and spinal cord) and ventral endoderm (foregut)
    - Failure of separation ⇒ split notochord or notochord deviated to side of adhesion
    - Incomplete separation of notochord layer from the endoderm (primitive foregut) layer hinders development of mesoderm; a small piece of primitive gut becomes trapped in developing spinal canal
    - Embryo growth, adhesion may lengthen or partially obliterate; enteric and spinal structures connected through persistent canal of Kovalevsky in severe cases
- Epidemiology: Rare: 0.3-0.5% of spinal "tumors"
- Associated abnormalities
  - Vertebral anomalies (≤ 50%): Anterior or posterior dysraphism, small dysplastic vertebral bodies, vertebral fusion, butterfly or hemivertebra, diastematomyelia (31%), lipoma (31%), dermal sinus tract, or tethered spinal cord (23%)
    - Implies earlier developmental "error" than cases without vertebral anomalies
    - More common if mediastinal or abdominal cysts
  - Klippel-Feil syndrome
  - Cutaneous stigmata
  - Alimentary duplication or fistulae, VACTERL syndrome

NEURENTERIC CYST

Gross Pathologic & Surgical Features
- Single smooth unilocular (rarely multilocular) cyst containing clear or proteinaceous fluid (milky, cream-colored, yellowish, xanthochromic)
  - Demonstrable cyst connection with spinal cord, vertebrae, or both; dorsal spinal-enteric tract traverses cartilage-lined canal of Kovalevsky through small dysplastic vertebra

Microscopic Features
- Thin-walled cyst lined by simple, pseudostratified, stratified cuboidal, or columnar epithelium +/- ciliated epithelium, goblet cells
- Ultrastructurally similar to brain Rathke cleft cyst, colloid cyst

Staging, Grading or Classification Criteria
- World Health Organization (WHO) classification: "Other malformative tumors and tumor-like lesions"
- Three types based on histology (Wilkins and Odum)
  - Type A: Single layer or pseudostratified epithelium resembling respiratory (17%) or gastrointestinal (50%) epithelium, or both (33%)
  - Type B: Type A + mucous or serous glands, smooth muscle connective tissue, lymphoid tissue or nervous tissue
  - Type C: Type A + ependymal or other glial elements

CLINICAL ISSUES

Presentation
- Most common signs/symptoms
  - Back/radicular pain
  - Progressive paraparesis/paresthesias
  - Gait disturbance
  - Meningitis
    - Mollaret → rupture into CSF
    - Bacterial → seeding by enteric organisms
  - Other signs/symptoms
    - Chronic fever and myelopathy 2° to secretion of TNF-α (usually infants)
    - Congenital mirror movements of hands (very rare, seen in conjunction with diastematomyelia)
- Clinical profile
  - Children present more commonly with cutaneous stigmata, spinal dysraphism symptoms
  - Adults present primarily with pain, myelopathy

Demographics
- Age
  - 2nd → 4th decades (range 8 days → 72 years)
    - Cysts with associated malformations present earlier than isolated cysts
- Gender: M:F = 3:2 to 2:1

Natural History & Prognosis
- Some asymptomatic → diagnosis at autopsy
- Most show progressive neurological deterioration
- Significant symptomatic improvement following resection in many patients

Treatment
- Primary treatment goal is complete surgical excision

- Drainage, partial resection if complete excision not possible
- Subtotal excision ⇒ recurrence

DIAGNOSTIC CHECKLIST

Consider
- Degree of cord compression, size of cyst, and severity of associated anomalies determine disease course and prognosis

Image Interpretation Pearls
- Imaging appearance reflects cyst composition
- Look for associated mediastinal or abdominal cysts, connecting fistulae, or vertebral anomalies

SELECTED REFERENCES

1. Agrawal D et al: Intramedullary neurenteric cyst presenting as infantile paraplegia: a case and review. Pediatr Neurosurg. 37(2):93-6, 2002
2. Kapoor V et al: Neuroradiologic-pathologic correlation in a neurenteric cyst of the clivus. AJNR Am J Neuroradiol. 23(3):476-9, 2002
3. Graham D et al: Greenfield's Neuropathology. 7th ed. London, Arnold. 968-969, 2002
4. Kumar R et al: Intraspinal neurenteric cysts--report of three paediatric cases. Childs Nerv Syst. 17(10):584-8, 2001
5. Lippman CR et al: Intramedullary neurenteric cysts of the spine. Case report and review of the literature. J Neurosurg. 94(2 Suppl):305-9, 2001
6. Filho FL et al: Neurenteric cyst of the craniocervical junction. Report of three cases. J Neurosurg. 94(1 Suppl):129-32, 2001
7. Kadhim H et al: Spinal neurenteric cyst presenting in infancy with chronic fever and acute myelopathy. Neurology. 54(10):2011-5, 2000
8. Barkovich A: Pediatric neuroimaging. 3rd ed. Philadelphia, Lippincott-Raven. Pages 655-658, 2000
9. Paleologos TS et al: Spinal neurenteric cysts without associated malformations. Are they the same as those presenting in spinal dysraphism? Br J Neurosurg. 14(3):185-94, 2000
10. Lee SH et al: Thoracic neurenteric cyst in an adult: case report. Neurosurgery. 45(5):1239-42; disscussion 1242-3, 1999
11. Ellis AM et al: Intravertebral spinal neurenteric cysts: a unique radiographic sign--"the hole-in-one vertebra". J Pediatr Orthop. 17(6):766-8, 1997
12. Atlas S. Magnetic Resonance Imaging of the Brain and Spine. 2nd ed. Philadelphia, Lippincott-Ravin. 1314-1316, 1996
13. Prasad VS et al: Cervico-thoracic neurenteric cyst: clinicoradiological correlation with embryogenesis. Childs Nerv Syst. 12(1):48-51, 1996
14. Gao PY et al: Neurenteric cysts: pathology, imaging spectrum, and differential diagnosis. International Journal of Neuroradiology 1:17-27, 1995
15. Brooks BS et al: Neuroimaging features of neurenteric cysts: analysis of nine cases and review of the literature. AJNR Am J Neuroradiol. 14(3):735-46, 1993
16. Kropp J et al: Neurenteric cyst diagnosed by technetium-99m pertechnetate sequential scintigraphy. J Nucl Med. 28(7):1218-20, 1987
17. Wilkins RH et al: Spinal intradural cysts. in Handbook of clinical neurology. 20:55-102, 1976

NEURENTERIC CYST

IMAGE GALLERY

Typical

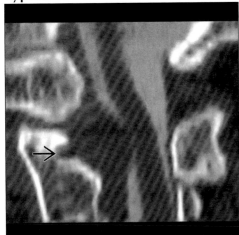

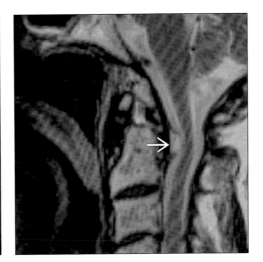

*(**Left**) Sagittal bone CT (Klippel-Feil syndrome) following myelography shows a sagittal vertebral cleft (arrow) in conjunction with a ventral cervical neurenteric cyst. Mild cord compression is present. (**Right**) Sagittal T2WI MR demonstrates a ventral neurenteric cyst (arrow) in conjunction with C2 vertebral cleft. Cyst produces mild ventral cord compression.*

Variant

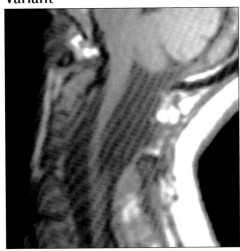

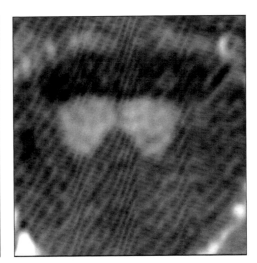

*(**Left**) Sagittal T1WI MR shows a dorsal cervical neurenteric cyst associated with cord myeloschisis and spinal canal remodeling. (**Right**) Axial T1WI MR depicts cervical dorsal diaschisis with associated dorsal neurenteric cyst. Spinal canal remodeling focally widens canal at cyst level. Cyst contents are slightly hyperintense to CSF.*

Variant

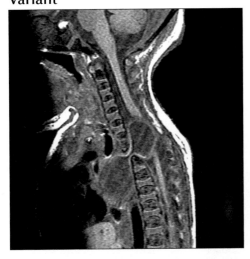

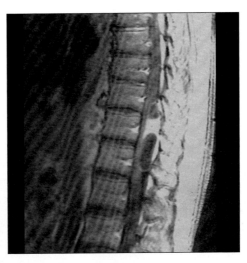

*(**Left**) Sagittal T1WI MR shows a large "dumbbell" neurenteric cyst extending from the mediastinum into the central canal through a patent canal of Kovalevsky causing cord compression (Courtesy S. Blaser, MD). (**Right**) Sagittal T1 C+ MR shows an atypical multilocular enhancing dorsal neurenteric cyst causing marked cord compression.*

FAILURE OF VERTEBRAL FORMATION

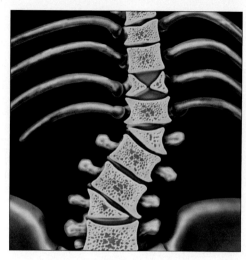

Coronal graphic shows segmented "balanced" L1 and L4 hemivertebra and a T11 butterfly vertebra.

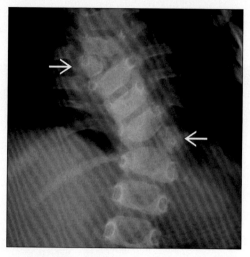

Anteroposterior radiography demonstrates segmented "balanced" right T7 and left T11 hemivertebrae (arrows) with resultant focal scoliotic curves.

TERMINOLOGY

Abbreviations and Synonyms
- Synonyms: Vertebral dysplasia, segmentation and fusion anomaly (SFA), "disorganized spine"

Definitions
- Partial or complete failure of vertebral formation
  - Partial formation failure ⇒ wedge vertebra
  - Complete formation failure ⇒ vertebral aplasia, hemivertebra, butterfly vertebra

IMAGING FINDINGS

General Features
- Best diagnostic clue: Sharply angulated, single curve, or focal scoliosis with deformed vertebral bodies
- Location: Thoracolumbar most common
- Size: Hemivertebra, butterfly vertebra generally smaller than normal vertebra
- Morphology: Incompletely formed vertebra; may be missing front, back, side, or middle of vertebral body

Radiographic Findings
- Radiography
  - Vertebral formation failure anomalies
  - +/- Scoliosis

- Paired bilateral hemivertebra ⇒ "balanced", scoliotic curves cancel out
- One or more unilateral hemivertebra ⇒ "unbalanced", uncompensated scoliotic curve
  - Best modality for "counting" vertebral levels, determining presence and severity of scoliosis

CT Findings
- Bone CT
  - Sagittal or coronal vertebral clefts, hemivertebra, butterfly vertebra
    - Abnormal vertebra difficult to evaluate in axial plane; sagittal, coronal reformats helpful
  - +/- Posterior element dysraphism, fusion anomalies
    - Most readily evaluated in axial plane
  - 3D CT reformatted images best demonstrate vertebral anomalies for surgical planning

MR Findings
- T1WI
  - Vertebral formation failure anomalies
  - Normal marrow, disc signal intensity
- T2WI
  - Similar findings to T1WI
  - +/- Lipoma, tethered cord, diastematomyelia, spinal cord compression

Imaging Recommendations
- Best imaging tool: MR imaging

DDx: Failure of Vertebral Formation

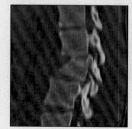

Burst Fracture

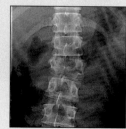

Burst Fracture

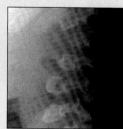

Hurler (MPS 1-H)

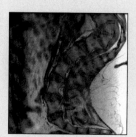

Achondroplasia

FAILURE OF VERTEBRAL FORMATION

Key Facts

Terminology
- Synonyms: Vertebral dysplasia, segmentation and fusion anomaly (SFA), "disorganized spine"
- Partial or complete failure of vertebral formation

Imaging Findings
- +/- Scoliosis
- Sagittal or coronal vertebral clefts, hemivertebra, butterfly vertebra
- +/- Lipoma, tethered cord, diastematomyelia, spinal cord compression

Top Differential Diagnoses
- Vertebral fracture
- Inherited spinal dysplasias

Pathology
- Abnormal vertebrae may be supranumerary or replace normal vertebral body
- More severe SFA ⇒ higher likelihood of associated visceral anomalies

Clinical Issues
- Abnormal spine curvature +/- neural deficits, limb or visceral abnormalities

Diagnostic Checklist
- Look for concurrent segmentation failure, other neural and visceral anomalies
- Type of deformity determines propensity for scoliosis progression

---

- Protocol advice
  - Long-cassette weightbearing radiographs ⇒ quantitate scoliosis, "counting" to definitively localize abnormal vertebral level
  - Multiplanar T1WI, T2WI MR ⇒ identify vertebral anomalies, evaluate spinal cord and soft tissues
    - Most vertebral and spinal cord anomalies seen best in coronal, sagittal planes
  - 3D Bone CT useful to characterize scoliosis and vertebral anomalies for pre-operative planning

DIFFERENTIAL DIAGNOSIS

Vertebral fracture
- Pathologic or traumatic; history critical
- Two pedicles per level
- Noncorticated irregular fracture margins +/- soft tissue edema, cord injury

Inherited spinal dysplasias
- Ex: Mucopolysaccharidosis, achondroplasia
- Distinguish by characteristic imaging, clinical, and laboratory findings

PATHOLOGY

General Features
- General path comments
  - Normal vertebral formation occurs over three sequential periods
    - Membrane development: Segmental formation of medial sclerotome (vertebral bodies) and lateral myotome (paraspinal muscles)
    - Chondrification: Sclerotomes separate transversely and join with adjacent sclerotomal halves ⇒ paired chondrification sites develop in vertebral bodies and neural arches
    - Ossification: Chondral skeleton ossifies from single ossification center
  - Segmentation and fusion anomalies result from aberrant vertebral column formation

- Abnormal vertebrae may be supranumerary or replace normal vertebral body
- More severe SFA ⇒ higher likelihood of associated visceral anomalies
  - Imaging appearance of vertebral formation failure determined by deficient vertebral body portion
    - Anterior formation failure (common) ⇒ sharply angulated kyphosis
    - Posterior formation failure (rare) ⇒ hyperlordotic curve
    - Lateral formation failure (common) ⇒ classic hemivertebrae of congenital scoliosis
  - Hemivertebra variants subclassified as incarcerated, nonincarcerated, segmented, nonsegmented, or semisegmented
    - Incarcerated: Vertebral bodies above and below shaped to accommodate hemivertebrae ⇒ do not generally produce scoliosis
    - Nonincarcerated: Found at scoliosis apex, curve magnitude depends on size of wedged segment
    - Segmented ("free"): Normal disks above and below hemivertebra ⇒ progressive scoliosis due to unbalanced growth
    - Nonsegmented: Lack disk spaces between wedged, normal adjacent vertebral bodies
    - Semisegmented: Normal disk space on one side, nonsegmented on other side
  - Segmental spinal dysgenesis (SSD) = rare congenital abnormality in which one segment of vertebral column/spinal cord fails to develop properly
    - Spinal cord thinned or indiscernible at abnormality level; bulky, low-lying cord segment caudad to focal abnormality in most cases
    - Severity of morphologic derangement correlates with residual spinal cord function, severity of clinical deficit
- Genetics
  - Deranged Pax-1 gene expression in developing vertebral column
  - Many syndromes manifest vertebral dysplasia
- Etiology
  - Total aplasia: Both chondral centers fail to develop early in development

FAILURE OF VERTEBRAL FORMATION

- ○ Lateral hemivertebra: One chondral center does not develop; ossification center subsequently fails to develop on that side
- ○ Sagittal cleft ("butterfly") vertebra: Separate ossification centers form (but fail to unite) in each paired paramedian chondrification center
- ○ Coronal cleft vertebra: Formation and persistence of separate ventral and dorsal ossification centers
- ○ Posterior hemivertebra: Later failure during ossification stage
- • Epidemiology
  - ○ Isolated or syndromal, singular or multiple
  - ○ Incidence increased with parental consanguinity, concurrent multisystem anomalies
- • Associated abnormalities
  - ○ Dysraphism, split notochord syndromes
    - ▪ Diastematomyelia, syrinx, tethered cord/fatty filum, congenital tumor, visceral organ anomalies
  - ○ Other developmental vertebral abnormalities
    - ▪ Partial duplication (supernumerary hemivertebra)
    - ▪ Segmentation failure (block vertebra, posterior element dysraphism, pediculate bar, neural arch fusion)
  - ○ Visceral abnormalities; 61% of congenital scoliosis patients

Gross Pathologic & Surgical Features

- • Normal bone density unless concurrent metabolic abnormality
- • Surgical observations of vertebral configuration matches imaging findings

Microscopic Features

- • Normal bone histology unless concurrent metabolic abnormality

CLINICAL ISSUES

Presentation

- • Most common signs/symptoms
  - ○ Asymptomatic
  - ○ Abnormal spine curvature +/- neural deficits, limb or visceral abnormalities
  - ○ Other signs/symptoms
    - ▪ Respiratory failure (impeded chest movement 2° to fused ribs, kyphoscoliosis) ⇒ rare
- • Clinical profile
  - ○ Most are asymptomatic or detected during scoliosis evaluation
  - ○ Syndromal patients usually detected in infancy

Demographics

- • Age
  - ○ Usually diagnosed in infancy → early childhood
  - ○ Mild cases may present in adulthood
- • Gender: M ≈ F

Natural History & Prognosis

- • Scoliosis is frequently progressive
  - ○ Expectant watching, early intervention if warranted to prevent development of severe deformities

Treatment

- • Conservative in mild cases (orthotics, observation)

- • Surgical resection and/or fusion to arrest/reverse kyphoscoliosis in moderate to severe cases

DIAGNOSTIC CHECKLIST

Consider

- • Syndromal origin or association → important to look for and characterize visceral anomalies

Image Interpretation Pearls

- • Look for concurrent segmentation failure, other neural and visceral anomalies
- • Type of deformity determines propensity for scoliosis progression

SELECTED REFERENCES

1. Arlet V et al: Congenital scoliosis. Eur Spine J. 12(5):456-63, 2003
2. Isono M et al: Limited dorsal myeloschisis associated with multiple vertebral segmentation disorder. Pediatr Neurosurg. 36(1):44-7, 2002
3. Suh SW et al: Evaluating Congenital spine deformities for intraspinal anomalies with magnetic resonance imaging. J Pediatr Orthop 21(4): 525-31, 2001
4. Kim YJ et al: Surgical treatment of congenital kyphosis. Spine. 26(20):2251-7, 2001
5. Jaskwhich D et al: Congenital scoliosis. Curr Opin Pediatr 12(1): 61-6, 2000
6. McMaster MJ et al: Natural history of congenital kyphosis and kyphoscoliosis. A study of one hundred and twelve patients. J Bone Joint Surg Am 81(10): 1367-83, 1999
7. Tortori-Donati P et al: Segmental spinal dysgenesis: neuroradiologic findings with clinical and embryologic correlation. AJNR Am J Neuroradiol. 20(3):445-56, 1999
8. Hayman LA et al: Bony spine and costal elements, Part II. Int J Neurorad. 4(1):61-68, 1998
9. McMaster MJ: Congenital scoliosis caused by a unilateral failure of vertebral segmentation with contralateral hemivertebrae. Spine. 23(9):998-1005, 1998
10. Aslan Y et al: Multiple vertebral segmentation defects. Brief report of three patients and nosological considerations. Genet Couns. 8(3):241-8, 1997
11. Lopez BC et al: Inadequate PAX-1 gene expression as a cause of agenesis of the thoracolumbar spine with failure of segmentation. Case report. J Neurosurg. 86(6):1018-21, 1997
12. Martinez-Frias ML: Multiple vertebral segmentation defects and rib anomalies. Am J Med Genet. 66(1):91, 1996
13. Mortier GR et al: Multiple vertebral segmentation defects: analysis of 26 new patients and review of the literature. Am J Med Genet. 61(4):310-9, 1996
14. Mayfield JK et al: Congenital kyphosis due to defects of anterior segmentation. J Bone Joint Surg Am. 62(8):1291-301, 1980
15. MacEwen GD et al: Scoliosis--a deforming childhood problem. Clin Pediatr (Phila). 6(4):210-6, 1967

FAILURE OF VERTEBRAL FORMATION

IMAGE GALLERY

Typical

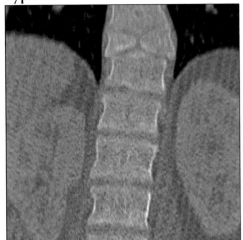
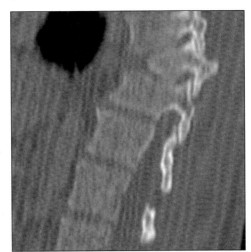

(Left) Coronal bone CT demonstrates a typical thoracic butterfly vertebra. Characteristic shape, corticated margins distinguish from fracture. *(Right)* Sagittal bone CT depicts a posterior thoracic hemivertebra producing focal kyphotic deformity.

Variant

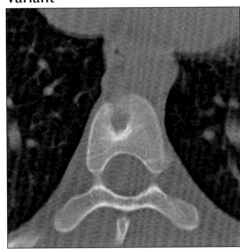
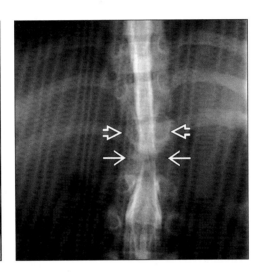

(Left) Axial bone CT depicts a partial sagittal cleft of a thoracic vertebra. This deformity would not be expected to produce scoliosis. *(Right)* Anteroposterior myelography shows T12 hypoplasia (open arrows) and aplasia of L1, producing spinal stenosis (arrows) and lateral cord compression (Courtesy R. Boyer, MD).

Variant

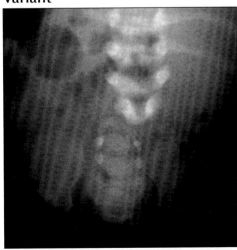
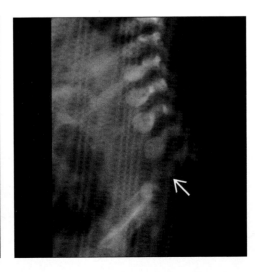

(Left) Anteroposterior radiography demonstrates segmental lumbar hypogenesis of L2 and agenesis of L3 (Courtesy R. Boyer, MD). *(Right)* Lateral radiography of lumbar segmental spinal dysgenesis shows hypogenesis of L2 (arrow) & agenesis of L3, w/posterior positioning of the lumbar spine relative to the sacrum (Courtesy R. Boyer, MD).

PARTIAL VERTEBRAL DUPLICATION

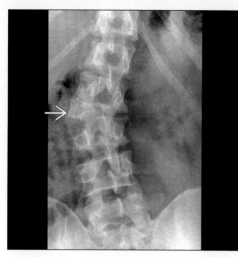

Anteroposterior radiography depicts a supernumerary hemivertebra (arrow) between the right L2 and L3 vertebral levels that produces a convex right scoliotic curve.

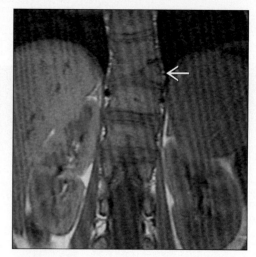

Coronal T1WI MR shows a typical left thoracic supernumerary hemivertebra (arrow) producing minimal scoliosis.

TERMINOLOGY

Abbreviations and Synonyms
- Synonym: Supranumerary vertebra

Definitions
- Partial duplication of vertebral column produces one or more supranumerary ("extra") vertebra

IMAGING FINDINGS

General Features
- Best diagnostic clue: Atypical scoliosis (sharply angulated, single curve, or focal) with one or more "extra" hemivertebra
- Location: Thoracolumbar > cervical
- Size: Hemivertebra is smaller than normal vertebra
- Morphology: "Extra" hemivertebra frequently associated with focal scoliotic curve

Radiographic Findings
- Radiography
  - Supranumerary hemivertebra with scoliosis
  - Plain films best for "counting" to definitively localize abnormal vertebral level
  - Long-cassette erect weightbearing radiographs quantitate scoliosis

CT Findings
- Bone CT: Supranumerary lateral hemivertebra

MR Findings
- T1WI: Supranumerary lateral hemivertebra +/- dysraphism, spinal cord anomalies
- T2WI: Same as T1WI

Imaging Recommendations
- Plain films for counting, quantitating scoliosis
- Multiplanar MR imaging to evaluate vertebral anatomy, assess for associated abnormalities
- CT with 3D reconstructions - demonstrates hemivertebra AND scoliosis

DIFFERENTIAL DIAGNOSIS

Butterfly vertebra
- Two pedicles; looks like "bilateral hemivertebra" with central cleft
- Separate bilateral ossification centers form, fail to unite

Vertebral fracture
- Pathologic or traumatic; history critical
- Noncorticated irregular margins +/- soft tissue edema, cord injury
- Two pedicles at level, unlike hemivertebra

DDx: Partial Vertebral Duplication

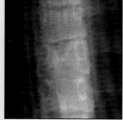
Butterfly Vertebra

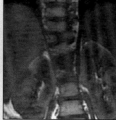
Butterfly Vertebra

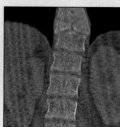
Butterfly Vertebra

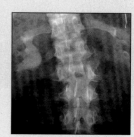
Vertebral Fracture

PARTIAL VERTEBRAL DUPLICATION

Key Facts

Terminology
- Synonym: Supranumerary vertebra
- Partial duplication of vertebral column produces one or more supranumerary ("extra") vertebra

Imaging Findings
- Plain films best for "counting" to definitively localize abnormal vertebral level
- Bone CT: Supranumerary lateral hemivertebra

- T1WI: Supranumerary lateral hemivertebra +/- dysraphism, spinal cord anomalies

Top Differential Diagnoses
- Butterfly vertebra
- Vertebral fracture

Diagnostic Checklist
- Supranumerary hemivertebra "missing" a pedicle on hypoplastic side; distinguishes from fracture

PATHOLOGY

General Features
- General path comments: Derangement of normal vertebral ossification, chondrification, and membrane formation
- Etiology
  - Disordered vertebral column formation produces hemivertebra
  - Cervicothoracic or thoracolumbar junction segmentation variation ⇒ "extra" hemivertebra
- Epidemiology
  - Isolated or syndromal, singular or multiple
    - Many syndromes are associated with segmentation and fusion anomalies (SFA)
    - Increased incidence when other multisystem congenital anomalies, parental consanguinity present
- Associated abnormalities: Dysraphism, split notochord syndromes, caudal regression, other vertebral SFA, congenital tumors, visceral organ anomalies

Gross Pathologic & Surgical Features
- Hemivertebra may be incorporated into adjacent vertebra to form unbalanced block vertebra

Microscopic Features
- Normal cortical and cancellous bone

CLINICAL ISSUES

Presentation
- Most common signs/symptoms
  - Asymptomatic
  - Neuromuscular scoliosis; usually progressive
  - Other signs/symptoms
    - Neural deficits, limb/visceral defects
    - Respiratory failure 2° to impeded chest movement, severe scoliosis (rare)
- Clinical profile: May appear normal, or present with scoliosis +/- stigmata of congenital disorder

Demographics
- Age
  - More severe cases detected in infancy or childhood
  - Milder cases detected in adolescence during school scoliosis checks, by pediatrician, or incidentally during imaging
- Gender: M = F

Natural History & Prognosis
- Variable; scoliosis may progress with growth, require treatment

Treatment
- Conservative in mild cases
- Surgical fusion to arrest/reverse scoliosis in more severe cases

DIAGNOSTIC CHECKLIST

Consider
- Scoliosis pattern
- Exclude associated abnormalities

Image Interpretation Pearls
- Supranumerary hemivertebra "missing" a pedicle on hypoplastic side; distinguishes from fracture

SELECTED REFERENCES

1. Jaskwhich D et al: Congenital scoliosis. Curr Opin Pediatr 12(1): 61-6, 2000
2. McMaster MJ et al: Natural history of congenital kyphosis and kyphoscoliosis. A study of one hundred and twelve patients. J Bone Joint Surg Am 81(10): 1367-83, 1999
3. McMaster MJ: Congenital scoliosis caused by a unilateral failure of vertebral segmentation with contralateral hemivertebrae. Spine. 23(9):998-1005, 1998

IMAGE GALLERY

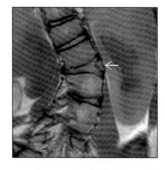 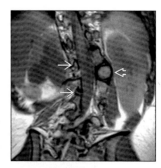

(Left) Coronal T1WI MR shows a small left supranumerary lumbar hemivertebra (arrow). *(Right)* Coronal T1WI MR centered at a left lumbar supranumerary hemivertebra (open arrow) shows normal right pedicles above and below hemivertebra (arrows) but not at hemivertebra level.

VERTEBRAL SEGMENTATION FAILURE

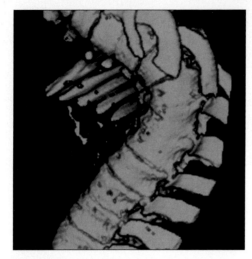

Coronal bone CT with 3D reformat shows hypogenesis and fusion of multiple mid-thoracic vertebrae. Developmental asymmetry produces rotational scoliotic curvature to the left.

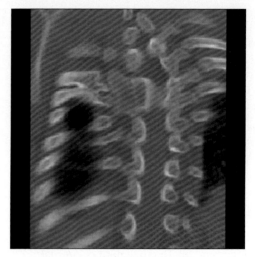

Coronal bone CT depicts bilateral interpedicular bars, with fusion of the posterior elements and ribs at multiple levels (Courtesy G. Hedlund, DO).

TERMINOLOGY

Abbreviations and Synonyms
- Segmentation anomaly, segmentation and fusion anomaly (SFA), "block vertebra", "disorganized spine"

Definitions
- Vertebral column malformations (block vertebra, pediculate bar, neural arch fusion) resulting from deranged embryological development ⇒ failure of normal segmentation

IMAGING FINDINGS

General Features
- Best diagnostic clue: Sharply angulated, single curve, or focal scoliosis with abnormal fused vertebra
- Location: Lumbar > cervical > thoracic
- Size
  ○ Range from focal ⇒ extensive involvement
  ○ Block vertebra usually larger than a single normal vertebral body
- Morphology: Incomplete vertebral body segmentation, fused posterior elements, and large misshapen vertebral bodies incorporating one or more levels

Radiographic Findings
- Radiography

○ Deformed, fused vertebra +/- scoliosis,
○ Upright images with lateral and AP bending assess weightbearing effect on scoliosis

CT Findings
- Bone CT
  ○ Incomplete vertebral body segmentation
    ▪ Large, misshapen vertebral bodies incorporating one or more levels
    ▪ +/- Fused pedicles, ribs, posterior elements

MR Findings
- T1WI
  ○ Deformed, fused vertebral bodies and posterior elements
  ○ +/- Scoliosis
  ○ Normal marrow signal intensity
- T2WI
  ○ Findings similar to T1WI
  ○ +/- Scoliosis, cord compression

Imaging Recommendations
- Weight bearing plain films to evaluate scoliosis, "count" to determine abnormal vertebral levels
- MR imaging
  ○ Multiplanar T1WI to evaluate vertebral anatomy
    ▪ Vertebral anomalies seen best in coronal, sagittal planes

DDx: Vertebral Segmentation Failure

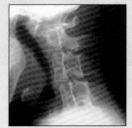
Juv. Chronic Arthritis

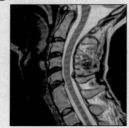
Surgical Fusion

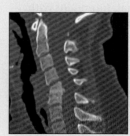
Chronic Discitis

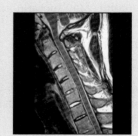
Ank. Spondylitis

VERTEBRAL SEGMENTATION FAILURE

Key Facts

Terminology
- Vertebral column malformations (block vertebra, pediculate bar, neural arch fusion) resulting from deranged embryological development ⇒ failure of normal segmentation

Imaging Findings
- Best diagnostic clue: Sharply angulated, single curve, or focal scoliosis with abnormal fused vertebra
- Location: Lumbar > cervical > thoracic
- +/- Fused pedicles, ribs, posterior elements
- +/- Scoliosis, cord compression

Top Differential Diagnoses
- Juvenile chronic arthritis
- Surgical fusion
- Chronic sequelae of discitis

- Ankylosing spondylitis

Pathology
- Mildest (and most common) form is indeterminate (transitional) vertebrae at thoracolumbar, lumbosacral transition

Clinical Issues
- Clinical profile: Asymptomatic incidental detection or presents for evaluation of abnormal spine curvature

Diagnostic Checklist
- Coronal MRI, AP radiography best for detecting and characterizing SFAs, "counting" to determine abnormal vertebral levels

---

- T2WI to evaluate spinal cord pathology, compression
- CT to characterize osseous structures
  - 3D CT useful for pre-operative planning

DIFFERENTIAL DIAGNOSIS

Juvenile chronic arthritis
- Difficult to distinguish from cervical block vertebra
- Search for other affected joints, appropriate history

Surgical fusion
- No "waist" at disc space level, facets infrequently ankylosed
- Surgical history key to making diagnosis

Chronic sequelae of discitis
- Cortical endplate margins irregular, "waist" absent
- Search for history of prior spinal infection

Ankylosing spondylitis
- Delicate contiguous syndesmophytes ("bamboo spine") + symmetric SI joint disease
- HLA - B27 positive (95%)

PATHOLOGY

General Features
- General path comments
  - Normal embryology: Vertebral formation occurs over three sequential periods
    - Membrane development: Segmental formation of medial sclerotome (vertebral bodies) and lateral myotome (paraspinal muscles)
    - Chondrification: Sclerotomes separate transversely and join with adjacent sclerotomal halves ⇒ paired chondrification sites develop in vertebral bodies and neural arches
    - Ossification: Chondral skeleton ossifies from single ossification center
  - Segmentation and fusion anomalies result from aberrant vertebral column formation

- Mildest (and most common) form is indeterminate (transitional) vertebrae at thoracolumbar, lumbosacral transition
- Genetics
  - Deranged Pax-1 gene expression ⇒ abnormal notochord signaling in developing vertebral column
  - Many syndromes associated with SFA
    - Klippel-Feil (cervical SFA): Common, gene locus 8q22.2
    - Spondylothoracic dysplasia (Jarcho-Levin): Uncommon, thoracic spine fusions in "crab-like" array with multiple rib fusions
- Etiology
  - Block vertebra: Segmentation failure of two or more vertebral somites
  - Posterior neural arch anomalies: Failure to unite in the midline ⇒ dysraphism +/- unilateral pedicle aplasia/hypoplasia
- Epidemiology
  - Isolated or syndromal, singular or multiple
  - SFAs account for 18% of scoliosis; incidence higher with multisystem abnormalities, parental consanguinity
- Associated abnormalities
  - Other neuraxis anomalies (40%)
    - Dysraphism, split notochord syndrome
    - Partial or complete failure of formation (vertebral aplasia, hemivertebra, butterfly vertebra)
    - Partial duplication (supernumerary hemivertebra)
  - Scoliosis
  - Renal, gastrointestinal (20%), congenital cardiac defects (10%)

Gross Pathologic & Surgical Features
- Normal bone density unless concurrent metabolic abnormality
- Surgical observations of vertebral configuration matches imaging findings

Microscopic Features
- Normal bone histology unless concurrent metabolic abnormality

VERTEBRAL SEGMENTATION FAILURE

Staging, Grading or Classification Criteria

- Block vertebra - failure of ≥ 2 vertebral somites to segment
  - Combined vertebrae may be normal height, short, or tall
  - Disc space frequently rudimentary or absent
  - Frequent association with hemivertebra/absent vertebra above or below block level, posterior element fusion
- Posterior neural arch anomalies
  - Failure to unite in the midline ⇒ dysraphism (+/- unilateral pedicle aplasia/hypoplasia)
  - Unfused spinous processes; L5, S1 > C1 > C7 > T1 > lower thoracic spine
  - Multiple level posterior fusion ⇒ congenital vertebral bar

CLINICAL ISSUES

Presentation

- Most common signs/symptoms
  - Asymptomatic
  - Kyphoscoliosis
  - Other signs/symptoms
    - Neural deficits (usually myelopathic), limb or visceral anomalies
    - Respiratory failure (rare, 2° impeded chest movement due to severe scoliosis, rib cage fusion)
- Clinical profile: Asymptomatic incidental detection or presents for evaluation of abnormal spine curvature

Demographics

- Age: Severe cases detected during infancy/childhood; mild cases may present as adults
- Gender: M ≈ F; dependent on syndromal association

Natural History & Prognosis

- Scoliosis frequently progressive
  - Unilateral unsegmented bar with contralateral hemivertebra ⇒ rapidly progressive, severely deforming congenital scoliosis
  - Isolated block vertebra rarely produce scoliosis
- Abnormal segments may continue to fuse

Treatment

- Conservative in mild cases (orthotics, observation)
- Surgical fusion to arrest/reverse kyphoscoliosis in moderate to severe cases

DIAGNOSTIC CHECKLIST

Consider

- Clinical manifestations variable, determined by type of SFA and syndromal association

Image Interpretation Pearls

- Coronal MRI, AP radiography best for detecting and characterizing SFAs, "counting" to determine abnormal vertebral levels

SELECTED REFERENCES

1. Arlet V et al: Congenital scoliosis. Eur Spine J. 12(5):456-63, 2003
2. Cornier AS et al: Controversies surrounding Jarcho-Levin syndrome. Curr Opin Pediatr. 15(6):614-20, 2003
3. Isono M et al: Limited dorsal myeloschisis associated with multiple vertebral segmentation disorder. Pediatr Neurosurg. 36(1):44-7, 2002
4. Suh SW et al: Evaluating Congenital spine deformities for intraspinal anomalies with magnetic resonance imaging. J Pediatr Orthop 21(4): 525-31, 2001
5. Kim YJ et al: Surgical treatment of congenital kyphosis. Spine. 26(20):2251-7, 2001
6. Nagashima H et al: No neurological involvement for more than 40 years in Klippel-Feil syndrome with severe hypermobility of the upper cervical spine. Arch Orthop Trauma Surg. 121(1-2):99-101, 2001
7. Jaskwhich D et al: Congenital scoliosis. Curr Opin Pediatr 12(1): 61-6, 2000
8. Yildiran A et al: Semantic and nosological confusions on multiple vertebral segmentation defects. Pediatr Neurosurg. 33(3):168, 2000
9. McMaster MJ et al: Natural history of congenital kyphosis and kyphoscoliosis. A study of one hundred and twelve patients. J Bone Joint Surg Am 81(10): 1367-83, 1999
10. McMaster MJ: Congenital scoliosis caused by a unilateral failure of vertebral segmentation with contralateral hemivertebrae. Spine. 23(9):998-1005, 1998
11. Anderson PJ et al: The cervical spine in Crouzon syndrome. Spine. 22(4):402-5, 1997
12. Lopez BC et al: Inadequate PAX-1 gene expression as a cause of agenesis of the thoracolumbar spine with failure of segmentation. Case report. J Neurosurg. 86(6):1018-21, 1997
13. Aslan Y et al: Multiple vertebral segmentation defects. Brief report of three patients and nosological considerations. Genet Couns. 8(3):241-8, 1997
14. Mortier GR et al: Multiple vertebral segmentation defects: analysis of 26 new patients and review of the literature. Am J Med Genet. 61(4):310-9, 1996
15. Jansen BR et al: Discitis in childhood. 12-35-year follow-up of 35 patients. Acta Orthop Scand. 64(1):33-6, 1993
16. Lee CK et al: Isolated congenital cervical block vertebrae below the axis with neurological symptoms. Spine. 6(2):118-24, 1981
17. Mayfield JK et al: Congenital kyphosis due to defects of anterior segmentation. J Bone Joint Surg Am. 62(8):1291-301, 1980

VERTEBRAL SEGMENTATION FAILURE

IMAGE GALLERY

Typical

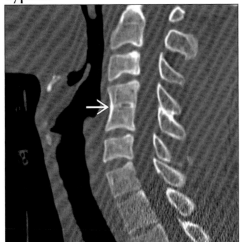
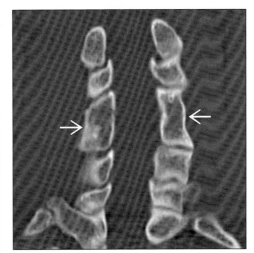

(Left) Sagittal bone CT (Klippel-Feil syndrome) shows mild single level congenital segmentation failure at C4-5. "Waist" (arrow) at the rudimentary disc space and fused spinous processes is typical. *(Right)* Coronal bone CT reveals solid bilateral facet fusion (arrows) in conjunction with congenital fusion. Mild degenerative facet changes are present above and below fusion reflecting altered biomechanics.

Variant

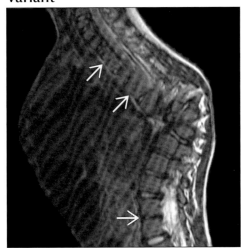
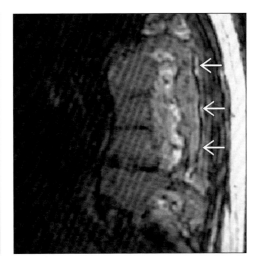

(Left) Sagittal T2WI MR (VACTERL syndrome) shows hypogenesis and fusion of multiple thoracic and lumbar vertebrae (arrows) producing kyphotic gibbus deformity (Courtesy R. Boyer, MD). *(Right)* Sagittal T2WI MR depicts multilevel vertebral segmentation failure with fusion of the facets and laminae (arrows) into an interlaminar bar (Courtesy R. Boyer, MD).

Variant

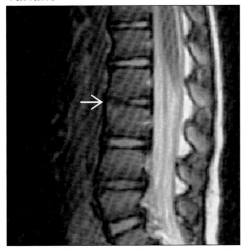
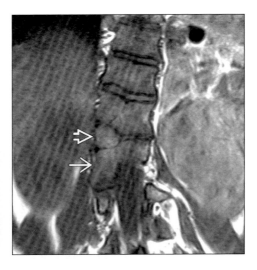

(Left) Sagittal T2WI MR shows partial fusion of the anterior L3 and L4 vertebral bodies (arrow), a mild variation of congenital block vertebra (Courtesy R. Boyer, MD). *(Right)* Coronal T1WI MR shows fusion of right L1 hemivertebra (open arrow) with the L2 vertebral body (arrow), producing focal scoliosis (Courtesy R. Boyer, MD).

KLIPPEL-FEIL SPECTRUM

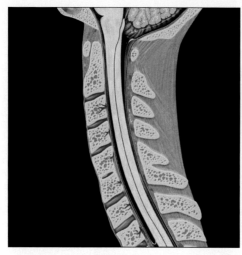

Sagittal graphic shows congenital fusion of the C5-6 vertebrae and spinous processes, with characteristic rudimentary disc space and distinctive "waist" typical of congenital fusion.

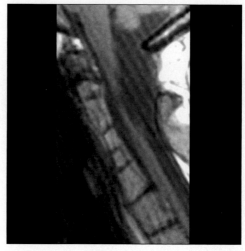

Sagittal T1WI MR (KFS type 1) shows congenital CVJ segmentation and fusion anomalies involving nearly the entire cervical spine. Diastematomyelic upper cervical cord is notably thinned.

TERMINOLOGY

Abbreviations and Synonyms
- Synonyms: KFS, Klippel-Feil syndrome

Definitions
- Congenital spinal malformation characterized by segmentation failure of two or more cervical vertebra

IMAGING FINDINGS

General Features
- Best diagnostic clue: Single or multiple level congenital cervical segmentation and fusion anomalies
- Location: C2-3 (50%) > C5-6 (33%) > CVJ, upper thoracic spine
- Size
  - Vertebral bodies < normal size with tapered contour at fused disc space
  - Rudimentary disc space reduced in height and diameter
- Morphology: Vertebral body narrowing ("wasp waist") at fused rudimentary disc space +/- fusion of posterior elements

Radiographic Findings
- Radiography

- One or more fused vertebral levels with rudimentary, narrow disc space(s)
  - Disc space always abnormal; frequently fused facets, spinous processes as well
  - Adjacent disc spaces at mobile levels +/- degenerative changes
- +/- Omovertebral bone
- Flexion/extension films → lack of motion between fused segments, increased mobility at non-fused levels

CT Findings
- Bone CT
  - Typical osseous findings +/- degenerative changes
  - Sagittal, transverse spinal canal diameter usually normal
    - Narrowing reflects secondary degenerative changes adjacent to fused segments
    - Canal enlargement ⇒ consider syringomyelia

MR Findings
- T1WI
  - Cervical fusion(s); vertebral bodies +/- facets, posterior elements
  - +/- Degenerative changes; spondylosis, disc herniations common (especially lower cervical spine)
  - +/- CVJ osseous anomalies, Chiari 1 malformation
- T2WI

DDx: Klippel-Feil Syndrome

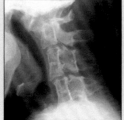

Juv. Chronic Arthritis

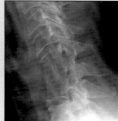

Surgical Fusion

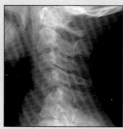

Chronic Discitis

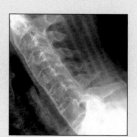

Ankylosing Spondylitis

KLIPPEL-FEIL SPECTRUM

Key Facts

Terminology
- Synonyms: KFS, Klippel-Feil syndrome

Imaging Findings
- Location: C2-3 (50%) > C5-6 (33%) > CVJ, upper thoracic spine
- Morphology: Vertebral body narrowing ("wasp waist") at fused rudimentary disc space +/- fusion of posterior elements
- +/- Omovertebral bone

Top Differential Diagnoses
- Juvenile chronic arthritis
- Surgical fusion
- Chronic sequelae of discitis
- Ankylosing spondylitis

Pathology
- Congenital cervical fusion 2° to failure of normal segmentation of cervical somites (3rd → 8th weeks)
- Sporadic; familial genetic component with variable expression identified in many patients

Clinical Issues
- Classic triad (33-50%): Short neck, low posterior hairline, and limited cervical motion
- Many patients have normal clinical appearance despite severity of involvement

Diagnostic Checklist
- Much KFS morbidity and nearly all mortality related to visceral system dysfunction
- Look for instability, progressive degenerative changes, cord/brainstem compression

---

- Osseous findings same as T1WI; normal marrow signal
- +/- Cord or nerve root compression, syringomyelia, brainstem abnormalities, myeloschisis

Imaging Recommendations
- Best imaging tool
  - Radiography to evaluate and follow instability, degenerative changes
  - MRI to exclude cord compression, detect degenerative changes
- Protocol advice
  - Serial neutral and flex/extend plain radiographs to detect progressive instability, degenerative disease
  - Multiplanar MRI to evaluate canal compromise, cord compression, soft tissue degenerative changes
  - Ultrasound or CECT to detect and characterize associated visceral organ abnormalities

DIFFERENTIAL DIAGNOSIS

Juvenile chronic arthritis
- Difficult to distinguish from cervical block vertebra
- Search for other affected joints, appropriate history

Surgical fusion
- No disc space "waist", facets infrequently ankylosed
- Surgical history key to making diagnosis

Chronic sequelae of discitis
- Irregular endplate margins, no "waist", +/- kyphosis
- Confirm history of prior spinal infection

Ankylosing spondylitis
- Delicate contiguous syndesmophytes ("bamboo spine") + symmetric SI joint disease
- HLA - B27 positive (95%)

PATHOLOGY

General Features
- General path comments

- "Klippel-Feil syndrome" colloquially used for all patients with cervical congenital fusion anomalies regardless of extent
- Congenital cervical fusion 2° to failure of normal segmentation of cervical somites (3rd → 8th weeks)
- Genetics
  - Sporadic; familial genetic component with variable expression identified in many patients
    - C2/3 fusion (type 2) ⇒ autosomal dominant with variable penetrance
    - C5/6 fusion (type 2) ⇒ autosomal recessive
  - SGMI (chromosome 8) ⇒ 1st Klippel-Feil gene identified; gene expression overlaps all 3 KFS types
- Etiology
  - No universally accepted etiology; embryonic insult postulated between 4th → 8th weeks
    - Putative environmental causative factors include teratogens, maternal alcoholism
    - Association with other syndromes (fetal alcohol, Goldenhar, Wildervanck - cervical/occulo/acoustic)
- Epidemiology: 1/42,000 births
- Associated abnormalities
  - Hemivertebrae, butterfly vertebrae, spina bifida
  - Scoliosis (usually congenital) +/- kyphosis (60%)
  - Odontoid dysplasia, basilar impression, C1 assimilation, occipito-cervical instability
  - Syringomyelia, diastematomyelia (20%), Chiari 1 malformation (8%), neurenteric cyst or dermoid (rare)
  - Cervicomedullary neuroschisis +/- synkinesis (20%)
  - Sprengel deformity +/- omovertebral bone (15-30%); unilateral or bilateral
  - Sensorineural hearing loss (30%), GU tract abnormalities (35%), congenital heart disease (14%), upper extremity deformity, facial anomalies

Gross Pathologic & Surgical Features
- Surgical observations correlate to imaging findings

Microscopic Features
- Histologically normal bone, disc

KLIPPEL-FEIL SPECTRUM

Staging, Grading or Classification Criteria

- Type 1 (9%): Massive fusion of cervical, upper thoracic spine → severe neurological impairment, frequent associated abnormalities
- Type 2 (84%): Fusion of one or more cervical vertebral interspaces
- Type 3 (7%): Fusions involve cervical and lower thoracic/lumbar vertebra

CLINICAL ISSUES

Presentation

- Most common signs/symptoms
  ○ Cosmesis complaints, neck or radicular pain, slowly progressive or acute myelopathy
    ■ Massive fusions often noted in infancy/early childhood 2° to cosmetic deformity
  ○ Neurologic problems in infancy, childhood usually 2° to CVJ abnormalities
  ○ Lower cervical fusions (unless massive) usually present ≥ 3rd decade when degenerative changes or instability of adjacent segments manifests
  ○ Other signs/symptoms
    ■ Vocal impairment (usually > 1 level fusion)
    ■ Synkinesia (mirror movements): 20%, upper > lower extremity, diminish with time
- Clinical profile
  ○ Classic triad (33-50%): Short neck, low posterior hairline, and limited cervical motion
  ○ Wide variation in clinical and anatomical expression
    ■ Many patients have normal clinical appearance despite severity of involvement
    ■ Cervical motion limitation is most consistent clinical finding

Demographics

- Age: 2nd → 3rd decade; spans entire range of life expectancy
- Gender: M ≤ F

Natural History & Prognosis

- Progressive accelerated degenerative changes adjacent to fused segments
- Three patterns at greatest risk for future instability
  ○ C0 → C3 fusion with occipitocervical synostosis
  ○ Long cervical fusion + abnormal C0/1 junction
  ○ Single open interspace between 2 fused segments
- ↑ Risk of neurological injury following minor trauma 2° hypermobility of cervical segments
  ○ High risk patients: Two sets of block vertebra, occipitalization of atlas + basilar invagination, and cervical fusion + spinal stenosis

Treatment

- Avoidance of contact sports, occupations and recreational activities at risk for head or neck trauma
- Activity modification, bracing, and traction may reduce symptoms
- Neurological lesion, significant pain despite conservative therapy, or progressive instability ⇒ decompression +/- spinal fusion

DIAGNOSTIC CHECKLIST

Consider

- Much KFS morbidity and nearly all mortality related to visceral system dysfunction

Image Interpretation Pearls

- Look for instability, progressive degenerative changes, cord/brainstem compression

SELECTED REFERENCES

1. Royal SA et al: Investigations into the association between cervicomedullary neuroschisis and mirror movements in patients with Klippel-Feil syndrome. AJNR Am J Neuroradiol. 23(4):724-9, 2002
2. Nagashima H et al: No neurological involvement for more than 40 years in Klippel-Feil syndrome with severe hypermobility of the upper cervical spine. Arch Orthop Trauma Surg. 121(1-2):99-101, 2001
3. Andronikou S et al: Klippel-Feil syndrome with cervical diastematomyelia in an 8-year-old boy. Pediatr Radiol. 31(9):636, 2001
4. Karasick D et al: The traumatized cervical spine in Klippel-Feil syndrome: imaging features. AJR Am J Roentgenol. 170(1):85-8, 1998
5. Clark et al: The Cervical Spine. 3rd ed. Philadelphia, Lippincott-Raven. 339-348, 1998
6. Clarke RA et al: Heterogeneity in Klippel-Feil syndrome: a new classification. Pediatr Radiol. 28(12):967-74, 1998
7. Rouvreau P et al: Assessment and neurologic involvement of patients with cervical spine congenital synostosis as in Klippel-Feil syndrome: study of 19 cases. J Pediatr Orthop B. 7(3):179-85, 1998
8. Thomsen MN et al: Scoliosis and congenital anomalies associated with Klippel-Feil syndrome types I-III. Spine. 22(4):396-401, 1997
9. Theiss SM et al: The long-term follow-up of patients with Klippel-Feil syndrome and congenital scoliosis. Spine. 22(11):1219-22, 1997
10. David KM et al: Split cervical spinal cord with Klippel-Feil syndrome: seven cases. Brain. 119 (Pt 6):1859-72, 1996
11. Baba H et al: The cervical spine in the Klippel-Feil syndrome. A report of 57 cases. Int Orthop. 19(4):204-8, 1995
12. Guille JT et al: The natural history of Klippel-Feil syndrome: clinical, roentgenographic, and magnetic resonance imaging findings at adulthood. J Pediatr Orthop. 15(5):617-26, 1995
13. Guggenbuhl P et al: Adult-onset Klippel-Feil syndrome with inaugural neurologic symptoms: two case reports. Rev Rhum Engl Ed. 62(11):802-4, 1995
14. Pizzutillo PD et al: Risk factors in Klippel-Feil syndrome. Spine. 19(18):2110-6, 1994
15. Ulmer JL et al: Klippel-Feil syndrome: CT and MR of acquired and congenital abnormalities of cervical spine and cord. J Comput Assist Tomogr. 17(2):215-24, 1993
16. Ritterbusch JF et al: Magnetic resonance imaging for stenosis and subluxation in Klippel-Feil syndrome. Spine. 16(10 Suppl):S539-41, 1991

IMAGE GALLERY

Typical

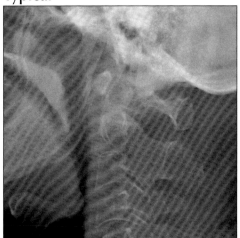
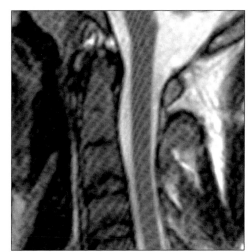

(Left) Lateral radiography (KFS type 2) demonstrates typical C2/3 congenital fusion. The disc space is rudimentary, and the facets and spinous processes are fused. (Right) Sagittal T2WI MR (KFS type 2) reveals uncomplicated congenital fusion of C2/3, with rudimentary disc space and fusion of the spinous processes.

Variant

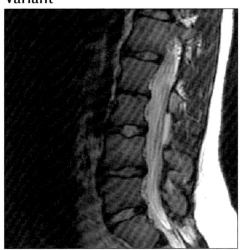
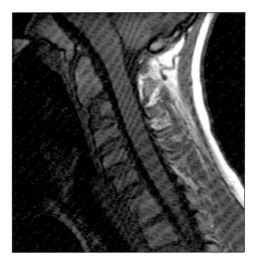

(Left) Sagittal T2WI MR (KFS type 3) shows congenital L2/3 fusion with narrow rudimentary disc space and normal AP canal diameter. (Right) Sagittal T1WI MR (KFS type 1) shows atlanto-occipital assimilation, dens hypoplasia, and partial segmentation failure at C7/T1 (Courtesy G. Hedlund, DO).

Variant

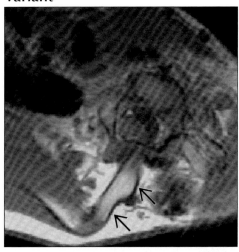
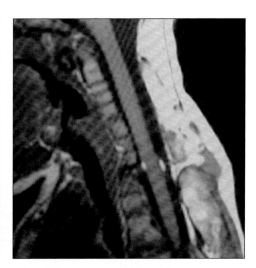

(Left) Axial T1WI MR (KFS type 1) depicts an omovertebral bone (arrows) connecting the lamina to the scapula (Courtesy G. Hedlund, DO). (Right) Sagittal T1WI MR (KFS type 1) shows multilevel cervical segmentation failure with two hyperintense intradural lipomas affixed to the spinal cord (Courtesy B. Chong, MD).

CRANIOVERTEBRAL JUNCTION VARIANTS

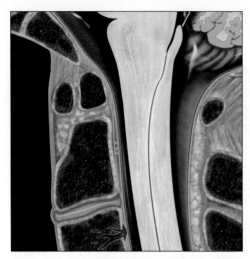

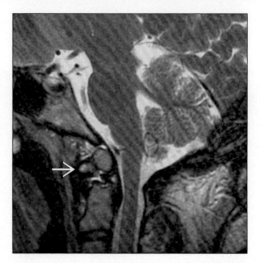

Sagittal graphic shows an os odontoideum and enlarged anterior C1 ring suggesting a congenital origin. No static instability or CVJ stenosis in this case.

Sagittal T2WI MR depicts a large os odontoideum in conjunction with enlargement of the anterior C1 ring (arrow). Static alignment is normal.

TERMINOLOGY

Abbreviations and Synonyms
- Synonyms: CVJ anomalies, craniocervical junction (CCJ) variants or anomalies

Definitions
- Anatomical variations of skull base-cervical spine articulation

IMAGING FINDINGS

General Features
- Best diagnostic clue: Flattening or malformation of clivus, anterior C1 ring, or odontoid process
- Location: Craniovertebral junction (CVJ)
- Size: Variable with specific anatomical variation
- Morphology: Variable: Platybasia, segmentation and fusion anomalies, C1 or C2/dens anomalies

Radiographic Findings
- Radiography: Platybasia, basilar invagination, C1 ring assimilation, asymmetrical C1/2 articulation, backward tilt, hypoplasia/aplasia, or os odontoideum of odontoid process, C2/3 fusion (Klippel-Feil)
- Fluoroscopy: Variable instability of C0/1, C1/2 articulations with dynamic flexion and extension

CT Findings
- CECT
  - +/- Enhancing granulation tissue mass ("pannus")
    - Patients with reducible abnormalities have largest pannus
- Bone CT
  - Similar findings to plain radiographs; sagittal and coronal reformats minimize effect of overlapping structures

MR Findings
- T1WI: Osseous anomalies +/- soft tissue granulation tissue, cord compression, hindbrain anomalies
- T2WI: Similar to T1WI; best shows spinal cord status
- T1 C+: +/- Enhancing "pannus"

Imaging Recommendations
- Best imaging tool: Bone CT with multiplanar reformats
- Protocol advice
  - Dynamic flex/extend plain films to demonstrate biomechanics, uncover instability
  - Multiplanar T1WI, T2WI to evaluate cord, soft tissues; flex/extend MRI optimally delineates effect of position on neural compression
  - CT with multiplanar reformats to evaluate osseous structures for surgical planning

DDx: Congenital CVJ Variants

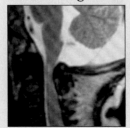

Mucopolysaccharidosis

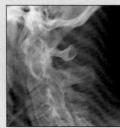

Psoriatic Arthritis

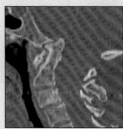

Juv. Chronic Arthritis

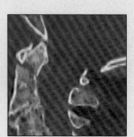

Type II Dens Fx

CRANIOVERTEBRAL JUNCTION VARIANTS

Key Facts

Terminology
- Synonyms: CVJ anomalies, craniocervical junction (CCJ) variants or anomalies

Imaging Findings
- Best diagnostic clue: Flattening or malformation of clivus, anterior C1 ring, or odontoid process
- +/- Enhancing granulation tissue mass ("pannus")
- Best imaging tool: Bone CT with multiplanar reformats

Top Differential Diagnoses
- Developmental CVJ anomalies
- Inflammatory and degenerative arthritides
- Acquired basilar impression
- Trauma

Pathology
- Severity ranges from benign, asymptomatic to potentially fatal instability ⇒ cord/brainstem compression

Clinical Issues
- Neurological symptoms usually gradual onset with localizing signs; some patients asymptomatic throughout life
- Occasionally neurological presentation is fulminant ⇒ quadriplegia, sudden death
- Undetected anomalies at risk for injury during minor trauma, anesthesia

Diagnostic Checklist
- Dynamic flex-extend imaging determines stability, reducibility of abnormality

DIFFERENTIAL DIAGNOSIS

Developmental CVJ anomalies
- CVJ stenosis or atlanto-axial instability 2° to achondroplasia, mucopolysaccharidosis, Down syndrome, or inborn errors of metabolism

Inflammatory and degenerative arthritides
- Rheumatoid, reactive, or psoriatic arthritides, ankylosing spondylitis, degenerative arthritis (osteoarthritis)
- +/- CVJ fusion, anterior displacement of C1 ring from dens, basilar invagination → possible cord compression 2° to canal stenosis
- Clinical manifestations include myelopathy, pain, extremity deformity
  - Elicit characteristic clinical, historical, and laboratory abnormalities to confirm diagnosis

Acquired basilar impression
- Upward displacement of occipital condyles above plane of foramen magnum, radiological protrusion of dens tip above Chamberlain line
- 2° to bone softening; Paget disease, osteogenesis imperfecta, rickets, rheumatoid arthritis, hyperparathyroidism

Trauma
- Fracture and/or ligamentous injury; CVJ injuries relatively uncommon but high morbidity/mortality
- Sharp, non-corticated margins argue against congenital anomaly
- Elicit appropriate history, clinical findings

PATHOLOGY

General Features
- General path comments
  - Congenital CVJ abnormalities are relatively uncommon

- Severity ranges from benign, asymptomatic to potentially fatal instability ⇒ cord/brainstem compression
  - Type and severity of anomaly determined by anatomy relative to one or more standard "lines of reference"
    - Chamberlain line: Line drawn from opisthion to dorsal margin of hard palate
    - McGregor line: Line drawn from upper posterior hard palate to most caudad point of occiput
- Etiology: Congenital insult to developing CVJ neural and osseous tissue between 4th → 7th intrauterine weeks ⇒ hypoplasia, segmentation/fusion anomalies, CVJ ankylosis
- Epidemiology: Relatively uncommon: 0.14-0.25% pediatric population
- Associated abnormalities: Dwarfism, jaw anomalies, cleft palate, congenital ear deformities, short neck, Sprengel deformity, funnel chest, pes cavus, and syndactyly

Gross Pathologic & Surgical Features
- Solid ankylosis or fibrous union in many irreducible anomalies
- Granulation tissue proliferation around motion areas in unstable or reducible anomalies

Microscopic Features
- Variable components of histologically normal bone, fibrous tissue, and granulation tissue

Staging, Grading or Classification Criteria
- Occipital sclerotome malformations
  - Most occiput anomalies associated with ↓ skull base height +/- basilar invagination (odontoid tip > 4.5 mm above McGregor line)
    - Condylus tertius, condylar hypoplasia, basiocciput hypoplasia, atlanto-occipital assimilation, bifid clivus
    - Platybasia = congenital flattening of craniocervical angle > 135°
    - Associated with hindbrain herniation, syringomyelia (≤ 30%)
- C1 ring anomalies

CRANIOVERTEBRAL JUNCTION VARIANTS

- o C1 assimilation ("occipitalized C1"): Segmentation failure → fibrous or osseous union between 1st spinal sclerotome and 4th occipital sclerotome
  - +/- Occipitocervical synostosis; most C1 ring assimilations asymptomatic, more likely to be symptomatic if retro-odontoid AP canal diameter < 19 mm
- o C1 malformation: Aplasia, hypoplasia, cleft C1 arch, "split atlas" (anterior and posterior arch rachischisis)
- o Association with Klippel-Feil, basilar invagination, Chiari 1 malformation
- C2 anomalies: C1/2 segmentation failure, dens dysplasia
  - o Majority confined to odontoid process; partial (hypoplasia) → complete absence (aplasia), ossiculum terminal persistens, os odontoideum
    - Ossiculum terminale persistens: Ossification failure of terminal ossicle → incidental "notch" in dens tip
    - Os odontoideum: Well-defined ossicle at dens tip + anterior C1 arch enlargement
  - o Odontoid anomalies in association with ligamentous laxity → atlantoaxial instability; most common in Down syndrome, Morquio syndrome, Klippel-Feil syndrome, and skeletal dysplasias
    - Incompetence of cruciate ligament → C1/2 instability, possible neurologic deficit or death

CLINICAL ISSUES

Presentation
- Most common signs/symptoms
  - o Posterior occipital headache exacerbated by flexion/extension
  - o Sub-occipital neck pain (85%); may clinically mimic "basilar migraine"
  - o Myelopathy, brainstem/cranial nerve deficits, weakness, lower extremity ataxia
  - o Vascular symptoms (15-20%); TIA, vertigo, visual symptoms with rotation or head manipulation
- Clinical profile
  - o Usually normal clinical appearance; obvious clinical dysmorphism implies syndromal association
  - o Symptomatic presentation following mild trauma common

Demographics
- Age: Infancy → late adulthood depending on severity
- Gender: M = F

Natural History & Prognosis
- Neurological symptoms usually gradual onset with localizing signs; some patients asymptomatic throughout life
- Occasionally neurological presentation is fulminant ⇒ quadriplegia, sudden death
- Undetected anomalies at risk for injury during minor trauma, anesthesia
- Early diagnosis permits treatment before symptoms or permanent neurological sequelae

Treatment
- Conservative approach initially unless unstable or neural deficits
  - o Traction, cervical orthosis, activity restriction
- Symptomatic, refractory to conservative management
  - o Skeletal traction to distinguish reducible from irreducible abnormalities, relieve symptoms pre-operatively
  - o Correction of underlying biomechanical abnormality with decompression +/- fusion

DIAGNOSTIC CHECKLIST

Consider
- Look for combinations of anomalies based on known association patterns
- Impact of diagnosis must be customized to individual patient to develop best treatment approach

Image Interpretation Pearls
- Dynamic flex-extend imaging determines stability, reducibility of abnormality
- CT with reformats indispensable to evaluate osseous abnormalities

SELECTED REFERENCES

1. Naderi S et al: Anatomical and computed tomographic analysis of C1 vertebra. Clin Neurol Neurosurg. 105(4):245-8, 2003
2. Perez-Vallina JR et al: Congenital anomaly of craniovertebral junction: atlas-dens fusion with C1 anterior arch cleft. J Spinal Disord Tech. 15(1):84-7, 2002
3. Taitz C: Bony observations of some morphological variations and anomalies of the craniovertebral region. Clin Anat. 13(5):354-60, 2000
4. Smoker WR: MR imaging of the craniovertebral junction. Magn Reson Imaging Clin N Am. 8(3):635-50, 2000
5. Kim FM: Developmental anomalies of the craniocervical junction and cervical spine. Magn Reson Imaging Clin N Am. 8(3):651-74, 2000
6. Iwata A et al: Foramen magnum syndrome caused by atlanto-occipital assimilation. J Neurol Sci. 154(2):229-31, 1998
7. Menezes AH: Craniovertebral junction anomalies: diagnosis and management. Semin Pediatr Neurol. 4(3):209-23, 1997
8. Menezes AH: Craniovertebral junction anomalies. In: Tindall et al (ed): The Practice of Neurosurgery. Baltimore, Williams and Wilkins, 2729-2740, 1996
9. Menezes AH: Primary craniovertebral anomalies and the hindbrain herniation syndrome (Chiari I): data base analysis. Pediatr Neurosurg. 23(5):260-9, 1995
10. Erbengi A et al: Congenital malformations of the craniovertebral junction: classification and surgical treatment. Acta Neurochir (Wien). 127(3-4):180-5, 1994
11. Smoker WR: Craniovertebral junction: normal anatomy, craniometry, and congenital anomalies. Radiographics. 14(2):255-77, 1994
12. Chamberlain W: Basilar impression (platybasia). Yale J Biol Med 11:487, 1938-1939

CRANIOVERTEBRAL JUNCTION VARIANTS

IMAGE GALLERY

Variant

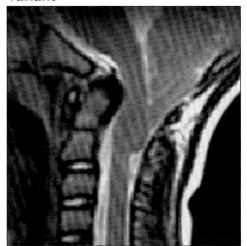 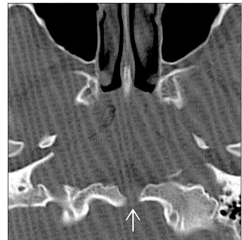

(Left) Sagittal T2WI MR *(Chiari 1 malformation) depicts a foreshortened clivus, platybasia, and a retroflexed odontoid in conjunction with severe tonsillar ectopia (Courtesy R. Boyer, MD).* *(Right)* *Axial bone CT demonstrates a flattened, bifid clivus (arrow).*

Variant

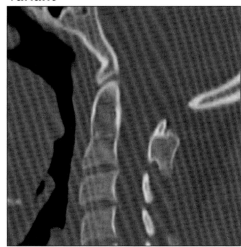 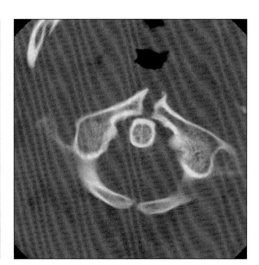

(Left) Sagittal bone CT shows variant C1 assimilation into the clivus and C2 spinous process, producing an aberrant articular facet between anterior C1 and odontoid process (Courtesy G. Hedlund, DO).* *(Right)* *Axial bone CT shows a congenital cleft of both anterior and posterior C1 rings ("split atlas"), with rounded corticated margins that distinguish from fracture (Courtesy G. Hedlund, DO).*

Variant

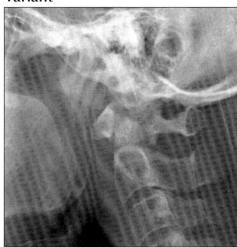 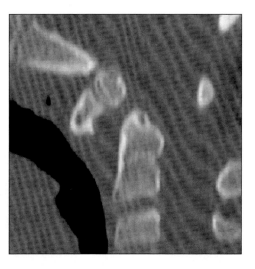

(Left) Lateral radiography shows mild dens hypoplasia. Anterior C1 ring enlargement suggests a congenital origin. Static alignment is normal, but dynamic imaging would be required to exclude instability.* *(Right)* *Sagittal bone CT shows os odontoideum, with hypertrophy of C1 anterior ring, platybasia, clival-os pseudoarticulation, and subluxation of the C0/C1/os complex indicating static C1/2 instability.*

LIMBUS VERTEBRA

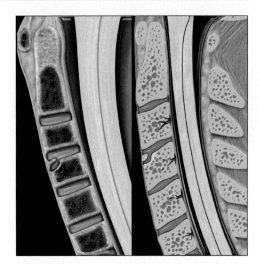

Disc herniation underneath the non-ossified apophysis in a pediatric patient (left) mimics a vertebral "defect", while subsequent ossification (right) produces a typical adult appearance.

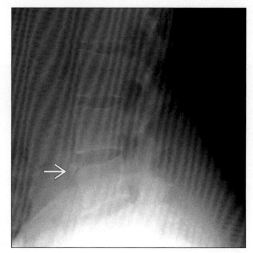

Lateral radiography shows a well corticated fragment (arrow) at anterosuperior L4 vertebral margin with matching vertebral donor site, typical of limbus vertebra (LV).

TERMINOLOGY

Abbreviations and Synonyms
- Synonyms: LV, slipped vertebral apophysis

Definitions
- Distinct type of cartilaginous node formation
  - Intraosseous disc penetration at junction of cartilaginous endplate, developing osseous rim apophysis

IMAGING FINDINGS

General Features
- Best diagnostic clue: Small corticated bone fragment matching osseous defect of anterosuperior vertebral margin
- Location
  - Mid-lumbar > mid-cervical
  - Anterior > > posterior
- Size: Small (≈ 1-3 mm)
- Morphology
  - Tiny unfused apophyseal fragment at vertebral margin
    - Lumbar LV: Anterosuperior > > posterior
    - Cervical LV: Anteroinferior > anterosuperior

Radiographic Findings
- Radiography
  - Children: Lucent defect in anterosuperior corner of vertebral body
    - Fragment may not be visible (non-ossified)
  - Adults: Triangular corticated bone fragment
    - Roughly matches corresponding donor site defect in adjacent vertebral body

CT Findings
- Bone CT
  - Osseous vertebral defect +/- matching corticated bone fragment
    - Fragment and donor site margins usually sclerotic when subacute/chronic
  - +/- Mild kyphosis
  - +/- Disc height loss

MR Findings
- T1WI
  - Hypointense bone fragment blends in with anterior ligaments
    - +/- Mild kyphosis
    - +/- Disc height loss
  - Mild hypointense marrow edema (if acute)
- T2WI
  - Hypointense bone fragment blends in with anterior ligaments

DDx: Limbus Vertebra

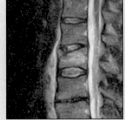

Acute Comp. Fx

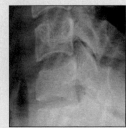

Acute Burst Fx

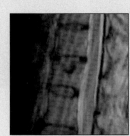

Schmorl Node

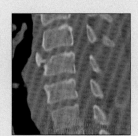

Acute Osteophyte Fx

LIMBUS VERTEBRA

Key Facts

Terminology
- Synonyms: LV, slipped vertebral apophysis

Imaging Findings
- Best diagnostic clue: Small corticated bone fragment matching osseous defect of anterosuperior vertebral margin
- Children: Lucent defect in anterosuperior corner of vertebral body
- Adults: Triangular corticated bone fragment
- Best imaging tool: Plain radiographs usually diagnostic
- MRI helpful (if necessary) to assess for edema or inflammation in context of acute symptoms

Top Differential Diagnoses
- Acute vertebral fracture

- Schmorl node
- Anterior osteophyte fragment
- Calcified disc herniation

Clinical Issues
- No further investigative procedures necessary following diagnosis
- LV may evolve into anterior Schmorl node in some patients

Diagnostic Checklist
- LV is sequel of remote injury in an immature skeleton
- Important to exclude other causes of back pain in a patient with LV
- LV fragment matches size of vertebral body defect

- ○ T2 hyperintense disc extends between fragment and vertebral body
  - ■ Caveat: Disc protrusion may be hypointense in adults with degenerative disc disease, but usually resembles intrinsic signal intensity within remainder of intervertebral disc
- STIR: Mild hyperintense marrow edema (if acute)

Other Modality Findings
- Discography: Intradiscal contrast flows between fragment and vertebral body, confirming diagnosis

Imaging Recommendations
- Best imaging tool: Plain radiographs usually diagnostic
- Protocol advice
  - ○ Plain radiographs to establish diagnosis
  - ○ MRI helpful (if necessary) to assess for edema or inflammation in context of acute symptoms

DIFFERENTIAL DIAGNOSIS

Acute vertebral fracture
- LV commonly misdiagnosed as fracture
- Look for trabecular smudging, soft tissue swelling

Schmorl node
- Schmorl node herniates more centrally into vertebral end plate than LV

Anterior osteophyte fragment
- Osteophyte fractures off, mimicking LV
- Usually no matching donor site on adjacent vertebral body

Calcified disc herniation
- No matching vertebral body defect
- Location usually not characteristic of LV

PATHOLOGY

General Features
- General path comments

- ○ Caused by herniation of nucleus pulposus beneath ring apophysis (junction of cartilaginous endplate, bony rim)
  - ■ Occurs prior to fusion of apophysis to vertebral body
  - ■ Apophysis remains separate from vertebral body
- ○ Anterosuperior vertebral margin may be more frequently affected because of adjacent vertebral body size difference (superior < inferior)
  - ■ During flexion, the anterior disc is forced down into superior end plate of larger inferior vertebra
  - ■ Pushes nucleus pulposis through the cartilage plate, isolating apophysis from main vertebral body
- Etiology
  - ○ Superior and inferior surface of developing vertebral body is covered by thin, peripherally thickened cartilage plate ⇒ cartilaginous marginal ridge
  - ○ Endochondral ossification of marginal ridge begins at age 7-9 years ⇒ forms rim apophysis (RA)
  - ○ RA separated from vertebral body by this thin cartilage layer until apophysis fuses to vertebral body at age 18-20 years
    - ■ Relative weak point in disc/vertebral body until fusion occurs
    - ■ LV occurs when nucleus pulposus herniates between RA and vertebral body, permanently isolating a small segment of vertebral rim
  - ○ Outermost fibers of anulus fibrosus (Sharpey fibers) embedded into RA fasten disc to spine
- Epidemiology
  - ○ Common radiologic finding in adults; relatively less common in children
  - ○ Trauma appears to be responsible for many cases
    - ■ LV more common in active, athletic children; traumatic insult may not be remembered
- Associated abnormalities
  - ○ Scheuermann Disease
  - ○ Schmorl nodes

Gross Pathologic & Surgical Features
- Small corticated bone fragment, separated from vertebral body by intervening disc material

LIMBUS VERTEBRA

Microscopic Features

- Cancellous bone, hyaline cartilage, and acellular hyaline tissue (disc)
- Basophilic degeneration, hemorrhagic foci in hyaline cartilage common

CLINICAL ISSUES

Presentation

- Most common signs/symptoms
  - Chronic back pain
  - Occasionally incidental finding
  - Inciting event rarely recognized or remembered
- Clinical profile
  - Variable symptomatology depending on location
    - Anterior defect ⇒ symptoms usually minor; stiffness or loss of physiologic lordosis
    - Posterior defect ⇒ symptoms mimic nerve root, cord compression
  - Physical exam generally shows decreased range of motion, +/- kyphosis, or pain on spinous process palpation

Demographics

- Age: Adults > children, adolescents
- Gender: M > F

Natural History & Prognosis

- No further investigative procedures necessary following diagnosis
  - Symptoms usually resolve over months to years
- LV may evolve into anterior Schmorl node in some patients

Treatment

- Conservative management
  - Analgesics
  - Physical therapy
  - Limitation of physical activity during acute phase
- Surgical management not indicated

DIAGNOSTIC CHECKLIST

Consider

- LV is sequel of remote injury in an immature skeleton
- Important to exclude other causes of back pain in a patient with LV

Image Interpretation Pearls

- Diagnosis of LV is less difficult in adults than children
  - Presence of characteristic, well formed triangular osseous fragment
- LV fragment matches size of vertebral body defect
  - Helps distinguish LV from other differential considerations such as calcified disc or osteophyte

SELECTED REFERENCES

1. Mupparapu M et al: Radiographic diagnosis of Limbus vertebra on a lateral cephalometric film: report of a case. Dentomaxillofac Radiol. 31(5):328-30, 2002
2. Mendez JS et al: Limbus lumbar and sacral vertebral fractures. Neurol Res. 24(2):139-44, 2002
3. Bonic EE et al: Posterior limbus fractures: five case reports and a review of selected published cases. J Manipulative Physiol Ther. 21(4):281-7, 1998
4. Swischuk LE et al: Disk degenerative disease in childhood: Scheuermann's disease, Schmorl's nodes, and the limbus vertebra: MRI findings in 12 patients. Pediatr Radiol. 28(5):334-8, 1998
5. Martinez-Lage JF et al: Avulsed lumbar vertebral rim plate in an adolescent: trauma or malformation? Childs Nerv Syst. 14(3):131-4, 1998
6. Talha A et al: Fracture of the vertebral limbus. Eur Spine J. 6(5):347-50, 1997
7. Carreon LY et al: Neovascularization induced by anulus and its inhibition by cartilage endplate. Its role in disc absorption. 1;22(13):1429-34, 1997
8. Henales V et al: Intervertebral disc herniations (limbus vertebrae) in pediatric patients: report of 15 cases. Pediatr Radiol. 23(8):608-10, 1993
9. Epstein NE: Lumbar surgery for 56 limbus fractures emphasizing noncalcified type III lesions. Spine. 17(12):1489-96, 1992
10. Cao LB et al: Imaging study of lumbar posterior marginal intraosseous node. An analysis of 36 cases. Chin Med J (Engl). 105(10):866-9, 1992
11. Epstein NE et al: Limbus lumbar vertebral fractures in 27 adolescents and adults. Spine. 16(8):962-6, 1991
12. Goldman AB et al: Posterior limbus vertebrae: a cause of radiating back pain in adolescents and young adults. Skeletal Radiol. 19(7):501-7, 1990
13. Hsu K et al: High lumbar disc degeneration. Incidence and etiology. Spine. 15(7):679-82, 1990
14. Banerian KG et al: Association of vertebral end plate fracture with pediatric lumbar intervertebral disk herniation: value of CT and MR imaging. Radiology. 177(3):763-5, 1990
15. McCarron RF: A case of mistaken identity, limbus annulare mimics fracture. Orthop Rev. 16(3):173-5, 1987
16. Kerns S et al: Annulus fibrosus calcification in the cervical spine: radiologic-pathologic correlation. Skeletal Radiol. 15(8):605-9, 1986
17. Yagan R: CT diagnosis of limbus vertebra. J Comput Assist Tomogr. 8(1):149-51, 1984
18. Kozlowski K: Anterior intervertebral disc herniations in children: unrecognised chronic trauma to the spine. Australas Radiol. 23(1):67-71, 1979
19. Ghelman B et al: The limbus vertebra: an anterior disc herniation demonstrated by discography. Am J Roentgenol. 127(5):854-5, 1976

LIMBUS VERTEBRA

IMAGE GALLERY

Typical

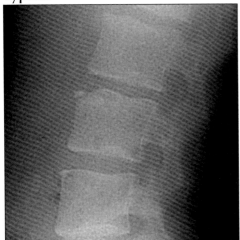
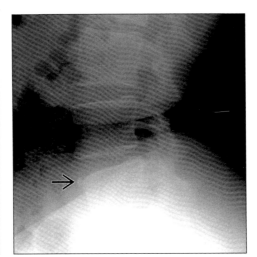

(Left) Lateral radiography depicts a classic L3 limbus vertebra in a young man with chronic back pain. (Right) Lateral radiography shows an L4 limbus vertebra, with typical anterosuperior corticated fragment (arrow).

Variant

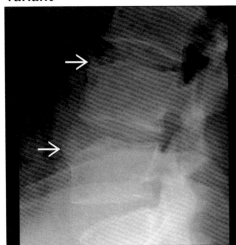
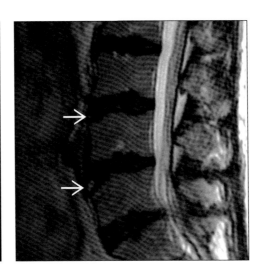

(Left) Lateral radiography shows LV at both L4 and L5 (arrows). L5 shows development of Schmorl node changes posterior to the corticated fragment. (Right) Sagittal T2WI MR demonstrates L4 and L5 LV (arrows), with variant Schmorl node changes posterior to the L5 corticated fragment.

Other

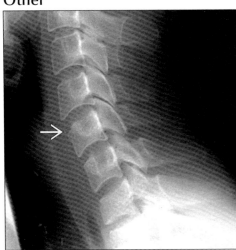
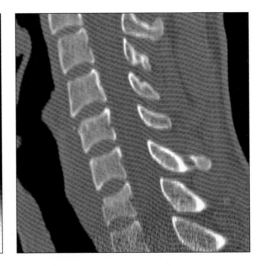

(Left) Lateral radiography demonstrates a typical LV of the C5 vertebra (arrow). Anterior wedging of C7 with small anterior defect, in comparison, reflects an acute vertebral fracture. (Right) Sagittal bone CT depicts a typical C5 LV. Anterior wedging of C7 vertebra, with anterior defect and dense trabecular compression, is compatible with clinical history of acute fracture.

CONJOINED NERVE ROOTS

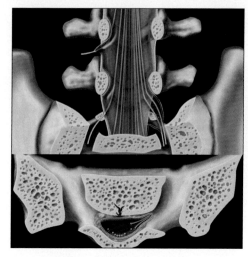

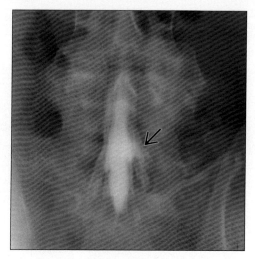

Composite graphic shows two nerve roots (left L5 and S1) exiting the dural sac through a single composite dural sleeve and neural foramen (left S1).

Anteroposterior myelography demonstrates typical conjoined root configuration, with an aberrant enlarged root sleeve (arrow) containing two roots (L5, S1).

TERMINOLOGY

Abbreviations and Synonyms
- Synonym: Composite nerve root sleeve

Definitions
- Asymmetric anomalous origin of an enlarged nerve root sleeve containing two nerve roots

IMAGING FINDINGS

General Features
- Best diagnostic clue: Enlarged root sleeve containing two roots originating midway between expected positions of two contributing nerve roots
- Location
  - Lumbar spine > > cervical, thoracic spine
    - L4/5 > L5/S1 > L3/4
- Size
  - Conjoined root sleeve larger than normal root sleeve
  - Nerve roots normal size (unless inflamed)
- Morphology
  - Asymmetric anomalous origin of enlarged nerve root sleeve
    - Roots usually exit separately at expected neural foraminal levels

- Occasionally both roots exit through same (usually lower) foramen

Radiographic Findings
- Radiography
  - Enlarged neural foramen
  - Ipsilateral hypoplastic or absent pedicle
- Myelography
  - Supernumerary nerve roots on CT myelography
    - Two nerve roots exit through single contrast filled sleeve midway between sleeve exit levels of contralateral side
    - Roots either exit separately through appropriate foramina or remain joined and exit through a single foramen
  - Most cases demonstrated equally well using MR imaging
    - Reserve myelography for problem solving, patients with MR imaging contraindications

CT Findings
- CECT
  - Enlarged neural foramen, +/- hypoplastic or absent pedicle
  - Asymmetric mild dilatation of ipsilateral osseous lateral recess
    - Not typically observed with extruded free intervertebral disk fragments
  - Normal dorsal root ganglion (DRG) enhancement

DDx: Conjoined Nerve Root

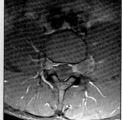

Neurofibroma

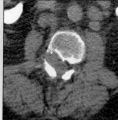

Schwannoma

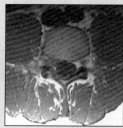

Disc Herniation

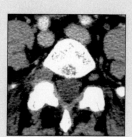

Synovial Cyst

CONJOINED NERVE ROOTS

Key Facts

Terminology
- Synonym: Composite nerve root sleeve
- Asymmetric anomalous origin of an enlarged nerve root sleeve containing two nerve roots

Imaging Findings
- Best diagnostic clue: Enlarged root sleeve containing two roots originating midway between expected positions of two contributing nerve roots
- Lumbar spine > > cervical, thoracic spine
- L4/5 > L5/S1 > L3/4
- Enlarged neural foramen
- Ipsilateral hypoplastic or absent pedicle

Top Differential Diagnoses
- Nerve sheath tumor (NST)
- Disc herniation

- Synovial cyst

Pathology
- Symptomatic (but undiagnosed) conjoined nerve roots are one cause of failed back syndrome
- Most commonly unilateral

Clinical Issues
- Usually asymptomatic
- Symptomatic patients present with radiculopathy

Diagnostic Checklist
- Important anatomical variant to identify prior to spinal surgery to prevent inadvertent nerve injury
- Dorsal root ganglia contrast-enhancement and enlargement of foraminal neural structures may lead to misdiagnosis as nerve sheath tumor

MR Findings
- T1WI
  - Enlarged neural foramen, +/- hypoplastic or absent pedicle
  - Nerve roots easily visualized in foramen surrounded by hyperintense fat
- T2WI
  - Similar osseous findings to T1WI MR
  - Supranumerary nerve roots identified within asymmetric enlarged root sleeve
- T1 C+
  - Normal dorsal root ganglion (DRG) enhancement
  - Remainder of nerve is nonenhancing (post-operatively nerves may enhance)

Ultrasonographic Findings
- Real Time: Two nerve roots within a single root sleeve

Imaging Recommendations
- Sagittal and axial MR imaging
  - Both T1WI and T2WI MR needed
    - Sagittal slice prescription must extend lateral to neural foramina
    - Contrast useful to locate DRG
- CT myelography demonstrates relationship of root sleeve to osseous structures well
  - Use for inconclusive MR imaging or when MR contraindications exist

DIFFERENTIAL DIAGNOSIS

Nerve sheath tumor (NST)
- Conjoined nerve root mimics appearance of schwannoma or neurofibroma
- Larger tumors show dumbbell configuration
- Entire NST usually enhances avidly; only DRG of conjoined nerve root normally enhances

Disc herniation
- Rim-enhancement of disc fragment, contiguity with disc space
- Neural sleeves exit dural sac at appropriate levels

Synovial cyst
- Severe degenerative facet disease
- Neural sleeves exit dural sac at appropriate levels

PATHOLOGY

General Features
- General path comments
  - More commonly recognized at autopsy or during surgery than on imaging studies
  - May produce sciatica without additional compressive impingement from disc herniation, spondylolisthesis, or lateral recess stenosis
  - Symptomatic (but undiagnosed) conjoined nerve roots are one cause of failed back syndrome
- Etiology: Unknown
- Epidemiology: Prevalence 0.3-2%; some studies as high as 10.6%
- Associated abnormalities: Occasionally developmental lumbar spinal stenosis

Gross Pathologic & Surgical Features
- Most commonly unilateral
- Composite root sleeve originates from the dural sac at point halfway between expected positions of the two sleeves it replaces, and is bigger than a normal sleeve
  - Conjoined nerve roots commonly leave spinal canal through separate neural foramina
  - Less commonly, the two roots exit through a single foramina (usually that of the lower root)
  - Failure to correctly appreciate this anatomical variant ⇒ misdiagnosis as nerve root tumor or operation at the wrong level for clinical radiculopathy

Microscopic Features
- Normal nerve, dural histology

CONJOINED NERVE ROOTS

CLINICAL ISSUES

Presentation
- Most common signs/symptoms
  - Usually asymptomatic
  - Symptomatic patients present with radiculopathy
    - Conjoined nerves prone to compression by discs, lateral bony stenosis along lateral recess
    - Herniated disc beneath the bifid root ⇒ pain, disability, signs of entrapment 2° to fixation of conjoined root within lateral recess, between pedicles
- Clinical profile: Patient presents with cervical or lumbar radiculopathy

Demographics
- Age: No age predilection
- Gender: M = F

Natural History & Prognosis
- Asymptomatic patients require no treatment
- Rare symptomatic patients referable to conjoined root level may require surgical therapy
- Symptomatic undiagnosed conjoined roots are one cause of failed back syndrome
  - Nerve root anomalies should be searched for in cases of failed disc surgery

Treatment
- Conservative non-operative observation unless symptomatic
- Surgical decompression in selected patients with documented concordant radiculopathy
  - Hemilaminectomy with foraminotomy, pediculectomy, and discectomy best alleviate symptomatology

DIAGNOSTIC CHECKLIST

Consider
- Important anatomical variant to identify prior to spinal surgery to prevent inadvertent nerve injury
- Exclude differential diagnoses such as nerve sheath tumor, disc herniation, or synovial cyst

Image Interpretation Pearls
- Dorsal root ganglia contrast-enhancement and enlargement of foraminal neural structures may lead to misdiagnosis as nerve sheath tumor

SELECTED REFERENCES

1. Bottcher J et al: Conjoined lumbosacral nerve roots: current aspects of diagnosis. Eur Spine J, 2003
2. Haijiao W et al: Diagnosis of lumbosacral nerve root anomalies by magnetic resonance imaging. J Spinal Disord. 14(2):143-9, 2001
3. Savas R et al: Hypoplastic lumbar pedicle in association with conjoined nerve root MRI demonstration. Comput Med Imaging Graph. 22(1):77-9, 1998
4. Sener RN: Sacral pedicle agenesis. Comput Med Imaging Graph. 21(6):361-3, 1997
5. Prestar FJ: Anomalies and malformations of lumbar spinal nerve roots. Minim Invasive Neurosurg. 39(4):133-7, 1996
6. Chu CR et al: Cervical conjoined nerve root variant: preoperative imaging and surgical conformation. Case report. J Neurosurg. 80(3):548-51, 1994
7. Phillips LH et al: The frequency of intradural conjoined lumbosacral dorsal nerve roots found during selective dorsal rhizotomy. Neurosurgery 33(1): 88-90, discussion 90-1, 1993
8. Firooznia H et al: Normal correlative anatomy of the lumbosacral spine and its contents. Neuroimaging clinics of North America 3(3): 411-24, 1993
9. Gomez JG et al: Conjoined lumbosacral nerve roots. Acta Neurochir (Wien). 120(3-4):155-8, 1993
10. Okuwaki T et al: Conjoined nerve roots associated with lumbosacral spine anomalies. A case report. Spine. 16(11):1347-9, 1991
11. Maiuri F et al: Anomalies of the lumbosacral nerve roots. Neurol Res. 11(3):130-5, 1989
12. Goffin J et al: Association of conjoined and anastomosed nerve roots in the lumbar region. A case report. Clin Neurol Neurosurg. 89(2):117-20, 1987
13. Torricelli P et al: CT diagnosis of lumbosacral conjoined nerve roots. Findings in 19 cases. Neuroradiology. 29(4):374-9, 1987
14. Peyster RG et al: Computed tomography of lumbosacral conjoined nerve root anomalies. Potential cause of false-positive reading for herniated nucleus pulposus. Spine. 10(4):331-7, 1985
15. Hoddick WK et al: Bony spinal canal changes that differentiate conjoined nerve roots from herniated nucleus pulposus. Radiology. 154(1):119-20, 1985
16. Rosner MJ et al: Anomalous exit of the C-6 nerve root via the C-6, C-7 foramen. Neurosurgery. 14(6):740-3, 1984
17. Gebarski SS et al: "Conjoined" nerve roots: a requirement for computed tomographic and myelographic correlation for diagnosis. Neurosurgery. 14(1):66-8, 1984
18. Cail WS et al: Conjoined lumbosacral nerve roots. Diagnosis with metrizamide myelography. Surg Neurol. 20(2):113-9, 1983
19. Neidre A et al: Anomalies of the lumbosacral nerve roots. Review of 16 cases and classification. Spine. 8(3):294-9, 1983
20. Coughlin JR et al: Metrizamide myelography in conjoined lumbosacral nerve roots. J Can Assoc Radiol. 34(1):23-5, 1983
21. Helms CA et al: The CT appearance of conjoined nerve roots and differentiation from a herniated nucleus pulposus. Radiology. 144(4):803-7, 1982
22. White JG 3rd et al: Surgical treatment of 63 cases of conjoined nerve roots. J Neurosurg. 56(1):114-7, 1982
23. Epstein JA et al: Conjoined lumbosacral nerve roots. Management of herniated discs and lateral recess stenosis in patients with this anomaly. J Neurosurg. 55(4):585-9, 1981
24. Bouchard JM et al: Preoperative diagnosis of conjoined roots anomaly with herniated lumbar disks. Surg Neurol. 10(4):229-31, 1978

IMAGE GALLERY

Typical

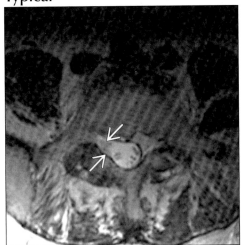
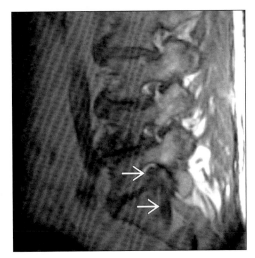

(Left) Axial T2WI MR demonstrates a large right nerve root sleeve, arising rostral to expected level, containing two different nerve roots *(arrows)*. *(Right)* Sagittal T1WI MR depicts conjoined L5 and S1 nerve roots *(arrows)* exiting independently through their appropriate neural foramen, the most common variation of conjoined nerve root anatomy.

Variant

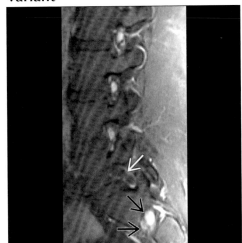
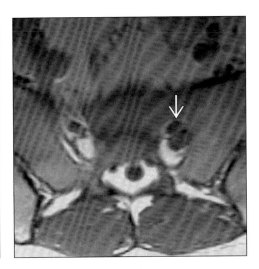

(Left) Sagittal T1 C+ MR shows normally enhancing DRG at all levels except left L5/S1 *(white arrow)*. Two enhancing DRGs are seen within the S1 foramen *(black arrows)*, an uncommon conjoined root variation. *(Right)* Axial T1WI MR of conjoined left L5 and S1 nerve roots reveals both DRGs within the left S1 neural foramen *(arrow)*, an uncommon conjoined root anatomical variation.

Variant

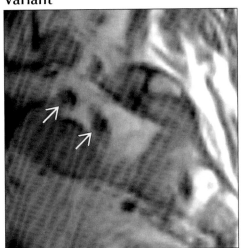
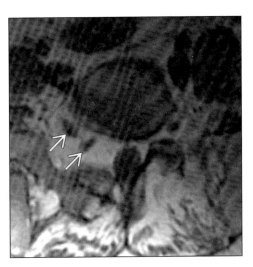

(Left) Sagittal T1WI MR shows two nerve roots *(arrows)* transiting a single aberrant enlarged neural foramen. *(Right)* Axial T1WI MR depicts both L5 and S1 nerve root DRGs *(arrows)* transiting a single enlarged neural foramen.

FILUM TERMINALE FIBROLIPOMA

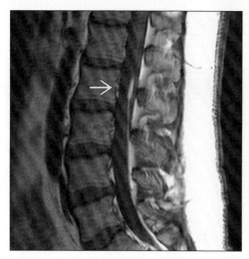

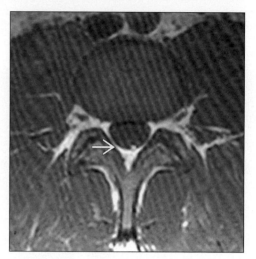

Sagittal T1WI MR shows linear high signal at L2-3 level (arrow). There is no thickening of filum, and conus is normal in position.

Axial T1WI MR at L3-4 level shows punctate high signal within dorsal thecal sac (arrow).

TERMINOLOGY

Abbreviations and Synonyms
- Synonyms: Fibrolipoma of filum terminale, fatty filum terminale, "fat in the filum"

Definitions
- Asymptomatic presence of fat within otherwise normal size filum terminale
- No tethered cord, conus normal position
- Symptomatic patient implies diagnosis of intraspinal lipoma, not asymptomatic fibrolipoma

IMAGING FINDINGS

General Features
- Best diagnostic clue: Linear fat signal within filum terminale on T1WI
- Location: Filum terminale (conus level to sacrum)
- Size: 1-5 mm
- Morphology: Linear, "stripe-like" high signal on T1WI

CT Findings
- NECT
  - Punctate fat attenuation in dorsal aspect of lumbar thecal sac
  - No associated dysraphism
- CECT: No enhancement

MR Findings
- T1WI
  - Linear high signal oriented in cranio-caudal direction on sagittal images
    - May occur anywhere from below conus to sacrum
  - Dorsal half of thecal sac in position of filum terminale
  - Low signal on fat suppressed sequence
- T2WI: Tracks fat signal
- T1 C+: No enhancement

Imaging Recommendations
- Best imaging tool: MR imaging: T1WI shows typical fat appearance, normal conus position and morphology
- Protocol advice: Add fat suppressed sequence if uncertain of T1WI signal etiology

DIFFERENTIAL DIAGNOSIS

Intraspinal lipoma
- Larger lipomatous mass (> few mm)
- Thickening of filum terminale (> 2 mm)
- Low lying or indistinct conus

Tethered cord
- Thick filum, indistinct conus termination, with smooth transition to filum

---

DDx: Intradural Hyperintensity on T1WI

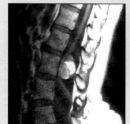

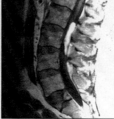

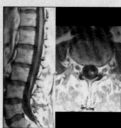

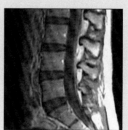

| *Epidermoid* | *Intraspinal Lipoma* | *Tethered Cord* | *SAH* |

FILUM TERMINALE FIBROLIPOMA

Key Facts

Terminology

- Synonyms: Fibrolipoma of filum terminale, fatty filum terminale, "fat in the filum"
- Asymptomatic presence of fat within otherwise normal size filum terminale
- No tethered cord, conus normal position
- Symptomatic patient implies diagnosis of intraspinal lipoma, not asymptomatic fibrolipoma

Imaging Findings

- Best imaging tool: MR imaging: T1WI shows typical fat appearance, normal conus position and morphology
- Protocol advice: Add fat suppressed sequence if uncertain of T1WI signal etiology

Pathology

- Epidemiology: Incidental in 4-6% of autopsy subjects

Lipomyelocele

- Dorsal dysraphism

Epidermoid/dermoid

- Complex intradural mass, variable fat suppression

Subarachnoid hemorrhage

- Typical acute history
- Fluid-fluid level in thecal sac

Tumor with paramagnetic effects

- Melanoma, melanotic meningioma, or schwannoma may show high signal on T1WI

PATHOLOGY

General Features

- General path comments: Fatty infiltration of filum
- Etiology: Congenital
- Epidemiology: Incidental in 4-6% of autopsy subjects
- Associated abnormalities: No cutaneous stigmata on lower back with asymptomatic filum fibrolipoma

Gross Pathologic & Surgical Features

- Small focus of fat within otherwise normal filum terminale

Microscopic Features

- Typical adipose tissue

CLINICAL ISSUES

Presentation

- Most common signs/symptoms: Asymptomatic by definition, incidental finding

Demographics

- Age: Children and adults
- Gender: M = F

Natural History & Prognosis

- Normal variant

Treatment

- None required for asymptomatic lesion

DIAGNOSTIC CHECKLIST

Consider

- Intraspinal lipoma if larger lesion and filum > 2 mm in thickness

SELECTED REFERENCES

1. Bulsara KR et al: Clinical outcome differences for lipomyelomeningoceles, intraspinal lipomas, and lipomas of the filum terminale. Neurosurg Rev. 24(4): 192-4, 2001
2. Xenos C et al: Spinal lipomas in children. Pediatr Neurosurg. 32(6): 295-307, 2000
3. Kujas M et al: Intradural spinal lipoma of the conus medullaris without spinal dysraphism. Clin Neuropathol. 19(1): 30-3, 2000
4. La Marca F et al: Spinal lipomas in children: outcome of 270 procedures. Pediatr Neurosurg. 26(1): 8-16, 1997
5. Brown E et al: Prevalence of incidental intraspinal lipoma of the lumbosacral spine as determined by MRI. Spine. 19(7): 833-6, 1994
6. Hawnaur JM et al: Investigation of children with suspected spinal dysraphism by magnetic resonance imaging. Eur J Pediatr Surg. 1 Suppl 1: 18-9, 1991
7. Okumura R et al: Fatty filum terminale: assessment with MR imaging. J Comput Assist Tomogr. 14(4): 571-3, 1990
8. Moufarrij NA et al: Correlation between magnetic resonance imaging and surgical findings in the tethered spinal cord. Neurosurgery. 25(3): 341-6, 1989

IMAGE GALLERY

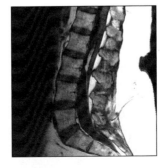 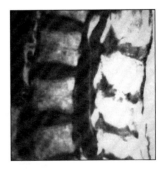

(Left) Sagittal T1WI MR shows large fibrolipoma of filum terminale as linear increased signal. Conus is normal in position. *(Right)* Sagittal T1WI MR shows large fibrolipoma of filum in asymptomatic patient.

BONE ISLAND

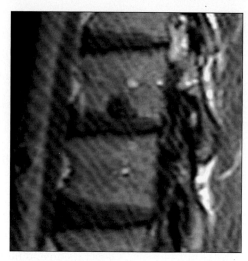

Sagittal T1 C+ MR demonstrates focal area of low signal in L1 vertebral body, without enhancement.

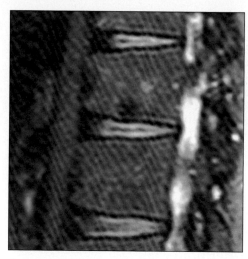

Sagittal STIR MR shows lesion with low T2 signal, with well-defined margins and no adjacent marrow hyperintensity.

TERMINOLOGY

Abbreviations and Synonyms
- Synonyms: Enostosis, sclerotic island, calcified island, compact island

Definitions
- Asymptomatic focal areas of bony sclerosis

IMAGING FINDINGS

General Features
- Best diagnostic clue: Small focal areas of sclerosis, with brush-like margins
- Location
  - Any bone may be involved
    - Vertebral body or posterior elements may be involved
  - Most common in pelvis, femur, ribs
- Size: 1 mm to several cm
- Morphology: Round, well-defined margins

Radiographic Findings
- Radiography
  - Single or multiple areas of focal homogeneously dense sclerosis in bone
  - Distinctive radiating bony streaks
    - "Thorny radiation"

- Blend with trabeculae of host bone with feathered or brush-like border

CT Findings
- NECT: Focal area(s) of high attenuation, well-defined margins, no soft tissue component

MR Findings
- T1WI: Focal low T1 signal
- T2WI: Focal low T2 signal
- T2* GRE: Low signal; may show slight blooming effect due to susceptibility artifact
- T1 C+: No enhancement

Nuclear Medicine Findings
- Bone Scan
  - Usually normal
  - Large lesions may show increased uptake

Imaging Recommendations
- Best imaging tool
  - Evaluation of solitary indeterminate lesion: CT
  - Evaluation of multiple lesions: MRI
- Protocol advice: Bone scan for definition of solitary lesion metastasis vs. bone island

DDx: Hypointense Bone Lesions

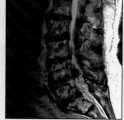

Prostate Metastases

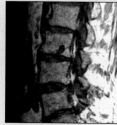

Schmorl Node

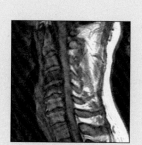

Type I Endplates

BONE ISLAND

Key Facts

Terminology
- Synonyms: Enostosis, sclerotic island, calcified island, compact island
- Asymptomatic focal areas of bony sclerosis

Imaging Findings
- Best diagnostic clue: Small focal areas of sclerosis, with brush-like margins
- Any bone may be involved

- Most common in pelvis, femur, ribs
- Size: 1 mm to several cm
- Usually normal

Pathology
- General path comments: Normal compact bone
- Etiology: Developmental
- Epidemiology: Spine involvement in up to 14% of subjects

DIFFERENTIAL DIAGNOSIS

Metastatic disease
- Multiple lesions, epidural extension

Schmorl node/degenerative endplates
- Adjacent to endplate, may enhance

Osteoid osteoma
- Bone expansion, central nidus

Osteopoikilosis
- Multiple bone islands

Bone infarct
- More ill-defined or patchy signal abnormality, may enhance

PATHOLOGY

General Features
- General path comments: Normal compact bone
- Etiology: Developmental
- Epidemiology: Spine involvement in up to 14% of subjects
- Associated abnormalities: Increased incidence in leprosy, particularly long disease duration

Gross Pathologic & Surgical Features
- Dense bony lesion

Microscopic Features
- Compact bone connected to adjacent bony trabeculae
- No cartilage or fibrous component

CLINICAL ISSUES

Presentation
- Most common signs/symptoms: Asymptomatic
- Clinical profile: Incidental finding in patient imaged for back pain

Demographics
- Age: All age groups
- Gender: M = F

Natural History & Prognosis
- Stable lesions
  ○ Rarely will increase or decrease in size over time

DIAGNOSTIC CHECKLIST

Consider
- Metastatic disease (prostate) will multiple small foci of low signal on MRI

SELECTED REFERENCES

1. White LM et al: Osteoid-producing tumors of bone. Semin Musculoskelet Radiol. 4(1):25-43, 2000
2. Leone A et al: Primary bone tumors and pseudotumors of the lumbosacral spine. Rays. 25(1):89-103, 2000
3. Carpintero P et al: Bone island and leprosy. Skeletal Radiol. 27(6):330-33, 1998
4. Murphey MD et al: From the archives of the AFIP. Primary tumors of the spine: radiologic pathologic correlation. Radiographics. 16(5):1131-58, 1996
5. Greenspan A: Bone island (enostosis): current concept--a review. Skeletal Radiol. 24(2):111-5, 1995
6. Greenspan A et al: Bone island: scintigraphic findings and their clinical application. Can Assoc Radiol J. 46(5):368-79, 1995
7. Greenspan A et al: Bone island (enostosis): clinical significance and radiologic and pathologic correlations. Skeletal Radiol. 20(2):85-90, 1991
8. Broderick TW et al: Enostosis of the spine. Spine. 3(2):167-70, 1978

IMAGE GALLERY

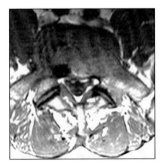 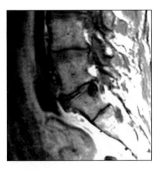

(Left) Axial T1WI MR shows focal low T1 signal in right S1 vertebral body without epidural soft tissue. *(Right)* Sagittal T1WI MR shows S1 vertebral lesion as focal T1 hypointensity.

VENTRICULUS TERMINALIS

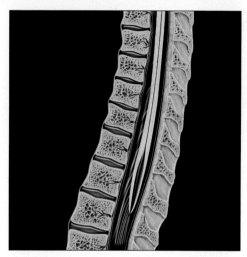

Sagittal graphic demonstrates uncomplicated fusiform dilatation of the distal central cord canal, typical of ventriculus terminalis.

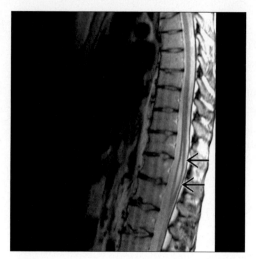

Sagittal T2WI MR shows mild dilatation of the central canal (arrows) limited to the conus, typical of classic ventriculus terminalis.

TERMINOLOGY

Abbreviations and Synonyms
- Synonyms: Terminal ventricle, fifth ventricle

Definitions
- CSF signal/density within central spinal cord, canal expansion at conus/proximal filum level

IMAGING FINDINGS

General Features
- Best diagnostic clue: Mild cystic dilatation of distal central spinal cord canal without cord signal abnormality or enhancement
- Location: Distal spinal cord, between conus medullaris tip and filum terminale origin
- Size: 2-4 mm (transverse); rarely exceeds 2 cms in length
- Morphology
  ○ Central intramedullary CSF signal/density dilatation with smooth regular margins and no mass
  ○ Conus terminates at normal level (T12 → L2)

CT Findings
- CECT
  ○ CSF density dilatation of distal spinal cord central canal

○ No mass lesion or enhancement

MR Findings
- T1WI
  ○ Hypointense CSF signal intensity dilatation of distal cord central canal
    ▪ Beware phase ghosting or truncation (Gibb) artifact imitating central canal dilatation
  ○ Conus terminates at normal level (T12 to L2)
  ○ No filum terminale thickening or lipoma
- T2WI
  ○ Hyperintense CSF signal intensity dilatation of distal cord central canal
  ○ No septation of dilated central canal
- T1 C+
  ○ No associated mass lesion or enhancement
    ▪ Differentiates from cystic cord neoplasm

Ultrasonographic Findings
- Real Time
  ○ Mild anechoic non-septated central canal dilatation within normally situated conus
  ○ Normal nerve root and conus pulsation
  ○ No filum terminale thickening (< 2 mm normal) or lipoma
- M-mode: Useful to confirm normal nerve root and conus pulsation

DDx: Ventriculus Terminalis

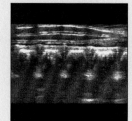
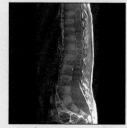
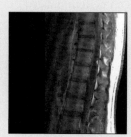
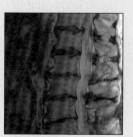

Transient Dilatation   Hydrosyringomyelia   Hemangioblastoma   Myelomalacia

VENTRICULUS TERMINALIS

Key Facts

Terminology
- Synonyms: Terminal ventricle, fifth ventricle

Imaging Findings
- Best diagnostic clue: Mild cystic dilatation of distal central spinal cord canal without cord signal abnormality or enhancement
- Size: 2-4 mm (transverse); rarely exceeds 2 cms in length
- Conus terminates at normal level (T12 → L2)

Top Differential Diagnoses
- Transient dilatation of the central canal
- Hydrosyringomyelia
- Cystic spinal cord neoplasm
- Myelomalacia

Pathology
- Simple CSF filled cavity of conus medullaris
- Normal cord microscopic histology

Clinical Issues
- Incidental finding on imaging performed for unrelated indications
- Clinical profile: Patient is asymptomatic or presents with nonspecific neurological symptoms

Diagnostic Checklist
- Most important imaging goal is to distinguish from cystic cord neoplasm or syrinx
- Isolated mild dilatation of distal central canal in a normally located conus is nearly always an incidental normal finding

Imaging Recommendations
- Newborns
  - Ultrasound to screen for congenital anomalies
    - Distinguish ventriculus terminalis from syrinx or cord neoplasm
    - Abnormal findings should be confirmed with MR imaging
- Children, adults, & infants (with positive ultrasound studies)
  - Thin-section sagittal T1WI & T2WI MR imaging (3 mm slice thickness)
  - Axial T1WI & T2WI (4 mm slice thickness) distal cord to sacrum
    - Best to exclude occult dysraphism, lipoma, or thick filum
  - T1 C+ MR in sagittal, axial planes to exclude mass

DIFFERENTIAL DIAGNOSIS

Transient dilatation of the central canal
- Normal variant
- Slight dilatation of central canal in a newborn
- Disappears in first weeks of life

Hydrosyringomyelia
- Cystic expansion of distal one-third (or more) of spinal cord
- Isolated finding, or associated with congenital spine anomalies (up to 30% of patients)

Cystic spinal cord neoplasm
- Astrocytoma, ependymoma, hemangioblastoma
- Differentiated by cord signal abnormality and expansion, contrast-enhancement in solid portions

Myelomalacia
- History of trauma, vascular accident, or other cord insult
- Cord atrophy, +/- T2 hyperintensity

PATHOLOGY

General Features
- General path comments
  - CSF-filled cavity at conus medullaris level
    - Enclosed by ependymal tissue
    - Normally present as either virtual cavity or ependymal residue
  - Size variable throughout life; smallest in middle-age and largest in early childhood, old age
- Etiology
  - Forms during embryogenesis (ninth week) via canalization and retrogressive differentiation of caudal spinal cord
    - Represents point of union between central canal portion formed by neurulation and portion formed by caudal cell mass canalization
    - Usually regresses in size during first weeks after birth; persistence leads to identification in children or adults
- Epidemiology
  - Identified at all ages, but most commonly before 5 years of age
    - 2.6% of normal children (under 5 years) have a visible ventriculus terminalis on MRI
    - Less commonly identified in adults; primarily an autopsy curiosity before widespread availability of MR imaging
- Associated abnormalities: Occasionally identified in conjunction with caudal regression or tethered cord

Gross Pathologic & Surgical Features
- Simple CSF filled cavity of conus medullaris
- No gliosis or neoplasm

Microscopic Features
- Normal cord microscopic histology
  - Cystic cavity lined by ependymal cells
  - No gliosis or neoplasm

VENTRICULUS TERMINALIS

CLINICAL ISSUES

Presentation

- Most common signs/symptoms
  - Incidental finding on imaging performed for unrelated indications
    - Usually identified during sciatica work-up
  - Rarely becomes abnormally dilated and symptomatic, necessitating treatment
    - Bilateral sciatica
    - Lower extremity weakness
    - Urinary retention
- Clinical profile: Patient is asymptomatic or presents with nonspecific neurological symptoms

Demographics

- Age: Most commonly identified under age 5; may occur at any age
- Gender: M = F

Natural History & Prognosis

- No effect on mortality or morbidity
  - Most commonly either stable in size or regresses; size progression not reported
- Rare symptomatic surgical cases show symptom improvement post-operatively

Treatment

- No treatment indicated for asymptomatic incidental finding
  - MRI follow-up if deemed necessary based on clinical findings
- Surgical decompression and management of associated abnormalities in rare symptomatic cases
  - Cyst fenestration +/- cyst shunting to the subarachnoid space, pleural cavity, or peritoneal cavity

DIAGNOSTIC CHECKLIST

Consider

- Most important imaging goal is to distinguish from cystic cord neoplasm or syrinx
- Asymptomatic patients require no further imaging evaluation
- Symptomatic patients should be monitored using clinical and MR follow-up unless degree of cyst expansion prompts surgical drainage

Image Interpretation Pearls

- Isolated mild dilatation of distal central canal in a normally located conus is nearly always an incidental normal finding
  - Calcification, septations, nodules, enhancement, or eccentric location all argue against ventriculus terminalis and prompt further evaluation
  - Beware of truncation or phase ghosting artifact mimicking a dilated terminal ventricle or syrinx
- Exclude other unsuspected abnormalities that may predispose to syrinx or cord tethering before attributing finding to incidental dilatation of ventriculus terminalis

SELECTED REFERENCES

1. Dullerud R et al: MR imaging of ventriculus terminalis of the conus medullaris. A report of two operated patients and a review of the literature. Acta Radiol. 44(4):444-6, 2003
2. Celli P et al: Cyst of the medullary conus: malformative persistence of terminal ventricle or compressive dilatation? Neurosurg Rev. 25(1-2):103-6, 2002
3. Kriss VM et al: Sonographic appearance of the ventriculus terminalis cyst in the neonatal spinal cord. J Ultrasound Med. 19(3):207-9, 2000
4. Tortori-Donati P et al: Spinal dysraphism: a review of neuroradiological features with embryological correlations and proposal for a new classification. Neuroradiology. 42(7):471-91, 2000
5. Unsinn KM et al: US of the spinal cord in newborns: spectrum of normal findings, variants, congenital anomalies, and acquired diseases. Radiographics. 20(4):923-38, 2000
6. Truong BC et al: Dilation of the ventriculus terminalis: sonographic findings. J Ultrasound Med. 17(11):713-5, 1998
7. Matsubayashi R et al: Cystic dilatation of ventriculus terminalis in adults: MRI. Neuroradiology. 40(1):45-7, 1998
8. Agrillo U et al: Symptomatic cystic dilatation of V ventricle: case report and review of the literature. Eur Spine J. 6(4):281-3, 1997
9. Unsinn KM et al: Sonography of the ventriculus terminalis in newborns. AJNR Am J Neuroradiol. 17(5):1003-4, 1996
10. Tindall et al: The Practice of Neurosurgery. Baltimore, Williams and Wilkins, 2797, 1996
11. Unsinn KM et al: Ventriculus terminalis of the spinal cord in the neonate: a normal variant on sonography. AJR Am J Roentgenol. 167(5):1341, 1996
12. Rypens F et al: Atypical and equivocal sonographic features of the spinal cord in neonates. Pediatr Radiol. 25(6):429-32, 1995
13. Coleman LT et al: Ventriculus terminalis of the conus medullaris: MR findings in children. AJNR Am J Neuroradiol. 16(7):1421-6, 1995
14. Kriss VM et al: The ventriculus terminalis of the spinal cord in the neonate: a normal variant on sonography. AJR Am J Roentgenol. 165(6):1491-3, 1995
15. Iskander BJ et al. Terminal hydrosyringomyelia and occult spinal dysraphism. J Neurosurg 81:513-19, 1994
16. Choi BH et al: The ventriculus terminalis and filum terminale of the human spinal cord. Hum Pathol. 23(8):916-20, 1992
17. Sigal R et al: Ventriculus terminalis of the conus medullaris: MR imaging in four patients with congenital dilatation. AJNR Am J Neuroradiol. 12(4):733-7, 1991
18. Stewart DH Jr et al: Surgical drainage of cyst of the conus medullaris. Report of three cases. J Neurosurg. 33(1):106-10, 1970

IMAGE GALLERY

Typical

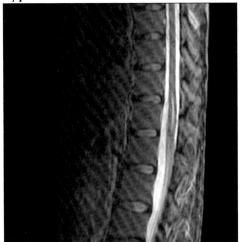
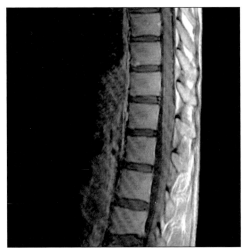

(Left) Sagittal T2WI MR shows mild focal dilation of the terminal ventricle limited to the conus, without cord signal abnormality that would imply a pathologic lesion. (Right) Sagittal T1 C+ MR shows no abnormal enhancement of the terminal ventricle.

Variant

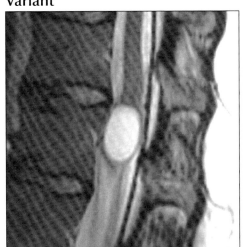
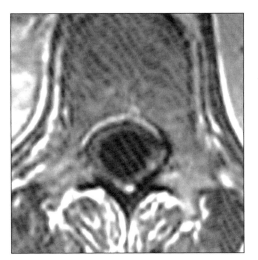

(Left) Sagittal T2WI MR demonstrates cystic enlargement of the terminal ventricle without other spinal cord abnormalities. (Right) Axial T1 C+ MR demonstrates cystic ventriculus terminalis enlargement. Absence of contrast enhancement helps to exclude cystic neoplasm.

Variant

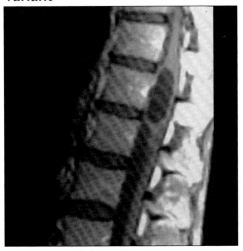
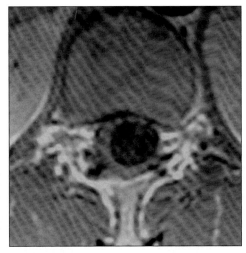

(Left) Sagittal T1 C+ MR shows a large hypointense ventriculus terminalis cyst within a normally located distal conus. The remainder of the spinal cord was normal (not shown). (Right) Axial T1 C+ MR demonstrates a mildly eccentric hypointense ventriculus terminalis cyst. Absence of contrast enhancement helps exclude cystic neoplasm.

CHIARI I MALFORMATION

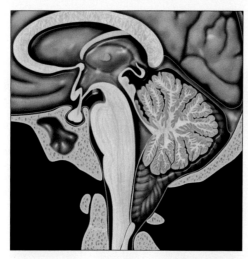

Sagittal graphic demonstrates pointed "peg-like" tonsils extending below foramen magnum, elongating the normally positioned IVth ventricle.

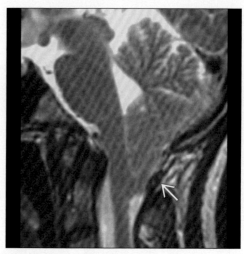

Sagittal T2WI MR depicts classic Chiari I changes. Elongated, "peg-shaped" tonsils extend below C1 ring (arrow), and display characteristic oblique cerebellar folia ("sergeant's stripes").

TERMINOLOGY

Abbreviations and Synonyms
- Synonyms: CM 1, Arnold-Chiari 1 malformation, AC1

Definitions
- Elongated, "peg-shaped" cerebellar tonsils extend below foramen magnum into cervical spinal canal

IMAGING FINDINGS

General Features
- Best diagnostic clue: Pointed cerebellar tonsils ≥ 5 mm below foramen magnum +/- syringohydromyelia (14-75%)
- Location: Craniovertebral junction (CVJ)
- Size: Tonsils > 5 mm below foramen magnum
- Morphology: Low-lying, pointed "peg-like" tonsils with oblique vertical sulci, elongated but normally located IVth ventricle

Radiographic Findings
- Radiography: Either normal or short clivus, CVJ segmentation/fusion anomalies, small posterior fossa (PF)
- Myelography: Low-lying tonsils efface CSF at foramen magnum

CT Findings
- NECT: Small posterior fossa ⇒ low torcular, "crowded" foramen magnum, tonsillar ectopia, flattened spinal cord
- Bone CT
  - Often normal; abnormal cases ⇒ short clivus, CVJ segmentation/fusion anomalies, small posterior fossa

MR Findings
- T1WI
  - Pointed (not rounded) tonsils ≥ 5 mm below foramen magnum
  - "Tight foramen magnum" with small/absent cisterns
  - +/- Elongation of IVth ventricle, hindbrain anomalies
- T2WI
  - Oblique tonsillar folia (like "sergeant's stripes")
  - +/- Short clivus ⇒ "apparent" descent of 4th ventricle, medulla
  - +/- Syringohydromyelia (14-75%)

Other Modality Findings
- Cine phase contrast (PC) MR: Disorganized CSF pulsation, ↑ brainstem/cerebellar tonsil motion ⇒ ↑ peak systolic velocity, ↓ flow through foramen magnum

---

DDx: Chiari I Malformation

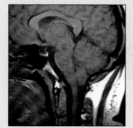
Normal Low Tonsils

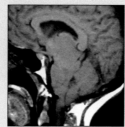
CSF Hypotension

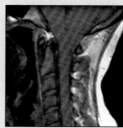
LP Overshunting

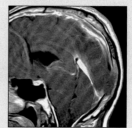
Downward Herniation

CHIARI I MALFORMATION

Key Facts

Terminology
- Synonyms: CM 1, Arnold-Chiari 1 malformation, AC1

Imaging Findings
- Best diagnostic clue: Pointed cerebellar tonsils ≥ 5 mm below foramen magnum +/- syringohydromyelia (14-75%)
- "Tight foramen magnum" with small/absent cisterns
- +/- Elongation of IVth ventricle, hindbrain anomalies
- Oblique tonsillar folia (like "sergeant's stripes")

Top Differential Diagnoses
- Normal tonsillar displacement below foramen magnum
- Acquired tonsillar herniation ("acquired Chiari 1")

Pathology
- Diagnostic criteria: Herniation of at least one cerebellar tonsil > 5 mm or herniation of both tonsils 3 mm to 5 mm below a line connecting the basion with opisthion

Clinical Issues
- Clinical profile: Clinical CM1 syndrome: Headache, pseudotumor-like episodes, Meniere disease-like syndrome, lower cranial nerve and spinal cord signs
- Increasing ectopia + time ⇒ ↑ likelihood symptoms

Diagnostic Checklist
- Unless tonsils > 5 mm and/or pointed, probably not clinically significant Chiari I malformation
- Tonsillar herniation > 12 mm nearly always symptomatic

Imaging Recommendations
- Best imaging tool: MR imaging
- Protocol advice: Multiplanar T1WI, T2WI of spinal axis and posterior fossa, PC MRI CSF flow study

DIFFERENTIAL DIAGNOSIS

Normal tonsillar displacement below foramen magnum
- Tonsils may normally lie below foramen magnum
- Unless tonsils > 5 mm and/or pointed, probably not clinically significant Chiari I malformation

Acquired tonsillar herniation ("acquired Chiari 1")
- Acquired basilar invagination (osteogenesis imperfecta, Paget disease, craniosynostosis, rickets, achondroplasia, acromegaly) ⇒ small posterior fossa
- "Pull from below" (LP shunt, CSF leak) 2° to intracranial hypotension
  - "Sagging" brainstem, tonsillar herniation, smooth dural enhancement, dilated epidural plexus, retrospinal C1/2 fluid collection, spinal hygroma
- "Push from above"
  - Chronic VP shunt; thick skull, premature sutural fusion, arachnoidal adhesions
  - ↑ ICP, intracranial mass

PATHOLOGY

General Features
- General path comments
  - Underdeveloped occipital enchondrium ⇒ small posterior fossa vault, downward hindbrain herniation
  - Foramen magnum obstruction ⇒ decreased communication between cranial, spinal CSF compartments
- Genetics
  - Autosomal dominant inheritance with reduced penetrance, or autosomal recessive inheritance
  - Syndromic/familial associations (velocardiofacial/microdeletion chromosome 22, Williams syndrome, craniosynostosis, achondroplasia, Hajdu-Cheney syndrome, and Klippel-Feil syndrome)
- Etiology
  - Hydrodynamic theory
    - Systolic piston-like descent of impacted tonsils/medulla ⇒ plugs CSF pathway at foramen magnum
    - During diastole, rapid recoil of brain stem/tonsils disimpacts foramen magnum, permits normal CSF diastolic pulsation
  - Posterior fossa underdevelopment theory
    - Underdevelopment of occipital somites of para-axial mesoderm produce diminutive posterior fossa ⇒ 2° tonsillar herniation
- Epidemiology: Incidence 0.01-0.6% all age groups, 0.9% pediatric patient groups
- Associated abnormalities
  - 4th occipital sclerotome syndromes (50%): Short clivus, craniovertebral segmentation/fusion anomalies
  - Osseous skull base/skeletal anomalies (25-50%)
    - Scoliosis +/- kyphosis (42%); left thoracic curve
    - Retroflexed odontoid process (26%)
    - Platybasia, basilar invagination (25-50%)
    - Klippel-Feil syndrome (5-10%)
    - Incomplete C1 ring ossification (5%)
    - Atlantooccipital assimilation (1-5%)
  - Syringomyelia (30-60%) ⇒ 60-90% in symptomatic CM1 patients
    - Most common C4-6; holocord hydrosyringomyelia, cervical/upper-thoracic syrinx, syringobulbia uncommon
  - Hydrocephalus (11%)

Gross Pathologic & Surgical Features
- Herniated, sclerotic tonsils grooved by opisthion
- Arachnoidal scarring and adhesions at foramen magnum

CHIARI I MALFORMATION

Microscopic Features
- Tonsillar softening or sclerosis with Purkinje/granular cell loss

Staging, Grading or Classification Criteria
- Diagnostic criteria: Herniation of at least one cerebellar tonsil > 5 mm or herniation of both tonsils 3 mm to 5 mm below a line connecting the basion with opisthion
  - Herniation of both tonsils 3-5 mm below foramen magnum + syrinx, cervicomedullary kinking, IVth ventricular elongation, or pointed tonsils ⇒ congenital CM 1
  - Tonsil herniation ≤ 5 mm does not exclude CM 1

CLINICAL ISSUES

Presentation
- Most common signs/symptoms
  - ≤ 50% asymptomatic (especially if ≤ 5 mm inferior displacement)
  - Symptomatic patients present with constellation of findings
    - Sudden death (rare)
    - Suboccipital headache, cranial nerve palsy, ocular disturbances, otoneurologic dysfunction, cord motor or sensory abnormalities, gait disturbance, neuropathic joint
    - Tonsillar herniation > 12 mm nearly always symptomatic; ≈ 30% with tonsils 5-10 mm below foramen magnum asymptomatic
    - CM 1 patients with syrinx nearly always present with symptoms referable to syrinx; if the syrinx extends into medulla, bulbar symptoms predominate
  - Trauma is a common precipitating event for symptom onset (24%)
- Clinical profile: Clinical CM1 syndrome: Headache, pseudotumor-like episodes, Meniere disease-like syndrome, lower cranial nerve and spinal cord signs

Demographics
- Age: 10 months → 65 years; syrinx, congenital CVJ anomalies hasten presentation
- Gender: F > M (3:2)

Natural History & Prognosis
- Natural history not clearly understood
  - Many patients asymptomatic for prolonged periods
  - Increasing ectopia + time ⇒ ↑ likelihood symptoms
- Children respond better to treatment than adults
- Degree of tonsillar herniation correlates with clinical severity

Treatment
- Treating asymptomatic patients is controversial
  - "Radiographic" CM 1 (no syrinx), no corresponding clinical signs/symptoms → conservative management
  - Asymptomatic Chiari I + syrinx → consider decompression

- Symptomatic patients: PF decompression/ resection of posterior arch C1, +/- duraplasty, cerebellar tonsil resection
  - > 90% ↓ brainstem signs
  - > 80% ↓ hydrosyringomyelia
  - +/- Scoliosis arrest
- Direct shunting of symptomatic syrinx obsolete; goal to restore normal CSF flow at foramen magnum

DIAGNOSTIC CHECKLIST

Consider
- Unless tonsils > 5 mm and/or pointed, probably not clinically significant Chiari I malformation

Image Interpretation Pearls
- Tonsillar herniation > 12 mm nearly always symptomatic

SELECTED REFERENCES

1. Milhorat TH et al: Tailored operative technique for Chiari type I malformation using intraoperative color Doppler ultrasonography. Neurosurgery. 53(4):899-905; discussion 905-6, 2003
2. Tubbs RS et al: Surgical experience in 130 pediatric patients with Chiari I malformations. J Neurosurg. 99(2):291-6, 2003
3. Eule JM et al: Chiari I malformation associated with syringomyelia and scoliosis: a twenty-year review of surgical and nonsurgical treatment in a pediatric population. Spine. 27(13):1451-5, 2002
4. Genitori L et al: Chiari type I anomalies in children and adolescents: minimally invasive management in a series of 53 cases. Childs Nerv Syst. 16(10-11):707-18, 2000
5. Milhorat TH et al: Chiari I malformation redefined: clinical and radiographic findings for 364 symptomatic patients. Neurosurgery. 44(5):1005-17, 1999
6. Nishikawa M et al: Pathogenesis of Chiari malformations: A morphometric study of the posterior cranial fossa. J Neurosurg 86: 40-7, 1997
7. Menezes AH: Primary craniovertebral anomalies and the hindbrain herniation syndrome (Chiari 1): Data base analysis. Pediatric Neurosurg 23: 260-69, 1995
8. Caldemeyer KS et al: Chiari I malformation: association with hypophosphatemic rickets and MR imaging appearance. Radiology. 195(3):733-8, 1995
9. Stovner LJ et al: Posterior cranial fossa dimensions in the Chiari I malformation: relation to pathogenesis and clinical presentation. Neuroradiology. 35(2):113-8, 1993
10. Elster AD et al: Chiari I malformations: clinical and radiologic reappraisal. Radiology. 183(2):347-53, 1992
11. Stovner LJ et al: Syringomyelia in Chiari malformation: relation to extent of cerebellar tissue herniation. Neurosurgery. 31(5):913-7; discussion 917, 1992
12. Pillay PK et al: Symptomatic Chiari malformation in adults: a new classification based on magnetic resonance imaging with clinical and prognostic significance. Neurosurgery. 28(5):639-45, 1991
13. Barkovich AJ et al: Significance of cerebellar tonsillar position on MR. AJNR Am J Neuroradiol. 7(5):795-9, 1986

IMAGE GALLERY

Typical

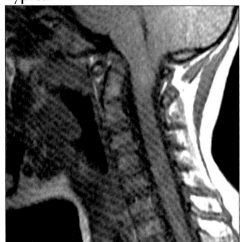 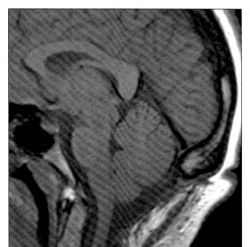

(Left) Sagittal T1WI MR shows clival foreshortening and flattening, retroflexed odontoid process, and mild tonsillar ectopia to the C2 level *(Courtesy G. Hedlund, DO)*. *(Right)* Sagittal T1WI MR shows expected post-operative findings following successful occipital craniectomy, duraplasty, and resection of posterior C1 ring.

Variant

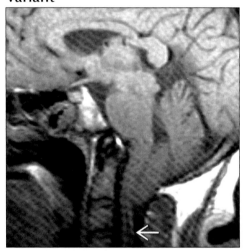 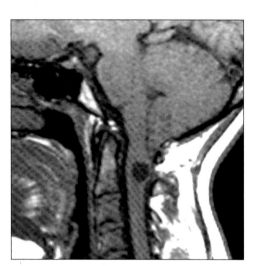

(Left) Sagittal T1WI MR *(congenital CM 1)* reveals large ectopic tonsils obliterating basilar CSF spaces. Associated findings include short, flattened clivus and cervical syringomyelia *(arrow)*. *(Right)* Sagittal T1WI MR depicts moderate tonsillar ectopia associated with variant focal cystic syringomyelia.

Variant

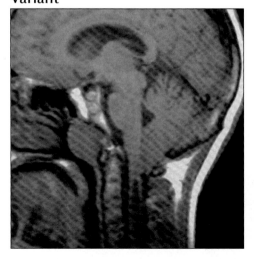 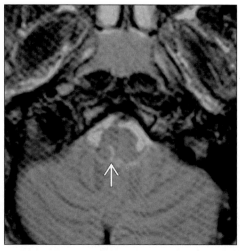

(Left) Sagittal T1WI MR shows "peg-like" tonsils descending inferiorly to posterior C1 level and a large cervical syringomyelia. *(Right)* Axial T2WI MR displays medullary extension *(arrow)* of cervical syringomyelia *(syringobulbia)* in a Chiari 1 patient with clinical brainstem symptoms.

LATERAL MENINGOCELE

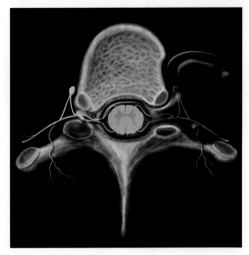

Axial graphic shows a large left lateral thoracic meningocele producing pedicular erosion, transverse process remodelling, and widening of the neural foramen.

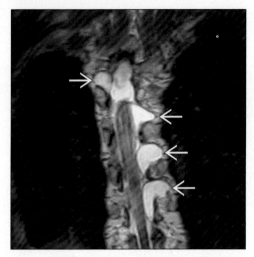

Coronal T2WI MR (Marfan syndrome) shows multiple lateral thoracic meningoceles (arrows).

TERMINOLOGY

Definitions
- Meningeal dysplasia ⇒ CSF filled dural/arachnoidal sac protrudes laterally through neural foramen

IMAGING FINDINGS

General Features
- Best diagnostic clue: CSF signal/density meningeal protrusion through neural foramen into adjacent intercostal/extrapleural space
- Location
  ○ Thoracic > lumbar spine
  ○ R > L; 10% bilateral
    ▪ Bilateral meningoceles nearly always associated with NF1, but may be seen in Marfan syndrome
- Size: Typical size 2-3 cm; range tiny ⇒ huge
- Morphology
  ○ CSF signal/density "cyst" adjacent to spine
    ▪ Contiguous with neural foramen
    ▪ +/- Sharply angled scoliosis at meningocele level

Radiographic Findings
- Radiography
  ○ Pedicular erosion +/- neural foraminal enlargement

- Often accompanied by scalloping of posterior vertebral bodies (dural ectasia)
- +/- Sharply angled kyphosis/scoliosis (meningocele is near apex of deformity on convex side)
- Myelography
  ○ Intrathecal contrast fills cyst from dural sac through an enlarged neural foramen
    ▪ Confirms contiguity with thecal sac
    ▪ Delayed imaging may be required
    ▪ Consider placing patient with meningocele(s) dependently to improve contrast filling

CT Findings
- CECT
  ○ CSF density mass extends through enlarged neural foramen
  ○ No enhancement; useful to distinguish from nerve sheath tumor, nerve inflammation (CIDP)
- CTA: +/- Aortic aneurysm, dissection in context of systemic connective tissue disorder
- Bone CT
  ○ Wide neural foramen; +/- pedicular thinning, posterior vertebral scalloping (usually)
  ○ Reformatted images may show focal scoliosis (coronal plane) and dural ectasia (sagittal plane)

MR Findings
- T1WI

DDx: Lateral Meningocele

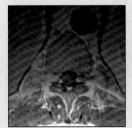

Neurofibroma

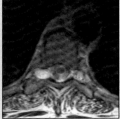

Radicular Cyst

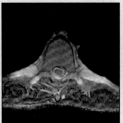

CIDP

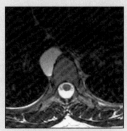

Foregut Dup. Cyst

LATERAL MENINGOCELE

Key Facts

Imaging Findings
- Best diagnostic clue: CSF signal/density meningeal protrusion through neural foramen into adjacent intercostal/extrapleural space
- Thoracic > lumbar spine
- R > L; 10% bilateral
- Wide neural foramen; +/- pedicular thinning, posterior vertebral scalloping (usually)
- T1 C+: No enhancement; distinguishes from nerve sheath tumor or inflammation (CIDP)

Top Differential Diagnoses
- Nerve sheath tumor
- Radicular (meningeal) cyst
- Chronic inflammatory demyelinating polyneuropathy

- Foregut duplication cyst

Pathology
- Strong association with neurofibromatosis type 1 (NF1) - 85%

Clinical Issues
- Age: Most commonly present during 4th ⇒ 5th decades of life
- Gender: M = F
- Most remain asymptomatic unless very large or scoliosis causes symptoms

Diagnostic Checklist
- Lateral meningocele prompts search for history/stigmata of NF1 or connective tissue disorder

---

- ○ CSF signal intensity (hypointense) mass in contiguity with thecal sac
- ○ Pedicular thinning, neural foraminal widening +/- posterior vertebral scalloping
- T2WI: CSF signal intensity (hyperintense) mass in contiguity with thecal sac; rarely see neural elements within meningocele
- T1 C+: No enhancement; distinguishes from nerve sheath tumor or inflammation (CIDP)

Ultrasonographic Findings
- Real Time
  - ○ Posterior mediastinal or lumbar hypoechoic paraspinal cystic mass contiguous with an expanded spinal canal
    - ■ Displaces and compresses adjacent spinal cord
  - ○ Ultrasound is primary diagnostic tool in utero, screening newborn infants
- Pulsed Doppler: No vascular flow pattern
- Color Doppler: Avascular hypoechoic mass

Imaging Recommendations
- Best imaging tool: MR imaging
- Protocol advice
  - ○ Consider sonography for newborn screening; follow-up with MRI to clarify positive ultrasound study
  - ○ MR imaging for diagnosis, pre-operative planning
  - ○ Bone CT to evaluate pedicles, vertebral bodies (particularly if surgery is contemplated)

DIFFERENTIAL DIAGNOSIS

Nerve sheath tumor
- Less hyperintense than CSF on T2WI, higher signal intensity than CSF on T1WI
- Contrast enhancement implies tumor
  - ○ Caveats: Some schwannomas may appear cystic, and some neurofibromas minimally enhance

Radicular (meningeal) cyst
- CSF signal intensity/density cyst within neural foramen

- ○ Cyst separate from dural sac, unlike meningocele
- Nerve root definable as discrete structure within or adjacent to cyst

Chronic inflammatory demyelinating polyneuropathy
- Solid fusiform nerve root enlargement, enhancement
- Clinical and laboratory findings characteristic

Foregut duplication cyst
- Bronchogenic most common; may contain GI mucosa
  - ○ Seldom contiguous with neural foramen
- Proximity to spinal canal +/- vertebral anomalies = neurenteric cyst

PATHOLOGY

General Features
- General path comments: Dural sac diverticulum, pedicular erosion, neural foraminal widening, and posterior vertebral scalloping
- Genetics
  - ○ Strong association with neurofibromatosis type 1 (NF1) - 85%
    - ■ Most common posterior mediastinal mass
  - ○ Less common with Ehlers-Danlos, Marfan syndromes
- Etiology
  - ○ Meningocele 2° to primary meningeal dysplasia
    - ■ Meningeal weakness permits dural sac to focally stretch in response to repetitive CSF pulsation ⇒ enlarges neural foramina
    - ■ Secondary osseous remodeling permits further herniation
  - ○ Posterior vertebral scalloping with dural dysplasia ⇒ same etiology
- Epidemiology: Uncommon in NF1 and inherited connective tissue disorders, but substantially more common than occurence as an isolated lesion
- Associated abnormalities
  - ○ Occasionally isolated finding

LATERAL MENINGOCELE

- ○ +/- Co-existent lumbar and thoracic lateral meningoceles
- ○ +/- Findings specific to hereditary disorder
  - ▪ NF1: Dural ectasia, nerve sheath tumors, CNS neoplasms, pheochromocytomas, interstitial pulmonary fibrosis, skin and subcutaneous neurofibromas
  - ▪ Marfan syndrome: Dural ectasia, vascular dissection/aneurysm, lens dislocation, joint laxity

Gross Pathologic & Surgical Features

- Scalloping of pedicles, laminae, and vertebral bodies adjacent to meningocele
- Enlarged central spinal canal, neural foramina
- Cord position variable; usually displaced away from meningocele
- Scoliosis convex toward meningocele

Microscopic Features

- Dura/arachnoid lined outpouching of thecal sac

CLINICAL ISSUES

Presentation

- Most common signs/symptoms
  - ○ Asymptomatic (most common)
  - ○ Nonspecific motor or sensory symptoms referable to cord/nerve root compression
  - ○ Other signs/symptoms
    - ▪ Respiratory embarrassment (neonates); very large meningocele fills thoracic cavity
- Clinical profile
  - ○ Asymptomatic patient (incidental discovery)
  - ○ +/- Scoliosis evaluation
  - ○ NF1: Cutaneous café-au-lait spots,cutaneous and subcutaneous neurofibromas, +/- kyphoscoliosis
  - ○ Connective tissue disorder: Frequently tall, joint hypermobility, lens dislocation, +/- normal intelligence, +/- scoliosis

Demographics

- Age: Most commonly present during 4th ⇒ 5th decades of life
- Gender: M = F

Natural History & Prognosis

- Most remain asymptomatic unless very large or scoliosis causes symptoms
- Most static in size; occasionally grow slowly
- May disappear after hydrocephalus shunting
- Excellent prognosis after surgical resection

Treatment

- Options, risks, complications
  - ○ Surgical ligation of dural sac neck, resection of meningocele
  - ○ Correction/stabilization of scoliosis

DIAGNOSTIC CHECKLIST

Consider

- Lateral meningocele prompts search for history/stigmata of NF1 or connective tissue disorder

Image Interpretation Pearls

- MR shows nonenhancing CSF signal intensity/density mass extending through an enlarged neural foramen

SELECTED REFERENCES

1. Kubota M et al: Lateral thoracic meningocele presenting as a retromediastinal mass. Br J Neurosurg. 16(6):607-8, 2002
2. Baysefer A et al: Lateral intrathoracic meningocele associated with a spinal intradural arachnoid cyst. Pediatr Neurosurg. 35(2):107-10, 2001
3. Zibis AH et al: Unusual causes of spinal foraminal widening. Eur Radiol. 10(1):144-8, 2000
4. Unsinn KM et al: US of the spinal cord in newborns: spectrum of normal findings, variants, congenital anomalies, and acquired diseases. Radiographics. 20(4):923-38, 2000
5. Barkovich A: Pediatric neuroimaging. 3rd ed. Philadelphia, Lippincott-Raven. 398, 667, 2000
6. Chen SS et al: Multiple bilateral thoracic meningoceles without neurofibromatosis: a case report. Zhonghua Yi Xue Za Zhi (Taipei). 61(12):736-40, 1998
7. Gripp KW et al: Lateral meningocele syndrome: three new patients and review of the literature. Am J Med Genet. 70(3):229-39, 1997
8. Strollo DC et al: Primary mediastinal tumors: part II. Tumors of the middle and posterior mediastinum. Chest. 112(5):1344-57, 1997
9. Ball W: Pediatric Neuroradiology. Philadelphia, Lippincott-Raven. 727, 1997
10. Gibbens DT et al: Chest case of the day. Lateral thoracic meningocele in a patient with neurofibromatosis. AJR Am J Roentgenol. 156(6):1299-300, 1991
11. Nakasu Y et al: Thoracic meningocele in neurofibromatosis: CT and MR findings. J Comput Assist Tomogr. 15(6):1062-4, 1991
12. Chee CP: Lateral thoracic meningocele associated with neurofibromatosis: total excision by posterolateral extradural approach. A case report. Spine. 14(1):129-31, 1989
13. Richaud J: Spinal meningeal malformations in children (without meningoceles or meningomyeloceles). Childs Nerv Syst. 4(2):79-87, 1988
14. Maiuri F et al: Lateral thoracic meningocele. Surg Neurol. 26(4):409-12, 1986
15. Weinreb JC et al: CT metrizamide myelography in multiple bilateral intrathoracic meningoceles. J Comput Assist Tomogr. 8(2):324-6, 1984
16. Erkulvrawatr S et al: Intrathoracic meningoceles and neurofibromatosis. Arch Neurol. 36(9):557-9, 1979
17. Booth AE: Lateral thoracic meningocele. J Neurol Neurosurg Psychiatry. 32(2):111-5, 1969
18. Bunner R: Lateral intrathoracic meningocele. Acta Radiol. 51(1):1-9, 1959

IMAGE GALLERY

Typical

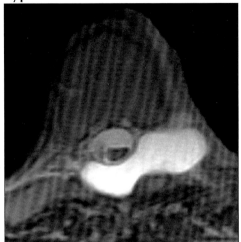
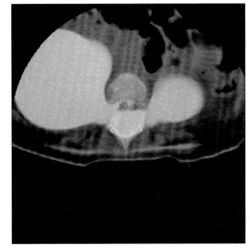

(Left) Axial T2WI MR *(Marfan syndrome)* demonstrates a large left lateral thoracic meningocele that displaces the thecal sac anteriorly. *(Right)* Axial NECT following myelography *(Marfan syndrome)* shows large lateral lumbar meningoceles bilaterally *(Courtesy R. Boyer, MD).*

Variant

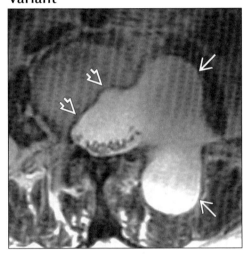
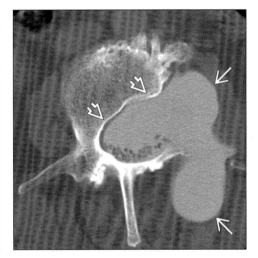

(Left) Axial T2WI MR *(neurofibromatosis type 1)* shows a large left lateral lumbar meningocele *(arrows)* in conjunction with extensive dural dysplasia *(open arrows)* and marked left pedicular erosion. *(Right)* Axial NECT following myelography *(NF1)* shows a large left lateral lumbar meningocele *(arrows)* and extensive dural dysplasia *(open arrows)* with marked left pedicular erosion.

Variant

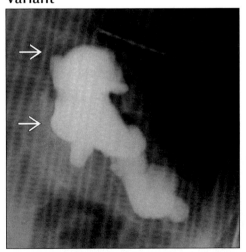
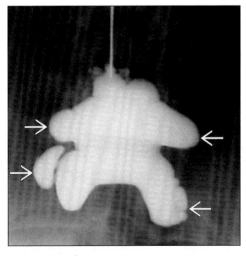

(Left) Lateral myelography *(neurofibromatosis type 1)* shows marked dural dysplasia with posterior vertebral scalloping *(arrows)* and multiple lumbar meningoceles. *(Right)* Anteroposterior myelography *(neurofibromatosis type 1)* demonstrates multiple bilateral lumbar meningoceles *(arrows).*

DORSAL SPINAL MENINGOCELE

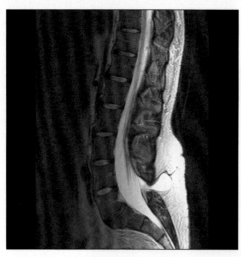

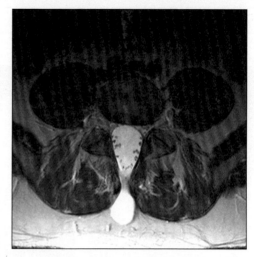

Sagittal T2WI MR shows a skin covered simple lumbar dorsal meningocele extending through a dorsal dysraphic defect into subcutaneous fat.

Axial T2WI MR demonstrates a simple dorsal meningocele protruding through a single-level posterior dysraphic defect into subcutaneous fat.

TERMINOLOGY

Abbreviations and Synonyms
- Synonyms: Simple meningocele, simple spinal meningocele, posterior meningocele

Definitions
- Dorsal herniation of dura, arachnoid, and CSF into spinal subcutaneous tissue

IMAGING FINDINGS

General Features
- Best diagnostic clue: Skin covered dorsal dural sac protruding thorough posterior osseous defect
- Location: Anywhere along dorsal spinal canal; lumbosacral junction, sacrum > > cervical, thoracic
- Size: Small and localized ⇒ large, encompassing multiple spinal levels
- Morphology
  - Sessile or pedunculated CSF intensity/density sac with spinal dysraphism
  - May (complex) or may not (simple) contain neural tissue

Radiographic Findings
- Radiography
  - Dorsal dysraphism; defect usually confined to one or two vertebrae
  - Widening of spinal canal, increased interpedicular distance
- Myelography
  - Dorsal dysraphism, widening of spinal canal, increased interpedicular distance
  - Dural sac herniates through dysraphic posterior elements
    - Dural sac communicates with subarachnoid space; may change size with position, Valsalva maneuver
    - +/- Neural elements, filum terminale within defect
  - Myelography mostly replaced by MRI
    - Primary utility is for patients with MRI contraindications and to answer discrepancies between MRI and clinical findings

CT Findings
- NECT
  - Hypodense CSF dural sac
  - Overlying skin intact; may be ulcerated
- Bone CT
  - Dysraphism +/- spinal canal widening, increased interpedicular distance
    - Mild cases may show only absent spinous process or localized spina bifida
    - More severe cases show multisegmental spina bifida, spinal canal enlargement

DDx: Dorsal Meningocele

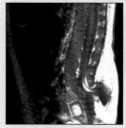
Lipomyelomeningocele

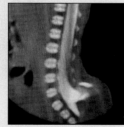
Lipomyelomeningocele

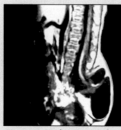
Term. Myelocystocele

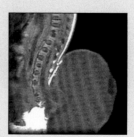
Myelomeningocele

DORSAL SPINAL MENINGOCELE

Key Facts

Terminology
- Synonyms: Simple meningocele, simple spinal meningocele, posterior meningocele

Imaging Findings
- Best diagnostic clue: Skin covered dorsal dural sac protruding thorough posterior osseous defect
- Best imaging tool: MR imaging best shows dural sac characteristics, associated vertebral or spinal cord anomalies

Top Differential Diagnoses
- Lipomyelomeningocele
- Terminal myelocystocele
- Myelomeningocele

Pathology
- Meningocele is always skin covered; skin may be dysplastic or ulcerated

Clinical Issues
- Palpable skin-covered mass or incidental discovery during imaging for other indications

Diagnostic Checklist
- Ultrasound for infants to determine cord level, presence or absence of neural elements in meningocele
- MR is best modality to definitively characterize meningocele, evaluate for other spinal abnormalities
- Imaging goals are lesion detection, determination of simple or complex morphology, and exclusion of other spinal anomalies

MR Findings
- T1WI
  - Skin-covered hypointense dural sac
  - Conus medullaris low or normal position
  - Occasional herniation of filum or nerve roots into defect
- T2WI
  - Hyperintense dural sac
  - Low or normal conus medullaris position
  - +/- Filum terminale or nerve roots within defect

Ultrasonographic Findings
- Real Time
  - Hypoechoic CSF-filled sac protrudes through posterior defect +/- entrapped nervous tissue
  - Demonstrates conus termination level and periodic motion
  - Primary utility for in utero or neonatal screening
    - Obstetrical ultrasound may detect large meningocele in utero → altered delivery planning
    - Less useful in older children, adults due to spinal column ossification → posterior acoustic shadowing

Imaging Recommendations
- Best imaging tool: MR imaging best shows dural sac characteristics, associated vertebral or spinal cord anomalies
- Protocol advice
  - Sagittal and axial T1WI and T2WI
    - Sagittal images useful to evaluate cord
    - Axial T1WI most helpful to evaluate size of dysraphic defect, exclude lipoma
    - Axial T2WI best for detecting nervous tissue within sac

DIFFERENTIAL DIAGNOSIS

Lipomyelomeningocele
- Distinguish by presence of neural tissue and fat within defect in addition to cyst

Terminal myelocystocele
- Hydromyelic, low-lying cord protrudes through meningocele

Myelomeningocele
- Open spinal dysraphism; clinical appearance is diagnostic

PATHOLOGY

General Features
- General path comments
  - Meningocele is always skin covered; skin may be dysplastic or ulcerated
  - Cervical lesions considered within cervical myelocystocele spectrum
  - Classically, simple meningoceles considered an isolated abnormality with normal conus termination level
  - However; some authors report low conus termination and other spinal anomalies with meningocele and question if meningocele is ever truly an isolated lesion
- Etiology: Unknown; no universally accepted unifying theory explains pathogenesis
- Epidemiology: 1/10,000 live births
- Associated abnormalities
  - +/- Hydromyelia, tethered cord, diastematomyelia
  - Chiari II malformation; much less common than with myelomeningocele

Gross Pathologic & Surgical Features
- Nearly always contain aberrant nerve roots, ganglion cells, and/or glial nodules at surgery, gross pathology
- Herniated meningocele sac contains both dura and arachnoid
- Overlying tissue intact unless secondary skin ulceration

DORSAL SPINAL MENINGOCELE

Microscopic Features
- Meningocele lined by arachnoid and thin-walled blood vessels; arachnoidal adhesions may obstruct neck of sac
- Overlying skin shows atrophic epidermis, lacks rete pegs and normal skin appendages

CLINICAL ISSUES

Presentation
- Most common signs/symptoms
  - Palpable skin-covered mass or incidental discovery during imaging for other indications
  - Other signs/symptoms
    - Back pain
    - Meningitis (ruptured or leaking meningocele)
    - Headache, other signs/symptoms of alternating high and low intracranial pressure
- Clinical profile
  - Patients are usually neurologically normal, and present for imaging of palpable back mass
  - Cervical, thoracic meningoceles more likely to be symptomatic than lumbar meningocele

Demographics
- Age: In utero ⇒ adult life
- Gender: M = F

Natural History & Prognosis
- Variable; depends on cyst size and contents, status of overlying skin, presence or absence of meningitis
- Skin covering permits more "elective" surgical correction, but most newborns require an operation before release from nursery to home

Treatment
- Asymptomatic patients may warrant conservative observation
- Symptomatic patients require surgical resection, repair of dural defect

DIAGNOSTIC CHECKLIST

Consider
- Ultrasound for infants to determine cord level, presence or absence of neural elements in meningocele
- MR is best modality to definitively characterize meningocele, evaluate for other spinal abnormalities

Image Interpretation Pearls
- Imaging goals are lesion detection, determination of simple or complex morphology, and exclusion of other spinal anomalies
  - Critical to determine whether neural elements reside within sac prior to surgery
- Meningocele may be most obvious abnormality that masks other less obvious but clinically more important lesions

SELECTED REFERENCES

1. Barazi SA et al: High and low pressure states associated with posterior sacral meningocele. Br J Neurosurg. 17(2):184-7, 2003
2. Bekavac I et al: Meningocele-induced positional syncope and retinal hemorrhage. AJNR Am J Neuroradiol. 24(5):838-9, 2003
3. Akay KM et al: The initial treatment of meningocele and myelomeningocele lesions in adulthood: experiences with seven patients. Neurosurg Rev. 26(3):162-7, 2003
4. Graham D et al: Greenfield's Neuropathology. 7th ed. London, Arnold. 380, 2002
5. Ersahin Y et al: Is meningocele really an isolated lesion? Childs Nerv Syst. 17(8):487-90, 2001
6. Tortori-Donati P et al: Spinal dysraphism: a review of neuroradiological features with embryological correlations and proposal for a new classification. Neuroradiology. 42(7):471-91, 2000
7. Unsinn KM et al: US of the spinal cord in newborns: spectrum of normal findings, variants, congenital anomalies, and acquired diseases. Radiographics. 20(4):923-38, 2000
8. Barkovich A: Pediatric neuroimaging. Philadelphia: Lippincott-Raven, 3rd ed, 666-667, 2000
9. Sattar TS et al: Pre-natal diagnosis of occult spinal dysraphism by ultrasonography and post-natal evaluation by MR scanning. Eur J Pediatr Surg. 8 Suppl 1:31-3, 1998
10. Ball W: Pediatric Neuroradiology. Philadelphia, Lippincott-Raven, 726-727, 1997
11. Tindall et al: The Practice of Neurosurgery. Baltimore, Williams and Wilkins, 2758-2760, 1996
12. Steinbok P et al: Cervical meningoceles and myelocystoceles: a unifying hypothesis. Pediatr Neurosurg. 23(6):317-22, 1995
13. DeLaPaz RL: Congenital anomalies of the lumbosacral spine. Neuroimaging Clinics of North America 3(3):429-31, 1993
14. Wolf YG et al: Thoraco-abdominal enteric duplication with meningocele, skeletal anomalies and dextrocardia. Eur J Pediatr. 149(11):786-8, 1990
15. Ebisu T et al: Neurenteric cysts with meningomyelocele or meningocele. Split notochord syndrome. Childs Nerv Syst. 6(8):465-7, 1990
16. Erkulvrawatr S et al: Intrathoracic meningoceles and neurofibromatosis. Arch Neurol. 36(9):557-9, 1979

IMAGE GALLERY

Typical

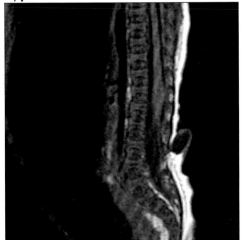 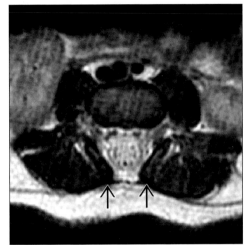

(Left) Sagittal T1WI MR shows a small lumbar dorsal meningocele, with borderline low-lying conus at L2/3 (Courtesy A. Illner, MD). *(Right)* Axial T2WI MR in a dorsal meningocele patient reveals wide (arrows) spinal dysraphism (Courtesy A. Illner, MD).

Variant

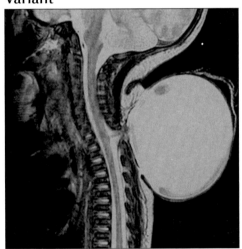 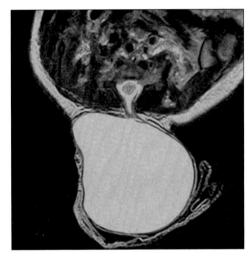

(Left) Sagittal T2WI MR depicts a large cervicothoracic dorsal meningocele extending into the subcutaneous tissues through a thin dysraphic isthmus (Courtesy S. Blaser, MD). *(Right)* Axial T2WI MR shows a large dorsal meningocele passing through a narrow posterior dysraphism (Courtesy S. Blaser, MD).

Variant

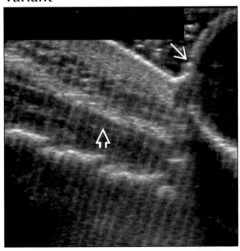 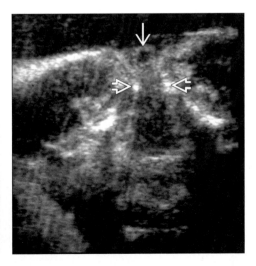

(Left) Sagittal ultrasound real time depicts a low-lying cord (open arrow) and the rostral portion (arrow) of a large dorsal meningocele (Courtesy R. Boyer, MD). *(Right)* Transverse ultrasound shows a small dorsal meningocele sac (arrow) extending through a wide posterior osseous defect (open arrows) (Courtesy R. Boyer, MD).

NEUROFIBROMATOSIS TYPE 1

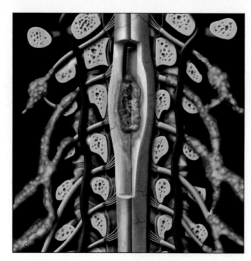

Coronal graphic shows bilateral spinal nerve root and brachial plexus neurofibromas. Intramedullary cervical glial tumor produces focal cord expansion, cystic central canal dilatation.

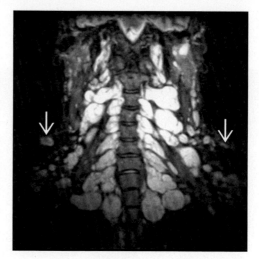

Coronal STIR MR demonstrates characteristic extensive bilateral hyperintense nerve root and brachial plexus neurofibromas. Small cutaneous neurofibromas (arrows) are also visible.

TERMINOLOGY

Abbreviations and Synonyms

- Synonyms: NF1, von Recklinghausen disease, peripheral neurofibromatosis
- Abbreviations: Nerve root neurofibroma (NF), plexiform neurofibroma (PNF), malignant peripheral nerve sheath tumor (MPNST)

Definitions

- Autosomal dominant mesodermal dysplasia characterized by plexiform and nerve root neurofibromas, spinal deformity, neoplastic and non-neoplastic brain lesions, and cutaneous stigmata

IMAGING FINDINGS

General Features

- Best diagnostic clue: Kyphoscoliosis +/- multiple nerve root tumors, plexiform neurofibroma, dural ectasia/lateral meningocele
- Location: Entire craniospinal axis
- Size: Tumors range tiny → very large
- Morphology
  - Kyphosis/kyphoscoliosis often severe and bizarre
  - Neurogenic tumors localized to nerve roots as well as within plexiform nerve masses, cutaneous lesions

Radiographic Findings

- Radiography: Kyphosis/scoliosis, scalloped vertebra, hypoplastic pedicles and posterior elements, ribbon ribs

CT Findings

- NECT
  - Hypodense fusiform or focal nerve root enlargement +/- heterogeneous spinal cord expansion (glial tumor)
  - Dural ectasia +/- CSF density lateral meningocele(s)
- CECT: Variable mild/moderate tumor enhancement
- Bone CT
  - Vertebral findings similar to radiography; canal, foraminal widening 2° dural ectasia +/- spinal cord tumor

MR Findings

- T1WI: NF, intramedullary glial cord tumors hypo- → isointense to normal spinal cord, nerve roots, muscle
- T2WI
  - NF, cord tumors hyperintense to normal spinal cord, nerve roots
    - NF "target sign" (hyperintense rim, low/intermediate signal intensity center) suggests neurogenic tumor; PNF > NF > MPNST
- STIR: NF, cord tumors hyperintense to normal nerve root, cord, muscle

DDx: Neurofibromatosis Type 1

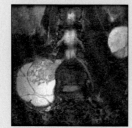

NF Type 2

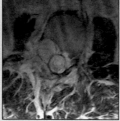

Solitary Schwannoma

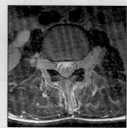

Inflam. Polyneuropathy

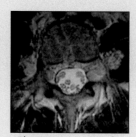

Charcot-Marie-Tooth

NEUROFIBROMATOSIS TYPE 1

Key Facts

Terminology
- Synonyms: NF1, von Recklinghausen disease, peripheral neurofibromatosis

Imaging Findings
- Best diagnostic clue: Kyphoscoliosis +/- multiple nerve root tumors, plexiform neurofibroma, dural ectasia/lateral meningocele

Top Differential Diagnoses
- Neurofibromatosis type 2 (NF2, central neurofibromatosis)
- Chronic inflammatory demyelinating polyneuropathy (CIDP)
- Congenital hypertrophic polyradiculoneuropathies

Pathology
- Plexiform neurofibroma is the hallmark of NF1

Clinical Issues
- Skeletal deformity common (25-40%)
- Palpable spinal or cutaneous mass
- Pigmentation anomalies (café-au-lait, axillary freckling, Lisch nodules) ≥ 90% NF1 patients

Diagnostic Checklist
- Multiple nerve sheath tumors, ≥ 1 plexiform neurofibroma, bizarre kyphoscoliosis with deformed vertebra → consider NF1
- Absence of visible stigmata does not exclude NF1
- Characteristic PNF imaging appearance best displayed using fat-saturated T2WI or STIR MR imaging

---

- T1 C+: Variable mild to moderate NF, cord tumor enhancement

Nuclear Medicine Findings
- PET: FDG standard uptake value (SUV) MPNST > benign tumors

Imaging Recommendations
- Best imaging tool: MR imaging
- Protocol advice
  - Radiography to quantitate and follow kyphosis, scoliosis
  - Multiplanar enhanced MRI (especially STIR, fat-saturated T2WI and T1 C+ MR) to evaluate cord, nerve pathology
  - Bone CT to optimally define osseous anatomy for surgical planning

DIFFERENTIAL DIAGNOSIS

Neurofibromatosis type 2 (NF2, central neurofibromatosis)
- Multiple intracranial schwannomas and meningiomas, spinal schwannomas and meningiomas
- Spinal deformity uncommon
- Clinical, laboratory, and genetic testing findings distinguish from NF1

Chronic inflammatory demyelinating polyneuropathy (CIDP)
- Repeated episodes of demyelination, remyelination ⇒ "onion skin" spinal, peripheral nerve enlargement
- Mimics PNF on imaging studies
- No cutaneous stigmata of NF1

Congenital hypertrophic polyradiculoneuropathies
- Charcot-Marie-Tooth, Dejerine-Sottas disease
- Nerve root enlargement mimics PNF on imaging studies
- No cutaneous stigmata of NF1

PATHOLOGY

General Features
- General path comments
  - Plexiform neurofibroma is the hallmark of NF1
  - Kyphoscoliosis is most common NF1 osseous abnormality; variable severity mild, nonprogressive → severe curvature
    - Dystrophic scoliosis: Short-segment, sharply angulated, < 6 spinal segments, tendency → severe deformity
    - Nondystrophic scoliosis: Similar to adolescent idiopathic curvature, usually 8-10 spinal segments, right convex
    - Severe cervical kyphosis highly suggestive of NF1
  - Dural ectasia: 1° bone dysplasia, some cases 2° pressure erosion from intraspinal tumors
  - "Ribbon" ribs 2° to bone dysplasia +/- intercostal NF
- Genetics
  - Autosomal dominant; chromosome 17q12, penetrance → 100%
    - NF gene product (neurofibromin) is a tumor suppressor
  - ≈ 50% new mutations (paternal germ line; paternal age (35 years ⇒ 2x ↑ in new mutations)
- Etiology: Postulated that NF1 tumor suppression gene "switched off" → tissue proliferation, tumor development
- Epidemiology: Common (1:4,000)
- Associated abnormalities
  - Brain abnormalities: Macrocephaly, focal areas of signal abnormality (FASI), sphenoid wing dysplasia, glial tumors, intellectual handicap, epilepsy, hydrocephalus, aqueductal stenosis
  - ↑ Risk other neuroendocrine tumors (pheochromocytoma, carcinoid tumor), CML
  - Congenital bowing, pseudoarthrosis of tibia and forearm, massive extremity overgrowth
  - ↑ Fibromuscular dysplasia, intracranial aneurysms, multiple sclerosis

Gross Pathologic & Surgical Features
- Three types of spinal NF recognized in NF1

NEUROFIBROMATOSIS TYPE 1

- ○ Localized NF (90% all NF)
  - Most common NF in both NF1, non-NF1 patients
  - Cutaneous and deep nerves, spinal nerve roots
  - NF1: Larger, multiple, more frequently involve large deep nerves (sciatic nerve, brachial plexus)
  - Malignant transformation rare
- ○ Diffuse NF
  - Infiltrating subcutaneous tumor; rarely affects spinal nerves, majority (90%) unassociated with NF1
- ○ Plexiform NF (pathognomonic for NF1)
  - Diffuse enlargement of major nerve trunks/branches ⇒ bulky rope-like ("bag of worms") nerve expansion with adjacent tissue distortion
  - Commonly large, bilateral, multilevel with predilection for sciatic nerve, brachial plexus
  - ≈ 5% risk malignant degeneration → sarcoma

Microscopic Features
- Neoplastic Schwann cells + perineural fibroblasts grow along nerve fascicles
  - ○ Collagen fibers, mucoid/myxoid matrix, tumor, nerve fascicles intermixed
  - ○ S-100 positive, mitotic figures rare unless malignant degeneration

Staging, Grading or Classification Criteria
- Consensus Development Conference on Neurofibromatosis (NIH, 1987) 2 or more of the following criteria
  - ○ > 6 café-au-lait spots measuring ≥ 15 mm in adults or 5 mm in children, ≥ 2 neurofibromas of any type or ≥ 1 plexiform neurofibroma, axillary or inguinal freckling, optic glioma, two or more Lisch nodules (iris hamartomas), distinctive bony lesion (sphenoid wing dysplasia, thinning of long bone +/- pseudoarthrosis, first-degree relative with NF1

CLINICAL ISSUES

Presentation
- Most common signs/symptoms
  - ○ Skeletal deformity common (25–40%)
    - Focal or acute angle kyphoscoliosis +/- myelopathy
    - Extremity bowing or overgrowth
  - ○ Palpable spinal or cutaneous mass
  - ○ Pigmentation anomalies (café-au-lait, axillary freckling, Lisch nodules) ≥ 90% NF1 patients
- Clinical profile
  - ○ Severity of clinical appearance highly variable
  - ○ Classic NF1 triad: Cutaneous lesions, skeletal deformity, and mental deficiency

Demographics
- Age: Childhood diagnosis; minimally affected patients may be diagnosed as adults
- Gender: M = F
- Ethnicity: ↑ Frequency in Arab-Israeli populations

Natural History & Prognosis
- Kyphosis, scoliosis frequently progressive

- NF growth usually slow; rapid growth associated with pregnancy, puberty, or malignant transformation

Treatment
- Conservative observation; intervention dictated by clinical symptomatology, appearance of neoplasm
- Surgical resection of symptomatic localized NF, spinal cord tumors
- PNF invasive, rarely resectable; observation +/- biological or chemotherapeutic (thalidomide, antihistamines, maturation agents, antiangiogenic drugs) intervention
- Spinal fusion reserved for symptomatic or severe kyphoscoliosis

DIAGNOSTIC CHECKLIST

Consider
- Multiple nerve sheath tumors, ≥ 1 plexiform neurofibroma, bizarre kyphoscoliosis with deformed vertebra → consider NF1
- Absence of visible stigmata does not exclude NF1

Image Interpretation Pearls
- Characteristic PNF imaging appearance best displayed using fat-saturated T2WI or STIR MR imaging

SELECTED REFERENCES

1. Cardona S et al: Evaluation of F18-deoxyglucose positron emission tomography (FDG-PET) to assess the nature of neurogenic tumours. Eur J Surg Oncol. 29(6):536-41, 2003
2. Iannicelli E et al: Radiol Med (Torino). English, Italian. MID: Apr;103(4):332-43, 2002
3. Packer RJ et al: Plexiform neurofibromas in NF1: toward biologic-based therapy. Neurology. 58(10):1461-70, 2002
4. Simoens WA et al: with radiologist's experience? Eur Radiol. 11(2):250-7, 2001
5. Lin J et al: Cross-sectional imaging of peripheral nerve sheath tumors: characteristic signs on CT, MR imaging, and sonography. AJR Am J Roentgenol. 176(1):75-82, 2001
6. Solomon SB et al: Positron emission tomography in the detection and management of sarcomatous transformation in neurofibromatosis. Clin Nucl Med. 26(6):525-8, 2001
7. Ferner RE et al: Evaluation of (18)fluorodeoxyglucose positron emission tomography ((18)FDG PET) in the detection of malignant peripheral nerve sheath tumours arising from within plexiform neurofibromas in neurofibromatosis 1. J Neurol Neurosurg Psychiatry. 68(3):353-7, 2000
8. von Deimling A et al: Neurofibromatosis Type 1. In: Kleihues P, Cavanee W (eds), Pathology and genetics of tumors of the nervous system. Lyon, IARC Press, 216-218, 2000
9. Mukonoweshuro W et al: Neurofibromatosis type 1: the role of neuroradiology. Neuropediatrics. 30(3):111-9, 1999
10. Murphey M et al: From the archives of the AFIP. Imaging of musculoskeletal neurogenic tumors: radiologic-pathologic correlation. Radiographics. 19(5):1253-80, 1999

IMAGE GALLERY

Typical

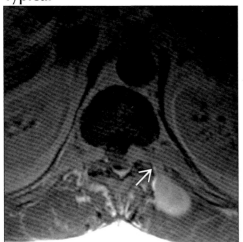
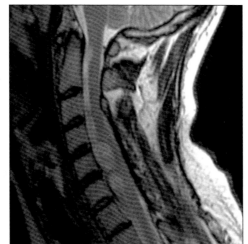

(Left) Axial T1 C+ MR shows bilateral nerve root localized neurofibromas; the left tumor extends along the dorsal primary ramus (arrow) into paraspinal muscle. (Right) Sagittal T2WI MR depicts multiple ventral intradural, extramedullary neurofibromas producing spinal cord compression (arrow).

Variant

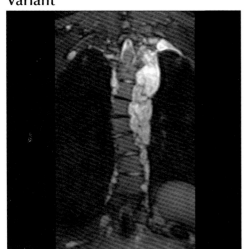
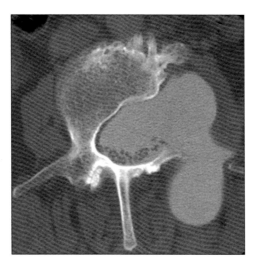

(Left) Coronal STIR MR reveals a large plexiform neurofibroma extending along the left paraspinal sympathetic chain, remodeling the adjacent vertebral bodies and contributing to scoliosis. (Right) Axial NECT following myelography shows marked dural dysplasia and left lumbar lateral meningocele. Posterior vertebral scalloping and erosion/hypoplasia of left pedicle are characteristic.

Variant

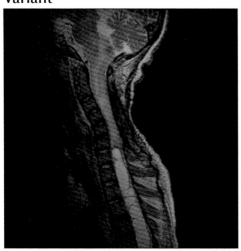
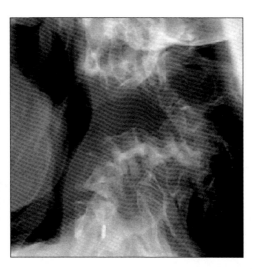

(Left) Sagittal T2WI MR shows a holocord astrocytoma extending into the brainstem with large neoplastic syrinx. Vertebral canal widening mimics that produced by dural dysplasia. (Right) Lateral radiography demonstrates bizarre acute angle cervical kyphosis with marked dural ectasia and neural foraminal enlargement, highly characteristic of NF1.

NEUROFIBROMATOSIS TYPE 2

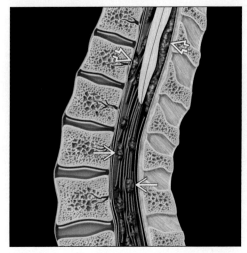

Sagittal graphic illustrates multiple rounded schwannomas (brown) (white arrows) along the cauda equina, as well as flat dural-based mengiomas (red) (open arrows) impinging the conus.

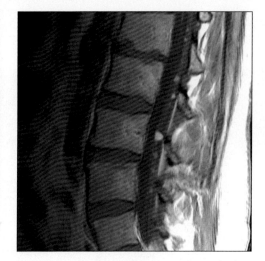

Sagittal T1 C+ MR shows numerous enhancing schwannomas. Note rounded morphology, close approximation to a nerve root for each lesion, and increased conspicuity with enhanced technique.

TERMINOLOGY

Abbreviations and Synonyms
- Neurofibromatosis type 2 (NF2), nonsyndromic (NS)
- Synonyms: Bilateral acoustic neurofibromatosis, central neurofibromatosis → all obsolete

Definitions
- Rare autosomal dominant disease from chromosomal 22 defect in which all patients develop CNS tumors
- Mnemonic for NF2 tumors = MISME; multiple inherited schwannomas, meningiomas, & ependymomas

IMAGING FINDINGS

General Features
- Best diagnostic clue: Multiple spinal tumors of various histologic types
- Location
  - Schwannomas
    - Intradural, extramedullary; occur anywhere
    - Rarely intramedullary; arise primarily or secondarily extend from nerve root tumor
    - May extend extradurally
  - Meningiomas: Intradural, extramedullary; typically involving thoracic spine but occur anywhere
  - Ependymomas: Intramedullary; typically upper cervical cord or conus but occur anywhere
- Size
  - Schwannomas: Tiny to several cms
  - Meningiomas: Vary from large to nodular studding
  - Ependymomas: Tiny to a few cms
- Morphology
  - Schwannomas
    - Rounded, cystic when large, near a nerve root
    - Dumbbell-shaped when extends extradurally
  - Meningiomas: Flattened with dural attachment
  - Ependymomas: Rounded

Radiographic Findings
- Radiography: Erosion & expansion 2° to tumor
- Myelography
  - Intradural filling defects and/or cord expansion
  - May have complete block

CT Findings
- NECT: Erosion & expansion 2° to tumor

MR Findings
- T1WI
  - Schwannomas
    - Well-delineated rounded intermediate signal mass
    - May undergo hemorrhage or cystic degeneration
    - Uncommon intramedullary, centrally located
  - Meningiomas: Mid to low intensity

DDx: Neurofibromatosis Type 2

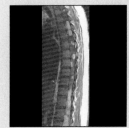
Drop Metastases

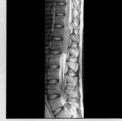
Drop Metastases

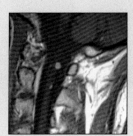
Hemangioblastomas

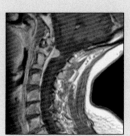
NS Meningioma

Key Facts

Terminology
- Mnemonic for NF2 tumors = MISME; multiple inherited schwannomas, meningiomas, & ependymomas

Imaging Findings
- Best diagnostic clue: Multiple spinal tumors of various histologic types
- Best imaging tool: MRI + gadolinium
- Protocol advice: Contrast-enhanced imaging is best method for detecting lesions regardless of size

Top Differential Diagnoses
- Metastases
- Hemangioblastomas
- Non-syndromic schwannoma, meningioma, ependymoma

Pathology
- 22q12 deletion correlates with loss of NF2 gene product "Merlin" (aka Schwannomin)

Clinical Issues
- Nearly half initially present with hearing loss
- Up to 45% with extramedullary tumors exhibit signs/symptoms of cord compression
- Few patients require therapeutic intervention for intramedullary tumors which often remain quiescent
- Intradural, extramedullary tumors frequently lead to surgical intervention

Diagnostic Checklist
- Presence of multiple & different pathologic types of spinal tumors is highly suggestive of NF2
- Screen using MRI C+ of brain & entire spine

- ○ Ependymomas
  - ■ Iso- to slightly hyperintense
  - ■ Centrally located with cord expansion
- T2WI
  - ○ Schwannomas
    - ■ Well-delineated rounded hyperintense mass
    - ■ May undergo hemorrhage or cystic degeneration
  - ○ Meningiomas
    - ■ May be heterogeneous
    - ■ Best defines high occurrence of cord compression
  - ○ Ependymomas: Hyperintense; centrally located with cord expansion
  - ○ Ill-defined hyperintense lesion may be low grade astrocytoma
  - ○ Any intramedullary lesion may have syrinx
- T1 C+
  - ○ Schwannomas: Enhance intensely; homogeneously when small, heterogeneously when large & cystic
  - ○ Meningiomas: Enhance intensely (often to a lesser degree than schwannomas) & homogeneously
  - ○ Ependymomas: Enhancing centrally located mass

Imaging Recommendations
- Best imaging tool: MRI + gadolinium
- Protocol advice: Contrast-enhanced imaging is best method for detecting lesions regardless of size

DIFFERENTIAL DIAGNOSIS

Metastases
- Originate from leptomeninges
- Eccentrically placed, rarely within center of cord

Hemangioblastomas
- Often associated with von-Hippel Lindau
- Originate from leptomeninges
- May have associated cyst

Non-syndromic schwannoma, meningioma, ependymoma
- Usually solitary
- Imaging appears identical to syndromic tumors

Lymphoma
- May coat spinal cord surface

PATHOLOGY

General Features
- General path comments: NF2 mostly associated with tumors of Schwann cells & meninges
- Genetics
  - ○ Inherited autosomal dominant syndrome
  - ○ 22q12 deletion correlates with loss of NF2 gene product "Merlin" (aka Schwannomin)
- Etiology
  - ○ Chromosomal 22 deletion with eventual inactivation of Merlin functionality
    - ■ 1st event is 22 chromosomal loss
    - ■ "Second hit theory": Remaining single NF2 copy is mutated; vast majority are null mutations
    - ■ Results in truncated, poorly or non-functional Merlin protein
- Epidemiology
  - ○ 1 in 50,000 live births worldwide
  - ○ Intradural spinal tumors are present in up to 65% patients at initial presentation for imaging
    - ■ 84% have intramedullary tumors
    - ■ 87% have intradural extramedullary tumors

Gross Pathologic & Surgical Features
- Multiple tumors of different histologic types

Microscopic Features
- Merlin associates at cell cytoskeleton near plasma membrane & inhibits cell proliferation, adhesion, and migration
- Merlin monoclonal antibody immunohistochemistry exhibits consistent immunostaining of Schwann cells
- NF2 histopathology no different than that of nonsyndromic tumors; exception is the multiplicity

Staging, Grading or Classification Criteria
- Definite diagnosis of NF2
  - ○ Bilateral CN8 (vestibular) schwannomas

NEUROFIBROMATOSIS TYPE 2

○ 1st degree relative with NF2 & either unilateral early onset vestibular schwannoma (age < 30 years) or any 2
  ▪ Meningioma, glioma, schwannoma, juvenile posterior subcapsular lenticular opacity
• Presumptive diagnosis of NF2
  ○ Early onset unilateral CN8 schwannomas (age < 30 years) and one of the following
    ▪ Meningioma, glioma, schwannoma, juvenile posterior subcapsular lenticular opacity
  ○ Multiple meningiomas (> 2) and unilateral vestibular schwannoma or one of the following
    ▪ Glioma, schwannoma, juvenile posterior subcapsular lenticular opacity
• Germline study findings support genotype-phenotype correlation of tumor grading
  ○ Nonsense & frameshift mutations
    ▪ Usually associated with severe disease phenotype
    ▪ A higher percentage of these patients have intramedullary tumors
    ▪ Have higher numbers of all spinal tumors; intramedullary & extramedullary
    ▪ Younger at the onset of symptoms, diagnosis of NF2, and presentation for imaging
  ○ Missense mutations & large gene deletions are found with mild phenotype
  ○ Splice-site mutations; severe or mild phenotype
    ▪ Dependent on intron involved and its affect on protein functionality
• Imaging classification of NF2 spinal tumors
  ○ Intradural, extramedullary tumors
    ▪ Schwannomas: Round & located near a nerve root
    ▪ Meningiomas: Flat surface of dural attachment
  ○ Three cardinal features of intramedullary tumors
    ▪ Central location within cord parenchyma
    ▪ Intense enhancement
    ▪ Multiplicity, often too many to count

CLINICAL ISSUES

Presentation
• Most common signs/symptoms
  ○ Nearly half initially present with hearing loss
  ○ Up to 45% with extramedullary tumors exhibit signs/symptoms of cord compression
    ▪ Varies depending on location
    ▪ Weakness & sensory loss at or below level
    ▪ Spasticity, pain, loss of bowel/bladder control
• Clinical profile
  ○ Detection rates for genetic testing ≈ 65%
  ○ Juvenile subcapsular lens opacities common
  ○ Retinal & choroidal hamartomas in 10-20%
  ○ Café-au-lait spots < 50%
  ○ Minimal to no cutaneous neurofibromas
  ○ Cutaneous schwannomas in 2/3rds

Demographics
• Age
  ○ Genetic disease present at conception
  ○ Become symptomatic 2nd-3rd decades
• Gender: M = F
• Ethnicity: No racial predilection

Natural History & Prognosis
• Many lead relatively normal lifespans
• Few patients require therapeutic intervention for intramedullary tumors which often remain quiescent
• Intradural, extramedullary tumors frequently lead to surgical intervention
  ○ Percentage of patients with extramedullary tumors who undergo surgery is about 5x higher than the percentage of patients with intramedullary tumors
  ○ Higher surgical rate is result of high number of tumors & frequent occurrence of cord compression
  ○ Schwannomas are present more often & in higher numbers than meningiomas and have more surgical procedures overall
  ○ Meningiomas account for a disproportionate number of symptomatic lesions
    ▪ Meningiomas comprise ≈ 12% of extramedullary tumors yet account for 37% of extramedullary tumors requiring excision
    ▪ Suggests NF2 meningiomas are more aggressive

Treatment
• Tumor resection is mainstay of NF2 treatment
• Intramedullary tumors: Monitor with regular imaging & appropriate clinical correlation
  ○ Relatively indolent course of most intramedullary tumors & anticipated burden from other spinal/intracranial tumors must be considered → standard aggressive management may not be warranted, even in symptomatic patient
• Intradural, extramedullary tumors: Early removal of rapidly growing or symptomatic tumors
• First-degree relatives need to be evaluated

DIAGNOSTIC CHECKLIST

Consider
• Presence of multiple & different pathologic types of spinal tumors is highly suggestive of NF2

Image Interpretation Pearls
• Screen using MRI C+ of brain & entire spine
• Imaging follow-up of patients with spinal tumors should be based on knowledge of tumor location, number, & suspected histologic type

SELECTED REFERENCES

1. Patronas NJ et al: Intramedullary and spinal canal tumors in patients with neurofibromatosis 2: MR imaging findings and correlation with genotype. Radiology. 218(2):434-42, 2001
2. Evans DG et al: Neurofibromatosis type 2. J Med Genet. 37(12):897-904, 2000
3. den Bakker MA et al: Expression of the neurofibromatosis type 2 gene in human tissues. J Histochem Cytochem. 47(11):1471-80, 1999
4. Kluwe L et al: Identification of NF2 germ-line mutations and comparison with neurofibromatosis 2 phenotypes. Hum Genet. 98(5):534-8, 1996
5. Mautner VF et al: The neuroimaging and clinical spectrum of neurofibromatosis 2. Neurosurgery. 38(5):880-5; discussion 885-6, 1996

IMAGE GALLERY

Typical

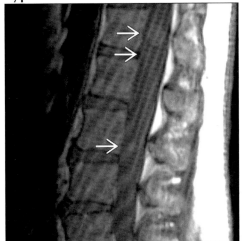 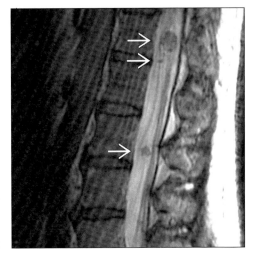

(Left) Sagittal T1WI MR shows numerous rounded intermediate intensity schwannomas (arrows). Without contrast they are difficult to distinguish. *(Right)* Sagittal T2WI MR demonstrates numerous rounded slightly iso- to hyperintense schwannomas (arrows), which are easier to see against bright CSF. Note approximation of each lesion to nerve root.

Typical

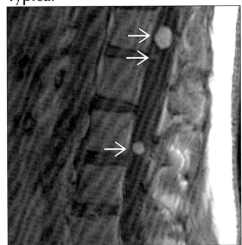 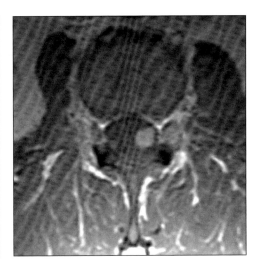

(Left) Sagittal T1 C+ MR demonstrates numerous rounded homogenously enhancing schwannomas (arrows). Contrast increases conspicuity. Note close approximation of each lesion to nerve root. *(Right)* Axial T1 C+ MR shows typical rounded homogeneously enhancing appearance of an intradural extramedullary schwannoma.

Typical

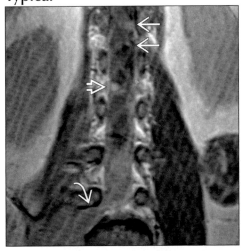 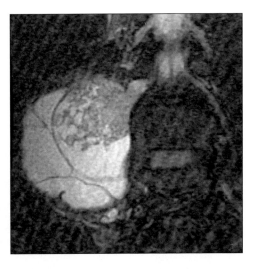

(Left) Coronal T1 C+ MR shows round enhancing schwannomas in close approximation to nerve roots (arrows), enhancing meningioma with broad dural base (open arrow), & dumbbell schwannoma (curved arrow). *(Right)* Coronal T2WI MR demonstrates large cystic hyperintense dumbbell-shaped schwannoma extending intradural to extradural through neural foramen.

DURAL DYSPLASIA

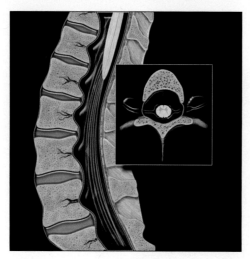

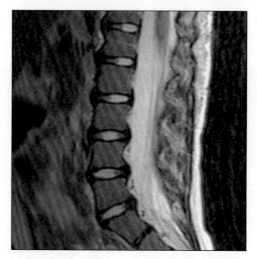

Sagittal graphic demonstrates scalloping of the posterior vertebral bodies with central canal enlargement. Also shown (inset) are bilateral lumbar lateral meningoceles.

Sagittal T2WI MR (neurofibromatosis type 1) shows classic posterior vertebral scalloping and patulous dural sac from L2 through S2 .

TERMINOLOGY

Abbreviations and Synonyms
- Synonym: Dural ectasia

Definitions
- Patulous dural sac with posterior vertebral scalloping

IMAGING FINDINGS

General Features
- Best diagnostic clue: Smooth "C" shaped scalloping of posterior vertebral bodies with patulous dural sac
- Location: Lumbar > cervical, thoracic
- Size: Mild ⇒ extensive deformity
- Morphology: Expansile dural sac, spinal canal remodeling with posterior vertebral scalloping

Radiographic Findings
- Radiography
  ○ Smooth remodeling of posterior vertebral body, expansion of osseous spinal canal, +/- kyphoscoliosis
  ○ Osteopenia (homocystinuria)
- Myelography: Posterior vertebral scalloping, contrast fills enlarged dural sac, +/- lateral meningocele(s)

CT Findings
- CECT

  ○ Posterior vertebral scalloping ⇒ spinal canal enlargement
    ■ Easiest to appreciate on sagittal images
  ○ Pedicular attenuation, widened interpediculate distance, erosion of anterior and posterior elements, patulous CSF density dural sac
- CTA: +/- Arterial dissection or aneurysm; implicates Marfan or Ehler-Danlos syndrome as underlying etiology

MR Findings
- T1WI
  ○ Posterior vertebral scalloping, expansion of osseous spinal canal, patulous dural sac, +/- kyphoscoliosis
  ○ +/- Pedicular thinning, lateral meningocele(s)
- T2WI
  ○ Similar findings to T1WI
  ○ Best evaluates position of neural elements relative to dural ectasia
- MRA: +/- Arterial dissection or aneurysm (Marfan, Ehler-Danlos syndrome)

Ultrasonographic Findings
- Real Time: Hypoechoic patulous dural sac, widening of spinal canal

Angiographic Findings
- Conventional

DDx: Dural Dysplasia

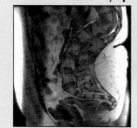

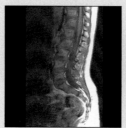

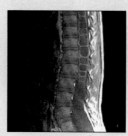

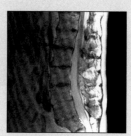

Achondroplasia   *Hurler (MPS 1-H)*   *Syringomyelia*   *Ankylosing Spondylitis*

DURAL DYSPLASIA

119

Key Facts

Terminology
- Synonym: Dural ectasia
- Patulous dural sac with posterior vertebral scalloping

Imaging Findings
- Best diagnostic clue: Smooth "C" shaped scalloping of posterior vertebral bodies with patulous dural sac
- Location: Lumbar > cervical, thoracic
- Posterior vertebral scalloping, expansion of osseous spinal canal, patulous dural sac, +/- kyphoscoliosis
- +/- Pedicular thinning, lateral meningocele(s)

Top Differential Diagnoses
- Congenital vertebral dysplasia
- Spinal tumor or syrinx
- Cauda equina syndrome of ankylosing spondylitis (AS)

Pathology
- General path comments: Genetic predisposition ⇒ primary meningeal dysplasia ⇒ weakness in meninges ⇒ expansion, secondarily remodeling of posterior vertebral body and pedicular thinning ⇒ further dural sac expansion
- NF1: Autosomal dominant (chromosome 17q12)
- Marfan: Autosomal dominant
- Homocystinuria: Autosomal recessive
- Ehler-Danlos: Autosomal dominant

Clinical Issues
- Moderate to severe back pain > 50% of Marfan patients; presence, degree of dural ectasia associated with back pain

---

- Not useful for imaging spine deformity; primary utility is detecting associated vascular anomalies
- Ascending aortic aneurysm ("tulip bulb configuration") suggests Marfan syndrome

Imaging Recommendations
- MRI shows osseous abnormalities well
- Additionally, MRI is most useful modality to exclude syrinx or tumor as cause of canal enlargement before attributing to dural ectasia

DIFFERENTIAL DIAGNOSIS

Congenital vertebral dysplasia
- Achondroplasia, mucopolysaccharidosis, osteogenesis inperfecta (tarda)
- Search for appropriate family history, clinical stigmata

Spinal tumor or syrinx
- Astrocytoma, ependymoma, nerve sheath tumor, syrinx
- Characteristic imaging findings lead to correct diagnosis

Cauda equina syndrome of ankylosing spondylitis (AS)
- Irregular lumbar canal expansion
- Proposed etiology for dural ectasia; proliferative inflammatory synovium ⇒ cauda equina symptoms
- Imaging and clinical stigmata of AS typically present

PATHOLOGY

General Features
- General path comments: Genetic predisposition ⇒ primary meningeal dysplasia ⇒ weakness in meninges ⇒ expansion, secondarily remodeling of posterior vertebral body and pedicular thinning ⇒ further dural sac expansion
- Genetics
  - NF1: Autosomal dominant (chromosome 17q12)
  - Marfan: Autosomal dominant

- Homocystinuria: Autosomal recessive
- Ehler-Danlos: Autosomal dominant
- Etiology
  - NF1: Primary mesenchymal disorder
  - Marfan syndrome: Primary connective tissue defect unknown
  - Ehlers-Danlos: > 10 different types of collagen synthesis defects
  - Homocystinuria: Cystathionine beta-synthetase deficiency
- Epidemiology
  - NF1: 1/4,000, 50% new mutations; dural ectasia common
  - Marfan: 1/5,000 (United States); dural ectasia present > 60% patients
  - Homocystinuria: 1/344,000 worldwide; dural dysplasia less common than Marfan
  - Ehler-Danlos: 1/400,000 (worldwide); dural dysplasia less common than Marfan
- Associated abnormalities
  - Lateral thoracic or lumbar meningocele, anterior sacral meningocele
  - Kyphoscoliosis
  - Joint hypermobility, lens abnormalities, aneurysm, arterial dissection (connective tissue disorders)
  - Peripheral and central neoplasms (NF1)

Gross Pathologic & Surgical Features
- Enlarged CSF thecal sac, remodeled posterior vertebral bodies
- Dura in ectatic areas is extremely thin, fragile

Microscopic Features
- Dural thinning in ectatic areas

CLINICAL ISSUES

Presentation
- Most common signs/symptoms
  - Back pain +/- radiculopathy

DURAL DYSPLASIA

- Moderate to severe back pain > 50% of Marfan patients; presence, degree of dural ectasia associated with back pain
- High prevalence of dural ectasia (41%) in Marfan patients without back pain however; mere presence of dural ectasia does not necessarily mean patient is symptomatic
  ○ Other signs/symptoms
    ▪ Headache
    ▪ Incontinence, pelvic symptoms
- Clinical profile
  ○ NF1: Plexiform neurofibromas, kyphoscoliosis, optic nerve gliomas and other astrocytomas, café-au-lait spots, axillary freckling, extremity pseudoarthrosis
  ○ Marfan syndrome: Tall, joint hypermobility, arachnodactyly, kyphoscoliosis, joint and lens dislocations
  ○ Homocystinuria: Tall, arachnodactyly, scoliosis, mental retardation, seizures, lens dislocations
  ○ Ehlers-Danlos: +/- Tall, thin hyperelastic skin, hypermobile joints, fragile connective tissue

Demographics
- Age: May present at any age depending on severity
- Gender: M = F
- Ethnicity
  ○ NF1: All ethnicities; higher in Arab-Israeli subpopulations
  ○ Marfan: All races, ethnicities
  ○ Homocystinuria: Northern European descent
  ○ Ehlers-Danlos: Caucasian, European descent

Natural History & Prognosis
- Variable; dependent on underlying etiology
- Morbidity and mortality primarily related to vascular pathology
  ○ Vascular fragility ⇒ predisposition to arterial dissection or aneurysm ⇒ premature death

Treatment
- Treatment directed toward addressing underlying etiology
- Meningocele repair, scoliosis surgery for more severe cases

DIAGNOSTIC CHECKLIST

Consider
- Three disease categories produce posterior vertebral scalloping
  ○ Dural ectasia
  ○ Increased intraspinal pressure
  ○ Congenital vertebral dysplasia
- Important to determine underlying disorder for treatment planning, genetic counseling and determining prognosis

Image Interpretation Pearls
- Recognition of specific imaging clues and integration of available clinical data permits a more specific diagnosis
- Look for imaging stigmata of etiological diseases
  ○ "Tulip bulb" aortic aneurysm ⇒ Marfan syndrome
  ○ Osteoporosis ⇒ homocystinuria

○ Pseudoarthrosis, CNS/PNS tumors ⇒ NF1

SELECTED REFERENCES
1. Nallamshetty L et al: Dural ectasia and back pain: review of the literature and case report. J Spinal Disord Tech. 15(4):326-9, 2002
2. Tubbs RS et al: Dural ectasia in neurofibromatosis. Pediatr Neurosurg. 37(6):331-2, 2002
3. Ahn NU et al: Dural ectasia and conventional radiography in the Marfan lumbosacral spine. Skeletal Radiol. 30(6):338-45, 2001
4. Oosterhof T et al: Quantitative assessment of dural ectasia as a marker for Marfan syndrome. Radiology. 220(2):514-8, 2001
5. Ahn NU et al: Dural ectasia in the Marfan syndrome: MR and CT findings and criteria. Genet Med. 2(3):173-9, 2000
6. Ahn NU et al: Dural ectasia is associated with back pain in Marfan syndrome. Spine. 25(12):1562-8, 2000
7. Schonauer C et al: Lumbosacral dural ectasia in type 1 neurofibromatosis. Report of two cases. J Neurosurg Sci. 44(3):165-8; discussion 169, 2000
8. Rose PS et al: A comparison of the Berlin and Ghent nosologies and the influence of dural ectasia in the diagnosis of Marfan syndrome. Genet Med. 2(5):278-82, 2000
9. Barkovich A: Pediatric neuroimaging. 3rd ed. Philadelphia, Lippincott-Raven, 398, 2000
10. Sponseller PD et al: Osseous anatomy of the lumbosacral spine in Marfan syndrome. Spine. 25(21):2797-802, 2000
11. Fattori R et al: Importance of dural ectasia in phenotypic assessment of Marfan's syndrome. Lancet. 354(9182):910-3, 1999
12. De Paepe A: Dural ectasia and the diagnosis of Marfan's syndrome. Lancet. 354(9182):878-9, 1999
13. Villeirs GM et al: Widening of the spinal canal and dural ectasia in Marfan's syndrome: assessment by CT. Neuroradiology. 41(11):850-4, 1999
14. Raff ML et al: Joint hypermobility syndromes. Curr Opin Rheumatol. 8(5): 459-66, 1996
15. Helfen M et al: Intrathoracic dural ectasia mimicking neurofibroma and scoliosis. A case report. Int Orthop. 19(3):181-4, 1995
16. Bensaid AH et al: Neurofibromatosis with dural ectasia and bilateral symmetrical pedicular clefts: report of two cases. Neuroradiology. 34(2):107-9, 1992
17. Stern WE: Dural ectasia and the Marfan syndrome. J Neurosurg. 69(2):221-7, 1988
18. Pyeritz RE et al: Dural ectasia is a common feature of the Marfan syndrome. Am J Hum Genet. 43(5):726-32, 1988
19. Katz SG et al: Thoracic and lumbar dural ectasia in a two-year-old boy. Pediatr Radiol. 6(4):238-40, 1978

IMAGE GALLERY

Variant

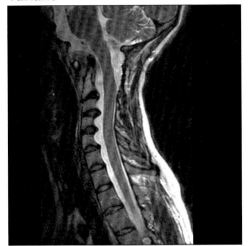
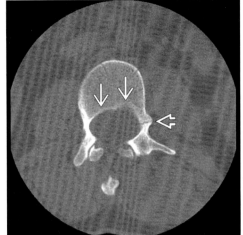

(Left) Sagittal T2WI MR *(neurofibromatosis type 1)* shows extensive scalloping of the posterior cervical vertebral bodies and clivus *(Courtesy G. Hedlund, DO).* *(Right)* Axial bone CT demonstrates posterior vertebral remodeling *(arrows)* and right pedicle thinning. The left pedicle demonstrates stress fracture with pseudoarthrosis *(open arrow).*

Variant

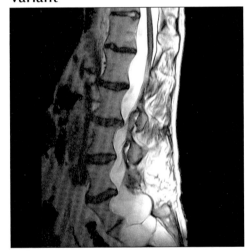
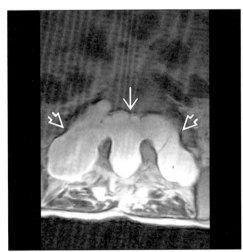

(Left) Sagittal T2WI MR *(Marfan syndrome)* shows striking posterior vertebral scalloping and dural ectasia. *(Right)* Axial T2WI MR *(Marfan syndrome)* depicts dural ectasia producing marked posterior vertebral scalloping *(arrow),* associated with large bilateral lumbar meningoceles *(open arrows).*

Typical

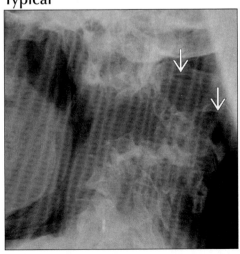
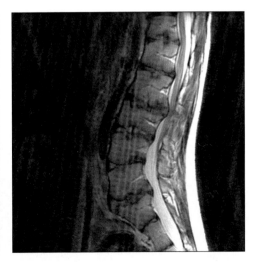

(Left) Lateral radiography *(neurofibromatosis type 1)* shows striking posterior vertebral scalloping, focal kyphosis, and marked foraminal enlargement *(arrows).* *(Right)* Sagittal T2WI MR *(homocystinuria)* in a young patient shows posterior vertebral scalloping, marked degenerative disc changes, and spinal stenosis *(Courtesy R. Boyer, MD).*

CONGENITAL SPINAL STENOSIS

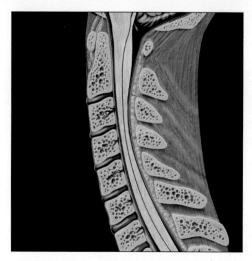

Sagittal graphic shows marked congenital AP narrowing of the central spinal canal.

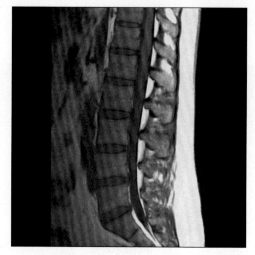

Sagittal T1WI MR demonstrates moderate congenital AP canal diameter reduction spanning L3 through the sacrum.

TERMINOLOGY

Abbreviations and Synonyms

- Synonyms: "Short pedicle" syndrome, congenital short pedicles, developmental spinal stenosis

Definitions

- Reduced AP canal diameter 2° to short, squat pedicles and laterally directed laminae

IMAGING FINDINGS

General Features

- Best diagnostic clue: Short, thick pedicles producing narrowed anteroposterior (AP) spinal canal diameter
- Location: Lumbar > cervical > thoracic spine
- Size
  - Central canal diameter is smaller than normal
    - Cervical spine: Absolute AP diameter < 14 mm
    - Lumbar spine: Absolute AP diameter < 15 mm
- Morphology
  - Short thick pedicles
  - "Trefoil-shaped" lateral recesses
  - Laterally directed laminae

Radiographic Findings

- Radiography

  - Shortened AP distance between posterior vertebral body and spinolaminar line
    - +/- Superimposed degenerative disc, facet disease
  - Lateral x-ray normally shows articular pillar ending before spinolaminar line
    - Imaging pearl: If articular pillar takes up entire AP canal dimension on lateral x-ray, central canal stenosis is present
- Myelography: Confirms shortened AP dimension, clarifies severity of neural compression

CT Findings

- Bone CT
  - Short thick pedicles, "trefoil-shaped" lateral recesses, and laterally directed laminae
    - +/- Acquired disc, facet degenerative changes
  - Sagittal plane useful to survey extent of congenital narrowing
  - Axial plane best demonstrates reduced AP canal diameter, short thick pedicles

MR Findings

- T1WI
  - Short AP diameter +/- superimposed acquired facet, disc degenerative changes
  - +/- Hypointense facet, vertebral body marrow changes indicative of superimposed degenerative changes
- T2WI

DDx: Congenital Spinal Stenosis

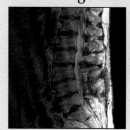

Acq. Lumbar Stenosis

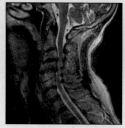

Acq. Cervical Stenosis

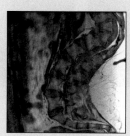

Achondroplasia

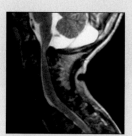

Mucopolysaccharidosis

CONGENITAL SPINAL STENOSIS

Key Facts

Terminology
- Synonyms: "Short pedicle" syndrome, congenital short pedicles, developmental spinal stenosis

Imaging Findings
- Location: Lumbar > cervical > thoracic spine
- Short thick pedicles, "trefoil-shaped" lateral recesses, and laterally directed laminae

Top Differential Diagnoses
- Acquired spinal stenosis
- Inherited spinal stenosis

Clinical Issues
- Low back pain, radiating leg pain (unilateral or bilateral), +/- bladder and bowel dysfunction

- Neurogenic claudication: Radiating leg pain with walking, relieved by rest, bending forward
- Cauda equina syndrome (rare): Bilateral leg weakness, urinary retention due to atonic bladder
- Progressive myelopathy (spinal cord dysfunction) or reversible acute neurologic deficits ("stingers")

Diagnostic Checklist
- Patients present at a younger age than typical for degenerative spine disease
- Congenital spinal stenosis may not produce symptoms until superimposed acquired degenerative changes accumulate
- Recognition of short thick pedicles, AP canal diameter reduction key to diagnosis

---

- ○ Similar osseous findings to T1WI MR
- ○ +/- Cord compression
- T2* GRE
  - ○ Best depicts osseous structures
  - ○ Caveat: Overestimates true degree of canal narrowing 2° to susceptibility "blooming" artifact

Imaging Recommendations
- CT with sagittal and coronal reformats to evaluate osseous structures
  - ○ Narrowed angle of laminae best appreciated in coronal plane
- MR imaging to assess degree/presence of spinal cord, dural sac compression
  - ○ Also demonstrates osseous anatomy well; permits complete imaging assessment with a single imaging study
  - ○ Sagittal MR best demonstrates AP canal narrowing, assesses for cord/cauda equina compression
  - ○ Axial MR images confirm pedicle configuration, assess severity of canal narrowing

DIFFERENTIAL DIAGNOSIS

Acquired spinal stenosis
- Normal pedicle length
- +/- Subluxation, spondylolysis, disc/facet degenerative changes

Inherited spinal stenosis
- Genetic predisposition
- Achondroplasia, mucopolysaccharidoses most common
- Frequently associated with characteristic brain, visceral, and/or extremity abnormalities enabling specific diagnosis

PATHOLOGY

General Features
- General path comments: Short, thickened pedicles
- Etiology: Idiopathic

- Epidemiology
  - ○ Prevalence in general population difficult to establish; up to 30% of surgically proven lumbar stenosis in one study
    - Not uncommonly seen in clinical practice during routine cervical or lumbar spine evaluation
    - Congenital cervical stenosis reported in 7.6% of 262 high school and college football players
  - ○ Symptomatic at earlier age than expected
- Associated abnormalities: Superimposed acquired (degenerative) stenosis

Gross Pathologic & Surgical Features
- Sagittal canal narrowed 2° to short pedicles, thick laminae, and protrusion of inferior facet articular processes
- Lateral recess often narrowed 2° to co-existent hypertrophic superior facet articular processes

Microscopic Features
- Histologically normal bone

Staging, Grading or Classification Criteria
- Cervical spine
  - ○ Torg ratio (AP canal diameter/AP vertebral body diameter) < 0.8
  - ○ Absolute diameter < 14 mm
    - Must take body habitus into account; relative dimension more important than absolute measurement
- Lumbar spine
  - ○ Absolute AP diameter < 15 mm
    - Body habitus influences significance of measurement

CLINICAL ISSUES

Presentation
- Most common signs/symptoms
  - ○ Lumbar
    - Low back pain, radiating leg pain (unilateral or bilateral), +/- bladder and bowel dysfunction

- Neurogenic claudication: Radiating leg pain with walking, relieved by rest, bending forward
    - Cauda equina syndrome (rare): Bilateral leg weakness, urinary retention due to atonic bladder
  ○ Cervical
    - Radiating arm pain or numbness
    - Progressive myelopathy (spinal cord dysfunction) or reversible acute neurologic deficits ("stingers")
- Clinical profile
  ○ Symptomatic cervical or lumbar stenosis symptoms at younger age than typical of degenerative stenosis
    - These patients typically lack complicating medical problems (diabetes or vascular insufficiency)
  ○ Athlete presents with temporary neurological deficit following physical contact that subsequently resolves

Demographics
- Age: Symptoms may arise in teens; more commonly in 4th-5th decade
- Gender: M ≥ F
- Ethnicity: No ethnic or racial predilection

Natural History & Prognosis
- May be incidental finding in younger patients
  ○ Borderline cases usually asymptomatic until superimposed acquired spinal degenerative disease occurs
- Many patients eventually develop symptomatic spinal stenosis
  ○ Minor superimposed acquired abnormalities (bulge, herniation, osteophyte) cause severe neurologic symptoms
- Early surgical treatment important for best outcome
  ○ Surgical decompression usually relieves symptoms effectively
  ○ Long term pain relief following surgery is common

Treatment
- Lumbar: Decompressive laminectomy, posterior foraminotomy at involved levels
  ○ Risk of complications increases with more levels of decompression, diabetes, and long term steroid use
- Cervical: Posterior cervical laminectomy or laminoplasty
  ○ Same risk factors for complication as lumbar decompression

DIAGNOSTIC CHECKLIST

Consider
- Patients present at a younger age than typical for degenerative spine disease
- Congenital spinal stenosis may not produce symptoms until superimposed acquired degenerative changes accumulate

Image Interpretation Pearls
- Recognition of short thick pedicles, AP canal diameter reduction key to diagnosis
- Look for superimposed degenerative changes

SELECTED REFERENCES

1. Brigham CD et al: Permanent partial cervical spinal cord injury in a professional football player who had only congenital stenosis. A case report. J Bone Joint Surg Am. 85-A(8):1553-6, 2003
2. Oguz H et al: Measurement of spinal canal diameters in young subjects with lumbosacral transitional vertebra. Eur Spine J. 11(2):115-8, 2002
3. Allen CR et al: Transient quadriparesis in the athlete. Clin Sports Med. 21(1):15-27, 2002
4. Boockvar JA et al: Cervical spinal stenosis and sports-related cervical cord neurapraxia in children. Spine. 26(24):2709-12; discussion 2713, 2001
5. Shaffrey CI et al: Modified open-door laminoplasty for treatment of neurological deficits in younger patients with congenital spinal stenosis: analysis of clinical and radiographic data. J Neurosurg. 90(4 Suppl):170-7, 1999
6. Bey T et al: Spinal cord injury with a narrow spinal canal: utilizing Torg's ratio method of analyzing cervical spine radiographs. J Emerg Med. 16(1):79-82, 1998
7. Yoshida M et al: Indication and clinical results of laminoplasty for cervical myelopathy caused by disc herniation with developmental canal stenosis. Spine. 23(22):2391-7, 1998
8. Torg JS et al: Suggested management guidelines for participation in collision activities with congenital, developmental, or postinjury lesions involving the cervical spine. Med Sci Sports Exerc. 29(7 Suppl):S256-72, 1997
9. Azhar MM et al: Congenital spine deformity, congenital stenosis, diastematomyelia, and tight filum terminale in a workmen's compensation patient: a case report. Spine. 21(6):770-4, 1996
10. Ducker TB: Post-traumatic progressive cervical myelopathy in patient with congenital spinal stenosis. J Spinal Disord. 9(1):76; discussion 77-81, 1996
11. Torg JS: Cervical spinal stenosis with cord neurapraxia and transient quadriplegia. Sports Med. 20(6):429-34, 1995
12. Lemaire JJ et al: Lumbar canal stenosis. Retrospective study of 158 operated cases. Neurochirurgie. 41(2):89-97, 1995
13. Smith MG et al: The prevalence of congenital cervical spinal stenosis in 262 college and high school football players. J Ky Med Assoc. 91(7):273-5, 1993
14. Major NM et al: Central and foraminal stenosis of the lumbar spine. Neuroimaging Clinics of North America 3(3):559-561, 1993
15. Moss A G et al: Computed tomography of the body. Vol two, Philadelphia: W.B.Saunders Company 496-500, 1992
16. Scher AT: Spinal cord concussion in rugby players. Am J Sports Med. 19(5):485-8, 1991
17. Torg JS: Cervical spinal stenosis with cord neurapraxia and transient quadriplegia. Clin Sports Med. 9(2):279-96, 1990
18. Dauser RC et al: Symptomatic congenital spinal stenosis in a child. Neurosurgery. 11(1 Pt 1):61-3, 1982
19. Reale F et al: Congenital stenosis of lumbar spinal canal: comparison of results of surgical treatment for this and other causes of lumbar syndrome. Acta Neurochir (Wien). 42(3-4):199-207, 1978
20. Dharker SR et al: Congenital stenosis of the lumbar canal. A study of 60 cases. Neurol India. 26(1):1-6, 1978
21. Hinck VC et al: Congenital stenosis of the cervical spinal canal. Northwest Med. 67(3):268-74, 1968

CONGENITAL SPINAL STENOSIS

IMAGE GALLERY

Typical

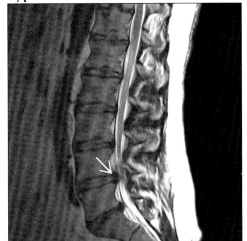
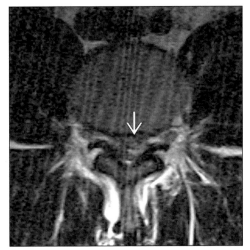

(Left) Sagittal T2WI MR reveals congenital lumbar AP canal diameter reduction complicated by superimposed degenerative disc disease. An L4/5 disc herniation (arrow) severely narrows central canal. *(Right)* Axial T2WI MR depicts moderate congenital AP canal reduction with superimposed left L4/5 disc herniation (arrow) that compresses transiting left L5 root.

Variant

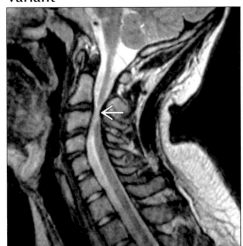
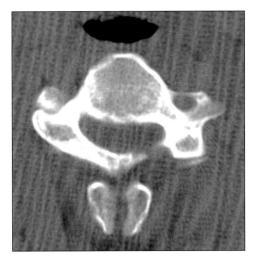

(Left) Sagittal T2WI MR shows marked congenital stenosis at C3 due to abnormally short pedicles. Cord T2 hyperintensity (arrow) corresponds to clinical myelopathy. *(Right)* Axial bone CT demonstrates marked AP canal reduction attributable to developmentally short pedicles and laterally oriented laminae.

Variant

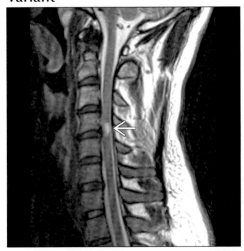
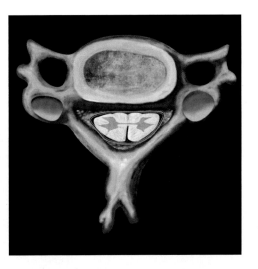

(Left) Sagittal T2WI MR reveals mild congenital AP canal narrowing exacerbated by C4/5 disc herniation that produces spinal cord T2 hyperintensity (arrow) corresponding to clinical myelopathy. *(Right)* Axial graphic depicts congenital cervical AP spinal narrowing. The pedicles are thick and laterally directed with resultant flattening of laminae.

SCOLIOSIS

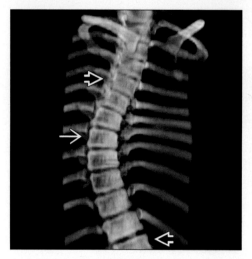

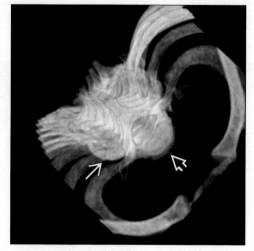

Anteroposterior bone CT 3D reformatted image of idiopathic scoliosis shows rotation as well as scoliosis to be present. Arrow on apical vertebra; open arrows on terminal vertebrae.

Axial bone CT 3D reformation shows the rotation of the apical vertebra (open arrow) compared to the terminal vertebrae (arrow). 3D CT is valuable in surgical planning.

TERMINOLOGY

Definitions
- General term for any lateral curvature of the spine
- Dextroscoliosis: Curve convex to the right
- Levoscoliosis: Curve convex to the left
- Kyphoscoliosis: Scoliosis with a component of kyphosis
- Rotoscoliosis: Scoliosis which includes rotation of the vertebrae
- S-curve scoliosis: Two adjacent curves, one to the right and one to the left
- C-curve scoliosis: Single curve
- Terminal vertebra: Most superior or inferior vertebra included in a curve
- Transitional vertebra: Vertebra between two curves
- Apical vertebra: Vertebra with greatest lateral displacement from the midline
- Primary curvature: Curvature with greatest angulation
- Secondary or compensatory curvature: Smaller curve which balances primary curvature

IMAGING FINDINGS

General Features
- Best diagnostic clue: Lateral curvature of the spine which returns to midline at ends of curve

- Location: Most commonly thoracic or thoracolumbar
- Size
  - Curve > 10 degrees
  - May be > 90 degrees
- Morphology
  - S-curve scoliosis
    - Idiopathic
    - Congenital
    - Syndromic
  - C-curve scoliosis
    - Neuromuscular
    - Neurofibromatosis
    - Scheuermann disease
    - Congenital
    - Syndromic
  - Short-curve scoliosis
    - Tumor
    - Trauma
    - Infection
    - Radiation
    - Congenital
    - Neuropathic

Radiographic Findings
- Radiography
  - Standing PA radiograph of the full thoracic and lumbar spine on single cassette
    - PA projection gives lower radiation dose to breasts than AP

DDx: Scoliosis

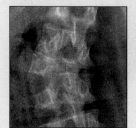

Congenital

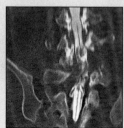

Osteomyelitis

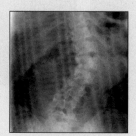

Tumor

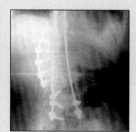

Radiation

SCOLIOSIS

Key Facts

Terminology
- General term for any lateral curvature of the spine

Imaging Findings
- Location: Most commonly thoracic or thoracolumbar
- Standing PA radiograph of the full thoracic and lumbar spine on single cassette
- Method of Cobb is standard for measuring scoliosis
- Lateral radiograph to show sagittal plane abnormalities
- MRI to screen for bone, cord abnormalities

Top Differential Diagnoses
- Idiopathic scoliosis
- Neuromuscular scoliosis
- Congenital scoliosis

- Scoliosis due to congenital syndromes without vertebral anomalies
- Scoliosis due to infection
- Scheuermann disease
- Scoliosis due to tumor
- Scoliosis due to trauma
- Degenerative scoliosis
- Compensatory scoliosis

Clinical Issues
- Idiopathic scoliosis asymptomatic
- Fusion for rapidly progressive curves, curves > 40°

Diagnostic Checklist
- Short-curve scoliosis usually has underlying abnormalities

- Lifts used to equalize limb lengths if needed
- Method of Cobb is standard for measuring scoliosis
  - Draw lines parallel to endplates of terminal vertebrae
  - If endplates difficult to see, use pedicles as landmarks
  - Cobb angle is angle between terminal endplates
  - Can also measure angle between two lines drawn perpendular to endplates
  - Second method is easier with small curves
- Choosing correct vertebrae to measure scoliosis critical to accuracy and monitoring
  - Terminal vertebra is one with greatest angle of endplate from horizontal
  - Rotoscoliosis: Terminal vertebra spinous process returns to midline
  - Interobserver variability 7-10 degrees
- Coned-down radiographs for better definition of vertebral abnormalities
- Lateral radiograph to show sagittal plane abnormalities
  - Usually alters normal thoracic kyphosis, lumbar lordosis
- Estimate rotational deformity by rib displacement on lateral radiograph

CT Findings
- Bone CT
  - Shows congenital bone anomalies, tumor, infection, post-operative complications

MR Findings
- Shows bone and spinal cord anomalies, syrinx, tumor, infection

Imaging Recommendations
- Best imaging tool: Radiography for initial diagnosis
- Protocol advice
  - MRI to screen for bone, cord abnormalities
    - Coronal and Sagittal T1WI and T2WI
    - Include craniocervical junction
    - Axial T2WI through areas of suspected abnormality
    - Axial T2WI through conus

  - CT for surgical planning
    - 1-3 mm multidetector CT with reformatted images
    - 3D helpful
  - CT for surgical complications
    - Thin, overlapping sections minimize artifact
    - Bone and soft tissue windows

DIFFERENTIAL DIAGNOSIS

Idiopathic scoliosis
- Classic S-curve scoliosis

Neuromuscular scoliosis
- Neurologic disorders
- Muscular dystrophies
- Usually C-curve

Congenital scoliosis
- Due to abnormal vertebral segmentation
- Morphology of curve highly variable

Scoliosis due to congenital syndromes without vertebral anomalies
- E.g., neurofibromatosis, Marfan, osteogenesis imperfecta, diastrophic dwarfism, Ehlers-Danlos syndrome
- Often complex curvatures

Scoliosis due to infection
- Painful
- Systemic signs may be absent
- Pyogenic bacteria, tuberculosis, fungi
- Usually short curve

Scheuermann disease
- 15% have scoliosis as well as kyphosis
- Scoliosis usually mild

Scoliosis due to tumor
- Painful
- Short curve
- Tumor may be occult on radiography
- Screen with MR

SCOLIOSIS

Scoliosis due to trauma
- Usually see post-traumatic deformity
- Stress fracture may be occult cause

Scoliosis due to radiation
- Usually avoided today by radiation port placement
- Radiation to entire vertebra rather than a portion preferred

Degenerative scoliosis
- Develops in adults
- Degenerative disc disease, facet arthropathy seen
- Can also have secondary degenerative disease from idiopathic scoliosis

Neuropathic spine
- Rapidly developing spine deformity
- Bony destruction seen on radiography

Compensatory scoliosis
- Due to limb length inequality
- Can be diagnosed on spine radiographs by position of iliac crests

Positional scoliosis
- Poor positioning by radiology technologist
- Present on supine radiographs
- Resolves on upright radiographs

Iatrogenic scoliosis
- Rib resection
- Level above lumbar fusion
- Hardware failure

PATHOLOGY

General Features
- Etiology: Causes listed above
- Epidemiology: Common

Gross Pathologic & Surgical Features
- Deformity of trunk visible on physical examination

Staging, Grading or Classification Criteria
- Etiology
- Direction of curve
- Severity of curve

CLINICAL ISSUES

Presentation
- Most common signs/symptoms
  - Visible deformity
  - Idiopathic scoliosis asymptomatic
  - Painful scoliosis indicates underlying abnormality

Demographics
- Age: Usually presents in childhood or adolescence
- Gender: Idiopathic M:F = 1:7

Natural History & Prognosis
- Most scoliosis is mild
- May progress rapidly, especially during growth spurts
- Degenerative disc disease common

- Greatest along concave aspect of scoliosis
- Severe scoliosis
  - Respiratory compromise
  - Neurologic symptoms
  - Instability

Treatment
- Options, risks, complications
  - Observation for minor curves
  - Bracing for curves > 25°
  - Fusion for rapidly progressive curves, curves > 40°

DIAGNOSTIC CHECKLIST

Consider
- Short-curve scoliosis usually has underlying abnormalities

SELECTED REFERENCES

1. Arlet V et al: Congenital scoliosis. Eur Spine J. 12(5):456-63, 2003
2. Daffner SD et al: Adult degenerative lumbar scoliosis. Am J Orthop. 32(2):77-82; discussion 82, 2003
3. Jones KB et al: Spine deformity correction in Marfan syndrome. Spine. 27(18):2003-12, 2002
4. Ahn UM et al: The etiology of adolescent idiopathic scoliosis. Am J Orthop. 31(7):387-95, 2002
5. Cassar-Pullicino VN et al: Imaging in scoliosis: what, why and how? Clin Radiol. 57(7):543-62, 2002
6. Berven S et al: Neuromuscular scoliosis: causes of deformity and principles for evaluation and management. Semin Neurol. 22(2):167-78, 2002
7. Lenke LG et al: Curve prevalence of a new classification of operative adolescent idiopathic scoliosis: does classification correlate with treatment? Spine. 27(6):604-11, 2002
8. Geijer H: Radiation dose and image quality in diagnostic radiology. Optimization of the dose-image quality relationship with clinical experience from scoliosis radiography, coronary intervention and a flat-panel digital detector. Acta Radiol Suppl. 43(427):1-43, 2002
9. Do T: Orthopedic management of the muscular dystrophies. Curr Opin Pediatr. 14(1):50-3, 2002
10. Redla S et al: Magnetic resonance imaging of scoliosis. Clin Radiol. 56(5):360-71, 2001
11. Thomson JD et al: Scoliosis in cerebral palsy: an overview and recent results. J Pediatr Orthop B. 10(1):6-9, 2001
12. Lowe TG et al: Etiology of idiopathic scoliosis: current trends in research. J Bone Joint Surg Am. 82-A(8):1157-68, 2000
13. Jaskwhich D et al: Congenital scoliosis. Curr Opin Pediatr. 12(1):61-6, 2000
14. Mohaideen A et al: Not all rods are Harrington - an overview of spinal instrumentation in scoliosis treatment. Pediatr Radiol. 30(2):110-8, 2000
15. Roach JW: Adolescent idiopathic scoliosis. Orthop Clin North Am. 30(3):353-65, vii-viii, 1999
16. Oestreich AE et al: Scoliosis circa 2000: radiologic imaging perspective. II. Treatment and follow-up. Skeletal Radiol. 27(12):651-6, 1998
17. Oestreich AE et al: Scoliosis circa 2000: radiologic imaging perspective. I. Diagnosis and pretreatment evaluation. Skeletal Radiol. 27(11):591-605, 1998
18. Kim HW et al: Spine update. The management of scoliosis in neurofibromatosis. Spine. 22(23):2770-6, 1997

SCOLIOSIS

IMAGE GALLERY

Typical

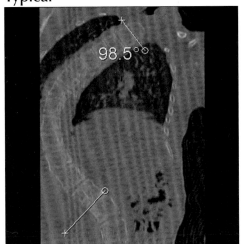
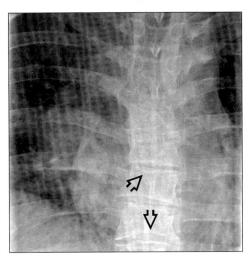

(Left) Coronal bone CT shows method of Cobb. Angle between endplates of terminal vertebrae is 98.5 degrees. Patient with neuromuscular scoliosis due to cerebral palsy. *(Right)* Anteroposterior radiography shows scoliosis due to Scheuermann kyphosis. Curvature is mild. Undulation of endplates can be seen (arrows) but is more readily apparent on lateral radiograph.

Typical

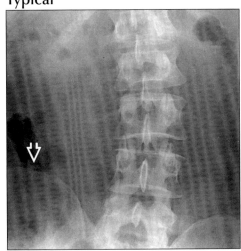
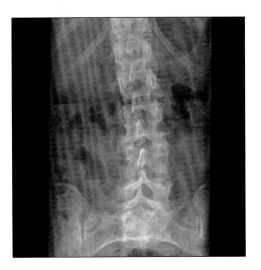

(Left) Posteroanterior radiography shows apparent levoscoliosis. However, right iliac crest (arrow) is higher than left, indicating scoliosis is compensatory for limb length inequality. *(Right)* Anteroposterior radiography shows mild scoliosis in patient with neurofibromatosis. Scoliosis is related to abnormal mesenchymal development not tumor.

Variant

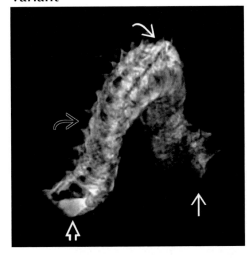
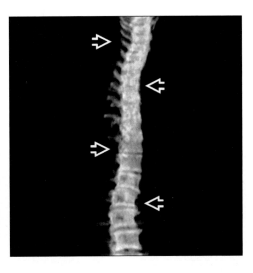

(Left) 3D CT shows complex kyphoscoliosis in Marfan syndrome. Open arrow is on T1 vertebra, white arrow at L5. Curved white arrow is at apex of kyphosis, curved black arrow at apex of thoracic scoliosis. *(Right)* AP 3D CT shows multiple curves in patient with Marfan syndrome. Four separate curves (arrows) are visible. Secondary degenerative changes are evident in the lumbar spine.

IDIOPATHIC SCOLIOSIS

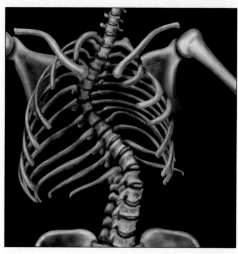

Coronal graphic shows S-curved scoliosis. Marked rotation is evident at apices of the curves, and is reflected in rib deformity.

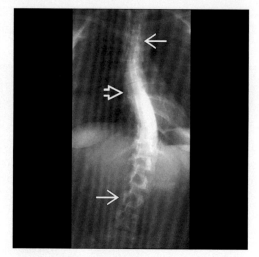

Posteroanterior radiography shows thoracic dextroscoliosis and thoracolumbar levoscoliosis. Arrows point to end vertebrae, open arrow to transitional vertebra.

TERMINOLOGY

Abbreviations and Synonyms
- S-curve scoliosis

Definitions
- Scoliosis of undetermined etiology, without underlying bony or neuromuscular abnormalities
- Primary curvature: Curvature with greatest angulation
- Secondary curvature: One more compensatory curvatures above or below the primary curvature
- Flexible curvature: Curvature which resolves when patient bends to contralateral side
- Structural curvature: Curvature which does not change when patient bends to contralateral side

IMAGING FINDINGS

General Features
- Best diagnostic clue: Smooth, S-shaped spinal curvature of thoracic and lumbar spine
- Location
  - Thoracic, lumbar most common
  - Occasionally involves cervical spine in addition
- Size
  - Curvature of at least 10 degrees
  - Can progress to > 90 degrees

- Morphology
  - Rotation as well as lateral curvature of spine always present
  - Most common pattern is thoracic dextroscoliosis with compensatory lumbar levoscoliosis
  - Usually see two curvatures, sometimes three
  - Thoracic levoscoliosis uncommon ⇒ increased association with underlying abnormalities

Radiographic Findings
- Radiography
  - Long, standing PA radiograph shows thoracic and lumbar spine together
  - Lift used to equalize limb lengths if needed
  - Wedging of vertebrae on concave aspect of curve common, does not indicate spinal anomaly
  - Curvature measured using the method of Cobb on frontal radiograph
  - Kyphosis, lordosis measured on lateral radiograph by angle between endplates
  - Severity of rotation can be only very approximately assessed
  - Lateral bending films distinguish between flexible and structural components of curve
    - Primary curve usually structural
    - Secondary curve usually flexible, but may become structural over time
  - Lateral radiograph important to show kyphosis and lordosis

DDx: Idiopathic Scoliosis

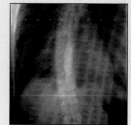

Neuromuscular

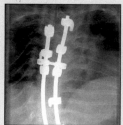

Osteogenesis

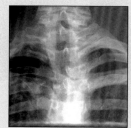

Congenital

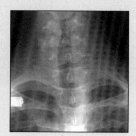

Osteoid Osteoma

IDIOPATHIC SCOLIOSIS

Key Facts

Terminology
- Scoliosis of undetermined etiology, without underlying bony or neuromuscular abnormalities

Imaging Findings
- Best diagnostic clue: Smooth, S-shaped spinal curvature of thoracic and lumbar spine
- Rotation as well as lateral curvature of spine always present
- Most common pattern is thoracic dextroscoliosis with compensatory lumbar levoscoliosis
- Usually see two curvatures, sometimes three
- Thoracic levoscoliosis uncommon ⇒ increased association with underlying abnormalities

Top Differential Diagnoses
- Neuromuscular scoliosis

- Scoliosis due to tumor
- Congenital scoliosis
- Scoliosis due to infection
- Scoliosis due to congenital syndromes
- Limb length inequality
- Degenerative scoliosis

Pathology
- Epidemiology: F:M = 7:1
- Spondylolysis at L5 common

Diagnostic Checklist
- Levoscoliosis of thoracic spine has higher incidence of syringomyelia, spinal cord tumors
- If scoliosis is painful, look for underlying cause; idiopathic scoliosis is not painful

---

- Often see loss of normal thoracic kyphosis and lumbar lordosis
- Thoracolumbar or lumbar kyphosis may be present
- Post-operative assessment
  - Evaluate correction of curvature
  - Monitor for loss of correction indicating failure of fusion
  - Posterolateral fusion mass best seen on concave aspect of curve
  - Fusion mass underestimated on radiographs, better seen on CT
  - Fracture of fixation rods indicates failure of fusion
  - Hooks may become dislodged from rods or from laminae

CT Findings
- Bone CT
  - Used to exclude vertebral anomalies, tumors
  - Rotary component of scoliosis can be assessed
    - 3D imaging shows rotary component most readily
  - Useful to evaluate success of spinal fusion
    - Bone graft matures to form cortex, medullary bone which merges with adjacent vertebral structures
    - Hardware fracture, gaps in fusion mass best seen on coronal, sagittal reformatted images

MR Findings
- T1WI
  - Used to exclude vertebral anomalies, bone tumor, or filum terminale lipoma
  - Fusion mass in postoperative patients poorly seen
- T2WI: Used to evaluate conus and exclude syrinx, tethered cord, or lipoma

Nuclear Medicine Findings
- Bone Scan: Used to exclude underlying bony abnormality, but nonspecific; CT or MR preferable

Imaging Recommendations
- Best imaging tool: Radiography
- Protocol advice: MRI should include coronal T1WI or PDWI to evaluate vertebral bodies

DIFFERENTIAL DIAGNOSIS

Neuromuscular scoliosis
- Usually single, long thoracolumbar curve

Scoliosis due to tumor
- Short curve, painful

Congenital scoliosis
- Vertebral anomalies present

Scoliosis due to infection
- Short curve, painful
- Infection may be in disc or paraspinous tissues
- Radiography shows endplate destruction, disc space narrowing

Scheuermann disease
- Scoliosis seen in 15%
- Lateral radiographs show kyphosis, endplate abnormalities and vertebral wedging

Scoliosis due to congenital syndromes
- E.g., Neurofibromatosis, Marfan, osteogenesis imperfecta, diastrophic dwarfism, Ehlers-Danlos syndrome

Scoliosis due to trauma
- Short curve scoliosis, characteristic vertebral body deformity

Scoliosis due to radiation
- Short curve scoliosis, vertebral hypoplasia, history of radiation

Limb length inequality
- Check heights of iliac wings on standing films

Degenerative scoliosis
- Arises later in adulthood, usually lumbar

IDIOPATHIC SCOLIOSIS

PATHOLOGY

General Features
- Genetics: Strong familial component with multifactorial inheritance
- Etiology: unknown, probably multifactorial
- Epidemiology: F:M = 7:1
- Associated abnormalities
  - Spondylolysis at L5 common
    - Important to identify pre-operatively to plan fusion levels

Gross Pathologic & Surgical Features
- Lateral curvature plus rotation
- Concave side of scoliosis often mildly hypoplastic
- Thoracic kyphosis and lumbar lordosis often straightened or reversed

Microscopic Features
- Bone normal histologically

Staging, Grading or Classification Criteria
- Infantile type: Onset before age of 4
  - Rare; usually resolves unless severe
- Juvenile type: Onset ages 4 to 9
  - Uncommon; almost always progresses
- Adolescent type: Onset 10 years to skeletal maturity
  - Most common type; usually diagnosed at puberty
- Since scoliosis usually will not progress after skeletal maturity, assessment of bone age important
- Skeletal maturity assessed by Risser method, based on apophysis of iliac wing
  - Apophysis not present = stage 0
  - Apophysis covers lateral 25% iliac wing = stage 1: Bone age 13 y, 8 mo (f); 14 y, 7 mo (m)
  - Apophysis covers lateral 50% iliac wing = stage 2: Bone age 14 y, 6 mo (f); 15 y, 7 mo (m)
  - Apophysis covers 75% iliac wing = stage 3: Bone age 15 y, 2 mo (f); 16 y, 2 mo (m)
  - Apophysis covers entire iliac wing = stage 4: Bone age 16 y, 2 mo (f); 17 y, 0 mo (m)
  - Apophysis fused = stage 5: Bone age 18 y, 1 mo (f); 18 y, 6 mo (m)
- Risser method less accurate than hand radiographs

CLINICAL ISSUES

Presentation
- Most common signs/symptoms
  - Asymptomatic
  - Diagnosed on physical exam with patient leaning forward

Demographics
- Age: Onset in infancy, childhood or adolescence
- Gender: F:M = 7:1

Natural History & Prognosis
- Curve often progresses during growth spurts
- Curve usually will not progress after skeletal maturity unless greater than 40-50 degrees
- Respiratory compromise seen with severe scoliosis
- Degenerative disc disease, sacroiliac arthritis develop in adults

Treatment
- Options, risks, complications
  - Observation used for curves < 20-25°
  - Bracing first treatment option
  - Fusion for severe or rapidly progressive scoliosis
    - Generally reserved for scoliosis of about 40° or greater
    - Posterior fusion with fixation rods
    - Most fixation rods currently in use are not Harrington rods; use generic term
    - Anterior fusion from lateral aspect of vertebral bodies
  - Complications of fusion include
    - Failure of fusion
    - Deformity, degenerative changes adjacent to fused levels
    - Infection
  - Crankshaft phenomenon
    - Posterior fusion in skeletally immature patients may act as a tether posteriorly
    - Growth continues anteriorly
    - Results in lordosis, progressive scoliosis
    - Change of > 10° diagnostic

DIAGNOSTIC CHECKLIST

Consider
- Levoscoliosis of thoracic spine has higher incidence of syringomyelia, spinal cord tumors

Image Interpretation Pearls
- If scoliosis is painful, look for underlying cause; idiopathic scoliosis is not painful

SELECTED REFERENCES

1. Bagchi K et al: Hardware complications in scoliosis surgery. Pediatr Radiol. 32(7):465-75, 2002
2. Redla S et al: Magnetic resonance imaging of scoliosis. Clin Radiol. 56(5):360-71, 2001
3. Lowe TG et al: Etiology of idiopathic scoliosis: current trends in research. J Bone Joint Surg Am. 82-A(8):1157-68, 2000
4. Mohaideen A et al: Not all rods are Harrington - an overview of spinal instrumentation in scoliosis treatment. Pediatr Radiol. 30(2):110-8, 2000
5. Roach JW: Adolescent idiopathic scoliosis. Orthop Clin North Am. 30(3):353-65, vii-viii, 1999
6. Oestreich AE et al: Scoliosis circa 2000: radiologic imaging perspective. II. Treatment and follow-up. Skeletal Radiol. 27(12):651-6, 1998
7. Oestreich AE et al: Scoliosis circa 2000: radiologic imaging perspective. I. Diagnosis and pretreatment evaluation. Skeletal Radiol. 27(11):591-605, 1998
8. Lee CS et al: The crankshaft phenomenon after posterior Harrington fusion in skeletally immature patients with thoracic or thoracolumbar idiopathic scoliosis followed to maturity. Spine. 22(1):58-67, 1997
9. Cordover AM et al: Natural history of adolescent thoracolumbar and lumbar idiopathic scoliosis into adulthood. J Spinal Disord. 10(3):193-6, 1997
10. Little DG et al: The Risser sign: a critical analysis. J Pediatr Orthop. 14(5):569-75, 1994

IMAGE GALLERY

Typical

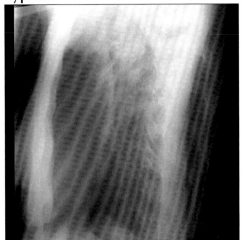
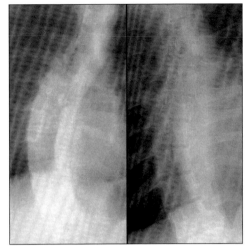

(Left) Lateral radiography shows thoracic lordosis in adult patient with idiopathic scoliosis. Note marked rotation of ribs reflecting vertebral body rotation. *(Right)* Posteroanterior radiography shows dextroscoliosis improves from neutral position (left image) when patient bends to right. Residual curve (right image) indicates structural component of scoliosis.

Typical

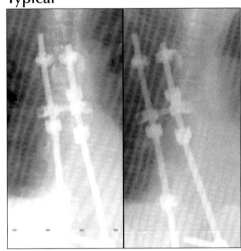
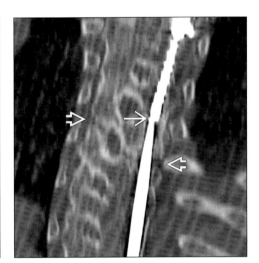

(Left) Anteroposterior radiography shows failure of posterior fusion for scoliosis. Left image shows appearance immediately postoperatively, right shows subsequent displacement of multiple laminar hooks. *(Right)* Coronal bone CT shows fracture (arrow) of unilateral posterior fixation rod. Failed bony fusion is readily apparent as a cleft (open arrows) in the otherwise solid fusion mass.

Variant

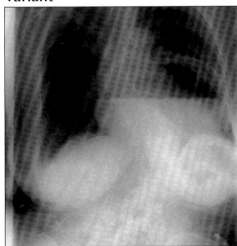
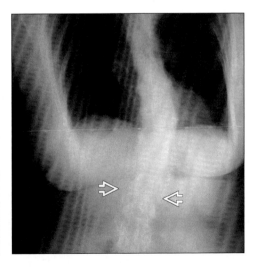

(Left) Anteroposterior radiography shows a 40 year old female with untreated idiopathic scoliosis and superimposed degenerative lumbar scoliosis. *(Right)* Posteroanterior radiography shows thoracolumbar levoscoliosis and lumbar dextroscoliosis. Left lateral listhesis at L1-L2 (arrows) is due to superimposed degenerative arthritis.

CONGENITAL SCOLIOSIS AND KYPHOSIS

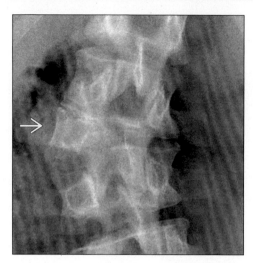

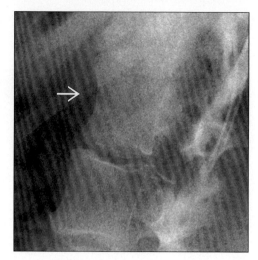

Anteroposterior radiography shows right-sided hemivertebra (arrow) at apex of focal scoliosis. It is fused to vertebra above it.

Lateral radiography demonstrates fused L1 and L2 vertebrae (arrow). Affected vertebrae are narrow in AP dimension and slightly wedged, and posterior elements are also fused.

TERMINOLOGY

Definitions
- Spinal curvature secondary to vertebral anomalies
- Hemivertebra: Unilateral or anterior vertebral hypoplasia
- Butterfly vertebra: Central vertebral cleft due to failure of central vertebral body development
- "Fused" vertebrae: Embryological failure of segmentation rather than fusion
  - Also called block vertebrae; may affect vertebral body, posterior elements, or both
  - Affected vertebrae narrow in mediolateral and anteroposterior dimensions
  - Rudimentary disc may be present
- Vertebral bar
  - Bony or cartilaginous connection between adjacent vertebrae
  - Often associated with rib fusions
- Klippel-Feil syndrome: Multiple cervical segmentation anomalies

IMAGING FINDINGS

General Features
- Best diagnostic clue: Vertebral anomaly in patient with scoliosis or kyphosis

- Location: Most common in thoracic spine, but can occur at any level
- Morphology
  - Usually short curve scoliosis
  - May have multiple curves if multiple anomalies present

Radiographic Findings
- Radiography
  - Screening with full spine PA and lateral radiographs
  - Vertebral anomalies often difficult to see; use coned-down radiographs, MR or CT to clarify

CT Findings
- Bone CT
  - Similar osseous findings to radiography
  - Coronal and sagittal reformatted images essential
  - 3D imaging helpful for surgical planning
    - Excellent correlation to surgical findings
  - Pearl: Vertebral bars may be cartilaginous in young children

MR Findings
- Coronal and sagittal images of entire spine necesary
  - Similar morphological findings to CT
- Use T1WI or PDWI to evaluate bone morphology, exclude tumor or Chiari I malformation
- T2WI, STIR to evaluate for tethered cord, syrinx, tumor

DDx: Congenital Scoliosis

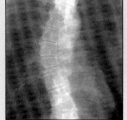

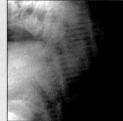

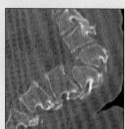

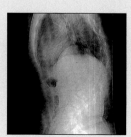

Idiopathic

Tuberculosis

Achondroplasia

Marfan Syndrome

CONGENITAL SCOLIOSIS AND KYPHOSIS

Key Facts

Terminology
- Spinal curvature secondary to vertebral anomalies

Imaging Findings
- Location: Most common in thoracic spine, but can occur at any level
- Usually short curve scoliosis
- May have multiple curves if multiple anomalies present
- Screening with full spine PA and lateral radiographs
- Vertebral anomalies often difficult to see; use coned-down radiographs, MR or CT to clarify

Top Differential Diagnoses
- Idiopathic scoliosis
- Neuromuscular scoliosis
- Scoliosis due to infection
- Scoliosis due to syndromes
- Scoliosis due to trauma
- Scoliosis due to radiation
- Limb length inequality
- Idiopathic kyphosis
- Scheuermann kyphosis
- Kyphosis due to tuberculosis
- Juvenile chronic arthritis

Pathology
- Abnormalities due either to failure of development and/or failure of segmentation

Clinical Issues
- Fusion of congenital kyphosis to prevent paralysis
- Surgery for scoliotic curves progressing more than 10 degrees per year

Imaging Recommendations
- Multiplanar MRI best modality to evaluate full spine in children
  - Avoids CT radiation dose, excludes associated neural axis abnormalites
- CT preferable for surgical planning in adults because of superior spatial resolution, 3D rendering capabilities

DIFFERENTIAL DIAGNOSIS

Idiopathic scoliosis
- S-shaped curve, no anomalies

Neuromuscular scoliosis
- Usually single, long thoracolumbar curve

Scoliosis due to infection
- Short curve, painful
- Infection may be in disc or paraspinous tissues
- May result in vertebral body fusion

Scoliosis due to syndromes
- E.g, neurofibromatosis, Marfan, osteogenesis imperfecta, diastrophic dwarfism, Ehlers-Danlos syndrome

Scoliosis due to trauma
- Short curve scoliosis, vertebral body deformity, soft tissue traumatic changes

Scoliosis due to radiation
- Short curve scoliosis, vertebral hypoplasia, history of radiation

Limb length inequality
- Check heights of iliac wings on standing films
- Use lifts under foot to equalize lengths, evaluate true scoliosis

Idiopathic kyphosis
- Vertebral anomalies absent

Scheuermann kyphosis
- Wedging of vertebral bodies, undulation of endplates
- 15% have scoliosis as well as kyphosis

Kyphosis due to tuberculosis
- Kyphosis may be severe ("gibbus") deformity
- Spinal fusion may develop
- Paraspinous cold abscess, endplate destruction

Juvenile chronic arthritis
- Fusion of vertebral bodies and facet joints
- Scoliosis or kyphosis may be present
- Onset later in childhood

Ankylosing spondylitis
- Syndesmophytes at anterior vertebral margin mimic congenital bar
- Kyphosis of upper thoracic spine
- Usually adult onset

PATHOLOGY

General Features
- General path comments
  - Abnormalities due either to failure of development and/or failure of segmentation
  - Failure of vertebral body development
    - Hypoplastic vertebra anteriorly or on one side (wedge vertebra)
    - Aplastic vertebra anteriorly or on one side (hemivertebra)
    - Butterfly vertebra: Central cleft
  - Failure of vertebral segmentation
    - Vertebral body forms from half of two adjacent sclerotomes
    - Therefore apparent congenital fusion of vertebrae is really failure of segmentation
    - May involve vertebral body, posterior elements, or both
  - Failure of development and of segmentation may both be present
    - Hemivertebra may be fused to adjacent vertebra

CONGENITAL SCOLIOSIS AND KYPHOSIS

- ○ Supernumerary hemivertebrae
- Genetics
  - ○ Sometimes associated with chromosomal abnormalities
  - ○ Usually not inherited
- Etiology: Fetal insult in 1st trimester causing abnormal development and/or segmentation of vertebrae
- Epidemiology: Sporadic, uncommon
- Associated abnormalities
  - ○ Klippel Feil associated with craniocervical anomalies, brainstem anomalies
  - ○ Syringohydromyelia
  - ○ Diastematomyelia
  - ○ Tethered spinal cord
  - ○ Caudal regression
  - ○ Component of VACTERL association
    - Incidence of VACTERL 1.6/10,000 live births
    - Defective mesodermal development in early embryogenesis
    - Some cases inherited, some due to fetal insult
    - Patients have at least 3 of the following: Vertebral anomalies (37%), anal atresia (63%), cardiac anomalies (77%), tracheo-esophageal fistula (40%), renal and genitourinary anomalies (72%), radial ray hypoplasia (58%)
    - Hydrocephalus may occur

Gross Pathologic & Surgical Features

- Bar between vertebrae may be either cartilaginous or bony

Microscopic Features

- Bone histologically normal

Staging, Grading or Classification Criteria

- Classified by types and number of segmentation abnormalities present

CLINICAL ISSUES

Presentation

- Most common signs/symptoms: Visible spinal axis deformity
- Clinical profile: May be isolated anomaly or associated with multisystem anomalies (VACTERL)

Demographics

- Age: Present at birth, but may not be evident clinically until later in childhood or adolescence
- Gender: M = F

Natural History & Prognosis

- Kyphosis
  - ○ Kyphosis tends to progress without treatment; fusion during childhood indicated
  - ○ May lead to cord compression, paralysis
- Scoliosis
  - ○ Difficult to predict which curves will progress
  - ○ Balanced anomalies may grow fairly normally
    - E.g., contralateral hemivertebrae at adjacent levels
  - ○ Hemivertebra not fused to adjacent levels causes rapidly progressive curve
  - ○ Hemivertebra with contralateral failure of segmentation causes rapidly progressive curve

Treatment

- Close clinical observation of scoliosis for progression
- Brace limited utility
- Fusion of congenital kyphosis to prevent paralysis
- Surgery for scoliotic curves progressing more than 10 degrees per year
  - ○ Anterior or posterior fusion with instrumentation
  - ○ Resection of vertebral bars, hemivertebrae
  - ○ Hemiepiphysiodesis: Fuse growth plate on one side to prevent progression of curve

DIAGNOSTIC CHECKLIST

Image Interpretation Pearls

- Bony bar probably present when see angular curve on radiography without hemivertebra: Evaluate with MR or CT
- Neural arch not fused in midline until approximately age 2; cleft on AP radiograph must not be confused with spinal anomaly
- Image entire spine to exclude additional bone or cord abnormalities, Chiari I malformation

SELECTED REFERENCES

1. Arlet V et al: Congenital scoliosis. Eur Spine J. 12(5):456-63, 2003
2. Hedequist DJ et al: The correlation of preoperative three-dimensional computed tomography reconstructions with operative findings in congenital scoliosis. Spine. 28(22):2531-4; discussion 1, 2003
3. Campbell RM Jr et al: Growth of the thoracic spine in congenital scoliosis after expansion thoracoplasty. J Bone Joint Surg Am. 85-A(3):409-20, 2003
4. Redla S et al: Magnetic resonance imaging of scoliosis. Clin Radiol. 56(5):360-71, 2001
5. Kim YJ et al: Surgical treatment of congenital kyphosis. Spine. 26(20):2251-7, 2001
6. Jaskwhich D et al: Congenital scoliosis. Curr Opin Pediatr. 12(1):61-6, 2000
7. Oestreich AE et al: Scoliosis circa 2000: radiologic imaging perspective. II. Treatment and follow-up. Skeletal Radiol. 27(12):651-6, 1998
8. Oestreich AE et al: Scoliosis circa 2000: radiologic imaging perspective. I. Diagnosis and pretreatment evaluation. Skeletal Radiol. 27(11):591-605, 1998
9. Rittler M et al: VACTERL association, epidemiologic definition and delineation. Am J Med Genet. 63(4):529-36, 1996
10. Levine F et al: VACTERL association with high prenatal lead exposure: similarities to animal models of lead teratogenicity. Pediatrics. 87(3):390-2, 1991
11. Evans JA et al: VACTERL with hydrocephalus: further delineation of the syndrome(s) Am J Med Genet. 34(2):177-82, 1989
12. Taybi H, Lachman RS: Radiology of syndromes, metabolic disorders, and skeletal dysplasias. 4th ed. St. Louis, Mosby. 510-12, 1996

CONGENITAL SCOLIOSIS AND KYPHOSIS

IMAGE GALLERY

Typical

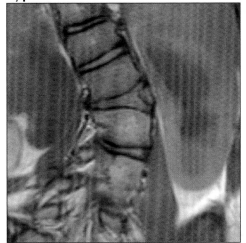
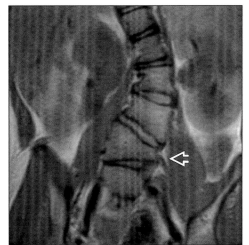

(Left) Coronal T1WI MR shows left hemivertebra with disc above and below, indicating high risk for curve progression. Hydronephrosis is also present in this patient with VACTERL. *(Right)* Coronal T1WI MR reveals a hypoplastic left L4 vertebral body (arrow) that balances left hemivertebra above it (not shown). Patient also had sacral hypoplasia (VACTERL).

Typical

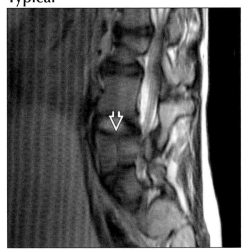
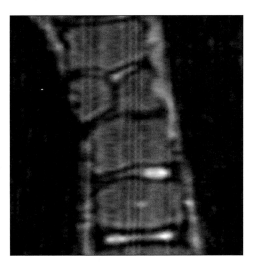

(Left) Sagittal T2WI MR depicts a coronal L4 vertebral body cleft (arrow) in young child. There is as yet no growth deformity and the child may be monitored clinically. *(Right)* Coronal T2WI MR shows butterfly thoracic vertebra in young child with multiple segmentation anomalies. No definite disc is seen below this vertebra, reflecting incomplete segmentation.

Typical

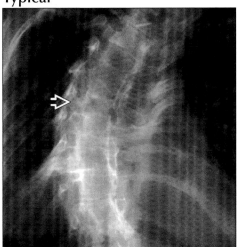
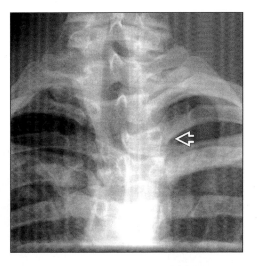

(Left) Anteroposterior radiography shows failure of segmentation of multiple thoracic vertebrae. Right sided hemivertebra (arrow) is present. There may be fusion of left-sided ribs. *(Right)* Anteroposterior radiography shows butterfly vertebra (arrow). Right side is fused to vertebra below, while left side has disc space above and below, indicating high risk for childhood progression.

NEUROMUSCULAR SCOLIOSIS

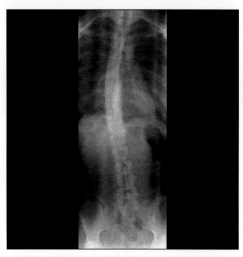

Anteroposterior radiography shows a mild, C-curve dextroscoliosis extending from upper thoracic to midlumbar region in a cerebral palsy patient.

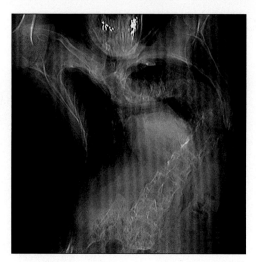

Anteroposterior radiography shows severe C-curve levoscoliosis in patient with cerebral palsy and paraplegia. Pelvic tilt reflects patient's sitting position. Note decreased lung volumes.

TERMINOLOGY

Abbreviations and Synonyms
- Neurogenic scoliosis

Definitions
- Scoliosis due to neurologic or myopathic diseases

IMAGING FINDINGS

General Features
- Best diagnostic clue: Long, single curve scoliosis
- Location: Thoracic and lumbar
- Size: > 10 degrees

Radiographic Findings
- Radiography
  - Single long curve, usually centered at thoracolumbar junction
  - Lateral radiograph often shows persistence of infantile kyphosis or thoracic lordosis

MR Findings
- Use to evaluate for cord, bone abnormalities

Imaging Recommendations
- Best imaging tool: Radiography and MRI
- Protocol advice
  - Sagittal T1WI and STIR, coronal T1WI through entire spine including craniocervical junction
  - Axial T2WI images through conus, syringomyelia (if present)

DIFFERENTIAL DIAGNOSIS

Idiopathic scoliosis
- S-shaped curve

Scoliosis due to tumor or infection
- Short curve, painful

Congenital scoliosis
- Vertebral anomalies present

Scheuermann disease
- Mild scoliosis, abnormal vertebral endplates

Scoliosis related to syndromes
- E.g., neurofibromatosis, Marfan, osteogenesis imperfecta, diastrophic dwarfism, Ehlers-Danlos syndrome

Scoliosis due to radiation
- Radiation history critical

DDx: Neuromuscular Scoliosis

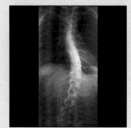

Idiopathic

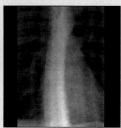

Scheuermann

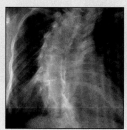

Congenital

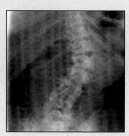

Neoplastic

NEUROMUSCULAR SCOLIOSIS

Key Facts

Terminology
• Scoliosis due to neurologic or myopathic diseases

Imaging Findings
• Single long curve, usually centered at thoracolumbar junction

Top Differential Diagnoses
• Idiopathic scoliosis

• Congenital scoliosis
• Scoliosis related to syndromes

Pathology
• Rigid curve

Clinical Issues
• Most difficult scoliosis to treat nonoperatively or surgically

---

Limb length inequality
• Compensatory scoliosis; look at iliac crest levels to diagnose

PATHOLOGY

General Features
• General path comments: Secondary to neurogenic causes or myopathy
• Etiology
  ○ Neurogenic causes
    ▪ Cerebral palsy
    ▪ Spinal cord tumor
    ▪ Syringomyelia
    ▪ Traumatic paralysis
    ▪ Poliomyelitis
    ▪ Myelomeningocele
    ▪ Charcot-Marie-Tooth disease
  ○ Myopathic causes
    ▪ Duchenne muscular dystrophy
    ▪ Spinal muscular atrophy
    ▪ Friedreich ataxia
    ▪ Arthrogryposis multiplex congenita
• Epidemiology: 20% of cerebral palsy patients
• Associated abnormalities
  ○ Syringomyelia, spinal dysraphism, tethered cord
  ○ Kyphosis or lordosis

Gross Pathologic & Surgical Features
• Rigid curve

Staging, Grading or Classification Criteria
• Minor curve: < 20 degrees
• Significant curve: > 20 degrees

CLINICAL ISSUES

Presentation
• Most common signs/symptoms
  ○ Rapidly progressive curvature
  ○ Other signs/symptoms
    ▪ Respiratory compromise

Demographics
• Age: Onset in infancy or childhood; may progress in adulthood
• Gender: M = F

Natural History & Prognosis
• Progresses rapidly → respiratory compromise
• Most difficult scoliosis to treat nonoperatively or surgically

Treatment
• Options, risks, complications
  ○ Bracing for minor curves; usually does not halt progression
  ○ Surgical fusion has higher complication rate than other scolioses

DIAGNOSTIC CHECKLIST

Consider
• Screening full spine MRI to exclude spinal cord or bony abnormalities

SELECTED REFERENCES

1. Do T: Orthopedic management of the muscular dystrophies. Curr Opin Pediatr. 14(1):50-3, 2002
2. Berven S et al: Neuromuscular scoliosis: causes of deformity and principles for evaluation and management. Semin Neurol. 22(2):167-78, 2002
3. Thomson JD et al: Scoliosis in cerebral palsy: an overview and recent results. J Pediatr Orthop B. 10(1):6-9, 2001
4. Redla S et al: Magnetic resonance imaging of scoliosis. Clin Radiol. 56(5):360-71, 2001

IMAGE GALLERY

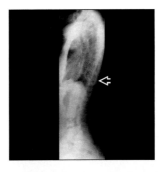 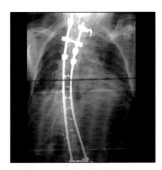

(Left) Lateral radiography shows loss of thoracic kyphosis and lumbar lordosis in cerebral palsy patient. Vertebral body rotation is reflected in posterior displacement of ribs on one side *(arrow)*. *(Right)* Anteroposterior radiography shows long segment fixation of scoliosis in cerebral palsy patient. Failure of fusion is more common than with idiopathic scoliosis, & close imaging follow-up is prudent.

IDIOPATHIC KYPHOSIS

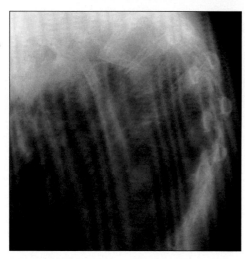

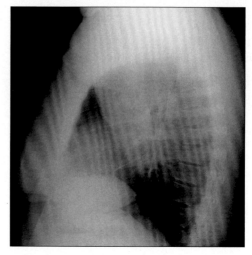

Lateral radiography shows marked kyphosis of the upper thoracic spine in 30 year old patient. Premature degenerative disc disease is present, with minimal wedging of vertebral bodies.

Lateral radiography shows patient with 35 degrees of kyphosis, near the upper limits of normal. Note that normal kyphosis is greatest in the upper thoracic spine.

TERMINOLOGY

Abbreviations and Synonyms
- Synonyms: Postural kyphosis, round back deformity

Definitions
- Thoracic kyphosis without underlying structural abnormality

IMAGING FINDINGS

General Features
- Best diagnostic clue: Thoracic kyphosis greater than approximately 40 degrees
- Location: Upper to mid-thoracic spine
- Size: > 40 degrees
- Morphology
  - Smooth, nonangular curvature
  - Rarely severe

Radiographic Findings
- Radiography
  - PA and lateral full spine or thoracic spine
    - Patient upright
    - PA to exclude scoliosis
  - Vertebral morphology usually normal
    - May have mild anterior wedging with normal endplates
  - Kyphosis measured from superior endplate of T3 to inferior endplate of T12
  - Wide variability in normal thoracic kyphosis
    - Kyphosis is normally less pronounced in children, increases in adolescence
    - Normal kyphosis in adolescence < 40 degrees
  - Interobserver variability measurement ≈ 9 degrees
  - Lateral radiograph in hyperextension to evaluate flexibility of curve

CT Findings
- Bone CT
  - Endplates are normal and vertebral anomalies are absent

MR Findings
- Premature degenerative disc disease
- Discogenic sclerosis common

Imaging Recommendations
- Best imaging tool: Radiography
- Protocol advice: MR or CT to exclude underlying bone abnormality

DIFFERENTIAL DIAGNOSIS

Scheuermann kyphosis
- Presents in adolescence

DDx: Idiopathic Kyphosis

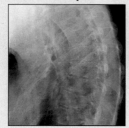

Scheuermann

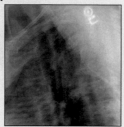

Ankylosing Spondylitis

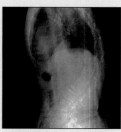

Marfan Syndrome

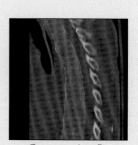

Compression Fx

IDIOPATHIC KYPHOSIS

Key Facts

Terminology
- Synonyms: Postural kyphosis, round back deformity

Imaging Findings
- Best diagnostic clue: Thoracic kyphosis greater than approximately 40 degrees
- Location: Upper to mid-thoracic spine
- Smooth, nonangular curvature

Top Differential Diagnoses
- Scheuermann kyphosis
- Congenital kyphosis
- Post-traumatic kyphosis

Pathology
- Curve usually flexible
- Curve may become structural if left unaddressed

- Wedging of 3 adjacent vertebral bodies, endplate irregularities, Schmorl nodes

Congenital kyphosis
- Anterior bony intervertebral bars may not present until adolescence

Post-traumatic kyphosis
- Vertebral body traumatic deformity

Insufficiency fractures
- Deformity of anterior vertebral cortex

Ankylosing spondylitis (AS)
- Thin syndesmophytes between vertebrae, facet ankylosis

Neuromuscular disease
- Persistence of infantile kyphosis

Infection
- Short curve +/- inflammatory mass

PATHOLOGY

General Features
- Etiology: Secondary to poor posture
- Epidemiology: Common

Gross Pathologic & Surgical Features
- Curve usually flexible
- Curve may become structural if left unaddressed

Microscopic Features
- Bone morphologically normal

CLINICAL ISSUES

Presentation
- Most common signs/symptoms
  - Asymptomatic
  - Stooped shoulders

Demographics
- Age: Adolescents
- Gender: More common in females

Natural History & Prognosis
- Premature development of thoracic degenerative disc disease

Treatment
- Exercise
- Brace decreases kyphosis, but kyphosis tends to recur

DIAGNOSTIC CHECKLIST

Consider
- A diagnosis of exclusion

Image Interpretation Pearls
- Congenital bars causing kyphosis may be occult on radiography; evaluate with MRI

SELECTED REFERENCES

1. Elder DA et al: Kyphosis in a Turner syndrome population. Pediatrics. 109(6):e93, 2002
2. Tala VT et al: Postural kyphosis and Scheuermann's disease. Seminars in Spine Surgery 4:216-24, 1992
3. Gutowski WT et al: Orthotic results in adolescent kyphosis. Spine. 13(5):485-9, 1988
4. Propst-Proctor SL et al: Radiographic determination of lordosis and kyphosis in normal and scoliotic children. J Pediatr Orthop. 3(3):344-6, 1983
5. Luque ER: The correction of postural curves of the spine. Spine. 7(3):270-5, 1982

IMAGE GALLERY

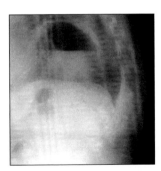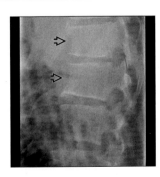

(Left) Lateral radiography shows idiopathic kyphosis compounded in an older patient by degenerative disc disease. (Right) Lateral radiography shows physiologic wedging (arrows), a normal phenomenon, at T12 and L1. Overall thoracic curvature was normal.

SCHMORL NODE

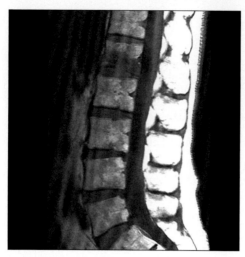

Sagittal T1WI MR shows focal undersurface end plate defect filled by disc material with low signal intensity of adjacent marrow suggesting recent event in patient with focal back pain.

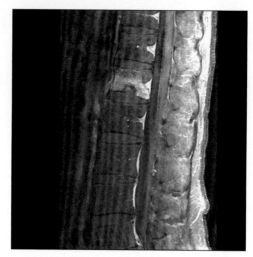

Sagittal T1 C+ MR with fat-saturation shows diffuse marrow enhancement surrounding disc extending through inferior end plate defect in patient with focal pain.

TERMINOLOGY

Abbreviations and Synonyms
- Intravertebral disc herniation

Definitions
- Node within vertebral body (VB) due to vertical disc extension through weakened VB endplate

IMAGING FINDINGS

General Features
- Best diagnostic clue: Focal invagination of endplate by disc material surrounded by either sclerotic (old), or abnormal (acute) bone
- Location: T-8 to L1 region most common
- Size: Varies from several millimeters to "giant"
- Morphology: Typically upwardly round or cone shaped defect contiguous with disc space

Radiographic Findings
- Radiography: Contour defect within endplate, extending from disc space into VB spongiosa with well-corticated margins

CT Findings
- NECT

  ○ Island of low density surrounded by condensed bone on axial slice through VB
  ○ Sagittal reformation shows end plate defect contiguous with disc space, capped by sclerotic bone
- Bone CT
  ○ Same as NECT
  ○ Schmorl node may calcify

MR Findings
- T1WI
  ○ Focal defect in end plate filled by disc
  ○ Low signal in adjacent marrow if acute
- T2WI: High signal in adjacent marrow if acute
- STIR: Accentuates edema if acute
- T1 C+
  ○ Localized marginal contrast-enhancement in subacute stage
  ○ Diffuse marrow enhancement in acute stage

Nuclear Medicine Findings
- Bone Scan: "Hot" in acute cases

Imaging Recommendations
- Analyze contiguity with parent disc on all sequences

DDx: Nodes Adjacent to Endplate

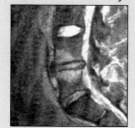
Type II Change

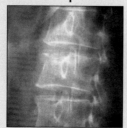
End Plate Fracture

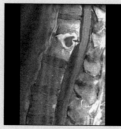
Discitis

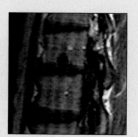
Bone Island

SCHMORL NODE

Key Facts

Terminology
- Intravertebral disc herniation

Imaging Findings
- Location: T-8 to L1 region most common
- Radiography: Contour defect within endplate, extending from disc space into VB spongiosa with well-corticated margins
- Low signal in adjacent marrow if acute
- T2WI: High signal in adjacent marrow if acute
- Localized marginal contrast-enhancement in subacute stage
- Diffuse marrow enhancement in acute stage

Top Differential Diagnoses
- Type II endplate change
- Discitis

- Limbus vertebrae
- Bone island

Pathology
- Developmental, degenerative, traumatic, and disease influences
- Typically repetitive stress of gravity on immature endplate
- Acute axial traumatic load can lead to Schmorl node formation with focal back pain
- Osteoporosis, neoplasm, and infection can weaken endplate
- Seen in up to 75% of all normal spines
- Most acute cases occur in 11-30 year old individuals

DIFFERENTIAL DIAGNOSIS

Acute compression fracture
- Simulates diffuse edema of acute Schmorl node, may in fact predispose to its ultimate formation
- Lacks imploded disc nodule within abnormal marrow

Type II endplate change
- Seen as reactive change to disc degeneration, typically both adjacent VBs affected
- Represent granulation tissue and edema incited by the degenerating disc
- Edema replaced by fat on follow-up studies
- No focal end plate defect

Discitis
- Both endplates show defect
- Disc signal diffusely abnormal

Limbus vertebrae
- Seen only at VB corners
- Truncated anterior margin of VB
- Bone fragments anterior to defect

Bone island
- Sclerotic nodule
- No endplate defect

Focal fatty marrow
- Hyperintense on T1WI

Focal metastasis
- Does not show contiguity with parent disc or its signal intensity

PATHOLOGY

General Features
- General path comments
  - Cartilaginous disc tissue with degenerative or inflammatory changes
    - The pathologic staging mirrors that of a focal endplate fracture

  - The typical Schmorl node is a healed focal endplate fracture
  - Embryology-anatomy
    - Anulus actually biomechanically more resistant to mechanical failure than endplate in young individuals
    - Focal weakness of endplate predisposes to Schmorl node formation
    - Associated with endplate weakening of Scheuermann disease
- Etiology
  - Developmental, degenerative, traumatic, and disease influences
  - Typically repetitive stress of gravity on immature endplate
  - Acute axial traumatic load can lead to Schmorl node formation with focal back pain
  - Osteoporosis, neoplasm, and infection can weaken endplate
- Epidemiology
  - Seen in up to 75% of all normal spines
  - Most acute cases occur in 11-30 year old individuals
  - Can occur with single traumatic episode

Gross Pathologic & Surgical Features
- Identical to end plate fracture

Microscopic Features
- Fibrocartilaginous tissue surrounded by marrow with sclerotic cancellous bone or inflammatory changes

Staging, Grading or Classification Criteria
- Edema of VB next to endplate with acute trauma, pain, no end plate defect on initial MR
- Subsequent formation of a chronic and asymptomatic Schmorl node on follow-up MR

CLINICAL ISSUES

Presentation
- Most common signs/symptoms
  - Sudden onset, localized, non-radiating pain and tenderness in acute cases

SCHMORL NODE

- Most cases found incidentally as chronic, "burned out" lesions
- Clinical profile
  - Teenager involved in axial-loading sports
  - Acute onset of localizing pain

Demographics

- Age: Adolescents and young adults
- Gender: M > F, up to 9:1 ratio

Natural History & Prognosis

- Self-limited
- Good, unless systemic osteoporosis leads to recurrent compression fractures

Treatment

- Observational, with pain management in symptomatic cases

DIAGNOSTIC CHECKLIST

Consider

- Follow-up MRI in cases of unexplained VB edema and localized pain

Image Interpretation Pearls

- Always contiguous with parent disc

SELECTED REFERENCES

1. Yamaguchi T et al: Schmorl's node developing in the lumbar vertebra affected with metastatic carcinoma: correlation magnetic resonance imaging with histological findings. Spine. 28(24):E503-5, 2003
2. Peng B et al: The pathogenesis of Schmorl's nodes. J Bone Joint Surg Br. 85(6):879-82, 2003
3. Hauger O et al: Giant cystic Schmorl's nodes: imaging findings in six patients. AJR Am J Roentgenol. 176(4):969-72, 2001
4. Wagner AL et al: Relationship of Schmorl's nodes to vertebral body endplate fractures and acute endplate disk extrusions. AJNR Am J Neuroradiol. 21(2):276-81, 2000
5. Wagner AL et al: Relationship of Schmorl's nodes to vertebral body endplate fractures and acute endplate disc extrusions. AJNR 21: 276-81, 2000
6. Grive E et al: Radiologic findings in two cases of acute Schmorl's nodes. AJNR Am J Neuroradiol. 20(9):1717-21, 1999
7. Silberstein M et al: Spinal Schmorl's nodes: sagittal sectional imaging and pathological examination. Australas Radiol. 43(1):27-30, 1999
8. Swischuk LE et al: Disk degenerative disease in childhood: Scheuermann's disease, Schmorl's nodes, and the limbus vertebra: MRI findings in 12 patients. Pediatr Radiol. 28(5):334-8, 1998
9. Seymour R et al: Magnetic resonance imaging of acute intraosseous disc herniation. Clin Radiol. 53(5):363-8, 1998
10. Tribus CB: Scheuermann's kyphosis in adolescents and adults: diagnosis and management. J Am Acad Orthop Surg. 6(1):36-43, 1998
11. Fahey V et al: The pathogenesis of Schmorl's nodes in relation to acute trauma. An autopsy study. Spine. 23(21):2272-5, 1998
12. Stabler A et al: MR imaging of enhancing intraosseous disk herniation (Schmorl's nodes). AJR Am J Roentgenol. 168(4):933-8, 1997
13. Takahashi K et al: Schmorl's nodes and low-back pain. Analysis of magnetic resonance imaging findings in symptomatic and asymptomatic individuals. Eur Spine J. 4(1):56-9, 1995
14. Takahashi K et al: A large painful Schmorl's node: a case report. J Spinal Disord. 7(1):77-81, 1994
15. Jensen MC et al: Magnetic resonance imaging of the lumbar spine in people without back pain. N Engl J Med. 331(2):69-73, 1994
16. Hamanishi C et al: Schmorl's nodes on magnetic resonance imaging. Their incidence and clinical relevance. Spine. 19(4):450-3, 1994
17. Magnetic resonance imaging of the lumbar spine in people without back pain: N Engl J Med. Jul 14;331(2):69-73, 1994
18. Sward L: The thoracolumbar spine in young elite athletes. Current concepts on the effects of physical training. Sports Med. 13(5):357-64, 1992
19. Walters G et al: Magnetic resonance imaging of acute symptomatic Schmorl's node formation. Pediatr Emerg Care. 7(5):294-6, 1991
20. Sward L et al: Back pain and radiologic changes in the thoraco-lumbar spine of athletes. Spine. 15(2):124-9, 1990
21. Mclain R et al: An unusual presentation of a Schmorl's node. Report of a case. Spine. 15(3):247-50, 1990
22. Roberts S et al: Biochemical and structural properties of the cartilage end-plate and its relation to the intervertebral disc. Spine. 14(2):166-74, 1989
23. McFadden KD et al: End-plate lesions of the lumbar spine. Spine. 14(8):867-9, 1989
24. Yasuma T et al: Schmorl's nodes. Correlation of X-ray and histological findings in postmortem specimens. Acta Pathol Jpn. 38(6):723-33, 1988
25. Kagen S et al: Focal uptake on bone imaging in an asymptomatic Schmorl's node. Clin Nucl Med. 13(8):615-6, 1988
26. Kornberg M: MRI diagnosis of traumatic Schmorl's node. A case report. Spine. 13(8):934-5, 1988
27. Malmivaara A et al: Plain radiographic, discographic, and direct observations of Schmorl's nodes in the thoracolumbar junctional region of the cadaveric spine. Spine. 12(5):453-7, 1987
28. Saluja G et al: Schmorl's nodes (intravertebral herniations of intervertebral disc tissue) in two historic British populations. J Anat. 145:87-96, 1986
29. Lipson SJ et al: Symptomatic intravertebral disc herniation (Schmorl's node) in the cervical spine. Ann Rheum Dis. 44(12):857-9, 1985
30. Resnick D et al: Intravertebral disk herniations: cartilaginous (Schmorl's) nodes. Radiology. 126(1):57-65, 1978
31. Deeg HJ: Schmorl's nodule. N Engl J Med. 298(1):57, 1978
32. Resnick D et al: Intervertebral disc abnormalities associated with vertebral metastasis: observations in patients and cadavers with prostatic cancer. Invest Radiol. 13(3):182-90, 1978
33. Resnick D et al: Intravertebral disc herniations: Cartilaginous (Schmorl's) nodes. Radiology 126: 57-65, 1978
34. Hilton RC et al: Vertebral end-plate lesions (Schmorl's nodes) in the dorsolumbar spine. Ann Rheum Dis. 35(2):127-32, 1976
35. Smith DM: Acute back pain associated with a calcified Schmorl's node: a case report. Clin Orthop. (117):193-6, 1976
36. Boukhris R et al: Schmorl's nodes and osteoporosis. Clin Orthop. 0(104):275-80, 1974

SCHMORL NODE

IMAGE GALLERY

Typical

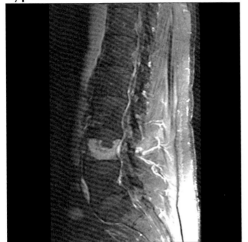
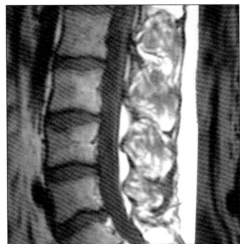

(Left) Sagittal T1 C+ MR with fat-saturation shows diffuse enhancement of marrow around focal disc incursion into superior end plate of L4 in patient with recent axial load trauma, non-lateralizing pain. *(Right)* Sagittal T1WI MR shows small, blister-like incursion into superior end plate. Note low signal border suggestive of condensed bone. No history of recent trauma, non-focal pain.

Typical

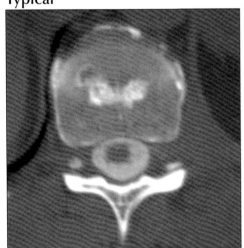
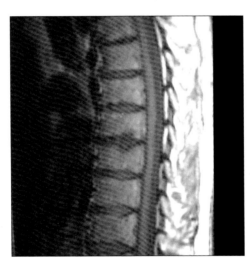

(Left) Axial NECT following myelogram shows sclerotic rim of bone surrounding low density material within the vertebral body just above interspace. *(Right)* Sagittal T1WI MR shows small focal node of disc encroaching into lower thoracic vertebral body's superior endplate. Note minimal "mirror" change in inferior end plate of suprajacent vertebral body.

Variant

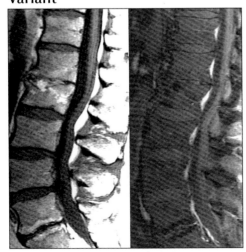
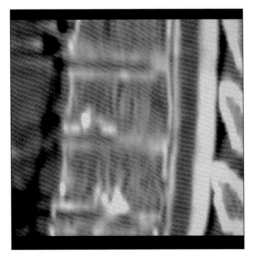

(Left) Sagittal T1WI MR (L) and T1 C+ (R) (fat-saturated) sections depict focal disc incursion into upper endplate of L2; fat signal (ossified disc) fades with fat-saturation (as do L5-S1 type II changes). *(Right)* Sagittal NECT shows sclerotic margins bordering a small, focal disc incursion into inferior end plate of a low-thoracic vertebral body. Note calcified node in the vertebral body immediately below.

SCHEUERMANN DISEASE

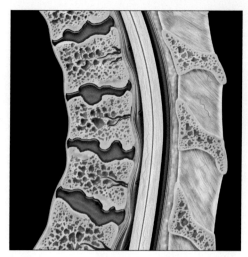

Sagittal graphic shows herniation of disc material through vertebral endplates creating focal subcortical bone defects. Undulation of endplates reflects bony reparative process.

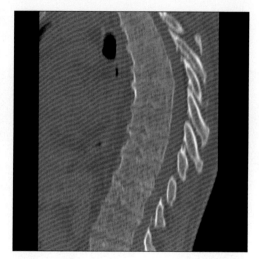

Sagittal bone CT shows multiple Schmorl nodes, irregular vertebral endplates, and anterior wedging of multiple thoracic vertebral bodies typical of Scheurmann disease.

TERMINOLOGY

Abbreviations and Synonyms
• Juvenile kyphosis

Definitions
• Kyphosis secondary to multiple Schmorl nodes → vertebral body wedging
• Schmorl node: Invagination of disc material through vertebral body endplate

IMAGING FINDINGS

General Features
• Best diagnostic clue: Three or more wedged thoracic vertebrae with irregular endplates
• Location
  ○ 75% thoracic
  ○ 20-25% thoracolumbar
  ○ < 5% lumbar only
  ○ Rarely cervical
• Size
  ○ Normal kyphosis of the thoracic spine increases with age
  ○ Kyphosis > 40 degrees considered abnormal

Radiographic Findings
• Radiography

○ 3 or more contiguous vertebrae, each showing ≥ 5 degrees of kyphosis
○ Undulation of endplates secondary to extensive disc invaginations
○ Disc spaces narrowed, with greatest narrowing anteriorly
○ Well-defined Schmorl nodes
○ Thoracic spine: Measure kyphosis from T3 to T12
○ Thoracolumbar or lumbar involvement
  ▪ Measure sagittal plane deformity from one vertebra above affected vertebrae to one vertebra below
  ▪ This method of measuring gives better estimate of functional kyphosis
  ▪ Loss of normal lumbar lordosis functionally significant
○ +/- Limbus vertebrae
○ 15% have scoliosis as well as kyphosis
  ▪ Hyperextension lateral radiograph to assess flexibility of kyphosis

CT Findings
• Bone CT
  ○ Endplate abnormalities more apparent than on radiography

MR Findings
• T1WI
  ○ Schmorl nodes, disc herniations low signal intensity

DDx: Scheurmann Disease

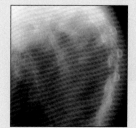

Idiopathic

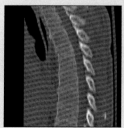

Compression Fx

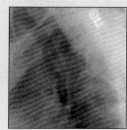

Ankylosing Spondylitis

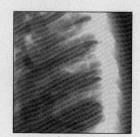

Spond. Dysplasia

SCHEUERMANN DISEASE

Key Facts

Terminology
- Kyphosis secondary to multiple Schmorl nodes → vertebral body wedging

Imaging Findings
- Best diagnostic clue: Three or more wedged thoracic vertebrae with irregular endplates
- 75% thoracic
- 15% have scoliosis as well as kyphosis

Top Differential Diagnoses
- Postural kyphosis
- Wedge compression fractures
- Congenital kyphosis
- Osteogenesis imperfecta tarda
- Ankylosing spondylitis (AS)
- Spondyloepiphyseal dysplasia tarda (SED)

Pathology
- Chronic repetitive trauma in a skeletally immature person
- Disc extrusions through weakened regions of vertebral end plates
- Prevalence: 0.4-8%
- Peak incidence: 13-17 years

Clinical Issues
- Thoracic spine pain and tenderness worsened by activity

Diagnostic Checklist
- Schmorl nodes without anterior wedging are not indicative of Scheuermann disease
- Radiography may show undulating endplates rather than discrete Schmorl nodes

---

  ○ +/- Discogenic sclerosis
- T2WI
  ○ Disc degeneration seen in 50% of involved discs
  ○ Disc herniations
  ○ Schmorl nodes may be low or high signal intensity
    ▪ +/- Bone marrow edema adjacent to Schmorl nodes

Nuclear Medicine Findings
- Bone Scan: May be normal or show increased activity

Other Modality Findings
- Bone mineral density normal (DEXA, CT bone densitometry)

Imaging Recommendations
- Plain film for diagnosis
- MRI to exclude disc herniations

DIFFERENTIAL DIAGNOSIS

Postural kyphosis
- Vertebral endplates normal
- Deformity usually corrects in hyperextension unless long-standing

Wedge compression fractures
- May involve contiguous levels
- Anterior vertebral cortex often shows angular deformity
- MR shows fracture lines, bone marrow edema

Congenital kyphosis
- Vertebral anomalies present

Tuberculosis
- Kyphosis often severe
- Endplate destruction +/- vertebral fusion

Osteogenesis imperfecta tarda
- Platyspondyly
- Severe osteopenia

Neuromuscular disease
- Persistence of infantile thoracolumbar kyphosis in nonambulatory patients
- Kyphoscoliosis

Ankylosing spondylitis (AS)
- Fusion of vertebral bodies
- Abnormalities of sacroiliac joints

Spondyloepiphyseal dysplasia tarda (SED)
- Platyspondyly throughout spine
- Epiphyses abnormal

PATHOLOGY

General Features
- Genetics: Familial tendency
- Etiology
  ○ Chronic repetitive trauma in a skeletally immature person
    ▪ Weight lifting, gymnastics, and other spine loading sports
    ▪ Hard physical labor
  ○ Disc extrusions through weakened regions of vertebral end plates
    ▪ Disc space loss
    ▪ Limbus vertebrae
    ▪ Schmorl node
  ○ Delayed growth in anterior portion of vertebrae causes wedging
- Epidemiology
  ○ Prevalence: 0.4-8%
  ○ Peak incidence: 13-17 years

Gross Pathologic & Surgical Features
- Schmorl nodes invaginate into vertebral bodies through fissures in weakened growth plates
- Limbus vertebrae occur when disc material protrudes through growth plate of ring apophysis

Microscopic Features
- Vertebral body growth plates

SCHEUERMANN DISEASE

- ○ Abnormal chondrocytes
- ○ Loose cartilage matrix
- ○ Diminished number or thickness of collagen fibers
- ○ Increased proteoglycan content
- Osteonecrosis, osteochondrosis not seen

CLINICAL ISSUES

Presentation
- Most common signs/symptoms
  - ○ Kyphosis
  - ○ Other signs/symptoms
    - Thoracic spine pain and tenderness worsened by activity
    - Neurologic symptoms from kyphosis or from disc herniations
    - Fatigue

Demographics
- Age: Develops in adolescence, may present later in life
- Gender: Slight male predominance

Natural History & Prognosis
- Increases in magnitude during adolescent growth spurt
- Mild progression after growth is complete
- Severe deformity uncommon
- Kyphosis greater than 70 degrees has poor functional result
- Premature disc degeneration
- Disc herniations related to degeneration, mechanical stress from spine deformity

Treatment
- Observation
  - ○ Indications
    - Growth still remains
    - Kyphotic deformity less than 50 degrees
  - ○ Elimination of the specific strenuous activity
  - ○ Analgesics
  - ○ Spine exercises
  - ○ Follow-up until growth-plate fuses, age 25
- Brace treatment
  - ○ Indications
    - At least one year of growth remains
    - < 70 degree kyphosis
    - At least partial correction of kyphosis on hyperextension
- Surgical treatment
  - ○ Uncommonly felt to be necessary
  - ○ Indications
    - > 75 degree kyphosis in a skeletally immature person
    - > 60 degree kyphosis in mature person
    - Excessive pain
    - Neurologic deficit
  - ○ Posterior instrumentation and fusion
  - ○ Anterior and posterior fusion for more severe kyphosis

DIAGNOSTIC CHECKLIST

Image Interpretation Pearls
- Schmorl nodes without anterior wedging are not indicative of Scheuermann disease
- Radiography may show undulating endplates rather than discrete Schmorl nodes

SELECTED REFERENCES

1. Soo CL et al: Scheuermann kyphosis: long-term follow-up. Spine J. 2(1):49-56, 2002
2. Stotts AK et al: Measurement of spinal kyphosis: implications for the management of Scheuermann's kyphosis. Spine. 27(19):2143-6, 2002
3. Wenger DR et al: Scheuermann kyphosis. Spine. 24(24):2630-9, 1999
4. Swischuk LE et al: Disk degenerative disease in childhood: Scheuermann's disease, Schmorl's nodes, and the limbus vertebra: MRI findings in 12 patients. Pediatr Radiol. 28(5):334-8, 1998
5. Tribus CB: Scheuermann's kyphosis in adolescents and adults: diagnosis and management. J Am Acad Orthop Surg. 6(1):36-43, 1998
6. Platero D et al: Juvenile kyphosis: effects of different variables on conservative treatment outcome. Acta Orthop Belg. 63(3):194-201, 1997
7. Chiu KY et al: Cord compression caused by multiple disc herniations and intraspinal cyst in Scheuermann's disease. Spine. 20(9):1075-9, 1995
8. Murray PM et al: The natural history and long-term follow-up of Scheuermann kyphosis. J Bonc Joint Surg Am. 75(2):236-48, 1993
9. Mandell GA et al: Bone scintigraphy in patients with atypical lumbar Scheuermann disease. J Pediatr Orthop. 13(5):622-7, 1993
10. Tala VT et al: Postural kyphosis and Scheuermann's disease. Seminars in Spine Surgery 4:216-24, 1992
11. Farsetti P et al: Juvenile and idiopathic kyphosis. Long-term follow-up of 20 cases. Arch Orthop Trauma Surg. 110(3):165-8, 1991
12. Findlay A et al: Dominant inheritance of Scheuermann's juvenile kyphosis. J Med Genet. 26(6):400-3, 1989
13. Gilsanz V et al: Vertebral bone density in Scheuermann disease. J Bone Joint Surg Am. 71(6):894-7, 1989
14. Paajanen H et al: Disc degeneration in Scheuermann disease. Skeletal Radiol. 18(7):523-6, 1989
15. Blumenthal SL et al: Lumbar Scheuermann's. a clinical series and classification. Spine 12:929-32, 1987
16. Ippolito E et al: Juvenile kyphosis; histological and histochemical studies. J Bone Joint Surg 63: 175-82, 1981
17. Fon GT et al: Thoracic kyphosis: range in normal subjects. AJR Am J Roentgenol. 134(5):979-83, 1980

IMAGE GALLERY

Typical

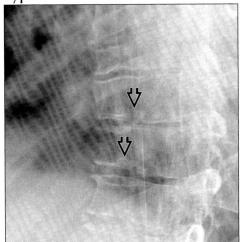 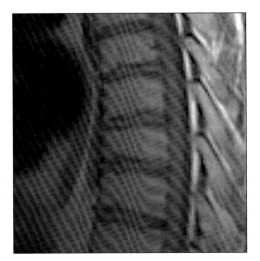

(Left) Lateral radiography demonstrates wedging deformity and undulation of vertebral endplates due to multiple Schmorl nodes at each level. Arrows point to two Schmorl nodes. *(Right)* Sagittal T1WI MR shows mild involvement of thoracic spine. There is diffuse irregularity of endplates due to disc invagination rather than discrete Schmorl nodes.

Typical

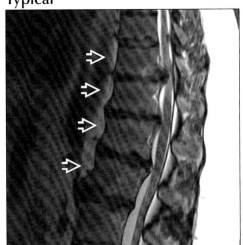 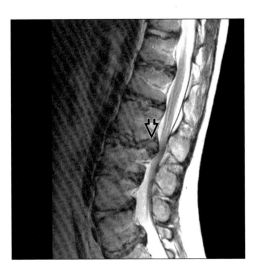

(Left) Sagittal T2WI MR depicts Schmorl nodes and disc degeneration throughout visualized spine. Contiguous levels of wedging are marked with arrows. *(Right)* Sagittal T2WI MR shows diffuse loss of intervertebral disc signal, wedging of vertebral bodies, undulation of endplates, and discrete Schmorl nodes. Large disc herniation is marked by arrow.

Variant

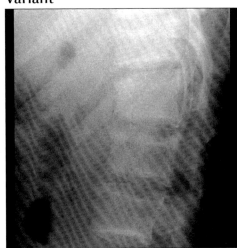 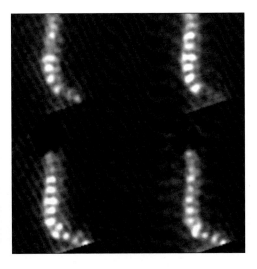

(Left) Lateral radiography reveals focal kyphosis secondary to isolated thoracolumbar Scheuermann disease. Scalloped contour of endplates distinguishes from multiple compression fractures. *(Right)* Sagittal bone scan SPECT images show increased radionuclide uptake throughout lumbar spine in adolescent patient with lumbar Scheuermann disease.

THANATOPHORIC DWARFISM

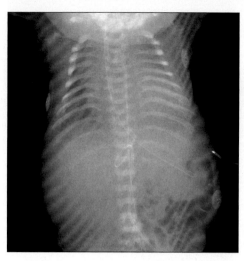

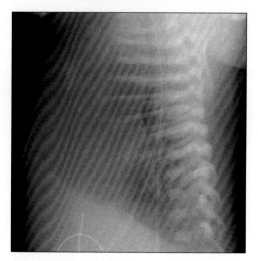

Anteroposterior radiography of a term infant shows short ribs, bell-shaped thorax, and platyspondyly. Lungs are hypoinflated.

Lateral radiography demonstrates short ribs and hypoplastic sternum. Vertebral morphology is often difficult to seen on CXR because of obscuration by pulmonary opacities.

TERMINOLOGY

Abbreviations and Synonyms
- Thanatophoric dysplasia

Definitions
- Lethal short-limbed dysplasia

IMAGING FINDINGS

General Features
- Best diagnostic clue: Severe dwarfism with narrow chest and short ribs
- Location: Entire spine affected
- Morphology: Severe flattening of vertebral bodies

Radiographic Findings
- Radiography
  - Flattened vertebral bodies
  - Short ribs
  - Severe limb shortening
  - Cloverleaf skull variably present

Ultrasonographic Findings
- Real Time
  - Diagnosis often possible in 2nd trimester
  - Short femurs, curved or straight
  - Enlarged skull

- Small, narrow thorax

Imaging Recommendations
- Best imaging tool: Antenatal ultrasound

DIFFERENTIAL DIAGNOSIS

Achondroplasia
- Deformities similar but less severe

Spondyloepiphyseal dysplasia
- Barrel shaped thorax
- Delayed ossification of epiphyses

Spondylocostal dysostosis
- Vertebral anomalies
- Thin, elongated bones of extremities

Osteogenesis imperfecta congenita
- Short, thick bones of extremities
- Fractures at birth

Asphyxiating thoracic dysplasia
- Short ribs
- "Trident" appearance iliac bones

DDx: Severe Dwarfism at Birth

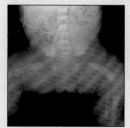

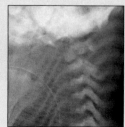

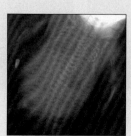

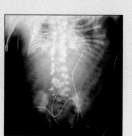

Achondroplasia   *Achondroplasia*   *SED Congenita*   *Spondylocostal*

THANATOPHORIC DWARFISM

Key Facts

Terminology
- Lethal short-limbed dysplasia

Imaging Findings
- Best diagnostic clue: Severe dwarfism with narrow chest and short ribs
- Morphology: Severe flattening of vertebral bodies
- Best imaging tool: Antenatal ultrasound

Top Differential Diagnoses
- Achondroplasia
- Osteogenesis imperfecta congenita

Clinical Issues
- Most common signs/symptoms: Respiratory distress in neonate with dwarfism
- Usually fatal shortly after birth; may survive several years

PATHOLOGY

General Features
- Genetics
  - Spontaneous mutation
  - Autosomal dominant
  - Allelic to same gene as achondroplasia and hypochondroplasia on chromosome 4p
- Etiology: Abnormality of fibroblast growth factor receptor
- Epidemiology
  - 1.7-3.8/100,000 births
  - Most common lethal neonatal skeletal dysplasia
- Associated abnormalities
  - Maternal polyhydramnios
  - Genitourinary abnormalities
  - Compression of cervical spinal cord

Gross Pathologic & Surgical Features
- Large skull, severe dwarfism

Microscopic Features
- Disruption of enchondral ossification of the growth plate

Staging, Grading or Classification Criteria
- Type 1: Without cloverleaf skull
- Type 2: Cloverleaf skull

CLINICAL ISSUES

Presentation
- Most common signs/symptoms: Respiratory distress in neonate with dwarfism

Demographics
- Age: Congenital
- Gender: M = F

Natural History & Prognosis
- Usually fatal shortly after birth; may survive several years

Treatment
- Options, risks, complications
  - Ventriculoperitoneal shunt
  - Tracheostomy

DIAGNOSTIC CHECKLIST

Consider
- Cloverleaf skull can occur with a wide variety of dysplasias or as an isolated anomaly

SELECTED REFERENCES

1. Lemyre E et al: Bone dysplasia series. Achondroplasia, hypochondroplasia and thanatophoric dysplasia: review and update. Can Assoc Radiol J. 50(3):185-97, 1999
2. Schild RL et al: Antenatal sonographic diagnosis of thanatophoric dysplasia: a report of three cases and a review of the literature with special emphasis on the differential diagnosis. Ultrasound Obstet Gynecol. 8(1):62-7, 1996
3. Taybi H, Lachman RS: Radiology of syndromes, metabolic disorders, and skeletal dysplasias. 4th ed. St. Louis, Mosby. 939-943, 1996
4. Rouse GA et al: Short-limb skeletal dysplasias: evaluation of the fetal spine with sonography and radiography. Radiology. 174(1):177-80, 1990

IMAGE GALLERY

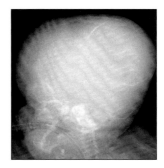 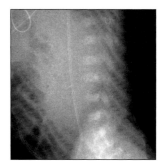

(Left) Lateral radiography depicts the cloverleaf skull abnormality which is often associated with thanatophoric dysplasia, as well as other congenital syndromes. *(Right)* Lateral radiography shows platyspondyly and wide intervertebral disc spaces. No other vertebral anomalies are present. Mineralization appears normal.

ACHONDROPLASIA

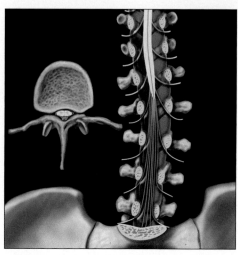

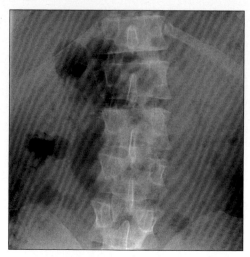

Graphic shows progressive narrowing of interpediculate distance in caudad direction. Axial insert image shows spinal stenosis related to short pedicles & decreased interpediculate distance.

Anteroposterior radiography depicts caudally decreasing interpediculate distance and mild levoscoliosis in an adult achondroplasia patient.

TERMINOLOGY

Abbreviations and Synonyms
- Achondroplastic dwarfism

Definitions
- Autosomal dominant dwarfism affecting spine and extremities
- Rhizomelic dwarfism; most severe growth disturbance in proximal portions of limbs

IMAGING FINDINGS

General Features
- Best diagnostic clue: Interpediculate distance decreases in caudal direction in lumbar spine (reversal of normal relationship)
- Location: Spine, skull, pelvis, extremities
- Morphology
  - Severe dwarfism involves trunk and extremities
  - Vertebral bodies mildly flattened
  - Pedicles short
  - Lumbar hyperlordosis
  - Thoracolumbar kyphosis

Radiographic Findings
- Radiography

- Lumbar interpedicular distance progressively decreases in caudad direction
- Vertebral bodies slightly flattened with short pedicles
- +/- Bullet-shaped vertebral bodies
  - Usually seen in childhood, resolve by adulthood
- Thoracolumbar kyphosis
  - Initially flexible deformity
  - May progress to fixed gibbus deformity or resolve as child grows
- Lumbar hyperlordosis
- Mild scoliosis may be present
- C1-2 instability rare
- Extraspinal findings
  - "Champagne glass" pelvis: Pelvic inlet is flat and broad
  - Squared iliac wings
  - Shortened long bones, most prominent in proximal long bones ("rhizomelic")
  - Short ribs
  - "Trident hand": 2nd, 3rd and 4th digits equal in length
  - Enlarged skull
- Bone mineral density normal
- Myelography
  - Spinal stenosis
  - Disc herniations common
- Ultrasound

DDx: Achondroplasia

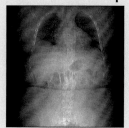

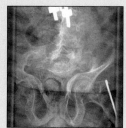

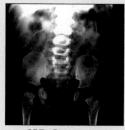

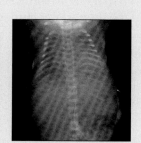

Hypochondroplasia   *Osteogenesis*   *SED Congenita*   *Thanatophoric*

ACHONDROPLASIA

Key Facts

Terminology

- Autosomal dominant dwarfism affecting spine and extremities
- Rhizomelic dwarfism; most severe growth disturbance in proximal portions of limbs

Imaging Findings

- Lumbar interpedicular distance progressively decreases in caudad direction
- Vertebral bodies slightly flattened with short pedicles
- +/- Bullet-shaped vertebral bodies
- Thoracolumbar kyphosis
- Bony spinal stenosis due to degenerative disease superimposed on short pedicles
- Best imaging tool: Single AP "babygram" at birth shows skull, spine, pelvic abnormalities

Top Differential Diagnoses

- Pseudoachondroplasia
- Hypochondroplasia
- Diastrophic dysplasia
- Spondyloepiphyseal dysplasia (SED) congenita
- Thanatophoric dysplasia
- Osteogenesis imperfecta (OI)

Pathology

- Autosomal dominant
- Epidemiology: Most common nonlethal skeletal dysplasia (1:26,000 live births)

Diagnostic Checklist

- Most likely cause of short limbed dwarfism with normal ossification detected in 3rd trimester

---

- ○ Growth disturbance evident in third trimester ultrasound
- ○ Ossification normal
- ○ Homozygous form can be diagnosed in second trimester

CT Findings

- NECT: Communicating hydrocephalus (uncommon)
- Bone CT
  - ○ Mildly flattened vertebral bodies
  - ○ Bullet shaped vertebral bodies
  - ○ Posterior vertebral body scalloping
  - ○ Bony spinal stenosis due to degenerative disease superimposed on short pedicles
  - ○ Deformity may lead to stress fractures
  - ○ Small foramen magnum

MR Findings

- Morphologic changes as described for CT
- Disc herniations common
- Compression of cervicomedullary junction, spinal cord, nerve roots ⇒ myelomalacia

Imaging Recommendations

- Best imaging tool: Single AP "babygram" at birth shows skull, spine, pelvic abnormalities
- Protocol advice
  - ○ 2-3 mm multidetector CT
  - ○ Coronal and sagittal reformations for surgical planning
  - ○ Axial, sagittal MR through foramen magnum in all infants and children to assess for stenosis

DIFFERENTIAL DIAGNOSIS

Pseudoachondroplasia

- Facial features and skull normal
- Usually detected in early childhood rather than at birth
- Vertebral body flattening variably seen

Hypochondroplasia

- Midface hypoplasia

- Similar to but milder than achondroplasia

Diastrophic dysplasia

- Facial features marked by micrognathia
- Flattened vertebral bodies; narrowed interpediculate distances
- Scoliosis and kyphosis
- C1-2 instability
- Subluxations in extremities ("hitchhiker's thumb")
- Clubfoot

Spondyloepiphyseal dysplasia (SED) congenita

- Facial features and skull normal
- Severe vertebral body flattening
- C1-2 instability and odontoid hypoplasia
- Delayed ossification of epiphyses
- Flattened epiphyses
- Shortened long bones
- Absent pubic ossification in infants

Thanatophoric dysplasia

- Lethal dwarfism
- Severe platyspondyly
- Long, narrow trunk
- Bell-shaped thorax
- May have "cloverleaf" skull

Osteogenesis imperfecta (OI)

- Infantile form has short, thick bones, multiple fractures
- Milder forms present in childhood or adulthood with short stature, platyspondyly, osteopenia, fractures, bone deformities

PATHOLOGY

General Features

- Genetics
  - ○ Autosomal dominant
  - ○ Gene mapped to chromosome 4p16.3
  - ○ Same allele as hypochondroplasia, thanatophoric dwarfism

ACHONDROPLASIA

○ Homozygous form rare, much more severe than heterozygous
- Etiology
  ○ Usually a spontaneous mutation
  ○ Fibroblast growth factor receptor abnormality
- Epidemiology: Most common nonlethal skeletal dysplasia (1:26,000 live births)
- Associated abnormalities
  ○ Sleep apnea
  ○ Sudden infant death
  ○ Chest wall deformity may lead to respiratory difficulties
  ○ Limb lengthening procedures can lead to neurologic symptoms

Gross Pathologic & Surgical Features

- Spinal stenosis
  ○ Premature fusion of neural arch synchondroses
  ○ Short pedicles, thickened laminae
  ○ Disc bulges and herniations contribute to stenosis
  ○ Can occur at all spinal levels
  ○ Significant cause of morbidity in adults
- Foramen magnum stenosis
  ○ Found in almost all children with achondroplasia
  ○ Often resolves functionally as child grows
- Thoracolumbar kyphosis
  ○ Related to hypotonia in infants
  ○ Often resolves but may develop fixed deformity
  ○ Seen in 30% of adults

Microscopic Features

- Disruption of growth plate enchondral ossification

CLINICAL ISSUES

Presentation

- Most common signs/symptoms
  ○ Dwarfism, characteristic facies evident at birth
  ○ Other signs/symptoms
    ▪ Infants hypotonic
    ▪ Sleep apnea in infants and children due to compression of cord at foramen magnum
    ▪ Thoracolumbar kyphosis
    ▪ Spinal stenosis
- Clinical profile
  ○ Rhizomelic dwarfism apparent at birth
  ○ Frontal bossing and depressed nasal bridge characteristic
  ○ Intelligence normal
  ○ Obesity a common clinical problem
  ○ Probably overdiagnosed clinically

Demographics

- Age: Congenital; diagnosis usually made in infancy
- Gender: M = F

Natural History & Prognosis

- High morbidity from spinal stenosis

Treatment

- Options, risks, complications
  ○ Growth hormone can promote growth of long bones

○ Kyphosis may be preventable by not allowing hypotonic infant to sit unassisted
○ Surgical decompression of foramen magnum in severe cases; usually symptoms resolve
○ Surgical decompression for spinal stenosis
○ Bracing, fusion for thoracolumbar kyphosis
- Extraspinal: Ilizarov limb lengthening procedure controversial

DIAGNOSTIC CHECKLIST

Consider

- Most likely cause of short limbed dwarfism with normal ossification detected in 3rd trimester

Image Interpretation Pearls

- Stress fracture or disc herniation may present acutely and can be evaluated with CT or MR
- Spine imaging must include foramen magnum to evaluate for stenosis

SELECTED REFERENCES

1. Tanaka N et al: The comparison of the effects of short-term growth hormone treatment in patients with achondroplasia and with hypochondroplasia. Endocr J. 50(1):69-75, 2003
2. Park HW et al: Correction of lumbosacral hyperlordosis in achondroplasia. Clin Orthop. (414):242-9, 2003
3. Thomeer RT et al: Surgical treatment of lumbar stenosis in achondroplasia. J Neurosurg. 96(3 Suppl):292-7, 2002
4. Gordon N: The neurological complications of achondroplasia. Brain Dev. 22(1):3-7, 2000
5. Lemyre E et al: Bone dysplasia series. Achondroplasia, hypochondroplasia and thanatophoric dysplasia: review and update. Can Assoc Radiol J. 50(3):185-97, 1999
6. Keiper GL Jr et al: Achondroplasia and cervicomedullary compression: prospective evaluation and surgical treatment. Pediatr Neurosurg. 31(2):78-83, 1999
7. Lachman RS: Neurologic abnormalities in the skeletal dysplasias: a clinical and radiological perspective. Am J Med Genet. 69(1):33-43, 1997
8. Taybi H, Lachman RS: Radiology of syndromes, metabolic disorders, and skeletal dysplasias. 4th ed. St. Louis, Mosby. 748-55, 1996
9. Hall JG: Information update on Achondroplasia. Pediatrics. 95(4):620, 1995
10. Ryken TC et al: Cervicomedullary compression in achondroplasia. J Neurosurg. 81(1):43-8, 1994
11. Hecht JT et al: Neurologic morbidity associated with achondroplasia. J Child Neurol. 5(2):84-97, 1990
12. Kao SC et al: MR imaging of the craniovertebral junction, cranium, and brain in children with achondroplasia. AJR Am J Roentgenol. 153(3):565-9, 1989
13. Fortuna A et al: Narrowing of thoraco-lumbar spinal canal in achondroplasia. J Neurosurg Sci. 33(2):185-96, 1989
14. Thomas IT et al: Magnetic resonance imaging in the assessment of medullary compression in achondroplasia. Am J Dis Child. 142(9):989-92, 1988
15. Beighton P et al: Gibbal achondroplasia. J Bone Joint Surg Br. 63-B(3):328-9, 1981

ACHONDROPLASIA

IMAGE GALLERY

Typical

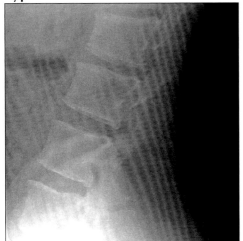 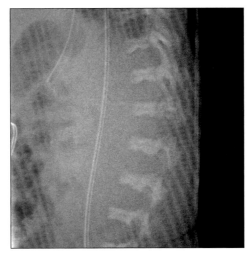

(Left) Lateral radiography demonstrates mild vertebral body flattening and posterior scalloping with short pedicles in an adult patient. (Right) Lateral radiography shows platyspondyly in a neonate. Endplates are notched, an abnormality which resolves in childhood.

Typical

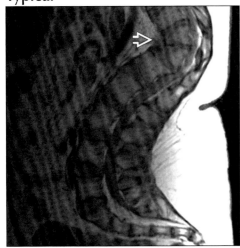 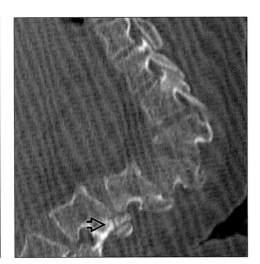

(Left) Sagittal T1WI MR shows a severe thoracolumbar junction kyphosis (arrow) and lumbosacral hyperlordosis in a 12 year old girl. T11 and T12 vertebrae are bullet-shaped. (Right) Sagittal bone CT depicts a stress fracture of the superior L2 articular process (arrow), probably due to increased stress from kyphosis. Patient complained of severe, focal pain.

Typical

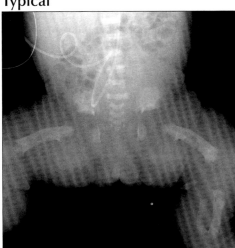 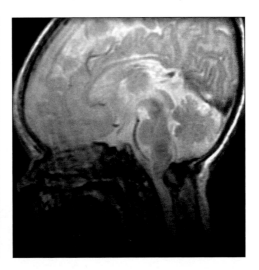

(Left) Anteroposterior radiography shows characteristic findings at birth. Vertebral bodies are flat, interpediculate distance narrows caudally, and deformity of pelvis and long bones is evident. (Right) Sagittal T2WI MR demonstrates foramen magnum stenosis in a neonate with compression of the cervicomedullary junction.

MUCOPOLYSACCHARIDOSES

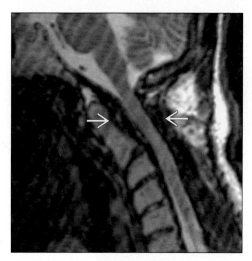

Sagittal T2WI MR (Hurler-Scheie, MPS 1-H/S) shows marked hypointense ligamentous thickening (arrows) and craniocervical junction stenosis.

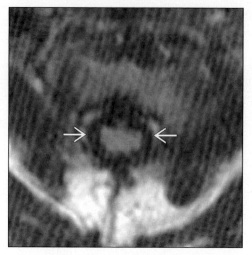

Axial T2WI MR (Hurler-Scheie, MPS 1-H/S) depicts classic marked hypointense ligamentous thickening (arrows).

TERMINOLOGY

Abbreviations and Synonyms
- Synonyms: MPS, lysosomal storage disorder, "gargoylism"

Definitions
- Inherited lysosomal storage disorders
  - Specific enzyme deficiency ⇒ inability to breakdown specific glycosaminoglycans (GAG)
  - Failure to break down GAG ⇒ intracellular accumulation and toxicity

IMAGING FINDINGS

General Features
- Best diagnostic clue: Dens hypoplasia, craniovertebral junction (CVJ) stenosis, and thickened dural ring at foramen magnum
- Location
  - Spine: CVJ, thoracolumbar spine, pelvis
  - Extraspinal: Brain, visceral organ deposition
- Size: Odontoid soft tissue mass varies from small to large; larger masses usually found in older patients
- Morphology
  - Craniocervical spine

  - Skull base thickening, occipital hypoplasia, short posterior C1 arch, odontoid hypoplasia +/- os odontoideum, ligamentous laxity, dural sac stenosis, and atlantoaxial instability
  - Thoracolumbar spine
    - Kyphosis, kyphoscoliosis
    - Platyspondyly, anterior beaking + thoracolumbar gibbus deformity (MPS I H and IV)

Radiographic Findings
- Radiography
  - Odontoid dysplasia +/- atlanto-axial subluxation
  - Dysplastic blunted spinous processes, wedged vertebral bodies, and spinal canal stenosis
  - Thoracolumbar inferior (MPS I-H) or central (MPS IV) vertebral beaking, gibbus deformity
- Fluoroscopy: +/- Dynamic CVJ instability on flexion-extension

CT Findings
- CECT: CVJ central and foraminal narrowing, marked dural thickening without abnormal enhancement
- Bone CT
  - Abnormal dens ossification, marked laminar thickening, enlargement of medullary cavity

MR Findings
- T1WI: Hypo- to isointense peri-odontoid soft tissue mass, hypointense thickened dura

DDx: Mucopolysaccharidosis

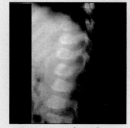

GM1 Gangliosidosis

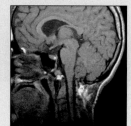

Achondroplasia

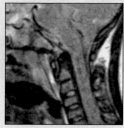

Down Syndrome

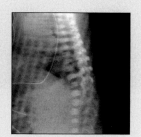

Spond. Dysplasia

MUCOPOLYSACCHARIDOSES

Key Facts

Terminology
- Synonyms: MPS, lysosomal storage disorder, "gargoylism"
- Inherited lysosomal storage disorders
- Specific enzyme deficiency ⇒ inability to breakdown specific glycosaminoglycans (GAG)

Imaging Findings
- Best diagnostic clue: Dens hypoplasia, craniovertebral junction (CVJ) stenosis, and thickened dural ring at foramen magnum
- Platyspondyly, anterior beaking + thoracolumbar gibbus deformity (MPS I-H and IV)

Top Differential Diagnoses
- GM1 gangliosidosis
- Mucolipidosis III (pseudo-Hurler polydystrophy)
- Achondroplasia
- Down syndrome
- Spondyloepiphyseal dysplasia

Pathology
- Odontoid hypoplasia, GAG deposition, +/- ligamentous laxity with reactive change produce soft tissue mass around dens

Clinical Issues
- Premature death the rule; rate of deterioration depends on specific enzymatic deficiency

Diagnostic Checklist
- Dens hypoplasia with mass and dural thickening suggests MPS syndrome

---

- T2WI
  - Hypoplastic dens and peri-odontoid soft tissue mass
  - Hypointense, thickened dura +/- cyst formation due to meningeal thickening (MPS 1-H, II)
  - +/- Cord compression with hyperintense signal abnormality
- T1 C+: No abnormal enhancement, even if mass present
- MRS: Brain proton MRS may show diminished NAA/choline ratio, elevated glutamine/glutamate and inositol peak areas

Imaging Recommendations
- Best imaging tool: MR imaging
- Protocol advice
  - Spine MR imaging to elucidate cause/site of cord compression
  - Plain radiographs to characterize osseous spine and limb abnormalities
  - Flexion-extension radiographs or fluoroscopy to detect craniovertebral instability

DIFFERENTIAL DIAGNOSIS

GM1 gangliosidosis
- Shares features of vertebral beaking, upper lumbar gibbus, and dens hypoplasia
- Distinguish on clinical, genetic criteria

Mucolipidosis III (pseudo-Hurler polydystrophy)
- Shares features of vertebral beaking, upper lumbar gibbus, and dens hypoplasia
- Distinguish on clinical, genetic criteria

Achondroplasia
- Autosomal dominant disorder of enchondral bone formation
- Short broad pedicles and thickened laminae ⇒ spinal stenosis
- Distinguish on genetic, clinical criteria

Down syndrome
- +/- Dens hypoplasia without soft tissue dens mass or marrow deposition features
- Distinguish using genetic and clinical information

Spondyloepiphyseal dysplasia
- Autosomal dominant; presents at birth
- Flattening of vertebral bodies, dens hypoplasia, scoliosis
- Minimal hand and foot involvement

PATHOLOGY

General Features
- General path comments
  - GAG accumulates in most organs and ligaments
    - Coarse facies (hence the name "gargoylism")
    - Hepatosplenomegaly, umbilical hernia,
    - Skeletal dysotosis multiplex, joint contractures
    - Arterial wall (mid-aortic stenosis), cardiac valve thickening
    - Upper airway obstruction (38%); very difficult intubations
  - Odontoid hypoplasia, GAG deposition, +/- ligamentous laxity with reactive change produce soft tissue mass around dens
  - Biconvex ovoid, bullet shaped or rectangular vertebral bodies, vertebral beaking, posterior vertebral slip (MPS IV), large disc protrusions (MPS VI)
- Genetics: Autosomal recessive (except MPS II Hunter's; X-linked recessive)
- Etiology: Inherited lysosomal enzyme deficiency
- Epidemiology: MPS I-H (1:10,000 births), MPS IV (1:40,000 births) most common

Gross Pathologic & Surgical Features
- CVJ stenosis ⇒ neurovascular compression, altered CSF dynamics ⇒ hydrocephalus, hydrosyringomyelia
- Dilated enlarged laminae medullary cavities
- Thickened dura may appear normal at surgery

MUCOPOLYSACCHARIDOSES

Microscopic Features
- Epidural/dural mucopolysaccharide deposition with elastic and collagenous proliferation

Staging, Grading or Classification Criteria
- Hurler (MPS I-H), Hurler-Scheie (MPS 1-H/S): α-L-iduronidase (4p16.3)
- Hunter (MPS II): Iduronate 2-sulfatase (Xq28)
- Sanfillipo (MPS III): Heparin N-sulfatase (17q25.3)
- Morquio (MPS IV): Galactose 6-sulfatase (16q24.3)
- Scheie (MPS V)
- Maroteaux-Lamy (MPS VI): Arylsulfatase B (5q11-q13)
- Sly (MPS VII)

CLINICAL ISSUES

Presentation
- Most common signs/symptoms
  - Gradual subtle progressive myelopathy (often falsely attributed to lower extremity deformities)
    - Common with MPS I-H, II, III, and VII; uncommon with MPS IV, I H/S, VI unless associated with musculoskeletal deformities
    - Reduced exercise tolerance; may be earliest symptom
  - Clinical neurologic symptoms attributable to brain GAG deposition, myelination abnormalities, spinal deformities, and peripheral nerve entrapment
- Clinical profile
  - Coarse facies with macroglossia, bushy eyebrows, flat nasal bridge (mild in MPS VI, VII)
  - Corneal clouding (except MPS II)
  - Significant mental retardation (except in MPS I H/S, IIb, IV)
  - Joint contractures, dysostosis multiplex (dominates in MPS IV, VI)
- Laboratory diagnosis: Measurement of specific urinary glycosaminoglycans
- Clinical diagnostic algorithm
  - Age, IQ, +/- corneal clouding, urinary GAG excretion, and specific clinical findings

Demographics
- Age: Usually diagnosed in childhood; occasional mild cases diagnosed as adults
- Gender: M = F except MPS II (boys only ⇒ X-linked)

Natural History & Prognosis
- Premature death the rule; rate of deterioration depends on specific enzymatic deficiency
- Slowly progressive cord compression ⇒ quadriparesis, sensory loss without treatment
  - Surgical results poor when performed late in disease course
- High spinal cord compression is major spinal cause of MPS complications and death
  - Apnea and sudden death may follow relatively minor trauma

Treatment
- Options, risks, complications
  - Conservative (mild symptoms): External spinal bracing
  - Surgical (more severe symptoms)
    - Posterior occipitocervical decompression/stabilization
    - Transoral odontoid resection/posterior stabilization for symptomatic dens mass
  - Bone marrow transplant (BMT) or intravenous recombinant human enzyme
    - Decreases GAG accumulation in organs; ameliorates some but not all manifestations

DIAGNOSTIC CHECKLIST

Consider
- Successful diagnosis requires combination of clinical, imaging, and genetic/biochemical information

Image Interpretation Pearls
- Dens hypoplasia with mass and dural thickening suggests MPS syndrome
- Vertebral beaking pattern may permit specific diagnosis

SELECTED REFERENCES

1. Chirossel JP et al: Management of craniocervical junction dislocation. Childs Nerv Syst. 16(10-11):697-701, 2000
2. Barkovich A: Pediatric neuroimaging. 3rd ed. Philadelphia, Lippincott-Raven, 121-22, 2000
3. Kim FM et al. Neuroimaging of scoliosis in childhood. Neuroimaging Clinics of North America. 9(1):213 14, 1999
4. Levin TL et al: Lumbar gibbus in storage diseases and bone dysplasias. Pediatr Radiol. 27(4): 289-94, 1997
5. Piccirilli CB et al: Cervical kyphotic myelopathy in a child with Morquio syndrome. Childs Nerv Syst. 12(2):114-6, 1996
6. Vinchon M et al: Cervical myelopathy secondary to Hunter syndrome in an adult. AJNR Am J Neuroradiol. 16(7):1402-3, 1995
7. Crockard HA et al: Craniovertebral junction anomalies in inherited disorders: part of the syndrome or caused by the disorder? Eur J Pediatr. 154(7):504-12, 1995
8. Blaser S et al: Neuroradiology of lysosomal disorders. Neuroimaging Clin NA 4:283-98, 1994
9. Stevens JM et al: The odontoid process in Morquio-Brailsford's disease. The effects of occipitocervical fusion. J Bone Joint Surg Br. 73(5):851-8, 1991
10. Murata R et al: MR imaging of the brain in patients with mucopolysaccharidosis. AJNR Am J Neuroradiol. 10(6):1165-70, 1989
11. Nelson J et al: Clinical findings in 12 patients with MPS IV A (Morquio's disease). Further evidence for heterogeneity. Part I: Clinical and biochemical findings. Clin Genet. 33(2):111-20, 1988
12. Banna M et al: Compressive meningeal hypertrophy in mucopolysaccharidosis. AJNR Am J Neuroradiol. 8(2):385-6, 1987
13. Kulkarni MV et al: Magnetic resonance imaging in the diagnosis of the cranio-cervical manifestations of the mucopolysaccharidoses. Magn Reson Imaging. 5(5):317-23, 1987
14. Edwards MK et al: CT metrizamide myelography of the cervical spine in Morquio syndrome. AJNR Am J Neuroradiol. 3(6):666-9, 1982

MUCOPOLYSACCHARIDOSES

IMAGE GALLERY

Typical

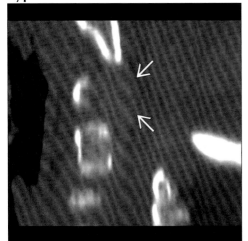
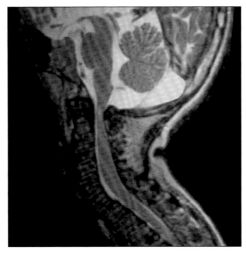

(Left) Sagittal NECT (Morquio, MPS IV) shows typical short posterior C1 arch, odontoid hypoplasia, and mildly hyperdense pannus (arrows) in an 11 year old male with clinical cord compression symptoms. (Right) Sagittal T2WI MR (Morquio, MPS IV) demonstrates odontoid hypoplasia with markedly hypointense pannus producing cord compression and abnormal cord hyperintensity at the craniocervical junction.

Typical

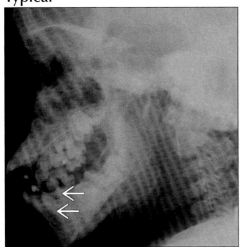
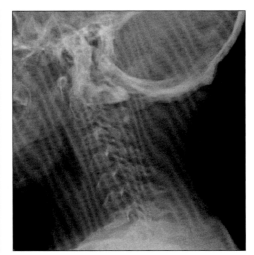

(Left) Lateral radiography (Morquio, MPS IV) shows characteristic central vertebral body beaking (arrows) and jaw abnormalities (Courtesy G. Hedlund, DO). (Right) Lateral radiography (Hurler, MPS I-H) shows characteristic inferior vertebral body beaking (Courtesy G. Hedlund, DO).

Variant

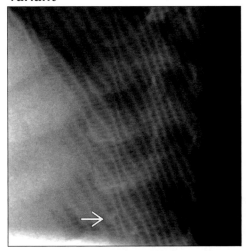
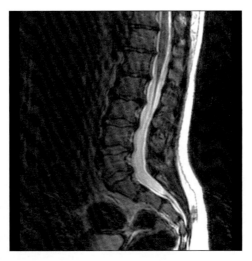

(Left) Lateral radiography (Hurler, MPS I-H) shows a hypoplastic thoracic vertebral body (arrow) with central beaking producing gibbus deformity (Courtesy R. Boyer, MD). (Right) Sagittal T2WI MR (Hurler, MPS I-H) shows variant dural dysplasia and pronounced degenerative disc changes (Courtesy R. Boyer, MD).

SICKLE CELL

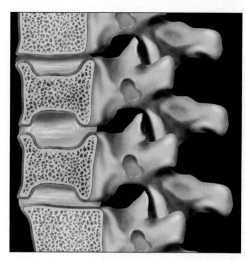

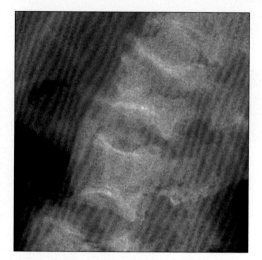

Infarcts due to sickle cell tend to affect central portion of vertebral body, causing focal collapse with preservation of height peripherally, yielding an "H-shaped" vertebra.

Lateral radiography shows central depression of the vertebral endplates, with normal height of anterior and posterior vertebral margins.

TERMINOLOGY

Abbreviations and Synonyms
- Synonyms: Sickle cell anemia, hemoglobin HbSS disease, HbSC disease, SS disease

Definitions
- Hereditary hemoglobin abnormality resulting in anemia, deformed (sickle) red cells which occlude blood vessels
- Homozygous: HbSS (sickle cell anemia)
- Heterozygous: HbSA (sickle cell trait, asymptomatic), HbSC (less severe form)
- Sickle cell crisis: Acute episode of severe bone, abdomen, chest pain

IMAGING FINDINGS

General Features
- Best diagnostic clue: H-shaped vertebral bodies
- Location: Spine: 43-70% of patients

Radiographic Findings
- Radiography
  - Marrow hyperplasia: Osteopenia, cupping of vertebral endplates
  - Bone infarction
    - Sclerosis, "bone-within-bone" appearance

- H-shaped vertebrae: Vertebra flattened centrally
  - Osteomyelitis: Rare in spine

CT Findings
- Bone CT
  - Mottled areas of sclerosis

MR Findings
- T1WI: Low signal intensity marrow due to hyperplastic hematopoietic marrow, infarction, infection
- T2WI
  - Hematopoietic marrow: Intermediate signal intensity
  - Infarct: Irregularly shaped areas of high signal intensity
  - Osteomyelitis: Rounded area of high signal intensity
- T1 C+
  - Infarct: Thin, linear rim-enhancement in serpentine contour
  - Osteomyelitis: Round area of enhancement, diffuse or rim

Imaging Recommendations
- Best imaging tool: Radiography

DDx: Sickle Cell Anemia

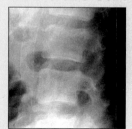

Renal Osteodystrophy

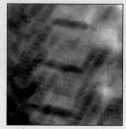

Osteopetrosis

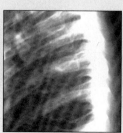

Spond. Dysplasia

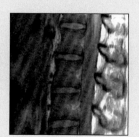

Leukemia

SICKLE CELL

Key Facts

Terminology
- Synonyms: Sickle cell anemia, hemoglobin HbSS disease, HbSC disease, SS disease

Imaging Findings
- Best diagnostic clue: H-shaped vertebral bodies

Top Differential Diagnoses
- Thalassemia

Pathology
- 1% of African-Americans homozygous HbSS, 8-13% HbSA (asymptomatic)

Clinical Issues
- Most common signs/symptoms: Sickle cell crisis
- High incidence of infections
- Pneumococcal septicemia, meningitis

DIFFERENTIAL DIAGNOSIS

Thalassemia
- Avascular necrosis less common than in sickle cell anemia

Other diagnoses may mimic radiographically, but not clinically
- Renal osteodystrophy
  - Thickened, dense vertebral endplates
- Osteopetrosis
  - Diffuse bone sclerosis
- Spondyloepiphyseal dysplasia (SED)
  - Vertebrae with cup shaped endplates
- Diffuse marrow replacement
  - Diffuse low signal marrow on T1WI MRI

PATHOLOGY

General Features
- Genetics
  - Autosomal recessive inheritance
  - Structural defect in hemoglobin HbS: Glutamic acid in position 6 substituted with valine
- Etiology
  - Altered shape and plasticity of red blood cells
  - Sickled cells occlude small blood vessels, producing multisystem infarcts
- Epidemiology
  - 1% of African-Americans homozygous HbSS, 8-13% HbSA (asymptomatic)
  - 3% of African-Americans are HbC carrier

Gross Pathologic & Surgical Features
- Infarction: Dense, hard, sclerotic bone

Microscopic Features
- Infarction: Thickened trabeculae, acellular necrotic bone, fibrotic healing response

CLINICAL ISSUES

Presentation
- Most common signs/symptoms: Sickle cell crisis
- Clinical profile
  - Recurrent crises, jaundice, growth retardation, stroke
  - High incidence of infections
    - Pneumococcal septicemia, meningitis
    - Osteomyelitis usually seen in children

Demographics
- Age: Children protected during first 6 months by elevated levels of fetal Hb (HbF)
- Ethnicity: African, Middle Eastern and Eastern Mediterranean ethnic heritage

Natural History & Prognosis
- Death < 50 years in homozygous form

Treatment
- Sickle cell crisis: Oxygen, hydration, pain management

DIAGNOSTIC CHECKLIST

Image Interpretation Pearls
- MRI to distinguish acute infarction from osteomyelitis

SELECTED REFERENCES

1. Lonergan GJ et al: Sickle cell anemia. Radiographics. 21:971-94, 2001
2. States LJ: Imaging of metabolic bone disease and marrow disorders in children. Radiol Clin North Am. 39:749-72, 2001
3. Umans H et al: The diagnostic role of gadolinium enhanced MRI in distinguishing between acute medullary bone infarct and osteomyelitis. Magn Reson Imaging. 18:255-62, 2000

IMAGE GALLERY

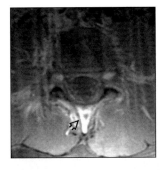 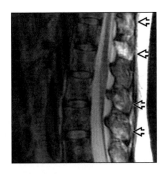

(Left) Axial T1 C+ MR with fat-saturation shows peripheral enhancement (arrow) of infarct of lumbar spinous process. Angular contour of enhancement differs from rounded morphology of infection. *(Right)* Sagittal STIR MR displays low signal in vertebral bodies due to marrow hyperplasia. High signal in multiple spinous processes (arrows) is consistent with bone infarctions.

OSTEOPETROSIS

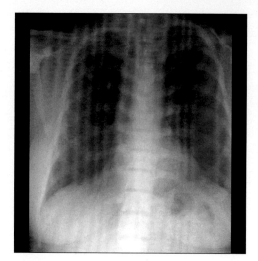

Posteroanterior radiography shows severe sclerosis of all visualized bones. Cortices are thickened and medullary cavities are narrow.

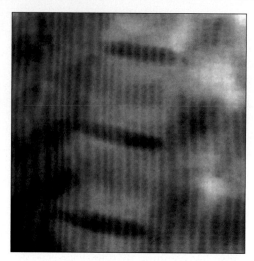

Lateral radiography shows sclerosis of vertebral bodies, ribs and sternum, creating a "rugger jersey" appearance similar to renal osteodystrophy.

TERMINOLOGY

Abbreviations and Synonyms
• Synonym: "Marble bone disease"

Definitions
• Heterogeneous grouping of hereditary osteoclast disorders

IMAGING FINDINGS

General Features
• Best diagnostic clue: Diffuse increase in bone density
• Location: Involves entire skeleton
• Morphology: Thickening of bone cortex

Radiographic Findings
• Radiography
  ○ Bowing deformity of bones
  ○ Frequent fractures
  ○ Infantile form: Dense bones, marrow space obliteration
  ○ Delayed form: Thickened bone cortex, "bone-within-bone" appearance

CT Findings
• CECT: Extramedullary hematopoiesis
• Bone CT

  ○ Severe cortical thickening

MR Findings
• Sclerotic bone low signal intensity on T1WI, T2WI
• Extramedullary hematopoiesis

Imaging Recommendations
• Best imaging tool: Radiography

DIFFERENTIAL DIAGNOSIS

Normal newborn
• "Sandwich" appearance of sclerotic endplates

Renal osteodystrophy
• "Rugger-jersey" spine
• Soft tissue calcification

Blastic metastatic disease
• Prostate > breast > colon; may be widespread

Paget disease
• Thickened, irregular trabeculae

Pycnodysostosis
• Dense bones, dwarfism

Hypervitaminosis A or D
• Dense, brittle bones

DDx: Multiple Dense Bones

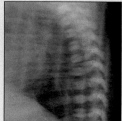

Normal Neonate

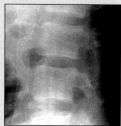

Renal Osteodystrophy

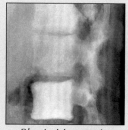

Blastic Metastasis

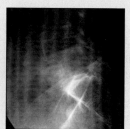

Paget Disease

OSTEOPETROSIS

Key Facts

Terminology
- Synonym: "Marble bone disease"
- Heterogeneous grouping of hereditary osteoclast disorders

Imaging Findings
- Best diagnostic clue: Diffuse increase in bone density
- Infantile form: Dense bones, marrow space obliteration
- Delayed form: Thickened bone cortex, "bone-within-bone" appearance

Top Differential Diagnoses
- Normal newborn
- Renal osteodystrophy
- Blastic metastatic disease
- Paget disease

Myelofibrosis
- Spine sclerosis but peripheral bones spared

PATHOLOGY

General Features
- General path comments: Heterogeneous grouping of genetic defects with similar appearance
- Genetics
  - Infantile types: Autosomal recessive
  - Intermediate, delayed types: Autosomal dominant
- Etiology: Abnormal osteoclastic activity
- Epidemiology: Up to 5.5/100,000 births
- Associated abnormalities
  - Renal tubular acidosis
  - Hepatosplenomegaly
  - Cranial nerve abnormalities secondary to cranial foramina narrowing
  - Cerebral calcifications ("marble brain syndrome")

Gross Pathologic & Surgical Features
- Dense, brittle bones with increased fracture risk

Microscopic Features
- Disorganized, dense bone

Staging, Grading or Classification Criteria
- Infantile presentation ("congenita")
- Intermediate presentation
- Adult presentation ("tarda")

CLINICAL ISSUES

Presentation
- Most common signs/symptoms
  - Growth disturbance in infantile forms
  - Other signs/symptoms
    - Fractures, pain, neurologic symptoms

Demographics
- Age: Severe forms present in infancy; mild forms may be asymptomatic with incidental detection

Natural History & Prognosis
- Infantile forms lethal
- Milder forms have increased fracture risk

Treatment
- Options, risks, complications

- Medical: Calcium restriction, calcitriol, steroids, parathyroid hormone
- Bone marrow transplantation for infantile form
  - Radiographic abnormalities regress 1-2 years following successful transplantation

DIAGNOSTIC CHECKLIST

Consider
- Osteopetrosis in differential for dense bones

Image Interpretation Pearls
- "Bone-within-bone" appearance not pathognomonic; may also be seen in young children during growth spurts

SELECTED REFERENCES

1. Kocher MS et al: Osteopetrosis. Am J Orthop. 32(5):222-8, 2003
2. Steward CG: Neurological aspects of osteopetrosis. Neuropathol Appl Neurobiol. 29(2):87-97, 2003
3. Stoker DJ: Osteopetrosis. Semin Musculoskelet Radiol. 6(4):299-305, 2002
4. Senel K et al: Type II autosomal dominant osteopetrosis. Rheumatol Int. 22(3):116-8, 2002
5. Cheow HK et al: Imaging of malignant infantile osteopetrosis before and after bone marrow transplantation. Pediatr Radiol. 31(12):869-75, 2001

IMAGE GALLERY

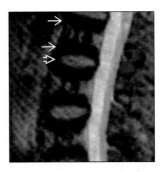 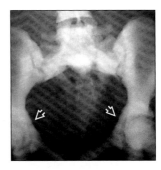

(Left) Sagittal T2WI MR demonstrates thick bands of sclerosis (arrows) at vertebral endplates, as well as sclerotic islands centrally. Intervertebral discs (open arrow), fatty marrow are high signal. *(Right)* Anteroposterior radiography shows severe cortical thickening throughout pelvis. Protrusio acetabulae (arrows) is secondary to weakened bone structure.

OCHRONOSIS

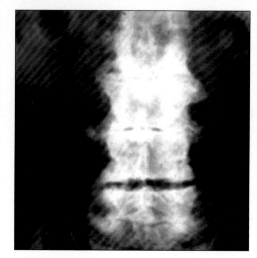

Lateral radiography shows linear calcification of intervertebral disc in lower thoracic spine. Bones are osteopenic (Courtesy M. Gelman, MD).

Anteroposterior radiography shows advanced degenerative disc disease overshadowing disc calcifications in young patient with ochronosis (Courtesy M. Gelman, MD).

TERMINOLOGY

Abbreviations and Synonyms
- Synonyms: Alkaptonuria, alcaptonuria

Definitions
- Deposition of homogentisic acid and its metabolites secondary to absence of homogentisic acid oxidase enzyme
- Ochronosis: Abnormal pigmentation caused by deposition of homogentisic acid
- Alkaptonuria: Homogentisic acid in urine

IMAGING FINDINGS

General Features
- Best diagnostic clue: Calcified intervertebral discs
- Location: Lumbar spine > thoracic > cervical
- Morphology: Linear intervertebral disc calcification

Radiographic Findings
- Radiography
  - Calcified intervertebral discs
  - Premature degenerative disc disease
  - Ankylosis of spine
  - Osteopenia
  - Scoliosis and kyphosis
  - Sacroiliac osteoarthritis

  - Extraspinal findings
    - Premature osteoarthritis of axial skeleton large joints
    - Calcification of pubic symphysis fibrocartilage
    - Chondrocalcinosis rare in peripheral skeleton
    - +/- Involvement of ear cartilage

Imaging Recommendations
- Best imaging tool: Radiography

DIFFERENTIAL DIAGNOSIS

Degenerative disc disease
- Degenerated discs may calcify
- Discogenic vertebral body sclerosis

Ankylosing spondylitis
- Calcification of annular ligament (not disc) + facet ankylosis

Osteoarthritis
- May have identical appearance in appendicular skeleton large joints

Gout
- Rare in spine; positive cases show endplate destruction, tophi

DDx: Ochronosis

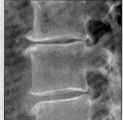

Disc Calcification

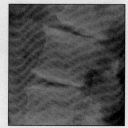

Disc Degeneration

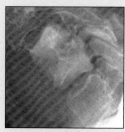

Hemodialysis

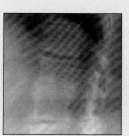

CPPD

OCHRONOSIS

Key Facts

Terminology
- Synonyms: Alkaptonuria, alcaptonuria
- Deposition of homogentisic acid and its metabolites secondary to absence of homogentisic acid oxidase enzyme

Imaging Findings
- Best diagnostic clue: Calcified intervertebral discs
- Calcified intervertebral discs

- Premature degenerative disc disease
- Ankylosis of spine
- Osteopenia
- Scoliosis and kyphosis
- Sacroiliac osteoarthritis

Top Differential Diagnoses
- Degenerative disc disease
- Ankylosing spondylitis
- Osteoarthritis

Hemodialysis arthropathy
- Deposition of crystals and/or amyloid
- Usually involves cervical spine
- Endplate destruction, peridiscal calcifications

Calcium pyrophosphate deposition disease (CPPD)
- Often spares spine; most commonly involves hips, pubic symphysis, shoulder, knees, wrists
- Calcification of hyaline and fibrocartilage, periarticular structures

PATHOLOGY

General Features
- General path comments
  - Homogentisic acid in urine causes urine to darken when exposed to air
  - Not all patients with alkaptonuria develop ochronotic arthritis
    - Arthritis caused by accumulation of homogentisic acid ⇒ brittleness, degeneration of cartilage
- Genetics: Autosomal recessive
- Etiology: Deficiency of enzyme homogentisic acid oxidase
- Epidemiology: 1:1,000,000
- Associated abnormalities: Cardiac ochronosis → accelerated coronary disease

Gross Pathologic & Surgical Features
- Brown or black pigmentation of skin, mucosa, sclerae, connective tissues, sweat, urine

Microscopic Features
- Intracellular pigment
- Cartilage pigmentation and degeneration

CLINICAL ISSUES

Presentation
- Most common signs/symptoms
  - Dark urine
  - Other signs/symptoms
    - Back pain
    - Arthritis of large peripheral joints

Demographics
- Age: Arthritis usually develops in adulthood

- Gender: M:F = 2:1

Natural History & Prognosis
- Accelerated degenerative disease of spine, hips, knees, shoulders
- Coronary artery disease

Treatment
- Nitisinone can reduce homogentisic acid production, but long term efficacy not known

DIAGNOSTIC CHECKLIST

Consider
- Extremely rare; consider other causes of disc calcification, severe degenerative spine first

SELECTED REFERENCES
1. Farzannia A et al: Alkaptonuria and lumbar disc herniation. Report of three cases. J Neurosurg. 98(1 Suppl):87-9, 2003
2. Nas K et al: Ochronosis: a case of severe ochronotic arthropathy. Clin Rheumatol. 21(2):170-2, 2002
3. Phornphutkul C et al: Natural history of alkaptonuria. N Engl J Med. 347(26):2111-21, 2002

IMAGE GALLERY

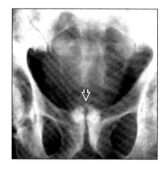 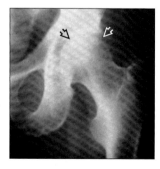

(Left) Anteroposterior radiography shows osteoarthritis-like changes due to ochronosis of sacroiliac joints. Chondrocalcinosis is present in pubic symphysis (arrow) (Courtesy M. Gelman, MD). (Right) Anteroposterior radiography shows joint space narrowing and minimal chondrocalcinosis (white arrow). Contour of femoral head is irregular (black arrow) (Courtesy M. Gelman, MD).

CONNECTIVE TISSUE DISORDERS

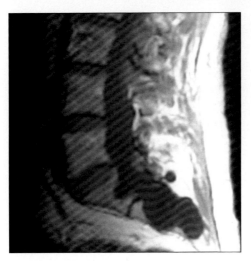

Sagittal T1WI MR shows marked dural ectasia eroding sacrum in patient with Marfan syndrome.

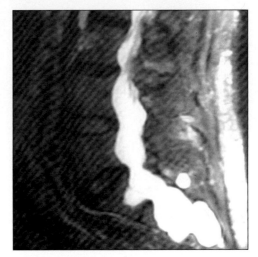

Sagittal T2WI MR shows homogeneously high signal intensity CSF in Marfan patient with severe dural ectasia.

TERMINOLOGY

Abbreviations and Synonyms
- Most common types are Marfan, Ehlers-Danlos (EDS), Stickler syndrome
- Ehlers-Danlos also known as cutis hyperelastica

Definitions
- Group of congenital disorders with similar imaging findings

IMAGING FINDINGS

General Features
- Best diagnostic clue: Dural ectasia
- Location: Most commonly lumbar spine and sacrum

Radiographic Findings
- Radiography
  - Tremendous overlap in appearance of connective tissue disorders
    - Rely on physical examination, other organ system findings for specific diagnosis
  - Dural ectasia
    - Scalloping posterior margins vertebral bodies
    - Widened interpediculate distance
    - Thinned, eroded pedicles
    - Erosion of sacrum

  - Scoliosis
    - Usually S-curve, same appearance as idiopathic scoliosis
    - Sometimes complex curve
    - Kyphosis often present
  - Osteopenia
    - Often said to be absent in Marfan syndrome, but documented by bone densitometry
  - Marfan syndrome
    - Increased anterior translation C1-C2
    - Rotary subluxation C1-C2
    - Increased height of odontoid process
    - Basilar invagination
    - Biconcave vertebrae
  - Ehlers-Danlos syndrome
    - Platyspondyly

CT Findings
- Bone CT
  - Dural ectasia
    - Width of dural sac > at L5 than L4
    - Scalloping posterior margins vertebral bodies
    - Anterior sacral meningocele
    - Perineural cysts
- CT myelogram
  - Delineates extent of ectasia
  - May show diverticula in spinal canal
    - Spinal cord compression can occur
  - Contrast diluted by large CSF space

DDx: Connective Tissue Disorders

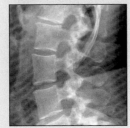

Neurofibromatosis

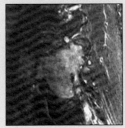

Neurofibroma T2WI

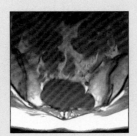

Tarlov Cyst T1WI

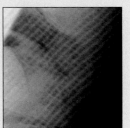

OI

CONNECTIVE TISSUE DISORDERS

Key Facts

Terminology
- Most common types are Marfan, Ehlers-Danlos (EDS), Stickler syndrome
- Group of congenital disorders with similar imaging findings

Imaging Findings
- Tremendous overlap in appearance of connective tissue disorders
- Dural ectasia
- Scalloping posterior margins vertebral bodies
- Widened interpediculate distance
- Scoliosis
- Osteopenia
- Best imaging tool: MRI

- Protocol advice: Include entire sacrum on sagittal images

Top Differential Diagnoses
- Neurofibromatosis
- Nerve sheath tumor
- Tarlov cyst
- Osteogenesis imperfecta (OI)

Pathology
- Variety of genetic defects in connective tissue
- Aortic root dilation
- Mitral valve prolapse
- Unusually tall, slender body habitus
- Joint hypermobility
- Arachnodactyly

- o May not have homogeneous filling of presacral meningocele or diverticula

MR Findings
- T1WI
  - o Enlarged CSF space
  - o Presacral meningocele may be difficult to see (mimicking bowel)
  - o Bone erosion
- T2WI
  - o Enlarged CSF space
  - o May have some heterogeneity of signal due to flow
  - o Presacral meningocele better seen than on T1WI
  - o May see spinal cord compression in thoracic spine due to diverticula
  - o May see cysts posterior to spinal canal
- STIR: Similar to T2WI
- T1 C+: No abnormal enhancement

Imaging Recommendations
- Best imaging tool: MRI
- Protocol advice: Include entire sacrum on sagittal images

DIFFERENTIAL DIAGNOSIS

Neurofibromatosis
- Scoliosis
- Dural ectasia
- Nerve sheath tumors
- Gracile bones

Nerve sheath tumor
- Posterior vertebral body scalloping
- Thinning of pedicles
- Heterogeneous SI on T2WI
- Enhance with gadolinium

Tarlov cyst
- Perineural cyst in sacrum
- Incidental finding on MR or CT

Osteogenesis imperfecta (OI)
- Scoliosis
- Vertebral deformities and fractures
- Short body habitus

Homocystinuria
- Scoliosis
- Osteopenia
- Arachnodactyly
- Ligamentous laxity
- Mental retardation
- Ectopia lentis

Seronegative spondyloarthropathy
- Rarely see scalloping posterior vertebral bodies
- Vertebral erosions progress to ankylosis

PATHOLOGY

General Features
- Genetics
  - o EDS: Heterogeneous group of genetic based disorders, with different modes of inheritance
    - EDS I,II (classic type), autosomal dominant, 80% of cases
    - EDS III (hypermobilty type), autosomal dominant
    - EDS IV (vascular type), dominant and recessive forms
    - EDS VII (arthrochalasia type), autosomal dominant
  - o Marfan: Autosomal dominant with wide range of clinical severity
    - Mutations in fibrillin-1 gene (FBN-1) on chromosome 15q21
    - > 90 different mutations of FBN-1
    - > 25% of cases are new mutations
  - o Stickler syndrome:
    - Autosomal dominant, osteoarthritis, joint hypermobility, mild spondyloepiphyseal dysplasia
- Etiology
  - o Variety of genetic defects in connective tissue

CONNECTIVE TISSUE DISORDERS

- Marfan: Fibrillin-1 protein important component of elastic + nonelastic connective tissues
  - EDS I-III linked to collagen type V mutations (COL5A1 ⇒ A3 genes)
  - EDS IV linked to collagen type III abnormality
  - EDS VII linked to collagen type I abnormality
  - Stickler syndrome: Most involve mutations of COL2A1 gene
- Epidemiology
  - Ehlers-Danlos: 1:20,000
  - Marfan: 1:10,000 ⇒ 20,000
- Associated abnormalities
  - Marfan, Ehlers Danlos and Stickler syndromes share following
    - Aortic root dilation
    - Mitral valve prolapse
    - Unusually tall, slender body habitus
    - Joint hypermobility
    - Arachnodactyly
    - Blue sclerae
  - Marfan
    - Ectopia lentis
    - Retinal detachment
    - Pectus carinatum or excavatum
    - Protrusio acetabulae
    - Leg length discrepancy
  - Ehlers Danlos syndrome
    - Hyperelastic, fragile skin
    - Fragile blood vessels
    - Aneurysms of multiple vessels
    - Peripheral neuropathy
    - Triphalangeal thumbs
    - Radioulnar synostosis
    - Some types have ectasia, perforation of bowel
  - Stickler Syndrome distinguished by
    - Midface hypoplasia, micrognathia

Staging, Grading or Classification Criteria

- Many types of Ehlers-Danlos

CLINICAL ISSUES

Presentation

- Most common signs/symptoms
  - Dural ectasia often asymptomatic
  - Cord symptoms if thoracic spine dural ectasia
  - High prevalence back pain in patients with connective tissue disorders
  - Other signs/symptoms
    - Headaches, sciatica
- Clinical profile: "Marfanoid" body habitus not specific to Marfan syndrome

Demographics

- Age
  - Usually becomes apparent in early childhood
  - May not present until adulthood
- Gender
  - Marfan: M = F
  - Ehlers-Danlos: More common in males

Natural History & Prognosis

- Premature death from cardiac disease common
  - Average life expectancy < 40 if untreated
- Bone and joint injuries common because of hypermobility

Treatment

- Options, risks, complications
  - Surgery for scoliosis has increased complication rate compared to idiopathic scoliosis
  - Surgical treatment of aortic dilation allows near normal life expectancy
    - Lifespan for Marfan syndrome ↑ from 32 years in 1972 ⇒ 61 years in 1996
  - Surgical treatment for Ehlers-Danlos complicated by skin and connective tissue fragility
- Injuries can be reduced by lifestyle alteration to avoid overly stressing joints

DIAGNOSTIC CHECKLIST

Image Interpretation Pearls

- Check for aortic dilation on all thoracic spine MR and CT of scoliosis

SELECTED REFERENCES

1. Giampietro PF et al: Marfan syndrome: orthopedic and genetic review. Curr Opin Pediatr. 14(1):35-41, 2002
2. Jones KB et al: Leg-length discrepancy and scoliosis in Marfan syndrome. J Pediatr Orthop. 22(6):807-12, 2002
3. Nallamshetty L et al: Plain radiography of the lumbosacral spine in Marfan syndrome. Spine J. 2(5):327-33, 2002
4. Rose PS et al: Thoracolumbar spinal abnormalities in Stickler syndrome. Spine. 26(4):403-9, 2001
5. Ahn NU et al: Dural ectasia and conventional radiography in the Marfan lumbosacral spine. Skeletal Radiol. 30(6):338-45, 2001
6. Herzka A et al: Atlantoaxial rotatory subluxation in patients with Marfan syndrome. A report of three cases. Spine. 25(4):524-6, 2000
7. Carter N et al: Bone mineral density in adults with Marfan syndrome. Rheumatology (Oxford). 39(3):307-9, 2000
8. Letts M et al: The spinal manifestations of Stickler's syndrome. Spine. 24(12):1260-4, 1999
9. Villeirs GM et al: Widening of the spinal canal and dural ectasia in Marfan's syndrome: assessment by CT. Neuroradiology. 41(11):850-4, 1999
10. Hobbs WR et al: The cervical spine in Marfan syndrome. Spine. 22(9):983-9, 1997
11. Raff ML et al: Joint hypermobility syndromes. Curr Opin Rheumatol. 8(5):459-66, 1996
12. Raftopoulos C et al: Anterior sacral meningocele and Marfan syndrome: a review. Acta Chir Belg. 93(1):1-7, 1993
13. Kozlowski K et al: Lumbar platyspondyly--characteristic sign of Ehlers-Danlos syndrome. Skeletal Radiol. 20(8):589-90, 1991

CONNECTIVE TISSUE DISORDERS

IMAGE GALLERY

Typical

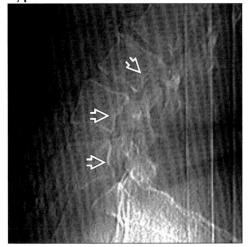
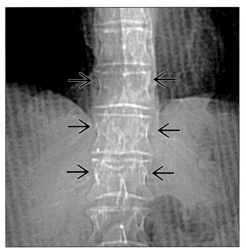

(Left) Lateral radiography shows posterior scalloping (arrows) of vertebral bodies due to dural ectasia in patient with Ehlers-Danlos syndrome. *(Right)* Anteroposterior radiography shows widened interpediculate distances and thinned pedicles at multiple levels (arrows) due to large thecal diverticulum in patient with Marfan syndrome.

Typical

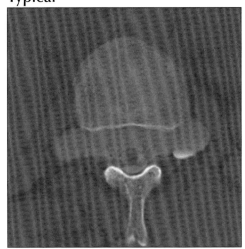
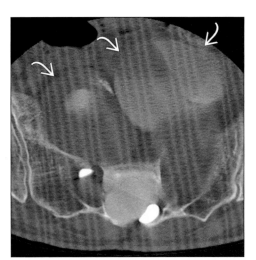

(Left) Axial CT myelogram shows contrast filling bilateral nerve root sleeve cysts in patient with Marfan syndrome. *(Right)* Axial CT myelogram shows large, multilocular presacral meningocele (arrows) in patient with Marfan syndrome. Note dilution of contrast due to size of meningocele.

Typical

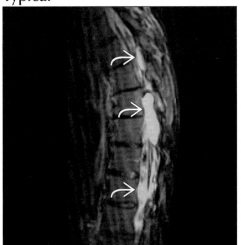
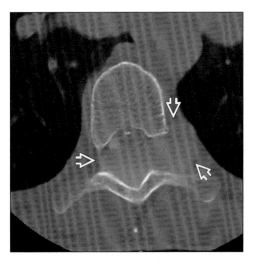

(Left) Sagittal STIR MR shows dural diverticula (arrows) in thoracic spine. *(Right)* Axial CT myelogram shows large dural diverticulum (arrow) compressing spinal cord in patient with Marfan syndrome.

OSTEOGENESIS IMPERFECTA

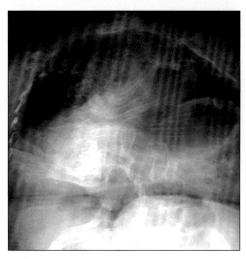

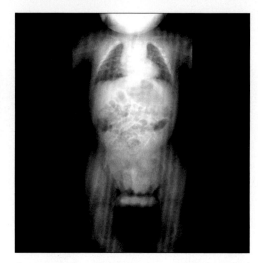

Anteroposterior radiography demonstrates severe kyphoscoliosis, as well as rib and clavicle fractures in adult patient with type I osteogenesis imperfecta.

Anteroposterior radiography shows relatively normal trunk length and short, deformed lower extremities in a 4 month old with type II disease.

TERMINOLOGY

Abbreviations and Synonyms

- Synonyms: Osteogenesis imperfecta (OI) "brittle bone disease"

Definitions

- Genetic disorder of type 1 collagen resulting in bone fragility
- Codfish vertebra: Cupping of superior and inferior vertebral body endplates
- Terms "congenita" and "tarda" no longer used

IMAGING FINDINGS

General Features

- Best diagnostic clue: Severe osteopenia and multiple fractures
- Location: Entire skeleton
- Morphology: Multiple skeletal fractures

Radiographic Findings

- Radiography
  - Vertebral fractures, vertebra plana, "codfish vertebrae"
  - Kyphoscoliosis
  - Osteoporosis
    - Cortical thinning, resorption of secondary trabeculae with prominent primary trabeculae
  - Multiple fractures of long bones and ribs
    - Bowing deformity due to microfractures as well as radiographically evident fractures
  - Enlarged epiphyses
  - "Popcorn" calcifications in metaphyses
    - Calcified cartilage nodules; due to fragmentation of growth plate from trauma
  - Growth retardation
  - Pelvis: Protrusio acetabulae, coxa vara
  - Increased anteroposterior chest diameter
  - Classified into 4 types based on clinical, genetic and radiographic criteria (see below)
    - Severe forms: Bones may be short, thickened due to multiple fractures in utero and early childhood
    - Milder forms: Bones thin and gracile

CT Findings

- Bone CT
  - Thin bony cortices
  - Medullary cavity almost entirely filled with fat
    - Primary trabeculae sparse, but normally oriented
    - Secondary trabeculae almost absent
  - Basilar invagination
  - Kyphoscoliosis
  - Otosclerosis

DDx: Diffuse Vertebral Loss of Height

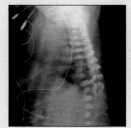

Spond. Dysplasia

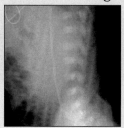

Thanatophoric

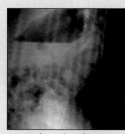

Achondroplasia

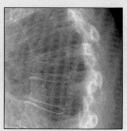

Osteoporosis

OSTEOGENESIS IMPERFECTA

Key Facts

Terminology
- Synonyms: Osteogenesis imperfecta (OI) "brittle bone disease"
- Genetic disorder of type 1 collagen resulting in bone fragility
- Terms "congenita" and "tarda" no longer used

Imaging Findings
- Best diagnostic clue: Severe osteopenia and multiple fractures
- Vertebral fractures, vertebra plana, "codfish vertebrae"
- Classified into 4 types based on clinical, genetic and radiographic criteria (see below)

Top Differential Diagnoses
- Nonaccidental trauma (NAT)
- Dwarfisms

- Osteoporosis

Pathology
- Nearly all cases autosomal dominant
- Inherited or spontaneous mutation
- Epidemiology: 4/100,000 births

Clinical Issues
- Multiple fractures
- Scoliosis
- +/- Deafness, blue sclerae
- Severe forms previously lethal now may survive to adulthood
- Fractures often less common after puberty
- Growth retardation varies with severity of disease

MR Findings
- Kyphoscoliosis
- Hydromyelia
- Abnormal marrow signal intensity due to fractures
- May be used to augment ultrasound for antenatal diagnosis

Ultrasonographic Findings
- Real Time
  - Antenatal diagnosis in 2nd trimester
  - Poorly ossified skull
  - Short ribs
  - Short, deformed limbs

Nuclear Medicine Findings
- Bone Scan: Positive at fracture sites

Other Modality Findings
- Bone densitometry with dual energy x-ray absorptiometry (DEXA) or CT
  - Used to aid diagnosis in mild forms, follow response to treatment

Imaging Recommendations
- Best imaging tool: Radiography
- Protocol advice: Low kVp technique to compensate for osteoporosis

DIFFERENTIAL DIAGNOSIS

Nonaccidental trauma (NAT)
- Normal bone mineral density
- Fractures may otherwise appear identical
- Careful history, family evaluation needed
- Genetic testing may be useful

Dwarfisms
- Loss of vertebral body height
- Short stature
- Scoliosis
- Bone density variable
- Common causes
  - Thanatophoric dwarfism

  - Achondroplasia
  - Spondyloepiphyseal dysplasia (SED)

Osteoporosis
- Thinned bone cortices, accentuation of primary trabeculae, resorption of secondary trabeculae
- Radiography insensitive for diagnosis; better evaluated by bone densitometry
- Codfish vertebrae, compression fractures
- Causes
  - Senile
  - Cushing disease
  - Hyperparathyroidism
  - Premature menopause
  - Cerebral palsy
  - Paralysis
  - Disuse
  - Malabsorption syndromes

PATHOLOGY

General Features
- General path comments
  - Abnormal type I collagen
  - Type I collagen found in bone, skin, sclerae
- Genetics
  - Nearly all cases autosomal dominant
  - Inherited or spontaneous mutation
- Etiology: Numerous type I collagen mutations ⇒ "brittle" bone
- Epidemiology: 4/100,000 births
- Associated abnormalities
  - Blue sclerae
  - Early hearing loss
  - Brittle teeth
  - Thin, fragile skin
  - Joint laxity
  - Respiratory, cardiac problems

Gross Pathologic & Surgical Features
- Thin, eggshell-like bone cortices
- Decreased medullary trabeculae

OSTEOGENESIS IMPERFECTA

- Recent or healed fractures
- Bowing, angulation of bones
- Overgrowth of epiphyses

Microscopic Features
- Lack of organized trabeculae
- Prominent osteoid seams
- Morphologically normal osteoblasts, increased in number
- Growth-plate fragmentation
  - Due to trauma
  - Results in "popcorn" calcifications in metaphyses seen on radiographs
  - Contributes to growth disturbance

Staging, Grading or Classification Criteria
- Type I: Most common type
  - Thin, gracile long bones
  - High fracture risk in childhood, decreases after puberty
  - Kyphoscoliosis, wormian bones
  - Blue sclerae
- Type II: Often lethal early in life
  - Short, broad, deformed bones at birth due to multiple fractures
- Type III: Autosomal recessive; rare
  - Fractures at birth, kyphoscoliosis
- Type IV: Similar to type I
  - Kyphoscoliosis, wormian bones
  - Sclerae usually normal in adulthood, may be blue in childhood
- Recently types V-VII have been proposed, not distinguishable radiographically
  - These types do not localize to genes for type I collagen; etiology unknown

CLINICAL ISSUES

Presentation
- Most common signs/symptoms
  - Multiple fractures
  - Scoliosis
  - +/- Deafness, blue sclerae
  - Short stature secondary to fractures, kyphoscoliosis, growth plate abnormalities
- Clinical profile
  - Diagnosis suggested by radiographs, confirmed with
    - Skin biopsy
    - Genetic testing
    - Caveat: Both tests may be false negative

Demographics
- Age
  - Often evident at birth
  - Mild cases may present in adulthood
- Gender: M = F

Natural History & Prognosis
- Severe forms previously lethal now may survive to adulthood
- Fractures often less common after puberty
- Growth retardation varies with severity of disease

Treatment
- Conservative management
  - Bisphosphonates used for medical therapy with some success
  - Prolonged immobilization avoided because of resultant worsening of osteoporosis
- Surgical management
  - Intramedullary rod placement for long bone fractures
    - Least invasive internal fixation for rapid mobilization
    - Helps prevent progression of deformity, further fractures
  - Spinal fusion for scoliosis
  - High risk of hardware mechanical failure

DIAGNOSTIC CHECKLIST

Consider
- Main differential diagnosis is nonaccidental trauma

SELECTED REFERENCES

1. Falk MJ et al: Intravenous bisphosphonate therapy in children with osteogenesis imperfecta. Pediatrics. 111(3):573-8, 2003
2. Teng SW et al: Initial experience using magnetic resonance imaging in prenatal diagnosis of osteogenesis imperfecta type II. a case report. Clin Imaging. 27(1):55-8, 2003
3. Zeitlin L et al: Modern approach to children with osteogenesis imperfecta. J Pediatr Orthop B. 12(2):77-87, 2003
4. Iwamoto J et al: Increased bone resorption with decreased activity and increased recruitment of osteoblasts in osteogenesis imperfecta type I. J Bone Miner Metab. 20(3):174-9, 2002
5. Cole WG: Advances in osteogenesis imperfecta. Clin Orthop. (401):6-16, 2002
6. Ward LM et al: Osteogenesis imperfecta type VII: an autosomal recessive form of brittle bone disease. Bone. 31(1):12-8, 2002
7. Marlowe A et al: Testing for osteogenesis imperfecta in cases of suspected non-accidental injury. J Med Genet. 39(6):382-6, 2002
8. Glorieux FH et al: Osteogenesis imperfecta type VI: a form of brittle bone disease with a mineralization defect. J Bone Miner Res. 17(1):30-8, 2002
9. Glorieux FH et al: Type V osteogenesis imperfecta: a new form of brittle bone disease. J Bone Miner Res. 15(9):1650-8, 2000
10. Mulpuri K et al: Intramedullary rodding in osteogenesis imperfecta. J Pediatr Orthop. 20(2):267-73, 2000
11. Bischoff H et al: Type I osteogenesis imperfecta: diagnostic difficulties. Clin Rheumatol. 18(1):48-51, 1999
12. Widmann RF et al: Spinal deformity, pulmonary compromise, and quality of life in osteogenesis imperfecta. Spine. 24(16):1673-8, 1999
13. Moore MS et al: The role of dual energy x-ray absorptiometry in aiding the diagnosis of pediatric osteogenesis imperfecta. Am J Orthop. 27(12):797-801, 1998
14. Kocher MS et al: Osteogenesis imperfecta. J Am Acad Orthop Surg. 6(4):225-36, 1998
15. Tongsong T et al: Prenatal diagnosis of osteogenesis imperfecta type II. Int J Gynaecol Obstet. 61(1):33-8, 1998

OSTEOGENESIS IMPERFECTA

IMAGE GALLERY

Typical

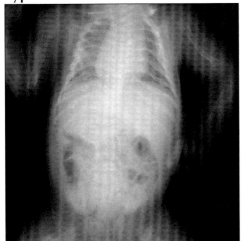
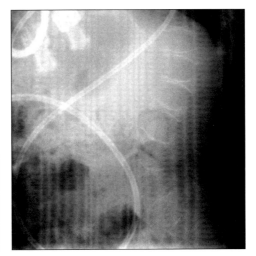

(Left) Anteroposterior radiography shows 1 year old with type II disease. Scoliosis, not present at birth, has developed. Left humerus is gracile, right is broad; both show fractures. *(Right)* Lateral radiography demonstrates flattened vertebrae throughout lumbar spine. Disc spaces are much taller than vertebrae.

Typical

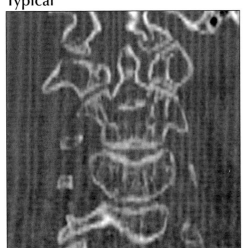
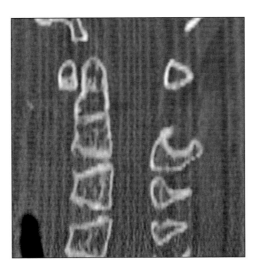

(Left) Coronal bone CT (type 1 osteogenesis imperfecta) shows paucity of trabeculae and cortical thinning in cervical spine. *(Right)* Sagittal bone CT (type I osteogenesis imperfecta) depicts wedging of cervical vertebral bodies at multiple levels. Secondary trabeculae are not seen, and primary trabeculae are sparse.

Typical

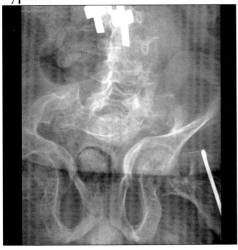
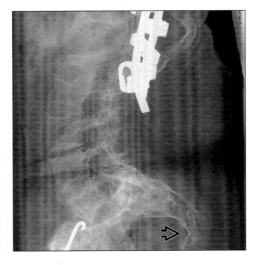

(Left) Anteroposterior radiography reveals typical type I osteogenesis imperfecta pelvic deformity, with gracile bones and severe protrusio acetabulae. *(Right)* Lateral radiography (type 1 osteogenesis imperfecta) shows cupping of vertebral endplates throughout lumbar spine. Sacral insufficiency fracture is also evident (arrow).

PART II

Trauma, Degeneration, and Inflammatory Arthritides

Trauma **1**

Degenerative Disease and Inflammatory Arthritides **2**

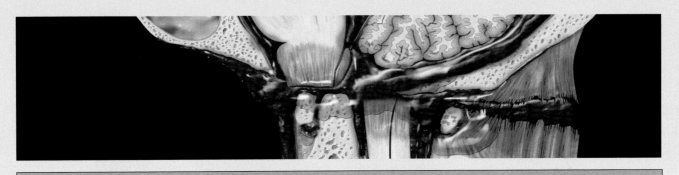

SECTION 1: Trauma

Introduction and Overview

Vertebral Column, Discs, and Paraspinal Muscle

Cord, Dura, and Vessels

SPINE ANATOMY

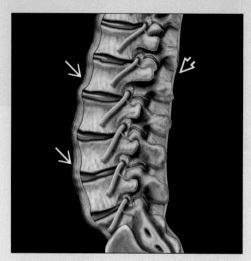

Lateral graphic of lumbar spine shows disc, vertebral body, and exiting root relationships. Note normal anterior longitudinal ligament (arrows) and interspinous ligaments (open arrow).

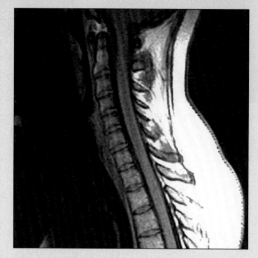

Sagittal T1WI MR shows normal cervical spine vertebral marrow signal slightly hyperintense to disc, with normal alignment and prevertebral soft tissues.

TERMINOLOGY

Abbreviations and Synonyms
- C1 (atlas), C2 (axis)
- Atlanto-occipital (AO)
- Anterior longitudinal ligament (ALL)
- Posterior longitudinal ligament (PLL)

IMAGING ANATOMY

- 33 spinal vertebrae
  - Two components
    - Cylindrical ventral bone mass - body; dorsal arch
  - 7 cervical, 12 thoracic, 5 lumbar
  - 5 fused elements form sacrum
  - 4-5 irregular ossicles form coccyx
- Arch
  - 2 pedicles, 2 laminae, 7 processes (1 spinous, 4 articular, 2 transverse)
  - Pedicles attach to dorsolateral aspect of body
  - Pedicles unit with pair of arched flat laminae
  - Lamina capped by dorsal projection – spinous process
  - Transverse process arise from sides of arches
  - Articular processes (zygapophyses)
    - Diarthrodial joints
    - Superior process bear facet with surface directed dorsally
    - Inferior process bear facet with surface directed ventrally
  - Pars interarticulares
    - Part of arch that lie between superior and inferior articular facets of all subatlantal movable elements
    - Position to receive biomechanical stress of translational forces displacing superior facets ventrally, while inferior facets remain attached to dorsal arch (spondylolysis)

- C2 unique anterior relation of superior facet with posterior placed inferior facet giving elongated C2 pars interarticularis which is site of hangman's fracture
- Cervical
  - Cervical bodies small, thin relative to size of arch, foramen
    - Transverse diameter > AP
    - Lateral edges of superior surface of body turned upward to form uncinate processes
    - Transverse foramen perforate transverse processes
  - C1: No body, circular
    - Superior facet large ovals, facing upwards
    - Inferior facets, circular
    - Large transverse processes with fused anterior and posterior tubercles
  - C2: Axis body with dens/odontoid process
    - Odontoid embryologically arises from centrum of first cervical vertebrae
  - C7: Transitional body with spinous process prominent
- Thoracic
  - Bodies increase in size from superior to inferior, heart-shaped
  - Facets for rib articulations, laminae broad/thick
  - Spinous processes long, directed obliquely caudally
  - Superior facets thin, directed posteriorly
  - T1 shows complete facet for capitulum of first rib, and inferior demifacet for capitulum of second rib
  - T12 resembles upper lumbar bodies with inferior facet directed more laterally
- Lumbar
  - Body large, wide, thick
  - Lack of transverse foramen or of costal articular facets
  - Pedicles strong, directed posteriorly
  - Superior articular processes directed dorsomedial (almost face each other)
  - Inferior articular processes directed anteriorly, laterally
- Joints

DIFFERENTIAL DIAGNOSIS

Extradural disease
- Trauma/fracture
- Congenital segmentation anomalies
- Degenerative disc disease/herniation
- Facet degenerative arthropathy/central stenosis
- Metastatic disease
- Primary bone tumors
- Disc space infection/vertebral osteomyelitis/epidural abscess
- Epidural hemorrhage

Intradural extramedullary disease
- Schwannoma
- Meningioma
- Leptomeningeal metastatic disease
- Granulomatous disease (sarcoid)
- Infectious/meningitis
- Subdural/subarachnoid hemorrhage

Intramedullary disease
- Infectious - primary viral or bacterial infection
- Demyelinating diseases
- Astrocytoma
- Ependymoma
- Hemangioblastoma
- Metastatic disease
- Infarction
- Vascular malformations
- Metabolic (B12 deficiency)
- Trauma

- ○ Synarthrosis
  - During development and 1st decade of life
  - Immovable joint of cartilage
  - Neurocentral joint occurs at union point of two centers of ossification for two halves of vertebral arch and centrum
- ○ Diarthrosis
  - True synovial joints
  - Articular processes, costovertebral joints
  - Atlantoaxial and sacroiliac articulations
  - Pivot type joint at median atlantoaxial articulation
  - All others are gliding joints
- ○ Amphiarthroses
  - Nonsynovial, movable connective tissue joints
  - Symphysis – fibrocartilage of intervertebral disc
  - Syndesmosis – ligamentous connections
  - → Paired syndesmoses include ligamenta flava, intertransverse ligaments, interspinous ligaments
  - → Unpaired syndesmosis: Supraspinous ligament
- ○ Atlanto-occipital articulation
  - Diarthrosis between lateral mass of atlas and occipital condyles
  - Syndesmoses of atlanto-occipital membranes
  - → Anterior AO membrane is extension of ALL
  - → Posterior AO membrane is homologous to ligamenta flava
- ○ Atlantoaxial articulation - pivot joint
  - Transverse ligament maintain relationship of odontoid to anterior arch of atlas
  - Synovial cavities between transverse ligament/odontoid, and atlas/odontoid junctions
- Disc
  - ○ Nucleus pulposus - remnant of notochordal tissue
    - Eccentric position within confines of annulus, more dorsal with respect to center of vertebral body
    - Loose fibrous strands with gelatinous matrix
    - Scattered chondrocytes
    - Proteoglycans form major macromolecular component, including chondroitin 6-sulfate, keratan sulfate, hyaluronic acid

- Proteoglycans consists of protein core with multiple attached glycosaminoglycan chains
- Nucleus consists of 85-90% water, along with extracellular matrix of collagen and proteoglycans
- ○ Annulus fibrosus
  - Blends gradually with nucleus pulposus
  - Concentric series of fibrous lamellae constraining nucleus
  - Type I collagen predominates at periphery of annulus, type II predominating in the inner annulus
- Anterior longitudinal ligament
  - ○ Ventral surface of spine from skull to sacrum
  - ○ Narrowest in cervical spine
  - ○ Firmly attached at ends of each vertebral body
  - ○ Loosely attached at midsection of disc
- Posterior longitudinal ligament
  - ○ Dorsal surface of bodies from skull to sacrum
  - ○ Segmental denticulate configuration
- Craniocervical ligaments
  - ○ Located anterior to spinal cord, in three layers
  - ○ Anterior - odontoid ligaments
    - Apical ligament - small fibrous band extending from dens tip to basion
    - Alar ligaments - thick, horizontally directed ligaments extending from lateral surface of dens tip to anteromedial occipital condyles
  - ○ Middle - cruciate ligament
    - Transverse ligament is strong horizontal component of cruciate ligament extending from behind dens to medial aspect of C1 lateral masses
    - Craniocaudal component consists of fibrous band running from transverse ligament superiorly to foramen magnum and inferiorly to C2
  - ○ Posterior - tectorial membrane
    - Continuation of PLL and attaches to anterior rim foramen magnum
- Vertebral artery
  - ○ First branch of subclavian on both sides
  - ○ Travels within foramen transversarium within transverse processes
  - ○ 10% of cases the artery passes through C7 foramen
  - ○ Nerve roots pass posterior to vertebral artery

SPINE ANATOMY

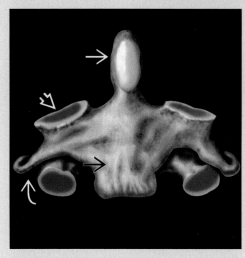

Normal axis anterior view shows odontoid with articular facet (arrow), superior articulating process (open arrow), body (black arrow), transverse process (curved arrow).

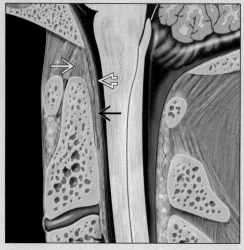

Sagittal view through C1-2 articulation shows apical ligament (arrow), cruciate ligament (black arrow), and tectorial membrane (open arrow) being superior extension of PLL.

- o At C2 level, artery loops and turns lateral to ascend in C1 transverse foramen
- o Turns medial crossing on top of C1 in groove
- o Artery then perforates the dura and arachnoid at lateral edge of posterior occipitoatlantal membrane, coursing ventrally on the medulla
- Vertebral column blood supply
  - o Paired segmental arteries (intercostals, lumbar arteries) arise from aorta and extend dorsolaterally around middle of vertebral body
  - o Near transverse process segmental artery divides into lateral and dorsal branches
  - o Lateral branch supplies dorsal musculature
  - o Dorsal branch
    - ▪ Passes lateral to foramen giving off branch(es) providing major vascular supply to bone and vertebral canal contents
    - ▪ Posterior central branch supplying disc and vertebral body
    - ▪ Prelaminal branch supplies inner surface of arch and ligamenta flava, regional epidural tissue
    - ▪ Neural branch entering neural foramen supplies pia, arachnoid, cord
    - ▪ Postlaminar branch supplies musculature overlying lamina and branches to bone
- Nerves
  - o Spinal nerves arranged in 31 pairs grouped regionally: 8 cervical, 12 thoracic, 5 lumbar, 5 sacral, 1 coccygeal
  - o Ascensus spinalis - apparent developmental rising of cord related to differential spinal growth
    - ▪ Course of nerve roots becomes longer and more oblique at lower segments
    - ▪ C1 nerve from C1 segment and exits above C1
    - ▪ C8 nerve from C7 segment and exits ⇒ C7-T1
    - ▪ T6 nerve from T5 segment and exits ⇒ T6-T7
    - ▪ T12 nerve from T8 segment and exits ⇒ T12-L1
    - ▪ L2 nerve from T10 segment and exits ⇒ L1-L2
    - ▪ S3 nerve from T12 segment and exits S3 foramen
- Meninges

- o Dura - dense tough covering, corresponding to meningeal layer of cranial dura
  - ▪ Epidural space filled with fat, loose connective tissue, veins
  - ▪ Dura continues with spinal nerves through foramen to fuse with epineurium
  - ▪ Cephalic attachment at foramen magnum, caudal attachment at back of coccyx
- o Arachnoid - middle covering, thin and delicate, continuous with cranial arachnoid
  - ▪ Separated from dura by potential subdural space
- o Pia - inner covering of delicate connective tissue closely applied to cord
  - ▪ Longitudinal fibers laterally concentrated as denticulate ligaments lying between posterior and anterior roots, and attach at 21 points to dura
  - ▪ Longitudinal fibers concentrated dorsally as septum posticum attaching dorsal cord to dorsal midline dura

CUSTOM DIFFERENTIAL DIAGNOSIS

Disease localization
- Extradural disease encompasses disease of vertebral bodies, arch, facets, paravertebral and epidural soft tissues and disc/annulus complex
- Intradural extramedullary disease encompasses dura, arachnoid and intrathecal nerve roots, vessels
- Intramedullary encompasses intrinsic spinal cord abnormalities of grey and white matter, vessels

SELECTED REFERENCES

1. White ML: Cervical spine: MR imaging techniques and anatomy. Magn Reson Imaging Clin N Am. 8(3):453-70, 2000
2. Bowen BC et al: Vascular anatomy and disorders of the lumbar spine and spinal cord. Magn Reson Imaging Clin N Am. 7(3):555-71, 1999

SPINE ANATOMY

IMAGE GALLERY

Typical

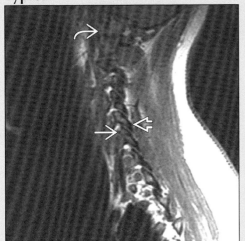
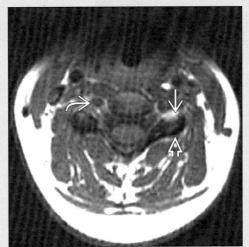

(Left) Sagittal T1WI MR shows normal parasagittal anatomy. Note smooth articulation of superior (arrow) and inferior (open arrow) articular facets, occipital condyle relationship to C1 (curved arrow). *(Right)* Axial T1WI MR shows normal anatomy at 1.5T. Superior facet is anterior (arrow), and inferior facet posterior (open arrow). Vertebral artery at neural foramenal level shows flow void (curved arrow).

Typical

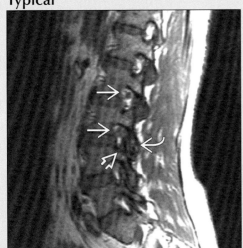
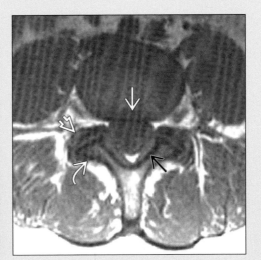

(Left) Sagittal T1WI MR shows parasagittal anatomy. Lumbar foramen (arrows) are well evaluated with direct sagittal view. Superior facet reside anterior (open arrow) to inferior facet (curved arrow). *(Right)* Axial T1WI MR shows normal disc contour (arrow), superior facet (open arrow), posterior facet (curved arrow) and ligamentum flavum (black arrow).

Typical

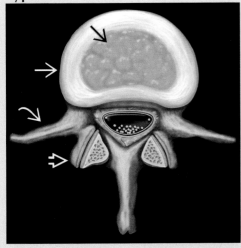
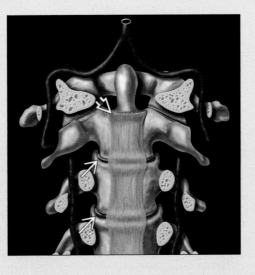

(Left) Axial graphic shows normal lumbar disc level, with annulus fibrosus (white arrow), nucleus pulposus (black arrow), facets (open arrow), transverse process (curved arrow). *(Right)* Posterior view of cervical spine with posterior elements removed shows relationship of uncovertebral joints (arrows), PLL (open arrow), and vertebral arteries in transverse foramen.

SPINE FRACTURE CLASSIFICATION-MODELS

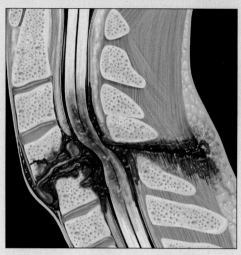

Sagittal graphic shows unstable cervical hyperflexion injury involving anterior and posterior longitudinal ligaments, disc and interspinous ligaments, epidural hemorrhage/cord compression.

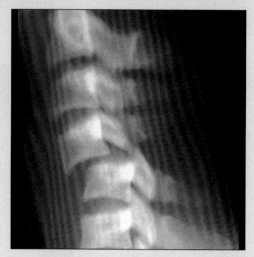

Lateral radiography shows C4-5 flexion facet dislocation with bilateral "jumped" facets. There is disruption of all three columns by this injury.

TERMINOLOGY

Abbreviations and Synonyms
- Abbreviations
  - Anterior longitudinal ligament (ALL)
  - Posterior longitudinal ligament (PLL)
  - Atlantodental interval (ADI)
- Synonyms
  - Chance fracture (seat belt fracture)
  - A1 fracture (wedge fracture, compression fracture)
  - A3 fracture (burst fracture, axial loading)
  - Clay shoveler's (coal shoveler's)
  - Hangman's fracture (traumatic spondylolisthesis)
  - Bilateral facet dislocation (bilateral locked facets)
  - Jefferson fracture (atlas burst fracture)
  - Articular mass (facets)
  - Atlas (C1), axis (C2), odontoid (dens)

IMAGING ANATOMY

- Occipital condyle fractures
  - Type I = comminuted fractures due to axial loading (stable if contralateral side intact)
  - Type II = occipital condyle with skull base fractures (most are stable)
  - Type III = avulsion fracture due to tensile force on alar ligaments (may show occipitocervical instability)
- C1 fractures
  - Anterior arch = vertical or transverse with avulsion from longus colli
  - Anterior arch bilateral fractures with posterior atlantoaxial dislocation = plow fracture
  - Lateral mass = stable if lateral ring intact, rare
  - Posterior arch = common
  - Jefferson = combined lateral mass displacement relative to C2 of 6.9 mm indicates disruption of transverse ligament and potential for instability
- Atlantoaxial instability
  - Nonphysiologic motion between C1-C2

- Wide variety of causes
  - Transverse ligament rupture (most common)
  - Odontoid fracture
  - Unstable Jefferson fracture
  - Fracture of lateral mass of C1 or C2
  - Unilateral alar ligament rupture
  - Alar and tectorial membrane rupture
- Classification (Fielding 1977)
  - Type I = rotation about dens without anterior translation (no increase in ADI)
  - Type II = rotation about one lateral mass with anterior translation of 3-5 mm (ADI) (transverse ligament injury)
  - Type III = rotation about lateral mass with anterior translation > 5 mm (transverse and alar ligament injury)
  - Type IV = posterior dislocation of C1 behind dens (rare, usually fatal)
- Odontoid
  - Type I = avulsion at tip of odontoid
  - Type II = transverse fracture of dens above C2 body
  - Type III = fracture involving superior portion of C2 body
- C2 ring fractures (Effendi 1981)
  - Type I = bilateral pars fractures with < 3 mm anterior subluxation (stable)
  - Type II = displacement of pars fracture + anterior translation of C2 with discoligamentous injury
  - Type III = pars fractures with C2-3 facet dislocations
- C2 body fractures (Fujimura 1996)
  - Type I = extension teardrop fracture of anterior inferior endplate of C2
  - Type II = horizontal shear fracture through body (more caudal than type III odontoid fracture)
  - Type III = C2 body burst fracture
  - Type IV = unstable sagittal cleavage fractures
- Cervical fracture classification
  - Hyperflexion
    - Anterior subluxation - posterior ligament disruption
    - Bilateral interfacetal dislocation - unstable

DIFFERENTIAL DIAGNOSIS

Clinical implications
- Denis classification unstable injuries includes
- 1) Three column disruption
- 2) > 50% collapse of anterior cortex
- 3) > 25 degrees focal kyphosis
- 4) Extending neurologic deficit

Thoracolumbar fractures
- Compression or wedging fracture involve only anterior column, stable
- Burst fracture involve anterior, middle +/- posterior columns, unstable or possibly unstable
- Seat belt or Chance fractures involve posterior and middle columns, unstable
- Fracture dislocation involve all columns and are highly unstable

- Stable injuries can be treated non-operatively
- Not all unstable injuries need operative treatment

Odontoid fractures
- Mortality rate of elderly with odontoid fractures up to 25%
- Type I odontoid fractures should be evaluated for occipitoatlantal instability
- Nonunion of odontoid bony injuries uncommon, except for type II odontoid fractures
- Type III odontoid fractures show broad surface of trabecular bone and good prognosis for healing

---

- Simple compression fracture
- Clay shoveler's fracture - avulsion of spinous process of C7 ⇒ T1
- Flexion teardrop fracture - unstable
- Hyperflexion and rotation
  - Unilateral facet dislocation (locked facet)
  - May have associated facet fracture
  - Radiograph shows forward displacement of vertebra < 1/2 AP diameter of cervical vertebral body
- Hyperextension and rotation
  - Pillar fracture
- Vertical compression
  - Jefferson fracture = fractures of both anterior and posterior rings with 2, 3, or 4 parts with radial displacement
  - Burst fracture = middle column involvement with bony retropulsion
- Hyperextension
  - Hyperextension dislocation
  - C1 anterior arch avulsion fracture = longus colli insertion around anterior tubercle of C1
  - Extension teardrop fracture of C2
  - C1 posterior arch fracture = compressed between occiput and C2 spinous process
  - Lamina fracture = between articular mass and spinous process
  - Hangman's fracture = bilateral pars fractures of C2
  - Hyperextension fracture - dislocation = bilateral facet fracture +/- dislocation
- Lateral flexion
  - Uncinate process fracture
- Atlanto occipital disassociation (dislocation)
- Thoracolumbar fracture classification
  - Holdsworth two column model (1963)
    - Superseded by Denis classification
    - Anterior column = ALL, vertebral body, disc, PLL
    - Posterior column = skeletal and ligamentous structures posterior to PLL
  - Denis three column model (1983)
    - Anterior – ALL, anulus, anterior vertebral body
    - Middle – posterior wall of vertebral body, anulus, PLL

- Posterior – facets, posterior elements, posterior ligaments
- Three column model also relevant to lower cervical injuries
- Denis subclassification of burst fracture (1984)
- Denis type A
  - Axial load force, anterior and middle columns involved, unstable
  - Upper and lower endplates involved
- Denis type B and C
  - Flexion and axial load, anterior and middle columns, possibly unstable
  - B upper endplate involved (most common)
  - C lower endplate involved
- Denis type D
  - Axial load and rotation, all columns, unstable
  - Atlas modification of D injuries (1986)
  - D1 burst lateral translation, D2 burst sagittal translation
- Denis type E
  - Lateral compression, all columns, possibly unstable
- Magerl AO pathomorphologic system (1994)
  - A, B, C types reflecting common injury patterns
  - Each type has three groups, each with three subgroups (3-3-3 scheme)
  - Type A vertebral compression fractures due to axial loading without soft tissue disruption in transverse plane (66%)
  - Type B distraction of anterior and posterior elements with soft tissue disruption in axial plane (14.5%)
  - Type C with axial torque forces giving anterior and posterior element disruption with rotation (19%)
    - Severity progresses through type A to C, as well as within types, groups, and subdivisions
    - Stable type A1 most common (wedge fracture)
    - A3 corresponds to "burst fracture" of Denis classification
  - Unstable – A3.2, A3.3, B, C types
- McCormack "load-sharing" classification (1994)
  - Specifically designed to evaluate need for anterior column reconstruction following pedicle screw stabilization

SPINE FRACTURE CLASSIFICATION-MODELS

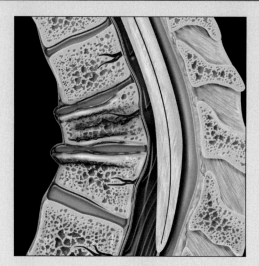

Sagittal graphic of thoracolumbar junction shows compression (wedge) fractures involving primarily anterior column, with normal middle and posterior columns.

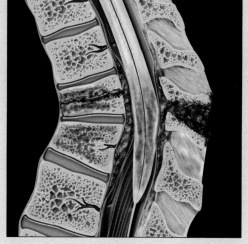

Sagittal graphic showing Chance (seat belt) fracture of thoracolumbar junction extending in horizontal plane through body and posterior elements (three column involvement).

- ○ Also useful as more generic guide to magnitude of comminution and biomechanical instability
- ○ Comminution graded
  - ▪ Amount of vertebral body damage
  - ▪ Fragment spread at fracture site
  - ▪ Degree of corrected kyphosis

CLINICAL IMPLICATIONS

Clinical Importance
- Fracture types and stability
  - ○ Stability is difficult to define, changes over time (immediate, subacute, chronic)
  - ○ Compression or wedging fractures involve only anterior column (stable)
  - ○ Burst fracture involve anterior, middle +/- posterior columns (unstable or possibly unstable)
  - ○ Seat belt or Chance fractures involve posterior and middle columns (unstable)
  - ○ Fracture dislocations involve all columns and are highly unstable

CUSTOM DIFFERENTIAL DIAGNOSIS

Imaging Considerations
- Differential considerations related to specific column involvement (stability), degree of cord/root compromise
- Multirow CT: 1.5-2 mm thick-sections, foramen Magnum to T1 level, with sagittal and coronal reformats
  - ○ Reformats critical for proper evaluation of C1-2 articulation and odontoid integrity
- MR: "Trauma technique" should include high-resolution T1/T2 images for ligament integrity, presence of traumatic herniation, degree of cord compromise
  - ○ Fat suppressed T2WI, STIR for definition of posterior ligamentous disruption

SELECTED REFERENCES

1. Leone A et al: Occipital condylar fractures: a review. Radiology. 216(3):635-44, 2000
2. Oner FC et al: MRI findings of thoracolumbar spine fractures: a categorisation based on MRI examinations of 100 fractures. Skeletal Radiol. 28(8):433-43, 1999
3. Vollmer DG et al: Classification and acute management of thoracolumbar fractures. Neurosurg Clin N Am. 8(4):499-507, 1997
4. Brandser EA et al: Thoracic and lumbar spine trauma. Radiol Clin North Am. 35(3):533-57, 1997
5. Fujimura Y et al: Classification and treatment of axis body fractures. J Orthop Trauma. 10(8):536-40, 1996
6. Noble ER et al: The forgotten condyle: the appearance, morphology, and classification of occipital condyle fractures. AJNR Am J Neuroradiol. 17(3):507-13, 1996
7. Dickman CA et al: Injuries involving the transverse atlantal ligament: classification and treatment guidelines based upon experience with 39 injuries. Neurosurgery. 38(1):44-50, 1996
8. Magerl F et al: A comprehensive classification of thoracic and lumbar injuries. Eur Spine J. 3(4):184-201, 1994
9. Benzel EC et al: Fractures of the C-2 vertebral body. J Neurosurg. 81(2):206-12, 1994
10. McCormack T et al: The load sharing classification of spine fractures. Spine. 19(15):1741-4, 1994
11. Atlas SW et al: The radiographic characterization of burst fractures of the spine. AJR Am J Roentgenol. 147(3):575-82, 1986
12. Denis F: The three column spine and its significance in the classification of acute thoracolumbar spinal injuries. Spine. 8(8):817-31, 1983

Typical

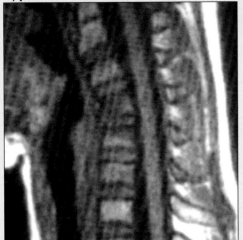
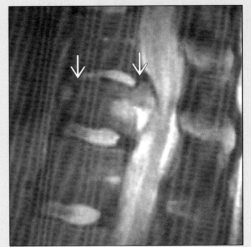

(Left) Sagittal T1WI MR shows simple wedge or compression fracture of C4 body, with no evidence of middle or posterior column involvement. *(Right)* Sagittal T2WI MR shows typical burst fracture of thoracolumbar junction, involving both anterior and middle columns (arrows). Posterior ligaments are preserved, and without T2 hyperintensity.

Typical

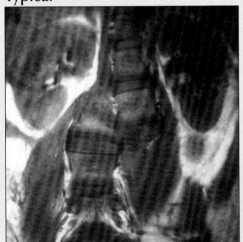
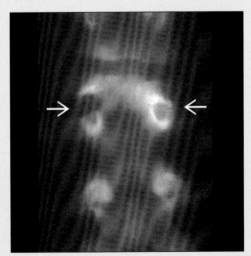

(Left) Coronal T1WI MR shows complete thoracolumbar dislocation with gross disruption of all three columns. *(Right)* Coronal tomogram of Chance fracture shows horizontal fractures through the pedicles bilaterally (arrows).

Typical

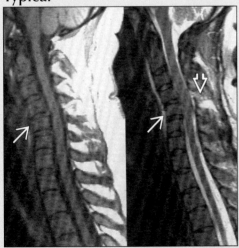
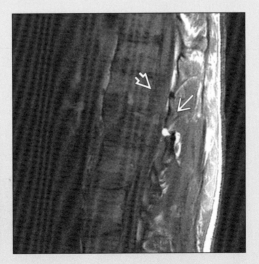

(Left) Sagittal T1WI MR (left) and T2WI (right) show disruption of ALL (arrows) with prevertebral edema, and disruption of interspinous ligaments (open arrow). *(Right)* Sagittal T1WI MR shows three column disruption with flexion dislocation injury to thoracolumbar junction. There is off-set of the posterior elements (arrow) and large epidural hematoma (open arrow).

ATLANTO-OCCIPITAL DISLOCATION

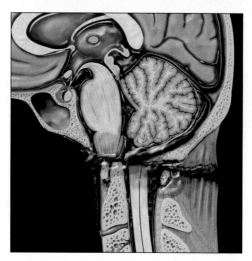

Sagittal graphic shows fatal atlanto-occipital dissociation, with cord transection at craniocervical junction. C1 is displaced posteriorly relative to skull base.

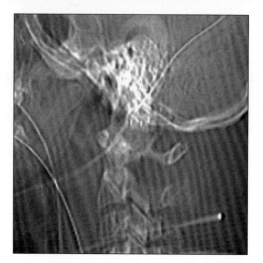

Lateral radiography shows increased distance between basion and C1, & abnormal Powers' ratio. Prevertebral soft tissues are too wide, even allowing for possible bleeding related to tubes.

TERMINOLOGY

Abbreviations and Synonyms
- Craniocervical dissociation
- Atlanto-occipital (AO) dislocation

Definitions
- Disruption of stabilizing ligaments between occiput, C1

IMAGING FINDINGS

General Features
- Best diagnostic clue: Widened distance between odontoid, C1

Radiographic Findings
- Radiography
  ○ Increased distance from basion to odontoid
    - Normal < 4-5 mm
    - Children < 10 mm
  ○ Powers' ratio > 1.15
    - BC = distance from tip of clivus (basion) to anterior cortex of posterior arch of C1
    - AO = distance from anterior arch C1 to posterior margin foramen magnum (opisthion)
    - If BC/AO > 1.15, then anterior atlanto-occipital dislocation is present

- Normal BC/AO = 0.77
  ○ Odontoid view
    - Increased space between occipital condyles & C1
  ○ Widened prevertebral soft tissues (nonspecific)

CT Findings
- Bone CT
  ○ Axial: May see portions of C1 on same image as occipital condyles
  ○ Coronal, sagittal: Widened space between occipital condyles + lateral masses of C1

MR Findings
- Displacement seen on coronal, sagittal images
- STIR best shows ligamentous injury
- MRA for vertebral artery injury

Imaging Recommendations
- Best imaging tool: CT scan with coronal + sagittal reformations
- Protocol advice: 1 mm helical multidetector CT

DIFFERENTIAL DIAGNOSIS

Occipital condyle fracture
- Best seen on CT
- May be associated with atlanto-occipital dislocation

DDx: Craniocervical Junction Instability

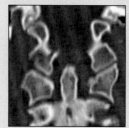
Occipital Fracture

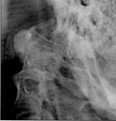
Down Syndrome

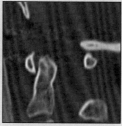
AO Dislocation

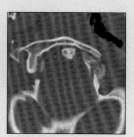
Occipital Fracture

ATLANTO-OCCIPITAL DISLOCATION

Key Facts

Terminology
- Disruption of stabilizing ligaments between occiput, C1

Imaging Findings
- Increased distance from basion to odontoid
- Powers' ratio > 1.15
- Best imaging tool: CT scan with coronal + sagittal reformations

Pathology
- Etiology: High speed motor vehicle accident

Clinical Issues
- Often immediately fatal

Diagnostic Checklist
- Only sign of injury on radiographs may be widened prevertebral soft tissues

---

Down syndrome
- Nontraumatic atlanto-occipital instability

PATHOLOGY

General Features
- Etiology: High speed motor vehicle accident
- Epidemiology: < 1% acute cervical spine injuries
- Associated abnormalities
  - Brainstem, cranial nerve injuries
  - Multilevel cervical injuries

Gross Pathologic & Surgical Features
- Rupture of ligaments between C1 and skull, dens and skull
  - Tectorial membrane
    - Continuation posterior longitudinal ligament
    - Attaches inner surface of clivus
    - Prime stabilizer of occiput to C1
  - Alar ligaments
    - Tip of dens superolaterally to foramen magnum
    - Rotational stability
  - Anterior atlanto-occipital ligament
    - Continuation anterior longitudinal ligament
    - From anterior arch of C1 to anterior cortex clivus
  - Posterior atlanto-occipital membrane
    - Posterior arch C1 to opisthion
  - Apical ligament
    - Tip of dens to basion; minor stabilizer

Staging, Grading or Classification Criteria
- Anterior or posterior
- Distraction
- Most anterior or posterior dislocations also have distraction component

CLINICAL ISSUES

Presentation
- Most common signs/symptoms
  - Cranial nerve injuries
  - Peripheral motor deficit

Demographics
- Age: More common in children

Natural History & Prognosis
- Often immediately fatal
- High incidence neurologic deficits in survivors

- Poor prognosis unless fused

Treatment
- Options, risks, complications: Occiput to C2 fusion needed

DIAGNOSTIC CHECKLIST

Consider
- Only sign of injury on radiographs may be widened prevertebral soft tissues

SELECTED REFERENCES

1. Saeheng S et al: Traumatic occipitoatlantal dislocation. Surg Neurol. 55(1):35-40; discussion 40, 2001
2. Harris JH Jr et al: Radiologic diagnosis of traumatic occipitovertebral dissociation: 2. Comparison of three methods of detecting occipitovertebral relationships on lateral radiographs of supine subjects. AJR Am J Roentgenol. 162(4):887-92, 1994
3. Dickman CA et al: Traumatic occipitoatlantal dislocations. J Spinal Disord. 6(4):300-13, 1993

IMAGE GALLERY

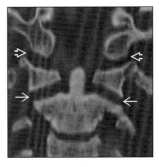 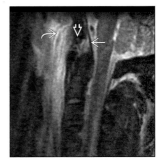

(Left) Coronal bone CT shows disruption of both occiput-C1 (open arrows) and C1-C2 (arrows) facet joints. (Right) Sagittal STIR MR shows disrupted apical ligament (open arrow) and anterior atlanto-occipital membrane (curved arrow). Tectorial membrane (arrow) appears intact.

OCCIPITAL CONDYLE FRACTURE

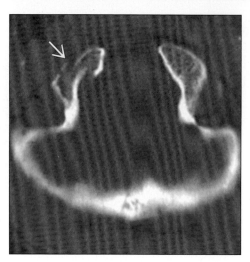

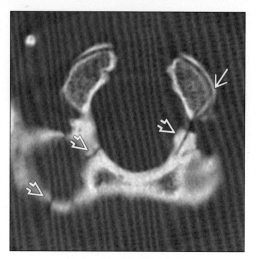

Axial bone CT demonstrates minimally displaced right occipital condyle fracture without comminution (arrow).

Axial bone CT shows nondisplaced left occipital condyle fracture (arrow) as involvement from skull base fracture (open arrows).

TERMINOLOGY

Abbreviations and Synonyms
- Occipital condyle (OC) fracture (OCFx)

Definitions
- Occipital condylar Fx 2° high-energy blunt trauma

IMAGING FINDINGS

General Features
- Best diagnostic clue: OCFx on CT
- Location: Uni- or bilateral occipital condyle(s)
- Morphology: Linear, comminuted, or avulsion type Fx
- OC anatomy
  - Project below the anterior third of foramen magnum
  - Oriented obliquely forward and inward
  - Narrowest at midportion, slopes caudally from lateral to medial
    - Makes 25–28° angle to mid-sagittal plane in adults
  - Occipitoatloid articulations are "cup-shaped" joints = convex OC surfaces + concave superior surfaces of atlas articular facets
    - In coronal plane, joint slopes downward medially
  - Inferolateral plane of occipitoatloid joint allows for 25° of flexion/extension, 5° lateral bending to one side, & 5° axial rotation to one side

- Within the base of each OC lie hypoglossal (anterior condyloid) canals containing CN12
- Lateral to OC & hypoglossal canal, posterior to carotid canal, is jugular foramen
  - Pars nervosa contains CN9 (Jacobson nerve)
  - Pars vascularis contains CN10 (Arnold nerve), CN11
- Joint has fibrous capsule that blends into the antero- & postero- atlanto-occipital membranes
  - Connecting margins of foramen magnum & upper border of atlantal ring
  - Leaves an arch posteriorly for vertebral arteries, venous plexus, & first cervical nerve
- Alar ligaments extend laterally from superolateral dens to medial OC
  - Very strong, bone often fails before these do
  - Checks lateral flexion & rotation, limiting cranial rotation with respect to atlas
- Tectorial membrane is attached to dorsal surfaces of the C-3 & C-2 vertebral bodies, dens body, & anterior occipital bone
  - Cephalad extension of posterior longitudinal lig.
  - Checks extension, flexion, & vertical translation
- Occipitoatloid articulation is less stable in young children due to small occipital condyles & horizontally oriented atlanto-occipital joints
- Relationship of multiple neurovascular structures explains symptomatologies from OCFx

DDx: Occipital Condyle Fracture Mimics

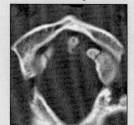

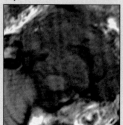

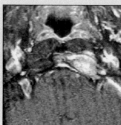

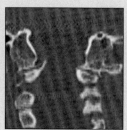

Accessory Centers *Osteomyelitis* *Metastasis* *Rheumatoid Arthritis*

OCCIPITAL CONDYLE FRACTURE

Key Facts

Terminology
- Occipital condylar Fx 2° high-energy blunt trauma

Imaging Findings
- Best diagnostic clue: OCFx on CT
- Morphology: Linear, comminuted, or avulsion type Fx
- CT: Thin-section with sagittal, coronal reformats
- MRI: Sagittal & coronal STIR

Top Differential Diagnoses
- Accessory ossification center(s)
- Marrow space abnormality

Pathology
- May be as high as 19% of patients with high-energy blunt trauma

Clinical Issues
- Presenting symptoms usually related to severity of head injury rather than to OCFx itself
- Cranial nerve (CN) deficit(s) (up to 30%)
- No specific predictors of OCFx
- Generally inconsistent
- Head injury is main determinant of outcomes
- Surgical therapy is controversial
- Follow-up CT is recommended 10-12 weeks after injury to document fracture healing

Diagnostic Checklist
- Suspect OCFx in all patients sustaining high-energy blunt trauma to head, upper cervical spine
- Search for OCFx in presence of unexplained neck pain, lower CN deficit(s)

- Via nerve root compression or stretching
- Direct brain stem injury or vascular compromise

Radiographic Findings
- Radiography
  - Very insensitive (0/51 in one study) due to
    - AP → superimposition of maxilla and occiput
    - Lateral → superimposition of mastoid processes
    - Open mouth → difficult or impossible to obtain in unconscious, intubated, severely injured patients
  - May see prevertebral soft tissue swelling
- Fluoroscopy
  - Flexion/extension fluoroscopy to assess for ligamentous injury, instability
    - Only after triaging injury with CT
    - Displacement of a Fx during flexion/extension could result in grave consequences

CT Findings
- CTA: Evaluate vertebrobasilar patency/injury
- Bone CT
  - Uni- or bilateral OCFx, occipitoatloid subluxation
  - Associated skull base Fx
    - Extension to hypoglossal and/or jugular foramen
  - Associated C1 or C2 Fx(s)

MR Findings
- STIR
  - Occipitoatloid joint subluxation, alar lig. disruption
  - Marrow edema
  - Prevertebral or nuchal ligament edema
  - Cord edema or hemorrhage
  - Foramen magnum extradural, subdural hemorrhage
- MRA: Evaluate vertebrobasilar patency/injury

Angiographic Findings
- Conventional: Replaced by CTA, MRA

Imaging Recommendations
- Best imaging tool
  - Bone CT for Fx
  - MRI for soft tissues
- Protocol advice
  - CT: Thin-section with sagittal, coronal reformats

- MRI: Sagittal & coronal STIR

DIFFERENTIAL DIAGNOSIS

Accessory ossification center(s)
- Anterior to OCD
- Well corticated

Marrow space abnormality
- Infectious: Osteomyelitis
- Neoplastic: Primary or metastatic neoplasms
- Inflammatory: Rheumatoid arthritis

PATHOLOGY

General Features
- Etiology
  - High-energy blunt trauma, most often MVA
  - Deployment of air bags has been associated with craniocervical junction injury
- Epidemiology
  - May be as high as 19% of patients with high-energy blunt trauma
    - True incidence, prevalence remains unknown
  - Increasingly being reported likely related to widespread use of CT & MR imaging
- Associated abnormalities
  - Subdural/epidural hematoma, subarachnoid hemorrhage, intra-axial contusion
  - Cervical spine fracture, usually C1 or C2
  - Thoracic, abdominal, & limb injuries

Staging, Grading or Classification Criteria
- Anderson & Montesano classification (1988)
  - Type I: Least common
    - Produced by axial load injury with a component of ipsilateral flexion; considered an impaction OCFx
    - Results in a comminuted Fx without displacement
  - Type II
    - Basilar skull fracture involving occipital condyle, usually from a direct blow to skull

- Linear Fx that may involve both OC
- Intact tectorial membrane & alar ligaments preserve stability
  - Type III: Most common (75%)
    - Avulsion Fx of inferomedial OC, usually result of severe contralateral flexion & rotation
    - May have medially displaced Fx fragment, & partial or complete disruption of tectorial membrane & contralateral alar ligament
    - Inferior clivus may also be involved
- Tulli classification (1997)
  - Type 1: Most common: Nondisplaced OCFx; stable
  - Type 2A: Displaced OCFx with intact ligaments; stable
  - Type 2B: Displaced OCFx with any one or move criteria of radiographic instability
    - > 8° of axial occipitoatloid rotation to one side
    - > 1 mm of occipitoatloid translation
    - > 7 mm of overhang of C1 on C2
    - > 45° of axial rotation of C1-C2 to one side
    - > 4 mm of C1-C2 translation
    - < 13 mm distance between posterior body of C2 to posterior ring of C1
    - Avulsed transverse ligament with MR evidence of ligamentous disruption
- Hanson classification (2001)
  - Uses A & M classification as a base
  - Subdivides type III into stable & unstable

CLINICAL ISSUES

Presentation

- Most common signs/symptoms
  - Presenting symptoms usually related to severity of head injury rather than to OCFx itself
  - Cranial nerve (CN) deficit(s) (up to 30%)
    - One or more CN9-12 (most often 12)
    - 40% manifest days to months after trauma, possibly fragment migration or callus formation
    - Collet-Sicard syndrome = full 9th through 12th CN deficits
  - Spasmodic torticollis from concomitant atlantoaxial rotatory fixation
  - Dysphagia from retropharyngeal hematoma
  - Hemi- or quadriparesis
  - Vertebrobasilar ischemia
  - High cervical pain, impaired skull mobility
- Clinical profile
  - No specific predictors of OCFx
  - Generally inconsistent
  - Most patients have mild/moderate ↓ GCS

Demographics

- Age: Infants to elderly
- Gender: M:F = 3:1

Natural History & Prognosis

- Functional recovery after unilateral CN deficit(s) is generally good
- Head injury is main determinant of outcomes

- 35% who survive to discharge have poor outcomes at 1 month requiring continued nursing support, tube feeding, or tracheostomy care; 35% of these gain functional independence with rehabilitation
- Remaining 65% have good outcomes becoming independently mobile & self-caring within 1 month
- Limited & painful mobility of craniocervical junction can persist after OCFx despite good osseous consolidation, especially when type III
  - Children generally have good osseous consolidation with normal & painless craniocervical mobility

Treatment

- By A & M classification
  - Type I & II OCFx are considered stable (tectorial membrane & contralateral alar ligament intact)
    - Treated conservatively → semirigid or rigid collar
  - Type III OCFx is a potentially unstable injury if ligamentous injury present
    - Assess for instability → flexion/extension
    - Treated with rigid collar, halo traction vest, or surgical fixation
- By Tulli classification
  - Type 1: Require no specific treatment
  - Type 2A: May be treated with a rigid collar
  - Type 2B: Surgical instrumentation or halo traction
- Surgical therapy is controversial
  - Possible indications → neurovascular decompression and/or stabilization
  - Usually posterior fusion (occipitoatlantoaxial arthrodesis)
- Follow-up CT is recommended 10-12 weeks after injury to document fracture healing

DIAGNOSTIC CHECKLIST

Consider

- Suspect OCFx in all patients sustaining high-energy blunt trauma to head, upper cervical spine

Image Interpretation Pearls

- Search for OCFx in presence of unexplained neck pain, lower CN deficit(s)

SELECTED REFERENCES

1. Momjian S et al: Occipital condyle fractures in children. Case report and review of the literature. Pediatr Neurosurg. 38(5):265-70, 2003
2. Hanson JA et al: Radiologic and clinical spectrum of occipital condyle fractures: retrospective review of 107 consecutive fractures in 95 patients. AJR Am J Roentgenol. 178(5):1261-8, 2002
3. Hadley et al: Occipital condyle fractures. Neurosurgery. 50(3 Suppl):S114-9, 2002
4. Demisch S et al: The forgotten condyle: Delayed hypoglossal nerve palsy caused by fracture of the occipital condyle. Clin Neurol Neurosurg. 100(1):44-5, 1998
5. Tuli S et al: Occipital condyle fractures. Neurosurgery. 41(2):368-76; discussion 376-7, 1997
6. Bloom AI et al: Fracture of the occipital condyles and associated craniocervical ligament injury: incidence, CT imaging and implications. Clin Radiol. 52(3):198-202, 1997

OCCIPITAL CONDYLE FRACTURE

IMAGE GALLERY

Typical

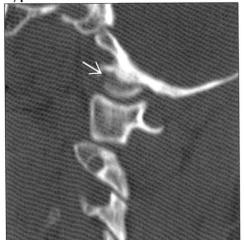 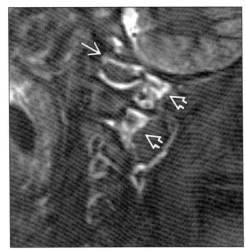

(Left) Sagittal bone CT reformat demonstrates minimally displaced right occipital condyle fracture without comminution (arrow). *(Right)* Sagittal STIR MR in the same case shows hyperintense edema along occipital condyle fracture (arrow) as well as associated hyperintense soft tissue injury to both ligaments & muscle (open arrows).

Typical

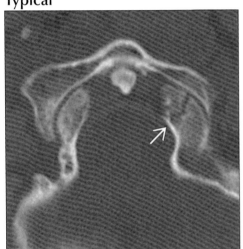 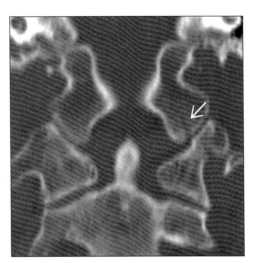

(Left) Axial bone CT shows nondisplaced left occipital condyle fracture (arrow). *(Right)* Coronal bone CT reformat demonstrates nondisplaced left occipital condyle fracture (arrow).

Typical

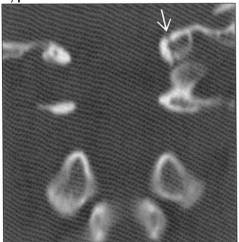 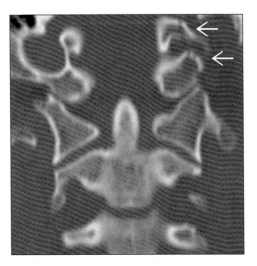

(Left) Coronal bone CT reformat demonstrates nondisplaced left occipital condyle fracture (arrow) contiguous with hypoglossal canal/skull base fracture (not shown). *(Right)* Coronal bone CT reformat shows hypoglossal canal involvement (arrows) from contiguous occipital condyle & skull base fracture (not shown).

JEFFERSON C1 FRACTURE

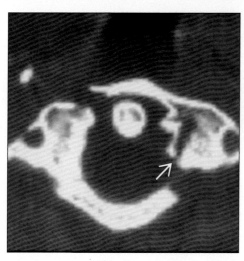 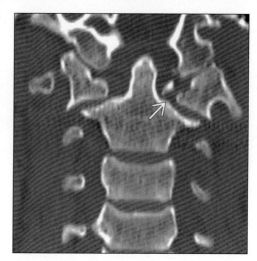

Axial bone CT shows fracture of C1 arch and avulsion of inner lateral mass at attachment of transverse ligament (arrow).

Coronal reformation shows avulsion Fx of C1 pillar (arrow) at attachment of transverse ligament, thus instability. Lateral offset of C1 vs. C2 pillars: C1 arch fracture seen on axial cut.

TERMINOLOGY

Abbreviations and Synonyms
- Atlas burst fracture

Definitions
- Compression fracture of C1 arch

IMAGING FINDINGS

General Features
- Best diagnostic clue: Lateral displacement of both articular masses of C1 from those of C2 on open-mouth radiograph

Radiographic Findings
- Radiography
  ○ Bony defects C1 arch on lateral/oblique views
  ○ Both articular pillars of C1 offset laterally vs. those of C2 on open mouth view
    ▪ One pillar may be offset with normal rotation, simulating fracture
  ○ Can see separation between dens & anterior arch of C1
  ○ May see anterior subluxation of C1 vs. C2
    ▪ Unstable C1 fracture
    ▪ Associated C2 fracture, especially Hangman's
  ○ Prevertebral soft tissue swelling at C1 level

  ○ Fractures at lower levels not uncommon
- Fluoroscopy: Subluxation if unstable

CT Findings
- NECT
  ○ CT defines components of fracture to best advantage
  ○ May see various patterns of arch disruption
  ○ May see hyperdensity in epidural space if bleeding occurs
- CTA: Look for loss of vertebral artery integrity if vertebrobasilar vascular syndrome present
- Bone CT
  ○ Disrupted ring of C1 arch
  ○ Multiple fractures of C1 arch typical
  ○ Both anterior, posterior arch fractures are seen in minority
  ○ Posterior arch fractured more often than anterior
  ○ Lateral masses alone may be fractured
  ○ A single site of arch fracture may occur
  ○ Look for avulsion fragment off inner pillar at insertion of transverse ligament
    ▪ ⇒ Indicates instability
  ○ Evaluate lower levels for additional fractures

MR Findings
- T1WI: Prevertebral soft tissue swelling anterior to C1
- T2WI: High signal in soft tissue anterior to C1; cord swelling, high or low signal if edema or hemorrhagic contusion

DDx: Congenital Variants

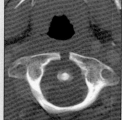 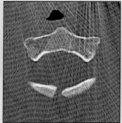 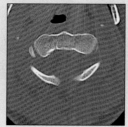 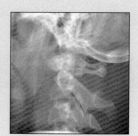

Congenital Cleft   *Posterior Cleft*   *Hypoplastic Arch*   *Hypoplastic C1 Arch*

JEFFERSON C1 FRACTURE

Key Facts

Terminology
- Atlas burst fracture
- Compression fracture of C1 arch

Imaging Findings
- Fluoroscopy: Subluxation if unstable
- CT defines components of fracture to best advantage
- May see various patterns of arch disruption
- Look for avulsion fragment off inner pillar at insertion of transverse ligament
- ⇒ Indicates instability
- Any lateral spread of C1 pillars on open-mouth x-ray view requires CT
- Evaluate entire cervical spine (and even upper thoracic) as associated fractures occur in 24-48% of cases

Top Differential Diagnoses
- Pseudospread of the atlas in children
- Congenital variants, clefts, malformations of atlas
- Rotational malalignment of atlas, axis pillars
- ⇒ Generally seen unilaterally, with rotation and abduction of head

Diagnostic Checklist
- Routine CT of cervical spine in every trauma victim complaining of severe neck pain
- Careful not to overcall 1-2 mm offset of C1 lateral masses vs. those of C2 on open mouth view in infants

---

- PD/Intermediate: Prevertebral soft tissue swelling
- MRA
  - May show vertebral artery occlusion
  - MRA useful if delayed cerebellar or brainstem signs appear

Angiographic Findings
- Conventional: Only needed if CTA or MRA findings are inconclusive

Imaging Recommendations
- Any lateral spread of C1 pillars on open-mouth x-ray view requires CT
- CT bone reconstruction algorithm details sites of fracture
  - Distinguishes well-corticated margins of congenital clefts from jagged edges of fracture defect
- Thin-section (1 mm) cuts mandatory, reformations very helpful
- Evaluate integrity of VBA foramina
- Evaluate entire cervical spine (and even upper thoracic) as associated fractures occur in 24-48% of cases

DIFFERENTIAL DIAGNOSIS

Pseudospread of the atlas in children
- Common finding in many children 3 months to four years of age evaluated for minor trauma
- Seen in 90% or more of two year olds
- Caused by disparity in growth rates of the atlas and axis
- Jefferson fracture rare in young children - greater plasticity, synchondroses of C1 arch serve as "buffer"

Congenital variants, clefts, malformations of atlas
- May show 1-2 mm offset of C1 pillars from those of C2
- Clefts found in 4% of posterior arches, 0.1% of anterior arches

- 97% of posterior clefts are midline, 3% through sulcus of vertebral artery
- Various deficiencies of arch development can be seen
- Most are partial hemiaplasias of posterior arch
- Clefts, congenital defects show smooth or well-corticated edges

Rotational malalignment of atlas, axis pillars
- ⇒ Generally seen unilaterally, with rotation and abduction of head

PATHOLOGY

General Features
- General path comments
  - Rough-edge fragmentation of C1 arch at one or more sites
  - Typically a stable fracture, unless transverse ligament avulsed, more than 7 mm offset a clue to such avulsion and instability
    - Unstable fractures occur if transverse or posterior longitudinal ligaments disrupted
    - Or if anterior arch is severely comminuted
    - And are more often associated with severe neurological deficits, lower levels of injury
  - Combined fractures occur, especially those of C2
- Etiology
  - Axial compressive force applied to skull vertex
  - Force transmitted down through occipital condyles onto C1 pillars with head + neck rigidly erect
- Epidemiology
  - C1 fractures represent 6% of all vertebral injuries
  - One-third of C1 fractures conform to classic burst Jefferson fracture
  - Rare in infants, young children
- Associated abnormalities
  - Fractures at other levels
  - VBA injury; dissection or occlusion

JEFFERSON C1 FRACTURE

CLINICAL ISSUES

Presentation
- Most common signs/symptoms
  - Upper neck pain after compression trauma (e.g., diving)
  - Other signs/symptoms
    - Neurologic signs uncommon, unless unstable fracture or associated fractures are present, or if VBA injured
- Clinical profile
  - Upper neck pain
  - Trauma victim
  - Fracture can be missed on plain films

Natural History & Prognosis
- Stable fracture with healing in majority of isolated cases

Treatment
- Immobilization, fusion if gross instability

DIAGNOSTIC CHECKLIST

Consider
- Routine CT of cervical spine in every trauma victim complaining of severe neck pain
- Evaluate lower levels for additional Fxs (present in 25-50% of cases)

Image Interpretation Pearls
- Well-corticated edges of midline C1 arch defects are likely congenital clefts
- Careful not to overcall 1-2 mm offset of C1 lateral masses vs. those of C2 on open mouth view in infants

SELECTED REFERENCES

1. Lustrin ES et al: Pediatric cervical spine: normal anatomy, variants, and trauma. Radiographics. 23(3): 539-60, 2003
2. Torreggiani WC et al: Musculoskeletal case 20. Jefferson fracture (C1 burst fracture). Can J Surg. 45(1):16, 65-6, 2002
3. Harris JH: The cervicocranium: its radiographic assessment. Radiology 218:337-51, 2001
4. Connor SE et al: Congenital midline cleft of the posterior arch of atlas: a rare cause of symptomatic cervical canal stenosis. Eur Radiol. 11(9): 1766-9, 2001
5. Sharma A et al: Partial aplasia of the posterior arch of the atlas with an isolated posterior arch remnant: findings in three cases. AJNR Am J Neuroradiol. 21(6): 1167-71, 2000
6. Guiot B et al: Complex atlantoaxial fractures. J Neurosurg. 91(2 Suppl): 139-43, 1999
7. Haakonsen M, Gudmundsen TE, Histol O. Midline anterior and posterior atlas clefts may simulate a Jefferson fracture. A report of 2 cases. Acta Orthop Scand. 66(4):369-71, 1995
8. Currarino G et al: Congenital defects of the posterior arch of the atlas: a report of seven cases including an affected mother and son. AJNR Am J Neuroradiol. 15(2):249-54, 1994
9. Kesterson L et al: Evaluation and treatment of atlas burst fractures (Jefferson fractures). J Neurosurg. 75(2):213-20, 1991
10. Lee C et al: Unstable Jefferson variant atlas fractures: an unrecognized cervical injury. AJNR Am J Neuroradiol. 12(6):1105-10, 1991
11. Gehwiler JA et al: Malformations of the atlas simulating the Jefferson fracture. AJNR 4:187-90, 1983
12. Jefferson G: Fracture of the atlas vertebra. Report of four cases and a review of those previously recorded. Br J Surg 7:407-11, 1920

JEFFERSON C1 FRACTURE

IMAGE GALLERY

Typical

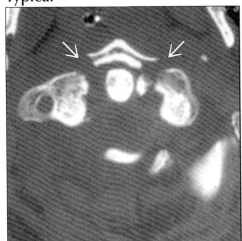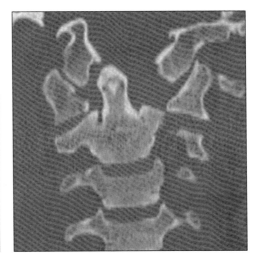

(Left) Axial bone CT shows fractures of anterior C1 arch (arrows). *(Right)* Coronal reformation, bone windows, shows lateral offset of C1 vs. C2 lateral mass. Axial slices showed anterior & posterior left sided C1 arch fractures, right side of arch was intact.

Variant

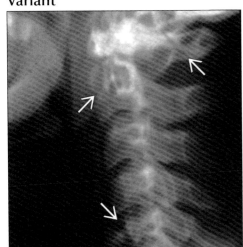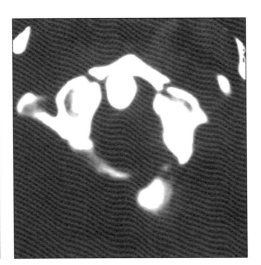

(Left) Lateral radiography shows fractures of C1, C2, C5 (arrows) in patient with diving injury (axial load and flexion). Note prevertebral swelling. *(Right)* Axial bone CT shows anterior arch components of Jefferson fracture in this patient with multiple fractures (C1 fracture being subtle on radiography). Lower slices showed C2 & C5 fractures.

Typical

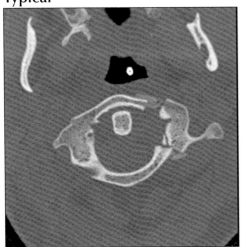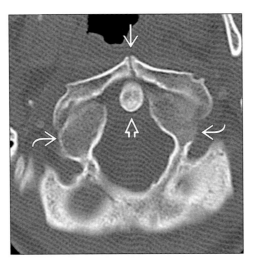

(Left) Axial bone CT window shows left-sided C1 arch fractures. *(Right)* Axial bone CT shows developmental midline defect (arrow) in C1 arch; note sclerotic, corticated edges. Foramen magnum level includes occipital condyles (curved arrows) & tip of dens (open arrow).

ODONTOID C2 FRACTURE

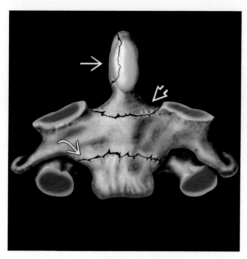

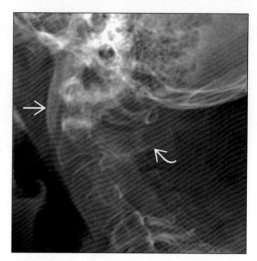

Anterior graphic shows three fractures through C2: Type I odontoid (arrow); type III odontoid (open arrow) & horizontal axis body fracture (curved arrow).

Lateral radiography shows defect at base of dens and prevertebral swelling (arrow), with posterior displacement of dens and C1 arch vs. C2 (curved arrow). Note osteopenia.

TERMINOLOGY

Abbreviations and Synonyms
• Dens fracture

Definitions
• Traumatic bony disruption of odontoid process

IMAGING FINDINGS

General Features
• Best diagnostic clue: Lateral radiograph shows anterior or posterior displacement of C1 arch vs. C2, + swelling of prevertebral soft tissue

Radiographic Findings
• Radiography
  ○ Classic imaging appearance: Lucent linear defect through base of dens, with posterior displacement of dens arch of C1 relative to C2 body/arch
  ○ Open-mouth frontal radiograph depicts transverse or oblique defect through dens
  ○ May be difficult to depict in elderly with osteoporosis
• Fluoroscopy: Used to evaluate stability of fusion

CT Findings
• NECT: Soft tissue swelling anterior to C2 in acute cases

• CTA: Used if vertebral artery injury is suspected
• Bone CT
  ○ Comminuted bone at level of dens on axial views, fracture line on reformations, displacement at base of dens or tip of odontoid
  ○ Axial (source) images may miss fracture if its plane parallels slice orientation
  ○ Coronal, sagittal reformations are mandatory!

MR Findings
• T1WI
  ○ Loss of dens/C2 body contiguity
  ○ Replacement of normal marrow's high signal from fat, by low signal of edema
  ○ Displacement of dens from C2 body, typically anterior subluxation
• T2WI: High signal of edema in marrow, + prevertebral soft tissues

Nuclear Medicine Findings
• Bone Scan: Can be used to detect old fracture with non-union

Imaging Recommendations
• Plain x-rays (especially lateral, open-mouth views) initially suggest need for CT if any of above mentioned clues are present

DDx: Altered Dens Morphology

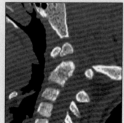

Os Odontoideum

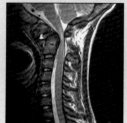

Os Odontoideum MR

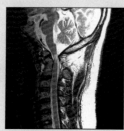

Third Condyle

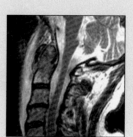

Dens Met Fracture

ODONTOID C2 FRACTURE

Key Facts

Terminology
- Traumatic bony disruption of odontoid process

Imaging Findings
- Best diagnostic clue: Lateral radiograph shows anterior or posterior displacement of C1 arch vs. C2, + swelling of prevertebral soft tissue
- Classic imaging appearance: Lucent linear defect through base of dens, with posterior displacement of dens arch of C1 relative to C2 body/arch
- Open-mouth frontal radiograph depicts transverse or oblique defect through dens
- May be difficult to depict in elderly with osteoporosis
- Axial (source) images may miss fracture if its plane parallels slice orientation

Top Differential Diagnoses
- Congenital nonunion of odontoid tip (Os odontoideum)
- Metastatic or other pathologic C2 fracture

Pathology
- Three ossification centers form C2
- Os odontoideum represents unfused ossification center atop dens C2
- Type III fracture follows embryologic line of union between dens and body of C2
- Type I: Avulsion of tip
- Type II: Transverse fracture at base of dens
- Type III: Fracture extending into body of C2

- Thin-section (1 mm) axial slices with bone reconstruction algorithm with fastest possible scan times for optimal reformation into sagittal, coronal planes
- MRI with T1WI in sagittal/coronal planes (3 mm slices), T2WI in sagittal plane to evaluate canal size, cord injury
- GRE imaging to detect blood in cord if myelopathy is present

DIFFERENTIAL DIAGNOSIS

Congenital nonunion of odontoid tip (Os odontoideum)
- Well-corticated ossification center above rudimentary dens
- No soft tissue swelling
- No history of trauma, or pain

Congenital variation - 3rd occipital condyle
- One of several anomalous bony structures which may form at foramen magnum as remnant of first sclerotome
- This midline bony peg off anterior lip of foramen magnum may articulate to dens, simulate odontoid fracture

Rheumatoid arthritis - C1/C2 subluxation
- Synovial proliferation erodes dens, leads to laxity & subluxation

Metastatic or other pathologic C2 fracture
- Can produce pathologic odontoid fracture

PATHOLOGY

General Features
- General path comments
  - Embryology-anatomy
    - Three ossification centers form C2
    - Os odontoideum represents unfused ossification center atop dens C2

- Type III fracture follows embryologic line of union between dens and body of C2
- Etiology
  - Caused by sudden forward or backward movement of the head, with neck rigidly erect & articulations locked
  - Osteoporosis in elderly predisposes to type II fracture + nonunion

Staging, Grading or Classification Criteria
- Type I: Avulsion of tip
- Type II: Transverse fracture at base of dens
- Type III: Fracture extending into body of C2

CLINICAL ISSUES

Presentation
- Most common signs/symptoms
  - Neck pain
  - Other signs/symptoms
    - Myelopathy
- Clinical profile
  - Often in elderly, osteoporotic patients
  - Fluctuating long tract signs, spasticity may be the only presentation in older patients whose initial trauma was minor & not well diagnosed

Natural History & Prognosis
- Chronic nonunion or fibrous union in elderly
- Nonunion common in elderly without primary fusion
  - May stabilize by fibrous union with prolonged immobilization
- Fusion produces stability

Treatment
- Fracture pattern dictates management
  - Type I fracture is an avulsion of the dens tip ⇒ considered stable, treated with simple immobilization
  - Type II is the most common ⇒ most likely to go on to non-union; primary fusion may be indicated to prevent myelopathy
  - Type III involves the C2 body

ODONTOID C2 FRACTURE

○ Nonunion uncommon after treatment with traction followed by bracing

DIAGNOSTIC CHECKLIST

Consider
- T2WI serve to verify edematous marrow, and better depict associated soft tissue edema in prevertebral space (missing in chronic nonunion)
- T1WI sagittal and coronal images best depict the disruption of bone contiguity, and degree of displacement
  ○ Marrow shows signal loss from edema in acute cases, normal signal indicates chronic nonunion
- Flexion/extension films or fluoroscopy for evaluating stability

Image Interpretation Pearls
- Sclerotic margins of ununited dens indicate chronic non-union of old fracture

SELECTED REFERENCES

1. Muller EJ et al: Non-rigid immobilisation of odontoid fractures. Eur Spine J. 12(5):522-5, 2003
2. v Ludinghausen M et al: The third occipital condyle, a constituent part of a median occipito-atlanto-odontoid joint: a case report. Surg Radiol Anat. 24(1):71-6, 2002
3. Rao PV: Median (third) occipital condyle. Clin Anat. 15(2):148-51, 2002
4. Sanderson SP et al: Fracture through the C2 synchondrosis in a young child. Pediatr Neurosurg. 36(5):277-8, 2002
5. Martin-Ferrer S: Odontoid fractures. J Neurosurg. 95(1 Suppl):158-9, 2001
6. Weisskopf M et al: CT scans versus conventional tomography in acute fractures of the odontoid process. Eur Spine J. 10(3):250-6, 2001
7. Sasso RC: C2 dens fractures: treatment options. J Spinal Disord. 14(5):455-63, 2001
8. Teo EC et al: Biomechanical study of C2 (Axis) fracture: effect of restraint. Ann Acad Med Singapore. 30(6):582-7, 2001
9. Vaccaro AR et al: Contemporary management of adult cervical odontoid fractures. Orthopedics. 23(10):1109-13; quiz 1114-5, 2000
10. Ziai WC et al: A six year review of odontoid fractures: the emerging role of surgical intervention. Can J Neurol Sci. 27(4):297-301, 2000
11. Govender S et al: Fractures of the odontoid process. J Bone Joint Surg Br. 82(8):1143-7, 2000
12. Swischuk LE et al: Is the open-mouth odontoid view necessary in children under 5 years? Pediatr Radiol. 30(3):186-9, 2000
13. Brant-Zawadzki M et al:CT in the evaluation of spine trauma. AJR. 136: 369, 1981
14. Charlton OP et al: Roentgenographic evaluation of cervical spine trauma. JAMA. 242:1073-5, 1979
15. Anderson et al: Fractures of the odontoid process of the axis. J Bone and Joint Surg 56A: 1663-74, 1974

IMAGE GALLERY

Typical

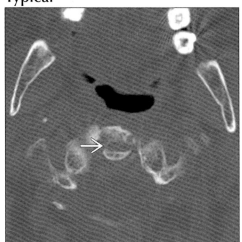
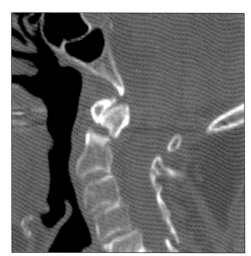

(Left) Axial bone CT shows fracture at base of dens (arrow); oblique plane of anatomy vs. slice orientation makes for confusing finding. *(Right)* Sagittal bone CT reformation shows true plane of fracture, displacement of dens & C1 arch posteriorly to better advantage.

Variant

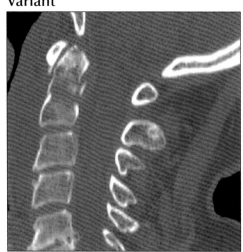
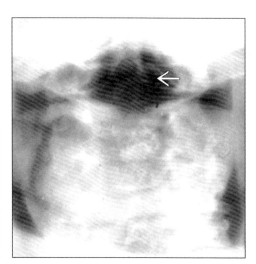

(Left) Sagittal bone CT reformation shows fracture through base of dens, with permeative bony destruction of dens, C2 body, and extensive prevertebral soft tissue mass due to metastatic disease. *(Right)* Anteroposterior radiography (open mouth) shows transverse type II fracture only vaguely (arrow) due to osteopenia.

Variant

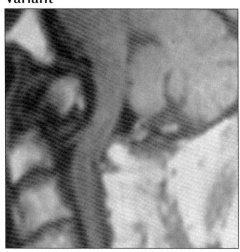
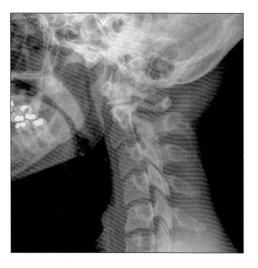

(Left) Sagittal T1WI MR shows fracture at base of dens with low signal margins indicating bony sclerosis, & normal C2 marrow signal (also seen on T2WI), indicative of chronic fracture nonunion. *(Right)* Lateral radiography shows sclerotic bony defect at base of dens. Note lack of prevertebral swelling, no subluxation suggesting fibrous fusion. Nonunion of old fracture versus os odontoideum.

BURST FRACTURE, C2

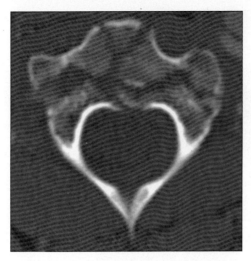

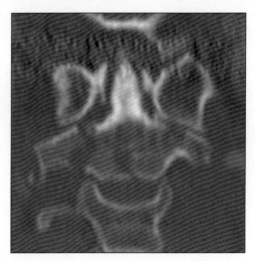

Axial bone CT demonstrates comminuted C2 burst fracture with centrifugal displacement of fragments and involvement of bilateral transversarium foramen.

Coronal bone CT reformat reveals comminuted C2 burst fracture with laterally displaced fragments & involvement of bilateral transversarium foramen.

TERMINOLOGY

Abbreviations and Synonyms
- Fracture (Fx)
- Dispersion or axial loading Fx

Definitions
- Compression injury often with displaced fracture fragments causing cord compromise
  - Highly associated with hangman fracture
    - 100% by one report

IMAGING FINDINGS

General Features
- Best diagnostic clue: Comminuted fracture of C2 body with multiple fragments dislocated anteroposteriorly
- Location: C2 body
- Size: May involve entire vertebral body
- Morphology: Minimal to severe deformity

Radiographic Findings
- Radiography
  - Variable range
    - Minimal compression with minimal fragment displacement
    - Severe comminution
    - Marked posteriorly retropulsed fragments

- Frontal radiograph
  - May see vertical Fx line within C2 body, either midline or eccentric
  - Magnitude indicated by degree of lateral fragment displacement, disruption of Luschka joints
- Lateral radiograph
  - Vertebral body comminution
  - Posteriorly retropulsed fragments
  - Intact facets
  - Focal prevertebral soft tissue swelling > 6 mm
- Associated hangman
  - Bilateral pars Fx
  - C2/3 anterolisthesis
  - Disruption C1/2 spinolaminar line
  - Disruption C2/3 posterior vertebral line
- Myelography: Demonstrates canal narrowing from fragment retropulsion

CT Findings
- CTA
  - Quickly, easily evaluates for vertebral artery injury if Fx involves transversarium foramen
    - Normal
    - Mass effect impinging luminal diameter
    - Dissection
    - Occlusion
- CT Bone
  - Axial images

DDx: C2 Burst Fracture Mimics

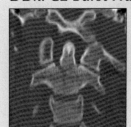

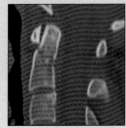

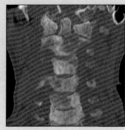

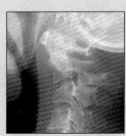

Type 3 Odontoid Fx   Type 3 Odontoid Fx   Pathologic Fx   Flexion Teardrop Fx

BURST FRACTURE, C2

Key Facts

Terminology
- Compression injury often with displaced fracture fragments causing cord compromise
- Highly associated with hangman fracture

Imaging Findings
- Best diagnostic clue: Comminuted fracture of C2 body with multiple fragments dislocated anteroposteriorly
- Morphology: Minimal to severe deformity
- Posteriorly retropulsed fragments
- Focal prevertebral soft tissue swelling > 6 mm
- May have acute cord injury
- Best imaging tool: CT Bone
- CT: Acquire axially with sagittal & coronal reformats
- MRI: Add sagittal STIR & GRE

Top Differential Diagnoses
- Odontoid type 3 Fx
- Pathologic Fx
- Flexion teardrop Fx

Pathology
- Associated abnormalities: Hangman Fx, cord contusion/hematoma, vertebral artery injury

Clinical Issues
- Symptoms are variable from no deficit to quadriplegia
- Age: C-spine injury: 80% of patients are 18-25 yrs
- Gender: C-spine injury: M:F = 4:1
- Considered unstable injury given high frequency of association with hangman fractures
- Steroids if neurologic symptoms & < 8 hrs in onset
- There is no standard surgical therapy

- Characterized by centrifugal displacement of Fx fragments
- CT best shows degree of spinal encroachment from retropulsed fragments
- Intact facets
- CT best evaluates possible involvement of transversarium foramen
- Associated hangman: Bilateral pars Fx
  - Sagittal reformat
    - Characterizes both comminuted body Fx and degree of fragment retropulsion
    - Demonstrates normal appearance of facet joints
    - Focal prevertebral soft tissue swelling > 6 mm
    - Associated hangman: C2/3 anterolisthesis, disruption C1/2 spinolaminar line, disruption C2/3 posterior vertebral line
  - Coronal reformat
    - Characterizes vertical Fx line within C2 body, either midline or eccentric
    - Defines well the degree of disruption of Luschka joints

MR Findings
- T1WI
  - Hypointense marrow edema
    - Chronic Fx: Marrow signal normalizes with time
  - May have acute cord injury
    - Edema: Iso- to slightly hypointense
    - Hematoma: Isointense
- T2WI
  - Hyperintense marrow edema
    - Chronic Fx: Marrow signal normalizes with time
  - Effacement of CSF anterior to cord from retropulsed fragments
  - Acute cord injury
    - Edema: Hyperintense
    - Hematoma: Hyperintense quickly changing to hypointense
  - May see traumatic disc herniation as disc signal material effacing CSF
- STIR
  - STIR best to visualize hyperintense marrow edema
    - Chronic Fx: Marrow signal normalizes with time

- Acute cord injury: Hyperintense edema
- STIR best evaluates any related soft tissue injury
- T2* GRE: Best shows acute cord hematoma → hypointense "blooming"
- MRA: Evaluate for vertebral artery injury if Fx involves transversarium foramen

Angiographic Findings
- Replaced by CTA/MRA for evaluating vertebral artery integrity

Nuclear Medicine Findings
- Bone Scan
  - 80% show ↑ activity at Fx site 24 hrs, 95% by 72 hrs
  - Patients > 75 yrs or debilitated may not show activity for several days to as much as 2 wks

Imaging Recommendations
- Best imaging tool: CT Bone
- Protocol advice
  - CT: Acquire axially with sagittal & coronal reformats
  - MRI: Add sagittal STIR & GRE
  - MRA: Add axial fat-saturated T1 to evaluate for luminal hematoma

DIFFERENTIAL DIAGNOSIS

Odontoid type 3 Fx
- Fx through base of dens (Anderson & D'Alonzo classification)
- Not a true dens Fx, but a superior C2 body Fx
- No fragment retropulsion
- No vertical Fx line within C2 body
- Superior articulating facets usually involved, disrupted

Pathologic Fx
- Normal or minimal trauma through pathologic bone
- Most often metastatic disease

Flexion teardrop Fx
- Clinically important to distinguish from burst
  - Difference in stability, management
  - May be difficult by radiologic criteria

BURST FRACTURE, C2

- Abnormal flexed alignment
- Anteroinferior body "teardrop" fragment
- Distraction of posterior column
  - Facet subluxation/distraction
  - Spinous process splaying
- Most severe & unstable C-spine type of Fx

PATHOLOGY

General Features
- General path comments
  - Since spinal canal diameter is greatest at C2, cord injury from retropulsed fragment compression is the exception
  - Considered a "major" Fx type
- Etiology
  - MVAs, falls cause most C2 fractures
  - Mechanism of burst
    - Compression forces cause axial loading
    - C2/3 nucleus pulposus is driven through C2 inferior endplate, into vertebral body
    - Sudden "explosive" pressure ↑ causes vertebral body comminution
    - Fragments undergo centrifugal dispersion
    - Posteriorly retropulsed fragments enter canal & may impact, compress cord
  - Hangman: Hyperextension injury
- Epidemiology
  - 25% of C2 fractures cannot be classified as odontoid or hangman Fxs → vertebral body, laminae, spinous processes
    - C2 burst is an uncommon Fx
  - Up to 10% of unconscious patients presenting to the ED following MVA have C-spine pathology
  - 1/3 C-spine injuries involve C2
  - C-spine injuries cause estimated 6,000 deaths & 5,000 new cases of quadriplegia each yr
- Associated abnormalities: Hangman's Fx, cord contusion/hematoma, vertebral artery injury

Gross Pathologic & Surgical Features
- Comminuted Fx
- Extruded blood, cellular debris, fragments of tissue envelope Fx site in hematoma
- Inflammation begins within hrs & continues for several days until replaced by developing soft callus

Microscopic Features
- Periosteal disruption
- Cortical bone displacement & separation
- Disruption of vessels within Haversian canals at Fx site
- Extrusion of marrow contents into Fx gap

Staging, Grading or Classification Criteria
- Classification of axis body fractures: Avulsion, transverse, burst, & sagittal

CLINICAL ISSUES

Presentation
- Most common signs/symptoms
  - Symptoms are variable from no deficit to quadriplegia

- May have transient symptoms
- With cord injury
  - Spinal shock: Flaccidity, areflexia, loss of anal sphincter tone, fecal incontinence, priapism, loss of bulbocavernosus reflex
  - Neurogenic shock: Hypotension, paradoxical bradycardia, flushed/dry/warm peripheral skin
  - Autonomic dysfunction: Ileus, urinary retention, poikilothermia
- Clinical profile: C-spine injury: Clinical evaluation is unreliable → 46% sensitivity

Demographics
- Age: C-spine injury: 80% of patients are 18-25 yrs
- Gender: C-spine injury: M:F = 4:1
- High risk activities: Diving, equestrian activities, football, gymnastics, skiing, hang gliding

Natural History & Prognosis
- Considered unstable injury given high frequency of association with hangman's fractures

Treatment
- Traction with cervical tongs if > 25% loss of height, fragment retropulsion, neurologic deficit
- Steroids if neurologic symptoms & < 8 hrs in onset
- Surgical treatment
  - There is no standard surgical therapy
    - Per Congress of Neurological Surgeons standards
  - Spontaneous interbody fusion between C2 & C3 can occur → conservative immobilization
  - Consider surgical C2/3 anterior interbody fusion

SELECTED REFERENCES

1. Congress of Neurological Surgeons: Isolated fractures of the axis in adults. Neurosurgery. 50(3 Suppl):S125-39, 2002
2. Daffner RH et al: A new classification for cervical vertebral injuries: influence of CT. Skeletal Radiol. 29(3):125-32, 2000
3. Fujimura Y et al: Classification and treatment of axis body fractures. J Orthop Trauma. 10(8):536-40, 1996
4. Lozano-Requena JA et al: Sagittal fracture of the second cervical vertebral body. Int Orthop. 18(2):114-5, 1994
5. Burke JT et al: Acute injuries of the axis vertebra. Skeletal Radiol. 18(5):335-46, 1989
6. Hadley MN et al: Acute axis fractures: a review of 229 cases. J Neurosurg. 71(5 Pt 1):642-7, 1989
7. Baba H et al: Burst fracture of the body of the axis; a case report [Japanese]. Orthop Surg Traumatol 32:1659-62, 1989
8. Jakim I et al: Transverse fracture through the body of the axis. J Bone Joint Surg Br. 70(5):728-9, 1988
9. Guerra J Jr et al: Vertebral burst fractures: CT analysis of the retropulsed fragment. Radiology. 153(3):769-72, 1984
10. Kobayashi K: Axis body fracture [Japanese]. Seikei Geka 28:1145-1153, 1977
11. Brashear R Jr et al: Fractures of the neural arch of the axis. A report of twenty-nine cases. J Bone Joint Surg Am. 57(7):879-87, 1975

BURST FRACTURE, C2

IMAGE GALLERY

Typical

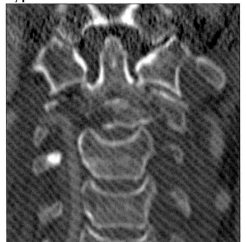 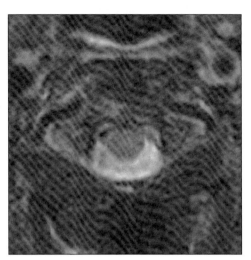

(Left) Coronal CTA shows patency of right vertebral artery to C2 level. Both right & left vertebral arteries were shown to be patent on adjacent images. *(Right)* Axial T2WI MR shows slight C2 body marrow edema hyperintensity no cord findings in patient with C2 burst fracture.

Typical

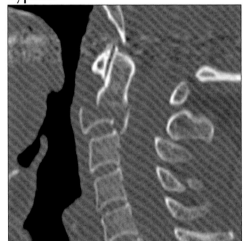 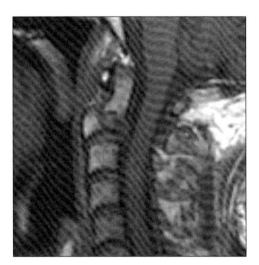

(Left) Sagittal bone CT reformat reveals centrifugal displacement of C2 burst fracture fragments with associated retropulsion into the spinal canal. *(Right)* Sagittal T1WI MR demonstrates hypointensity within fracture marrow as well as retropulsed fragment entering canal. Cord signal intensity isointense appears normal.

Typical

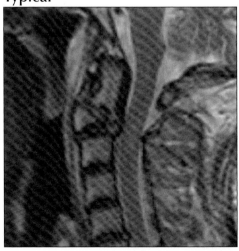 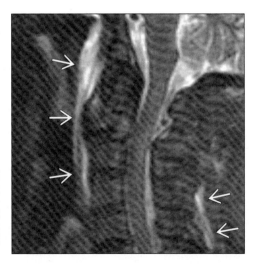

(Left) Sagittal T2WI MR better demonstrates retropulsed fragment entering canal effacing anterior CSF. Cord edema/contusion hyperintensity can be seen. *(Right)* Sagittal STIR MR confirms cord hyperintensity from contusion as well as hyperintense soft tissue ligamentous injury anteriorly and posteriorly (arrows).

HANGMAN'S C2 FRACTURE

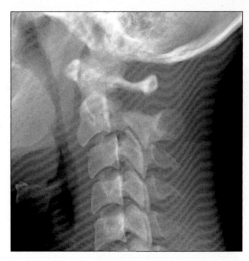

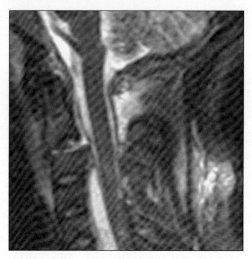

Lateral radiography shows lucent gap in pedicles of C2, its laminal line aligned with C3, but its body and C1 anteriorly displaced vs. C3.

Sagittal T2WI MR shows the anterior subluxation of C2 vb, edema in the disc interspace and anteriorly, preservation of anteroposterior canal dimension and cord integrity.

TERMINOLOGY

Abbreviations and Synonyms
- Traumatic spondylolisthesis of axis (TSA)

Definitions
- Bilateral avulsion of C2 vertebral body (vb) from its arch

IMAGING FINDINGS

General Features
- Best diagnostic clue
  - Anterior displacement of C2 vb, C1, & skull vs. C3 on lateral x-ray
  - Classic imaging appearance: Defects through pedicles of C2, C2 vertebral body (vb) anterior to C3 vb, laminae aligned
    - CT defines components of fracture to best advantage
    - May see various patterns of arch, vb disruption
    - Soft tissue swelling anterior to vb common
    - May not see malalignment despite pedicle disruption
    - C1 & skull ride with anteriorly subluxed C2 vb
- Location: Both pedicles of C2

Radiographic Findings
- Radiography
  - C2 vb anteriorly subluxed vs. C3
  - Radiolucent gap in pedicles of C2
  - Prevertebral soft tissue swelling
  - C1 arch and skull ride forward with C2 vb
  - Posterior elements and laminal line of C2 and C3 remain aligned
- Fluoroscopy
  - Flexion exaggerates C2-C3 subluxation
  - Useful for verifying stability of therapeutic fusion

CT Findings
- NECT
  - Bone window CT
    - Multiple bilateral fractures of C2 arch, including pedicles
    - Axial slice shows disrupted ring of C2
    - Variation of fracture sites, including extension into body, not uncommon
    - Dens typically spared
    - Extension into vertebral artery foramen raises possibility of vertebral artery (VBA) damage
    - Additional fracture levels seen in 33% of cases, C1 most commonly
    - Canal at C2 enlarged
  - Soft tissue windows
    - Prevertebral soft tissue swelling

DDx: Hangman's Mimics

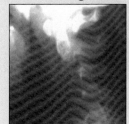

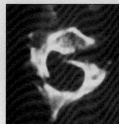

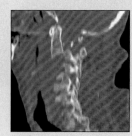

Pseudosubluxation

Variant Hangman's

C2-3 Fx, Rotation

HANGMAN'S C2 FRACTURE

Key Facts

Terminology
- Traumatic spondylolisthesis of axis (TSA)

Imaging Findings
- Anterior displacement of C2 vb, C1, & skull vs. C3 on lateral x-ray
- Classic imaging appearance: Defects through pedicles of C2, C2 vertebral body (vb) anterior to C3 vb, laminae aligned
- Axial slice shows disrupted ring of C2
- Variation of fracture sites, including extension into body, not uncommon
- Dens typically spared
- Extension into vertebral artery foramen raises possibility of vertebral artery (VBA) damage

- Additional fracture levels seen in 33% of cases, C1 most commonly
- Canal at C2 enlarged
- Any anterior subluxation of C2 vs. C3 on lateral x-ray deserves CT
- Evaluate entire cervical spine (and even upper thoracic) as associated fractures occur in 33% of cases
- MR if neurologic symptoms are present

Top Differential Diagnoses
- Pseudosubluxation
- Rotatory subluxation of C2-C3
- Primary spondylolysis

- May show high density (blood) in spinal canal
- CTA: If VBA foramen fractured, CTA shows loss of VBA integrity

MR Findings
- T1WI: Low signal in pedicles of C2
- T2WI: High signal in thickened prevertebral soft tissue
- STIR: High signal in pedicles of C2
- T2* GRE: Blood products in canal or cord may be depicted
- MRA: VBA signal loss if foramen fracture or significant subluxation occurred

Imaging Recommendations
- Any anterior subluxation of C2 vs. C3 on lateral x-ray deserves CT
- Thin-section (1 mm) cuts mandatory, reformations very helpful to assess degree of subluxation, canal status
- Evaluate entire cervical spine (and even upper thoracic) as associated fractures occur in 33% of cases
- MR if neurologic symptoms are present
- Get MRA, CTA, or conventional angiogram if fracture line involves transverse foramen

DIFFERENTIAL DIAGNOSIS

Pseudosubluxation
- Seen in young children
- Affects multiple upper cervical levels
- Occurs on lateral x-ray view when mild flexion present
- No associated soft tissue swelling
- Due to ligamentous laxity of youth
- Laminal line remains aligned

Rotatory subluxation of C2-C3
- Unilateral fracture(s) of C2 arch, pedicle

Primary spondylolysis
- Rare anomaly
- Persistent embryonic synchondrosis

PATHOLOGY

General Features
- General path comments
  - Classical hanging with knot in submental position produces complete disruption of C2, C3 disc & ligaments
  - Sudden contusion or tearing of upper cord & brainstem by hyperextension and distraction
  - Traumatic TSA has different mechanism (e.g., chin vs. dashboard), similar results in bony spine
- Etiology: Traumatic TSA results from hyperextension with axial loading, or forced hyperflexion with compression in falls or MVAs
- Epidemiology
  - TSA represents 4-7% of all cervical fractures and/or dislocations
  - Isolated TSA represented 7% of all craniovertebral fractures in one series
  - Almost all modern cases represent sequelae of accidents rather than hanging
    - Only a minority of judicial hanging victims show C2 arch fracture
- Associated abnormalities
  - Fractures at other (not always contiguous) levels
  - Associated C1 fracture is most common of other levels involved

Staging, Grading or Classification Criteria
- Type I: Non-displaced, no angulation
- Type II: Significant angulation and translation
- Type III: Type II plus unilateral or bilateral facet dislocations

CLINICAL ISSUES

Presentation
- Most common signs/symptoms
  - Acute neck pain
  - Other signs/symptoms
    - Neurological deficits

HANGMAN'S C2 FRACTURE

- Cerebellar findings suggest stroke due to vertebral artery dissection or occlusion
- Clinical profile
  ○ Pain upper neck after trauma
  ○ Neurological sequelae in minority of traumatic cases, as canal wide here and further decompressed by fracture
  ○ Nevertheless, neurological sequelae occur in 25%
  ○ Vertebral artery injury may cause delayed neurological signs

Natural History & Prognosis
- Depends on presence of neurological damage
- Delayed stroke a possibility if vertebral artery damaged
- Accelerated degenerative changes

Treatment
- Immobilization
- Fusion

DIAGNOSTIC CHECKLIST

Consider
- Check vb alignment, soft tissue thickness (4 mm or less) on lateral x-ray and get CT if abnormal
- Evaluate transverse foramen for integrity; get MRA if any question to exclude vertebral artery injury

Image Interpretation Pearls
- C2-C3 vb anterior subluxation with laminal line normally aligned requires CT even without fracture shown on x-ray

SELECTED REFERENCES
1. Ranjith RK, Mullett JH, Burke TE. Hangman's fracture caused by suspected child abuse. A case report. J Pediatr Orthop B. 11(4):329-32, 2002
2. Management of combination fractures of the atlas and axis in adults. Neurosurgery. 50(3 Suppl):S140-7, 2002
3. Harrop JS, Vaccaro A, Przybylski GJ. Acute respiratory compromise associated with flexed cervical traction after C2 fractures. Spine. 15;26(4):E50-4, 2001
4. Isolated fractures of the axis in adults. Neurosurgery. 50(3 Suppl):S125-39, 2002
5. Samaha C et al: Hangman's fracture: the relationship between asymmetry and instability. J Bone Joint Surg Br. 82(7):1046-52, 2000
6. Williams JP 3rd et al: CT appearance of congenital defect resembling the Hangman's fracture. Pediatr Radiol. 29(7):549-50, 1999
7. Guiot B et al: Complex atlantoaxial fractures. J Neurosurg. 91(2 Suppl):139-43, 1999
8. Agrillo U et al: Hangman's fracture. Spine. 24(22):2412, 1999
9. Greene KA et al: Acute axis fractures. Analysis of management and outcome in 340 consecutive cases. Spine. 22(16):1843-52, 1997
10. Nunez DB et al: Cervical spine trauma: How much more do we learn by routinely using helical CT? Radiographics 16: 1307-18, 1996
11. Starr JK et al: Atypical hangman's fractures. Spine. 18(14):1954-7, 1993
12. James R et al: The occurrence of cervical fractures in victims of judicial hanging. Forensic Sci Int. 54(1):81-91, 1992
13. Parisi M et al: Hangman's fracture or primary spondylolysis: a patient and a brief review. Pediatr Radiol. 21(5):367-8, 1991
14. Burke JT et al: Acute injuries of the axis vertebra. Skeletal Radiol. 18(5):335-46, 1989
15. Fielding JW et al: Traumatic spondylolisthesis of the axis. Clin Orthop. (239):47-52, 1989
16. Mivris SE et al: Hangman's fracture: radiologic assessment in 27 cases. Radiology 163: 713-7, 1987
17. Baumgarten M et al: Computed axial tomography in C1-C2 trauma. Spine. 10(3):187-92, 1985
18. Hadley MN et al: Axis fractures: a comprehensive review of management and treatment in 107 cases. Neurosurgery. 17(2):281-90, 1985
19. Sherk HH et al: Clinical and pathologic correlations in traumatic spondylolisthesis of the axis. Clin Orthop. (174):122-6, 1983
20. Bucholz RW: Unstable hangman's fractures. Clin Orthop. (154):119-24, 1981
21. Pepin JW et al: Traumatic spondylolisthesis of the axis: Hangman's fracture. Clin Orthop. (157):133-8, 1981
22. Seljeskog EL et al: Spectrum of the hangman's fracture. J Neurosurg. 45(1):3-8, 1976
23. Marar BC: Fracture of the axis arch. "Hangman's fracture" of the cervical spine. Clin Orthop. (106):155-65, 1975
24. Williams TG: Hangman's fracture. J Bone Joint Surg Br. 57(1):82-8, 1975

IMAGE GALLERY

Typical

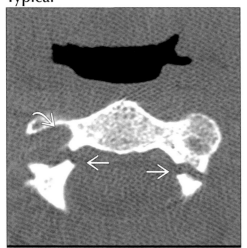 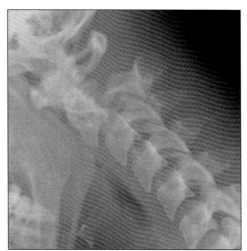

(Left) Axial bone CT at level of pedicles (1 mm section does not include laminae) shows their cleavage (arrows) from body of C2. Note relationship of fracture line to VBA foramen (curved arrow). *(Right)* Lateral radiography in flexion shows exaggerated gap at level of pedicular fracture and maximal subluxation. Note increased anteroposterior canal dimension at level of fracture.

Typical

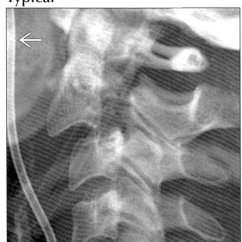 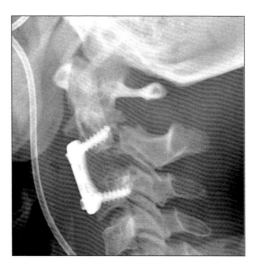

(Left) Lateral radiography shows classic features of Hangman's fracture, including prevertebral swelling delineated by anteriorly displaced nasogastric tube (arrow). *(Right)* Lateral radiography after anterior internal plate/screw fixation shows re-alignment of C2 & C3. Note the hypoplastic arch of C1simulates persistent anterior subluxation of C1 & dens.

Variant

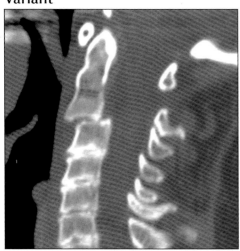 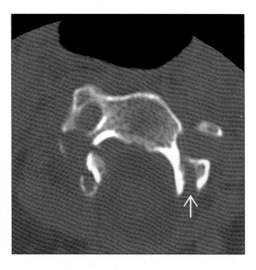

(Left) Sagittal bone CT reformation shows anterior displacement of C2 vb, C1, skull; C2 arch stays with C3-finding typical of Hangman's. *(Right)* Axial bone CT shows transverse right C2 pedicle fracture, sagittal left pedicle fracture entering vertebral foramen (arrow).

HYPERFLEXION INJURY, CERVICAL

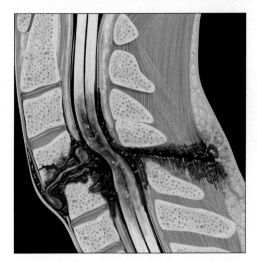

Sagittal graphic shows flexion injury at C4-5 with subluxation, disc herniation, ligamentous disruption, cord compression & epidural hemorrhage.

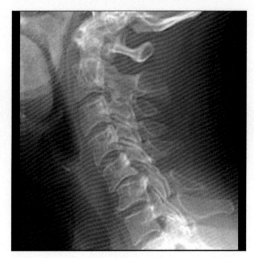

Sagittal radiography shows focal kyphosis, separation of spinous processes, and anterior subluxation of facets at C5-6 in patient with pain, no neurologic defect. Note wide canal.

TERMINOLOGY

Abbreviations and Synonyms
• Traumatic anterior subluxation

Definitions
• Flexion force disrupting capsular and posterior ligaments, with anterior vertebral displacement/angulation

IMAGING FINDINGS

General Features
• Best diagnostic clue: Focal kyphosis, abnormal vertical separation of facets/spinous processes
• Location: Mid or lower cervical spine

Radiographic Findings
• Radiography: Focal angulation of adjacent vertebral bodies with increased space between adjacent facets, spinous processes
• Fluoroscopy: Increased laxity on flexion at the involved level

CT Findings
• Sagittal reformation shows separation between adjacent facets, spinous processes

• May see mild compression of superior end plate or wedging of vertebral bodies (vb) at involved interspace

MR Findings
• T1WI: Focal kyphosis, abnormal separation of facets/spinous processes in sagittal plane
• T2WI
  ○ Increased signal in interspinous ligament
  ○ Sagittal plane shows canal compromise, ventral cord edema (if central cord syndrome present)

Angiographic Findings
• Conventional: Done only to verify suspected arterial dissection

Imaging Recommendations
• High-resolution CT best shows facet relationships
• Fluoroscopy helpful to show lax ligaments in flexion

DIFFERENTIAL DIAGNOSIS

Burst fracture
• Axial force a major component, flexion secondary

Flexion-rotation injury
• Facet subluxation typically unilateral, with facet fracture more common

DDx: Fractures with Flexion Components

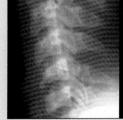
Burst Fracture

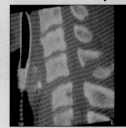
Whiplash Fracture

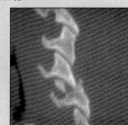
Flexion Rotation

HYPERFLEXION INJURY, CERVICAL

Key Facts

Terminology
- Flexion force disrupting capsular and posterior ligaments, with anterior vertebral displacement/angulation

Imaging Findings
- Best diagnostic clue: Focal kyphosis, abnormal vertical separation of facets/spinous processes

Pathology
- Anatomy of C-spine predisposes to instability once ligaments are disrupted
- Associated abnormalities: Central cord syndrome

Diagnostic Checklist
- Fluoroscopy with appropriate history of severe flexion injury, but only minimal separation on static films

Whiplash fracture
- Extension component leads to laminar fracture, flexion causes vb compression

PATHOLOGY

General Features
- General path comments
  - Disruption of middle column of the spine causes mechanical instability
  - Neurological compromise subsequent to injury may occur if unstable nature of fracture not recognized
  - Disc displacement can occasionally contribute to cord compression
- Etiology
  - Small, flat, articular processes of C-spine, their almost horizontal articulation, little overlap of articular surfaces
  - Ligaments (capsular as well as ligamentum flavum and nuchae) provide considerable stability
  - Anatomy of C-spine predisposes to instability once ligaments are disrupted
- Associated abnormalities: Central cord syndrome

CLINICAL ISSUES

Presentation
- Most common signs/symptoms
  - History of trauma with flexion components (e.g., diving)
  - Acute neck pain without or with neurologic deficit

Natural History & Prognosis
- Depends on presence and degree of neurologic compromise
- Good if no neurologic damage, and stabilization achieved
- Accelerated degenerative disease may be seen
- Fixed neurologic deficit if cord shows hemorrhagic contusion

Treatment
- If no neurological injury, treatment is aimed at immobilization (halo), correction of any deformity
- If neurologic signs present, & compression found, acute decompression
- If cord is edematous, high dose steroids (first 24 hours)

DIAGNOSTIC CHECKLIST

Consider
- Fluoroscopy with appropriate history of severe flexion injury, but only minimal separation on static films

Image Interpretation Pearls
- Evaluate other levels carefully, as non contiguous injury or fracture may occur

SELECTED REFERENCES

1. Laporte C et al: Severe hyperflexion sprains of the lower cervical spine in adults. Clin Orthop. (363):126-34, 1999
2. Murakami H et al: Central cord syndrome secondary to hyperflexion injury of the cervical spine in a child. J Spinal Disord. 8(6):494-8, 1995
3. Barquet A et al: Occult severe hyperflexion sprain of the lower cervical spine. Can Assoc Radiol J. 44(6):446-9, 1993
4. Fazl M et al: Posttraumatic ligamentous disruption of the cervical spine, an easily overlooked diagnosis: presentation of three cases. Neurosurgery. 26(4):674-8, 1990
5. Braakman M et al: Hyperflexion sprain of the cervical spine. Follow-up of 45 cases. Acta Orthop Scand. 58(4):388-93, 1987
6. Green JD et al: Anterior subluxation of the cervical spine: hyperflexion sprain. AJNR Am J Neuroradiol. 2(3):243-50, 1981

IMAGE GALLERY

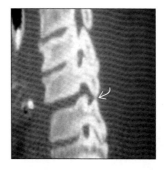 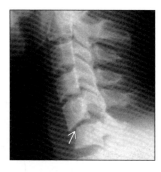

(Left) Sagittal Oblique bone CT reformation shows perched facet (arrow) at C5-6 in patient with flexion injury. *(Right)* Sagittal radiography shows C5 subluxed anteriorly on C6 in patient with flexion injury & central cord syndrome (arrow).

HYPEREXTENSION INJURY, CERVICAL

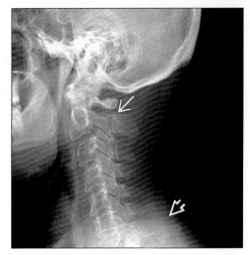

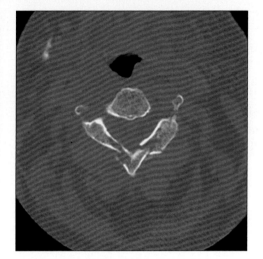

Lateral radiography shows ill-defined defect in C2 arch (arrow), with slight anterior C2 vb displacement. Note old C7 spinous process (clay shoveler) Fx (open arrow), from previous trauma.

Axial bone CT windowed section shows disruption of both laminae just anterior to spinous process in this patient with traumatic hyperextension.

TERMINOLOGY

Abbreviations and Synonyms
- Arch fracture (Fx)
- Posterior element Fx

Definitions
- Fracture of the laminae due to forceful posterior displacement of head and/or upper cervical spine

IMAGING FINDINGS

General Features
- Best diagnostic clue: Bony defect through posterior arch with posterior element malalignment
- Location: Typically mid- or lower cervical spine
- Morphology: May see distraction or rotational malalignment

Radiographic Findings
- Radiography
  - Fracture through posterior elements on lateral or oblique views
  - Malalignment of posterior laminal line at level of fracture
  - Fullness of prevertebral soft tissues
- Fluoroscopy
  - Laxity at level of fracture

- Performed only under controlled conditions

CT Findings
- NECT
  - Axial slices show defect best
  - Bone windows demonstrate fracture lines through laminae
- CTA
  - Done when vertebral artery injury suspected
  - Absence of enhancement within vertebral artery indicates injury
- Bone CT
  - High-resolution algorithm best for non-displaced fracture
  - Arch defect best shown on axial views
  - Sagittal reformation shows listhesis, facet relationships

MR Findings
- T1WI: Difficult to see non-displaced Fx
- T2WI
  - Shows cord edema if myelopathy present
  - May see soft tissue edema in retrospinal tissues
  - Shows edema of anterior longitudinal ligament
  - MR has low sensitivity but high specificity for posterior element fracture
- STIR: Delineates soft tissue edema
- T2* GRE: Best depicts associated hemorrhagic cord contusion

---

DDx: Posterior Element Defects

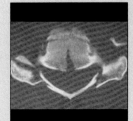

Whiplash Fx

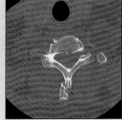

Clay Shoveler Fx

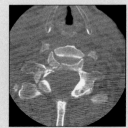

Rotational Fx

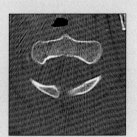

Congenital Cleft

HYPEREXTENSION INJURY, CERVICAL

Key Facts

Terminology
• Fracture of the laminae due to forceful posterior displacement of head and/or upper cervical spine

Imaging Findings
• Best diagnostic clue: Bony defect through posterior arch with posterior element malalignment
• Bone CT
• High-resolution algorithm best for non-displaced fracture
• Arch defect best shown on axial views
• Sagittal reformation shows listhesis, facet relationships
• Shows cord edema if myelopathy present
• T2* GRE: Best depicts associated hemorrhagic cord contusion

• Must obtain CT once plain film findings suggest fracture
• MR vital if neurologic signs present to evaluate cord injury, compression

Top Differential Diagnoses
• Whiplash fracture
• Rotational fracture-subluxation
• Clay shoveler fracture
• Congenital cleft

Diagnostic Checklist
• CT in any case, particularly when shoulder density precludes evaluation of cervico-thoracic junction
• Using CTA or MRA to exclude vertebral artery injury

• MRA: Can show vertebral artery disruption
• T2WI demonstrates cord edema or hemorrhage, anterior longitudinal ligament disruption, & may show nuchal ligament injury
• GRE sequences most sensitive to blood in cord which heralds irreversible damage

Angiographic Findings
• Conventional
  ○ Done if CTA or MRA suggests dissection or occlusion
  ○ Missing arterial dissection risks delayed neurologic damage

Imaging Recommendations
• Must obtain CT once plain film findings suggest fracture
• CT may show more fractures at other levels
• Thin-section (max 1 mm) cuts mandatory
• Reformations very helpful
• MR vital if neurologic signs present to evaluate cord injury, compression
• Consider CTA, MRA to exclude dissection

DIFFERENTIAL DIAGNOSIS

Whiplash fracture
• Associated vb fracture
• Malalignment more common

Rotational fracture-subluxation
• May have associated laminar fracture

Clay shoveler fracture
• Spinous process avulsion from sudden severe force placed on ligamentum nuchae
• Laminae typically spared

Congenital cleft
• Typically midline

PATHOLOGY

General Features
• General path comments
  ○ Disruption of posterior column of the spine causes mechanical instability
  ○ Neurological compromise subsequent to the injury may occur if unstable nature of fracture not recognized
  ○ Disc fragment displacement, though uncommon, can contribute to cord compression
• Etiology
  ○ Hyperextension force during traumatic event
  ○ Some degree of axial load usually present as well
  ○ Disrupted ligaments (anterior, posterior longitudinal and capsular add to considerable instability
• Epidemiology: Sports are a common setting
• Associated abnormalities
  ○ Cord contusion
  ○ Vertebral artery dissection
  ○ Other fractures

Gross Pathologic & Surgical Features
• Typical traumatic bone disruption

CLINICAL ISSUES

Presentation
• Most common signs/symptoms: Severe neck pain with transient or lasting myelopathic signs
• Clinical profile: History of trauma with extension components and/or axial loading (e.g., diving)

Natural History & Prognosis
• Depends on presence/degree of neurologic compromise
• Good if no neurologic damage and stabilization achieved
• Accelerated degenerative disease may be seen
• Neurologic recovery can occur if only mild edema is seen in cord acutely

HYPEREXTENSION INJURY, CERVICAL

- Fixed neurologic deficit if cord shows hemorrhagic contusion
- Progression of fixed deficit superiorly if post-traumatic syrinx appears late

Treatment

- If no neurological injury, treatment is aimed at immobilization (halo) and correction of any deformity
- If neurologic signs present, and compression found, acute decompression
- If cord is edematous, high dose steroids (first 24 hours) may help
- If cord demonstrates hemorrhage or transection, immobilization to prevent further deformity

DIAGNOSTIC CHECKLIST

Consider

- CT in any case, particularly when shoulder density precludes evaluation of cervico-thoracic junction
- Evaluation of upper thoracic spine for associated fractures, as non-contiguous fractures can be seen
- Using CTA or MRA to exclude vertebral artery injury

Image Interpretation Pearls

- Subtle malalignment of posterior laminal line on lateral radiograph should prompt CT
- Multiple, non-contiguous fractures may be seen

SELECTED REFERENCES

1. Ranger GS: "Radiographic clearance of blunt cervical spine injury: plain radiograph or computed tomography scan?", by Griffen MM, et al. J Trauma. 56(2):457; author reply 457, 2004
2. Berlin L: CT versus radiography for initial evaluation of cervical spine trauma: what is the standard of care? AJR Am J Roentgenol. 180(4):911-5, 2003
3. Cothren CC et al: Cervical spine fracture patterns predictive of blunt vertebral artery injury. J Trauma. 55(5):811-3, 2003
4. Hayes KC et al: Retropulsion of intervertebral discs associated with traumatic hyperextension of the cervical spine and absence of vertebral fracture: an uncommon mechanism of spinal cord injury. Spinal Cord. 40(10):544-7, 2002
5. Maiman DJ et al: Preinjury cervical alignment affecting spinal trauma. J Neurosurg. 97(1 Suppl):57-62, 2002
6. Hanson JA et al: Cervical spine injury: a clinical decision rule to identify high-risk patients for helical CT screening. AJR Am J Roentgenol. 174(3):713-7, 2000
7. Matar LD et al: "Spinolaminar breach": an important sign in cervical spinous process fractures. Skeletal Radiol. 29(2):75-80, 2000
8. Biffl WL et al: The devastating potential of blunt vertebral arterial injuries. Ann Surg. 231(5):672-81, 2000
9. Klein GR et al: Efficacy of magnetic resonance imaging in the evaluation of posterior cervical spine fractures. Spine. 24(8):771-4, 1999
10. Zhu Q et al: Traumatic instabilities of the cervical spine caused by high-speed axial compression in a human model. An in vitro biomechanical study. Spine. 24(5):440-4, 1999
11. Brady WJ et al: ED use of flexion-extension cervical spine radiography in the evaluation of blunt trauma. Am J Emerg Med. 17(6):504-8, 1999
12. Klein GR et al: Efficacy of magnetic resonance imaging in the evaluation of posterior cervical spine fractures. Spine. 24(8):771-4, 1999
13. Makan P: Neurologic compromise after an isolated laminar fracture of the cervical spine. Spine. 24(11):1144-6, 1999
14. Kinoshita H: Pathology of hyperextension injury of the cervical spine: a case report. Spinal Cord. 35(12):857-8, 1997
15. Plezbert JA et al: Fracture of a lamina in the cervical spine. J Manipulative Physiol Ther. 17(8):552-7, 1994
16. Kinoshita H: Pathology of hyperextension injuries of the cervical spine. Paraplegia. 32(6):367-74, 1994
17. Lukhele M: Fractures of the vertebral lamina associated with unifacet and bifacet cervical spine dislocations. S Afr J Surg. 32(3):112-4, 1994
18. Plezbert JA et al: Fracture of a lamina in the cervical spine. J Manipulative Physiol Ther. 17(8):552-7, 1994
19. Kang JD et al: Sagittal measurements of the cervical spine in subaxial fractures and dislocations. An analysis of two hundred and eighty-eight patients with and without neurological deficits. J Bone Joint Surg Am. 76(11):1617-28, 1994
20. Kiwerski J: Hyperextension-dislocation injuries of the cervical spine. Injury. 24(10):674-7, 1993
21. Silberstein M et al: Prevertebral swelling in cervical spine injury: identification of ligament injury with magnetic resonance imaging. Clin Radiol. 46(5):318-23, 1992
22. Goldberg AL et al: Hyperextension injuries of the cervical spine. Magnetic resonance findings. Skeletal Radiol. 18(4):283-8, 1989
23. Barquet A et al: An unusual extension injury to the cervical spine. A case report. J Bone Joint Surg Am. 70(9):1393-5, 1988
24. Edeiken-Monroe B et al: Hyperextension dislocation of the cervical spine. AJR Am J Roentgenol. 146(4):803-8, 1986
25. Coin CG et al: Diving type injury of the cervical spine: Contribution of CT to management. J Comput Assist Tomogr. 3: 362-5, 1979
26. Calenoff L et al: Multiple level spinal injuries: importance of early recognition. AJR Am J Roentgenol. 130(4):665-9, 1978
27. Penning L: Functional pathology of the cervical spine. Baltimore, Williams and Wilkins, 1968

HYPEREXTENSION INJURY, CERVICAL

IMAGE GALLERY

Typical

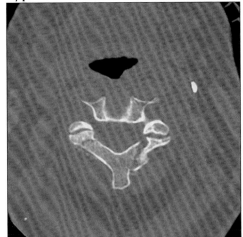 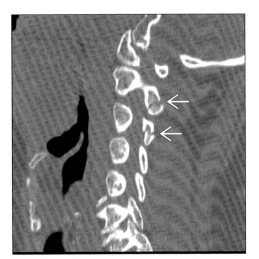

(Left) Axial bone CT shows fracture through right anterior lamina & left posterior laminae, with slight subluxation of left facet joint. *(Right)* Sagittal bone CT reformation shows fractures of C2 and C3 laminae (arrows), with minimal displacement.

Typical

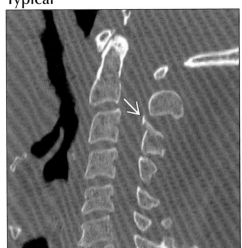 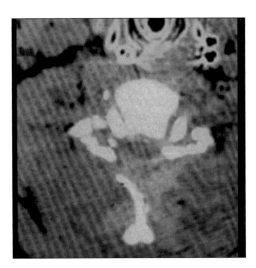

(Left) Sagittal bone CT shows displaced laminar fragment at C3, midline, as well as slight anterior subluxation of C2 on C3; both C2 and C3 showed laminar fractures on axial views. *(Right)* Axial NECT shows blood within and behind the canal in a patient rendered paraplegic by extension trauma. Note disrupted bony arch.

Typical

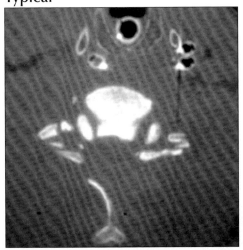 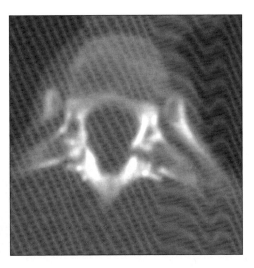

(Left) Axial NECT shows "sprung" C7 arch in patient with paralysis after extension trauma. *(Right)* Axial NECT shows fractures of T4 laminae in patient who also showed mid-cervical extension fracture.

HYPERFLEXION-ROTATION INJURY, CERVICAL

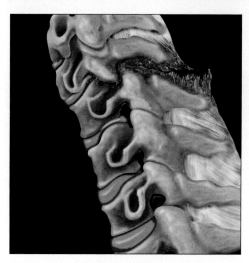

Lateral graphic shows disrupted facet and posterior ligaments, with facet subluxation.

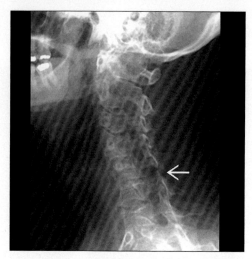

Sagittal Oblique radiography shows offset of facets at C5-6 (arrow), inferior C5 facet perched on superior C6 facet.

TERMINOLOGY

Abbreviations and Synonyms
- Jumped facet(s)
- Rotatory subluxation of vertebral bodies (vb), posterior elements in the cervical spine (C-spine)

Definitions
- Traumatic disruption of cervical spine (ligaments alone, or together with bony elements) causing facet subluxation

IMAGING FINDINGS

General Features
- Best diagnostic clue: Malalignment of adjacent facets and spinous processes on lateral x-ray, with focal vertebral body angulation
- Location: Typically mid- or lower C-spine

Radiographic Findings
- Radiography
  - Altered adjacent facet relationship on lateral radiograph
  - Spinous process malalignment, esp. vertical offset on anteroposterior view
  - Focal vb kyphosis

CT Findings
- CTA: Done to detect vertebral artery dissection or occlusion
- Bone CT
  - Normally, lower vb facet (superior facet) is anteriorly oriented in respect to its upper neighbor's inferior facet
  - Axial: "Naked" inferior facet; its subjacent neighbor, superior facet of the lower vb, not seen at joint interface
  - Sagittal: Affected lateral mass "perched" on or jumped anterior to subjacent partner
  - May see fracture of facet tip
  - May see fracture of vb if significant flexion component
  - Axial views show rotated relationship between lower vb with its upper neighbor

MR Findings
- T1WI
  - Shows the malalignment
  - Insensitive to associated fractures
- T2WI
  - Depicts edema of disrupted ligaments
  - Demonstrates cord compromise, contusion when present
- STIR: More sensitive to fracture than T1WI, but not as sensitive as CT

DDx: Cervical Subluxation Injury

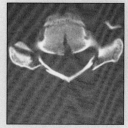

Whiplash Fx

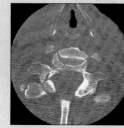

Rotary Extension Fx

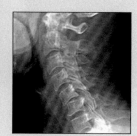

Whiplash Fx

HYPERFLEXION-ROTATION INJURY, CERVICAL

Key Facts

Terminology
- Jumped facet(s)
- Rotatory subluxation of vertebral bodies (vb), posterior elements in the cervical spine (C-spine)

Imaging Findings
- 5 view cervical spine series starts work-up
- CT with thin axial sections & reformations recommended with serious trauma, or if patient cannot cooperate
- Always evaluate the following relationships when examining C-spine trauma x-rays
- Anterior vb edges should trace gentle C-like lordosis
- Posterior edges of vb should parallel the anterior curve
- Facets should align on lateral and oblique views

- Posterior laminal line (point of junction of the laminae) should show the same gentle lordotic curve as anterior + posterior vb edges on lateral view
- Prevertebral soft tissue should show ½ thickness of AP vb diameter or less
- AP x-ray should show regular spacing between spinous processes, all vertically aligned in midline
- Disc space height loss can be clue (in absence of degenerative changes)

Pathology
- Rotatory shear forces tear capsular, annular, longitudinal ligaments; allows even intact bony elements to sublux

---

- T2* GRE: More sensitive to cord hemorrhage
- MRA: Done to detect vertebral or carotid artery damage

Angiographic Findings
- Conventional: Done to verify suspected arterial damage

Imaging Recommendations
- 5 view cervical spine series starts work-up
- CT with thin axial sections & reformations recommended with serious trauma, or if patient cannot cooperate
- Always evaluate the following relationships when examining C-spine trauma x-rays
  - Anterior vb edges should trace gentle C-like lordosis
  - Posterior edges of vb should parallel the anterior curve
  - Facets should align on lateral and oblique views
  - Posterior laminal line (point of junction of the laminae) should show the same gentle lordotic curve as anterior + posterior vb edges on lateral view
  - Prevertebral soft tissue should show ½ thickness of AP vb diameter or less
  - AP x-ray should show regular spacing between spinous processes, all vertically aligned in midline
  - Disc space height loss can be clue (in absence of degenerative changes)

DIFFERENTIAL DIAGNOSIS

Whiplash fracture
- No facet malalignment
- Some rotational component may be present

Burst or tear drop fracture
- May see slight separation of facet joints
- Less rotational malalignment

Rotatory extension fracture
- Similar, but greater disruption of posterior arch

PATHOLOGY

General Features
- General path comments
  - Capsular, other ligaments provide considerable support to relatively small facets of cervical vbs
  - Near horizontal articulation of cervical facets predisposes to easy subluxation once ligaments are torn
  - Rotatory shear forces tear capsular, annular, longitudinal ligaments; allows even intact bony elements to sublux
    - Once facets "jump" each other and lock, fracture is stable
    - Considerable traction necessary to restore normal relationships
- Etiology: Sudden, forceful rotational + flexion force on skull/spine
- Associated abnormalities
  - Spinal cord damage
  - Dissection of vertebral or carotid arteries

Gross Pathologic & Surgical Features
- Torn ligaments
- Displacement of inferior facet (articular pillar) on top of or anterior to its inferior neighbor

Staging, Grading or Classification Criteria
- Facet subluxation may vary from mild (perched facets) with threat of further damage, to severe (locking) a fixed injury
- Fracture-subluxation combine to produce considerable instability

CLINICAL ISSUES

Presentation
- Most common signs/symptoms: Severe neck pain, often associated with neurological compromise
- Clinical profile: Major trauma victim with neck pain, may have neurologic deficit

Natural History & Prognosis
- Dictated by type and degree of neurological deficit
- Mild cord contusion can regress
- Cord hematoma heralds grave prognosis

Treatment
- Traction
- Decompression and stabilization as necessary
- Fusion

DIAGNOSTIC CHECKLIST

Consider
- CT in any case of malalignment of vbs, facets on radiograph of C-spine

Image Interpretation Pearls
- Check facet surface relationships on every lateral radiograph
- Obtain sagittal reformations through both left + right lateral mass columns on every CT done for spine trauma
- Look for associated vascular injury

SELECTED REFERENCES

1. Vaccaro AR et al: Is magnetic resonance imaging indicated before reduction of a unilateral cervical facet dislocation? Spine. 27(1):117-8, 2002
2. Crawford NR et al: Unilateral cervical facet dislocation: injury mechanism and biomechanical consequences. Spine. 27(17):1858-64; discussion 1864, 2002
3. Hart RA: Cervical facet dislocation: when is magnetic resonance imaging indicated? Spine. 27(1):116-7, 2002
4. Sim E et al: In vitro genesis of subaxial cervical unilateral facet dislocations through sequential soft tissue ablation. Spine. 26(12):1317-23, 2001
5. Lingawi SS: The naked facet sign. Radiology. 219(2):366-7, 2001
6. Razack N et al: The management of traumatic cervical bilateral facet fracture-dislocations with unicortical anterior plates. J Spinal Disord. 13(5):374-81, 2000
7. Daffner RH et al: A new classification for cervical vertebral injuries: influence of CT. Skeletal Radiol. 29(3):125-32, 2000
8. Argenson C et al: Traumatic rotatory displacement of the lower cervical spine. Bull Hosp Jt Dis. 59(1):52-60, 2000
9. An HS et al: Cervical Spine Trauma. Spine. Vol 23:2713-29, 1998
10. Andreshak JL et al: Management of unilateral facet dislocations: a review of the literature. Orthopedics. 20(10):917-26, 1997
11. Halliday AL et al: The management of unilateral lateral mass/facet fractures of the subaxial cervical spine: the use of magnetic resonance imaging to predict instability. Spine. 22(22):2614-21, 1997
12. Leite CC et al: MRI of cervical facet dislocation. Neuroradiology. 39(8):583-8, 1997
13. Korres DS et al: The significance of rotation in fracture-separation of the articular pillar of a lower cervical vertebra. A clinical and cadaveric study. Acta Orthop Scand Suppl. 275:17-20, 1997
14. Sim E: Vertical facet splitting: a special variant of rotary dislocations of the cervical spine. J Neurosurg. 82(2):239-43, 1995
15. Shanmuganathan K et al: Rotational injury of cervical facets: CT analysis of fracture patterns with implications for management and neurologic outcome. AJR Am J Roentgenol. 163(5):1165-9, 1994
16. Willis BK et al: The incidence of vertebral artery injury after midcervical spine fracture or subluxation. Neurosurgery. 34(3):435-41; discussion 441-2, 1994
17. Shapiro SA: Management of unilateral locked facet of the cervical spine. Neurosurgery. 33(5):832-7; discussion 837, 1993
18. Hadley MN et al: Facet fracture-dislocation injuries of the cervical spine. Neurosurgery. 30(5):661-6, 1992
19. Roy-Camille R et al: Treatment of lower cervical spinal injuries--C3 to C7. Spine. 17(10 Suppl):S442-6, 1992
20. Beyer CA et al: Unilateral facet dislocations and fracture-dislocations of the cervical spine: a review. Orthopedics. 15(3):311-5, 1992
21. Myers BS et al: The role of torsion in cervical spine trauma. Spine. 16(8):870-4, 1991
22. Young JW et al: The laminar space in the diagnosis of rotational flexion injuries of the cervical spine. AJR Am J Roentgenol. 152(1):103-7, 1989
23. Rorabeck CH et al: Unilateral facet dislocation of the cervical spine. An analysis of the results of treatment in 26 patients. Spine. 12(1):23-7, 1987
24. Yetkin Z et al: Uncovertebral and facet joint dislocations in cervical articular pillar fractures: CT evaluation. AJNR Am J Neuroradiol. 6(4):633-7, 1985
25. Brant-Zawadzki M et al: Trauma, Computed Tomography of the Spine and Spinal Cord. Newton TH, Potts DG, Clavadal Press, 149-86, 1983
26. O'Callaghan JP et al: CT of facet distraction in flexion injuries of the thoracolumbar spine: the "naked" facet. AJR Am J Roentgenol. 134(3):563-8, 1980
27. Pick RY et al: C7--T1 bilateral facet dislocation: a rare lesion presenting with the syndrome of acute anterior spinal cord injury. Clin Orthop. (150):131-6, 1980
28. Ravichandran G: Traumatic single facet subluxation of cervical spine without neurological damage. A new clinical sign. Arch Orthop Trauma Surg. 92(2-3):221-4, 1978
29. Scher AT: Unilateral locked facet in cervical spine injuries. AJR Am J Roentgenol. 129(1):45-8, 1977
30. Babcock JL: Cervical spine injuries. Diagnosis and classification. Arch Surg. 111(6):646-51, 1976
31. Holdsworth FW et al: Fractures, Dislocations and Fracture-Dislocations of the Spine. Journal of Bone and Joint Surgury. 45B: 6-20, 1963

IMAGE GALLERY

Typical

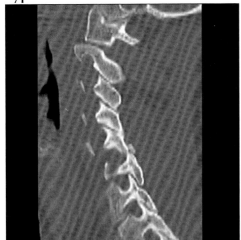 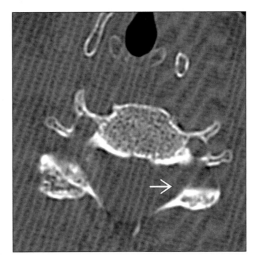

(Left) Sagittal bone CT shows anterior subluxation of C5 facet anterior to that of C6, with chip fracture of latter's superior tip, in patient with rotatory flexion injury. *(Right)* Axial bone CT shows naked left inferior facet of C5 (arrow), missing its anterior counterpart (superior facet of C6) in patient with rotatory flexion injury.

Typical

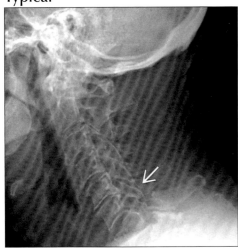 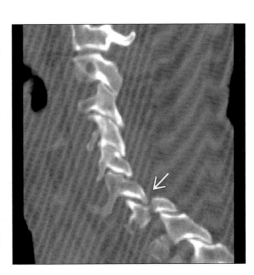

(Left) Lateral radiography shows facet offset at C6-7. Note anterior displacement of laminal line of C6 versus C7 (arrow), slight compression fracture of C7 superior endplate. *(Right)* Sagittal CECT shows fractured lateral mass of C7 due to anterior rotatory subluxation of C6 facet (arrow).

Typical

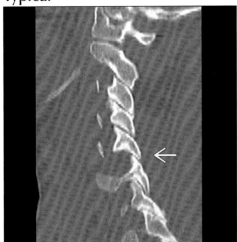 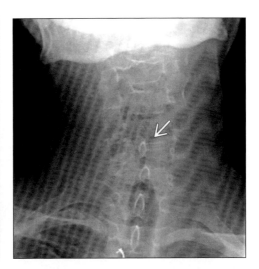

(Left) Sagittal bone CT reformation shows perched facet of C5 atop C6 (arrow). *(Right)* Anteroposterior radiography shows offset of C6 spinous process vs. C7 (arrow) with flexion-rotation injury. CT showed jumped right facets (note indistinct lateral mass region on the right at C6-7).

BURST FRACTURE, CERVICAL

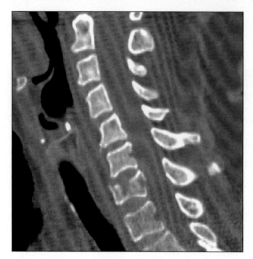

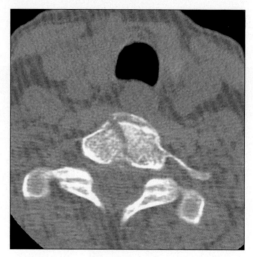

Sagittal bone CT window reformation shows vertical cleavage plane of C7 burst fracture. Pedicles + arch were intact.

Axial bone CT shows fracture plane through C7 vertebral body, which extended from superior to inferior end plate.

TERMINOLOGY

Abbreviations and Synonyms
- Shattered vertebral body (vb)
- Teardrop fracture

Definitions
- Comminuted fracture (Fx) of vb extending through both endplates due to axial compression

IMAGING FINDINGS

General Features
- Best diagnostic clue: Wedged lower cervical vb with end plate defect, focal gibbus on lateral radiograph
- Location: Typically mid- or lower cervical spine

Radiographic Findings
- Radiography: Cleavage of vb extending through end plate with focal flexion or gibbus deformity

CT Findings
- NECT: Fragmented vb without posterior element Fx
- Bone CT
  - Fracture lines extend through end plates, anterior and/or posterior vb margins

MR Findings
- T1WI: Low signal and loss of height of vb
- T2WI
  - High signal, loss of vb height with soft tissue edema in prevertebral region
  - May see canal compromise, even cord compression if retropulsed fragment present
- T2* GRE: May show cord contusion

Angiographic Findings
- Conventional: Only done if vertebral artery foramen fractured, or signs of vertebrobasilar insufficiency suggest dissection

Imaging Recommendations
- Always obtain CT if Fx of cervical vb seen on radiographs
- Thin-section axial slices with sagittal reformations, bone and soft tissue windows
- MR vital if neurologic symptoms/signs present
- MRA or CTA if Fx involves vertebral artery foramen

DIFFERENTIAL DIAGNOSIS

Benign compression fracture
- No endplate-to-endplate comminution
- No retropulsion of fragments or pedicular widening

DDx: Other Types of Vertebral Body Fractures

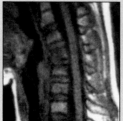

Compression Fracture

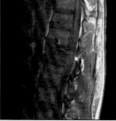

Dislocation Fracture

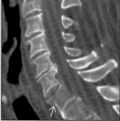

Flexion Fracture

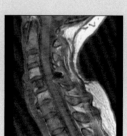

Pathologic Fracture

BURST FRACTURE, CERVICAL

II

1

43

Key Facts

Terminology
- Comminuted fracture (Fx) of vb extending through both endplates due to axial compression

Imaging Findings
- Best diagnostic clue: Wedged lower cervical vb with end plate defect, focal gibbus on lateral radiograph

Top Differential Diagnoses
- Benign compression fracture
- Flexion fracture

Clinical Issues
- Severe neck pain after trauma with axial load
- Radiculopathy or myelopathy may be present

Pathologic compression fracture
- Soft tissue mass replacing major portion of vb on MR
- No branching fracture lines on CT
- Focal lesion within vb

Flexion fracture
- Posterior element fracture also present
- Obvious malalignment at Fx site

PATHOLOGY

General Features
- General path comments: Instability of anterior/middle column
- Etiology: Axial compression, mild flexion combine to produce the Fx

Gross Pathologic & Surgical Features
- Fragmented vertebral body

CLINICAL ISSUES

Presentation
- Most common signs/symptoms
  - Severe neck pain
  - Other signs/symptoms
    - Myelopathy or radiculopathy if canal or foraminal compromise by fragments
- Clinical profile
  - Severe neck pain after trauma with axial load
  - Radiculopathy or myelopathy may be present

Natural History & Prognosis
- Self-limited unless neurologic injury becomes permanent

Treatment
- Surgical stabilization and (if needed) canal decompression
  - Bed rest may be sufficient with immobilization if comminution is minimal

DIAGNOSTIC CHECKLIST

Consider
- CT or MR angiography to exclude vertebral artery dissection

Image Interpretation Pearls
- Absence of posterior arch or pedicle fractures doesn't exclude instability if vb itself is shattered

SELECTED REFERENCES

1. Fisher CG et al: Comparison of outcomes for unstable lower cervical flexion teardrop fractures managed with halo thoracic vest versus anterior corpectomy and plating. Spine. 27(2):160-6, 2002
2. Kiwerski JE: Early anterior decompression and fusion for crush fractures of cervical vertebrae. Int Orthop. 17(3):166-8, 1993
3. Schweighofer F et al: Complications after an unusual procedure in the treatment of a cervical spine burst fracture. A case report. Langenbecks Arch Chir. 377(4):235-6, 1992
4. Ripa DR et al: Series of ninety-two traumatic cervical spine injuries stabilized with anterior ASIF plate fusion technique. Spine. 16(3 Suppl):S46-55, 1991
5. Cabanela ME et al: Anterior plate stabilization for bursting teardrop fractures of the cervical spine. Spine. 13(8):888-91, 1988
6. Mazur JM et al: Unrecognized spinal instability associated with seemingly "simple" cervical compression fractures. Spine. 8(7):687-92, 1983
7. Johnson JL et al: Nonoperative treatment of the acute tear-drop fracture of the cervical spine. Clin Orthop. (168):108-12, 1982

IMAGE GALLERY

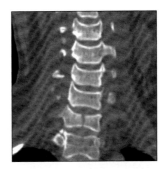 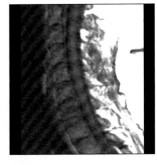

(Left) Coronal bone CT reformation shows vertical cleavage component of C7 burst fracture. No posterior element fractures were seen. *(Right)* Sagittal T1WI MR shows compression of C7, and low signal intensity within marrow; however, true burst nature of fracture was much better appreciated on CT exam.

HYPEREXTENSION-ROTATION, CERVICAL

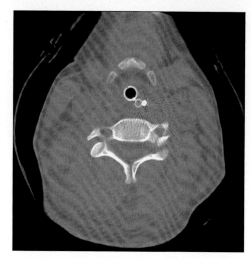

Axial bone CT shows linear fracture extending from lateral mass into left vertebral foramen in patient after motor vehicle accident. CT angiogram showed dissected vertebral artery.

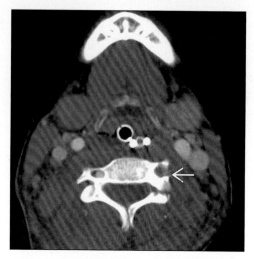

Axial CECT shows disrupted left vertebral artery (arrow), & left lateral mass fracture after vehicular accident. Adjacent slice showed fracture line into foramen.

TERMINOLOGY

Abbreviations and Synonyms
- Variation of hyperextension fracture

Definitions
- Unilateral facet or laminar fracture due to hyperextension + rotation combined, typically with ligament disruption

IMAGING FINDINGS

General Features
- Best diagnostic clue: Unilateral posterior element fracture
- Location: Below C2

Radiographic Findings
- Radiography: Mild rotational subluxation on anteroposterior + lateral views
- Fluoroscopy: Focal instability

CT Findings
- NECT: Fractured pedicle, articular pillar or laminar strut
- CECT: May show absent filling of vertebral artery
- CTA: Used to verify disruption of vertebral artery
- Bone CT

- High-resolution of bony disruption depicted best with bone algorithm

MR Findings
- T1WI: May see disc extrusion
- T2WI
  - May see edematous annulus, or ligaments
  - Effusion within facet joint
  - Will show cord edema or contusion, if present
- STIR: Shows ligamentous injury more sensitively, especially in facet capsular ligamentous complex
- T2* GRE: More sensitive to blood products when hemorrhagic cor contusion present
- MRA: Can be used to show vertebral artery disruption

Angiographic Findings
- Conventional: Verifies suspected arterial dissection

Imaging Recommendations
- Best imaging tool: CT
- Protocol advice: Thin-section slices with bone algorithm for reconstruction of axial and reformatted images

DIFFERENTIAL DIAGNOSIS

Hyperextension fracture
- Usually multifocal arch disruption

DDx: Posterior Element Fractures

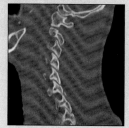

Jumped Facet

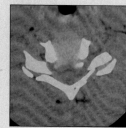

Hyperextension Fx

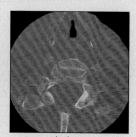

Lateral Flexion Fx

Key Facts

Terminology
- Variation of hyperextension fracture
- Unilateral facet or laminar fracture due to hyperextension + rotation combined, typically with ligament disruption

Imaging Findings
- Best diagnostic clue: Unilateral posterior element fracture

- NECT: Fractured pedicle, articular pillar or laminar strut
- CECT: May show absent filling of vertebral artery
- May see edematous annulus, or ligaments
- Effusion within facet joint
- Will show cord edema or contusion, if present

Diagnostic Checklist
- MRA or CTA in any case of unilateral posterior element fracture

---

- Cord injury more frequent
- Greater degree and incidence of prevertebral swelling

Flexion rotation injury
- Jumped or perched facet, with fracture
- More obvious focal malalignment of spinous processes, vertebral bodies

Lateral flexion injury
- Vertebral body fracture present

PATHOLOGY

General Features
- General path comments: Unilateral pedicle, facet complex, and/or lamina fracture, with anterior annular and capsular ligament disruption
- Etiology: Rotational and extension forces combined
- Epidemiology: Unusual fracture category
- Associated abnormalities: Mandibular fracture can predispose (upper cut-like force to chin)

CLINICAL ISSUES

Presentation
- Most common signs/symptoms: Neck pain, without or with neurological signs
- Clinical profile: Major force to head or chin from anterolateral direction

Natural History & Prognosis
- Depends on presence and extent of neurologic damage

Treatment
- Options, risks, complications: Anterior fusion mandatory

DIAGNOSTIC CHECKLIST

Consider
- MRA or CTA in any case of unilateral posterior element fracture

Image Interpretation Pearls
- MRI best evaluates associated disc extrusion, cord injury

SELECTED REFERENCES

1. Berlin L: CT versus radiography for initial evaluation of cervical spine trauma: what is the standard of care? AJR Am J Roentgenol. 180(4):911-5, 2003
2. Lifeso RM et al: Anterior fusion for rotationally unstable cervical spine fractures. Spine. 25(16):2028-34, 2000
3. Biffl WL et al: The devastating potential of blunt vertebral arterial injuries. Ann Surg. 231(5):672-81, 2000
4. Klein GR et al: Efficacy of magnetic resonance imaging in the evaluation of posterior cervical spine fractures. Spine. 24(8):771-4, 1999
5. Makan P: Neurologic compromise after an isolated laminar fracture of the cervical spine. Spine. 24(11):1144-6, 1999
6. London PS: Extension injuries of the neck. Injury. 18(4):223, 1987
7. Woodring JH et al: Fractures of the articular processes of the cervical spine. AJR Am J Roentgenol. 139(2):341-4, 1982
8. Dolan KD: Cervical spine injuries below the axis. Radiol Clin North Am. 15(2):247-59, 1977
9. Nieminen R: Fractures of the articular processes of the lower cervical spine. An analysis of 28 cases treated conservatively. Ann Chir Gynaecol Fenn. 63(3):204-11, 1974
10. Frankel H et al: Closed injuries of the cervical spine and spinal cord: results of conservative treatment of extension rotation injuries of the cervical spine with tetraplegia. Proc Veterans Adm Spinal Cord Inj Conf. (19):52-5, 1973

IMAGE GALLERY

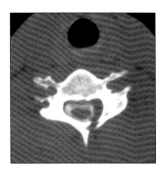 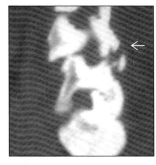

(Left) Axial bone CT after intrathecal contrast injection shows unilateral left laminar fracture in patient with rotational extension injury. *(Right)* Sagittal oblique CT reformation shows fragmented lateral mass (arrow) in patient with rotational extension injury.

LATERAL FLEXION INJURY, CERVICAL

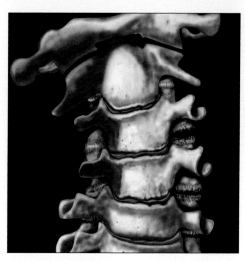

Anterior graphic shows disrupted left facets & ligaments from lateral flexion injury.

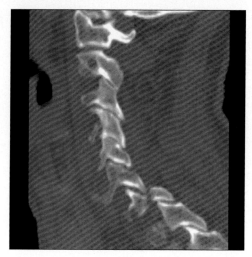

Sagittal bone CT reformation shows vertical cleavage of C7 lateral mass. Axial view showed fracture of uncovertebral process. AP radiograph showed slight rotation.

TERMINOLOGY

Abbreviations and Synonyms
• Articular mass fracture, pillar fracture

Definitions
• Fracture of articular mass, often associated with fracture of transverse, uncinate processes + vertebral body (vb)

IMAGING FINDINGS

General Features
• Best diagnostic clue: Fracture of articular pillar on AP view with widening of uncovertebral joint
• Location: Mid, lower cervical spine
• Morphology: Sagittal cleavage of lateral mass

Radiographic Findings
• Radiography
  ○ Slight malalignment maybe only clue on lateral view
  ○ Triangular appearance of lateral mass on oblique view
  ○ "Pillar" view (cephalad angled AP view) shows fracture lines in articular mass

CT Findings
• NECT

  ○ Sagittal fracture of pillar
  ○ Malaligned, impacted lateral masses best shown on sagittal reformation
  ○ Associated transverse process fracture, or vb fracture
• Bone CT
  ○ High-resolution, thin-section, bone algorithm with multiplanar reformations

MR Findings
• T1WI: Lowered signal in affected pillar
• T2WI
  ○ Increased signal in pillar
  ○ High signal in torn ligaments

Angiographic Findings
• Conventional: Done for suspected dissection

Imaging Recommendations
• Best imaging tool: High-resolution CT with bone algorithm for reconstruction of axial and reformatted slices
• Protocol advice: 1 mm slices are best

DIFFERENTIAL DIAGNOSIS

Flexion/rotation fracture
• Different mechanism with rotational component
• Often see unilateral "jumped" facet

DDx: Lateral Mass Fracture/Subluxation

"Jumped" Facet   "Floating" Pillar   Flexion-Extension

LATERAL FLEXION INJURY, CERVICAL

Key Facts

Terminology
- Articular mass fracture, pillar fracture

Imaging Findings
- Slight malalignment maybe only clue on lateral view
- Sagittal fracture of pillar
- Associated transverse process fracture, or vb fracture

Top Differential Diagnoses
- Flexion/rotation fracture
- Fracture isolation of lateral mass

Diagnostic Checklist
- CT in any serious spine injury or persistent post-traumatic neck pain

---

Fracture isolation of lateral mass
- Complete separation of articular mass from vb & ipsilateral lamina ("floating" lateral mass)
- Produces 3 levels of instability

PATHOLOGY

General Features
- General path comments: Comminuted lateral mass, ipsilateral + contralateral capsular ligamentous injury
- Etiology: Lateral flexion forces during trauma
- Epidemiology: Sporadic traumatic injury
- Associated abnormalities: Neurological deficits (plegia, radiculopathy) in almost 50%

Gross Pathologic & Surgical Features
- Fracture instability at affected level

CLINICAL ISSUES

Presentation
- Most common signs/symptoms
  - Post-traumatic neck pain
  - Other signs/symptoms
    - Quadriplegia
    - Hemiplegia
    - Radiculopathy

Natural History & Prognosis
- Depends on neurological damage

Treatment
- Options, risks, complications: Fusion necessary in cases of gross instability

DIAGNOSTIC CHECKLIST

Consider
- CT in any serious spine injury or persistent post-traumatic neck pain

Image Interpretation Pearls
- Unilateral displacement of one facet versus its neighbor suggests fracture

SELECTED REFERENCES

1. Halliday AL et al: The management of unilateral lateral mass/facet fractures of the subaxial cervical spine: the use of magnetic resonance imaging to predict instability. Spine. 22(22):2614-21, 1997
2. Nunez DB Jr et al: Cervical spine trauma: how much more do we learn by routinely using helical CT? Radiographics. 16(6):1307-18; discussion 1318-21, 1996
3. Shanmuganathan K et al: Traumatic isolation of the cervical articular pillar: imaging observations in 21 patients. AJR Am J Roentgenol. 166(4):897-902, 1996
4. Shanmuganathan K et al: Rotational injury of cervical facets: CT analysis of fracture patterns with implications for management and neurologic outcome. AJR Am J Roentgenol. 163(5):1165-9, 1994
5. Woodring JH et al: Limitations of cervical radiography in the evaluation of acute cervical trauma. J Trauma. 34(1):32-9, 1993
6. Lee C et al: Sagittally oriented fractures of the lateral masses of the cervical vertebrae. J Trauma. 31(12):1638-43, 1991
7. Woodring JH et al: Fractures of the articular processes of the cervical spine. AJR Am J Roentgenol. 139(2):341-4, 1982
8. Scher AT: Radiological assessment of lateral flexion injuries of the cervical spine. S Afr Med J. 60(26):983-5, 1981
9. Smith GR et al: Articular mass fracture: a neglected cause of post-traumatic neck pain? Clin Radiol. 27(3):335-40, 1976

IMAGE GALLERY

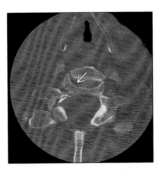 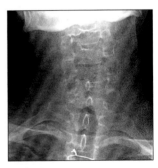

(Left) Axial bone CT shows fractures of right lateral mass, uncovertebral process (arrow) and transverse process at C7. *(Right)* Anteroposterior radiography shows step-off at C6-7 in spinous processes alignment, separation of left uncovertebral joint, compression of C7 right lateral mass suggesting its fracture (shown by CT).

POSTERIOR COLUMN INJURY, CERVICAL

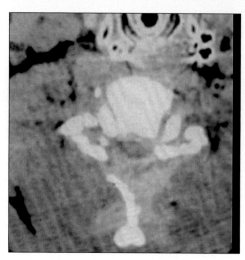

Axial NECT shows disrupted posterior arch, with blood in epidural space & within posterior ligaments indicative of severe posterior column injury.

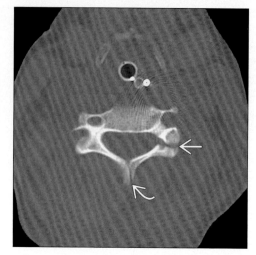

Axial bone CT shows unilateral fracture of left lateral mass (arrow) a stable fracture within the posterior column. Note congenital cleft at laminal line (curved arrow).

TERMINOLOGY

Abbreviations and Synonyms
- Vertebral body (vb)
- Posterior longitudinal ligament (PLL)
- Fracture (Fx)

Definitions
- Posterior column: Spinal architecture beyond PLL, anulus, posterior vb margin
  - Includes facets, their joint ligaments, laminae, ligamentum flavum, interspinous ligaments, spinous processes

IMAGING FINDINGS

General Features
- Best diagnostic clue: Disrupted alignment, relationships of posterior arch in adjacent vertebral levels

Radiographic Findings
- Radiography
  - Fracture lines through laminae, facets, or spinous process
  - Malaligned posterior elements

CT Findings
- NECT: Fx of laminae or articular pillar, may see blood in epidural space
- Bone CT
  - High-resolution algorithm better at detecting non-displaced Fx

MR Findings
- T2WI
  - Increased signal in muscles, ligaments
  - Depicts cord edema when contusion present
- STIR: Best for showing soft tissue edema, marrow edema of fractured vb or arch

Imaging Recommendations
- Best imaging tool: CT with soft tissue + bone windows, reformations
- Protocol advice: 1 mm slice thickness, bone algorithm reconstruction of CT slices, isotropic reformations

DIFFERENTIAL DIAGNOSIS

Multicolumn fractures with element of posterior column involvement
- Flexion-extension Fx
- Flexion-rotation Fx
- Extension-rotation Fx

DDx: Combined Posterior Column Injuries

Flexion-Extension Fx   *Flexion-Rotation*   *Jumped Facets*

POSTERIOR COLUMN INJURY, CERVICAL

II

1

49

Key Facts

Terminology
- Posterior column: Spinal architecture beyond PLL, anulus, posterior vb margin

Pathology
- Tear of ligaments bridging spinous processes + laminae
- Fractures of laminae, facets, or spinous processes

- Posterior column fracture thought to be generally stable, as anterior/middle columns intact and prevent subluxation
- Exception: If capsular ligaments torn, facets and/or laminae both fractured, rotational instability may exist

Diagnostic Checklist
- Flexion extension films or fluoroscopy to assess degree of instability

---

- Jumped facets

PATHOLOGY

General Features
- General path comments
  - Tear of ligaments bridging spinous processes + laminae
  - Fractures of laminae, facets, or spinous processes
  - Posterior column fracture thought to be generally stable, as anterior/middle columns intact and prevent subluxation
    - Exception: If capsular ligaments torn, facets and/or laminae both fractured, rotational instability may exist
- Associated abnormalities: May have associated disruption of middle or anterior column, which results in instability

CLINICAL ISSUES

Presentation
- Most common signs/symptoms
  - Neck pain
  - Other signs/symptoms
    - Neurological disturbance
- Clinical profile: Post-traumatic neck pain and loss of mobility

Treatment
- Options, risks, complications
  - Immobilization
  - Surgical fusion

DIAGNOSTIC CHECKLIST

Consider
- Flexion extension films or fluoroscopy to assess degree of instability

Image Interpretation Pearls
- Even minor degrees of malalignment may indicate sever ligamentous disruption

SELECTED REFERENCES

1. Maiman DJ et al: Preinjury cervical alignment affecting spinal trauma. J Neurosurg. 97(1 Suppl):57-62, 2002
2. Matar LD et al: "Spinolaminar breach": an important sign in cervical spinous process fractures. Skeletal Radiol. 29(2):75-80, 2000
3. Brady WJ et al: ED use of flexion-extension cervical spine radiography in the evaluation of blunt trauma. Am J Emerg Med. 17(6):504-8, 1999
4. Zhu Q et al: Traumatic instabilities of the cervical spine caused by high-speed axial compression in a human model. An in vitro biomechanical study. Spine. 24(5):440-4, 1999
5. Plezbert JA et al: Fracture of a lamina in the cervical spine. J Manipulative Physiol Ther. 17(8):552-7, 1994
6. Goldberg AL et al: Hyperextension injuries of the cervical spine. Magnetic resonance findings. Skeletal Radiol. 18(4):283-8, 1989
7. Denis, F: The three column spine and its significance in the classification of acute thoracolumbar spinal injuries. Spine. 8(8):817-31, 1983

IMAGE GALLERY

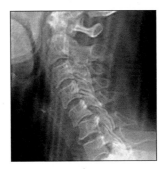 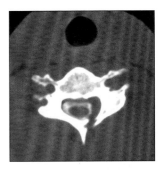

(Left) Lateral radiography shows anterior subluxation of C5-C6. Gross separation of spinous processes, facets of C5 perched on those of C6 indicate ligamentous disruption in the posterior column. *(Right)* Axial bone CT with intrathecal contrast shows fractured lamina - a stable posterior column injury.

ANTERIOR COMPRESSION FRACTURE, THORACIC

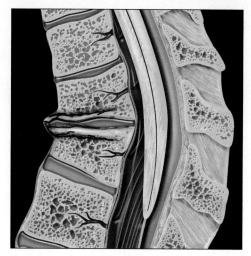 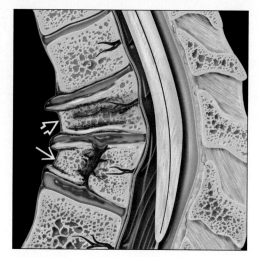

Sagittal graphic shows 2 compression fractures. Most common type is compression of superior endplate. Compression of inferior endplate alone is rare.

Sagittal graphic shows 2 additional types of compression fracture. Open arrow shows common type involving both endplates. Arrow shows rare type with coronally oriented cleft.

TERMINOLOGY

Abbreviations and Synonyms
• Wedge compression

Definitions
• Vertebral body fracture compressing anterior cortex, sparing middle/posterior columns

IMAGING FINDINGS

General Features
• Best diagnostic clue: Wedge-shaped vertebral body
• Location
   ○ May occur at multiple levels, contiguous or noncontiguous
   ○ Mid-/lower thoracic most common

Radiographic Findings
• Radiography
   ○ Anteroposterior radiography
      ▪ Paraspinous hematoma apparent
      ▪ Loss of vertebral height difficult to see
   ○ Diagnostic signs primarily visible on lateral radiography
   ○ Wedge-shaped vertebral body
   ○ Distinct fracture line usually not visible
   ○ Kyphosis common

○ Almost always involves superior endplate
   ▪ Most commonly superior endplate alone
   ▪ May involve both endplates
   ▪ < 5% involve inferior endplate only
○ Endplate depression may be cup-like or angular
○ Angular deformity, stepoff anterior cortex
○ Rarely, coronal fracture through vertebral body
○ Normal posterior elements
○ < 40-50% loss of height in patients with normal density
   ▪ If greater loss of height, probably Chance fracture
○ In osteoporotic patients, may develop vertebra plana
○ Upper thoracic vertebrae less commonly involved
   ▪ Difficult to see on radiographs

CT Findings
• Bone CT
   ○ Multiple fracture lines often visible
   ○ May extend to posterior cortex of vertebral body
   ○ Posterior cortical displacement absent
   ○ Fractures of posterior elements absent
   ○ Alignment of posterior elements normal on reformatted images

MR Findings
• T1WI
   ○ Low signal intensity fracture line may or may not be seen
   ○ Band-like or triangular region of low signal

DDx: STIR MRI Compressed Thoracic Vertebrae Due to Different Causes

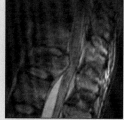 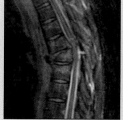 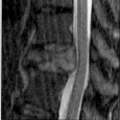 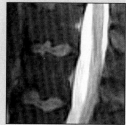

Burst   *Chance*   *Metastasis*   *Scheuermann*

Key Facts

Terminology
- Vertebral body fracture compressing anterior cortex, sparing middle/posterior columns

Imaging Findings
- Best diagnostic clue: Wedge-shaped vertebral body
- May occur at multiple levels, contiguous or noncontiguous
- May extend to posterior cortex of vertebral body
- Fractures of posterior elements absent
- Best imaging tool: CT best to differentiate from Chance, burst fractures

Top Differential Diagnoses
- Compression-distraction injury (Chance fracture)
- Burst fracture
- Pathologic fracture due to tumor

- Scheuermann kyphosis
- Physiologic vertebral wedging

Pathology
- Axial load with or without flexion component
- Two distinct populations: Major trauma, insufficiency fracture

Clinical Issues
- Patients with normal bone mineral density heal well with conservative management
- Osteoporotic patients may have progressive fracture

Diagnostic Checklist
- Compression fracture involving inferior endplate with normal superior endplate raises suspicion for pathologic fracture

---

- ○ Posterior cortex intact
- ○ Paraspinous hematoma mimics tumor
- T2WI
  - ○ High signal in vertebral body
  - ○ Usually has band-like or triangular morphology
  - ○ Ligaments intact
- STIR
  - ○ Shows marrow edema most prominently
  - ○ Fracture line may or may not be seen
- T1 C+: May have diffuse or linear enhancement

Nuclear Medicine Findings
- Bone Scan
  - ○ Positive in all three phases if acute
  - ○ Indistinguishable from infection, tumor, Charcot arthropathy, degenerative instability

Imaging Recommendations
- Best imaging tool: CT best to differentiate from Chance, burst fractures
- Protocol advice
  - ○ Multidetector CT with thin overlapping helical sections
  - ○ Sagittal/coronal reformations essential to detect signs of ligament injuries
  - ○ If patient undergoing thoracic multidetector CT because of trauma, dedicated spine CT not needed
    - Small field of view coronal/sagittal reformations obtained from original data set
    - Bone (edge-enhancing) algorithm can be applied after scanning in soft tissue algorithm

DIFFERENTIAL DIAGNOSIS

Compression-distraction injury (Chance fracture)
- Chance fracture involves middle, posterior columns
- If more than 50% loss of vertebral body height and bone density normal, probably Chance fracture
- Horizontally oriented posterior element fractures OR
- Disruption of facet joints and interspinous ligaments

Burst fracture
- Loss of height anterior + posterior vertebral body
- Retropulsion of posterior vertebral cortex
- Less common in thoracic spine because of stabilizing effect of ribs

Pathologic fracture due to tumor
- Cortical destruction
- Trabecular destruction (best seen on CT)
- Rounded mass in medullary bone seen on CT or MR
- More likely to involve inferior cortex of vertebral body
- Metastases often involve posterior elements as well as vertebral body
- Paraspinous mass may be due to hematoma (benign compression fracture) or tumor extension
- Often see tumor at other levels away from fracture

Scheuermann kyphosis
- 3 contiguous levels
- Schmorl nodes
- Undulation of vertebral endplates

Physiologic vertebral wedging
- Seen at T12-L1
- Loss of height is mild
- Usually involves both superior, inferior endplates

PATHOLOGY

General Features
- General path comments: Most common type of thoracic spine fracture due to blunt trauma
- Etiology
  - ○ Axial load with or without flexion component
  - ○ Because of normal thoracic kyphosis, axial load affects anterior portion of vertebral body more than posterior
- Epidemiology
  - ○ Two distinct populations: Major trauma, insufficiency fracture
  - ○ Young patients: Due to significant fall
  - ○ Osteoporotic patients: Insufficiency fracture

ANTERIOR COMPRESSION FRACTURE, THORACIC

- Associated abnormalities
  - Other spine fractures, contiguous or not contiguous
  - Fractures of the pelvis + lower extremities

CLINICAL ISSUES

Presentation

- Most common signs/symptoms
  - Acute trauma with focal back pain
  - Insidious back pain in elderly patients
  - Other signs/symptoms
    - Radiculopathy
    - Kyphotic deformity

Demographics

- Age
  - Bimodal
  - Young trauma patients and
  - Elderly osteoporotic patients

Natural History & Prognosis

- Patients with normal bone mineral density heal well with conservative management
- Increased risk of premature degenerative disc disease in young patients
- Osteoporotic patients may have progressive fracture
  - Chronic pain
- Kyphotic deformity often progressive in osteoporotic patients
- Patients with 1 osteoporotic compression fracture at increased risk for other fractures
- May have delayed onset of neurologic symptoms

Treatment

- Options, risks, complications: Conservative management usually successful
- Vertebroplasty & kyphoplasty used for chronic pain, kyphotic deformity
  - Usually affords immediate pain relief
  - May increase risk of compression fractures of adjacent vertebrae
- Bisphosphonates, calcitonin decrease pain & risk of further osteoporotic fracture

DIAGNOSTIC CHECKLIST

Image Interpretation Pearls

- Compression fracture involving inferior endplate with normal superior endplate raises suspicion for pathologic fracture

SELECTED REFERENCES

1. Folman Y et al: Late outcome of nonoperative management of thoracolumbar vertebral wedge fractures. J Orthop Trauma. 17(3):190-2, 2003
2. Wintermark M et al: Thoracolumbar spine fractures in patients who have sustained severe trauma: depiction with multi-detector row CT. Radiology. 227(3):681-9, 2003
3. Naves M et al: The effect of vertebral fracture as a risk factor for osteoporotic fracture and mortality in a Spanish population. Osteoporos Int. 14(6):520-4, 2003
4. Hsu JM et al: Thoracolumbar fracture in blunt trauma patients: guidelines for diagnosis and imaging. Injury. 34(6):426-33, 2003
5. Haba H et al: Diagnostic accuracy of magnetic resonance imaging for detecting posterior ligamentous complex injury associated with thoracic and lumbar fractures. J Neurosurg. 99(1 Suppl):20-6, 2003
6. Phillips FM: Minimally invasive treatments of osteoporotic vertebral compression fractures. Spine. 28(15):S45-53, 2003
7. Sheridan R et al: Reformatted visceral protocol helical computed tomographic scanning allows conventional radiographs of the thoracic and lumbar spine to be eliminated in the evaluation of blunt trauma patients. J Trauma. 55(4):665-9, 2003
8. Hiwatashi A et al: Increase in vertebral body height after vertebroplasty. AJNR Am J Neuroradiol. 24(2):185-9, 2003
9. Sapkas GS et al: Thoracic spinal injuries: operative treatments and neurologic outcomes. Am J Orthop. 32(2):85-8, 2003
10. Wintermark M et al: Thoracolumbar spine fractures in patients who have sustained severe trauma: depiction with multi-detector row CT. Radiology. 227(3):681-9, 2003
11. Haba H et al: Diagnostic accuracy of magnetic resonance imaging for detecting posterior ligamentous complex injury associated with thoracic and lumbar fractures. J Neurosurg. 99(1 Suppl):20-6, 2003
12. Wittenberg RH et al: Noncontiguous unstable spine fractures. Spine. 27(3):254-7, 2002
13. Zhou XJ et al: Characterization of benign and metastatic vertebral compression fractures with quantitative diffusion MR imaging. AJNR Am J Neuroradiol. 23(1):165-70, 2002
14. Lane JM et al: Minimally invasive options for the treatment of osteoporotic vertebral compression fractures. Orthop Clin North Am. 33(2):431-8, viii, 2002
15. Baur A et al: Acute osteoporotic and neoplastic vertebral compression fractures: fluid sign at MR imaging. Radiology. 225(3):730-5, 2002
16. Robertson A et al: Spinal injury patterns resulting from car and motorcycle accidents. Spine. 27(24):2825-30, 2002
17. Parisini P et al: Treatment of spinal fractures in children and adolescents: long-term results in 44 patients. Spine. 27(18):1989-94, 2002
18. Robertson A et al: Spinal injury patterns resulting from car and motorcycle accidents. Spine. 27(24):2825-30, 2002
19. Parisini P et al: Treatment of spinal fractures in children and adolescents: long-term results in 44 patients. Spine. 27(18):1989-94, 2002
20. O'Connor PA et al: Spinal cord injury following osteoporotic vertebral fracture: case report. Spine. 27(18):E413-5, 2002
21. Lindsay R et al: Risk of new vertebral fracture in the year following a fracture. JAMA. 285(3):320-3, 2001
22. Holmes JF et al: Epidemiology of thoracolumbar spine injury in blunt trauma. Acad Emerg Med. 8(9):866-72, 2001
23. Vaccaro AR et al: Post-traumatic spinal deformity. Spine. 26(24 Suppl):S111-8, 2001
24. van Beek EJ et al: Upper thoracic spinal fractures in trauma patients - a diagnostic pitfall. Injury. 31(4):219-23, 2000
25. Kerttula LI et al: Post-traumatic findings of the spine after earlier vertebral fracture in young patients: clinical and MRI study. Spine. 25(9):1104-8, 2000
26. Rechtine GR 2nd et al: Treatment of thoracolumbar trauma: comparison of complications of operative versus nonoperative treatment. J Spinal Disord. 12(5):406-9, 1999

IMAGE GALLERY

Typical

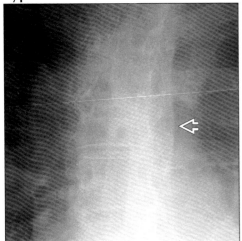 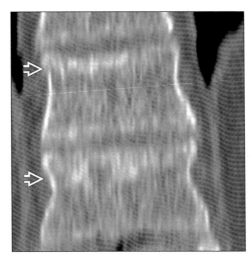

(Left) Anteroposterior fluoroscopy shows widening of paraspinous line (arrow) due to hematoma from compression fracture. Scoliosis was due to muscle spasm. (Right) Coronal bone CT shows mild endplate depression and linear bands of sclerosis at T10 and T11 (arrows) from mild compression fractures at both levels. Normal trabecular pattern excludes tumor.

Typical

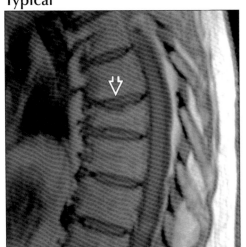 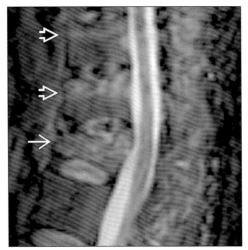

(Left) Sagittal T1WI MR shows cup-shaped depression (arrow) of superior vertebral cortex in osteoporotic patient. Low signal intensity fracture line is immediately beneath cortex. (Right) Sagittal STIR MR shows T12 burst (arrow) compared to T10, T11 compressions (open arrows). Note band-like configuration of edema, & preserved posterior cortices of compression fractures.

Variant

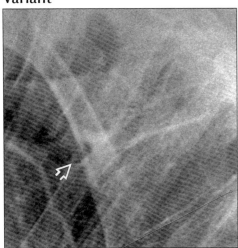 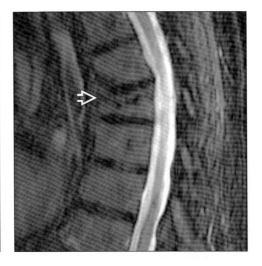

(Left) Lateral radiography shows T3 compression fracture (arrow). Fractures at this level are difficult to see on routine radiography due to overlap from shoulders, + swimmer's view is needed. (Right) Sagittal STIR MR shows chronic compression fracture. Bone marrow edema is absent. Transversely oriented callus (arrow) is very low signal intensity. Focal kyphosis is present.

LATERAL COMPRESSION FRACTURE, THORACIC

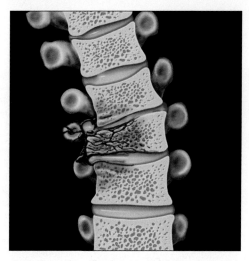

Coronal graphic illustrates a right lateral thoracic compression fracture. Note associated endplate injuries to both vertebral bodies above + below.

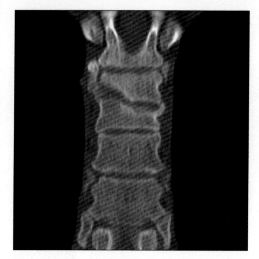

Coronal bone CT reformat reveals right lateral T5 compression & left lateral T6 compression fractures. Posterior vertebral body & facets were intact (not shown).

TERMINOLOGY

Abbreviations and Synonyms
- Vertebral compression fracture (VCF)

Definitions
- Thoracic vertebral body Fx with ↓ vertebral height, predominantly lateral location

IMAGING FINDINGS

General Features
- Best diagnostic clue: Lateral wedge deformity of affected thoracic spine (TS) vertebral body
- Location: Bimodal: Larger peak at thoracolumbar junction, smaller peak at T6-T7
- Size: Deformity graded in degrees of body height loss
- Morphology
  ○ Prominent lateral wedge deformity
  ○ Partial or no loss of posterior vertebral body height nor subluxation

Radiographic Findings
- Radiography
  ○ Entire spinal evaluation important as up to 20% of all VCF are multiple
  ○ AP: Lateral predominance of VCF deformity
  ○ Lateral: ↓ Vertebral body height; kyphosis

  ○ Intravertebral clefts seen as vacuum phenomenon

CT Findings
- Bone CT
  ○ Intact posterior body wall, no fragment retropulsion
  ○ Arc of irregular bone fragments circumferentially from vertebral body

MR Findings
- T1WI
  ○ Acute: Hypointense marrow edema
  ○ Chronic: Marrow signal normalizes with time
- STIR
  ○ Acute: STIR best visualizes hyperintense marrow edema which CAN extend into pedicles
  ○ Acute: May reveal fluid filled intravertebral cleft = "fluid sign"
    ▪ Detected in a slightly over 25% VCF
    ▪ More indicative of acute benign osteoporotic VCF
    ▪ Most often adjacent to the site of end-plate Fx
  ○ Chronic: Marrow signal normalizes with time
- DWI
  ○ Controversial: May be helpful for differentiating acute benign from pathologic VCF
    ▪ T2 shine-through confuses pattern
  ○ ADC mapping improves distinction between benign + malignant lesions
    ▪ Mean ADC for benign 68% > than for metastases
    ▪ May ↑ specificity of MR for acute VCF

DDx: Non-Lateral Compression Deformities

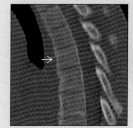

Compression Fx

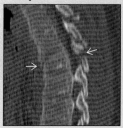

Chance Fx

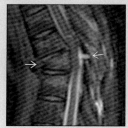

Chance Fx

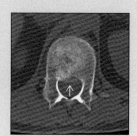

Burst Fx

Key Facts

Terminology

- Thoracic vertebral body Fx with ↓ vertebral height, predominantly lateral location

Imaging Findings

- Best diagnostic clue: Lateral wedge deformity of affected thoracic spine (TS) vertebral body
- Acute: STIR best visualizes hyperintense marrow edema which CAN extend into pedicles
- CT > > radiography

Top Differential Diagnoses

- Chance Fx ("seat belt Fx")
- Burst Fx

Pathology

- Lateral TS VCF correlated with seat belt injury

- Thoracic VCF may be result of single event trauma or ongoing chronic microfractures
- 11% of VCF are lateral

Clinical Issues

- Many experience severe & prolonged pain that can markedly alter activities of daily living
- 84% of VCF are painful, on average lasting 4-6 wks
- Main VCF risk factor is osteoporosis
- Women with VCF have higher mortality rates as compared to age-matched control subjects without Fx
- Early intervention with vertebroplasty may be indicated given low complication rates

Diagnostic Checklist

- VCF in elderly patient with unrelenting back pain
- Up to 20% of VCF are multiple → screen entire spine

- T1 C+
  - Both benign + malignant processes may enhance!
  - Paraspinal, epidural enhancing tissue suggests malignant pathology
- MRS: Vertebral body percent fat fraction is significantly ↑ in weakened bone controls

Nuclear Medicine Findings

- Bone Scan: ↑ Activity on bone scan highly predictive of positive outcome after vertebroplasty
- Fluorine-18 deoxyglucose (FDG) PET
  - No ↑ uptake in acute vertebral fractures originating from osteoporosis or preclinical osteoporosis
  - High FDG uptake is characteristic for malignant & inflammatory processes
  - FDG-PET may have potential value differentiating osteoporotic from pathologic VCF

Imaging Recommendations

- Best imaging tool
  - CT > > radiography
  - MRI for neurologic deficit(s)
- Protocol advice
  - CT: Sagittal & coronal reformats
  - MRI: STIR & fat-saturation T1 C+

DIFFERENTIAL DIAGNOSIS

Compression Fx

- Anterior without lateral component

Chance Fx ("seat belt Fx")

- Horizontal splitting of spinous process, laminae, pedicles, superior vertebral body
- Disc and facet distraction with ligament disruption

Burst Fx

- Abnormal posterior vertebral body wall
- Fragment retropulsion into spinal canal

PATHOLOGY

General Features

- General path comments
  - Anatomic-pathologic correlation
    - Thoracic cage provides ↑ structural stability to TS
    - Kyphosis & extensive overlap of articulating facets limits extension injuries
    - Trauma forces translate into flexion vector
    - Results in wedging or compression deformities
    - Posterior elements, ligaments often remain intact
  - VCF occur when combined axial & bending loads exceed strength of vertebral body
  - Lateral TS VCF correlated with seat belt injury
- Genetics
  - Inherited bone disorders (i.e., NF1, Gaucher)
  - Vitamin D receptor polymorphism may influence bone mineral density & osteoporotic
- Etiology
  - Typically result of flexion, axial forces, or both
  - Trauma, osteopenia, metabolic bone disease, genetic disorders, neoplasm (primary or metastatic)
    - Metastatic vertebral lesions account for 39% of bony mets in patients with primary neoplasms
    - Myeloma appears similar to benign VCF
    - Benign vertebral lesions occur in approximately 1/3 of cancer patients
  - Seat belt injury
    - Result of shoulder-lap belt assemblies
    - Results in anterolateral wedge compression of thoracolumbar vertebra
    - Lateral compression occurs on side opposite restrained shoulder
    - Posterior elements may be disrupted contralateral to anterolateral body compression
    - Postulated mechanism, referred to as "roll-out phenomenon" = flexion & rotation about axis of shoulder strap
  - Thoracic VCF may be result of single event trauma or ongoing chronic microfractures
- Epidemiology
  - 11% of VCF are lateral

LATERAL COMPRESSION FRACTURE, THORACIC

- 16% of postmenopausal women suffer one or more VCF during their lifetime
- Osteoporosis is most common cause of VCF in US
- Prevalence of radiographic VCF has been reported as high as 26% in women ≥ 50 yrs
- Frequency of radiographic evidence of VCF increases from 500/100,000 person years (py) in women aged 50-54 yrs to 2,960/100,000 py in women > 85 yrs
- In the U.S., VCF account for 150,000 hospital admissions, 161,000 physician office visits, & > 5 million restricted activity days annually
- Associated abnormalities
  - Immobility makes more susceptible to pneumonia, deep vein thrombosis, & pulmonary embolism
  - Patients with osteoporotic VCF have significantly lower vital capacity and forced expiratory volume

Microscopic Features
- Inflammatory phase: Hematoma, osteocytic death, intense inflammatory response
- Reparative phase: Hematoma organizes with fibrovascular invasion, callus forms on collagen matrix
- Remodeling phase: Resorption of unnecessary callus, trabecular proliferation along lines of stress

CLINICAL ISSUES

Presentation
- Many experience severe & prolonged pain that can markedly alter activities of daily living
  - 84% of VCF are painful, on average lasting 4-6 wks
  - Subgroup of patients has subacute or chronic pain that is refractory to conservative therapy
- Numbness, tingling, & weakness may indicate nerve compression; may be asymptomatic

Demographics
- Age
  - Atraumatic: ↑ Frequency with age
  - Traumatic: Usually younger patient population
- Gender: M:F ≈ 2:1, yet high male incidence contradicts misconception that osteoporosis is women's health problem

Natural History & Prognosis
- Main VCF risk factor is osteoporosis
  - Severity of osteoporosis is worsened by smoking, physical inactivity, use of prednisone & other medications, poor nutrition
  - In males all above risk factors apply as well as low testosterone levels
- Women with VCF have higher mortality rates as compared to age-matched control subjects without Fx
  - Women with 1 or more VCF have a 1.23-fold greater age-adjusted mortality rate
  - Mortality rises as the number of VCF increases; women with ≥ 5 Fxs have a > twofold increase

Treatment
- Conservative therapy
  - Consists of analgesic use, rest, & external bracing
  - Immobilization accelerates bone loss, which may contribute to further VCF
- Vertebroplasty

- Direct injection of polymethylmethacrylate into collapsed body
- Can be performed throughout all thoracic levels without need of small diameter needles
- Alleviates pain & prevents further collapse
  - Achieves 90% efficacy in pain relief
- Highly efficacious regardless of Fx age, even with severe deformity (> 70%)
- May see opacifying intravertebral clefts
- Antecedent venography does not improve effectiveness or safety
- Early intervention with vertebroplasty may be indicated given low complication rates
  - Complications reported include transitory fever, transient worsening of pain, radiculopathy, rib Fx, cement pulmonary embolism, infection, & spinal cord compression
  - With osteoporotic VCF, complication rate is 1-2%
  - With malignant tumors, the complication rate ↑ 2° to cement leakage from destruction
  - MR is preferred for guiding vertebroplasty as it offers anatomic detail and concurrent information about other abnormalities (i.e., spinal stenosis)
  - If tumor suspected it may be appropriate to precede vertebroplasty with biopsy after cannula placed
    - Vertebroplasty cement presence does not hinder the therapeutic result of subsequent or concomitant radiation or chemotherapy
- Surgery when neurologic dysfunction and/or instability occurs as result of VCF
- Kyphoplasty = vertebroplasty variation in which an inflatable balloon is first placed inside compressed vertebral body into which cement is instilled

DIAGNOSTIC CHECKLIST

Consider
- VCF in elderly patient with unrelenting back pain

Image Interpretation Pearls
- Up to 20% of VCF are multiple → screen entire spine

SELECTED REFERENCES

1. Jung HS et al: Discrimination of metastatic from acute osteoporotic compression spinal fractures with MR imaging. Radiographics. 23(1):179-87, 2003
2. Kallmes DF et al: Vertebroplasty in the mid/upper thoracic spine. AJNR Am J Neuroradiol. 23(7):1117-20, 2002
3. Schmitz A et al: FDG-PET findings of vertebral compression fractures in osteoporosis: preliminary results. Osteoporos Int. 13(9):755-61, 2002
4. Baur A et al: Acute osteoporotic and neoplastic vertebral compression fractures: fluid sign at MR imaging. Radiology. 225(3):730-5, 2002
5. Herneth AM et al: Vertebral metastases: assessment with ADC. Radiology. 225(3):889-94, 2002
6. Miniaci A et al: Anterolateral compression fracture of the thoracolumbar spine. A seat belt injury. Clin Orthop. (240):153-6, 1989

LATERAL COMPRESSION FRACTURE, THORACIC

IMAGE GALLERY

Typical

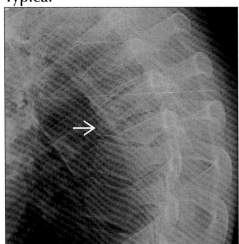

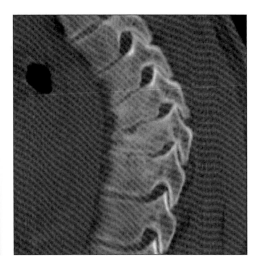

(Left) Lateral radiography shows T6 anterior compression deformity (arrow) confirmed as a lateral compression fracture on coronal & axial CT (not shown). *(Right)* Left parasagittal bone CT reformat reveals compression deformity of T6; note intact pedicle & facet. Axial CT and other reformatted images verified this as lateral compression fracture.

Typical

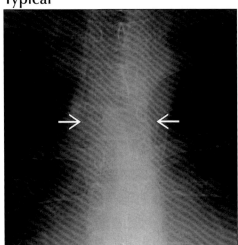

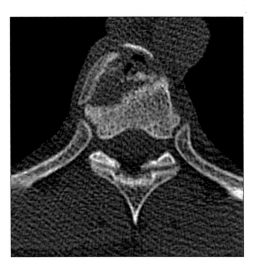

(Left) Anteroposterior radiography shows right lateral T5 compression fracture (arrows) which was verified with CT imaging. *(Right)* Axial bone CT demonstrates right lateral circumferential arc of bone fragments from thoracic lateral compression fracture. Note intact posterior vertebral body & facets.

Typical

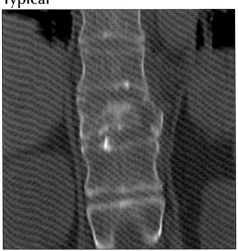

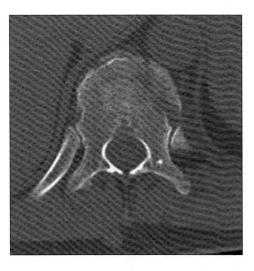

(Left) Coronal bone CT reformat demonstrates left lateral thoracic compression fracture. Posterior vertebral body & facets were intact (not shown). *(Right)* Axial bone CT shows left lateral circumferential arc of bone fragments from thoracic lateral compression fracture. Note intact posterior vertebral body & pedicles.

BURST THORACOLUMBAR FRACTURE

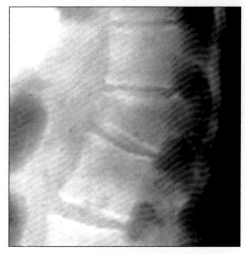

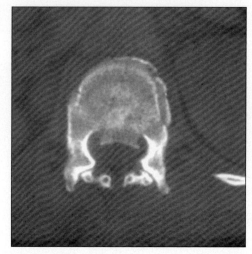

Lateral radiography shows wedge compression of L1 vertebral body. Pedicles were widened on AP view. Patient had jumped off garage roof, experienced neck and lower back pain.

Axial bone CT, same case as on left, shows comminuted vertebral body Fxs, outward rotation of pedicles, retropulsed fragment not seen on x-ray.

TERMINOLOGY

Abbreviations and Synonyms
• Unstable compression fracture (Fx)

Definitions
• Comminuted fracture of vertebral body (vb) extending through both superior and inferior endplates

IMAGING FINDINGS

General Features
• Best diagnostic clue: Compressed thoracic vb with fractured endplates, widened pedicles
• Location: Typically mid- or lower thoracic spine, upper lumbar spine
• Morphology: Anterior wedging of vb on lateral or sagittal views

Radiographic Findings
• Radiography
  ○ Widened pedicles on anteroposterior view
  ○ Wedge-shaped vb on lateral v view
  ○ May see malalignment
• Myelography: ± Epidural mass

CT Findings
• NECT

  ○ Soft tissue swelling surrounding vb
  ○ May see blood in canal
  ○ Stellate pattern of fractures through vb
• Bone CT
  ○ Comminuted vb on axial, reformatted views
  ○ Posterior displacement of bone into canal
  ○ Malalignment of vb and/or facets

MR Findings
• T1WI
  ○ Low signal within wedged vb
  ○ Surrounding soft tissue swelling
• T2WI
  ○ High signal within disrupted vb, surrounding soft tissue
  ○ May see cord contusion
• STIR: As with T2WI
• T2* GRE
  ○ As with T2WI
  ○ May see susceptibility changes in soft tissue from blood products
• T1 C+: Enhancing disrupted vb and nearby soft issue

Imaging Recommendations
• Thin-section axial slices with sagittal reformations, bone and soft tissue windows
• MR vital if neurologic symptoms/signs present

DDx: Thoracolumbar Fractures

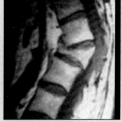

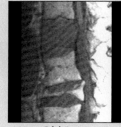

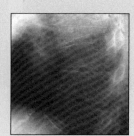

Old Compression Fx *New, Old Porotic Fxs* *Scheuermann*

BURST THORACOLUMBAR FRACTURE

Key Facts

Terminology
- Unstable compression fracture (Fx)
- Comminuted fracture of vertebral body (vb) extending through both superior and inferior endplates

Imaging Findings
- Location: Typically mid- or lower thoracic spine, upper lumbar spine
- Widened pedicles on anteroposterior view
- Wedge-shaped vb on lateral v view
- May see malalignment
- Posterior displacement of bone into canal
- Low signal within wedged vb
- High signal within disrupted vb, surrounding soft tissue
- May see cord contusion

DIFFERENTIAL DIAGNOSIS

Benign compression fracture
- No retropulsion of fragments or pedicular widening

Pathologic compression fracture
- Soft tissue mass replacing major portion of vb on MR

Scheuermann syndrome
- Three contiguous wedged vbs

PATHOLOGY

General Features
- General path comments: Typically due to vertical force trauma (jumping, landing on buttock)
- Etiology: Trauma
- Associated abnormalities
  - Epidural hematoma
  - Cord contusion

Gross Pathologic & Surgical Features
- Disrupted vb
- Column instability

Microscopic Features
- Microtrabecular disruption, hemorrhage

CLINICAL ISSUES

Presentation
- Most common signs/symptoms
  - Acute, focal pain after trauma
  - Other signs/symptoms
    - Lower extremity weakness, with or without sphincter disruption
- Clinical profile: Focal back pain after trauma with vertical force component; may have neurologic deficit or radiculopathy

Natural History & Prognosis
- Self-limited unless neurologic injury becomes permanent

Treatment
- Surgical stabilization ± canal decompression

DIAGNOSTIC CHECKLIST

Consider
- Underlying neoplasm, osteoporosis if vb Fx occurs with only minor trauma

Image Interpretation Pearls
- Widened pedicles relative to vb above is strong clue to burst vb, instability

SELECTED REFERENCES

1. Verlaan JJ et al: Operative compared with nonoperative treatment of a thoracolumbar burst fracture without neurological deficit. J Bone Joint Surg Am. 86-A(3):649-50; author reply 650-1, 2004
2. Kim NH et al: Neurologic injury and recovery in patients with burst fracture of the thoracolumbar spine. Spine. 24(3):290-3; discussion 294, 1999
3. Saifuddin A et al: The role of imaging in the diagnosis and management of thoracolumbar burst fractures: current concepts and a review of the literature. Skeletal Radiol. 25(7):603-13, 1996
4. McAffee PC et al: The unstable burst fracture. Spine 7: 365-73, 1982
5. Holdsworth FW: Fractures, dislocations, and fracture-dislocations of the spine. J Bone and Joint Surg Br. 45: 6-20, 1963

IMAGE GALLERY

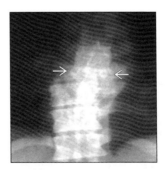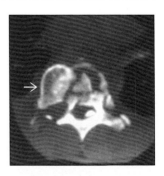

(Left) Anteroposterior radiography shows severe compression of mid-thoracic vb & translational displacement in patient who fell from third floor. Pedicles are widened (arrows) compared to vb above. (Right) Axial bone CT shows comminuted mid thoracic vb with severe dislocation from vb below (arrow), retropulsed fragment. Patient fell from third floor.

FACET-LAMINA FRACTURE, THORACIC

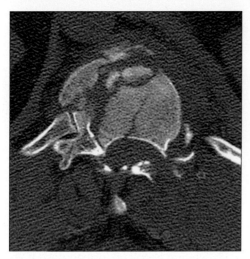

Axial bone CT shows comminuted fractures involving a thoracic vertebral body and its posterior elements.

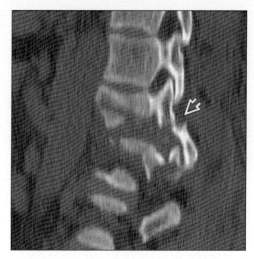

Axial bone CT with sagittal reformation shows fractures through vertebral body & lamina (arrow).

TERMINOLOGY

Abbreviations and Synonyms
- Neural (vertebral) arch fracture
- Posterior column fracture

Definitions
- Fracture through thoracic vertebral arch

IMAGING FINDINGS

General Features
- Best diagnostic clue: Cortical disruption/discontinuity through laminae, facet joints of thoracic vertebrae
- Location
  - Uncommon in upper/mid-thoracic spine
    - T1-T10 stabilized by ribs
    - 60% of thoracolumbar fractures occur between T12 and L2
    - 90% of fractures involve T11 to L4
- Size: Multiple thoracic levels involved

Radiographic Findings
- Radiography
  - Widened paraspinal line
    - Paraspinal hematoma
  - Vertebral height loss

- Posterior column usually not involved in compression fractures
  - Increased interpediculate distance
    - Vertebral arch disrupted only in severe burst fractures
  - Facet dislocation/subluxation; vertebral dislocation; increased interspinous distance
    - Indicates ruptured posterior ligamentous complex often with concomitant neural arch fractures
- Myelography
  - Limited role in acute trauma
  - Evaluation of spinal cord morphology when MRI not feasible

CT Findings
- NECT: Paraspinal hematoma on total body trauma CT
- CTA
  - Evaluation of thoracic aorta and arch vessels
    - Especially in presence of upper thoracic and rib fractures
- Bone CT
  - Widened, comminuted neural arch
  - Fracture through facet joints
  - Facet subluxation/dislocation
    - "Naked facet" sign: Partially or completely uncovered articulating processes on axial imaging
    - Locked facets: Inferior facets of vertebra above anterior to superior facets of vertebra below
  - Vertebral body comminution

DDx: Vertebral Arch Marrow Edema

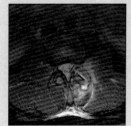

Septic Facet Arthritis

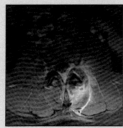

Septic Facet Arthritis

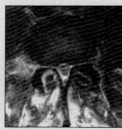

Septic Facet Arthritis

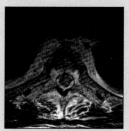

Metastases

FACET-LAMINA FRACTURE, THORACIC

II

1

61

Key Facts

Terminology
- Neural (vertebral) arch fracture

Imaging Findings
- Best diagnostic clue: Cortical disruption/discontinuity through laminae, facet joints of thoracic vertebrae
- 60% of thoracolumbar fractures occur between T12 and L2
- Widened paraspinal line
- Increased interpediculate distance
- Facet subluxation/dislocation
- Vertebral body comminution
- Vertebral subluxation/dislocation
- Hyperintense marrow edema
- Posterior soft tissue edema
- Cord edema

- Paraspinal and intraspinal hematoma
- Thin-section bone CT most effective in characterizing posterior column fractures
- MRI best for cord evaluation
- Sagittal reformation from axial CT
- Sagittal STIR or T2WI with fat suppression for posterior ligamentous injury

Top Differential Diagnoses
- Septic facet arthritis and osteomyelitis
- Pathologic fracture

Diagnostic Checklist
- Look for paraspinal soft tissue hematoma as clue to spinal fractures on CT

- Retropulsed bony fragments within spinal canal
  - Vertebral subluxation/dislocation
    - "Double body" sign: Overlapping vertebrae on axial imaging

MR Findings
- T1WI
  - Acute intraspinal hemorrhage hyperintense
  - Hypointense fracture lines
  - Separated osseous fragments
- T2WI
  - Hyperintense marrow edema
  - Posterior soft tissue edema
    - Ligamentous tear with widened interspinous gap
  - Cord edema
    - Swelling
    - Compression
    - Distraction
- STIR: Hyperintense marrow edema accentuated
- Herniated disc
- Paraspinal and intraspinal hematoma

Ultrasonographic Findings
- Disrupted supraspinous and interspinous ligaments
  - Difficult to visualize between T10 and T12 due to overlapping spinous processes

Nuclear Medicine Findings
- Bone Scan
  - Focal increased uptake of radiotracer in posterior elements
    - Limited role in acute trauma: Positive 24 hours after fracture
    - Useful in occult injuries with chronic back pain

Imaging Recommendations
- Best imaging tool
  - Thin-section bone CT most effective in characterizing posterior column fractures
  - MRI best for cord evaluation
    - Must be included in imaging workup of patients with neurologic deficit
- Protocol advice
  - Sagittal reformation from axial CT

- Demonstrates extent of canal compromise
- Shows horizontal fractures through posterior elements
  - Sagittal STIR or T2WI with fat suppression for posterior ligamentous injury

---

DIFFERENTIAL DIAGNOSIS

Septic facet arthritis and osteomyelitis
- Marrow edema in facet articular processes & adjacent laminae on MRI
- Fluid intensity within facet joint
- Surrounding soft tissue edema, enhancement and abscess

Pathologic fracture
- Underlying lytic or sclerotic lesion on CT
- Bony expansion
- Soft tissue mass
- More commonly associated with vertebral body

PATHOLOGY

General Features
- Etiology
  - Motor vehicle accidents
  - Falls
  - Sports
  - Penetrating injuries
- Epidemiology
  - Prevalence of thoracolumbar injuries
    - Approximately 6% in blunt trauma patients
- Associated abnormalities
  - Intracranial hemorrhage
  - Other fractures
  - Injury to visceral organs
  - Vascular trauma
- Anatomy
  - Neural (vertebral) arch
    - Pedicles, laminae, articular processes, base of spinous process

FACET-LAMINA FRACTURE, THORACIC

- Posterior ligamentous complex
  - Ligamentum flavum, facet joint capsule, interspinous ligament, supraspinous ligament
- Three column concept of thoracic spine
  - Anterior column: Anterior longitudinal ligament (ALL), anterior one half of vertebral body and annulus fibrosis
  - Middle column: Posterior longitudinal ligament (PLL), posterior one half of vertebral body and annulus fibrosis
  - Posterior column: Neural arch, facet joints, spinous process, transverse process, ligamentous complex
- Mechanism of injury
  - Neural arch often fractured in following mechanisms
    - Extension
    - Flexion-distraction: Horizontal fracture through vertebral body, PLL, posterior elements
    - Flexion-rotation: Ruptured posterior ligamentous complex, fractures, dislocation
    - Shear: All ligaments disrupted with listhesis in all three directions
  - Neural arch usually not involved in following mechanisms
    - Flexion: Posterior ligaments may rupture
    - Compression: Except in severe burst fractures
    - 75% of thoracolumbar fractures

Staging, Grading or Classification Criteria

- Mechanical stability of fractures depend on number of columns involved
- Stable: One or two columns injured
  - Anterior column: Compression fracture
  - Anterior and middle columns: Most burst fractures
  - Middle and posterior columns: Chance flexion-distraction injury
- Unstable: Three columns involved
  - Some burst and Chance fractures
  - All fracture dislocations

CLINICAL ISSUES

Presentation

- Most common signs/symptoms
  - Back pain
  - Neurologic deficits
  - Other signs/symptom
    - Multisystemic injury

Demographics

- Age: Mean age between 25-40 years
- Gender
  - M:F ratio
    - 9:1 in motorcycle accidents
    - 3:2 in car accidents
- Ethnicity: No race predilection

Natural History & Prognosis

- Residual neurologic deficits in 15-20% of thoracolumbar trauma
  - Complete paraplegia at time of injury rarely improves despite therapy

- Incomplete cord injury may achieve neurologic recovery

Treatment

- Initial IV high-dose steroids if cord injury present
- Conservative treatment if mechanically stable
  - One or two column injuries
  - Stabilization with bracing
  - Early mobilization
- Surgery to prevent instability and deformity, preserve neural function
  - Indicated in three column injuries, kyphosis > 20 degrees, and progressive neurologic deficits
  - Anterior and/or posterior fusion
  - Spinal decompression may be indicated

DIAGNOSTIC CHECKLIST

Consider

- Use bone windows to evaluate entire spine on total body trauma CT
  - Retro-reconstruction to thinner collimation if spinal fractures detected
    - Sagittal and coronal reformation through area of interest
  - Evaluate spinal canal for hematoma & cord compromise

Image Interpretation Pearls

- Look for paraspinal soft tissue hematoma as clue to spinal fractures on CT

SELECTED REFERENCES

1. Sheridan R et al: Reformatted visceral protocol helical computed tomographic scanning allows conventional radiographs of the thoracic and lumbar spine to be eliminated in the evaluation of blunt trauma patients. J Trauma. 55(4):665-9, 2003
2. Haba H et al: Diagnostic accuracy of magnetic resonance imaging for detecting posterior ligamentous complex injury associated with thoracic and lumbar fractures. J Neurosurg. 99(1 Suppl):20-6, 2003
3. Wintermark M et al: Thoracolumbar spine fractures in patients who have sustained severe trauma: depiction with multi-detector row CT. Radiology. 227(3):681-9, 2003
4. Sapkas GS et al: Thoracic spinal injuries: operative treatments and neurologic outcomes. Am J Orthop. 32(2):85-8, 2003
5. Moon SH et al: Feasibility of ultrasound examination in posterior ligament complex injury of thoracolumbar spine fracture. Spine. 27(19):2154-8, 2002
6. Trivedi JM: Spinal trauma: therapy--options and outcomes. Eur J Radiol. 42(2):127-34, 2002
7. Holmes JF et al: Epidemiology of thoracolumbar spine injury in blunt trauma. Acad Emerg Med. 8(9):866-72, 2001
8. Denis F: Spinal instability as defined by the three-column spine concept in acute spinal trauma. Clin Orthop. (189):65-76, 1984
9. Denis F: The three column spine and its significance in the classification of acute thoracolumbar spinal injuries. Spine. 8(8):817-31, 1983

Typical

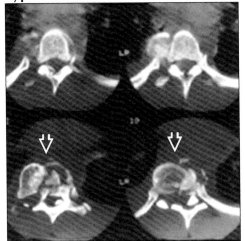
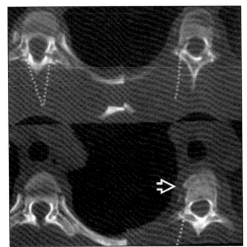

(Left) Axial NECT series shows fracture-dislocation of thoracic vertebral bodies & posterior elements. A "double body" sign is present (arrows). (Right) Axial bone CT series shows bilateral lamina & right pedicle fractures at T3. Comminuted fractures (arrow) are present at T4.

Typical

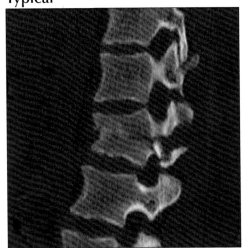
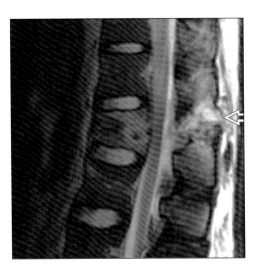

(Left) Axial bone CT with sagittal reformation shows horizontal fracture through thoracic vertebral body, pedicle, and lamina (Chance flexion-distraction injury). (Right) Sagittal T2WI MR with fat suppression shows ruptured posterior ligamentous complex (arrow). There is marrow edema with mild anterior wedging in vertebral body.

Typical

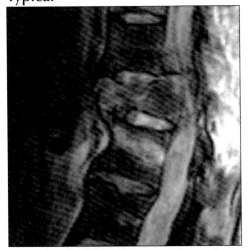
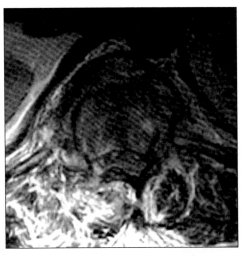

(Left) Sagittal T2WI MR with fat suppression shows comminuted vertebral fractures. Retropulsed bony fragments severely narrow central canal. (Right) Axial T2WI MR shows comminuted vertebral body & arch fractures with central canal stenosis.

CHANCE FRACTURE, THORACIC

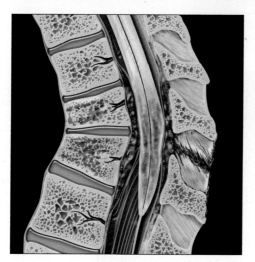

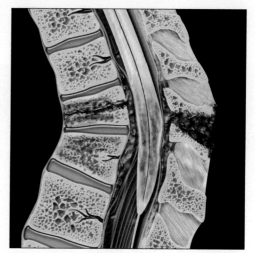

Sagittal graphic shows soft tissue Chance injury through PLL, ligamentum flavum, facet joints (not shown) & interspinous ligaments, with cord contusion.

Sagittal graphic shows bony Chance injury through vertebral body, pedicles (not shown) and spinous process with cord contusion.

TERMINOLOGY

Abbreviations and Synonyms
• Flexion-distraction injury

Definitions
• Injury involving compression of anterior column with distraction of middle and posterior columns
• Anterior column: Anterior longitudinal ligament (ALL), anterior 1/2 vertebral body & anterior anulus fibrosis
• Middle column: Posterior longitudinal ligament (PLL), posterior 1/2 vertebral body & posterior anulus fibrosis
• Posterior column: Posterior neural arch, facet joint capsular ligaments, ligamentum flavum, inter- & supra-spinous ligaments
• Spine mechanical instability: Involvement of 2 out of 3 columns
• Spine neurologic instability: Neurologic injury, especially to spinal cord
• Transitional zone: T11 to L1 vertebrae, highly susceptible to fracture

IMAGING FINDINGS

General Features
• Best diagnostic clue: Wedging anterior vertebral body + increased interspinous distance or spinous process fracture
• Location
  ○ Usually occurs at T11-L3
  ○ Occasionally at mid-thoracic spine

Radiographic Findings
• Radiography
  ○ Wedging anterior vertebral body
    ▪ Usually more than 40-50% loss of vertebral body height
  ○ Focal kyphosis
  ○ Transversely oriented posterior element fracture OR
  ○ Separation of facet joints
  ○ Increased interspinous distance
  ○ Posterior element injury may be hard to see on radiographs
  ○ Listhesis of vertebral body absent
  ○ Retropulsion of posterior vertebral body cortex absent

CT Findings
• Fracture vertebral body, often comminuted
• Transversely oriented posterior element fracture OR

DDx: Unstable Thoracic Spine Injuries

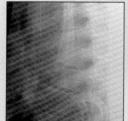

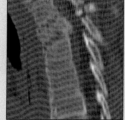

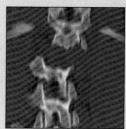

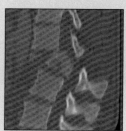

Shear Injury   *Burst Fracture*   *Distraction*   *Shear Injury*

CHANCE FRACTURE, THORACIC

Key Facts

Terminology
- Flexion-distraction injury

Imaging Findings
- Best diagnostic clue: Wedging anterior vertebral body + increased interspinous distance or spinous process fracture
- Usually occurs at T11-L3
- Occasionally at mid-thoracic spine
- Disruption of posterior longitudinal ligament (PLL), interspinous ligaments
- Anterior longitudinal ligament (ALL) usually intact
- More likely to be disrupted in midthoracic injuries than lower thoracic

Top Differential Diagnoses
- Shear injury

- Distraction injury
- Burst fracture
- Traumatic compression fracture
- Osteoporotic compression fracture

Pathology
- Less common than burst & compression fractures

Clinical Issues
- Long term kyphotic deformity common without surgical fusion

Diagnostic Checklist
- Consider Chance fracture whenever radiography shows severe compression fracture in patient with normal bone density

---

- Separation of facet joints and
- Increased interspinous distance
- Focal kyphosis

MR Findings
- T1WI: Discrete fractures as for CT or amorphous low signal in vertebral body
- T2WI
  - Disruption of posterior longitudinal ligament (PLL), interspinous ligaments
  - Anterior longitudinal ligament (ALL) usually intact
    - More likely to be disrupted in midthoracic injuries than lower thoracic
    - ALL may be stripped from vertebra inferior to the fracture
  - Vertebral edema +/- discrete fracture line
  - May see cord contusion
  - Syringomyelia may develop chronically
- STIR: Appearance similar but injuries more conspicuous compared to T2WI

Imaging Recommendations
- Best imaging tool
  - CT scan for surgical planning
  - Allows distinction between Chance, burst, compression fractures to be most reliably made
- Protocol advice
  - 1-3 mm overlapping helical multidetector CT
  - Coronal/sagittal reformations reformations essential
  - If multidetector CT performed for evaluation of chest, abdomen injuries, obviates need for dedicated spine CT
    - Reformatted images coned to spine
    - Expedites treatment of multitrauma patients

DIFFERENTIAL DIAGNOSIS

Shear injury
- Cause: Transverse shearing force
- All three columns disrupted
- Anterior, posterior or lateral listhesis of vertebra

Distraction injury
- Cause: Vertical distraction or hyperextension
- All three columns disrupted
- Distraction and/or listhesis of vertebra

Burst fracture
- Cause: Axial load force
- Retropulsion of posterior vertebral cortex
- Vertically oriented fractures of posterior elements
- Normal interspinous distance

Traumatic compression fracture
- Cause: Axial load force +/- flexion
- < 40% loss of vertebral body height
- No posterior element fracture
- Normal interspinous distance

Osteoporotic compression fracture
- Cause: Normal weight-bearing stress or minor trauma
- May have complete loss of vertebral body height
- Pedicles may be involved
- Often at multiple levels
- Osteoporosis usually apparent on radiographs

Neoplastic compression fracture
- Cause: Normal weight-bearing stress or minor trauma
- May have complete loss vertebral body height
- Trabecular destruction on CT
- Ovoid region of marrow replacement on MRI
- Tumor may be difficult to see at fracture site
- Often see marrow replacement at other levels on CT or MRI (use STIR sequence)

PATHOLOGY

General Features
- General path comments
  - All fractures more common in lower thoracic spine
    - Ribs, sternum stabilize upper thoracic spine
    - Coronally oriented thoracic facet joints resist motion more than sagittally oriented lumbar facets

CHANCE FRACTURE, THORACIC

- Usually see medial rib, transverse process fractures in mid-thoracic Chance
- Etiology
  - Motor vehicle accident or fall
  - Anterior compression, posterior distraction around fulcrum
  - Injury patterns depend on position of fulcrum
  - Classic pattern: Lap seat belt
    - Seat belt fulcrum anterior to vertebral column
    - Compression anterior column, distraction posterior column
    - May have compression failure of anterior column, or functionally intact column
  - Midthoracic Chance fractures have fulcrum in middle column
    - Posterior column tension failure
    - Anterior column compression failure
  - Anterior longitudinal ligament (ALL) is usually intact
    - In severe fractures, ALL may be stripped from vertebral body
- Epidemiology
  - Less common than burst & compression fractures
  - Decreased prevalence after institution of automobile shoulder belts
- Associated abnormalities: 65% have significant abdominal injuries (bowel most common)

Staging, Grading or Classification Criteria

- Osseous Chance fracture
  - Fracture of vertebral body,
  - Posterior element fractures: Pedicles, transverse processes, laminae, spinous process
- Ligamentous Chance injury
  - Intervertebral disc
  - Facet dislocation
  - Rupture interspinous ligaments
- Osteoligamentous Chance injury
  - Variable combination of fracture + ligament injury

CLINICAL ISSUES

Presentation

- Most common signs/symptoms
  - Back pain following high speed injury
  - Other signs/symptoms
    - Neurologic injury may be present
- Clinical profile
  - High speed motor vehicle accident
  - Fall
  - Has been reported through pedicle screw at lower level of surgical fusion

Natural History & Prognosis

- Long term kyphotic deformity common without surgical fusion
- Osseous injury
  - Acutely unstable
  - May require fixation if reduction cannot be maintained
- Osteoligamentous, ligamentous injury
  - Poor prognosis for healing unless fusion performed

Treatment

- Options, risks, complications: Osteoligamentous & ligamentous injuries usually require spinal fusion

DIAGNOSTIC CHECKLIST

Image Interpretation Pearls

- Consider Chance fracture whenever radiography shows severe compression fracture in patient with normal bone density

SELECTED REFERENCES

1. Sapkas GS et al: Thoracic spinal injuries: operative treatments and neurologic outcomes. Am J Orthop. 32(2):85-8, 2003
2. Wintermark M et al: Thoracolumbar spine fractures in patients who have sustained severe trauma: depiction with multi-detector row CT. Radiology. 227(3):681-9, 2003
3. Hsu JM et al: Thoracolumbar fracture in blunt trauma patients: guidelines for diagnosis and imaging. Injury. 34(6):426-33, 2003
4. Haba H et al: Diagnostic accuracy of magnetic resonance imaging for detecting posterior ligamentous complex injury associated with thoracic and lumbar fractures. J Neurosurg. 99(1 Suppl):20-6, 2003
5. Sheridan R et al: Reformatted visceral protocol helical computed tomographic scanning allows conventional radiographs of the thoracic and lumbar spine to be eliminated in the evaluation of blunt trauma patients. J Trauma. 55(4):665-9, 2003
6. Liu YJ et al: Flexion-distraction injury of the thoracolumbar spine. Injury. 34(12):920-3, 2003
7. Bouliane MJ et al: Instability resulting from a missed Chance fracture. Can J Surg. 44(1):61-2, 2001
8. Beaunoyer M et al: Abdominal injuries associated with thoraco-lumbar fractures after motor vehicle collision. J Pediatr Surg. 36(5):760-2, 2001
9. Levine DS et al: Chance fracture after pedicle screw fixation. A case report. Spine. 23(3):382-5; discussion 386, 1998
10. Greenwald TA et al: Pediatric seatbelt injuries: diagnosis and treatment of lumbar flexion-distraction injuries. Paraplegia. 32(11):743-51, 1994
11. Anderson PA et al: Flexion distraction and chance injuries to the thoracolumbar spine. J Orthop Trauma. 5(2):153-60, 1991
12. Reid AB et al: Pediatric Chance fractures: association with intra-abdominal injuries and seatbelt use. J Trauma. 30(4):384-91, 1990
13. Denis F: Spinal instability as defined by the three-column spine concept in acute spinal trauma. Clin Orthop. (189):65-76, 1984
14. Rogers LF: The roentgenographic appearance of transverse or chance fractures of the spine: the seat belt fracture. Am J Roentgenol Radium Ther Nucl Med. 111(4):844-9, 1971

CHANCE FRACTURE, THORACIC

IMAGE GALLERY

Typical

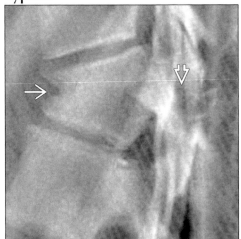 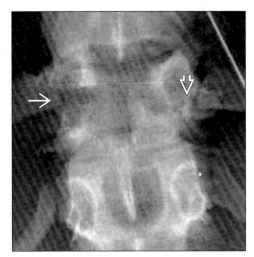

(Left) Lateral radiography shows anterior compression of T11 *(arrow)*, widely distracted fracture of pars interarticularis *(open arrow)*. *(Right)* Anteroposterior radiography shows loss of vertebral body height at T11, & horizontal fractures through right pedicle *(arrow)*, left pars interarticularis *(open arrow)*.

Variant

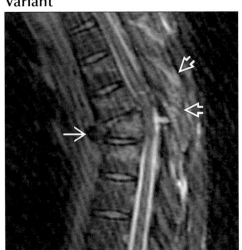 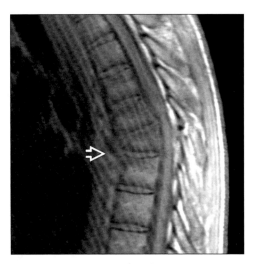

(Left) Sagittal STIR MR shows mid-thoracic Chance. There are extensive interspinous ligament injuries *(open arrows)*. ALL is partially disrupted at fracture site *(arrow)*. *(Right)* Sagittal T1WI MR shows 50% height loss and diffuse low signal intensity in T6 vertebra. ALL is amorphous *(arrow)* & attached to anterior vertebral fragment.

Typical

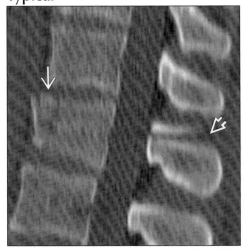 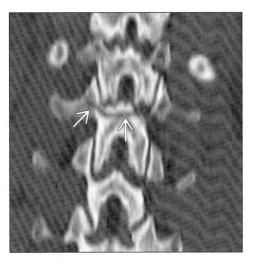

(Left) Sagittal bone CT shows comminuted fracture of anterior portion of T12 vertebral body *(arrow)*, & horizontal fracture through spinous process *(open arrow)*. *(Right)* Coronal bone CT shows T12 Chance fracture extending through right pars interarticularis & laminae *(arrows)*.

DISTRACTION FX, LOW THORACIC

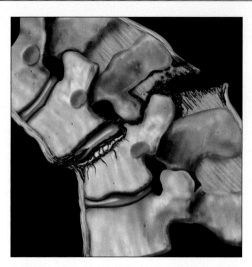

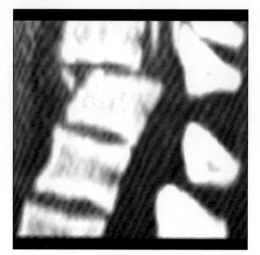

Sagittal graphic shows thoracic complex fracture with anterior compression, posterior ligament disruption with distraction.

Sagittal bone CT reformation, intrathecal contrast, shows T11-12 chance Fx with fragment off T12, anterior subluxation T11/12, no caudal flow of contrast & canal kink.

TERMINOLOGY

Abbreviations and Synonyms
- Seat belt fracture; Chance fracture; flexion-distraction fracture

Definitions
- Vertebral body (vb) wedge compression & anterior displacement of spine above fracture with facet subluxation

IMAGING FINDINGS

General Features
- Best diagnostic clue: Focal kyphosis at thoraco-lumbar junction with wedging of vb
- Location: Typically thoracolumbar junction or upper lumbar spine

Radiographic Findings
- Radiography: Anterior wedging of low thoracic or upper lumbar vb with focal kyphosis, facet and vb subluxation

CT Findings
- Bone CT
  - Fx of anterior endplate of vb , with little overlap of, or "naked" facets (typically bilateral)
  - Sagittal reformations show vb compression, anterior slippage of vb above, perched or jumped facets

MR Findings
- T2WI: High signal in interspinous ligaments, compromised canal due to subluxation

Imaging Recommendations
- Must obtain CT once plain film findings suggest fracture, or show focal kyphosis; look for intra-abdominal injury
- MR to evaluate cord injury, compression

DIFFERENTIAL DIAGNOSIS

Other vb fractures at thoracolumbar junction
- Burst fracture
- Simple compression fracture
- Scheuermann disease

PATHOLOGY

General Features
- General path comments
  - Disruption of anterior, middle and posterior columns of the spine causes mechanical instability

DDx: Other Thoracolumbar Fractures

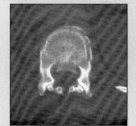

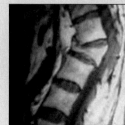

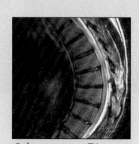

Burst Fracture　　　*Compression Fx*　　　*Scheuermann Disease*

DISTRACTION FX, LOW THORACIC

Key Facts

Terminology
- Seat belt fracture; Chance fracture; flexion-distraction fracture

Imaging Findings
- Radiography: Anterior wedging of low thoracic or upper lumbar vb with focal kyphosis, facet and vb subluxation

Pathology
- Lap belt restraint of torso during violent deceleration in car accident
- Stabilizing ligaments (anterior, posterior longitudinal, capsular, ligamenta flavum) are torn with this mechanism
- Up to 65% have intra-abdominal injury, especially bowel
- Neurological damage in 30%

- ○ Neurological compromise subsequent to the injury caused by canal compromise at time of subluxation
- Etiology
  - ○ Lap belt restraint of torso during violent deceleration in car accident
  - ○ Thoracic curvature, rib cage translate most thoracic traumatic forces into flexion component
  - ○ Considerable force needed to displace the broad, coronally overlapped thoracic facets
  - ○ Stabilizing ligaments (anterior, posterior longitudinal, capsular, ligamenta flavum) are torn with this mechanism
- Associated abnormalities
  - ○ Up to 65% have intra-abdominal injury, especially bowel
  - ○ Neurological damage in 30%

CLINICAL ISSUES

Presentation
- Most common signs/symptoms
  - ○ Back pain
  - ○ Other signs/symptoms
    - ▪ Hypotension, rigid abdomen (intra-abdominal vascular, bowel injury)
- Clinical profile: Lap-belted car accident victim

Natural History & Prognosis
- Depends on neurologic damage, extent of intra-abdominal injury
- Persistent kyphosis common

Treatment
- Correction of deformity with traction & stabilization with Harrington rod fusion
- If neurologic signs present + compression found, acute decompression

DIAGNOSTIC CHECKLIST

Consider
- Always check for associated intra-abdominal damage

Image Interpretation Pearls
- > 15 degrees of kyphosis ⇒ indicates instability

SELECTED REFERENCES

1. Voss L et al: Pediatric chance fractures from lapbelts: unique case report of three in one accident. J Orthop Trauma. 10(6):421-8, 1996
2. Sturm PF et al: Lumbar compression fractures secondary to lap-belt use in children. J Pediatr Orthop. 15(4):521-3, 1995
3. Triantafyllou SJ et al: Flexion distraction injuries of the thoracolumbar spine: a review. Orthopedics. 15(3):357-64, 1992
4. Anderson PA et al: Flexion distraction and chance injuries to the thoracolumbar spine. J Orthop Trauma. 5(2):153-60, 1991
5. LeGay DA et al: Flexion-distraction injuries of the lumbar spine and associated abdominal trauma. J Trauma. 30(4):436-44, 1990
6. Taylor GA et al: Lap-belt injuries of the lumbar spine in children: a pitfall in CT diagnosis. AJR Am J Roentgenol. 150(6):1355-8, 1988
7. Brant-Zawadzki M et al: High-resolution CT of thoracolumbar fractures. AJNR 3:69-72, 1982 Contribution of CT to management. J Comput Assist Tomogr. 3: 362-65, 1979
8. Burke DC et al: The management of thoracic and thoracolumbar injuries of the spine with neurologic involvement. J Bone and Joint Surg 58B:72-5, 1976
9. Rogers LF: The roentgenographic appearance of transverse or chance fractures of the spine: the seat belt fracture. Am J Roentgenol Radium Ther Nucl Med. 111(4):844-9, 1971

IMAGE GALLERY

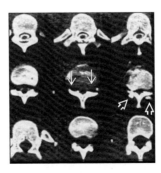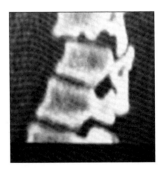

(Left) Axial bone CT consecutive slice set shows block of intrathecal contrast at T11-12 Chance Fx. Note naked facets (arrows) of T11, jumped anterior to T12 (open arrows) in paraplegic post MVA. *(Right)* Sagittal bone CT shows jumped T11-12 facets in lap-belted MVA victim with paraplegia resulting from Chance Fx. T12 showed anterior wedging on mid-sagittal view, which also showed kyphotic canal kink.

ANTERIOR COMPRESSION FRACTURE, LUMBAR

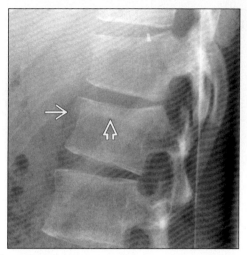

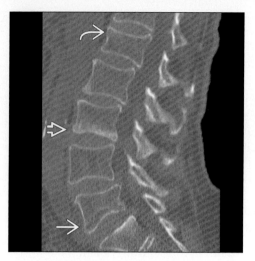

Lateral radiography shows compression fractures at T12 and L1; normal bone mineral density. Note anterior cortical break (arrow) and sclerotic trabecular compression (open arrow).

Sagittal bone CT shows multiple compression fractures with differing features: Cup-like depression L1 (curved arrow), sclerotic band L3 (open arrow), sclerotic line L5 (arrow).

TERMINOLOGY

Abbreviations and Synonyms
- Wedge fracture, wedge compression fracture

Definitions
- Fracture of anterior cortex of vertebral body without displacement of posterior wall or involvement of neural arch

IMAGING FINDINGS

General Features
- Best diagnostic clue: Loss of height of anterior portion of vertebral body
- Location
  - Trauma: Most common upper lumbar
  - Osteoporosis: Any level

Radiographic Findings
- Radiography
  - Depression of vertebral endplate, usually superior only
    - May be cup-shaped or angular
  - +/- Stepoff anterior cortex
  - Variant: Coronal fracture of vertebral body
  - Abnormalities much more prominent on lateral than anteroposterior radiography

CT Findings
- Bone CT
  - Band of sclerosis due to trabecular impaction
  - Endplate depression
  - +/- Stepoff anterior cortex
  - Rarely see extension of fracture to posterior cortex, but posterior displacement absent

MR Findings
- T1WI: Low signal intensity, band-like or triangular configuration
- T2WI
  - High signal intensity, band-like or triangular configuration
  - Obscured by fatty marrow unless fat-saturation pulse used
- STIR
  - Greatest conspicuity of edema
  - Differentiate acute from old fractures

Imaging Recommendations
- Best imaging tool
  - Earliest diagnosis by MRI
  - CT may better distinguish from pathologic fracture
- Protocol advice: Sagittal T1WI, STIR

DDx: Loss of Vertebral Body Height

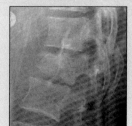
Burst Fracture

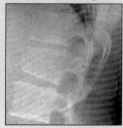
Chance Fracture

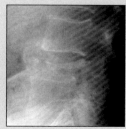
Pathologic Fracture

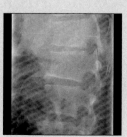
Physiologic

Key Facts

Terminology
- Fracture of anterior cortex of vertebral body without displacement of posterior wall or involvement of neural arch

Imaging Findings
- Depression of vertebral endplate, usually superior only
- Variant: Coronal fracture of vertebral body

- Earliest diagnosis by MRI
- CT may better distinguish from pathologic fracture

Top Differential Diagnoses
- Chance fracture
- Burst fracture
- Pathologic fracture due to tumor
- Physiologic wedging
- Scheuermann disease

DIFFERENTIAL DIAGNOSIS

Chance fracture
- > 40-50% wedging usually Chance fracture if bone density normal
- Posterior element fracture or widening interspinous distance

Burst fracture
- Retropulsion posterior cortex
- Widening of interpediculate distance usually present

Pathologic fracture due to tumor
- Cortical, trabecular destruction on XR or CT
- Rounded mass on MRI

Physiologic wedging
- At T12 or L1 level
- Slight wedging with normal cortical contour

Scheuermann disease
- Wedging of 3 or more adjacent vertebrae
- Schmorl nodes and/or undulation vertebral endplate

PATHOLOGY

General Features
- Etiology: Axial load with flexion
- Epidemiology
  - Bimodal
    - Young patients with motor vehicle accident, fall
    - Insufficiency fracture in osteoporotic patients
- Associated abnormalities: Other spine, pelvis, lower extremity fractures

CLINICAL ISSUES

Presentation
- Most common signs/symptoms
  - Post-traumatic back pain
  - Other signs/symptoms
    - Insidious onset back pain

Natural History & Prognosis
- Heals well in young patients
  - Increased incidence disc degeneration
- May progress in osteoporotic patients

Treatment
- Options, risks, complications
  - Conservative management
  - Vertebroplasty or kyphoplasty for deformity, chronic pain

DIAGNOSTIC CHECKLIST

Image Interpretation Pearls
- L5 compression fracture in young patient suspicious for bone tumor

SELECTED REFERENCES

1. Folman Y et al: Late outcome of nonoperative management of thoracolumbar vertebral wedge fractures. J Orthop Trauma. 17(3):190-2, 2003
2. Wintermark M et al: Thoracolumbar spine fractures in patients who have sustained severe trauma: depiction with multi-detector row CT. Radiology. 227(3):681-9, 2003
3. Lane JM et al: Minimally invasive options for the treatment of osteoporotic vertebral compression fractures. Orthop Clin North Am. 33(2):431-8, viii, 2002
4. Lindsay R et al: Risk of new vertebral fracture in the year following a fracture. JAMA. 285(3):320-3, 2001
5. Kerttula LI et al: Post-traumatic findings of the spine after earlier vertebral fracture in young patients: clinical and MRI study. Spine. 25(9):1104-8, 2000

IMAGE GALLERY

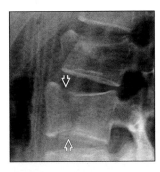 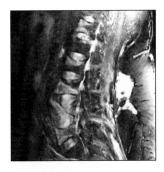

(Left) Lateral radiography shows compression fractures at L2 & L3 from skiing accident. L3 vertebral fracture is less common pattern, with vertical fracture (arrows) as well as endplate depression. *(Right)* Sagittal STIR MR shows compression fractures from T12 to L5. Configuration of edema is band-like or triangular. There is cupping of superior endplates but no discrete fracture lines.

LATERAL COMPRESSION FRACTURE, LUMBAR

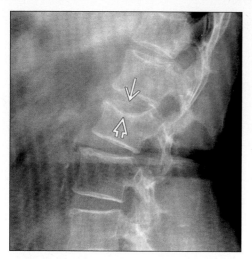

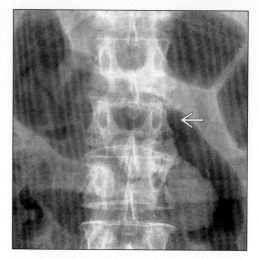

Lateral radiography shows L2 lateral compression fracture. The lateral nature is evident by one normal superior end-plate (arrow) & one abnormal superior endplate (open arrow).

Anteroposterior radiography confirms left lateral compression fracture of L2 (arrow).

TERMINOLOGY

Abbreviations and Synonyms
- Vertebral compression fracture (VCF)

Definitions
- Lumbar vertebral body fracture (Fx) with ↓ vertebral height, predominantly lateral

IMAGING FINDINGS

General Features
- Best diagnostic clue: Lateral wedge deformity of affected lumbar spine (LS) vertebral body
- Location: 50-65% VCF are between T12 & L2
- Size: Deformity graded in degrees of body height loss
- Morphology
  - Prominent lateral wedge deformity
  - Partial or no loss of posterior vertebral body height nor subluxation

Radiographic Findings
- Radiography
  - Entire spinal evaluation important as up to 20% of all VCF are multiple
  - AP: Lateral predominance of VCF deformity
  - Lateral: ↓ Vertebral body height; kyphosis

  - Intravertebral clefts seen as intraosseous vacuum phenomenon

CT Findings
- Bone CT
  - Arc of irregular bone fragments circumferentially from vertebral body
  - Intact posterior body wall, no fragment retropulsion

MR Findings
- T1WI
  - Acute: Hypointense marrow edema
  - Chronic: Marrow signal normalizes with time
- STIR
  - Acute: STIR best visualizes hyperintense marrow edema which CAN extend into pedicles
  - Acute: May reveal fluid filled intravertebral cleft = "fluid sign"
    - Detected in slightly over 25% VCF
    - More indicative of acute benign osteoporotic VCF
    - Most often adjacent to site of end-plate Fx
  - Chronic: Marrow signal normalizes with time
- DWI
  - Controversial: May be helpful for differentiating acute benign osteoporotic from pathologic VCF
    - T2 shine-through confuses pattern
  - ADC mapping improves distinction between benign, malignant lesions
    - Mean ADC for benign 68% > than for metastases

DDx: Non-Lateral Compression Lumbar Deformity

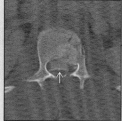

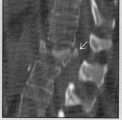

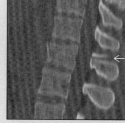

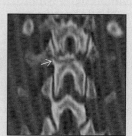

Burst Fracture   *Burst Fracture*   *Chance Fracture*   *Chance Fracture*

Key Facts

Terminology
- Lumbar vertebral body Fx with ↓ vertebral height, predominantly lateral

Imaging Findings
- Best diagnostic clue: Lateral wedge deformity of affected lumbar spine (LS) vertebral body
- Location: 50-65% VCF are between T12 & L2
- Arc of irregular bone fragments circumferentially from vertebral body
- Acute: STIR best visualizes hyperintense marrow edema which CAN extend into pedicles
- CT > > radiography

Top Differential Diagnoses
- Burst Fx
- Chance Fx ("seat belt Fx")

Pathology
- Lateral VCF of thoracolumbar spine is correlated with seat belt injury
- 11% of VCF are lateral
- LS VCF is most common spine fracture, comprising nearly 50% of all spine fractures

Clinical Issues
- Many experience severe & prolonged pain that can markedly alter activities of daily living
- Main VCF risk factor is osteoporosis
- Early intervention with vertebroplasty may be indicated given low complication rates

Diagnostic Checklist
- VCF in elderly patient with unrelenting back pain
- Up to 20% of VCF are multiple → screen entire spine!

- May ↑ specificity of MR for acute VCF
- T1 C+
  ○ Both benign, malignant processes may enhance
  ○ Paraspinal epidural enhancing tissue suggests malignant pathology
- MRS: ¹H MRS measurements of vertebral body percent fat fraction significantly ↑ in weakened bone compared with controls

Nuclear Medicine Findings
- Bone Scan: ↑ Activity on bone scan highly predictive of positive outcome after vertebroplasty
- Fluorine-18 deoxyglucose (FDG) PET
  ○ No ↑ uptake in acute vertebral fractures originating from osteoporosis or preclinical osteoporosis
  ○ High FDG uptake is characteristic for malignant & inflammatory processes
  ○ FDG-PET may have potential value differentiating osteoporotic from pathologic VCF

Imaging Recommendations
- Best imaging tool
  ○ CT > > radiography
  ○ MRI for neurologic deficit(s)
- Protocol advice
  ○ CT: Sagittal & coronal reformats
  ○ MRI: STIR & fat-saturation T1 C+

DIFFERENTIAL DIAGNOSIS

Burst Fx
- Abnormal posterior vertebral body wall
- Fragment retropulsion into spinal canal

Chance Fx ("seat belt Fx")
- Horizontal splitting of spinous process, laminae, pedicles, superior vertebral body
- Disc and facet distraction with ligament disruption

PATHOLOGY

General Features
- General path comments
  ○ VCF occur when combined axial & bending loads exceed the strength of the vertebral body
  ○ Lateral VCF of thoracolumbar spine is correlated with seat belt injury
- Genetics
  ○ Inherited bone disorders (i.e., NF1, Gaucher)
  ○ Vitamin D receptor polymorphism may influence bone mineral density & osteoporotic VCF
- Etiology
  ○ Typically result of flexion, axial forces, or both
  ○ Trauma, osteopenia, metabolic bone disease, genetic disorders, neoplasm (primary or metastatic)
    ▪ Benign vertebral lesions occur in approximately 1/3 of cancer patients
    ▪ Metastatic vertebral lesions account for 39% of bony mets in patients with primary neoplasms
    ▪ Myeloma appears similar to benign VCF
  ○ Seat belt injury
    ▪ Result of shoulder-lap belt assemblies
    ▪ Results in anterolateral wedge compression of thoracolumbar vertebra
    ▪ Lateral compression occurs on side opposite restrained shoulder
    ▪ Posterior elements may be disrupted contralateral to anterolateral body compression
    ▪ Postulated mechanism, referred to as "roll-out phenomenon" = flexion & rotation about axis of shoulder strap
- Epidemiology
  ○ 11% of VCF are lateral
  ○ LS VCF is most common spine fracture, comprising nearly 50% of all spine fractures
  ○ 16% of postmenopausal women suffer one or more VCF during their lifetime
  ○ Osteoporosis is most common cause of VCF in US
  ○ Prevalence of radiographic VCF has been reported as high as 26% in women ≥ 50 yrs

LATERAL COMPRESSION FRACTURE, LUMBAR

- ○ Frequency of radiographic evidence of VCF increases from 500/100,000 person years (py) in women aged 50-54 yrs to 2,960/100,000 py in women > 85 yrs
- ○ In the US, VCF account for 150,000 hospital admissions, 161,000 physician office visits, & > 5 million restricted activity days annually
- Associated abnormalities
  - ○ Immobility makes more susceptible to pneumonia, deep vein thrombosis, & pulmonary embolism
  - ○ Patients with osteoporotic VCF have significantly lower vital capacity and forced expiratory volume

Microscopic Features

- Inflammatory phase: Hematoma, osteocytic death, intense inflammatory response
- Reparative phase: Hematoma organized by fibrovascular tissue, callus forms on collagen matrix
- Remodeling phase: Resorption of unnecessary callus, trabecular proliferation along lines of stress

CLINICAL ISSUES

Presentation

- Many experience severe & prolonged pain that can markedly alter activities of daily living
  - ○ 84% of VCF are painful, on average lasting 4-6 wks
  - ○ Subgroup of patients has subacute or chronic pain that is refractory to conservative therapy
- Numbness, tingling, & weakness may indicate nerve compression
- May be asymptomatic

Demographics

- Age
  - ○ Osteoporotic: ↑ Frequency with age
  - ○ Traumatic: Usually younger patient population
- Gender
  - ○ M:F ≈ 2:1
  - ○ Yet male incidence is high contradicting common misconception that osteoporosis is women's health problem

Natural History & Prognosis

- Main VCF risk factor is osteoporosis
  - ○ Severity of osteoporosis is worsened by smoking, physical inactivity, use of prednisone & other medications, poor nutrition
  - ○ In males all above risk factors apply as well as low testosterone levels
- Women with VCF have higher mortality rates as compared to age-matched control subjects without Fx
  - ○ Women with 1 or more VCF have a 1.23-fold greater age-adjusted mortality rate
  - ○ Mortality rises as the number of VCF increases; women with ≥ 5 Fxs have a > twofold increase

Treatment

- Conservative therapy usually consists of analgesic use, rest, & external bracing
  - ○ Immobilization accelerates bone loss, which may contribute to further VCF
- Early intervention with vertebroplasty may be indicated given low complication rates

- ○ Complications reported include transitory fever, transient worsening of pain, radiculopathy, rib Fx, cement pulmonary embolism, infection, & spinal cord compression
- ○ With osteoporotic VCF, complication rate is 1-2%
- ○ With malignant tumors, the complication rate ↑ 2° to cement leakage resulting from vertebral body destruction caused by the malignant process
- ○ MR is preferred for guiding vertebroplasty as it offers anatomic detail and concurrent information about other abnormalities (i.e., spinal stenosis)
- ○ If tumor is suspected, it may be appropriate to precede vertebroplasty with biopsy after the cannula is placed but before cement is injected
  - ▪ Vertebroplasty cement presence does not hinder the therapeutic result of subsequent or concomitant radiation or chemotherapy
- Surgery when neurologic dysfunction and/or instability occurs as a result of VCF
- Vertebroplasty
  - ○ Direct injection of polymethylmethacrylate into collapsed body
  - ○ Alleviates pain & prevents further collapse
    - ▪ Achieves 90% efficacy in pain relief
  - ○ Highly efficacious regardless of Fx age, even with severe deformity (> 70%)
  - ○ May see opacifying intravertebral clefts
  - ○ Antecedent venography does not improve effectiveness or safety
- Kyphoplasty = vertebroplasty variation in which an inflatable balloon is first placed inside compressed vertebral body into which cement is instilled

DIAGNOSTIC CHECKLIST

Consider

- VCF in elderly patient with unrelenting back pain

Image Interpretation Pearls

- Up to 20% of VCF are multiple → screen entire spine!

SELECTED REFERENCES

1. Jung HS et al: Discrimination of metastatic from acute osteoporotic compression spinal fractures with MR imaging. Radiographics. 23(1):179-87, 2003
2. Schmitz A et al: FDG-PET findings of vertebral compression fractures in osteoporosis: preliminary results. Osteoporos Int. 13(9):755-61, 2002
3. Baur A et al: Acute osteoporotic and neoplastic vertebral compression fractures: fluid sign at MR imaging. Radiology. 225(3):730-5, 2002
4. Herneth AM et al: Vertebral metastases: assessment with ADC. Radiology. 225(3):889-94, 2002
5. Kaufmann TJ et al: Age of fracture and clinical outcomes of percutaneous vertebroplasty. AJNR Am J Neuroradiol. 22(10):1860-3, 2001
6. Miniaci A et al: Anterolateral compression fracture of the thoracolumbar spine. A seat belt injury. Clin Orthop. (240):153-6, 1989

Typical

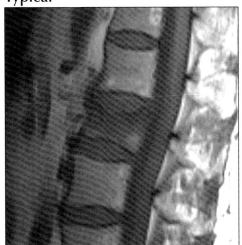 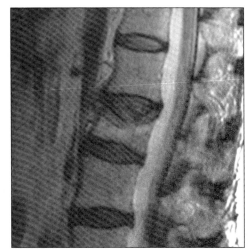

(Left) Sagittal T1WI MR shows deformity as well as marrow hypointensity from edema following lateral L2 compression fracture. Note intact posterior vertebral body cortex. *(Right)* Sagittal T2WI MR shows deformity as well as mild marrow hyperintensity from edema following lateral L2 compression fracture. Note intact posterior vertebral body cortex.

Typical

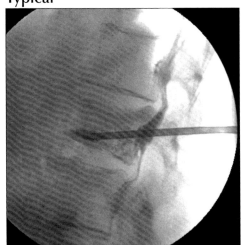 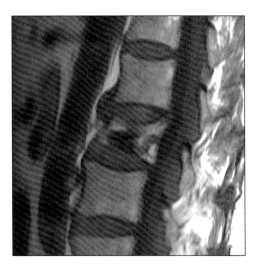

(Left) Lateral spot radiography during vertebroplasty demonstrates transpedicular cannula placement & early methyl-methacrylate instillation (prior intrathecal contrast administration). *(Right)* Sagittal T1WI MR following vertebroplasty shows hypointense methyl-methacrylate and slight superior end-plate elevation.

Typical

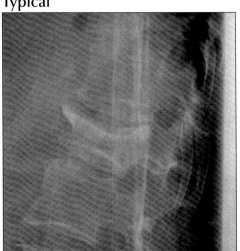 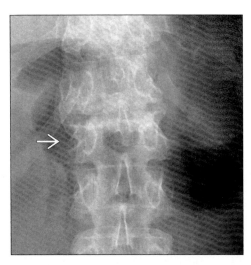

(Left) Lateral radiography shows L1 lateral compression Fx. *(Right)* Anteroposterior radiography confirms right lateral compression fracture of L1 (arrow).

BURST FRACTURE, LUMBAR

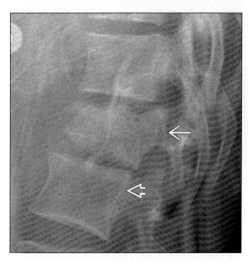

Lateral radiography shows burst fracture of L1 with retropulsed fragment (arrow) in spinal canal. White arrow shows normal posterior cortex of L2 body for comparison.

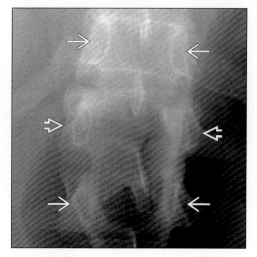

Anteroposterior radiography shows widened L1 interpediculate distance (open arrows) due to burst fracture. Compare normal interpediculate distance at levels above & below (arrows).

TERMINOLOGY

Definitions
- Vertebral fracture due to axial load, involving all 3 columns
- Anterior column: Anterior longitudinal ligament, anterior 1/2 vertebral body & anterior anulus fibrosis
- Middle column: Posterior longitudinal ligament, posterior 1/2 vertebral body & posterior anulus fibrosis
- Posterior column: Posterior neural arch, facet joint capsulare ligaments, ligamentum flavum, inter- & supra-spinous ligaments
- Spine mechanical instability: Involvement of 2 of 3 columns
- Spine neurologic instability: Neurologic injury, especially to spinal cord
- Transition zone: T11 to L1 vertebrae; highly susceptible to injury, including burst fracture

IMAGING FINDINGS

General Features
- Best diagnostic clue: Retropulsion of posterior vertebral body cortex
- Location
  - Most common upper lumbar

  - 60% of thoracolumbar spine injuries of all types occur between T11 and L1
  - Thoracic spine relatively stabilized by ribs/sternum, coronal alignment of facet joints
- Morphology: May involve superior endplate, inferior endplate or both

Radiographic Findings
- Radiography
  - Compression of the vertebral body on anteroposterior, lateral radiography
    - Usually anterior portion of body compressed more than posterior
  - Posterior displacement of posterior vertebral body cortex on lateral radiography
    - Usually superior portion of body is displaced
    - Normally, see concave contour of vertebral body posteriorly
    - Entire posterior vertebral body cortex should be seen on lateral radiography
    - Nutrient groove in central portion of posterior cortex
  - Widening interpediculate distance on anteroposterior radiography
    - Axial load fractures pedicles, displaces them laterally
    - Pedicle displacement absent in mild burst fractures
  - Posterior element fractures often not visible

DDx: Lumbar Fractures

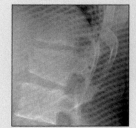
Chance

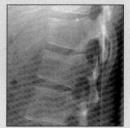
Compression

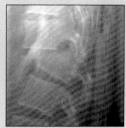
Fracture-Dislocation

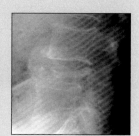
Pathologic

BURST FRACTURE, LUMBAR

Key Facts

Terminology
- Vertebral fracture due to axial load, involving all 3 columns

Imaging Findings
- Most common upper lumbar
- Morphology: May involve superior endplate, inferior endplate or both
- Compression of the vertebral body on anteroposterior, lateral radiography
- Posterior displacement of posterior vertebral body cortex on lateral radiography
- Widening interpediculate distance on anteroposterior radiography
- Multidetector abdomen CT scan obviates need for dedicated spine CT

Top Differential Diagnoses
- Compression fracture
- Chance fracture
- Pathologic fracture due to tumor
- Fracture-dislocation

Pathology
- Degree of neurologic injury with lumbar burst highly dependent on position of conus
- Lower lumbar burst fractures may have minimal or no neurologic signs

Diagnostic Checklist
- High association with lower extremity & pelvis fractures

    - Vertically oriented
  o May have compression fractures at adjacent levels

CT Findings
- Bone CT
  o Retropulsed bone fragments in spinal canal
    - Percent narrowing of spinal canal should be reported
  o Vertically oriented posterior element fractures
  o Widening interpediculate distance
- Can be diagnosed on routine CT scan of abdomen in multitrauma patients
- Multidetector abdomen CT scan obviates need for dedicated spine CT
  o Expedites care of patients with multiple injuries already undergoing abdomen CT
  o Thin slices can be fused for evaluation of abdomen, unfused for spine
  o Small field of view coronal and sagittal images reformatted from original data set

MR Findings
- T1WI: Visualization of retropulsed fragments
- T2WI
  o Evaluate position of conus relative to fracture
  o Evaluate cord contusion
- STIR: Cord abnormalities more conspicuous
- Posterior element fractures often difficult to see on all sequences

Imaging Recommendations
- Best imaging tool: CT for surgical planning
- Protocol advice
  o 1-3 mm overlapping helical images
  o Coronal, sagittal reformations

DIFFERENTIAL DIAGNOSIS

Compression fracture
- Posterior vertebral body cortex intact
- Posterior element fractures absent
- Less than 40-50% loss of height in patients with normal bone density

Chance fracture
- Anterior vertebral body compression
- Horizontal fractures posterior elements OR
- Separation of spinous processes

Pathologic fracture due to tumor
- More commonly compression fracture, but sometimes burst fracture
- Mass may be obscured by fracture and hematoma
- CT may show trabecular, cortical destruction
- MR may show tumor at other levels

Fracture-dislocation
- Due to shear injury or distraction
- Vertebra displaced relative to vertebra above or below

PATHOLOGY

General Features
- General path comments
  o Position of vertebral fragments in canal on CT not true measure of displacement at time of injury
    - Fragments tend to move forward after initial posterior excursion
  o Posterior element fracture may be greenstick fracture in adolescents
  o Degree of neurologic injury with lumbar burst highly dependent on position of conus
  o Lower lumbar burst fractures may have minimal or no neurologic signs
- Etiology
  o Most commonly due to falls from height
  o Twisting or lateral flexion component may be present
- Epidemiology
  o Construction workers
  o Mountain climbers
  o Sky divers
  o Skiers
  o Sometimes osteoporotic insufficiency fracture
  o Occasionally pathologic fracture due to tumor
- Associated abnormalities

BURST FRACTURE, LUMBAR

○ Dural laceration
○ Other spine fractures
  ■ Contiguous or noncontiguous levels
○ Pelvic fractures
○ Lower extremity fractures
  ■ Calcaneus
  ■ Tibial plateau
  ■ Tibial plafond

Staging, Grading or Classification Criteria
• Denis classification
  ○ Type A: Fracture of both superior and inferior endplates
    ■ Primarily seen in lower lumbar region
  ○ Type B: Fracture of superior endplate
    ■ Most common type
    ■ Primarily seen at thoracolumbar junction
  ○ Type C: Fracture of inferior endplate
  ○ Type D: Burst plus malrotation due to rotary force as well as axial load
  ○ Type E: Burst plus lateral compression due to lateral flexion as well as axial load

CLINICAL ISSUES

Presentation
• Most common signs/symptoms
  ○ Traumatic back pain
  ○ Other signs/symptoms
    ■ Lower extremity neurologic deficits

Natural History & Prognosis
• Fragments in spinal canal remodel over time
  ○ Canal narrowing decreases significantly in size within one year following injury
  ○ Best seen on CT scan, but can be evaluated on lateral radiography

Treatment
• Options, risks, complications
  ○ Systemic steroids generally given at time of injury
  ○ Conservative management for
    ■ Mild fractures
    ■ Lower lumbar fractures
    ■ Long term outcomes similar to fusion in neurologically intact patients
  ○ Laminectomy and posterior fusion used if there is
    ■ Neurologic dysfunction
    ■ Greater than 20-30 degree kyphosis
    ■ Subluxation of facet joints
    ■ Greater than 50% loss of vertebral body height

DIAGNOSTIC CHECKLIST

Consider
• High association with lower extremity & pelvis fractures

Image Interpretation Pearls
• Plain radiographic diagnosis possible in most cases
  ○ Look carefully at lateral radiograph for retropulsed fragments

○ Widening of interpediculate distance on anteroposterior view may be subtle or absent

SELECTED REFERENCES

1. Chipman JG et al: Early surgery for thoracolumbar spine injuries decreases complications. J Trauma. 56(1):52-7, 2004
2. Wilcox RK et al: A dynamic study of thoracolumbar burst fractures. J Bone Joint Surg Am. 85-A(11):2184-9, 2003
3. Sheridan R et al: Reformatted visceral protocol helical computed tomographic scanning allows conventional radiographs of the thoracic and lumbar spine to be eliminated in the evaluation of blunt trauma patients. J Trauma. 55(4):665-9, 2003
4. Mulkern RV et al: In re: characterization of benign and metastatic vertebral compression fractures with quantitative diffusion MR imaging. AJNR Am J Neuroradiol. 24(7):1489-90; author reply 1490-1, 2003
5. Haba H et al: Diagnostic accuracy of magnetic resonance imaging for detecting posterior ligamentous complex injury associated with thoracic and lumbar fractures. J Neurosurg. 99(1 Suppl):20-6, 2003
6. Leferink VJ et al: Burst fractures of the thoracolumbar spine: changes of the spinal canal during operative treatment and follow-up. Eur Spine J. 12(3):255-60, 2003
7. Wood K et al: Operative compared with nonoperative treatment of a thoracolumbar burst fracture without neurological deficit. A prospective, randomized study. J Bone Joint Surg Am. 85-A(5):773-81, 2003
8. Wintermark M et al: Thoracolumbar spine fractures in patients who have sustained severe trauma: depiction with multi-detector row CT. Radiology. 227(3):681-9, 2003
9. Nguyen HV et al: Osteoporotic vertebral burst fractures with neurologic compromise. J Spinal Disord Tech. 16(1):10-9, 2003
10. Parisini P et al: Treatment of spinal fractures in children and adolescents: long-term results in 44 patients. Spine. 27(18):1989-94, 2002
11. McLain RF et al: Segmental instrumentation for thoracic and thoracolumbar fractures: prospective analysis of construct survival and five-year follow-up. Spine J. 1(5):310-23, 2001
12. Aydinli U et al: Dural tears in lumbar burst fractures with greenstick lamina fractures. Spine. 26(18):E410-5, 2001
13. Lalonde F et al: An analysis of burst fractures of the spine in adolescents. Am J Orthop. 30(2):115-20, 2001
14. Dai LY: Remodeling of the spinal canal after thoracolumbar burst fractures. Clin Orthop. (382):119-23, 2001
15. Kuklo TR et al: Measurement of thoracic and lumbar fracture kyphosis: evaluation of intraobserver, interobserver, and technique variability. Spine. 26(1):61-5; discussion 66, 2001
16. Carl AL et al: Anterior dural laceration caused by thoracolumbar and lumbar burst fractures. J Spinal Disord. 13(5):399-403, 2000

BURST FRACTURE, LUMBAR

IMAGE GALLERY

Typical

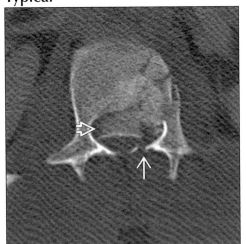
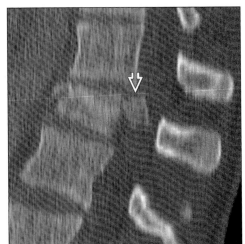

(Left) Axial bone CT shows left laminar fracture (arrow) and retropulsed fragment (open arrow) from vertebral body filling 90% of spinal canal. *(Right)* Sagittal bone CT shows L1 burst fracture with superior endplate depression and large retropulsed fragment (arrow) from superior vertebral body. There is about 50% loss of vertebral body height.

Typical

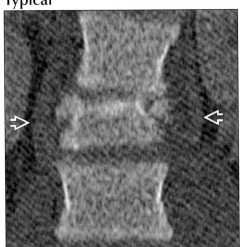
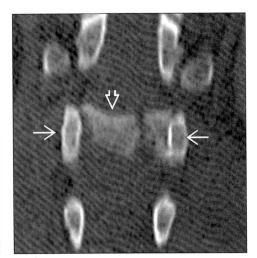

(Left) Coronal bone CT shows comminution of vertebral body & loss of height. Paraspinous hematoma (arrows) is evident. *(Right)* Coronal bone CT shows widened interpediculate distance (arrows) at level of burst fracture. Large fragments of bone are present in spinal canal (open arrow).

Variant

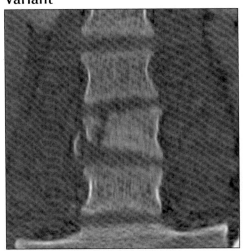
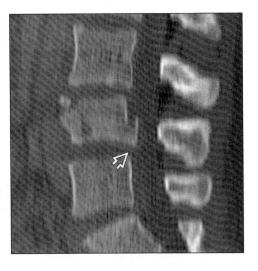

(Left) Coronal bone CT shows burst fracture of L4 with right lateral compression due to axial load plus lateral flexion. Fracture extends to both superior and inferior vertebral endplates. *(Right)* Sagittal bone CT shows L4 burst fracture with superior and inferior endplate involvement and retropulsion of inferior portion of posterior cortex (arrow).

FACET-POSTERIOR FRACTURE, LUMBAR

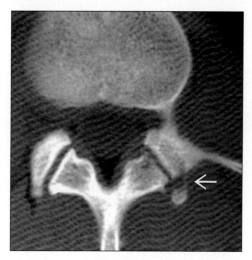

Axial bone CT shows an L3 superior facet fracture (arrow) in a young hockey player who experienced sudden onset low back pain while playing (Courtesy William O. Shaffer, MD).

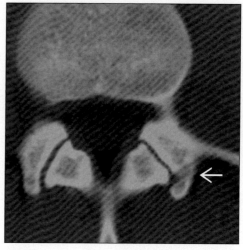

Axial bone CT obtained two months later demonstrates interval healing (arrow) following brace therapy and abstaining from play (Courtesy William O. Shaffer, MD).

TERMINOLOGY

Definitions
- Fracture (Fx) involving lumbar facet(s)

IMAGING FINDINGS

General Features
- Best diagnostic clue: Lumbar facet Fx line +/- facet joint distraction

Radiographic Findings
- Radiography
  - Often negative, may see joint space widening
  - Oblique radiographs best for facet subluxation

CT Findings
- Bone CT: Traumatic facet fracture dislocation
  - Three major patterns
    - Anterior vertebral body subluxation with anteriorly locked facets
    - Lateral vertebral body subluxation with laterally locked facets
    - Acute kyphosis with little vertebral body subluxation but superiorly dislocated facets
  - Best seen on reformated images
- Bone CT: Post-operative spine
  - Axial

- Often reveal no abnormality other than slight widening of the joint on the affected side
- Lamina uncommonly affected
  - Sagittal reformat: Lucent defect similar to pars interarticularis Fx
  - Coronal reformat: Best shows inferior facet Fx at a different location than pars interarticularis Fx
- Bone CT: Back pain in athletes
  - L5 facet Fx
  - Type II sacral Fx

MR Findings
- STIR
  - Hyperintense facet fluid
    - Sign of capsular disruption
    - With subluxation suggests facet Fx
  - Hyperintensity within facet capsular ligaments
  - Hyperintense edema along erector spinal muscle adjacent to affected facet

Nuclear Medicine Findings
- Bone Scan: ↑ Uptake at involved facet

Other Modality Findings
- Normal facet axial anatomy
  - Joint has a mushroom appearance
  - "Cap" = superior articular facet
  - "Stem" = inferior articular facet & spinal lamina
- Normal facet sagittal anatomy

DDx: Lumbar Facet Fracture Mimic

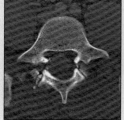

Bilateral Pars Fx

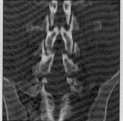

Bilateral Pars Fx

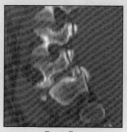

Pars Fx

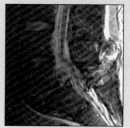

Pars Fx

FACET-POSTERIOR FRACTURE, LUMBAR

Key Facts

Terminology
- Fracture (Fx) involving lumbar facet(s)

Imaging Findings
- Best diagnostic clue: Lumbar facet Fx line +/- facet joint distraction
- Best imaging tool: Bone CT
- Protocol advice: Sagittal + coronal reformats

Clinical Issues
- Most common signs/symptoms: Most common symptom: Low back pain
- Majority heal with conservative therapy

Diagnostic Checklist
- Consider facet Fx in athlete experiencing acute pain after an inciting event

---

- ○ More pointed superior articular facet above
- ○ Somewhat rounded inferior articular facet below
- ○ Pars interarticularis lies between

Imaging Recommendations
- Best imaging tool: Bone CT
- Protocol advice: Sagittal + coronal reformats

DIFFERENTIAL DIAGNOSIS

Pars interarticularis Fx (spondylolysis)
- Doesn't involve facets
- "Double facet" sign on axial imaging

PATHOLOGY

General Features
- Etiology
  - ○ Trauma: Most often MVA
  - ○ Athletes: When athlete's torso is in rotation, facets become loaded & additional external force (e.g., checking in hockey) can cause facet Fx
  - ○ Post-Op
    - Facetectomy & pars excision destabilize & add to pre-operative risk factors for instability
    - Thinning of the inferior facet at location of facetectomy predisposes it to stress Fx
- Associated abnormalities: Type II sacral Fx have L5/S1 facet Fx in 20%
- Anatomy of lumbar facet (aka zygapophyseal joint)
  - ○ Diarthrodial synovial joint between superior, inferior facets of adjacent vertebrae
  - ○ Joint space = 2-4 mm (cartilage + joint space)

CLINICAL ISSUES

Presentation
- Most common signs/symptoms: Most common symptom: Low back pain
- Clinical profile
  - ○ Athlete: Acute pain after inciting event, often hidden out of desire to "keep playing"
  - ○ Post-Op: New pain pattern, local tenderness, pain on unusual movements, relief with recumbency suggest facet Fx versus recurrent disk herniation

Natural History & Prognosis
- Majority heal with conservative therapy

Treatment
- Conservative therapy → bracing & pain control
  - ○ Utilize follow-up CT to evaluate healing
- Spinal fusion is standard treatment for instability

DIAGNOSTIC CHECKLIST

Consider
- Consider facet Fx in athlete experiencing acute pain after an inciting event

SELECTED REFERENCES

1. Kaya RA, Aydin Y. Modified transpedicular approach for the surgical treatment of severe thoracolumbar or lumbar burst fractures. Spine J. 4(2):208-17, 2004
2. Tsirikos AI, Saifuddin A, Noordeen MH, Tucker SK. Traumatic lumbosacral dislocation: report of two cases. Spine. 14;29(8):E164-8, 2004
3. Mori K, Hukuda S, Katsuura A, Saruhashi Y, Asajima S. Traumatic bilateral locked facet at L4-5: report of a case associated with incorrect use of a three-point seatbelt. Eur Spine J. 11(6):602-5, 2002
4. Malberg MI. A new system of classification for spinal injuries. Spine J. 1(1):18-25, 2001
5. Mann DC et al: Unusual causes of back pain in athletes. J Spinal Disord. 4(3):337-43, 1991
6. Hopp E et al: Postdecompression lumbar instability. Clin Orthop. 227:143-51, 1988
7. Manaster BJ et al: CT patterns of facet fracture dislocations in the thoracolumbar region. AJR Am J Roentgenol. 148(2):335-40, 1987

IMAGE GALLERY

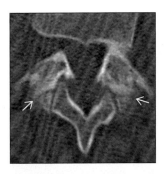 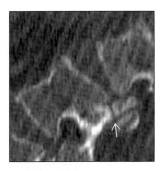

(Left) Axial bone CT demonstrates bilateral superior lumbar facet fractures (arrows). *(Right)* Sagittal bone CT reformat shows lumbar superior facet fracture (arrow).

SACRAL TRAUMATIC FRACTURE

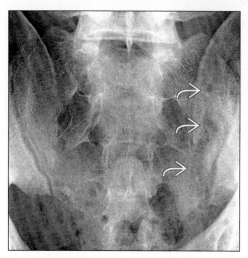 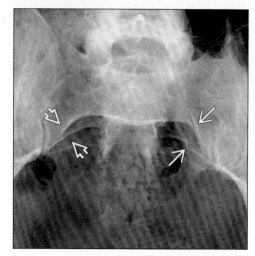

Anteroposterior radiography shows vertically oriented fracture through zone 1 of the sacrum (arrows). Mechanism of injury was anteroposterior force or open-book.

Anteroposterior radiography shows zone 2 fracture due to lateral compression. Note angular deformity of arcuate lines on left (arrows) compared to normal right side (open arrows).

TERMINOLOGY

Definitions
- Pelvic ring: Pelvic bones form hollow, obliquely horizontal ring-shaped structure around pelvic organs
- Pelvic ring disruption: Fractures and/or ligament injuries through anterior and posterior portions of pelvis
  - Posterior ring fracture: Behind ischial spine; usually sacrum or sacroiliac joint
  - Anterior ring fracture: Anterior to ischial spine, usually pubic rami

IMAGING FINDINGS

General Features
- Best diagnostic clue: Disruption of sacral arcuate lines
- Location
  - 95% vertical or oblique
  - 5% horizontal
- Morphology
  - Pelvic ring disruption: Vertically or obliquely oriented fracture
  - Isolated sacral fracture: Horizontally oriented fracture

Radiographic Findings
- Radiography
  - Difficult to see on routine radiography
    - Up to 60% reportedly missed prior to institution of CT scanning
  - Disruption of arcuate line of neural foramina
    - Normally see smooth curve above neural foramen
    - Angular contour of arcuate line indicates fracture
  - Lateral compression causes decreased width of sacrum on affected side
  - Displacement of fracture line uncommonly visible
  - Lateral radiography shows angular deformity of transverse fractures
  - Anteroposterior radiography
    - Inlet view of pelvis: 25 degree caudad angulation
    - Outlet view of pelvis: 25 degree cephalad angulation
    - Ferguson view sacrum: 15 degree cephalad angulation
  - Fracture seen best on outlet, Ferguson views
  - L5 transverse process fracture raises suspicion for sacral fracture
  - Children may have "greenstick" fracture of sacrum
  - Sacro-coccygeal junction fractures
    - Angular deformity at junction (but may be normal variant in this location)
    - Transverse fracture line on Ferguson view

DDx: Sacral Traumatic Fracture

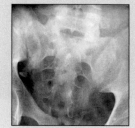 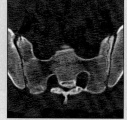 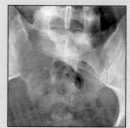 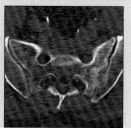

Sacroiliac Dislocation *Normal Ossification* *Tumor* *Insufficiency*

SACRAL TRAUMATIC FRACTURE

Key Facts

Imaging Findings
- Best diagnostic clue: Disruption of sacral arcuate lines
- Pelvic ring disruption: Vertically or obliquely oriented fracture
- Isolated sacral fracture: Horizontally oriented fracture
- Difficult to see on routine radiography
- Best imaging tool: Multidetector CT scan

Top Differential Diagnoses
- Sacroiliac joint disruption/dislocation
- Stress fracture
- Tumor
- Accessory centers of ossification

Pathology
- 95% occur in association with pelvic fractures

- Neurologic injury may be masked by concurrent injuries at higher levels
- Denis classification
- Divides fracture by involvement of 3 different zones
- Zone 1: Lateral to neural foramina
- Zone 2: Through neural foramina
- Zone 3: Through spinal canal

Clinical Issues
- Posterior pelvic pain or tenderness following high velocity trauma

Diagnostic Checklist
- High velocity injuries in adults always involve anterior pelvic ring when sacrum is fractured

CT Findings
- Bone CT
  - Shows displacement not apparent on radiography
  - Defines position of fracture relative to neural foramina, spinal canal
  - Fracture may be subtle even on high resolution CT scan

MR Findings
- Because sacrum is thin and obliquely positioned, fracture may be missed or mistaken for tumor
  - Oblique coronal T1WI, STIR along plane of sacrum useful
  - 3 mm thick slices
- Generally not used in acute trauma setting
- Used to evaluate for nerve root injury
  - Traumatic avulsion may be masked acutely by surrounding hematoma
  - Can see injury of sacral plexus on STIR sequences

Imaging Recommendations
- Best imaging tool: Multidetector CT scan
- Protocol advice: 1-3 mm overlapping helical images, coronal & sagittal reformations

DIFFERENTIAL DIAGNOSIS

Sacroiliac joint disruption/dislocation
- May require CT scan to differentiate from fracture

Stress fracture
- Back pain of insidious onset, disabling severity
- No history or trauma
- Usually insufficiency fracture due to osteoporosis
- May be fatigue fracture in athletes
- Vertically oriented fracture through sacral ala
  - Unilateral or bilateral
  - Horizontal component connecting two vertical fractures in < 50%
- Vacuum phenomenon often seen in anterior portion of fracture

- Wide rectilinear bands of abnormal signal on MRI may be mistaken for tumor

Tumor
- Loss of arcuate lines on radiography
- Round or oval region of trabecular destruction on CT scan
- Round or oval region of high T2WI signal on MRI

Traumatic lumbosacral dislocation
- Due to high speed injury, motor vehicle accident or fall
- Extremely rare
- Diagnosed with lateral radiograph or CT scan

Accessory centers of ossification
- Seen at lateral margins of sacrum in children
- Undulating contour, bilaterally symmetric

PATHOLOGY

General Features
- General path comments
  - 95% occur in association with pelvic fractures
  - Neurologic injury may be masked by concurrent injuries at higher levels
- Etiology
  - Sacral fractures without pelvic ring disruption
    - Often suicidal jumpers
    - Transverse fracture may occur if patient lands in seated or supine position
    - Fractures at sacro-coccygeal junction due to minor falls
  - 3 major mechanisms of pelvic ring disruption
  - Anteroposterior compression ("open book")
    - Vertically oriented sacral fracture, often slightly diastatic
  - Lateral compression ("T-bone injury")
    - Vertically oriented fracture
    - May see sclerotic rather than lucent line due to impaction
    - Impaction at sacral fracture causes decreased mediolateral dimension sacral ala

SACRAL TRAUMATIC FRACTURE

○ Vertical shear (fall from a height)
  ▪ Usually vertically oriented fracture
  ▪ Vertical displacement may be present or may have spontaneously reduced
  ▪ Fractures of L5 transverse processes sometimes present
- Epidemiology: Common injury
- Associated abnormalities
  ○ Lumbosacral junction injury
    ▪ Seen in up to 1/3 of sacral fractures with pelvic ring involvement
    ▪ Facet joint injury or L5-S1 disc injury
  ○ Fracture of L5 transverse process indicates unstable fracture
    ▪ Fracture due to avulsion of lumbosacral ligament
  ○ Fractures anterior pelvic ring
  ○ Lumbar spine fractures
    ▪ Spine fracture with neurologic deficit may cause sacral fracture to be overlooked clinically
  ○ Neurologic injuries in 40% of displaced fractures
    ▪ Nerve roots or sacral plexus
    ▪ Transection or stretch injury
  ○ Vascular injuries
    ▪ Therapeutic embolization may be needed
    ▪ Active bleeding often seen on contrast-enhanced CT scan at time of trauma
  ○ Injury bladder or urethra
  ○ Lower extremity fractures
  ○ Degloving injury of posterior soft tissues

Staging, Grading or Classification Criteria
- Denis classification
  ○ Divides fracture by involvement of 3 different zones
- Zone 1: Lateral to neural foramina
  ○ 50% of sacral fractures
  ○ Vertical or oblique orientation
  ○ Neurologic deficit in 6-24%
  ○ L5 nerve root may be entrapped in fracture
- Zone 2: Through neural foramina
  ○ 34% of sacral fractures
  ○ Vertical or oblique
  ○ Neurologic deficit in 28%
  ○ Traumatic "far out syndrome"
    ▪ L5 root caught between sacral alar fragment and transverse process
- Zone 3: Through spinal canal
  ○ 16% of sacral fractures
  ○ Transverse zone 3 fracture
    ▪ 35% have associated avulsion of nerve roots
    ▪ "Sacral burst fracture": Transverse fracture with retropulsion of bone into spinal canal
    ▪ Fracture-dislocation may occur through rudimentary disc at S1-S2
    ▪ Neurologic deficit in 57-60%
    ▪ May have fracture below lumbosacral fusion
  ○ Vertical zone 3 fracture
    ▪ Majority have neurologic deficit
    ▪ Bowel, bladder, sexual dysfunction

CLINICAL ISSUES

Presentation
- Most common signs/symptoms

○ Posterior pelvic pain or tenderness following high velocity trauma
○ Other signs/symptoms
  ▪ Neurologic deficit
  ▪ Bowel, bladder symptoms

Natural History & Prognosis
- Unstable injuries require open reduction internal fixation (ORIF)
- Neurologic injury
  ○ S1, S2 deficits tend to improve within 1 year regardless of treatment
  ○ Dural laceration may lead to cerebrospinal fluid leak

Treatment
- Options, risks, complications
  ○ Bed rest, slow progression to weightbearing if stable
  ○ Stabilization of unstable fractures with transalar screws
  ○ Role of surgical decompression controversial
    ▪ Neurologic recovery improved with early compared to late decompression
  ○ Neural canal or neural foraminal obstruction may be removed
  ○ Significant post-operative infection rate

DIAGNOSTIC CHECKLIST

Image Interpretation Pearls
- High velocity injuries in adults always involve anterior pelvic ring when sacrum is fractured
- If see L5 transverse process fracture, suspect sacral fx

SELECTED REFERENCES
1. Bellabarba C et al: Midline sagittal sacral fractures in anterior-posterior compression pelvic ring injuries. J Orthop Trauma. 17(1):32-7, 2003
2. Rubel IF et al: Description of a rare type of posterior pelvis traumatic involvement: the green-stick fracture of the sacrum. Pediatr Radiol. 31(6):447-9, 2001
3. Verlaan JJ et al: Traumatic lumbosacral dislocation: case report. Spine. 26(17):1942-4, 2001
4. Kim MY et al: Transverse sacral fractures: case series and literature review. Can J Surg. 44(5):359-63, 2001
5. Leone A et al: Lumbosacral junction injury associated with unstable pelvic fracture: classification and diagnosis. Radiology. 205(1):253-9, 1997
6. Templeman D et al: Internal fixation of displaced fractures of the sacrum. Clin Orthop. (329):180-5, 1996
7. Rodriguez-Fuentes AE: Traumatic sacrolisthesis S1-S2. Report of a case. Spine. 18(6):768-71, 1993
8. Albert TJ et al: Concomitant noncontiguous thoracolumbar and sacral fractures. Spine. 18(10):1285-91, 1993
9. Gibbons KJ et al: Neurological injury and patterns of sacral fractures. J Neurosurg. 72(6):889-93, 1990
10. Denis F et al: Sacral fractures: an important problem. Retrospective analysis of 236 cases. Clin Orthop. 227:67-81, 1988

SACRAL TRAUMATIC FRACTURE

IMAGE GALLERY

Typical

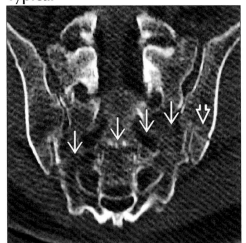 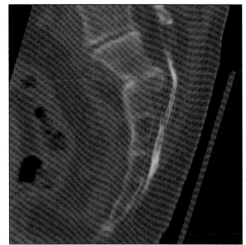

(Left) Axial oblique bone CT shows transverse fracture of sacrum (arrows) in unrestrained passenger in motor vehicle accident. Fracture continues through parasacral iliac bone (open arrow). *(Right)* Sagittal bone CT shows transversely oriented S2 fracture with 50% anterior displacement in patient who fell from height.

Typical

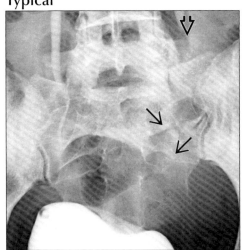 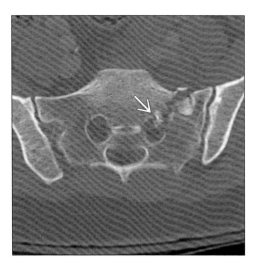

(Left) Anteroposterior radiography shows vertical shear zone 2 fracture through S1 & S2 neural foramina (arrows). L5 transverse process fracture (open arrow) indicates pelvic instability. *(Right)* Axial bone CT shows extension of sacral fracture into S1 neural foramen (arrow).

Variant

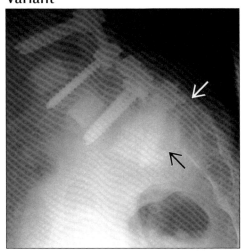 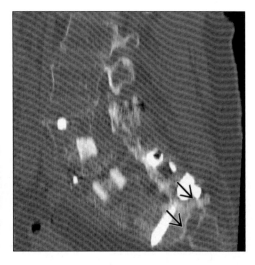

(Left) Lateral radiography shows displaced traumatic fracture occurring at S1/2 level (arrows), below spinal fusion. This fracture can also occur as an insufficiency fracture. *(Right)* Sagittal bone CT shows traumatic fracture (arrows) at S1/S2 level, below fusion. Fracture is through rudimentary disc at this level.

SACRAL INSUFFICIENCY FRACTURE

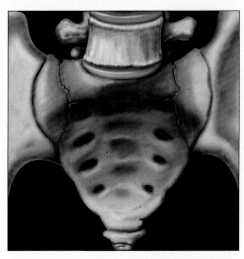

Sagittal graphic depicts the characteristic "H" shaped sacral insufficiency fractures, with bilateral vertical sacral alar and horizontal upper sacral fractures.

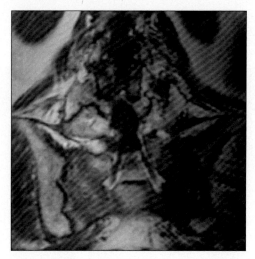

Coronal T1WI MR shows bilateral (L > R) ill-defined sacral marrow hypointensities adjacent to sacroiliac joints.

TERMINOLOGY

Abbreviations and Synonyms
- Sacral stress fracture

Definitions
- Stress fracture resulting from normal physiological stress on demineralized bone with decreased elastic resistance

IMAGING FINDINGS

General Features
- Best diagnostic clue: Bilateral or unilateral sacral marrow edema adjacent to sacroiliac joint(s) on MRI
- Location
  - Sacral alae
    - May be unilateral
  - Nearby sacroiliac joints
- Size: Variable extent of sacral involvement
- Morphology
  - Sclerotic bands or regions parallel to sacroiliac joints on CT and plain film
  - Curvilinear lines with associated ill-defined marrow signal abnormality on MRI
  - "H" shaped pattern of increased radiotracer uptake in sacrum on bone scintigraphy

- Horizontal component and/or one of two vertical components may be absent

Radiographic Findings
- Radiography
  - Approximately half will be normal at time of presentation
  - Osteopenia
  - Sacral alar vertical sclerotic bands
    - Healing fractures seen weeks to months after onset of symptoms
  - Disruption of sacral alae
  - Lucent fracture lines rare
  - Concomitant insufficiency fractures in lumbar spine and pelvis

CT Findings
- Bone CT
  - Presence of fracture lines
    - Early stage
    - May or may not extend to anterior sacral cortex
  - Sclerotic bands or irregular zones in sacral alae
    - Healing phase
    - Adjacent to sacroiliac joints
  - Ventral cortical disruption
  - Vacuum phenomena may be present
    - Within sacroiliac joints
    - Within fractures
  - Sensitive & specific

DDx: Sacral Marrow Abnormalities

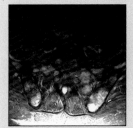
Metastases

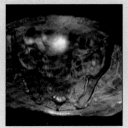
Osteomyelitis

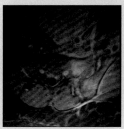
Infectious Sacroiliitis

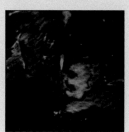
Infl. Sacroiliitis

SACRAL INSUFFICIENCY FRACTURE

Key Facts

Terminology
- Stress fracture resulting from normal physiological stress on demineralized bone with decreased elastic resistance

Imaging Findings
- Best diagnostic clue: Bilateral or unilateral sacral marrow edema adjacent to sacroiliac joint(s) on MRI
- Sclerotic bands or regions parallel to sacroiliac joints on CT and plain film
- "H" shaped pattern of increased radiotracer uptake in sacrum on bone scintigraphy
- Concomitant insufficiency fractures in lumbar spine and pelvis
- May be overlooked on MRI of lumbar spine

Top Differential Diagnoses
- Sacral metastases
- Sacral osteomyelitis
- Sacroiliitis

Clinical Issues
- High clinical suspicion required to make the diagnosis
- Favorable outcome and good prognosis

Diagnostic Checklist
- Make sure to evaluate sacrum on lumbar spine MRI
- Consider sacral insufficiency fractures when marrow edema adjacent to sacral iliac joints present

MR Findings
- T1WI: Hypointense linear or ill-defined marrow signal
- T2WI: Hyperintense linear or ill-defined marrow signal
- STIR: Patchy hyperintense marrow
- T1 C+: Curvilinear fracture lines better delineated
- Sacral marrow edema
  - Unilateral or bilateral
  - Ill-defined and irregular
  - Adjacent to sacroiliac joints
    - Not involving or crossing sacroiliac joints
  - Seen within three weeks after symptom onset
  - Resolves after three months
  - Associated cortical disruption
- Presence of discrete fracture lines
  - Usually visualized between three weeks and three months
  - Parallel to sacroiliac joints
- Lack of bony expansion
- Absent soft tissue mass
- Intact sacroiliac joints
- Sensitive and specific
- May be overlooked on MRI of lumbar spine
  - If no coronal sequence
  - If only limited axial imaging through sacrum

Nuclear Medicine Findings
- Bone Scan
  - Bilateral or unilateral sacral radiotracer uptake with or without a horizontal component
  - Characteristic "H" shaped pattern of radiotracer uptake only present in 19% of the cases
  - Sensitive but not specific

Other Modality Findings
- Osteoporosis on bone densitometry

Imaging Recommendations
- Fat suppression sequences valuable
  - STIR or FSE T2 with fat suppression accentuates marrow edema
- Imaging in oblique coronal plane better visualizes fracture lines
  - MRI
  - CT coronal reformation

DIFFERENTIAL DIAGNOSIS

Sacral metastases
- More discrete in morphology
- Random distribution
- Invasion of adjacent soft tissue and neural foramina
- Other sites involved

Primary sacral neoplasm
- Large and solitary
- Bony expansion
- Cortical breakthrough
- Soft tissue invasion

Sacral osteomyelitis
- Cutaneous and subcutaneous abnormalities present
  - Soft tissue edema
  - Abscess
- Ill-defined marrow edema
  - Contiguous with subcutaneous abnormality
  - Extending across sacroiliac joints
  - Associated with sacroiliitis
- No fracture lines

Sacroiliitis
- Signal alteration within sacroiliac joints
- Erosions at joints
- Joint ankylosis
- Marrow edema also present on iliac side of sacroiliac joints

Osteoarthritis
- Sclerosis on iliac side of sacroiliac joints
- Anterior bridging osteophyte

PATHOLOGY

General Features
- General path comments: Underlying abnormal bony mineralization

SACRAL INSUFFICIENCY FRACTURE

- Etiology
  - Predisposing factors
    - Osteoporosis
    - Rheumatoid arthritis
    - Renal osteodystrophy
    - Endogenous or exogenous corticosteroid excess
    - Radiation therapy
    - Other causes of osteopenia
    - Paget disease
  - Minor trauma
    - Often elicited after the diagnosis
  - No precipitating event in many instances
- Epidemiology
  - Incidence 0.14-1.8%
  - More common in women
- Associated abnormalities
  - Vertebral compression fractures
  - Other pelvic insufficiency fractures
    - Acetabular roof
    - Pubic rami
    - Parasymphysial pubic bone

Microscopic Features

- Organizing hematoma
- Trabecular condensation
- New bone and cartilage matrix
- Remodeling by osteoblasts and osteoclasts

CLINICAL ISSUES

Presentation

- Most common signs/symptoms
  - Acute or subacute pain
    - Low back
    - Buttock
    - Hip
    - Groin
    - Often in multiple sites
  - Sacral tenderness
  - Radiculopathy
  - Signs and symptoms mimic multiple medical conditions
    - Degenerative disc disease
    - Spinal stenosis
    - Vertebral compression fracture
    - Hip arthritis
    - Metastases
  - High clinical suspicion required to make the diagnosis
    - Women with postmenopausal osteoporosis
    - Elderly men with senile osteoporosis
- Clinical profile
  - Pain exacerbated by activity
  - Relieved by rest

Demographics

- Age: Sixth through eighth decades of life
- Gender
  - Elderly men
  - Postmenopausal women
- Ethnicity: No racial predilection

Natural History & Prognosis

- Favorable outcome and good prognosis
  - Symptoms resolve in as early as one month
    - Usually within 6-9 months
- May be limited by co-morbidities

Treatment

- Conservative
  - Bed rest
  - Protected weight bearing
  - Analgesics
  - Physical therapy
  - Treatment of underlying osteoporosis
- Sacroplasty
  - Injection of polymethylmethacrylate

DIAGNOSTIC CHECKLIST

Consider

- Including coronal T1WI on all lumbar spine MRI

Image Interpretation Pearls

- Make sure to evaluate sacrum on lumbar spine MRI
- Consider sacral insufficiency fractures when marrow edema adjacent to sacral iliac joints present

SELECTED REFERENCES

1. Pommersheim W et al: Sacroplasty: a treatment for sacral insufficiency fractures. AJNR Am J Neuroradiol. 24(5):1003-7, 2003
2. White JH et al: Imaging of sacral fractures. Clin Radiol. 58(12):914-21, 2003
3. Dasgupta B et al: Sacral insufficiency fractures: an unsuspected cause of low back pain. Br J Rheumatol. 37(7):789-93, 1998
4. Peh WC et al: Vacuum phenomena in the sacroiliac joints and in association with sacral insufficiency fractures. Incidence and significance. Spine. 22(17):2005-8, 1997
5. Grangier C et al: Role of MRI in the diagnosis of insufficiency fractures of the sacrum and acetabular roof. Skeletal Radio 26:517-24, 1997
6. Grasland A et al: Sacral insufficiency fractures: an easily overlooked cause of back pain in elderly women. Arch Intern Med 156:668-74, 1996
7. Peh WC et al: Imaging of pelvic insufficiency fractures.Radiographics 16:335-48, 1996
8. Stabler A et al: Vacuum phenomena in insufficiency fractures of the sacrum. Skeletal Radiology 24:31-35, 1995
9. Peh WC et al: Sacral insufficiency fractures. Spectrum of radiological features. Clin Imaging. 19(2):92-101, 1995
10. Baker RJ Jr et al: Sacral insufficiency fracture: half of an "H". Clin Nucl Med. 19(12):1106-7, 1994
11. West SG et al: Sacral insufficiency fractures in rheumatoid arthritis. Spine. 19(18):2117-21, 1994
12. Blomlie V et al: Radiation-induced insufficiency fractures of the sacrum: evaluation with MR imaging. Radiology. 188(1):241-4, 1993
13. Weber M et al: Insufficiency fractures of the sacrum. Twenty cases and review of the literature. Spine. 18(16):2507-12, 1993
14. Kayes K et al: Radiologic case study. Sacral insufficiency fracture. Orthopedics. 14(7):817-8, 820, 1991

SACRAL INSUFFICIENCY FRACTURE

IMAGE GALLERY

Typical

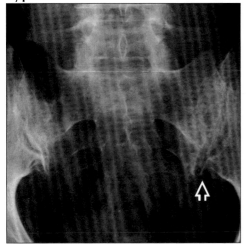
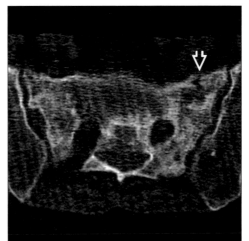

(Left) Coronal radiography shows left-sided sacral patchy sclerosis (arrow) next to sacroiliac joint. *(Right)* Axial bone CT shows bilateral sacral ill-defined sclerotic densities nearby sacroiliac joints. Left-sided fracture line extends to anterior cortex (arrow).

Typical

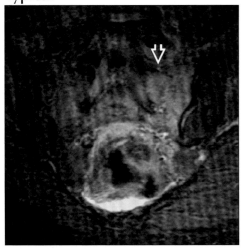
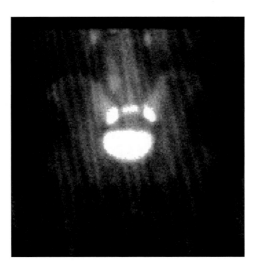

(Left) Coronal T2WI MR shows bilateral (L > R) sacral marrow edema with left-sided cortical disruption (arrow). Bilateral sacroiliac joints are intact. *(Right)* Coronal bone scan shows characteristic "H" pattern of radiotracer uptake in sacrum.

Typical

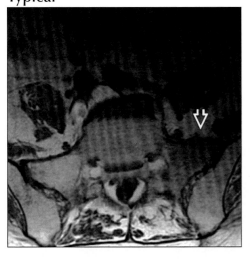
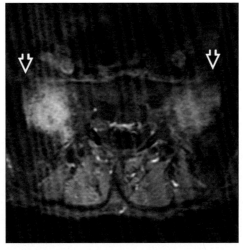

(Left) Axial T1WI MR shows left-sided sacral marrow edema extending to, but not involving, sacroiliac joint. Anterior cortical disruption is present (arrow). *(Right)* Axial T1 C+ MR shows bilateral sacral marrow enhancement with associated subtle cortical disruptions (arrows), sparring sacroiliac joints.

TRAUMATIC DISC HERNIATION

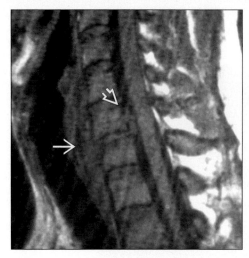

Sagittal T1WI MR shows C5-6 flexion injury with subluxation, prevertebral hemorrhage (arrow), disc extrusion touching ventral cord (open arrow).

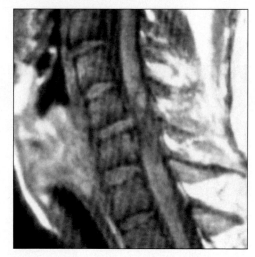

Sagittal T1WI MR shows C5-6 flexion injury with disc extrusion compressing cord with cord hemorrhage & edema.

TERMINOLOGY

Abbreviations and Synonyms
- Herniated nucleus pulposus (HNP)
  - Non-standard terminology
- Traumatic disc herniation (tHNP)
- Spinal cord injury (SCI)

Definitions
- Disc herniation induced by trauma

IMAGING FINDINGS

General Features
- Best diagnostic clue: Herniation of disc material most evident on T2WI
- Location
  - Cervical spine most frequently
  - 50% of tHNP occur at level of injury or one level below/above
- Size: Small to large
- Morphology: Appearance is the same as disc herniation unrelated to trauma

Radiographic Findings
- Radiography
  - Insensitive for disc pathology
  - Associated traumatic bone injuries

- Myelography
  - Extradural mass effacing anterior CSF-filled subarachnoid space
  - May see associated cord flattening
  - Distortion or obliteration of adjacent nerve root sleeve(s)

CT Findings
- NECT
  - Soft tissue density projecting into spinal canal
  - Obliteration of adjacent epidural fat
  - Narrowing of the disc space
- CTA: Quick screening for traumatic vascular injury
- Bone CT
  - tHNP often obscured by associated fractures, epidural hematoma
  - May also see locked facets, joint subluxation, Fxs

MR Findings
- T1WI
  - Disc material effacing anterior CSF perhaps compressing cord or cauda equina
    - Young: Hydrated mid-intensity disc material
    - Older: Desiccated hypointense material
- T2WI
  - Disc material effacing anterior CSF perhaps compressing cord or cauda equina
    - Young: Hydrated hyperintense disc material, may be more hyperintense than normal

DDx: Spinal Epidural Masses

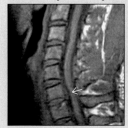

Nontraumatic HNP

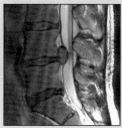

Nontraumatic HNP

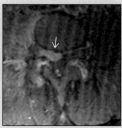

Epidural Abscess

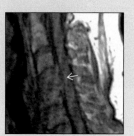

Epidural Metastasis

TRAUMATIC DISC HERNIATION

Key Facts

Terminology
- Disc herniation induced by trauma

Imaging Findings
- Best diagnostic clue: Herniation of disc material most evident on T2WI
- 50% of tHNP occur at level of injury or one level below/above
- Morphology: Appearance is the same as disc herniation unrelated to trauma
- MRI is modality of choice
- CT Bone depicts associated osseous injuries better

Top Differential Diagnoses
- Nontraumatic HNP
- Epidural abscess, phlegmon
- Epidural tumor

Pathology
- Pre-existing disc degeneration likely
- Epidemiology: Seen in 3-9% of all SCI patients, 33-48% of unstable cervical spine injuries

Clinical Issues
- Radicular syndrome (pain & segmental neurologic deficit) ($\approx$ 65%)
- Myeloradiculopathy ($\approx$ 30%)
- Medullary symptoms ($\approx$ 7%)
- Anterior cord syndrome is highly associated with traumatic disc herniation
- Good prognosis: Radiculopathy
- Poor prognosis: Myelopathy

Diagnostic Checklist
- tHNP in any patient who fails closed reduction

    ▪ Older: Desiccated hypointense material
  ○ Hyperintense cord contusion from compression
  ○ Stripping of posterior longitudinal ligament
- STIR: Associated ligamentous or soft tissue injury
- T2* GRE
  ○ Susceptibility from hemorrhage
  ○ Thin-section for cervical spine foraminal evaluation
- MRA: Quick screening for traumatic vascular injury

Angiographic Findings
- Conventional: Replaced by CTA, MRA

Imaging Recommendations
- Best imaging tool
  ○ MRI is modality of choice
  ○ CT Bone depicts associated osseous injuries better
- Protocol advice
  ○ Best seen with sagittal T2WI
  ○ Add GRE to assess for cord hemorrhage
  ○ STIR for ligamentous & soft tissue injury

DIFFERENTIAL DIAGNOSIS

Nontraumatic HNP
- Disc herniation with little or no trauma
- Appears similar to tHNP on imaging

Epidural abscess, phlegmon
- Usually from discitis
- Not as focal, may extend > 1 spinal segment
- Majority enhances, unlike disc material

Epidural tumor
- Usually back pain without trauma history
- Often enhances diffusely
- Look for extension from adjacent bony metastasis

PATHOLOGY

General Features
- General path comments

  ○ Discs allow movement between vertebral bodies & transmit loads from one vertebral body to the next
  ○ Annulus & nucleus disperse axial load pressure
  ○ When an axial load is applied to nucleus it shortens & radially expands exerting pressure on annulus
  ○ Annular resistance opposes this outward pressure
  ○ Axial loads up to 40 kg cause only 1 mm of vertical compression & 0.5 mm of radial expansion
  ○ During movement the annulus acts as ligament restraining movement & partially stabilizing interbody joint
- Genetics
  ○ Collagen type II gene deficiency, vitamin D receptor intragenic polymorphism both map to same region on chromosome 12q13
    ▪ Strong association with disc degeneration & herniation
    ▪ Established for nontraumatic HNP, however most agree that pre-existing disc degeneration predisposes to tHNP
    ▪ Thus same genes likely play some role in tHNP
- Etiology
  ○ Trauma-induced disruption of annulus → nucleus pulposus herniation
  ○ Pre-existing disc degeneration likely
- Epidemiology: Seen in 3-9% of all SCI patients, 33-48% of unstable cervical spine injuries
- Associated abnormalities
  ○ Bone Fxs, subluxations, dislocations
  ○ Cord contusion, hemorrhage
  ○ Ligamentous, soft tissue injury
  ○ Brain injury

Microscopic Features
- Fibrovascular tissue surrounds herniated disc material
- Vessels extend into annulus fibrosus but not endplate
- Scattered cartilage fragments & macrophages localize around disc margin
- Findings are similar to degenerated herniated discs & suggest an absorptive process

TRAUMATIC DISC HERNIATION

Staging, Grading or Classification Criteria

- Herniation = presence of nuclear material within or beyond the confines of an annular tear
  - Protrusion = focal or asymmetric disc extension beyond the interspace with a broader base than any other dimension of protrusion
  - Extrusion = focal or asymmetric disc extension beyond the interspace with base of origin narrower than the diameter of extruding material itself
  - Free fragment = herniation (extrusion) that has no connection with original disc
- Modifiers
  - Contained = restricted beneath an intact posterior longitudinal ligament
  - Noncontained = herniation extends through defective posterior longitudinal ligament

CLINICAL ISSUES

Presentation

- Most common signs/symptoms
  - Radicular syndrome (pain & segmental neurologic deficit) ($\approx$ 65%)
  - Myeloradiculopathy ($\approx$ 30%)
  - Medullary symptoms ($\approx$ 7%)
  - Anterior cord syndrome is highly associated with traumatic disc herniation
    - Injury to anterior 2/3 of cord
    - Pain & temperature affected
    - Touch & vibration intact
  - Brown-Sequard syndrome
    - Injury to 1/2 cord
    - Ipsilateral loss of touch & motor function
    - Contralateral loss of pain & temperature
    - Often superimposed on central cord syndrome
  - Central cord syndrome
    - Upper extremities involvement > lower
    - Older population, seen with spondylosis w/o Fx
    - Historically associated with central hematoma, predominantly white matter injury
  - Cauda equina syndrome: Pelvic & sacral pain due to compression of cauda equina spinal nerve roots
- Clinical profile: SCI patient, often with numerous injuries

Demographics

- Age: SCI: Mean age = 30.5 yrs, median = 26 yrs; 50% are 16-30
- Gender: SCI: > 80% male
- Ethnicity: SCI: More common in non-Caucasians
- Timing of SCI
  - Highest rate in July, lowest in February
  - 39% occur on Saturday or Sunday

Natural History & Prognosis

- Good prognosis: Radiculopathy
- Poor prognosis: Myelopathy

Treatment

- A number of large clinical series have failed to establish a relationship between tHNP & subsequent neurological deterioration with attempted closed traction-reduction in awake patients
  - There is no practice standard
- Surgical treatment often in association with repair of associated injuries

DIAGNOSTIC CHECKLIST

Consider

- tHNP in any patient who fails closed reduction

SELECTED REFERENCES

1. Martinez-Lage JF et al: Lumbar disc herniation in early childhood: case report and literature review. Childs Nerv Syst. 19(4):258-60, 2003
2. Tohme-Noun C et al: Imaging features of traumatic dislocation of the lumbosacral joint associated with disc herniation. Skeletal Radiol. 32(6):360-3, 2003
3. Hayes KC et al: Retropulsion of intervertebral discs associated with traumatic hyperextension of the cervical spine and absence of vertebral fracture: an uncommon mechanism of spinal cord injury. Spinal Cord. 40(10):544-7, 2002
4. Hadley MN: Initial closed reduction of cervical spine fracture-dislocation injuries. Neurosurgery. 50(3 Suppl):S44-50, 2002
5. Zortea M et al: Genetic mapping of a susceptibility locus for disc herniation and spastic paraplegia on 6q23.3-q24.1. J Med Genet. 39(6):387-90, 2002
6. Fuentes S et al: Traumatic thoracic disc herniation. Case illustration. J Neurosurg. 95(2 Suppl):276, 2001
7. Gray L et al: Thoracic and lumbar spine trauma. Semin Ultrasound CT MR. 22(2):125-34, 2001
8. Dai L et al: Central cord injury complicating acute cervical disc herniation in trauma. Spine. 25(3):331-5; discussion 336, 2000
9. Lee JY et al: Histological study of lumbar intervertebral disc herniation in adolescents. Acta Neurochir (Wien). 142(10):1107-10, 2000
10. Benedetti PF et al: MRI findings in spinal ligamentous injury. AJR Am J Roentgenol. 175(3):661-5, 2000
11. Katzberg RW et al: Acute cervical spine injuries: prospective MR imaging assessment at a level 1 trauma center. Radiology. 213(1):203-12, 1999
12. Vaccaro AR et al: Magnetic resonance evaluation of the intervertebral disc, spinal ligaments, and spinal cord before and after closed traction reduction of cervical spine dislocations. Spine. 24(12):1210-7, 1999
13. Bucciero A et al: Myeloradicular damage in traumatic cervical disc herniation. J Neurosurg Sci. 42(4):203-11, 1998
14. Rumana CS et al: Brown-Sequard syndrome produced by cervical disc herniation: case report and literature review. Surg Neurol. 45(4):359-61, 1996
15. Carreon LY et al: Histologic changes in the disc after cervical spine trauma: evidence of disc absorption. J Spinal Disord. 9(4):313-6, 1996
16. Doran SE et al: Magnetic resonance imaging documentation of coexistent traumatic locked facets of the cervical spine and disc herniation. J Neurosurg. 79(3):341-5, 1993

TRAUMATIC DISC HERNIATION

IMAGE GALLERY

Typical

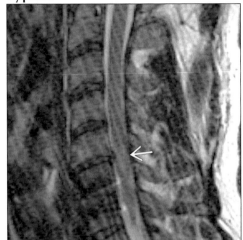
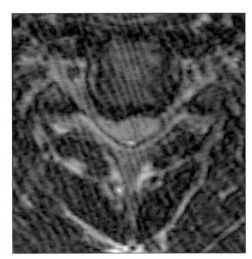

(Left) Sagittal T2WI MR demonstrates C5/6 disc herniation with hyperintense cord contusion (arrow) at level above pre-existing anterior fusion following diving accident. *(Right)* Axial T2WI MR confirms C5/6 disc herniation & hyperintense cord contusion.

Typical

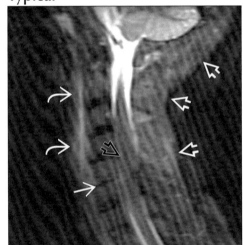
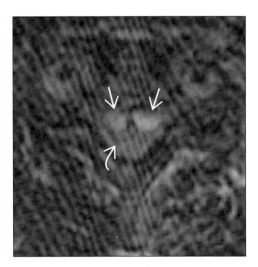

(Left) Sagittal STIR shows disc space height loss following C5/6 traumatic herniation (arrow), epidural blood (open black), ligamentous/muscle injury (open white) & prevertebral injury (curved white). *(Right)* Axial STIR MR on this ventilated patient confirms hyperintense epidural blood (arrows), right paracentral C5/6 relatively hypointense HNP (curved arrow), & diffuse soft tissue injury.

Typical

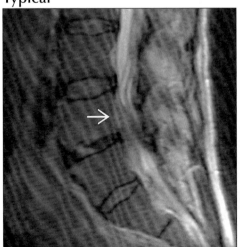
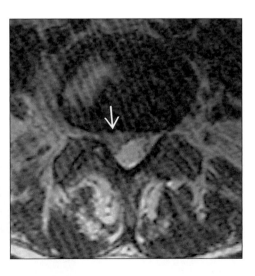

(Left) Sagittal T2WI MR demonstrates large L4/5 traumatic disc herniation as an extruded fragment posterior to L4 vertebral body (arrow). *(Right)* Axial T2WI MR confirms L4/5 traumatic disc herniation (arrow).

APOPHYSEAL RING FRACTURE

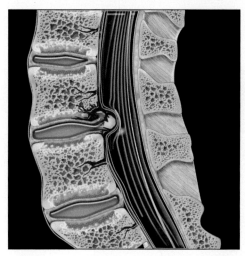

Sagittal graphic of young adult shows acute apophyseal ring fracture involving posterior inferior corner with displacement, associated hemorrhage & thecal sac compression.

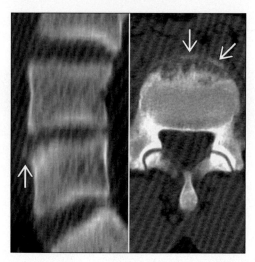

Sagittal bone CT reformation (L) and source axial cut (R) show sclerosed anterior margin of superior end plate with truncated corner, fragments displaced anteriorly (arrows).

TERMINOLOGY

Abbreviations and Synonyms
- Vertebral apophyseal Fx, limbus vertebra
- Endplate avulsion fracture (Fx), corner Fx, slipped vertebral apophysis, lumbar posterior marginal node

Definitions
- Fx or avulsion of vertebral ring apophysis (RA) due to injury in immature skeleton
  - Fx of anterior ring termed limbus vertebra (LV)
  - Fx of posterior ring termed posterior apophyseal ring Fx (PAR-Fx)

IMAGING FINDINGS

General Features
- Best diagnostic clue: Concentric bone fragment displaced from endplate margin
- Location
  - Lumbosacral spine most common; rare thoracic > cervical
  - L3-S1; PAR-Fx commonly L4, S1
  - Inferior or superior endplate may be involved; LV usually superior
  - Fractured apophyseal fragment usually midline
- Size: Fragment size can vary

- Morphology: Rim-like morphology typical, but fragment(s) may be amorphous

Radiographic Findings
- Radiography: Bone fragments displaced from corner defect of endplate; bone fragment not identified > 50%
- Myelography: Epidural defect on contrast column in PAR-Fx

CT Findings
- NECT
  - Acute
    - PAR-Fx: Arc-shaped or rectangular bone fragment posterior to dorsal endplate margin
    - Vertebral donor site occasionally not identified
    - LV: Same as PAR-Fx except located anteriorly, +/- mild kyphosis
    - Altered marrow signal (high on T2WI, low on T1WI)
  - Subacute - chronic
    - Sclerosis of fragment and donor site margins
    - Donor defect often enlarges, particularly LV

MR Findings
- T1WI
  - Corner defect in marrow of parent vb with disc extending into defect
  - Hypointense bone fragment

DDx: Limbus Simulators

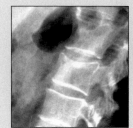

Flexion Fracture

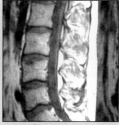

Schmorl Node

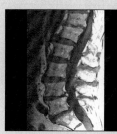

Ossified Disc 4/5

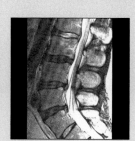

Disc Protrusion

APOPHYSEAL RING FRACTURE

Key Facts

Terminology
- Vertebral apophyseal Fx, limbus vertebra
- Endplate avulsion fracture (Fx), corner Fx, slipped vertebral apophysis, lumbar posterior marginal node
- Fx or avulsion of vertebral ring apophysis (RA) due to injury in immature skeleton

Imaging Findings
- Inferior or superior endplate may be involved; LV usually superior
- Corner defect in marrow of parent vb with disc extending into defect
- Hypointense bone fragment
- Defect in endplate; hyperintense disc between fragment and vb
- T1 C+: Enhancement of donor site marrow if acute Fx

- Best imaging tool: CT with bone as well as soft tissue windows
- Protocol advice: Thin-sections, sagittal reformations

Top Differential Diagnoses
- Schmorl node
- Compression/flexion fracture of anterior end plate corner
- Disc calcification or ossification
- Calcified disc fragment; posterior osteophyte

Pathology
- Stress on relative weak point described above in adolescent spine
- LV: Herniation of nucleus pulposus (NP) between RA and vertebral body

---

- T2WI
  - Defect in endplate; hyperintense disc between fragment and vb
  - High signal in subjacent marrow on T2WI in acute cases
- STIR: Same as T2WI, edema accentuated
- T2* GRE: Accentuation of sclerotic bone margins in chronic lesions
- T1 C+: Enhancement of donor site marrow if acute Fx
- ↓ T1/T2 merges with adjacent ligaments
- LV: T2
- PAR-Fx: Commonly associated variable-sized posterior disc protrusion
  - Disc between fragment and vertebral body uncommon finding
  - Fx fragment plus Sharpey fibers = "Y or 7" shape on sagittal MR
- Disc height loss common, +/- disc desiccation (↓ T2): Both ↑ over time

Nuclear Medicine Findings
- Bone Scan: "Hot" in acute lesions

Other Modality Findings
- Discography (LV): Contrasts enters space between fragment & vertebral body

Imaging Recommendations
- Best imaging tool: CT with bone as well as soft tissue windows
- Protocol advice: Thin-sections, sagittal reformations

DIFFERENTIAL DIAGNOSIS

Schmorl node
- End plate defect is within the interspace, not at endplate corner

Compression/flexion fracture of anterior end plate corner
- Seen in adults, after apophysis fused

Disc calcification or ossification
- Painful childhood nucleus pulposus calcification of unknown etiology
  - Multilevel common, cervical > thoracic, occasionally asymptomatic
  - Spontaneous resolution of calcifications and symptoms

Calcified disc fragment; posterior osteophyte
- Sequelae longstanding degenerative disc disease, usually adult
- Fragment at level of disc, not above or below
- May see marrow if ossified

PATHOLOGY

General Features
- General path comments
  - Embryology-anatomy
    - Superior & inferior surface of developing vb covered by thin, peripherally thickened, cartilage plate ⇒ cartilaginous marginal ridge
    - Endochondral ossification of marginal ridge begins 7-9 yrs ⇒ RA
    - RA seen as small bony triangles at corners of vertebral body (XR, sag/cor recon CT)
    - RA separated from vertebral body by thin cartilage layer until apophysis fuses to vertebral body at 18-20 yrs ⇒ relative weak point in disc/vertebral body complex until fusion occurs
    - Outermost fibers of annulus fibrosus (Sharpey fibers) embedded in RA, attaching disc to spine
- Genetics: Often seen with Scheuermann disease
- Etiology
  - Stress on relative weak point described above in adolescent spine
  - LV: Herniation of nucleus pulposus (NP) between RA and vertebral body
  - PAR-Fx: Two possible mechanisms described

APOPHYSEAL RING FRACTURE

- Same as LV or herniating NP spares Sharpey fibers & avulses RA
- Epidemiology: 20% prevalence PAR-Fx teen lumbar disc surgeries (33% in 14-17 yo)
- Associated abnormalities
  ○ Disc herniation
  ○ Kyphosis

Gross Pathologic & Surgical Features

- Displaced bony/cartilaginous rim fragment with or without disc material
- Sharpey fibers and posterior longitudinal ligament usually intact

Microscopic Features

- Cancellous bone, hyaline cartilage, & acellular hyaline tissue (disc)
- Basophilic degeneration & foci hemorrhage in hyaline cartilage common

Staging, Grading or Classification Criteria

- I: Avulsion posterior cortical vertebral rim (most common)
- II: Central cortical and cancellous bone Fxs
- III: Lateralized chip Fx
- IV: Spans entire posterior vertebral margin

CLINICAL ISSUES

Presentation

- Most common signs/symptoms: Back pain in acute (adolescent) cases
- Clinical profile: Adolescent athlete with acute low back pain
- PAR-Fx: Principal presentation
  ○ Acute > > prolonged history of central low back pain +/- sciatica
    ▪ 66% hx minor trauma or lifting event (weight-lifting, gymnastics)
  ○ Physical exam (PE) findings: Similar to herniated nucleus pulposus
- LV: No inciting event; chronic hx back pain; occasionally incidental finding
  ○ PE: ↓ ROM, +/- kyphosis & pain with palpation of spinous processes
- Majority patients with Par-Fx/LV report engagement in sporting activities

Demographics

- Age: Late childhood through adolescence
- Gender: M > F (up to 85% males in PAR-Fx group)

Natural History & Prognosis

- Reports document evolution LV into anteriorly located Schmorl node
- LV: Symptoms resolve months (usual) to years (rare)
- PAR-Fx: Good-excellent with surgery; occasional mild, short term deficits

Treatment

- LV: Conservative - analgesics & limitation physical activity in acute setting
- PAR-Fx: Surgical therapy mainstay, conservative rarely successful

○ Uni- or bilateral laminotomy with removal bone fragment, +/- disc

DIAGNOSTIC CHECKLIST

Consider

- Obtaining bone scan to ascertain chronicity

Image Interpretation Pearls

- If seen in adult, typically an incidental finding

SELECTED REFERENCES

1. Asazuma T et al: Lumbar disc herniation associated with separation of the posterior ring apophysis: analysis of five surgical cases and review of the literature. Acta Neurochir (Wien). 145(6):461-6; discussion 466, 2003
2. Mendez JS et al: Limbus lumbar and sacral vertebral fractures. Neurol Res. 24(2):139-44, 2002
3. Bonic EE et al: Posterior limbus fractures: five case reports and a review of selected published cases. J Manipulative Physiol Ther. 21(4):281-7, 1998
4. Swischuk LE et al: Disk degenerative disease in childhood: Scheuermann's disease, Schmorl's nodes, and the limbus vertebra: MRI findings in 12 patients. Pediatr Radiol. 28(5):334-8, 1998
5. Martinez-Lage JF et al: Avulsed lumbar vertebral rim plate in an adolescent: Trauma or malformation? Childs Nerv Syst. 14:131-4, 1998
6. Talha A et al: Fracture of the vertebral limbus. Eur Spine J. 6(5):347-50, 1997
7. Henales V et al: Intervertebral disc herniations (limbus vertebrae) in pediatric patients: Report of 15 cases. Pediatr Radiol. 23:608-10, 1993
8. Sward L et al: Vertebral ring apophysis injury in athletes. Is the etiology different in the thoracic and lumbar spine? Am J Sports Med. 21(6):841-5, 1993
9. Thiel HW et al: Lumbar apophyseal ring fractures in adolescents. J Manipulative Physiol Ther. 15(4):250-4, 1992
10. Wagner A et al: Diagnostic imaging in fracture of lumbar vertebral ring apophyses. Acta Radiol. 33(1):72-5, 1992
11. Leroux JL et al: Lumbar posterior marginal node (LPMN) in adults. Report of fifteen cases. Spine. 17(12):1505-8, 1992
12. Epstein NE: Lumbar surgery for 56 limbus fractures emphasizing noncalcified type III lesions. Spine. 17(12):1489-96, 1992
13. Epstein NE et al: Limbus lumbar vertebral fractures in 27 adolescents and adults. Spine. 16(8):962-6, 1991
14. Jonsson K et al: Avulsion of the cervical spinal ring apophyses: acute and chronic appearance. Skeletal Radiol. 20(3):207-10, 1991
15. Albeck MJ et al: Fracture of the lumbar vertebral ring apophysis imitating disc herniation. Acta Neurochir (Wien). 113(1-2):52-6, 1991
16. Banerian KG et al: Association of Vertebral End Plate Fracture with Pediatric Lumbar Intervertebral Disk Herniation: Value of CT and MR Imaging. Radiology. 177:763-5, 1990
17. Sward L et al: Acute injury of the vertebral ring apophysis and intervertebral disc in adolescent gymnasts. Spine. 15(2):144-8, 1990
18. Hellstrom M et al: Radiologic abnormalities of the thoraco-lumbar spine in athletes. Acta Radiol. 31(2):127-32, 1990
19. Goldman AB et al: Posterior limbus vertebrae: a cause of radiating back pain in adolescents and young adults. Skeletal Radiol. 19(7):501-7, 1990

APOPHYSEAL RING FRACTURE

IMAGE GALLERY

Typical

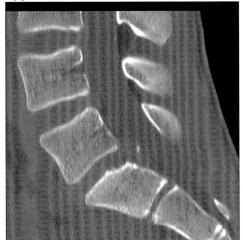
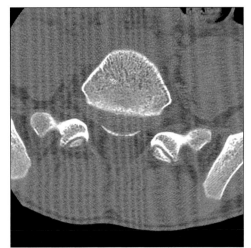

(Left) Sagittal bone CT reformation shows small bone fragment displaced posteriorly from truncated superior S1 endplate. Note sclerosis of donor site, & associated disc protrusion. *(Right)* Axial bone CT shows concentric bony rim displaced from superior margin of S1, with sclerosis of donor site.

Typical

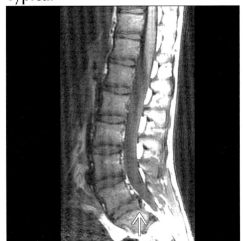
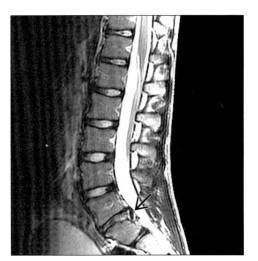

(Left) Sagittal T1WI MR shows distorted posterosuperior S1 corner (arrow), with disc protruding posteriorly, displacing iso-intense tissue. CT showed bone fragments corresponding to displaced tissue. *(Right)* Sagittal T2WI MR depicts bone fragment with low signal intensity (arrow) displaced from posterior superior S1 margin. Note truncated posterior vb corner.

Typical

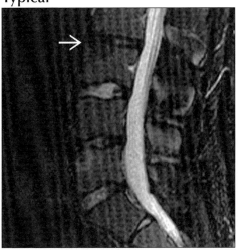
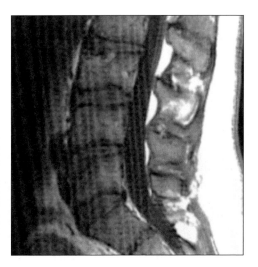

(Left) Sagittal FLAIR MR demonstrates edema subjacent to a distorted anterosuperior vb margin, typical of a subacute Limbus L5 injury. Note more chronic appearance of Limbus vb two levels above (arrow). *(Right)* Sagittal T1WI MR shows two limbus vb (L3, L5). The lower one demonstrates subjacent edema seen as low signal.

RHABDOMYOLYSIS

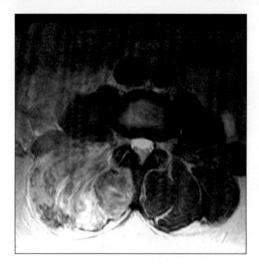

Axial T2WI MR shows diffuse hyperintensity of dorsal right paraspinal muscles with sharp ventral margin. Patient was in prolonged right decubitus position for surgery.

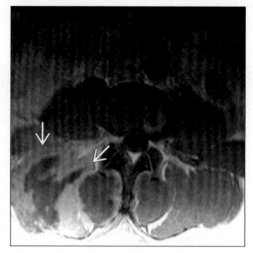

Axial T1 C+ MR shows diffuse and irregular muscle enhancement (arrows), with central nonenhancing component.

TERMINOLOGY

Abbreviations and Synonyms
- Rhabdomyolysis (RML), myonecrosis

Definitions
- Clinical and biochemical syndrome resulting from damage of integrity of skeletal muscle, with release of toxic muscle cell components into circulation

IMAGING FINDINGS

General Features
- Best diagnostic clue: Increased T2 signal within affected skeletal muscle group
- Location: Skeletal muscle
- Size: Large: May involve multiple paraspinal muscle groups
- Morphology: Diffuse abnormal signal

CT Findings
- NECT
  - Normal to slight low attenuation by CT
  - Skeletal muscle calcification may occur early in disease course
- CECT: Normal to slight enhancement

MR Findings
- T1WI: Isointense to hypointense T1 signal from affected muscle groups
- T2WI: Diffuse increased T2 signal with margins confined by facial boundaries
- STIR: Increased T2 signal
- T1 C+
  - May show patchy contrast enhancement
  - Severe disease with myonecrosis shows peripheral enhancement with no central enhancement

Nuclear Medicine Findings
- Bone Scan
  - Bone scan shows widespread, diffuse accumulation of the radioisotope in the affected muscles
  - Tc99-MDP 95% sensitive in early active stage (first 10 days)

Imaging Recommendations
- Best imaging tool
  - Bone scan to total body extent of damage
  - MRI for extent of focal muscle damage
- Protocol advice: T2WI in multiple planes

DDx: Rhabdomyolysis, Spine

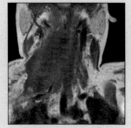

Myositis Ossif

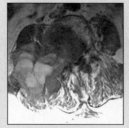

Sarcoma

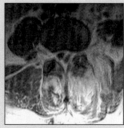

Septic Facet

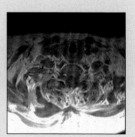

Abscess

RHABDOMYOLYSIS

Key Facts

Terminology
- Rhabdomyolysis (RML), myonecrosis
- Clinical and biochemical syndrome resulting from damage of integrity of skeletal muscle, with release of toxic muscle cell components into circulation

Imaging Findings
- Best diagnostic clue: Increased T2 signal within affected skeletal muscle group
- T1WI: Isointense to hypointense T1 signal from affected muscle groups
- T2WI: Diffuse increased T2 signal with margins confined by facial boundaries
- Bone scan shows widespread, diffuse accumulation of the radioisotope in the affected muscles

Pathology
- Common pathway of RML may be a disturbance in myocyte calcium homeostasis
- Elevated serum creatine kinase (CK) 5x normal value, 100% sensitive
- Genetic etiologies include glycolytic enzyme deficiencies (McArdle disease)
- Major etiologies include trauma (38%), including prolonged immobilization for surgical procedures, prolonged seizures, direct muscle injury

Clinical Issues
- Hydration with isotonic crystalloid
- Treatment of acute renal failure (mannitol, diuretics)
- Life threatening complications include acute renal failure, hyperkalemia and cardiac arrest

DIFFERENTIAL DIAGNOSIS

Hemorrhage/hematoma
- T1WI MR: Darker than fat
- T2WI MR: Brighter than fat
- Surrounding edema

Infection/abscess
- Reticular to circumscribed subcutaneous edema
- Peripheral enhancement with abscess

Myositis ossificans
- Localized soft tissue ossifications with circumscribed pattern

Soft tissue tumor
- Heterogeneous enhancement
- Prominent vessels
- Bone sclerosis/periosteal reaction

PATHOLOGY

General Features
- General path comments
  - Common pathway of RML may be a disturbance in myocyte calcium homeostasis
  - Elevated serum creatine kinase (CK) 5x normal value, 100% sensitive
    - CK-MM isoenzyme predominates
  - Urine + hemoglobin/myoglobin, negative does not exclude diagnosis
    - "Coke colored" urine
- Genetics
  - Multiple genetic predispositions
  - Genetic etiologies include glycolytic enzyme deficiencies (McArdle disease)
    - Autosomal recessive
  - Abnormal lipid metabolism (carnitine deficiency)
  - Malignant hyperthermia
    - Autosomal dominance with variable penetrance
    - Defect in receptor of calcium release channel of sarcoplasmic reticulum

- Episodes of hyperthermia/rhabdomyolysis triggered by exposure to volatile anesthetics
  - Neuroleptic malignant syndrome
    - Drug related development of hyperthermia, muscle rigidity, fluctuating consciousness, and autonomic instability
    - Phenothiazines, butyrophenones, other antipsychotics/antidepressants
    - Underlying defect may be presynaptic
- Etiology
  - Multiple etiologies
    - Major etiologies include trauma (38%), including prolonged immobilization for surgical procedures, prolonged seizures, direct muscle injury
    - Ischemia (14%), including compression and vascular occlusion
    - Polymyositis (8%)
    - Drug overdose (7%), and wide variety of drugs (including statins)
    - Exertion (6%), marathon running
    - Burns
    - Infections, both bacterial and viral
    - Wide variety of toxins, including alcohol
    - Metabolic disorders such as diabetic ketoacidosis and hypothyroidism
  - Accumulation of cell lysis products ⇒ microvascular damage, capillary leak, increased intracompartmental pressures, reduced tissue perfusion and ischaemia
- Epidemiology: 25 cases per 2.5 million population

Gross Pathologic & Surgical Features
- Swelling, edema of muscle groups

Microscopic Features
- Disruption of myofibrillar architecture and wide spread vacuolization
- Late: Atrophy

Staging, Grading or Classification Criteria
- Risk factors for acute renal failure due to RML
  - Presence of sepsis
  - Age > 70
  - Volume depletion

RHABDOMYOLYSIS

○ Initial uric acid levels elevated
○ Degree of elevation of CPK, potassium, phosphorus

CLINICAL ISSUES

Presentation
• Most common signs/symptoms
  ○ Muscle pain (50%)
  ○ Acute renal failure with myoglobinuria (30%)
  ○ Disseminated intravascular coagulation (DIC) near universal finding, although rarely symptomatic
  ○ Metabolic acidosis
  ○ Hyperkalemia
  ○ Hypovolemia
  ○ Other signs/symptoms
    ▪ Tense muscle compartment may be compartment syndrome
• Clinical profile: Muscle pain with tense swollen compartment following local trauma

Demographics
• Age: Any age group
• Gender: M > F

Natural History & Prognosis
• 5% mortality rate

Treatment
• Options, risks, complications
  ○ Hydration with isotonic crystalloid
  ○ Treatment of acute renal failure (mannitol, diuretics)
• Life threatening complications include acute renal failure, hyperkalemia and cardiac arrest

DIAGNOSTIC CHECKLIST

Consider
• Requires a high index of suspicion
• Clinical and laboratory findings give diagnosis, with imaging secondary role
• Statins cause < < 1 death/million users due to rhabdomyolysis

Image Interpretation Pearls
• Imaging findings nonspecific
• Clinical history, lab values critical

SELECTED REFERENCES

1.	Getachew E et al: Pathologic quiz case: a man with exertion-induced cramps and myoglobinuria. McArdle disease (glycogenosis type V or myophosphorylase deficiency). Arch Pathol Lab Med. 127(9):1227-8, 2003
2.	Torres-Villalobos G et al: Pressure-induced rhabdomyolysis after bariatric surgery. Obes Surg. 13(2):297-301, 2003
3.	Wiltshire JP et al: Lumbar muscle rhabdomyolysis as a cause of acute renal failure after Roux-en-Y gastric bypass. Obes Surg. 13(2):306-13, 2003
4.	Kisakol G et al: Rhabdomyolysis in a patient with hypothyroidism. Endocr J. 50(2):221-3, 2003
5.	Masaoka S et al: Malignant lymphoma in skeletal muscle with rhabdomyolysis: a report of two cases. J Orthop Sci. 7(6): 688-93, 2002
6.	Blanco JR et al: Rhabdomyolysis of infectious and noninfectious causes. South Med J. 95(5): 542-4, 2002
7.	Bocca G et al: Compartment syndrome, rhabdomyolysis and risk of acute renal failure as complications of the lithotomy position. J Nephrol. 15(2): 183-5, 2002
8.	Wexler RK: Evaluation and treatment of heat-related illnesses. Am Fam Physician. 65(11): 2307-14, 2002
9.	Criner JA et al: Rhabdomyolysis: the hidden killer. Medsurg Nurs. 11(3): 138-43, 155, 2002
10.	Lappa A et al: Successful treatment of a complicated case of neuroleptic malignant syndrome. Intensive Care Med. 28(7): 976-7, 2002
11.	Evans M et al: The myotoxicity of statins. Curr Opin Lipidol. 13(4): 415-20, 2002
12.	Atmaca H et al: Rhabdomyolysis associated with gemfibrozil-colchicine therapy. Ann Pharmacother. 36(11): 1719-21, 2002
13.	Kikuno N et al: Traumatic rhabdomyolysis resulting from continuous compression in the exaggerated lithotomy position for radical perineal prostatectomy. Int J Urol. 9(9): 521-4, 2002
14.	Kuang W et al: Rhabdomyolysis after laparoscopic donor nephrectomy. Urology. 60(5): 911, 2002
15.	Bolego C et al: Safety considerations for statins. Curr Opin Lipidol. 13(6): 637-44, 2002
16.	Modi JR et al: Fluvastatin-induced rhabdomyolysis. Ann Pharmacother. 36(12): 1870-4, 2002
17.	Kratz A et al: Effect of marathon running on hematologic and biochemical laboratory parameters, including cardiac markers. Am J Clin Pathol. 118(6): 856-63, 2002
18.	Black C et al: Etiology and frequency of rhabdomyolysis. Pharmacotherapy. 22(12): 1524-6, 2002
19.	Barahona MJ et al: Hypothyroidism as a cause of rhabdomyolysis. Endocr J. 49(6): 621-3, 2002

RHABDOMYOLYSIS

IMAGE GALLERY

Typical

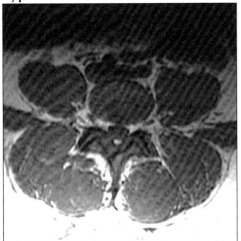 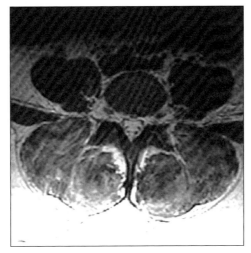

(Left) Axial T1WI MR shows no significant T1 signal change in this patient with severe bilateral dorsal muscle pain, following prolonged exertion. *(Right)* Axial T2WI MR shows diffuse hyperintensity from dorsal paraspinal muscles bilaterally, bounded by facial planes in this patient with severe bilateral dorsal muscle pain following prolonged exertion.

Typical

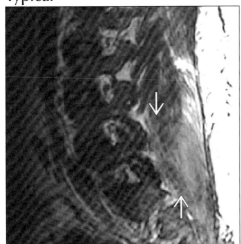 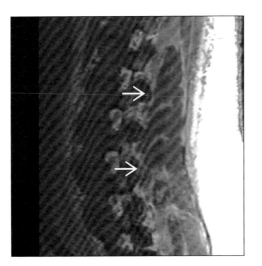

(Left) Sagittal T2WI MR shows hyperintensity from dorsal muscles (arrows), with normal adjacent posterior elements. *(Right)* Sagittal T1 C+ MR shows irregular peripheral enhancement within dorsal paraspinal muscles, with central nonenhancing necrosis (arrows).

Typical

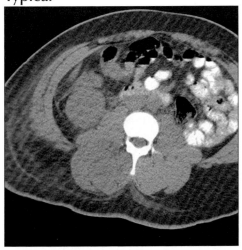 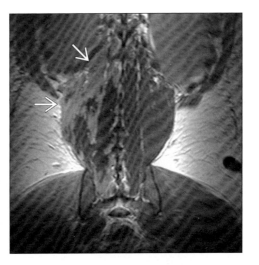

(Left) Axial NECT shows enlargement of the right paraspinal muscles, without abnormal attenuation. There is irregular reticulation of subcutaneous fat due to edema. *(Right)* Coronal T1 C+ MR shows irregular enhancement of right dorsal paraspinal muscles (arrows), in contrast to normal left muscle signal intensity.

TRAUMATIC SPINAL MUSCLE INJURY

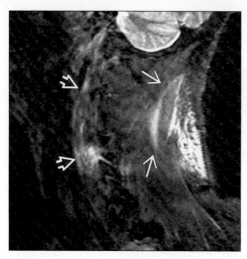

Parasagittal STIR shows splenius capitis muscle belly contusion & associated fascial injury (arrows). Also note prevertebral tissue & facet ligament injuries (open arrows).

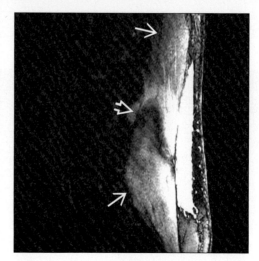

Parasagittal STIR shows diffuse paraspinal lumbar muscle hyperintense strain (arrows) with hypointense hemorrhage within muscle fiber disruption (open arrow).

TERMINOLOGY

Definitions
- Strain = muscle fiber disruption from indirect forces
- Sprain = ligamentous injury

IMAGING FINDINGS

General Features
- Best diagnostic clue: Muscle T2 hyperintensity
- Morphology: Laceration, contusion, strain

CT Findings
- NECT: Contusion: May form dense myositis ossificans

MR Findings
- T1WI
  - Contusion: ↑ Circumference
  - Laceration: Muscle defect, often transverse, usually with hemorrhage
  - Strain: Grade 3: Muscle discontinuity with hemorrhage at torn edge, may form hematoma
  - Muscle may herniate through fascial rent
- STIR
  - Contusion: Hyperintense edema
  - Contusion: Feathery interstitial pattern from fluid tracking between muscle fibers
  - Laceration: Edema, hemorrhage

  - Strain:
    - Grade 1 & 2: Edema +/- blood; initially center of affected muscle → entire muscle involvement
    - Grade 3: Edema & muscle discontinuity, may form hematoma
- T1 C+: May see enhancement acutely

Imaging Recommendations
- Best imaging tool: MRI
- Protocol advice: T2 + fat suppressing technique

DIFFERENTIAL DIAGNOSIS

Denervation-related muscle atrophy
- Acutely appears similar to injury
- Unlike injury becomes fatty replaced

Neoplasm, inflammation, or infection
- Appear similar to acute injury
- Fails to resolve with time

PATHOLOGY

General Features
- Etiology
  - Most commonly from MVA; also athletic injuries, blow from falling objects, direct injury

DDx: Traumatic Muscle Injury Mimics

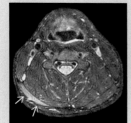

Denervation Atrophy

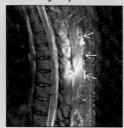

Infectious Myositis

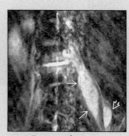

Psoas Abscess

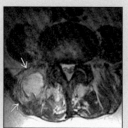

Psoas Abscess

TRAUMATIC SPINAL MUSCLE INJURY

Key Facts

Imaging Findings
- Best diagnostic clue: Muscle T2 hyperintensity
- Morphology: Laceration, contusion, strain
- Best imaging tool: MRI
- Protocol advice: T2 + fat suppressing technique

Top Differential Diagnoses
- Denervation-related muscle atrophy
- Neoplasm, inflammation, or infection

Pathology
- Most commonly from MVA; also athletic injuries, blow from falling objects, direct injury

Clinical Issues
- Most common signs/symptoms: Pain; symptoms may be delayed 2-3 days
- Clinical profile: Palpation often reveals spasm
- 20-90% may have persistent symptoms

- ○ Mechanism
  - ▪ Hyperextension > hyperflexion, lateral flexion
  - ▪ Excessive stretch and/or tension
- ○ Contusion
  - ▪ Muscle compression from direct trauma
  - ▪ Common in contact sports (aka "charleyhorse")
  - ▪ Muscle can still function, even with severe injury
- ○ Laceration: Result of penetrating trauma
- ○ Strain: Injury from single violent force
- • Epidemiology
  - ○ Lacerations are rare
  - ○ Contusions more frequent
- • Associated abnormalities: TMJ, cervical nerve-root, esophageal, tracheal, vascular injuries

Microscopic Features
- Contusion: Hematoma formation, inflammation, connective tissue scar replacing muscle fibers
- Laceration repair: Dense connective tissue, not normal muscle fibers, with ↓ ability to generate tension
- Strain: Muscle fiber disruption
  - ○ Usually myotendinous junction (weakest aspect)
  - ○ Often accompanied by hemorrhage, hematoma
  - ○ Damaged muscle fiber necrosis & breakdown
    - ▪ Proliferation of inflammatory cells
    - ▪ Inelastic scar predisposes to recurrent injury
  - ○ May form myositis ossificans during later healing

Staging, Grading or Classification Criteria
- Strain
  - ○ 1st degree: Microscopic muscle fiber disruption; similar appearance to contusion
  - ○ 2nd degree: Macroscopic disruption with preservation of structural integrity; may see mass, stellate defect, or both
  - ○ 3rd degree: Complete muscle disruption

CLINICAL ISSUES

Presentation
- Most common signs/symptoms: Pain; symptoms may be delayed 2-3 days
- Clinical profile: Palpation often reveals spasm

Natural History & Prognosis
- Hyperextension injuries more severe and take longer to recover
- 20-90% may have persistent symptoms
- Nearly 40% develop degenerative disc disease compared to 6% for age-matched controls

- • Rhabdomyolysis
  - ○ Fever, intense pain, weakness
  - ○ Myoglobulin may induce renal failure

Treatment
- Mobilization & activity leads to less scar in healing contusion with more rapid recovery of tensile strength
- As healing progresses, rehabilitation activity may become more aggressive
- Soft collar may be used for no more than 2-4 wks
- Brief therapy with analgesics +/- muscle relaxants

SELECTED REFERENCES

1. Jinkins JR: Lumbosacral interspinous ligament rupture associated with acute intrinsic spinal muscle degeneration. JBR-BTR. 86(4):226-30, 2003
2. Hayashi N et al: Accuracy of abnormal paraspinal muscle findings on contrast-enhanced MR images as indirect signs of unilateral cervical root-avulsion injury. Radiology. 223(2):397-402, 2002
3. Vaccaro AR et al: Magnetic resonance imaging analysis of soft tissue disruption after flexion-distraction injuries of the subaxial cervical spine. Spine. 26(17):1866-72, 2001

IMAGE GALLERY

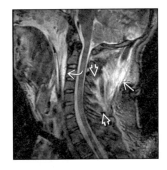 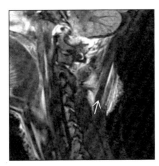

(Left) Sagittal STIR shows splenius capitis strain (arrow) containing fiber disruption (not shown). Also note interspinous/supraspinous ligament (open arrows) and prevertebral injuries (curved arrow). *(Right)* Parasagittal STIR reveals diffuse hyperintense muscle injury including trapezius (white arrow), splenius capitis, & other muscles. There are also diffuse fascial, ligament, & subcutaneous injuries.

PEDICLE INSUFFICIENCY FRACTURE

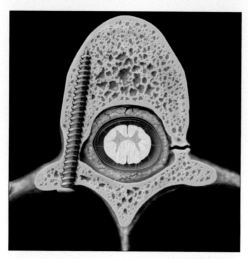

Axial graphic of lumbar body shows right pedicle screws, altering biomechanics to produce left pedicle stress fracture.

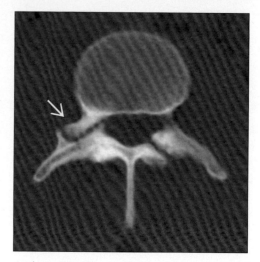

Axial NECT shows well-defined coronal oriented fracture through right pedicle (arrow), with bone production reflecting a chronic lesion. There is an old appearing fracture of left lamina.

TERMINOLOGY

Abbreviations and Synonyms
- Pedicle stress fracture (PSF)
- Pediculolysis

Definitions
- Fracture of spinal pedicle not related to direct acute trauma

IMAGING FINDINGS

General Features
- Best diagnostic clue: Linear low attenuation on CT through pedicle, well-defined margins
- Location: Lumbar pedicle > cervical > thoracic
- Size: Variable fracture size through pedicle, from partial to complete with separation
- Morphology
  - Linear fracture, vertically oriented
  - May be associated with sclerosis, hyperostosis

Radiographic Findings
- Radiography
  - Linear fracture through pedicle
  - Adjacent bony sclerosis

CT Findings
- NECT
  - Coronal oriented fracture through pedicle
  - Associated bony sclerosis
    - +/- Association with adjacent sclerosis
    - Sclerosis may be extensive, & mimic more aggressive lesion
  - Look for contralateral posterior element abnormality
    - Pedicle fracture
    - Spondylolysis
    - Pedicle aplasia, hypoplasia

MR Findings
- T1WI
  - Coronal or vertically oriented linear low signal through pedicle
  - May show larger area of low signal in pedicle due to bony sclerosis
  - Contralateral posterior element abnormality
  - Osteophyte and bony hyperplasia may complicate diagnosis by masking fracture site
  - Variable pedicle marrow signal
    - Low pedicle signal on T1WI due to sclerosis or edema
    - Chronic lesions may show fatty T1 marrow signal in pedicle adjacent to fracture site
- T2WI

DDx: Pedicle Insufficiency Fracture

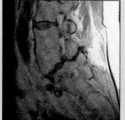
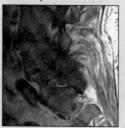
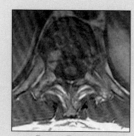
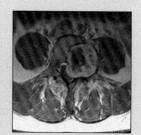

Pseudoarthrosis   Septic Facet   Paget Disease   Primary Bone Tumor

PEDICLE INSUFFICIENCY FRACTURE

Key Facts

Terminology
- Pedicle stress fracture (PSF)
- Pediculolysis
- Fracture of spinal pedicle not related to direct acute trauma

Imaging Findings
- Best diagnostic clue: Linear low attenuation on CT through pedicle, well-defined margins
- Coronal oriented fracture through pedicle
- Look for contralateral posterior element abnormality
- Osteophyte and bony hyperplasia may complicate diagnosis by masking fracture site
- Variable pedicle marrow signal
- Low pedicle signal on T1WI due to sclerosis or edema

Pathology
- Etiology: Altered biomechanics leads to stress fracture

Clinical Issues
- Back pain, radiculopathy if associated bony hypertrophy and nerve compression
- Symptomatic treatment for pain
- Surgical pedicle screw fixation of fracture

Diagnostic Checklist
- Look for contralateral posterior element disease such as pedicle hypoplasia, or aplasia
- Look for causative abnormality above or below fracture site

- Chronic lesions may show fatty T1 marrow signal in pedicle adjacent to fracture site

---

  - Coronal or vertically oriented linear low signal through pedicle
  - High signal intensity in adjacent pedicle due to edema, repair
- STIR
  - Coronal or vertically oriented linear low signal through pedicle
  - High signal intensity in adjacent pedicle due to edema, repair
- T2* GRE: Precise fracture site may be better defined on gradient echo images
- T1 C+: Patchy adjacent reactive marrow enhancement

Nuclear Medicine Findings
- Bone Scan
  - Increased uptake from fracture site
  - Increased uptake from associated abnormalities such as contralateral spondylolysis

Imaging Recommendations
- Best imaging tool: CT shows fracture, displacement, contralateral abnormality
- Protocol advice: Thin slice CT with multiplanar reformats

DIFFERENTIAL DIAGNOSIS

Metastatic disease
- Rounded mass lesion with enhancement
- Multiple lesions
- Associated pathologic fracture
- Bone destruction

Primary bone tumor
- Osteoblastoma, ABC, giant cell
- Mass lesion within pedicle, with expansion, enhancement
- Bone destruction or remodeling

Infection/septic facet
- Abnormal low signal from facet, with irregular adjacent soft tissue extension
- Joint effusion

- Enhancement of soft tissue and peripheral enhancement of epidural abscess

Paget disease
- Bone expansion with thickened cortex
- No bone destruction
- Thickened trabeculae, heterogeneous marrow signal may simulate fracture site on MR

Pseudoarthrosis
- Horizontal (axial) directed defect through prior surgical fusion site
- Pseudoarthrosis involving intervertebral disc level and posterior elements in a horizontal plane

PATHOLOGY

General Features
- General path comments: Fracture with new bone production, callus
- Etiology: Altered biomechanics leads to stress fracture
- Epidemiology
  - Related to prior spinal fusion surgery
  - Remote trauma may also be involved
- Associated abnormalities: Prior spinal fusion, with or without instrumentation

Gross Pathologic & Surgical Features
- Mixture of reparative processes, bone formation, collagen deposition, fibrosis

Microscopic Features
- Typical chronic fracture

CLINICAL ISSUES

Presentation
- Most common signs/symptoms
  - Back pain, radiculopathy if associated bony hypertrophy and nerve compression
  - Other signs/symptoms
    - May be asymptomatic finding

PEDICLE INSUFFICIENCY FRACTURE

- Clinical profile: Patient with back pain, prior spinal fusion

Demographics
- Age: Adult
- Gender: M = F

Natural History & Prognosis
- Chronic course if no relief of inducing stress
- May produce pseudoarthrosis

Treatment
- Options, risks, complications
  - Symptomatic treatment for pain
  - Surgical pedicle screw fixation of fracture

DIAGNOSTIC CHECKLIST

Consider
- Look for contralateral posterior element disease such as pedicle hypoplasia, or aplasia

Image Interpretation Pearls
- Look for causative abnormality above or below fracture site

SELECTED REFERENCES

1. Hollenberg GM et al: Imaging of the spine in sports medicine. Curr Sports Med Rep. 2(1):33-40, 2003
2. Bose B: Fracture of S1-2 after L4-S1 decompression and fusion. Case report and review of the literature. J Neurosurg. 99(3 Suppl):310-2, 2003
3. Slipman CW et al: Sacral stress fracture in a female field hockey player. Am J Phys Med Rehabil. 82(11):893-6, 2003
4. Sirvanci M et al: Pedicular stress fracture in lumbar spine. Clin Imaging. 26(3): 187-93, 2002
5. Shah MK et al: Sacral stress fractures: an unusual cause of low back pain in an athlete. Spine. 27(4):E104-8, 2002
6. Kraft DE: Low back pain in the adolescent athlete. Pediatr Clin North Am. 49(3):643-53, 2002
7. Reitman CA et al: Lumbar isthmic defects in teenagers resulting from stress fractures. Spine J. 2(4):303-6, 2002
8. Fourney DR et al: Early sacral stress fracture after reduction of spondylolisthesis and lumbosacral fixation: case report. Neurosurgery. 51(6):1507-10; discussion 1510-1, 2002
9. Macdessi SJ et al: Pedicle fracture after instrumented posterolateral lumbar fusion: a case report. Spine. 26(5): 580-2, 2001
10. Chong VF et al: Pedicular stress fracture in the lumbar spine. Australas Radiol. 41(3): 306-7, 1997
11. Heggeness MH et al: The trabecular anatomy of thoracolumbar vertebrae: implications for burst fractures. J Anat. 191 (Pt 2): 309-12, 1997
12. Gunzburg R et al: Stress fracture of the lumbar pedicle. Case reports of "pediculolysis" and review of the literature. Spine. 16(2): 185-9, 1991
13. Traughber PD et al: Bilateral pedicle stress fractures: SPECT and CT features. J Comput Assist Tomogr. 15(2): 338-40, 1991

PEDICLE INSUFFICIENCY FRACTURE

IMAGE GALLERY

Typical

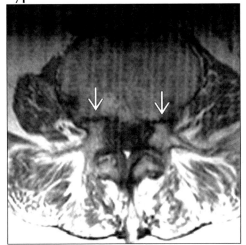 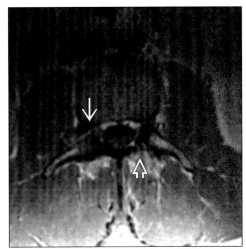

(Left) Axial T1WI MR shows bilateral pedicle fractures as linear low signal extending through pedicle/vertebral body junction (arrows). *(Right)* Axial T1WI MR shows fracture line as intermediate signal outline by low signal sclerotic pedicle (arrow). Left lamina fracture is present, but indistinct (open arrow).

Typical

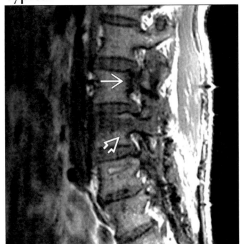 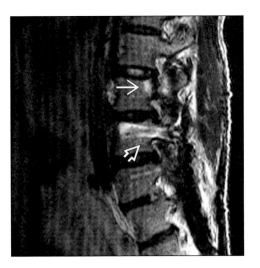

(Left) Sagittal T1WI MR shows pedicle fracture as line through L2 pedicle (arrow), with low signal adjacent low signal pedicle sclerosis. Patient is post removal of multilevel pedicle screws (open arrow). *(Right)* Sagittal T2WI MR shows pedicle fracture as low signal with adjacent edema (arrow). Pedicle screw tract from prior surgery (open arrow) also show high signal.

Variant

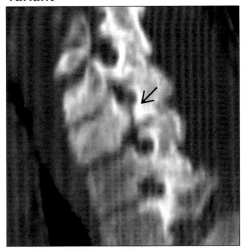 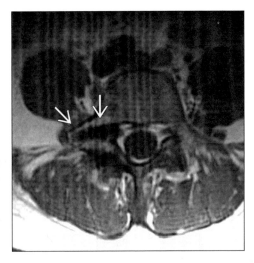

(Left) NECT Sagittal oblique shows lucent fracture line through C5-6 left pedicle (arrow) with sclerotic margins. Patient was post C5-6 discectomy & failed fusion. *(Right)* Axial T1WI MR shows chronic right pedicle fracture as linear low signal with large amount of bony hyperplasia (arrows).

POST-TRAUMATIC SYRINX

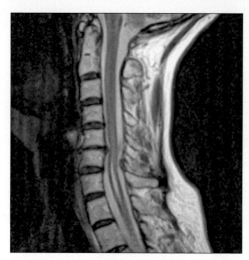

Sagittal T2WI MR demonstrates a syrinx which formed following a C5/6 disc herniation.

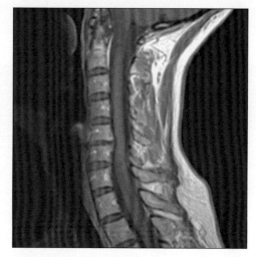

Sagittal T1 C+ MR shows no abnormal enhancement associated with syrinx which formed following C5/6 disc herniation. Same case as on left.

TERMINOLOGY

Abbreviations and Synonyms
- Post-traumatic syrinx (PTS)
- Syringomyelia, Syringohydromyelia

Definitions
- Cystic cord cavity that may (hydromyelia) or may not (syringomyelia) communicate with central canal
- Artificial distinction → many use syringohydromyelia

IMAGING FINDINGS

General Features
- Best diagnostic clue: Cystic expansile cord lesion
- Location: Rostral to injury site in 81%, caudal in 4%, both directions in 15%
- Size: Average length 6 cm; range 5 mm to entire cord
- Morphology
  - Longitudinal spinal cord cleft with CSF imaging characteristics
  - Frequently has a fusiform "beaded" appearance

Radiographic Findings
- Radiography
  - Spinal deformities: Fx, dislocations, kyphotic or lordotic changes
  - Flexion/extension evaluate spinal stability

- Myelography
  - Arachnoiditis & adhesions at level of injury
  - Focal changes in cord size
  - Delayed CT myelography
    - Syrinx fills in with delayed scanning
    - May change with position, characteristically ↓ in size when moving from prone to supine

CT Findings
- NECT
  - Cavitation with central CSF hypodensity
  - Normal or atrophied cord
  - May be difficult to appreciate central cavity on unenhanced imaging
- Bone CT
  - May see posterior vertebral body scalloping in longstanding lesions

MR Findings
- T1WI: Focal hypointensity
- T2WI
  - Focal hyperintensity
    - Myelomalacia precedes overt syrinx formation = "presyrinx state"
  - May begin as small cysts → coalesce into larger cysts
  - Adjacent cord may be normal or atrophied
    - May appear to be an "expansile" lesion, a relative finding in presence of cord atrophy
- CSF Flow

DDx: "Lesions" Appearing Similar to Post-Traumatic Syrinx

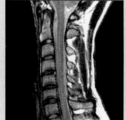

Gibbs Artifact

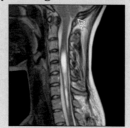

Chiari 1

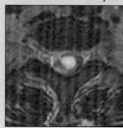

Glioma Associated

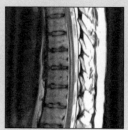

Idiopathic

POST-TRAUMATIC SYRINX

Key Facts

Imaging Findings
- Best diagnostic clue: Cystic expansile cord lesion
- Location: Rostral to injury site in 81%, caudal in 4%, both directions in 15%
- Frequently has a fusiform "beaded" appearance
- Arachnoiditis & adhesions at level of injury
- May begin as small cysts → coalesce into larger cysts
- Adjacent cord may be normal or atrophied
- Best imaging tool: T2WI, T1 C+ MR

Top Differential Diagnoses
- Gibbs artifact
- Myelitis
- Spinal cord tumor
- Myelomalacia
- Idiopathic

Pathology
- Trauma most common cause of secondary syrinx
- PTS incidence 0.3-4% of spinal cord injuries

Clinical Issues
- Most common symptom = pain which may increase with coughing, sneezing, or straining
- Classic presentation: Severe pain unrelieved by analgesics, ascending disassociated sensory loss
- Untreated syrinx is progressive
- Heralded by changing or new symptoms
- Shunting can arrest neurologic progression
- Followed post-operatively by physical exam & MRI

Diagnostic Checklist
- Main imaging goal is to exclude associated or causative lesions

---

- ○ Sagittal 2D cine phase-contrast technique for defining presence, direction of flow
- ○ May show abnormal CSF dynamics

Ultrasonographic Findings
- Intraoperative US: Delineates location, extent

Imaging Recommendations
- Best imaging tool: T2WI, T1 C+ MR
- Protocol advice
  - ○ Axial images confirm location and clarify relationship to adjacent anatomical structures
  - ○ Sagittal sequence most useful for defining craniocaudal extent
  - ○ Contrast essential to exclude neoplasm
  - ○ Consider cine PC CSF flow study if suspect obstruction to CSF flow (e.g., arachnoid adhesions)

DIFFERENTIAL DIAGNOSIS

Gibbs artifact
- Bright or dark lines parallel & adjacent to borders of abrupt intensity change
- Commonly seen when going from bright CSF to dark spinal cord on T2WI

Chiari I associated
- Cerebellar tonsillar herniation

Myelitis
- Demyelinating disease (e.g., MS)
- Acute disseminated encephalomyelitis
- Lateral myelitis

Spinal cord tumor
- Astrocytoma, ependymoma, hemangioblastoma
- Cord expansion; nearly always enhancing

Myelomalacia
- Cord volume loss, gliosis
- Do not see CSF signal central cavitation on T1WI

Idiopathic
- Nontraumatic hydromyelia

- Ventriculitis terminalis (distal cord)

PATHOLOGY

General Features
- General path comments
  - ○ Longitudinally oriented CSF-filled cavity with surrounding gliosis
    - Hydromyelia: Central canal dilatation
    - Syringomyelia: Cavity is lateral to or independent of central canal
    - Most cases show features of both on pathologic exam (e.g., syringohydromyelia)
  - ○ Medullary extension is termed syringobulbia
- Etiology
  - ○ May develop secondary to contusion, myelomalacia, or hemorrhage within cord
  - ○ Exact mechanism is unknown
  - ○ "One-way valve" theory: Phenomenon allowing CSF into, but not out of, cyst cavity
  - ○ "Slosh-and-suck" theory: ↑ Epidural venous flow during activity (e.g., coughing) ↑ pressure around cord which cannot be dissipated because of disruptions in CSF flow forcing CSF into cyst
    - Thus coughing, sneezing, straining can enlarge cavity over time
- Epidemiology
  - ○ Trauma most common cause of secondary syrinx
  - ○ PTS incidence 0.3-4% of spinal cord injuries
    - Idiopathic = 0.1%
    - With complete tetraplegia incidence = 8%
  - ○ Higher incidence following thoracolumbar SCI

Gross Pathologic & Surgical Features
- Cavitation of gray matter within spinal cord centrally or eccentrically

Microscopic Features
- Forms in partially damaged cord adjacent to area of complete injury
- Often begin as small areas of cavitation that coalesce into larger cysts

POST-TRAUMATIC SYRINX

- Tubular spinal cord cavitation surrounded by dense glial fibril wall (Rosenthal fibers)
- Most form in gray matter between dorsal horns & posterior columns
  - Predominantly affecting crossing pain & temperature fibers
- Hyalinized thickened vessels
- Aberrant nerve fibers in cavity wall
- Perivascular (Virchow Robin) spaces may be enlarged
- Adhesions often present tethering cord with local scarring
- Microinfarction is another possible cause
- Enlargement secondary to cavity fluid motion in response to pressure changes

CLINICAL ISSUES

Presentation
- Most common signs/symptoms
  - Spasticity, hyperhidrosis, pain, sensory loss, automotive hyperreflexia
  - May result in neurologic deterioration years after injury
    - Delays from 6 mos to 35 yrs reported
    - Mean interval ranges 9-13 yrs
  - Cervical: Rarely CN deficit(s), 25% have bulbar signs
  - Rarely new onset urinary dysfunction, neuropathic joint
- Clinical profile
  - Most common symptom = pain which may increase with coughing, sneezing, or straining
    - Axial > radicular pain
  - Classic presentation: Severe pain unrelieved by analgesics, ascending disassociated sensory loss
    - Loss to pain & temperature with preservation to touch
  - Uncommon in childhood
    - Most childhood syrinx is simple hydromyelia or Chiari-associated
    - More likely than adults to present with scoliosis
  - EMG → ↑ in polyphasic spikes with ↑ in motor unit action potential duration

Demographics
- Age: May occur at any age; average age at the time of injury ≈ 28 yrs (range, 16-67)
- Gender: M > F

Natural History & Prognosis
- Variable; dependent on underlying etiology
- PTS onset earlier with ↑ age, cervical & thoracic levels, dislocated Fx, spinal instrumentation without decompression, complete SCI
- Untreated syrinx is progressive
- As cavity enlarges
  - Involves previously unaffected neural tissue
  - Results in progressive myelopathy
  - Heralded by changing or new symptoms
- Muscle wasting +/- spasticity
- Neuropathic Charcot joints

Treatment
- Shunting can arrest neurologic progression

- Syringoperitoneal or syringosubarachnoid
- Shunt procedural goals
  - Associated scar dissection → promotes normal local CSF dynamics
  - Cyst drainage → ↓ abnormal intramedullary pressure
- Outcomes
  - Pain or motor recovery occurs in ≈ 50%
  - Sensory symptoms improve in 33%
  - Fails to halt symptom progression in 10%
  - Nearly 50% shunts non-functional at 6 yrs
- Often performed with somatosensory evoked potential monitoring to assess cord function during procedure
- Followed post-operatively by physical exam & MRI
  - Syrinx reduction postoperative MRI correlates with satisfactory clinical outcome in 85%
- Other surgical considerations
  - Laser syringotomy
  - Decompressive laminectomy with subarachnoid space reconstruction
  - Spinal cord transection
  - Pedicled omental graft transposition

DIAGNOSTIC CHECKLIST

Image Interpretation Pearls
- Main imaging goal is to exclude associated or causative lesions

SELECTED REFERENCES

1. Vannemreddy SS et al: Posttraumatic syringomyelia: predisposing factors. Br J Neurosurg. 16(3):276-83, 2002
2. Brugieres P et al: CSF flow measurement in syringomyelia. AJNR 21(10): 1785-92, 2000
3. Fischbein NJ et al: The "presyrinx" state: a reversible myelopathic condition that may precede syringomyelia. AJNR 20(1): 7-20, 1999
4. Perrouin-Verbe B et al: Post-traumatic syringomyelia and post-traumatic spinal canal stenosis: a direct relationship: review of 75 patients with a spinal cord injury. Spinal Cord. 36(2):137-43, 1998
5. Jinkins JR et al: MR of parenchymal spinal cord signal change as a sign of active advancement in clinically progressive posttraumatic syringomyelia. AJNR Am J Neuroradiol. 19(1):177-82, 1998
6. Kramer KM et al: Posttraumatic syringomyelia: a review of 21 cases. Clin Orthop. (334):190-9, 1997
7. Schurch B et al: Post-traumatic syringomyelia (cystic myelopathy): a prospective study of 449 patients with spinal cord injury. J Neurol Neurosurg Psychiatry. 60(1):61-7, 1996
8. Sgouros S et al: Management & outcome of posttraumatic syringomyelia. J Neurosurg. 85(2):197-205, 1996
9. Silberstein M et al: Delayed neurologic deterioration in the patient with spinal trauma: role of MR imaging. AJNR Am J Neuroradiol. 13(5):1373-81, 1992
10. Bronskill MJ et al: Syrinx-like artifacts on MR images of the spinal cord. Radiology. 166(2):485-8, 1988

IMAGE GALLERY

Typical

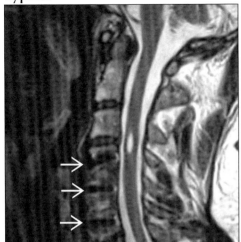 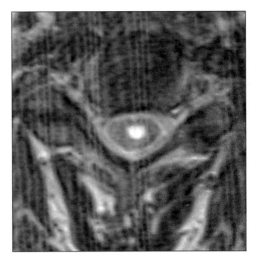

(Left) Sagittal T2WI MR demonstrates syrinx that followed cervical spine trauma with fracture (not shown); susceptibility can be seen from anterior fusion hardware (arrows). *(Right)* Axial T2WI MR confirms central location of this post-traumatic syrinx.

Typical

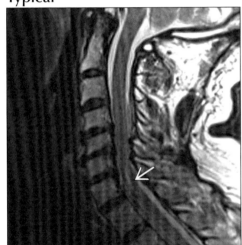 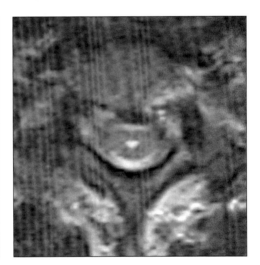

(Left) Sagittal T2WI MR shows a small syrinx (arrow) resulting from longstanding cervical spondylosis. Note multilevel posterior osteophyte-disc complexes & listhesis from C4/5 through C6/7 levels. *(Right)* Axial T2WI MR confirms central syrinx.

Typical

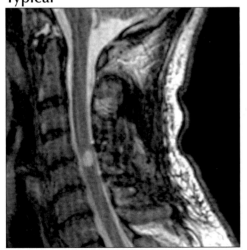 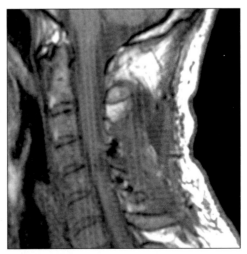

(Left) Sagittal T2WI MR reveals rounded syrinx following cervical trauma & ligament disruption; note changes in posterior tissues from placement of C4 to C5 cerclage wire. *(Right)* Sagittal T1WI MR also shows a rounded syrinx following cervical trauma and ligament disruption; note changes in posterior tissues from placement of C4 to C5 cerclage wire.

SPINAL CORD CONTUSION-HEMATOMA

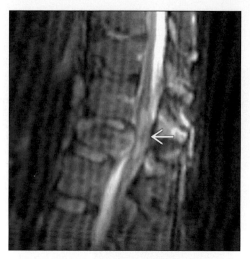

Sagittal T2WI MR demonstrates hyperintense cord contusion with focus of hypointense hemorrhage (arrow) following thoracic spine burst fracture.

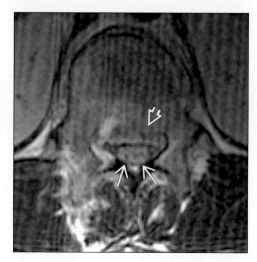

Axial T2WI MR shows foci of hypointense hemorrhage (arrows) within cord contusion. Note retropulsed fragments (open arrow) following thoracic spine burst fracture.

TERMINOLOGY

Abbreviations and Synonyms
- Spinal cord injury (SCI)

Definitions
- Traumatic cord edema, swelling, and/or hemorrhage

IMAGING FINDINGS

General Features
- Best diagnostic clue: Abnormal cord MR signal
- Location
  - Most common level of SCI is C5, then C4 & C6
  - In cases resulting in paraplegia, most common level is T12, then L1 & T10

Radiographic Findings
- Radiography: Associated Fx, subluxation
- Myelography
  - Contusion: Focal cord enlargement effacing contrast
  - Hematoma: May mimic syrinx containing contrast
    - 140-300 Hounsfield units (HU)
  - Transection: No cord visible in affected axial slice

CT Findings
- NECT
  - Contusion: May see cord hypodensity

  - Hematoma: Focal cord hyperdensity; 50-90 HU
- CTA: Quick screening for associated vascular injury
- Bone CT
  - Associated Fx, subluxation
  - Often find predisposing spondylosis, spinal stenosis

MR Findings
- T1WI
  - Acute contusion
    - Parenchymal iso- to hypointensity
    - May show cord swelling
  - Hematoma: Only positive days later when becomes hyperintense methemoglobin
  - Transection: Sagittal T1WI best sequence to show cord discontinuity
  - Chronic contusion: Focal to long segment atrophy
- T2WI
  - Acute contusion: Parenchymal T2 hyperintensity
  - Hematoma: Follows typical MR aging appearance
  - May see traumatic disc herniation
  - Chronic contusion: Focal to long segment residual hyperintense gliosis
  - Chronic hematoma: Hypointense hemosiderin scar
- STIR: Best for marrow edema & hyperintense ligamentous, soft tissue injury
- T2* GRE: Hematoma: ↑ Sensitivity 2° susceptibility "blooming"
- MRA: Quick screening for associated vascular injury

DDx: Cord Lesions With Edema +/- Hemorrhage

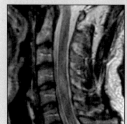

Multiple Sclerosis

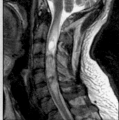

Ependymoma

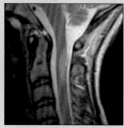

Hemangioblastoma

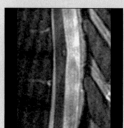

Cavernous Malform.

SPINAL CORD CONTUSION-HEMATOMA

Key Facts

Terminology
- Traumatic cord edema, swelling, and/or hemorrhage

Imaging Findings
- Best diagnostic clue: Abnormal cord MR signal
- Acute contusion: Parenchymal T2 hyperintensity
- Hematoma: Follows typical MR aging appearance
- May see traumatic disc herniation
- STIR: Best for marrow edema & hyperintense ligamentous, soft tissue injury
- T2* GRE: Hematoma: ↑ Sensitivity 2° susceptibility "blooming"
- Best imaging tool: MRI
- Protocol advice: Add STIR & GRE

Top Differential Diagnoses
- Myelitis
- Spinal cord tumor
- Myelomalacia

Pathology
- MVA (45%), falls (22%), acts of violence (16%), sports injury (13%)

Clinical Issues
- Mean age = 30.5 yrs, median = 26 yrs
- Gender: Over 80% male
- Chronic care best approached from rehabilitation team approach

Diagnostic Checklist
- Screening MRI for all symptomatic SCI
- Sagittal STIR key to diagnose marrow edema & ligamentous injury

Ultrasonographic Findings
- Intraoperative US
  - Acute cord lesions appear hyperechoic
  - Size of echoic abnormality correlates with severity of neurologic symptoms
  - Assists in shunt placement and/or drainage guidance

Angiographic Findings
- Conventional: Replaced by CTA, MRA

Imaging Recommendations
- Best imaging tool: MRI
- Protocol advice: Add STIR & GRE

DIFFERENTIAL DIAGNOSIS

Myelitis
- Demyelinating disease (e.g., MS), ADEM, lateral myelitis
- All may enhance

Spinal cord tumor
- Astrocytoma, ependymoma, hemangioblastoma
- Cord expansion; nearly always enhancing

Cavernous malformation
- Best seen with GRE
- May be multiple
- May be asymptomatic

Myelomalacia
- Cord volume loss, gliosis
- Do not see CSF signal central cavitation on T1WI

PATHOLOGY

General Features
- Etiology
  - MVA (45%), falls (22%), acts of violence (16%), sports injury (13%)
    - Most common act of violence is shooting
    - Most common sports injury results from diving
    - If > 45 yrs most likely from fall
    - In non-Caucasians most likely act of violence
  - Spondylosis is significant risk factor for SCI
- Epidemiology
  - 14,000 SCI occur each year, of which 10,000 survive to reach treatment facility
  - Estimated cost to society ≈ $2 billion each year

Gross Pathologic & Surgical Features
- Ranges in severity
  - Cord edema without hemorrhage
  - Cord petechial hemorrhage
  - Cord pulverization & bleeding
  - Complete transection

Microscopic Features
- Cord microcirculation alterations maximize 24-48 hrs
- Intramedullary edema +/- hemorrhage involving central gray matter
  - Edema peaks 3-6 days, subsides by 1-2 weeks
- Extends outward with severity of trauma
- Hemorrhagic necrosis & liquification may occur
- Demyelination & cystic myelomalacia ensues
  - Reactive gliosis, vascular proliferation at the margins

Staging, Grading or Classification Criteria
- American Spinal Injury Association (ASIA)
  - Grade A: No motor or sensory function preserved in sacral segments S4-S5
  - Grade B: Sensory, but not motor function is preserved below neurologic level; sacral S4-S5 function preserved
  - Grade C: Motor function preserved below neurologic level, > 50% key muscles below have muscle grade < 3/5
  - Grade D: Motor function preserved below neurologic level, > 50% key muscles below have muscle grade > 3/5
  - Grade E: Normal
  - (neurologic level of injury = most caudal cord segment with normal sensory & motor function on both sides of body)
- Kulkarni classification

SPINAL CORD CONTUSION-HEMATOMA

○ Type 1: Cord hemorrhage evident acutely as T1 inhomogeneity; poorest prognosis
○ Type 2 (most common): T2 hyperintense contusion & swelling with normal T1; good prognosis
○ Type 3 (uncommon): T2 central hypointensity, thick peripheral hyperintensity at focal cord enlargement with normal T1; intermediate pattern & prognosis

CLINICAL ISSUES

Presentation
- Anterior cord syndrome
  ○ Injury to anterior 2/3 of cord
  ○ Pain & temperature affected
  ○ Touch & vibration intact
  ○ Highly associated with traumatic disc herniation
- Central cord syndrome
  ○ Upper extremities involvement > lower
  ○ Older population, seen with spondylosis without Fx
  ○ Historically associated with central hematoma, predominantly a white matter injury
- Posterior cord syndrome: Uncommon; loss of dorsal column function
- Brown-Sequard syndrome
  ○ Injury to 1/2 the cord
  ○ Ipsilateral loss of touch & motor function
  ○ Contralateral loss of pain & temperature
  ○ Often superimposed on central cord syndrome
- Autonomic hyperreflexia
  ○ Arise in SCI above T6
  ○ Paroxysmal hypertension with agonizing headache
  ○ May result in intracerebral hemorrhage, seizure, cardiac arrhythmias, death
- Contusion may be present in asymptomatic patients

Demographics
- Age
  ○ Mean age = 30.5 yrs, median = 26 yrs
  ○ 50% are 16-30
- Gender: Over 80% male
- Ethnicity: More common in non-Caucasians
- Timing of injury
  ○ Highest rate in July, lowest in February
  ○ 39% occur on Saturday or Sunday

Natural History & Prognosis
- Contusion
  ○ Regresses over 1-2 weeks
  ○ Has good prognosis for neurologic recovery
- Hematoma: Poor prognosis, often without recovery
- Poor prognostic factors: C4, C5, C6 level injuries, age > 50 yrs
- Anterior cord syndrome: 70% regain ambulation
- Central cord syndrome: < 50 yrs 70% ambulate, > 50 yrs 40%
- Posterior column syndrome: Ambulation usually possible unless proprioception involved, which then makes it difficult
- Brown Sequard syndrome: 90% will ambulate
- Post-traumatic spinal cord syndrome (aka post-traumatic progressive myelopathy)
  ○ ≤ 2% post-traumatic SCI
  ○ Spinothalamic symptoms (i.e., pain, sensory loss)

○ Cysts may occur above or below original cord lesion
○ Cysts not related to site or severity of original lesion
○ May occur months to years following SCI

Treatment
- Surgical → stabilization
- Medical
  ○ Limit damaging processes → methylprednisolone bolus followed by infusion is standard
  ○ Respiratory support
  ○ Spinal shock
    ■ Loss of sympathetic tone below injury level
    ■ Unopposed vagal tone → asystole → atropine
  ○ Autonomic hyperreflexia
    ■ Occurs 85% patients with transection above T5
    ■ Lower blood pressure, sit patient upright to reduce intracranial pressures
    ■ Remove inciting factor, most often distended bladder; also bowel distension, renal stones, sexual activity, numerous other stimuli
  ○ Neurogenic bladder: Need bladder drainage practical for patient yet minimizes potential complications
    ■ Usually intermittent catheterization
- Chronic care best approached from rehabilitation team approach
  ○ Rehab specialist, physical/occupational therapy, pain management, psychosocial support
- Vascular endothelial growth factor improves functional outcome & ↓ secondary degeneration in experimental rat SCI

DIAGNOSTIC CHECKLIST

Consider
- Screening MRI for all symptomatic SCI

Image Interpretation Pearls
- Sagittal STIR key to diagnose marrow edema & ligamentous injury

SELECTED REFERENCES

1. Widenfalk J et al: Vascular endothelial growth factor improves functional outcome and decreases secondary degeneration in experimental spinal cord contusion injury. Neuroscience. 120(4):951-60, 2003
2. Collignon F et al: Acute traumatic central cord syndrome: magnetic resonance imaging and clinical observations. J Neurosurg. 96(1 Suppl):29-33, 2002
3. Katzberg RW et al: Acute cervical spine injuries: prospective MR imaging assessment at a level 1 trauma center. Radiology. 213(1):203-12, 1999
4. Flanders AE et al: The relationship between the functional abilities of patients with cervical spinal cord injury and the severity of damage revealed by MR imaging. AJNR Am J Neuroradiol. 20(5):926-34, 1999
5. Lipper MH et al: Brown-Sequard syndrome of the cervical spinal cord after chiropractic manipulation. AJNR Am J Neuroradiol. 19(7):1349-52, 1998
6. Quencer RM et al: Acute traumatic central cord syndrome: MRI-pathological correlations. Neuroradiology. 34(2):85-94, 1992

IMAGE GALLERY

Typical

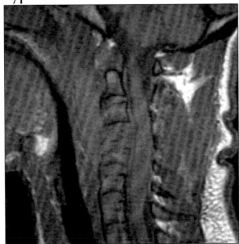 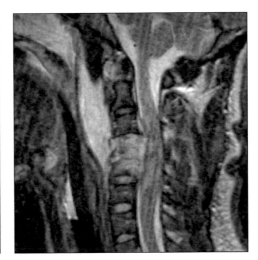

(Left) Sagittal T1WI MR demonstrates isointense cord contusion following multilevel cervical spine fractures including C4 burst. Note prevertebral soft tissue swelling. *(Right)* Sagittal T2WI MR shows hyperintense cord contusion with several hypointense hemorrhagic foci following multilevel cervical spine fractures including C4 burst. Note prevertebral soft tissue swelling.

Typical

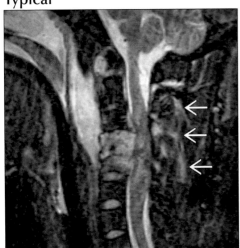 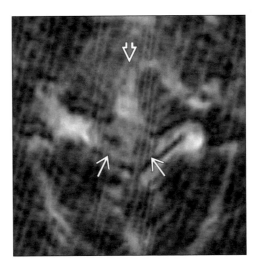

(Left) Sagittal STIR MR confirms hyperintense cord contusion & hypointense hemorrhagic foci. STIR best images associated hyperintense interspinous & supraspinous ligamentous injury (arrows). *(Right)* Axial T2WI MR shows two hypointense hemorrhagic foci (arrows) within cord contusion. Note horizontal cleft within vertebral body (open arrow), characteristic for burst fracture.

Typical

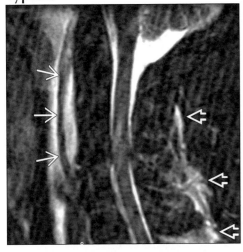 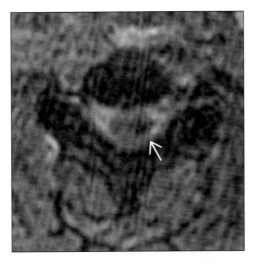

(Left) Sagittal STIR MR demonstrates hyperintense cord contusion with a suggestion of hypointense hemorrhage. Also note prevertebral (arrows) & ligamentous (open arrows) injuries. *(Right)* Axial T2* GRE MR confirms hemorrhage (arrow) within cord contusion.

CENTRAL SPINAL CORD SYNDROME

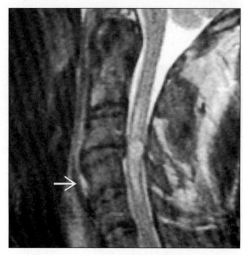

Sagittal T2WI MR shows flame-shaped high signal in cord centered on slight C3-4 disc protrusion. Note high signal in anterior longitudinal ligament (arrow).

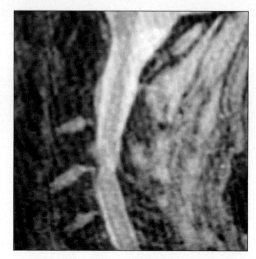

Sagittal T2* GRE MR of patient with cord edema seen on T2WI shows no evidence of hemorrhage in the cord; note poor sensitivity of GRE image to edema.

TERMINOLOGY

Abbreviations and Synonyms
- Acute traumatic central cord syndrome (ATCCS)
- Spinal cord injury without radiographic abnormality (SCIWORA)
- Synonyms
  - Spinal cord concussion
  - Transient traumatic cord apraxia

Definitions
- Acute post-traumatic paralysis affecting arms > legs, with bladder dysfunction, variable sensory loss

IMAGING FINDINGS

General Features
- Best diagnostic clue: T2WI shows high signal in cord
- Location: Predominates at C3-4 through C5-6 levels

Radiographic Findings
- Radiography
  - Typically negative
  - May show spondylosis or congenitally diminished canal diameter
- Myelography
  - Done only if no MRI available
  - Tight canal

CT Findings
- NECT: May show disc protrusion or extrusion
- Bone CT
  - Spondylosis or congenital canal stenosis
  - Typically no fracture
  - May be normal

MR Findings
- T1WI: Slight cord swelling
- T2WI
  - High signal
  - Typically C3-4 and/or C5-6 level
  - Disc protrusion or extrusion
  - Narrow canal
- T2* GRE
  - High intraparenchymal cord signal
  - Low signal indicates hemorrhage, and predicts permanent injury (not central cord syndrome)
  - Spondylosis exaggerated
  - Loss of CSF signal (narrow canal and/or swollen cord)

Imaging Recommendations
- MRI in any case of post-traumatic cord signs is mandatory

DDx: Acute Myelopathy

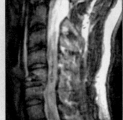

Cord Blood, C5 Fx

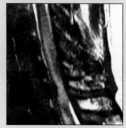

Transverse Myelitis

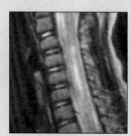

Cord Infarct

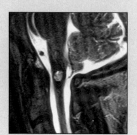

Cavernous Angioma

CENTRAL SPINAL CORD SYNDROME

Key Facts

Terminology
- Acute traumatic central cord syndrome (ATCCS)
- Acute posttraumatic paralysis affecting arms > legs, with bladder dysfunction, variable sensory loss

Imaging Findings
- Best diagnostic clue: T2WI shows high signal in cord
- Location: Predominates at C3-4 through C5-6 levels

Top Differential Diagnoses
- Cord contusion

Pathology
- Hyperextension force
- Compression of cervical cord by buckling of ligamenta flava
- With pre-existing canal narrowing

- Spur, disc or ligamentous ossification predispose
- May have normal canal
- Most often seen in young athletes
- Primary injury to lateral corticospinal tract with loss of axons; predominantly white matter injury
- No hemorrhage
- Central grey intact in acute, reversible cases

Clinical Issues
- Complete resolution to slight residual weakness and spasticity
- Cord compression or extensive edema on MRI indicate worse prognosis
- In general, conservative therapy produces equal outcomes to surgical intervention

DIFFERENTIAL DIAGNOSIS

Cord contusion
- Generally much slower recovery
- Greater residual deficit
- Swollen edematous cord on MRI with minimal blood

Cord hematoma
- No or little recovery long term
- Low signal from blood on T2WI and GRE

Spinal cord infarct
- No history of trauma

Transverse myelitis
- Subacute evolution rather than immediate traumatic onset

Cavernous angioma
- Incidental but striking finding in patient with minor trauma

PATHOLOGY

General Features
- General path comments
  - Spectrum of changes seen in experimental models
  - Cord may be normal: Kinetic energy reversibly blocks impulse transmission
  - May see slight edema
  - Axonal stretching analogous to "shear injury" in brain
  - Damage predominates in lateral corticospinal tracts
- Etiology
  - Hyperextension force
  - Compression of cervical cord by buckling of ligamenta flava
    - With pre-existing canal narrowing
  - Spur, disc or ligamentous ossification predispose
  - May have normal canal
  - Most often seen in young athletes
- Epidemiology

  - One study estimated that 1.3 of every 10,000 US football players sustained it
  - Up to 25% of traumatic paralysis associated with restricted canal
- Associated abnormalities
  - Spinal stenosis
  - Disc protrusion or extrusion

Gross Pathologic & Surgical Features
- Cord swelling or compression

Microscopic Features
- Primary injury to lateral corticospinal tract with loss of axons; predominantly white matter injury
- No hemorrhage
- Central grey intact in acute, reversible cases
- Wallerian degeneration distal to epicenter of injury
- Minimal degeneration within ventral corticospinal tract
- Neuronal loss in regions supplying hand musculature in cases of chronic injury

Staging, Grading or Classification Criteria
- Spinal cord concussion
  - Completely reversible
  - Seen most often in athletes
  - Functional rather than mechanical interruption of neuronal activity
  - Cord normal on MRI
- Central cord syndrome if cord shows edema as high signal on T2WI
- Cord contusion (not central cord syndrome) if blood in cord on MRI

CLINICAL ISSUES

Presentation
- Most common signs/symptoms
  - Acute posttraumatic arm weakness, especially hands, with bladder dysfunction
  - Other signs/symptoms
    - Varying degrees of leg weakness
    - Variable sensory loss

- Leg spasticity as residual
- Clinical profile: Post-traumatic cord signs in patient with underlying congenital or acquired spinal stenosis
- Variability of clinical post-traumatic cord syndromes which resolve to considerable degree within hours to days
  - Anterior cervical cord syndrome
    - Immediate complete paralysis, altered sensation
    - Preserved vibratory/positional sense
  - Posterior cervical cord syndrome
    - Pain and paresthesias in neck, upper arms and trunk
    - Symmetric and burning sensation
    - May have mild paresis of arms

Demographics
- Age: Children typically show some abnormality on radiographs, adults more often exhibit spinal cord injury without radiographic abnormality
- Gender: No differences
- Ethnicity: Asians have higher incidence of ossified posterior longitudinal ligament as predisposition

Natural History & Prognosis
- Complete resolution to slight residual weakness and spasticity
- Generally complete or near complete reversal of the acute paralysis
- Prognosis is age related
  - Most under age of fifty recover completely
  - Those over age of seventy usually have significant residual deficits
- Cord compression or extensive edema on MRI indicate worse prognosis

Treatment
- Initial stabilization if spinal instability suspected
- Decompression if focal stenosis from disc or focal spur
- Steroid therapy in first 24 hours may have a role
- In general, conservative therapy produces equal outcomes to surgical intervention

DIAGNOSTIC CHECKLIST

Consider
- Any cord signs after trauma are indication for MRI

Image Interpretation Pearls
- Hemorrhage on MRI in cord heralds lack of recovery

SELECTED REFERENCES

1. Hendey GW et al: Spinal cord injury without radiographic abnormality: results of the National Emergency X-Radiography Utilization Study in blunt cervical trauma. J Trauma. 53(1):1-4, 2002
2. Collignon F et al: Acute traumatic central cord syndrome: magnetic resonance imaging and clinical observations. J Neurosurg. 96(1 Suppl):29-33, 2002
3. Dai L: Magnetic resonance imaging of acute central cord syndrome: correlation with prognosis. Chin Med Sci J. 16(2):107-10, 2001
4. Kothari P et al: Injury to the spinal cord without radiological abnormality (SCIWORA) in adults. J Bone Joint Surg Br. 82(7):1034-7, 2000
5. Jimenez O et al: A histopathological analysis of the human cervical spinal cord in patients with acute traumatic central cord syndrome. Spinal Cord. 38(9):532-7, 2000
6. Newey ML et al: The long-term outcome after central cord syndrome: a study of the natural history. J Bone Joint Surg Br. 82(6):851-5, 2000
7. An HS: Cervical Spine trauma. Spine 23:2713-29, 1998
8. Chen TY et al: Efficacy of surgical treatment in traumatic central cord syndrome. Surg Neurol. 48(5):435-40; discussion 441, 1997
9. Massaro F et al: Acute traumatic central cord syndrome. Acta Neurol (Napoli). 15(2):97-105, 1993
10. Martin D et al: MRI-pathological correlations in acute traumatic central cord syndrome: case report. Neuroradiology. 34(4):262-6, 1992
11. Quencer RM et al: Acute traumatic central cord syndrome: MRI-pathological correlations. Neuroradiology. 34(2):85-94, 1992
12. Zwimpfer TJ et al: Spinal cord concussion. J Neurosurg 72:894-900, 1990
13. Riviello JJ Jr et al: Delayed cervical central cord syndrome after trivial trauma. Pediatr Emerg Care. 6(2):113-7, 1990
14. Fox JL et al: Central spinal cord injury: magnetic resonance imaging confirmation and operative considerations. Neurosurgery. 22(2):340-7, 1988
15. Torg JS et al: Neurapraxia of the cervical spinal cord with transient quadriplegia. J Bone Joint Surg (Am)68:1354-70, 1986
16. Merriam WF et al: A reappraisal of acute traumatic central cord syndrome. J Bone Joint Surg Br. 68(5):708-13, 1986

Typical

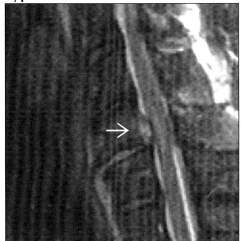
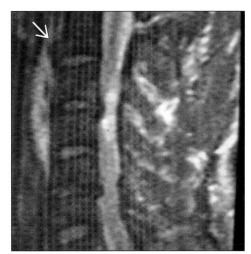

(Left) Sagittal T2WI MR shows cord edema due to disc herniation (arrow), note signal increase of anterior longitudinal ligament from hyperextension tear: Central cord syndrome. *(Right)* Sagittal T2WI MR shows canal stenosis, slight C3-4 disc protrusion, high signal in cord, and prominent prevertebral edema; note also inferior C2 fracture (arrow).

Typical

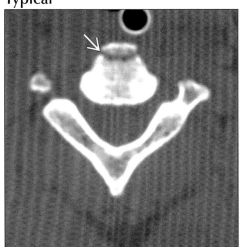
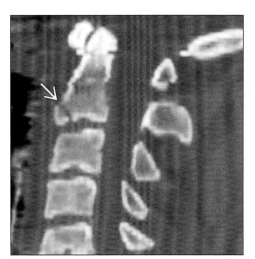

(Left) Axial bone CT shows C2 fracture in anteroinferior edge of the vertebral body (arrow) caused by surfing injury in patient with central cord syndrome. *(Right)* Sagittal bone CT reformation shows C2 fracture of anteroinferior vertebral body to better advantage (arrow) than did axial slices in this patient with central cord syndrome after a surfing injury.

Typical

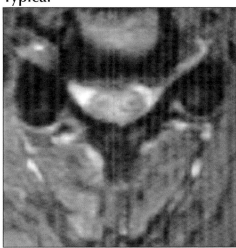
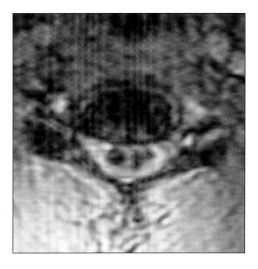

(Left) Axial T2* GRE MR shows high signal in cord in patient whose mild disc protrusion resulted in canal stenosis, central cord syndrome. *(Right)* Axial T2* GRE MR shows low signal from hemorrhage (due to magnetic susceptibility effects) in cord: Irreversible paralysis following spinal trauma.

SPINAL CORD HERNIATION

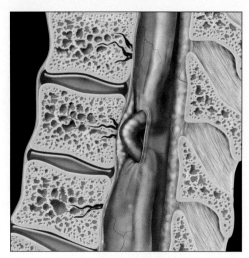

Sagittal graphic shows focal dural defect in thoracic spine allowing cord herniation. Note distinctive cord kink.

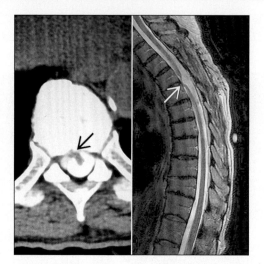

Axial CECT myelogram (L) and sagittal T2WI MR (R) show cord distortion, anterior displacement into extradural cavity (arrows), with focal expansion of dorsal sac.

TERMINOLOGY

Abbreviations and Synonyms
- Ventral cord herniation

Definitions
- Herniation of spinal cord through defect in dura of ventral canal

IMAGING FINDINGS

General Features
- Best diagnostic clue: Focal anterior displacement of cord with expansion of dorsal subarachnoid space
- Location: Typically in mid-thoracic spine
- Morphology: S-shaped or kinked, thinned cord

Radiographic Findings
- Myelography: Focal deformity of cord and subarachnoid space

MR Findings
- T1WI
  - Focal cord deformity
  - Cord displaced anteriorly against posterior edge of vertebral body
  - Increased dorsal subarachnoid sac
- T2WI
  - Focal dorsal spinal fluid pocket
  - Focal anterior cord displacement
  - Kink or s-shaped cord
- T2* GRE: Same as T2WI
- T1 C+: Excludes extramedullary mass

Other Modality Findings
- CT with intrathecal contrast (post-myelography)
  - Anterior displacement of cord
  - Focal cord deformity at level of displacement
  - Expanded dorsal subarachnoid space
  - May see secondary collection of contrast in extradural sac

Imaging Recommendations
- Best imaging tool: CT post-myelography
- Protocol advice
  - Thin-section slices
  - Sagittal reformations
  - Delayed scan to see filling of extradural sac

DIFFERENTIAL DIAGNOSIS

Arachnoid cyst
- Can produce identical findings if dorsal
- Usually lacks cord deformity
- Can accompany herniation (due to adhesions)

DDx: Focal Thecal Sac Deformities

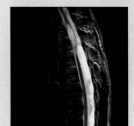

Arachnoid Cyst

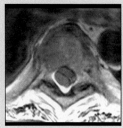

Epidural Bleed

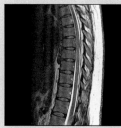

Epidural Abscess

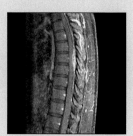

Epidural Abscess

Key Facts

Terminology
- Ventral cord herniation
- Herniation of spinal cord through defect in dura of ventral canal

Imaging Findings
- Best diagnostic clue: Focal anterior displacement of cord with expansion of dorsal subarachnoid space
- Location: Typically in mid-thoracic spine
- Focal cord deformity
- Cord displaced anteriorly against posterior edge of vertebral body
- Increased dorsal subarachnoid sac
- May see secondary collection of contrast in extradural sac
- Best imaging tool: CT post-myelography

Top Differential Diagnoses
- Arachnoid cyst
- Adhesions
- Epidural hematoma
- Epidural empyema

Pathology
- General path comments: Defect or diverticulum in ventral dural sheet with cord herniation into it
- Several proposed mechanisms ⇒
- Congenital weakening of ventral dural fibers
- Damage to ventral dura by disc herniation or other mechanism
- Abnormal adhesion of cord to anterior dural sleeve progressively wears down dura leading to herniation

---

Adhesions
- Simulates appearance of arachnoid cyst
- Cord adhesions usually present with herniation

Epidural hematoma
- Can produce focal cord displacement
- If subacute, will show high signal on T1WI
- Usually more diffuse

Epidural empyema
- Usually more extensive
- T1WI show enhancement

PATHOLOGY

General Features
- General path comments: Defect or diverticulum in ventral dural sheet with cord herniation into it
- Etiology
  - Several proposed mechanisms ⇒
    - Congenital weakening of ventral dural fibers
    - Damage to ventral dura by disc herniation or other mechanism
    - Abnormal adhesion of cord to anterior dural sleeve progressively wears down dura leading to herniation
    - Large nerve sleeve diverticulum
- Epidemiology: Rare
- Associated abnormalities: Arachnoid cyst

Gross Pathologic & Surgical Features
- Ventral dural defect or diverticulum
- Cord herniated into defect
- Adhesions
- May see arachnoid cyst

CLINICAL ISSUES

Presentation
- Most common signs/symptoms
  - Chronic leg pain

  - Leg weakness
  - Other signs/symptoms
    - Brown-Sequard syndrome
    - Spasticity
    - Sphincter dysfunction
- Clinical profile: Unexplained chronic, progressive leg pain with onset of myelopathy

Demographics
- Age: Most reported cases in middle-aged individuals
- Gender: No preference
- Ethnicity: All

Natural History & Prognosis
- Progressive neurologic symptoms and signs until diagnosis made

Treatment
- Options, risks, complications
  - Surgery
    - Repair of dural defect
    - Repositioning of cord
    - Excision of arachnoid cyst if present
    - Enlargement of dural defect with surgery, freeing cord also successful
- Symptoms improve or resolve after successful surgery

DIAGNOSTIC CHECKLIST

Consider
- Any focal cord displacement or subarachnoid space deformity as possible herniation
- Rare, but important to recognize sice represents curable cause of myelopathy

Image Interpretation Pearls
- Delayed filling of extradural sac on CT after myelography with focal filling defect contiguous with cord = herniation

SPINAL CORD HERNIATION

SELECTED REFERENCES

1. Sasaoka R et al: Idiopathic spinal cord herniation in the thoracic spine as a cause of intractable leg pain: case report and review of the literature. J Spinal Disord Tech. 16(3):288-94, 2003

2. Barbagallo GM et al: Thoracic idiopathic spinal cord herniation at the vertebral body level: a subgroup with a poor prognosis? Case reports and review of the literature. J Neurosurg. 97(3 Suppl):369-74, 2002

3. Miyaguchi M et al: Idiopathic spinal cord herniation associated with intervertebral disc extrusion: a case report and review of the literature. Spine. 26(9):1090-4, 2001

4. Aizawa T et al: Idiopathic herniation of the thoracic spinal cord: report of three cases. Spine. 26(20):E488-91, 2001

5. Eguchi T et al: Spontaneous thoracic spinal cord herniation--case report. Neurol Med Chir (Tokyo). 41(10):508-12, 2001

6. Watanabe M et al: Surgical management of idiopathic spinal cord herniation: a review of nine cases treated by the enlargement of the dural defect. J Neurosurg. 95(2 Suppl):169-72, 2001

7. Pereira P et al: Idiopathic spinal cord herniation: case report and literature review. Acta Neurochir (Wien). 143(4):401-6, 2001

8. Wada E et al: Idiopathic spinal cord herniation: report of three cases and review of the literature. Spine. 25(15):1984-8, 2000

9. Ewald C et al: Progressive spontaneous herniation of the thoracic spinal cord: case report. Neurosurgery. 46(2):493-5; discussion 495-6, 2000

10. Tekkok IH: Spontaneous spinal cord herniation: case report and review of the literature. Neurosurgery. 46(2):485-91; discussion 491-2, 2000

11. Marshman LA et al: Idiopathic spinal cord herniation: case report and review of the literature. Neurosurgery. 44(5):1129-33, 1999

12. Vallee B et al: Ventral transdural herniation of the thoracic spinal cord: surgical treatment in four cases and review of literature. Acta Neurochir (Wien). 141(9):907-13, 1999

13. Dix JE et al: Spontaneous thoracic spinal cord herniation through an anterior dural defect. AJNR Am J Neuroradiol. 19(7):1345-8, 1998

14. Henry A et al: Tethered thoracic cord resulting from spinal cord herniation. Arch Phys Med Rehabil. 78(5):530-3, 1997

15. Baur A et al: Imaging findings in patients with ventral dural defects and herniation of neural tissue. Eur Radiol. 7(8):1259-63, 1997

16. Sioutos P et al: Spontaneous thoracic spinal cord herniation. A case report. Spine. 21(14):1710-3, 1996

17. Kumar R et al: Herniation of the spinal cord. Case report. J Neurosurg. 82(1):131-6, 1995

SPINAL CORD HERNIATION

IMAGE GALLERY

Typical

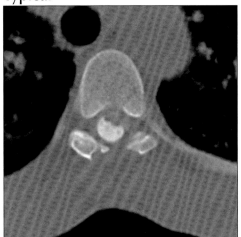

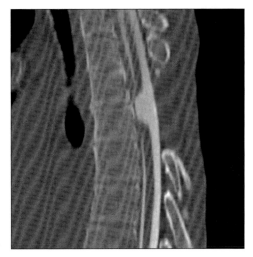

(Left) Axial CECT *(post-myelography)* shows expanded dorsal subarachnoid sac with distorted cord displaced against the back of vertebral body. *(Right)* Sagittal CECT *(post-myelography)* shows kink of thoracic cord & anterior adhesion to back of vertebral body. Expanded dorsal thecal sac mimics arachnoid cyst.

Typical

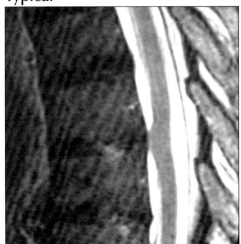

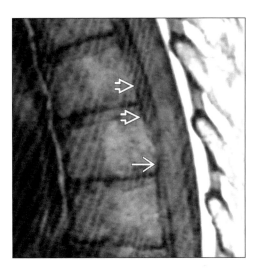

(Left) Sagittal T2WI MR depicts subtle s-shaped cord alteration with contact of cord apex to vertebral body. Surgery verified ventral dural defect and herniation in patient with leg weakness. *(Right)* Sagittal T1WI MR shows s-shaped, anteriorly displaced cord *(arrow)*. Note suggestion of second, extradural sac *(open arrows)*. Post-myelographic CT verified cord herniation, as did surgery.

Typical

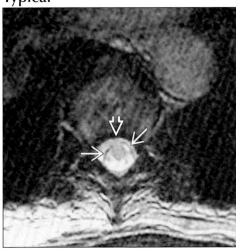

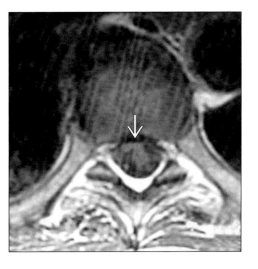

(Left) Axial T2WI MR shows defect in normal dural *(arrows)* sac, with extension of cord *(open arrow)* through it. *(Right)* Axial T1WI MR shows distorted, anteriorly displaced cord. Surgery confirmed the dural defect in patient with slowly progressive leg weakness.

LUMBAR FRACTURE WITH DURAL TEAR

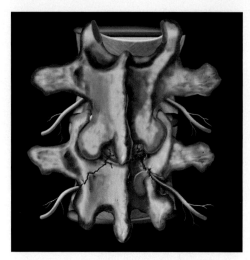

Posterior graphic shows bilateral lumbar posterior element fractures. Right fracture has caused dural tear, allowing nerve root entrapment with CSF leak.

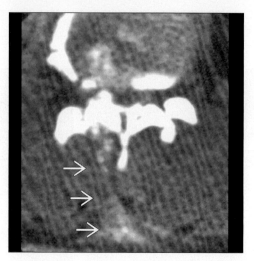

Axial bone CT myelogram shows facet joint subluxation, fracture fragments, with leak of intrathecal dye (arrows). Stabilization surgery verified suspected herniated nerve roots.

TERMINOLOGY

Abbreviations and Synonyms
- Traumatic dural laceration with nerve root (NR) entrapment

Definitions
- Vertebral body (vb) compression fracture (typically "burst" fracture) & laminar fracture with associated dural tear

IMAGING FINDINGS

General Features
- Best diagnostic clue: Wedged vb on lateral view with focal kyphosis, widened pedicles on AP view with vertical fracture through laminae
- Location: Thoracic or lumbar vb

Radiographic Findings
- Radiography: Burst Fx of vb, with widened pedicles on ap view, may see Fx through lamina on lateral view

CT Findings
- Bone CT
  - Comminuted Fx of vb involving endplates, lamina, +/- retropulsion

  - Sagittal reformation shows vb compression, slight listhesis

MR Findings
- T1WI: Compressed vb with low signal within
- T2WI: Compressed vb with high signal, may see increased signal in retrospinal soft tissues
- STIR: Accentuates high signal in vb and retrospinal tissues

Other Modality Findings
- CT myelography
  - Documents site of leakage

Imaging Recommendations
- Must obtain CT once plain film findings suggest fracture
  - Thin-section (1-3 mm) cuts mandatory, reformations very helpful
  - Intrathecal dye necessary to demonstrate dural tear
  - Dural tear warns surgeon to look for NR if posterior fusion planned

DIFFERENTIAL DIAGNOSIS

Other VB fractures without dural tear
- Isolated anterior column Fx unlikely to produce dural tear

DDx: Fractures without CSF Leak

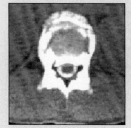

Burst Fracture

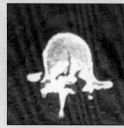

Arch, Vb Fracture

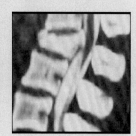

Fx, Retropulsion

LUMBAR FRACTURE WITH DURAL TEAR

Key Facts

Terminology

- Traumatic dural laceration with nerve root (NR) entrapment

Imaging Findings

- Intrathecal dye necessary to demonstrate dural tear
- Dural tear warns surgeon to look for NR if posterior fusion planned

Pathology

- CSF leak seen (if looked for) in up to 60% of thoracolumbar Fxs
- When neurological deficit present with lumbar Fx, 25% have dural tear
- L3 burst and laminar fx particularly common level to demonstrate CSF leak, NR herniation (65% in one series)

PATHOLOGY

General Features

- General path comments
  - Disruption of vb, arch
  - Dural tear, arch fracture allow NR to escape confines of canal, become entrapped
- Etiology: Severe axial force on lumbar region when it is rigid or extended
- Epidemiology
  - CSF leak seen (if looked for) in up to 60% of thoracolumbar Fxs
  - When neurological deficit present with lumbar Fx, 25% have dural tear
    - L3 burst and laminar fx particularly common level to demonstrate CSF leak, NR herniation (65% in one series)

Gross Pathologic & Surgical Features

- Nerve roots posterior to or within fractured lamina

CLINICAL ISSUES

Presentation

- Most common signs/symptoms: Back pain, radiculopathy

Natural History & Prognosis

- Depends on presence and degree of neurologic compromise
- Good if no neurologic damage, and stabilization achieved
- Accelerated degenerative disease may be seen

Treatment

- Treatment is aimed at immobilization, fixation (rods) and closing dura
  - If neurologic signs present, care taken not to transect NR on approach

DIAGNOSTIC CHECKLIST

Consider

- CT with intrathecal contrast injection for evaluating any patient with neurological signs & burst fracture prior to surgery

Image Interpretation Pearls

- Posterior VB fragment displaced into canal may be cause of anterior dural tear

SELECTED REFERENCES

1. Aydinli U et al: Dural tears in lumbar burst fractures with greenstick lamina fractures. Spine. 26(18):E410-5, 2001
2. Carl AL et al: Anterior dural laceration caused by thoracolumbar and lumbar burst fractures. J Spinal Disord. 13(5):399-403, 2000
3. Pau A et al: Can lacerations of the thoraco-lumbar dura be predicted on the basis of radiological patterns of the spinal fractures? Acta Neurochir (Wien). 129(3-4):186-7, 1994
4. Silvestro C et al: On the predictive value of radiological signs for the presence of dural lacerations related to fractures of the lower thoracic or lumbar spine. J Spinal Disord. 4(1):49-53, 1991
5. Suh PB: Dural laceration occurring with burst fractures and associated laminar fractures. J Bone Joint Surg Am. 73(2):314, 1991
6. Denis F et al: Diagnosis and treatment of cauda equina entrapment in the vertical lamina fracture of lumbar burst fractures. Spine. 16(8 Suppl):S433-9, 1991
7. Cammisa FP Jr et al: Dural laceration occurring with burst fractures and associated laminar fractures. J Bone Joint Surg Am. 71(7):1044-52, 1989
8. Brant-Zawadzki M et al: High resolution CT of thoracolumbar fractures. AJR Am J Roentgenol. 138(4):699-704, 1982

IMAGE GALLERY

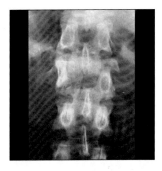 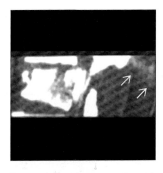

(Left) Anteroposterior radiography demonstrates "burst" L1 Fx with widened pedicles. CT myelography demonstrated CSF leak prior to stabilization surgery where suspected nerve root herniation was verified. *(Right)* Sagittal bone CT myelogram reformation shows comminuted fracture and leak of contrast (arrows) prior to surgical fixation which verified herniated nerve roots.

EPIDURAL-SUBDURAL HEMATOMA

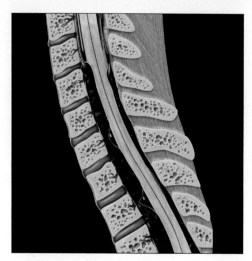

Sagittal graphic of cervico-thoracic junction shows extensive dorsal epidural & ventral subdural hemorrhage with cord compression.

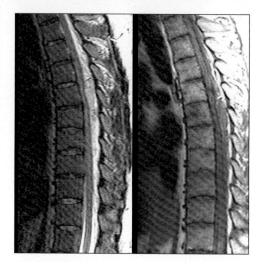

Sagittal T2WI MR (L) and T1WI MR (R) show lobulated collections pushing cord anteriorly. Patient had acute pain and leg weakness after minor exertion.

TERMINOLOGY

Abbreviations and Synonyms
- Intraspinal hemorrhage
  ○ Epidural hematoma (EDH)
  ○ Subdural hematoma (SDH)

Definitions
- Extravasation of blood into the epidural or subdural compartment of the spine

IMAGING FINDINGS

General Features
- Best diagnostic clue: Long segmental extra-axial mass encasing or displacing cord or cauda equina
- Location: Anywhere along spinal canal
- Size
  ○ Variable, typically multisegmental
    ■ Rarely focal, as when associated with focal fracture or disc extrusion
- Morphology: Typically fusiform, oval, or tubular

Radiographic Findings
- Myelography: Effaced or constricted subarachnoid space

CT Findings
- NECT: High density within canal
- CTA: May show arteriovenous malformation as rare cause

MR Findings
- T1WI
  ○ Hypo-, iso- or hyperintense (depending on age) eccentric, multilocular or inhomogeneous multisegmental collection
    ■ May conform symmetrically to subdural space cinching the CSF space if in subdural compartment
- T2WI: Long mass in extraaxial compartment with inhomogeneous low (if acute), or high signal (if subacute) intensity features
- PD/Intermediate: Iso- to high signal of long fusiform or oval mass in epidural space
- T2* GRE: Accentuates low signal of tubular, multisegmental extra-axial collection
- T1 C+: Marginal enhancement of collection

Angiographic Findings
- Conventional
  ○ Usually negative when searching for source
    ■ Rarely, may show AVM or vascular tumor as source

DDx: Extra-Axial Collections

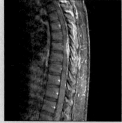
Epidural Abscess

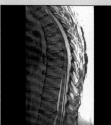
Lipomatosis

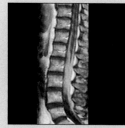
Tumor Spread

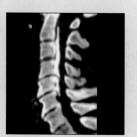
OPLL

EPIDURAL-SUBDURAL HEMATOMA

Key Facts

Terminology
- Epidural hematoma (EDH)
- Subdural hematoma (SDH)
- Extravasation of blood into the epidural or subdural compartment of the spine

Imaging Findings
- Best diagnostic clue: Long segmental extra-axial mass encasing or displacing cord or cauda equina
- Hypo-, iso- or hyperintense (depending on age) eccentric, multilocular or inhomogeneous multisegmental collection
- May conform symmetrically to subdural space cinching the CSF space if in subdural compartment

- T2WI: Long mass in extraaxial compartment with inhomogeneous low (if acute), or high signal (if subacute) intensity features

Top Differential Diagnoses
- Epidural abscess/empyema
- Epidural lipomatosis
- Epidural tumor

Pathology
- Minor exertion, e.g., sit-ups with Valsalva
- Therapeutic anticoagulation
- Instrumentation

Clinical Issues
- Intense, knife-like pain
- Extremity weakness

Imaging Recommendations
- Best imaging tool: MR, with T1WI, T2WI, multiple planes
- Protocol advice: Fat-saturation helps exclude lipomatosis as cause, outlines collection to better advantage

DIFFERENTIAL DIAGNOSIS

Epidural abscess/empyema
- Usually vivid enhancement
- Typically more focal, one or two segments
- Many have associated osteomyelitis or paraspinous infection
- Patient has constitutional signs; fever, pain, chills

Epidural lipomatosis
- Diffuse multisegmental epidural, almost always dorsal, mass
- Signal intensity matches fat on all sequences
- Fat saturation nulls signal
- Clinical picture of obesity or metabolic disturbance
  ○ Steroid use
  ○ Cushing syndrome
- Slow, as opposed to acute, onset of weakness

Epidural tumor
- Typically quite focal
- Adjacent bone often involved
- Lymphoma may simulate EDH
- Subdural (leptomeningeal) spread is isointense, enhances vividly

Extramedullary hematopoiesis
- Multifocal lobulated paravertebral & epidural masses
- Chronic anemia

Ossification (including marrow) of posterior longitudinal ligament
- Ventral location
- Typically cervical
- Bone easily shown with CT, or T2WI

PATHOLOGY

General Features
- General path comments: Clot characteristics depend on compartment, age of collection
- Genetics: Inherited bleeding diatheses are predisposing factors
- Etiology
  ○ Spontaneous in 1/3
    - Pressure elevation in vertebral venous plexus
    - Minor exertion, e.g., sit-ups with Valsalva
    - Chiropractic manipulation
  ○ Therapeutic anticoagulation
    - Coumadin
    - Anti platelet agents
  ○ Instrumentation
    - Epidural anesthetic
    - Nerve block
    - Facet joint injection
    - Lumbar puncture
  ○ Vascular malformation
- Epidemiology: Rare

Gross Pathologic & Surgical Features
- Clot in various stages

CLINICAL ISSUES

Presentation
- Most common signs/symptoms
  ○ Intense, knife-like pain
    - "Coup de poignard"
  ○ Other signs/symptoms
    - Extremity weakness
    - Sphincter disturbance
- Clinical profile
  ○ Predisposing strain with Valsalva maneuver
  ○ Recent instrumentation
  ○ Bleeding diathesis
  ○ Anticoagulation/antiplatelet therapy

EPIDURAL-SUBDURAL HEMATOMA

Demographics
- Age: Majority of afflicted aged 55-70
- Gender: 2/3 men
- Ethnicity: All

Natural History & Prognosis
- 40% recover completely

Treatment
- Options, risks, complications
  - Surgical
  - Non-surgical option exists for those with minor neurological signs

DIAGNOSTIC CHECKLIST

Consider
- Contrast injection & fat-saturation for complete characterization
  - Active bleed may enhance vividly

Image Interpretation Pearls
- CT may help identify hemorrhage when MRI confusing

SELECTED REFERENCES

1. Groen RJ: Non-operative treatment of spontaneous spinal epidural hematomas: a review of the literature and a comparison with operative cases. Acta Neurochir (Wien). 146(2):103-10, 2004
2. Liao CC et al: Experience in the surgical management of spontaneous spinal epidural hematoma. J Neurosurg. 100(1 Suppl):38-45, 2004
3. Kirwan R et al: Nontraumatic acute and subacute enhancing spinal epidural hematoma mimicking a tumor in a child. Pediatr Radiol, 2004
4. Steinmetz MP et al: Successful surgical management of a case of spontaneous epidural hematoma of the spine during pregnancy. Spine J. 3(6):539-42, 2003
5. Uribe J et al: Delayed postoperative spinal epidural hematomas. Spine J. 3(2):125-9, 2003
6. Lang SA et al: Spinal epidural hematoma and epidural analgesia. Can J Anaesth. 50(4):422-3, 2003
7. Chang FC et al: Contrast enhancement patterns of acute spinal epidural hematomas: a report of two cases. AJNR Am J Neuroradiol. 24(3):366-9, 2003
8. Muthukumar N: Chronic spontaneous spinal epidural hematoma -- a rare cause of cervical myelopathy. Eur Spine J. 12(1):100-3, 2003
9. Kreppel D et al: Spinal hematoma: a literature survey with meta-analysis of 613 patients. Neurosurg Rev. 26(1):1-49, 2003
10. Houten JK et al: Paraplegia after lumbosacral nerve root block: report of three cases. Spine J. 2(1):70-5, 2002
11. Clark MA et al: Spinal epidural hematoma complicating thrombolytic therapy with tissue plasminogen activator--a case report. J Emerg Med. 23(3):247-51, 2002
12. Stoll A et al: Epidural hematoma after epidural block: implications for its use in pain management. Surg Neurol. 57(4):235-40, 2002
13. Ravid S et al: Spontaneous spinal epidural hematoma: an uncommon presentation of a rare disease. Childs Nerv Syst. 18(6-7):345-7, 2002
14. Allison EJ Jr et al: Spinal epidural haematoma as a result of warfarin/fluconazole drug interaction. Eur J Emerg Med. 9(2):175-7, 2002
15. Dardik A et al: Subdural hematoma after thoracoabdominal aortic aneurysm repair: an underreported complication of spinal fluid drainage? J Vasc Surg. 36(1):47-50, 2002
16. Sung JM et al: Acute spontaneous spinal epidural hematoma in a hemodialysis patient with a bleeding tendency. Nephron. 91(2):358-60, 2002
17. Tseng SH et al: Cervical epidural hematoma after spinal manipulation therapy: case report. J Trauma. 52(3):585-6, 2002
18. Reitman CA et al: Subdural hematoma after cervical epidural steroid injection. Spine. 27(6):E174-6, 2002
19. Uber-Zak LD et al: Neurologic complications of sit-ups associated with the Valsalva maneuver: 2 case reports. Arch Phys Med Rehabil. 83(2):278-82, 2002

EPIDURAL-SUBDURAL HEMATOMA

IMAGE GALLERY

Typical

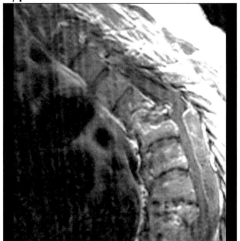 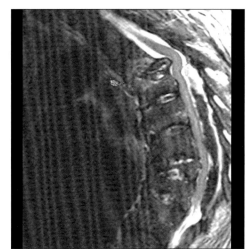

(Left) Sagittal T1 C+ MR depicts peripherally enhancing tubular collection dorsal to cord in patient with osteoporotic compression fracture following minor trauma. (Right) Sagittal T2WI MR depicts large low signal collection dorsal to cord in patient with osteoporotic fracture following minor trauma.

Typical

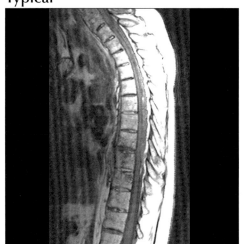 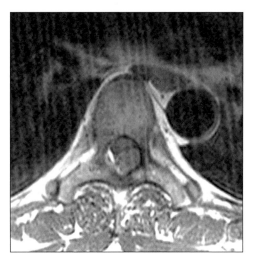

(Left) Sagittal T1WI MR shows inhomogeneous, diffuse thoracic EDH in patient with sudden onset of lancing pain, leg weakness. (Right) Axial T1WI MR shows focal isointense EDH in left dorsolateral spinal canal displacing cord anteriorly in patient with sudden onset of lancing pain & leg weakness.

Variant

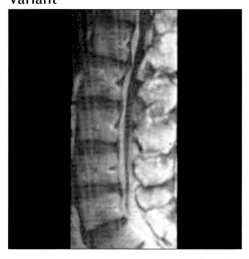 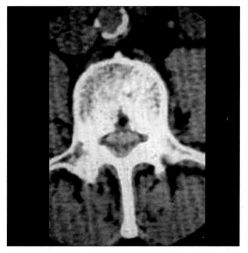

(Left) Sagittal T1WI MR shows high signal SDH conforming to subdural space in patient with platelet dysfunction, recent fall, onset of pain and leg weakness. Note cinching of CSF space. (Right) Axial NECT depicts hyperdense SDH cinching butterfly shaped low density CSF space in patient with fall, platelet dysfunction, onset of pain & leg weakness.

VERTEBRAL ARTERY DISSECTION

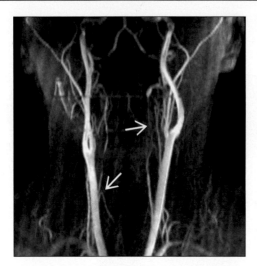

Coronal MRA shows diffuse bilateral vertebral artery narrowing due to bilateral vertebral artery dissections (arrows).

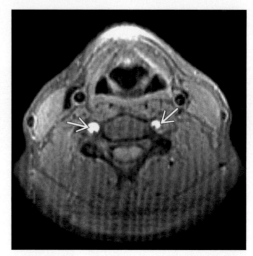

Axial T1WI MR with fat suppression shows crescentic hyperintense intramural hematomas in bilateral vertebral arteries, with significantly narrowed flow voids (arrows).

TERMINOLOGY

Abbreviations and Synonyms

- Vertebral artery dissection (VAD)

Definitions

- Hemorrhage into vessel wall with subsequent stenosis or pseudoaneurysm

IMAGING FINDINGS

General Features

- Best diagnostic clue: Intramural hematoma (IH): Crescentic T1 hyperintensity surrounding diminished flow void
- Location: Most common between C2 & C1 vertebrae
- Size: Variable length of dissection
- Morphology: IH crescentic, circumferential, or filling entire lumen on axial MRI

Radiographic Findings

- Radiography: Upper cervical subluxation may be present in children with VAD

CT Findings

- NECT
  - Subarachnoid hemorrhage (SAH) from intracranial extension of VAD: 10%
  - Brain stem and cerebellar infarcts
- CTA
  - 3D reformation
  - Tapered or abruptly occluded lumen
  - Irregular luminal surface
  - "Pearl and string" sign: Focal dilatation followed by narrowing
  - Double lumen
  - Aneurysmal dilation

MR Findings

- T1WI
  - Hyperintense IH
    - May be isointense initially
- T2WI: Hyperintense IH
- DWI: Restricted diffusion in posterior fossa infarcts
- T1 C+: IH ± enhance after intravenous gadolinium
- MRA
  - Luminal narrowing
  - Absent flow distal to dissection
  - Focal aneurysmal dilatation
  - IH intermediate signal intensity between flow-related enhancement & surrounding soft tissue
    - May be isointense to soft tissue
  - Less sensitive for vertebral artery dissection compared to conventional angiography
  - Equally sensitive for carotid artery dissection
- IH may spiral along artery
- Normal or narrowed flow void

DDx: Irregular Vertebral Lumen

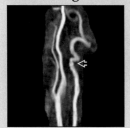

FMD

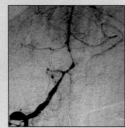

Vasospasm

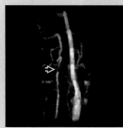

Atherosclerosis

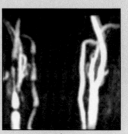

Artifacts

VERTEBRAL ARTERY DISSECTION

Key Facts

Terminology
- Hemorrhage into vessel wall with subsequent stenosis or pseudoaneurysm

Imaging Findings
- Best diagnostic clue: Intramural hematoma (IH): Crescentic T1 hyperintensity surrounding diminished flow void
- Location: Most common between C2 & C1 vertebrae
- Tapered or abruptly occluded lumen
- Irregular luminal surface
- "Pearl and string" sign: Focal dilatation followed by narrowing
- Double lumen
- Aneurysmal dilation

Pathology
- Causes 5-20% of all infarcts in young & middle-aged patients
- Associated abnormalities: Multi-vessel involvement up to two thirds of cases

Clinical Issues
- Clinical profile: Neurologic symptoms may be delayed up to one week or longer in 61% of cases
- Resolution or significant improvement of angiographic stenosis in 90% within first 2 to 3 months

Diagnostic Checklist
- Axial T1WI with fat-saturation to look for IH

- Thin, curvilinear, hypointense intimal flap

Ultrasonographic Findings
- Real Time
  - IH
  - Pseudoaneurysm
- Color Doppler
  - Narrowing and occlusion
  - Intimal flap with double lumen

Angiographic Findings
- Conventional
  - Smoothly or irregularly tapered luminal narrowing
    - Mild stenosis
    - "String" sign: Long segment of narrowing
    - Complete occlusion
  - Pseudoaneurysm: 25-35%
  - Intimal flap: 10%
  - Double lumen
  - Branch vessel occlusion from embolization
  - 4-vessel angiography required due to multi-vessel involvement

Imaging Recommendations
- CTA with 3D reformation from origin of neck vessels to vertex
- Intra- and extracranial MR angiogram if intravenous iodinated contrast contraindicated

DIFFERENTIAL DIAGNOSIS

Fibromuscular disease (FMD)
- Focal narrowing and/or dilatation
- Alternating narrowing & dilatation
- Vertebral artery involvement (7%) less common than carotid (85%)
- No intramural hematoma

Vasospasm
- Diffuse narrowing without dilatation
- May be present in intracranial dissection with associated SAH
- No intramural hematoma

Atherosclerotic disease
- Often at vertebral artery origin
- Focal or diffuse narrowing
- Lack of intramural hematoma

Artifacts
- Motion
- Adjacent hardware
  - Carotid stent

PATHOLOGY

General Features
- General path comments
  - Anatomy of AV segments
    - V1: Between origin in subclavian artery to C6 transverse processes
    - V2: Within transverse foramina from C6 to C2
    - V3: From C2 transverse foramen to before entering dura
    - V4: Intracranial; more prone to rupture due to thinner adventitia
    - Sites of greater mobility most susceptible to injury
- Genetics
  - Connective tissue disorder predisposing to spontaneous dissection
    - Present in up to 25% of patients with dissection
    - Ehlers-Danlos syndrome, Marfan syndrome, autosomal dominant polycystic kidney disease
  - Other arteriopathies
    - Fibromuscular dysplasia: 15%
    - Cystic medial necrosis
  - Hyperhomocysteinemia
- Etiology
  - Spontaneous
  - Hypertension
    - Primary or drug-induced, including over-the-counter, e.g., ephedrine
  - Major penetrating or blunt trauma
  - Cervical manipulative therapy
  - Trivial trauma

VERTEBRAL ARTERY DISSECTION

- Coughing, sneezing, roller-coaster ride
- Prolonged or sudden neck hyperextension or rotation may be precipitating factor
- Epidemiology
  - Estimate of 1 to 1.5 per 100,000
  - VAD responsible for 0.4-2.5% of all cerebrovascular accidents
    - Causes 5-20% of all infarcts in young & middle-aged patients
    - 40% of posterior fossa ischemic strokes
    - Carotid artery dissection 3-5x more common than VAD
- Associated abnormalities: Multi-vessel involvement up to two thirds of cases
- Pathophysiology
  - Intimal tear or ruptured vasa vasorum leading to intramural hematoma
    - Subintimal hematoma cases complete or partial vascular occlusion
    - Subadventitial dissection results in pseudoaneurysm: Potential rupture & SAH in intracranial VAD
  - Vascular stasis leading to emboli formation

Microscopic Features
- Hematoma within tunica media of vessel wall
  - Compressing intima, distending adventitia
  - May rupture back into vascular lumen: Double lumen
- Underlying atherosclerosis uncommon

CLINICAL ISSUES

Presentation
- Most common signs/symptoms
  - Posterior neck pain
    - Common in adults
    - Infrequent in children: 12%
  - Occipital headaches
    - 70% of patients
  - Neurologic deficits
    - Up to 85% of patients
    - Lateral medullary syndrome of Wallenberg
    - Ipsilateral Horner syndrome
    - Cerebellar signs
- Clinical profile: Neurologic symptoms may be delayed up to one week or longer in 61% of cases

Demographics
- Age
  - Mean age: 44.9 years
    - Range 16-76 years
- Gender
  - Male to female ratio
    - 6.6 to 1 in children
    - 1.3 to 1 in adults

Natural History & Prognosis
- Spontaneously healing or recanalization in most cases
- Resolution or significant improvement of angiographic stenosis in 90% within first 2 to 3 months
- Recurrent ischemic rate of 15%

- Rate of recurrent VAD: 8%
  - 50% within first month
  - 1% per year

Treatment
- May not be indicated in absence of neurologic symptoms
- Anticoagulation, unless SAH present
- Antiplatelet therapy
- If persistent ischemia, recurrent embolic events, or intracranial hemorrhage
  - Surgical ligation
  - Endovascular occlusion with coils or balloons
  - Stent-assisted angioplasty

DIAGNOSTIC CHECKLIST

Consider
- Axial T1WI with fat-saturation to look for IH

Image Interpretation Pearls
- Variable size and position of vertebral artery within transverse foramina as a normal variant on CTA

SELECTED REFERENCES

1. Cohen JE et al: Endovascular management of symptomatic vertebral artery dissection achieved using stent angioplasty and emboli protection device. Neurol Res. 25(4):418-22, 2003
2. Dziewas R et al: Cervical artery dissection--clinical features, risk factors, therapy and outcome in 126 patients. J Neurol. 250(10):1179-84, 2003
3. Sanelli PC et al: Normal variation of vertebral artery on CT angiography and its implications for diagnosis of acquired pathology. J Comput Assist Tomogr. 26(3):462-70, 2002
4. Hasan I et al: Vertebral artery dissection in children: a comprehensive review. Pediatr Neurosurg. 37(4):168-77, 2002
5. Schievink WI: Spontaneous dissection of the carotid and vertebral arteries. N Engl J Med 344:898-906, 2001
6. Nakatsuka M et al: Three-dimensional computed tomographic angiography in four patients with dissecting aneurysms of the vertebrobasilar system. Acta Neurochir (Wien). 142(9):995-1001, 2000
7. Ahmad HA et al: Cervicocerebral artery dissections. J Accid Emerg Med. 16(6):422-4, 1999
8. Barinagarrementeria F et al: Causes and mechanisms of cerebellar infarction in young patients. Stroke. 28(12):2400-4, 1997
9. Bartels E et al: Evaluation of extracranial vertebral artery dissection with duplex color-flow imaging. Stroke. 27(2):290-5, 1996
10. Provenzale JM: Dissection of the internal carotid and vertebral arteries: Imaging features. AJR 165: 1099-104, 1995
11. Schievink WI et al: Recurrent spontaneous cervical-artery dissection. N Engl J Med. 330(6):393-7, 1994
12. Levy C et al: Carotid and vertebral artery dissection: Three-dimensional time-of-flight MR angiography and MR imaging versus conventional angiography. Radiology 190:97-103, 1994
13. Hart RG et al: Cerebral infarction in young adults: a practical approach. Stroke. 14(1):110-4, 1983

IMAGE GALLERY

Typical

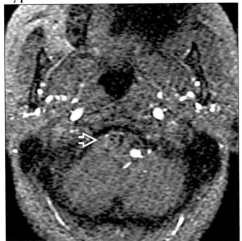 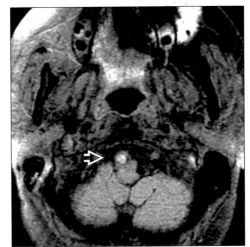

(Left) Axial MRA source image shows loss of flow related signal in distal intracranial right vertebral artery (arrow). *(Right)* Axial T1WI MR with fat suppression shows a hyperintense intramural hematoma in distal intracranial right vertebral artery (arrow).

Typical

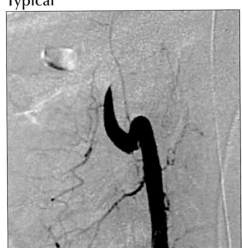 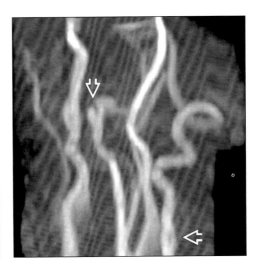

(Left) Sagittal angiography shows smoothly tapered complete occlusion in a vertebral artery. *(Right)* Coronal MRA shows subtle intimal flaps (arrows) in bilateral vertebral arteries.

Typical

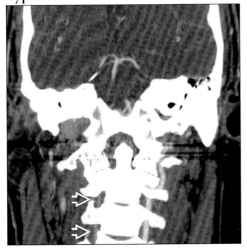 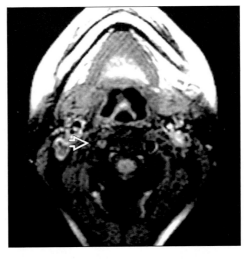

(Left) Coronal CTA shows diffusely narrowed right vertebral artery with minimal contrast in its lumen (arrows). *(Right)* Axial T1WI MR with fat suppression shows a narrowed flow void in right vertebral artery, surrounded by hyperintense intramural hematoma (arrow).

CAROTID ARTERY DISSECTION

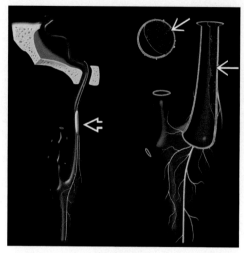

3D graphic illustrates internal carotid dissection with clot filling the false lumen (arrows). Injury of adjacent sympathetic ganglia (open arrow) can cause Horner syndrome.

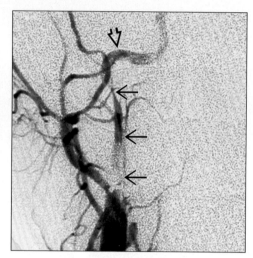

Common carotid DSA shows dissection at ICA origin as near total loss of flow & distal string sign (arrows); dissection stops at skull base without petrous extension (open arrow).

TERMINOLOGY

Abbreviations and Synonyms
- Internal carotid (ICA), common carotid (CCA)

Definitions
- Traumatic-induced injury to carotid intima resulting in blood dissecting into media creating false lumen

IMAGING FINDINGS

General Features
- Best diagnostic clue: Tapering luminal narrowing
- Location
  - ICA at or near the bifurcation is most common
  - ICA between bifurcation & base of skull
  - CCA proximal to bifurcation
  - ICA at base of skull is least common
  - Rarely extends intracranially
- Size: Extends a few centimeters
- Morphology: "Sting sign" = tapered luminal stenosis

CT Findings
- NECT: Secondary ischemia: Hypodense brain parenchyma
- CTA
  - Quick & easily accessible
  - Requires invasive contrast bolus administration

MR Findings
- T1WI
  - Eccentric crescentic thrombus within arterial wall
    - Most often hyperintense (subacute)
    - Best seen with fat-saturation technique applied
- DWI: Secondary ischemia: Restricted brain diffusion
- MRA
  - "String sign" (76%)
  - Abrupt luminal normalization upon entry into carotid canal (42%)
  - Intimal flap (29%)
  - Dissecting aneurysm: Saccular near skull base (40%)
  - Uncommon: Double lumen
  - Bilateral in 15%
  - Infrequently extends intracranially

Ultrasonographic Findings
- Duplex sonography less reliable than MRA as dissection is usually distal to region that can be seen well on sonograms
- May see echogenic intimal flap or echogenic thrombus
- Doppler waveforms may show highly resistive, obstructive pattern

Angiographic Findings
- Conventional
  - Replaced by CTA for quick trauma screening

DDx: Carotid Dissection Mimics

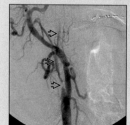

Atherosclerosis

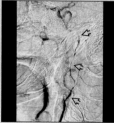

Atherosclerosis

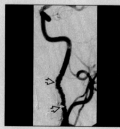

FMD

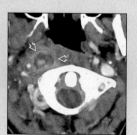

External Compression

CAROTID ARTERY DISSECTION

Key Facts

Terminology
- Traumatic-induced injury to carotid intima resulting in blood dissecting into media creating false lumen

Imaging Findings
- Best diagnostic clue: Tapering luminal narrowing
- Morphology: "Sting sign" = tapered luminal stenosis
- Best imaging tool: Neck CTA

Top Differential Diagnoses
- Atherosclerotic narrowing
- Spontaneous dissection
- External compression

Pathology
- Precise mechanism unclear; four mechanisms of craniocervical injury have been described

- High risk associations: MVA, boxing, hanging, chiropractic manipulation, coughing/sneezing
- Accounts for 0.4-2.5% of all strokes in general population but 5-20% of strokes among young patients (< 45 yrs)

Clinical Issues
- Most common symptom is unilateral anterior headache (86%)
- Many spontaneously heal in 7-30 days
- Primary therapy: Anticoagulation for 3-6 mos
- Consider endovascular treatment

Diagnostic Checklist
- Hyperintense hematoma mimics flow on routine MRA → add axial fat-saturation T1WI if dissection suspected

---

  - ○ Used to define complicated pathology, especially dissecting aneurysm
  - ○ May see slow intracranial ICA or MCA flow
- Interventional
  - ○ Stent angioplasty
    - Provides centrifugal force apposition of dissected segment to vessel wall obliterating false lumen
    - Can also provide mechanical support to serve as a scaffold for coil embolization of broadneck dissecting aneurysms
  - ○ Dissecting aneurysm therapy
    - Balloon or coil trapping → occludes parent vessel
    - Packing with coils (+/- stenting) → spares parent

Nuclear Medicine Findings
- Tc-HMPAO SPECT may show brain perfusion defects before diffusion restriction occurs

Imaging Recommendations
- Best imaging tool: Neck CTA
- Protocol advice: Add axial T1WI with fat-saturation to best image arterial wall hematoma

DIFFERENTIAL DIAGNOSIS

Atherosclerotic narrowing
- Often associated with dense calcifications
- In setting of trauma, collateralization suggests pre-existing disease & not acute dissection

Spontaneous dissection
- Cause may be unclear
- Often underlying arteriopathy such as FMD, Marfan, Ehler-Danlos, cystic medial necrosis

External compression
- Adjacent hematoma, tumor
- Often visible on trauma cervical CT

Iatrogenic dissection
- Catheter-induced dissection occurring during angiography

Vasospasm
- Catheter induced during angiography

Fibromuscular disease
- Beaded lumen in distal cervical internal carotid

PATHOLOGY

General Features
- General path comments
  - ○ An autopsy study evaluating the carotid artery in 200 consecutive MVA victims showed
    - Some degree of arterial disruption was present in nearly one-third
    - Cases with arterial disruption had dual or triple vessel involvement in 39%
    - There were large number of intimal disruptions, 44.7% of which showed extension along internal elastic lamina without breaching it
    - Tears along the media occurred in 52.6%, particularly at sites of bifurcation
    - Compound intimomedial tears occurred in almost two-thirds
    - Adventitial contusions occurred in 70%
    - Vessel wall transection occurred in 26%
    - Injuries were most common in left & right common carotid arteries, with a reduced frequency in internal & external carotid branches
- Etiology
  - ○ Blunt or penetrating trauma
    - Penetrating much more common
    - 3-5% from blunt trauma
  - ○ Precise mechanism unclear; four mechanisms of craniocervical injury have been described
    - Type 1 = direct blow to neck, proposed in ≈ 50% of cases, producing shear stresses damaging intima & media
    - Type 2 = lateral neck flexion with stretching of carotid against lateral mass of atlas & portions of second cervical vertebra

CAROTID ARTERY DISSECTION

- Type 3 = intraoral trauma (classically children running with items in their mouth)
- Type 4 = skull base Fx with intrapetrous thrombosis
  - Suggested that severe abdominal injuries may cause carotid injury by transmission of a pressure wave along the aorta
  - High risk associations: MVA, boxing, hanging, chiropractic manipulation, coughing/sneezing
  - If in setting of minimal/mild trauma, consider underlying arteriopathy: FMD, Marfan, Ehler-Danlos, cystic medial necrosis
- Epidemiology
  - Traumatic carotid dissection becoming increasingly recognized
  - Accounts for 0.4-2.5% of all strokes in general population but 5-20% of strokes among young patients (< 45 yrs)
  - Dissecting aneurysms occur in 25–35% of patients with carotid dissection
- Associated abnormalities: TIA, stroke, subarachnoid hemorrhage

Gross Pathologic & Surgical Features

- Vessel tortuosity may indicate structural wall anomaly predisposing to external mechanical injury

Microscopic Features

- Penetration of blood through intima into carotid wall
- This splits media creating a false lumen
- Dissects for varying distances
- Dissecting aneurysm = intramural hematoma expanding into adventitia
  - Distinguished from pseudoaneurysm by presence of retaining adventitial layer

CLINICAL ISSUES

Presentation

- Most common signs/symptoms
  - Most common symptom is unilateral anterior headache (86%)
  - Other signs/symptoms
    - TIA or stroke (58%)
    - Postganglionic Horner syndrome (52%)
    - Bruit (48%); neck pain (25%)
    - Amaurosis fugax (12%)
    - Lower cranial nerve deficit(s) (12%)
    - May be asymptomatic
  - Delayed neurologic event in patient with history of trauma is typical
    - Symptoms onset can range 4 hrs to 75 days
- Clinical profile
  - May not have any external sign of injury
  - May also be masked or misinterpreted in setting of associated head or neck trauma
  - Postganglionic Horner syndrome (aka oculosympathetic paresis)
    - Ptosis of upper eyelid & miosis
    - Elevation of lower eyelid (upside-down ptosis)
    - Loss of ipsilateral sweating of the face (anhidrosis)

Demographics

- Age: Most are 35-50 yrs
- Gender: All carotid dissection → M:F = 1.5:1

Natural History & Prognosis

- Prone to elaborate microemboli → TIA or stroke
  - Cerebral ischemia is most serious consequence
- Many spontaneously heal in 7-30 days
- Dissecting aneurysms remain stable, ↓ in size, or resolve, but do not ↑ in size
- Rarely result in death
- Blunt carotid artery injury has poorer prognosis
  - Associated with 20-40% mortality & permanent neurologic deficit in 40-80%

Treatment

- Primary therapy: Anticoagulation for 3-6 mos
  - In cases of residual aneurysm, persisting severe stenosis, or underlying arteriopathy, long term aspirin therapy is often used
- If embolic events occur while anticoagulated
  - Consider endovascular treatment
    - Circumvents need for blood flow occlusion required during surgical bypass
    - Long term efficacy & durability of stent placement for carotid dissection remains to be determined
  - Surgical options
    - Extracranial to intracranial bypass
    - Bypass grafting
    - Ligation of internal carotid artery for pseudoaneurysm repair
- Obtain follow-up study after a few months to evaluate healing

DIAGNOSTIC CHECKLIST

Image Interpretation Pearls

- Hyperintense hematoma mimics flow on routine MRA → add axial fat-saturation T1WI if dissection suspected

SELECTED REFERENCES

1. Payton TF et al: Traumatic dissection of the internal carotid artery. Pediatr Emerg Care. 20(1):27-9, 2004
2. Pride GL Jr et al: Stent-coil treatment of a distal internal carotid artery dissecting pseudoaneurysm on a redundant loop by use of a flexible, dedicated nitinol intracranial stent. AJNR Am J Neuroradiol. 25(2):333-7, 2004
3. Malek AM et al: Endovascular management of extracranial carotid artery dissection achieved using stent angioplasty. AJNR Am J Neuroradiol. 21(7):1280-92, 2000
4. Djouhri H et al: MR angiography for the long-term follow-up of dissecting aneurysms of the extracranial internal carotid artery. 174(4):1137-40, 2000
5. Nusbaum AO et al: Isolated vagal nerve palsy associated with a dissection of the extracranial internal carotid artery. AJNR Am J Neuroradiol. 19(10):1845-7, 1998
6. Leclerc X et al: Helical CT for the follow-up of cervical internal carotid artery dissections. AJNR Am J Neuroradiol. 19(5):831-7, 1998
7. Opeskin K: Traumatic carotid artery dissection. Am J Forensic Med Pathol. 18(3):251-7, 1997

IMAGE GALLERY

Typical

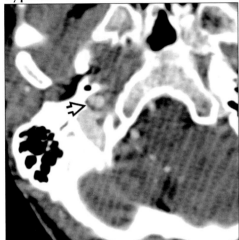
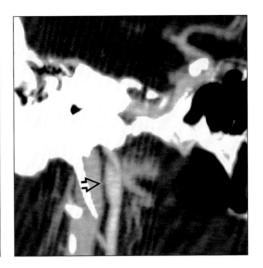

(Left) Axial CTA of internal carotid artery dissection (arrow) shows flow within both true and false lumen; dissection did not extend further into petrous portion (not shown). *(Right)* Oblique sagittal CTA reformat demonstrates a dissecting aneurysm (arrow) within distal internal carotid dissection at skull base.

Typical

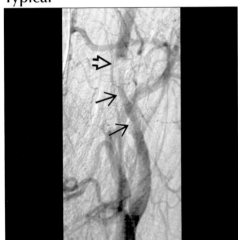
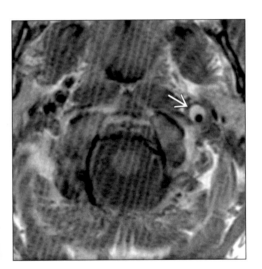

(Left) Common carotid DSA shows luminal narrowing from dissection (arrows) as well as a meniscus interface from luminal thrombus (open arrow). *(Right)* Axial T1WI MR demonstrates hyperintense clot within the false lumen of carotid dissection.

Typical

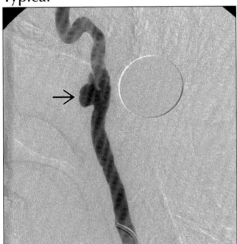
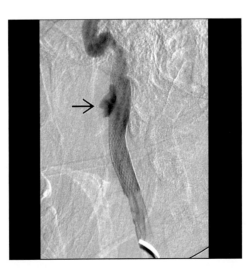

(Left) Internal carotid DSA shows contrast filling within dissecting aneurysm (arrow). *(Right)* Internal carotid DSA following stent placement reveals already decreased flow within dissecting aneurysm.

TRAUMATIC DURAL AV FISTULA

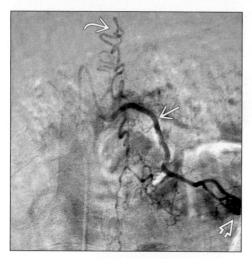

Superselected spinal DSA demonstrates single large arterial feeder (arrow), compact nidus (open arrow), & dilated venous outflow (curved arrow) of traumatic dural AVF.

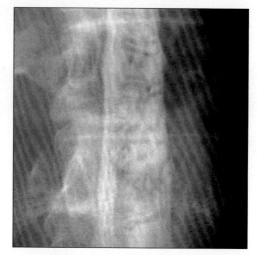

Supine radiograph obtained during myelography reveals numerous dilated veins resulting from a traumatic dural AVF.

TERMINOLOGY

Abbreviations and Synonyms
- Arteriovenous fistula (AVF)
- Traumatic dural AV fistula (tDAVF)
- Post-traumatic paraspinal (AVF)

Definitions
- Traumatic induced arteriovenous fistula

IMAGING FINDINGS

General Features
- Best diagnostic clue: DSA demonstration of AVF nidus with enlarged draining veins
- Location
  - Dural or extradural
  - Any segment; cervical > lumbar
- Size
  - Small nidus
  - May have extensive draining vein engorgement
- Morphology
  - Small, tight AVF nidus
  - Serpiginous veins

Radiographic Findings
- Myelography: Serpiginous dye column defects from enlarged perimedullary or epidural draining veins

MR Findings
- T1WI: Perimedullary or epidural flow voids from enlarged draining veins
- T2WI
  - Unlike spontaneous DAVF, often no cord enlargement/hyperintensity from congestive myelopathy
  - Perimedullary or epidural flow voids from enlarged draining veins
    - May compress cord or nerve roots
- T1 C+
  - May ↑ conspicuity of enlarged draining veins
  - Rarely demonstrates nidus
- MRA
  - Both time of flight & contrast techniques have been described
  - Performed as adjunct to MRI for helping guide DSA

Angiographic Findings
- Conventional
  - "Gold standard" for diagnosis and defining tDAVF
  - Angiographic protocol for evaluation of a suspected tDAVF includes selective injections of both external carotid + vertebral arteries, thyrocervical trunks, & paired segmental arteries
  - Demonstrates solitary AVF nidus & perimedullary or epidural enlarged draining veins
    - Angiographic appearance is same as sDAVF

DDx: Other Spinal Vascular Lesions

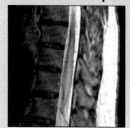

Spontaneous DAVF

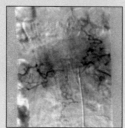

Spontaneous DAVF

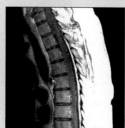

Spinal AVM

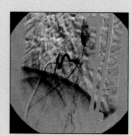

Spinal AVM

TRAUMATIC DURAL AV FISTULA

Key Facts

Terminology
• Traumatic induced arteriovenous fistula

Imaging Findings
• Best diagnostic clue: DSA demonstration of AVF nidus with enlarged draining veins

Top Differential Diagnoses
• Spontaneous dural AVF

• Spinal AVM

Pathology
• Usually caused by direct penetrating wounds
• Epidemiology: Rare lesions; much rarer than spontaneous DAVF

Clinical Issues
• Embolization preferred given decreased invasiveness

• Interventional
  ○ Embolization using N-butyl 2-cyanoacrylate, polyvinyl alcohol particles

Imaging Recommendations
• Best imaging tool: Digital subtraction angiography

DIFFERENTIAL DIAGNOSIS

Spontaneous dural AVF
• Typically older men who present with chronic progressive myelopathy
• Hyperintense conus expansion from congestive myelopathy
• Acquired vascular lesion preceded by venous thrombosis

Spinal AVM
• Intradural; on or within cord parenchyma
• Congenital vascular lesions

PATHOLOGY

General Features
• Etiology
  ○ Usually caused by direct penetrating wounds
    ▪ Stabbing, gunshot, or major trauma with bone Fx
• Epidemiology: Rare lesions; much rarer than spontaneous DAVF

CLINICAL ISSUES

Presentation
• Most common signs/symptoms
  ○ Radiculopathy as a result of enlarged epidural veins
  ○ Back pain

Demographics
• Gender: Unlike spontaneous DAVF, tDAVF not associated with males

Natural History & Prognosis
• Rapidly progressive without treatment

Treatment
• MRI with MRA provides improved screening for dural AVF guiding subsequent DSA studies by helping target fistula level

• Interventional radiology embolization or surgical ligation
  ○ Both are efficacious with low morbidity & mortality
  ○ Embolization preferred given decreased invasiveness

SELECTED REFERENCES

1. Kahara V et al: Presacral arteriovenous fistula: case report. Neurosurgery. 53(3):774-6; discussion 776-7, 2003
2. Saraf-Lavi E et al: Detection of spinal dural arteriovenous fistulae with MR imaging and contrast-enhanced MR angiography: sensitivity, specificity, and prediction of vertebral level. AJNR Am J Neuroradiol. 23(5):858-67, 2002
3. Song JK et al: N-butyl 2-cyanoacrylate embolization of spinal dural arteriovenous fistulae. AJNR Am J Neuroradiol. 22(1):40-7, 2001
4. Goyal M et al: Paravertebral arteriovenous malformations with epidural drainage: clinical spectrum, imaging features, and results of treatment. AJNR Am J Neuroradiol. 20(5):749-55, 1999
5. Cognard C et al: Paraspinal arteriovenous fistula with perimedullary venous drainage. AJNR Am J Neuroradiol. 16(10):2044-8, 1995

IMAGE GALLERY

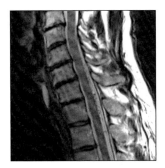 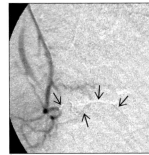

(Left) T2WI MR reveals flow voids on cord surface of dilated veins from traumatic DAVF. Unlike spontaneous DAVF, traumatic often has not formed cord engorgement/congestion at time of patient presentation. *(Right)* Embolization material can be seen (arrows) following successful interventional therapy of a traumatic dural AVF.

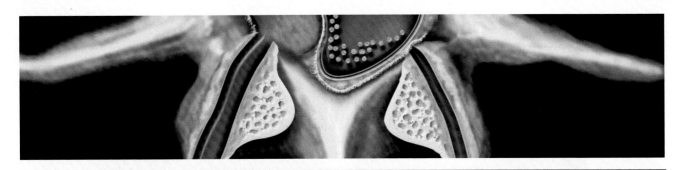

SECTION 2: Degenerative Disease and Inflammatory Arthritides

DEGENERATIVE DISC DISEASE NOMENCLATURE

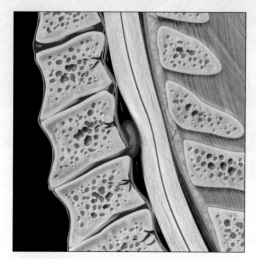

Sagittal graphic shows cervical disk extrusion, with the base of herniation smaller than component within epidural space.

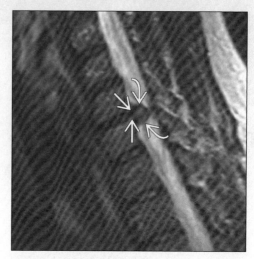

Sagittal T2WI MR shows C5-6 disc extrusion where the base of herniation (arrows) is smaller than rest of epidural component (curved arrows).

TERMINOLOGY

Abbreviations and Synonyms
- Anulus (annulus)
- Disc (disk)
- Tear (fissure)
- Extraforaminal (far lateral)

Definitions
- Nomenclature describes disc disease, leaves clinician with patient evaluation/description
- Definitions do not define or imply need for treatment, or cause of abnormality (such as trauma)
- Nomenclature was primarily developed for the lumbar spine, but may be utilized for thoracic and cervical disc disease

IMAGING ANATOMY

- Diagnostic categories of disc morphology
  - Normal
  - Congenital/developmental variation
  - Degenerative/traumatic
  - Inflammation/infection
  - Neoplasia
  - Morphologic variant of unknown significance
- Normal
  - Disc normally developed, free of trauma or ageing change
  - Only the disc morphology is defined, not the clinical context (normal does not imply patient does not hurt!)
  - Many minor abnormalities with no clinical import are considered "abnormal" by this strict criteria (minor osteophytes, minor bulging disc, etc.)
- Spondylosis deformans
  - Form of degeneration
  - Annulus fibrosus and adjacent apophyses
  - Vertebral body osteophytes
  - Largely result of ageing

- Term "spondylosis" used more generically for degenerative disease with osteophytes
- Intervertebral osteochondrosis
  - Degenerative change of nucleus pulposus and endplates
  - Involves nucleus pulposus, vertebral endplates; tears of anulus fibrosus, vacuum phenomenon, endplate sclerosis
  - Physiologic and pathologic change, but not necessarily symptomatic abnormalities
- Bulging anulus
  - Not a herniation
  - Disc tissue circumferentially beyond edges of apophyses involving > 180 degrees of circumference (50-100% of disc circumference)
  - Usually < 3 mm beyond edges of apophyses
  - Bulge has differential including normal variant, disc degeneration, vertebral body remodeling, ligamentous laxity, illusion of partial volume averaging
- Anular tear/fissure
  - Radial, transverse, or concentric separation of anular fibers
  - Both "tear" and "fissure" are appropriate
  - "Tear" does not imply traumatic etiology
  - In pure traumatic setting, "rupture" of annulus may be used
- Radial tear/fissure
  - Disruption of anulus
  - Disruption involving fibers extending from nucleus to periphery of anulus
  - Contrast with "concentric" tear
- Concentric tear
  - Disruption of anulus
  - Separation or breaking fibers in plane parallel to curve of disc periphery
  - Creation of fluid filled spaces between adjacent anular lamellae
- High intensity zone (HIZ)
  - T2 hyperintensity within outer anulus
  - May reflect anular tear/fissure

DEGENERATIVE DISC DISEASE NOMENCLATURE

DIFFERENTIAL DIAGNOSIS

Methods of defining disc disease - 1
- Normal
- Bulge
- Herniation (small, medium, large)

Methods of defining disc disease - 2
- Normal
- Bulge
- Herniation (size measurement in 3 planes)

Methods of defining disc disease - 3
- Normal
- Bulge
- Protrusion
- Extrusion
- Extrusion with free fragment

Locations
- Craniocaudal - disc level
- Craniocaudal - infra-pedicular level
- Craniocaudal - pedicular level
- Craniocaudal - supra-pedicular level
- Axial - central
- Axial - right (or left) central
- Axial - right (or left) sub-articular
- Axial - right (or left) foraminal
- Axial - right (or left) extra-foraminal

Canal compromise - axial images
- Compromise < 1/3 is "mild"
- Compromise between 1/3 and 2/3 of canal is "moderate"
- Compromise of > 2/3 is severe

- Does not imply etiology, symptomatology or need of treatment
- Herniated disc
  - Localized displacement of disc material beyond limits of disc space defined by vertebral body endplates (herniated material may be nucleus, cartilage, bone, anular tissue or combination)
  - Localized herniation < 50% of disc circumference (180°)
  - Herniation is "broad-based" if involves 90-180° of circumference (25-50% of circumference)
  - One intervertebral disc may have more than one herniation
  - Intervertebral disc may have co-existing bulge and herniation
- Protrusion
  - Category of disc herniation
  - Triangular shaped focal disc abnormality with base broader than apex
  - In craniocaudal direction the length of base cannot exceed the height of the intervertebral disc
- Extrusion
  - Category of disc herniation
  - Base of herniation is narrower than portion extending into epidural space (toothpaste sign)
  - Distance between of disc material beyond the disc space is greater than distance between edges of base in same plane, or if no continuity occurs between disc material beyond disc space and that within disc space
- Extrusion categorization
  - Sequestered or "free fragment" if no contiguity exists between herniated segment and parent disc
  - Migrated signifies displacement of disc away from level of parent disc
  - "Protrusions" cannot be migrated or sequestered by definition
  - Sequestered not the same as "uncontained"
- Chronic disc herniation
  - Herniation with calcification, ossification or gas suggesting herniation is not of recent origin
  - Term should not be used for "soft" disc herniations regardless of duration

- Contained
  - Herniations further categorized as "contained" if covered by outer annulus
  - Disc with contained herniation does not leak injected fluid into the vertebral canal
  - CT and MR not sensitive or specific in discriminating "contained" from "uncontained"
  - Discography separates only "leaking disc" from "non-leaking" disc
    - Containing capsule could be either PLL/anulus or only PLL
- Canal compromise (herniation)
  - Herniations also categorized by location, volume, content
  - Canal compromise defined by axial images
  - Compromise < 1/3 = "mild"
  - Compromise between 1/3 and 2/3 of canal = "moderate"
  - Compromise of > 2/3 = severe
  - Displaced material may be further categorized by terms such as "bony", "ossified", "dessicated", "gaseous"
- Canal compromise (foraminal stenosis)
  - Canal compromise defined by axial images
  - Compromise < 1/3 = "mild"
  - Compromise between 1/3 and 2/3 of canal = "moderate"
  - Compromise of > 2/3 = severe
- Location (craniocaudal)
  - Disc level
  - Infrapedicular level
  - Pedicular level
  - Suprapedicular level
- Location (axial or horizontal) moving from central to lateral location
  - Central
  - Right (or left) central (paracentral is discouraged since less precise)
  - Right (or left) sub-articular
  - Right (or left) foraminal
  - Right (or left) extra-foraminal (far lateral is synonymous)
- Intra-anular displacement (intra-discal herniation)

DEGENERATIVE DISC DISEASE NOMENCLATURE

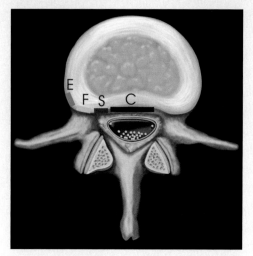

Axial view of lumbar disc showing right-left location classification: C (central), S (sub-articular), F (foraminal), E (extra-foraminal).

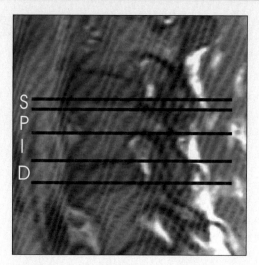

Sagittal view for level classification: S (suprapedicular), P (pedicular), I (infrapedicular), D (disc).

- Displacement of nuclear material to a more peripheral site in the disc space
- Form of internal disc disruption
- Avoid use of "herniation" since that implies extension beyond disc space
• Limbus fracture
- Traumatic separation of bone from edge of vertebral ring apophysis
- May have associated disc herniation
• Limbus vertebrae
- Separation of rim of vertebral body ring apophysis which may be traumatic or developmental
- Also called "rim lesion"
• Spondylosis
- Shortened form of "spondylosis deformans", a specifically defined sub-classification of degeneration
- Most commonly used in generic sense for any degenerative changes of spine including osteophytic enlargement of apophyseal bone
  ▪ As in "cervical spondylosis"
• Sub-ligamentous
- Underneath the PLL
- Distinct meaning from "sub-anular" (where disc herniation is contained by anulus)
- When distinction between sub-anular and sub-ligamentous cannot be made, then use term "sub-capsular"
• Peridural membrane
- Delicate membrane attaching undersurface of PLL extending laterally and posteriorly encircling canal outside dura
• Sub-membranous
- When characterizing herniation infers that displaced material is extruded beyond anulus and PLL, with only peridural membrane investing the material
• Degenerative endplate changes (Modic changes)
- MR signal abnormalities involving vertebral body endplates related to degenerative disc disease
- Type I: Hypointense on T1WI, hyperintense on T2WI (fibrovascular marrow + edema)

- Type II: Hyperintense on T1WI, isointense on T2WI (adipose tissue)
- Type III: Hypointense on T1WI and T2WI (discogenic sclerosis)
• Non standard disc terms to avoid
- Disc material beyond the interspace (DEBIT)
- Herniated nucleus pulposus (material other than nucleus may be herniated)
- Rupture (implied traumatic etiology)
- Prolapse (synonymous with protrusion)

CUSTOM DIFFERENTIAL DIAGNOSIS

Bulging disc
• Disc tissue circumferentially beyond edges of apophyses involving > 180 degrees of circumference (50-100% of disc circumference)
• Bulge is term that needs a differential diagnosis
• Bulge may be normal variant
• Bulge associated with advanced disc degeneration
• Bulge associated with vertebral body remodeling (related to osteoporosis, trauma)
• Bulge in response to loading or angular motion with ligamentous laxity
• Bulge as fake out from central sub-ligamentous disc herniation

SELECTED REFERENCES

1.   Fardon DF et al: Nomenclature and classification of lumbar disc pathology. Recommendations of the Combined task Forces of the North American Spine Society, American Society of Spine Radiology, and American Society of Neuroradiology. Spine. 26(5):E93-E113, 2001
2.   Milette PC: The proper terminology for reporting lumbar intervertebral disk disorders. AJNR Am J Neuroradiol. 18(10):1859-66, 1997

DEGENERATIVE DISC DISEASE NOMENCLATURE

IMAGE GALLERY

Typical

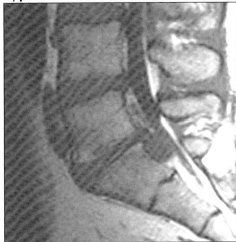
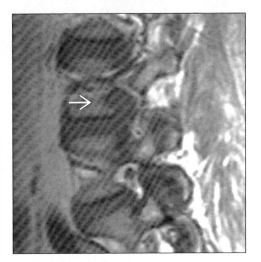

(Left) Sagittal T1WI MR shows extrusion where base of herniation is narrower than portion extending into epidural space. There is inferior migration of herniation consistent with free fragment. *(Right)* Sagittal T1WI MR shows large L3-4 disc extrusion which is located within the neural foramen (foraminal herniation)(arrow).

Typical

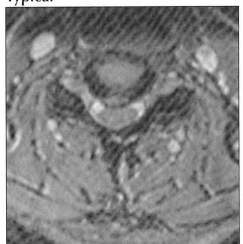
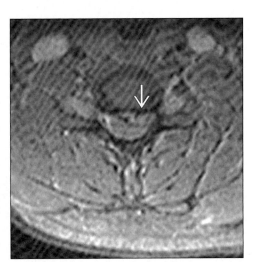

(Left) Axial T2* GRE MR shows a focal central disc protrusion with mild effacement of the thecal sac, and mild cord compression. *(Right)* Axial T2* GRE MR shows left central disc extrusion with moderate compression of thecal sac and cord (arrow).

Typical

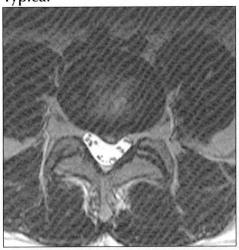
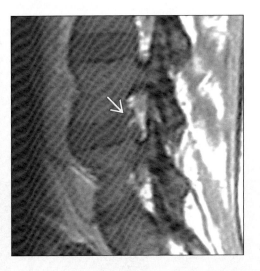

(Left) Axial T2WI MR shows triangular shaped focal disc abnormality with base broader than apex, reflecting disc protrusion. *(Right)* Sagittal T1 C+ MR shows anular tear/fissure as focal enhancement within the posterolateral anulus fibrosus (arrow).

DEGENERATIVE DISC DISEASE

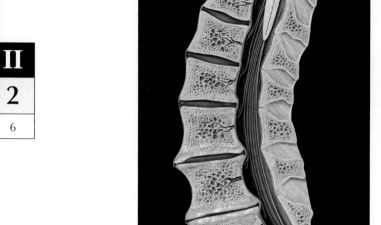

Sagittal graphic shows degeneration of L4-5 and L5-S1 intervertebral discs with loss of disc height, associated type II fatty endplate change, and osteophyte formation.

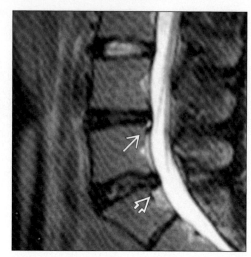

Sagittal T2WI MR shows low signal at L4-5, L5-S1 compared to normal disc signal at L3-4. Loss of disc height at L4-5, disc herniation at L5-S1 (open arrow), and anular tear at L4-5 (arrow).

TERMINOLOGY

Abbreviations and Synonyms
- Degenerative disc disease (DDD), disc degeneration, spondylosis

Definitions
- Generalized and multifactorial process affecting the discovertebral unit leading to biomechanical/morphologic alterations
- Asymptomatic or associated with back/neck pain +/- radiculopathy

IMAGING FINDINGS

General Features
- Best diagnostic clue: Decreased signal of intervertebral disc on T2WI
- Location: Intervertebral disc, adjacent endplates
- Size: Normal disc height with mild signal loss to marked loss of height
- Morphology: Nucleus/anulus alteration, with adjacent facet/foramina osteoarthritic degenerative change

Radiographic Findings
- Radiography: Late disease shows loss of disc space height, osteophyte formation, bony endplate eburnation "discogenic sclerosis", vacuum phenomenon
- Fluoroscopy: Instability shows with abnormal motion segment
- Myelography: Nonspecific extradural defects associated with central stenosis, osteophyte formation, herniation

CT Findings
- NECT: Useful for assessment of bulge, focal disc herniation, osteophyte formation with facet arthropathy, central stenosis

MR Findings
- T1WI
  - Loss of disc space height, vacuum phenomenon seen as low signal within disc
  - Degenerative endplate changes I ⇒ III
- T2WI
  - T2 show loss of signal from nucleus, loss of horizontal nuclear cleft
  - Degenerative endplate changes I ⇒ III
- T1 C+: Disc may show linear enhancement with DDD, enhancement within Schmorl nodes

DDx: Degenerative Endplate Changes

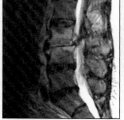

Disc Space Infection

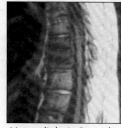

Hemodialysis Spondy.

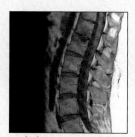

Ankylosing Spondylitis

DEGENERATIVE DISC DISEASE

Key Facts

Terminology

- Degenerative disc disease (DDD), disc degeneration, spondylosis
- Generalized and multifactorial process affecting the discovertebral unit leading to biomechanical/morphologic alterations
- Asymptomatic or associated with back/neck pain +/- radiculopathy

Imaging Findings

- Loss of disc space height, vacuum phenomenon seen as low signal within disc
- Degenerative endplate changes I ⇒ III

Pathology

- Etiology of symptomatic DDD not fully known

- Some studies show strong familial predisposition to discogenic back pain
- Individuals involved in manual materials handling, with repeated heavy lifting at increased risk
- More controversial associations of back pain with psychosocial factors
- Lifetime incidence of back pain in United States 50-80%
- Prevalence among adults range from 15-30%
- Back pain most common cause of disability in persons younger than 45 years
- 1998 total health care expenditures for back pain in United States ~ $90 billion dollars

Clinical Issues

- LBP symptoms self limited and resolve spontaneously (< 2 weeks)

Nuclear Medicine Findings

- Bone Scan: Generalize increased uptake with DDD, osteophyte formation and facet degenerative arthropathy

Other Modality Findings

- Discography role limited in patients with DDD
  - Used in a confirmatory role, and to evaluate adjacent level disc degeneration
  - Provocative discography used for determination of levels included in fusion surgery

Imaging Recommendations

- Best imaging tool: MR shows intrinsic disc signal changes, anular tears, bulge, herniation, and stenosis
- Protocol advice: Standard T1WI and T2WI in sagittal/axial planes (4 mm maximum slice thickness)

DIFFERENTIAL DIAGNOSIS

Disc space infection

- Endplate destruction

Hemodialysis spondyloarthropathy

- Low signal on T1WI, may be indistinguishable from pyogenic infection

Seronegative spondyloarthropathy

- Inflammatory endplate changes may mimic type I degenerative endplate changes

PATHOLOGY

General Features

- General path comments
  - Etiology of symptomatic DDD not fully known
  - Multiple abnormalities can be present in symptomatic patients such as disc space narrowing, endplate sclerosis, osteophytes, vacuum phenomenon
- Genetics

  - Two collagen IX alleles associated with sciatica and disc herniation
  - Disc degeneration associated with aggrecan gene polymorphism, matrix metalloproteinase 3, 7 gene alleles
  - Some studies show strong familial predisposition to discogenic back pain
- Etiology
  - Etiology of disc degeneration multifactorial
  - Individuals involved in manual materials handling, with repeated heavy lifting at increased risk
  - More controversial associations of back pain with psychosocial factors
    - Depression, mental stress, job dissatisfaction, high work pace, lack of job support
  - Cigarette smoking and obesity linked to back pain in some studies
  - Evidence of dose response relationship between physical workload and long duration LBP
- Epidemiology
  - Overall incidence of back pain ~ 45 per 1,000 person-year
  - Lifetime incidence of back pain in United States 50-80%
  - Prevalence among adults range from 15-30%
  - 2-5% of population receives medical care every year from back pain
  - 15 million physician visits in 1990 for back pain
  - 1% of population disabled because of back pain
  - Back pain most common cause of disability in persons younger than 45 years
  - Highest prevalence of back pain 40-60 years of age
  - 1998 total health care expenditures for back pain in United States ~ $90 billion dollars
- Associated abnormalities
  - Bulging anulus, disc herniation, osteophyte formation, central and foraminal stenosis
  - Degenerative spondylolisthesis
    - M < F, occurs after age 40 years, 3x more common in African-American women than Caucasian women, L4-5 level

DEGENERATIVE DISC DISEASE

Gross Pathologic & Surgical Features
- Disc abnormalities
  - Disc dessication with decreased proteoglycan water binding
  - Collagen content increases
  - Loss of negatively charged proteoglycan side chains
  - Loss of hydrostatic properties of disc with loss of disc space height
  - Bulging of anulus with anular tears/herniation
  - Loss of boundary between anulus and nucleus
  - Nucleus becomes progressively disorganized and fibrous with fibrocartilage replacing distinct nucleus/anulus
  - Decrease in anular cells, with shift to more type II collagen
- Endplate abnormalities
  - Endplates show progressive thinning and hyalinization
  - Loss of nutritional function of endplate with decreased diffusion ability
  - Endplate marrow conversion to type I-III, endstage of endplate bony eburnation
  - Osteophyte formation
- Facet joints
  - Loss of disc space height ⇒ rostrocaudal subluxation of facets with capsule laxity, ligamentous buckling/thickening
  - Shift of axial load pattern leading to increased facet degenerative arthropathy, osteophyte formation

Microscopic Features
- Nucleus becomes progressively disorganized and fibrous, cracks and fissures throughout nucleus
- Endplate fragmentation and disruption with new bone formation, granulation tissue
- Marrow conversion from hematopoietic to fat, or fibrous (type II, type I endplate change respectively)

Staging, Grading or Classification Criteria
- Classification systems
  - MR disc grading scheme I ⇒ V (Pfirrmann et al)
  - Histologic classification system of age related changes (Boos et al)

CLINICAL ISSUES

Presentation
- Most common signs/symptoms
  - Commonly asymptomatic with normal neurologic exam
  - Low back or neck pain
    - +/- Radiculopathy
  - Other signs/symptoms
    - Range of motion restricted
    - Extension may exacerbate pain
- Clinical profile: Middle-aged person engaged in manual lifting with chronic back pain

Demographics
- Age: Back pain peak 45-65 years
- Gender: M = F

Natural History & Prognosis
- LBP has benign natural history
- LBP symptoms self limited and resolve spontaneously (< 2 weeks)
- 7% of patients with acute symptoms develop chronic pain
- Of patients complaining of chronic pain (> 3 months), 1/3 have disabling symptoms
- Over 5 year period, ~ 70% have clinical improvement

Treatment
- Nonoperative treatment with bedrest, exercise, drug therapy, manipulation
  - Manipulation effective in treatment of LBP of short duration
- Operative treatment
  - Surgical treatment for axial pain from DDD most commonly involves fusion

DIAGNOSTIC CHECKLIST

Consider
- 30% of normal individuals have abnormal signal in lumbar discs

Image Interpretation Pearls
- Discography should consist of 4 data points
  - Morphology of disc injected
  - Disc pressure/volume of fluid accepted
  - Patient subjective pain response
  - Lack of pain response at adjacent levels

SELECTED REFERENCES

1. Boos N et al: Classification of age-related changes in lumbar intervertebral discs: 2002 Volvo Award in basic science. Spine. 27(23):2631-44, 2002
2. Moore KR et al: Degenerative disc disease treated with combined anterior and posterior arthrodesis and posterior instrumentation. Spine. 27(15):1680-6, 2002
3. Frobin W et al: Height of lumbar discs measured from radiographs compared with degeneration and height classified from MR images. Eur Radiol. 11(2):263-9, 2001
4. Weishaupt D et al: Painful Lumbar Disk Derangement: Relevance of Endplate Abnormalities at MR Imaging. Radiology. 218(2): 420-7, 2001
5. Pfirrmann CW et al: Magnetic resonance classification of lumbar intervertebral disc degeneration. Spine. 26(17):1873-8, 2001
6. Luoma K et al: Low back pain in relation to lumbar disc degeneration. Spine. 25(4):487-92, 2000
7. Beattie PF et al: Associations between patient report of symptoms and anatomic impairment visible on lumbar magnetic resonance imaging. Spine. 25(7):819-28, 2000
8. Jensen MC et al: Magnetic resonance imaging of the lumbar spine in people without back pain. N Engl J Med. 331(2):69-73, 1994
9. Modic MT et al: Magnetic resonance imaging in the evaluation of low back pain. Orthop Clin North Am. 22(2):283-301, 1991
10. Modic MT et al: Degenerative disk disease: assessment of changes in vertebral body marrow with MR imaging. Radiology. 166(1 Pt 1):193-9, 1988

DEGENERATIVE DISC DISEASE

IMAGE GALLERY

Typical

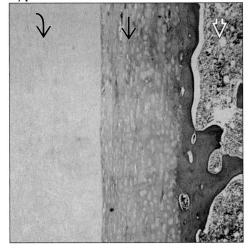 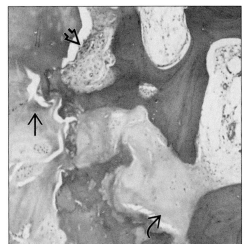

(Left) Micropathology, low power, H&E shows normal endplate with nucleus (curved arrow), smooth cartilage junction (arrow), thin bony trabeculae and normal hematopoietic marrow (open arrow). (Right) Micropathology, low power, H&E shows degenerated endplate with disruption of cartilage, fissures in nucleus (arrow), granulation tissue (open arrow) and cartilage endplate herniation (curved arrow).

Typical

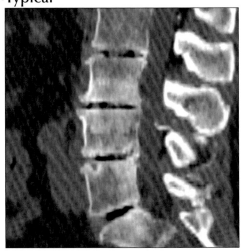 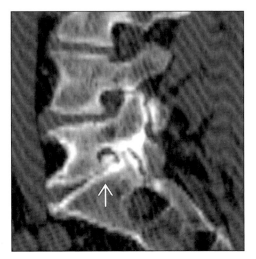

(Left) Sagittal NECT reformat shows multilevel severe loss of disc height and vacuum phenomenon. Endplate eburnation present at L3-4, L4-5. Osteophyte present at several levels. (Right) Sagittal NECT shows loss of disc height at L5-S1 with resultant rostrocaudal subluxation of facets, foraminal stenosis. Osteophyte causes further stenosis extending into foramen (arrow).

Typical

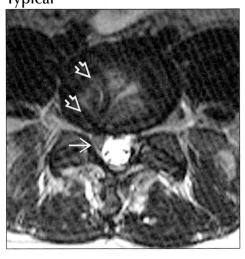 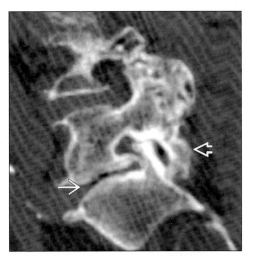

(Left) Axial T2WI MR shows protrusion (arrow) compressing exiting root. Degeneration of disc shows low signal centrally, with disrupted internal disc contents pointing to herniation (open arrows). (Right) Sagittal NECT reformat shows loss of disc space height L5-S1 with vacuum phenomenon (arrow), facet hypertrophic degenerative arthropathy (open arrow) giving severe foraminal stenosis.

DEGENERATIVE ENDPLATE CHANGES

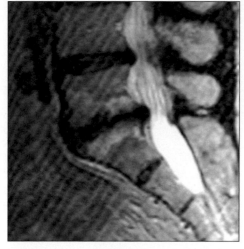

Sagittal T2WI MR shows type I degenerative endplate changes as increased signal at L5-S1. There is disc degeneration with loss of signal from intervertebral disc.

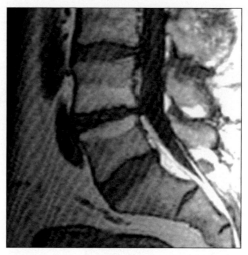

Sagittal T1WI MR shows classic type II endplate changes due to fatty marrow replacement at L4-5.

TERMINOLOGY

Abbreviations and Synonyms
- Vertebral endplate change, modic changes
- Type I, II, III endplate change

Definitions
- MR signal abnormalities involving vertebral body endplates related to degenerative disc disease
  - Type I: Hypointense on T1WI, hyperintense on T2WI
  - Type II: Hyperintense on T1WI, isointense on T2WI
  - Type III: Hypointense on T1WI and T2WI

IMAGING FINDINGS

General Features
- Best diagnostic clue: Parallel signal alteration of vertebral endplates, associated with evidence of disc degeneration
- Location: Most common in lumbar spine, may occur in any vertebral body
- Size: Variable: Small linear bands to near complete vertebral body involvement
- Morphology: Linear, parallel to intervertebral disc

Radiographic Findings
- Radiography: Insensitive to early changes, type III change seen as "discogenic" sclerosis of endplates

CT Findings
- NECT: Insensitive to early changes, type III seen as endplate sclerosis

MR Findings
- T1WI
  - Type I: Hypointense horizontal bands involving endplates
  - Type II: Hyperintense bands
  - Type III: Hypointense bands
- T2WI
  - Type I: Hyperintense horizontal bands involving endplates
  - Type II: Isointense to slightly hyperintense bands
    - Signal tracks fat on all pulse sequences
  - Type III: Hypointense bands involving endplates
- T1 C+
  - Type I: May show prominent enhancement
  - Commonly associated with linear intervertebral disc enhancement

Nuclear Medicine Findings
- Bone Scan: Nonspecific increased uptake with all degenerative disc disease

DDx: Low Signal Endplate on T1WI

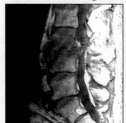
Disc Infection

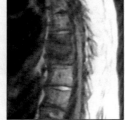
Hemodialysis

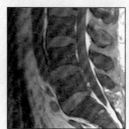
Mets

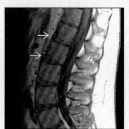
Ankylosing Spondy

DEGENERATIVE ENDPLATE CHANGES

Key Facts

Terminology

- Vertebral endplate change, modic changes
- Type I, II, III endplate change
- MR signal abnormalities involving vertebral body endplates related to degenerative disc disease
- Type I: Hypointense on T1WI, hyperintense on T2WI
- Type II: Hyperintense on T1WI, isointense on T2WI
- Type III: Hypointense on T1WI and T2WI

Top Differential Diagnoses

- Disk space infection
- Hemodialysis spondyloarthropathy
- Seronegative spondyloarthropathy
- Metastatic disease
- Gout

Pathology

- Type I: Replacement with fibrovascular marrow
- Type II: Replacement by fatty marrow
- Type III: Replacement by bony sclerosis with little residual marrow
- Type I: Present in 4% of patients undergoing MR for disc disease
- Type II: Present in 16% of patients undergoing MR for disc disease
- Type III: Least common, approximately 1%

Clinical Issues

- Relationship of type I endplate changes to low back pain (discogenic pain) controversial

- PET
  - Hypometabolic with degenerative endplate changes
  - Hypermetabolic with disc space infection or vertebral osteomyelitis
  - PET accurate and specific to differentiate degenerative endplate change from infection
- Gallium Scan
  - No increased uptake with degenerative endplate changes

Imaging Recommendations

- Best imaging tool: MRI
- Protocol advice: Sagittal T1WI and T2WI defines lesions and classification

DIFFERENTIAL DIAGNOSIS

Disk space infection

- Low signal involving endplates similar to type I change
- Endplate destruction
- Hyperintense intervertebral disc on T2WI
- Paravertebral or epidural soft tissue phlegmon/abscess

Hemodialysis spondyloarthropathy

- Low signal on T1WI involving endplates similar to pyogenic disc space infection
- May be indistinguishable from pyogenic disc space infection

Seronegative spondyloarthropathy

- Inflammatory endplate changes (Anderson lesions) may mimic type I degenerative endplates
- Typical squaring of vertebral bodies
- Late changes with fusion of bodies and posterior elements

Metastatic disease

- Focal low signal on T1WI with bone destruction ± epidural extension
- Low signal does not parallel endplates as in type I change

Gout

- Rarely vertebral involvement with low signal involving endplates, similar to disc space infection

PATHOLOGY

General Features

- General path comments
  - Replacement of normal hematopoietic marrow
    - Type I: Replacement with fibrovascular marrow
    - Type II: Replacement by fatty marrow
    - Type III: Replacement by bony sclerosis with little residual marrow
- Genetics: None known
- Etiology
  - Unknown
    - Type I: Probably reflects sequelae of acute disc degeneration
    - Type I: Present in 30% of chymopapain treated discs (good model for acute disc degeneration)
    - Type II: Probably reflects sequelae of chronic disc degeneration
- Epidemiology
  - Adult with disc degeneration
  - Type I: Present in 4% of patients undergoing MR for disc disease
  - Type II: Present in 16% of patients undergoing MR for disc disease
  - Type III: Least common, approximately 1%
- Associated abnormalities
  - Disc degeneration
    - Loss of disc space height
    - Loss of signal from disc on T2WI

Gross Pathologic & Surgical Features

- Disc degeneration with dessication of disc, bony endplate eburnation

Microscopic Features

- Type I: Spindle cells, capillaries (vascularized fibrous tissue) with prominent interstitial space, thickened trabeculae with new bone production

- Type II: Adipose cells, prominent trabeculae with new bone production (woven bone)
- Type III: Dense woven bone

CLINICAL ISSUES

Presentation
- Most common signs/symptoms
  - May be incidental or asymptomatic finding with disc degeneration
  - Nonspecific neck or back pain
  - Relationship of type I endplate changes to low back pain (discogenic pain) controversial
    - No significant correlation between concordant pain at discography and presence of endplate changes
    - Some studies suggest type I, II change have high specificity (> 90%), but low sensitivity (20-30%) for painful lumbar disc
- Clinical profile: Low back pain without major radicular component

Demographics
- Age: Adult
- Gender: M = F

Natural History & Prognosis
- Natural history variable
  - Type I change may convert to type II over course of months to years
  - Type II more stable change

Treatment
- Options, risks, complications
  - Degenerative endplate changes may be asymptomatic
  - Controversial as to role of endplate changes regarding spinal fusion
  - Endplate changes proposed as one criteria for spinal fusion for discogenic pain

DIAGNOSTIC CHECKLIST

Consider
- Disc space infection if high signal within disc on T2WI
- Disc degeneration may also show increased signal within disc on T2WI due to cracks, fissures

Image Interpretation Pearls
- Discrimination of early disc space infection and severe type I endplate changes may be difficult or impossible
- Degenerative endplate changes due not show paravertebral enhancing soft tissue, which is often present with disc space infection
- Use axial post-contrast fat suppressed T1WI to better define paravertebral soft tissues

SELECTED REFERENCES

1. Senegas J: Mechanical supplementation by non-rigid fixation in degenerative intervertebral lumbar segments: the Wallis system. Eur Spine J. 11 Suppl 2: S164-9, 2002
2. Stumpe KD et al: FDG positron emission tomography for differentiation of degenerative and infectious endplate abnormalities in the lumbar spine detected on MR imaging. AJR Am J Roentgenol. 179(5): 1151-7, 2002
3. Weishaupt D et al: Painful Lumbar Disk Derangement: Relevance of Endplate Abnormalities at MR Imaging. Radiology. 218(2): 420-7, 2001
4. Sandhu HS et al: Association between findings of provocative discography and vertebral endplate signal changes as seen on MRI. J Spinal Disord. 13(5): 438-43, 2000
5. Van Goethem JW et al: The value of MRI in the diagnosis of postoperative spondylodiscitis. Neuroradiology. 42(8): 580-5, 2000
6. Braithwaite I et al: Vertebral end-plate (Modic) changes on lumbar spine MRI: correlation with pain reproduction at lumbar discography. Eur Spine J. 7(5): 363-8, 1998
7. Ito M et al: Predictive signs of discogenic lumbar pain on magnetic resonance imaging with discography correlation. Spine. 23(11): 1252-8; discussion 1259-60, 1998
8. Ross JS et al: The postoperative lumbar spine: enhanced MR evaluation of the intervertebral disk. AJNR Am J Neuroradiol. 17(2): 323-31, 1996
9. Ulmer JL et al: Lumbar spondylolysis: reactive marrow changes seen in adjacent pedicles on MR images. AJR Am J Roentgenol. 164(2): 429-33, 1995
10. Modic MT et al: Contrast-enhanced MR imaging in acute lumbar radiculopathy: a pilot study of the natural history. Radiology. 195(2): 429-35, 1995
11. Ross JS et al: Current assessment of spinal degenerative disease with magnetic resonance imaging. Clin Orthop. (279): 68-81, 1992
12. Ross JS et al: Assessment of extradural degenerative disease with Gd-DTPA-enhanced MR imaging: correlation with surgical and pathologic findings. AJNR Am J Neuroradiol. 10(6):1243-9, 1989
13. Modic MT et al: Degenerative disk disease: assessment of changes in vertebral body marrow with MR imaging. Radiology. 166(1 Pt 1):193-9, 1988
14. Masaryk TJ et al: High-resolution MR imaging of sequestered lumbar intervertebral disks. AJR Am J Roentgenol. 150(5):1155-62, 1988
15. Hueftle MG et al: Lumbar spine: postoperative MR imaging with Gd-DTPA. Radiology. 167(3):817-24, 1988

DEGENERATIVE ENDPLATE CHANGES

IMAGE GALLERY

Typical

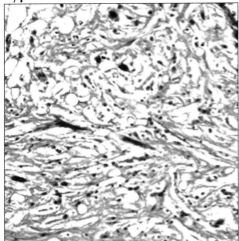 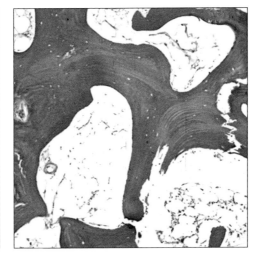

(Left) Micropathology, low power, H&E shows type I change with fibrovascular replacement of hematopoietic marrow. There are prominent interstitial spaces & scattered capillaries amongst spindle shaped cells. *(Right)* Micropathology, low power, H&E shows type II changes with fatty replacement of normal hematopoietic marrow. There is thickened trabeculae with new woven bone formation.

Typical

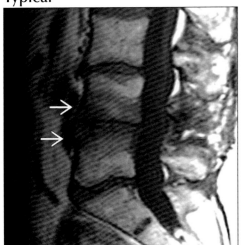 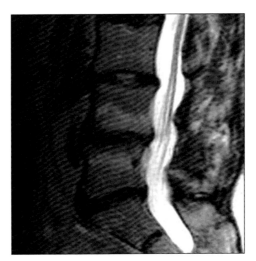

(Left) Sagittal T1WI MR shows low signal involving L4-5 endplates (arrow), with vacuum phenomena within several disc spaces. Low signal endplate margins appear intact. *(Right)* Sagittal T2WI MR shows high signal from L4-5 endplates. The disc at L4-5 is low signal reflecting disc degeneration. Note that endplates are intact.

Typical

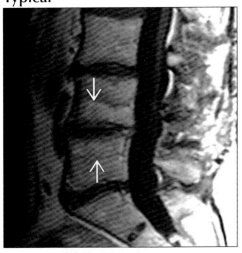 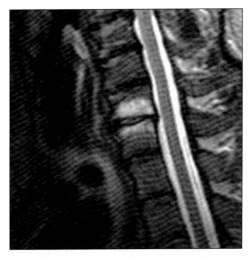

(Left) Sagittal T1 C+ MR shows prominent enhancement of the type I change at L4-5 (arrows). Mild linear enhancement due to disc degeneration present within the disc itself. *(Right)* Sagittal T2WI MR shows type I endplate changes at C5-6 level with increased signal. Slight increased signal present within disc itself due to disc degeneration with fissuring.

INSTABILITY

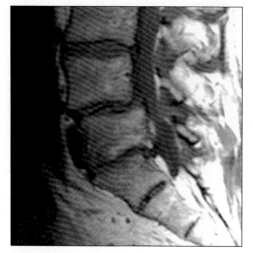

Sagittal T1WI MR shows anterolisthesis L4 on L5, with loss of disc height and vacuum phenomenon. Retrolisthesis present at L5-S1 with marked loss of disc height.

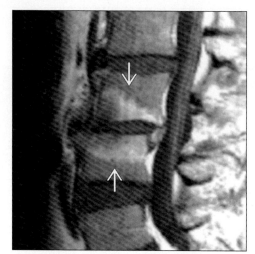

Sagittal T1 C+ MR shows loss of disc height at L3-4, with retrolisthesis. There is pronounced contrast-enhancement of type I degenerative endplate changes (arrows).

TERMINOLOGY

Abbreviations and Synonyms
- Spine instability (SI), segmental instability, abnormal spinal motion, degenerative instability

Definitions
- Loss of spine motion segment stiffness, where applied force produces greater displacement than normal, with pain/deformity

IMAGING FINDINGS

General Features
- Best diagnostic clue: Deformity which increases with motion and increases over time
- Location: Any spinal motion segment (comprised of two adjacent vertebrae, disc and connecting spinal ligaments)
- Size: Displacement may vary from few mm to width of vertebral body
- Morphology: Displacement of vertebral body with respect to adjacent body
- Stabilizing anatomic structures
  ○ Ligaments
    ▪ Anterior longitudinal ligament (resists hyperextension)
    ▪ Posterior longitudinal ligament
    ▪ Intertransverse ligaments (connect neighboring transverse processes)
    ▪ Interspinous ligaments (resists hyperflexion)
    ▪ Facet capsule
    ▪ Ligamentum flavum
  ○ Intervertebral disc: Main stabilizer of lumbar and thoracic spine
  ○ Muscular attachments: Both global (rectus and abdominal muscles) and local paraspinal muscle groups

Radiographic Findings
- Radiography
  ○ Various parameters used for degenerative instability by plain films
    ▪ Dynamic slip > 3 mm in flexion/extension
    ▪ Static slip of 4.5 mm or greater
    ▪ Angulation > 10-15° suggests need for surgical intervention
  ○ Traction spurs
  ○ Vacuum phenomenon
- Fluoroscopy: Increased motion with flexion/extension or translation

CT Findings
- NECT: Nonspecific findings of degenerative disc disease +/- spondylolisthesis

DDx: Causes of Instability

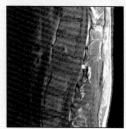

Trauma

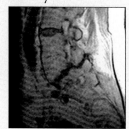

Pseudoarthosis

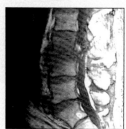

Infection

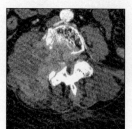

Tumor

INSTABILITY

Key Facts

Terminology
- Loss of spine motion segment stiffness, where applied force produces greater displacement than normal, with pain/deformity

Imaging Findings
- Best diagnostic clue: Deformity which increases with motion and increases over time
- Various parameters used for degenerative instability by plain films
- Dynamic slip > 3 mm in flexion/extension
- Static slip of 4.5 mm or greater
- Angulation > 10-15° suggests need for surgical intervention
- Traction spurs
- Vacuum phenomenon

Pathology
- Translational instability occurs 5-6x more often in women, 3x more common in African-American women than Caucasian women

Clinical Issues
- Nonspecific symptoms
- Low back pain with occasional radiation
- Nonspecific clinical findings leads to use of radiographic surrogate findings

Diagnostic Checklist
- Radiographic assessment begins with standing AP and lateral views of lumbar spine with flexion/extension views

MR Findings
- T1WI
  - Anterolisthesis, retrolisthesis, lateral translation
  - Nonspecific changes of degenerative disc disease
  - Controversial as to role in defining instability: Type I degenerative endplate changes
- T2WI: Loss of disc signal ± disc space height
- STIR: Type I endplate changes may be more evident on this sequence
- T1 C+
  - Nonspecific enhancement of disc due to degenerative disc disease
  - Enhancement of type I degenerative endplate changes

Imaging Recommendations
- Best imaging tool: Flexion/extension plain films
- Protocol advice: MR findings useful as secondary tool for degeneration, endplate changes, stenosis and herniation

DIFFERENTIAL DIAGNOSIS

Pseudoarthrosis
- Abnormal low T1 signal extending through disc, posterior elements and ligaments

Infection
- Endplate destruction, disc T2 hyperintensity

Tumor
- Enhancing soft tissue mass

Post-operative
- Following multilevel laminectomy or facetectomy

PATHOLOGY

General Features
- General path comments
  - Many causes of spinal instability
    - Fractures
    - Infection (especially anterior column involvement)
    - Primary bone and metastatic tumors (vertebral body destruction, neural compression, post resection)
    - Isthmic spondylolisthesis (L5-S1 progressive deformity in children)
    - Scoliosis
    - Degenerative instabilities
      - Axial rotational (recurrent pain worse with twisting); plain films show malaligned spinous processes and pedicle rotation
      - Translational (degenerative spondylolisthesis); plain films show spondylolisthesis, traction spurs, vacuum phenomenon
      - Retrolisthesis (posterior displacement of cephalad body, loss of posterior disc height, facet subluxation); plain films show increased retrolisthesis with extension
      - Degenerative scoliosis (low back pain +/- claudication, radiculopathy); imaging shows central and foraminal stenosis
      - Post laminectomy (resection of 50% of bilateral facets alters segmental stiffness); plain films show new or worsening segmental motion
      - Post fusion (altered biomechanics from fusion, but little correlation between radiographic findings and clinical symptoms)
- Etiology: Multifactorial
- Epidemiology
  - Translational instability occurs 5-6x more often in women, 3x more common in African-American women than Caucasian women
  - Facet joint angulation has been suggested as cause
- Associated abnormalities: Clinical and imaging relationship of disc degeneration to instability controversial

Gross Pathologic & Surgical Features
- Findings of degenerative disc disease

Microscopic Features
- Same as degenerative disc disease

INSTABILITY

CLINICAL ISSUES

Presentation
- Most common signs/symptoms
  - Nonspecific symptoms
  - Low back pain with occasional radiation
  - Physical signs suggesting instability include palpable step off deformity ± or spinous process lateral deviation
  - Paraspinal muscle spasms
  - Nonspecific clinical findings leads to use of radiographic surrogate findings
- Clinical profile: Elderly female with nonspecific back pain with evidence of L4-5 spondylolisthesis by plain films

Demographics
- Age: > 50 years
- Gender: M < F for degenerative anterior slip, especially at L4-5

Natural History & Prognosis
- 20% of subjects have instability resolve over 10 year time period
- Increased flexion by plain films does not adversely affect long term clinical outcome
- L5-S1 isthmic spondylolisthesis rarely unstable in adults

Treatment
- Conservative medical treatment of pain including exercise, physical therapy, NSAIDs
- Surgical treatment
  - Posterolateral fusion (+/- pedicle screw fixation)
    - Disadvantages include variable satisfactory outcomes (16-95%), pseudoarthrosis (14-70%), reoperation rates (25%)
  - Interbody fusions via anterior, posterior or circumferential approaches
    - Posterior lumber interbody fusion (PLIF)
    - Anterior lumbar interbody fusion (ALIF)
    - Transforaminal lumbar interbody fusion (TLIF)
- Risks: ALIF (retrograde ejaculation, cage displacement, iatrogenic herniation), PLIF (arachnoiditis, epidural hemorrhage, cage displacement)

DIAGNOSTIC CHECKLIST

Consider
- Findings of "mechanical back pain" present with degenerative instability
- Specificity of plain films limited by high prevalence of lumbar spondylosis in general population

Image Interpretation Pearls
- Radiographic assessment begins with standing AP and lateral views of lumbar spine with flexion/extension views

SELECTED REFERENCES

1. Tay BB et al: Indications, techniques, and complications of lumbar interbody fusion. Semin Neurol. 22(2):221-30, 2002
2. Kristof RA et al: Degenerative lumbar spondylolisthesis-induced radicular compression: nonfusion-related decompression in selected patients without hypermobility on flexion-extension radiographs. J Neurosurg. 97(3 Suppl):281-6, 2002
3. Haughton VM et al: Measuring the axial rotation of lumbar vertebrae in vivo with MR imaging. AJNR Am J Neuroradiol. 23(7):1110-6, 2002
4. Pitkanen MT et al: Segmental lumbar spine instability at flexion-extension radiography can be predicted by conventional radiography. Clin Radiol. 57(7):632-9, 2002
5. Kuroki H et al: Clinical results of posterolateral fusion for degenerative lumbar spinal diseases: a follow-up study of more than 10 years. J Orthop Sci. 7(3):317-24, 2002
6. Chen WJ et al: Surgical treatment of adjacent instability after lumbar spine fusion. Spine. 26(22):E519-24, 2001
7. Bendo JA et al: Importance of correlating static and dynamic imaging studies in diagnosing degenerative lumbar spondylolisthesis. Am J Orthop. 30(3):247-50, 2001
8. Nizard RS et al: Radiologic assessment of lumbar intervertebral instability and degenerative spondylolisthesis. Radiol Clin North Am. 39(1):55-71, v-vi, 2001
9. Gibson JN et al: Surgery for degenerative lumbar spondylosis. Cochrane Database Syst Rev. (2):CD001352, 2000
10. Gibson JN et al: Surgery for degenerative lumbar spondylosis. Cochrane Database Syst Rev. (3):CD001352, 2000
11. Mochida J et al: How to stabilize a single level lesion of degenerative lumbar spondylolisthesis. Clin Orthop. (368):126-34, 1999
12. Nakai S et al: Long-term follow-up study of posterior lumbar interbody fusion. J Spinal Disord. 12(4):293-9, 1999
13. Herkowitz HN et al: Management of degenerative disc disease above an L5-S1 segment requiring arthrodesis. Spine. 24(12):1268-70, 1999
14. Whitecloud TS 3rd et al: Operative treatment of the degenerated segment adjacent to a lumbar fusion. Spine. 19(5):531-6, 1994
15. Murata M et al: Lumbar disc degeneration and segmental instability: a comparison of magnetic resonance images and plain radiographs of patients with low back pain. Arch Orthop Trauma Surg. 113(6):297-301, 1994
16. Boden SD et al: Lumbosacral segmental motion in normal individuals. Have we been measuring instability properly? Spine. 15(6):571-6, 1990
17. Abumi K et al: Biomechanical evaluation of lumbar spinal stability after graded facetectomies. Spine. 15(11):1142-7, 1990
18. Weiler PJ et al: Numerical [corrected] analysis of the load capacity of the human spine fitted with L-rod instrumentation. Spine. 15(12):1285-93, 1990
19. Hayes MA et al: Roentgenographic evaluation of lumbar spine flexion-extension in asymptomatic individuals. Spine. 14(3):327-31, 1989
20. Johnsson KE et al: Postoperative instability after decompression for lumbar spinal stenosis. Spine. 11(2):107-10, 1986
21. Frymoyer JW et al: Segmental instability. Rationale for treatment. Spine. 10(3):280-6, 1985
22. Gertzbein SD et al: Centrode patterns and segmental instability in degenerative disc disease. Spine. 10(3):257-61, 1985

INSTABILITY

IMAGE GALLERY

Typical

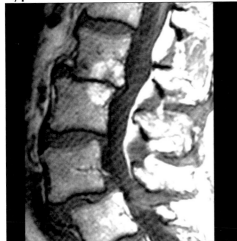 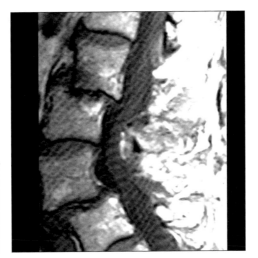

(Left) Sagittal T1WI MR shows retrolisthesis L2 on L3 with type II fatty degenerative endplate changes. Anterolisthesis present at L4-5 with vacuum phenomenon. *(Right)* Sagittal T1WI MR shows progressive retrolisthesis at L2-3, with loss of type II fatty endplate changes reflecting ongoing instability at that level.

Typical

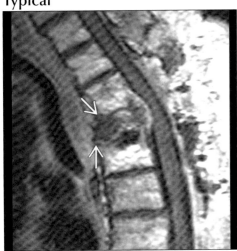 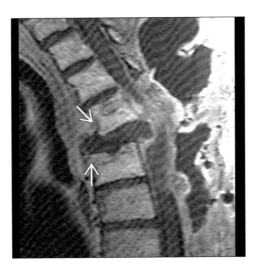

(Left) Sagittal T1 C+ MR shows upper thoracic retrolisthesis (arrows), following multilevel laminectomy/debridement for infection. *(Right)* Sagittal T1 C+ MR shows progressive deformity and retrolisthesis (arrows) at operative site, marked thecal sac compromise, and extensive pseudomeningocele.

Typical

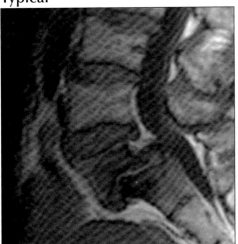 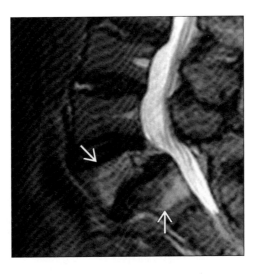

(Left) Sagittal T1WI MR in an adolescent shows severe spondylolisthesis L5 on S1, with disc degeneration and extensive type I endplate changes. *(Right)* Sagittal T2WI MR shows the extensive type I degenerative endplate changes (arrows), and severe lumbar spondylolisthesis.

VERTEBRAL DISC BULGE

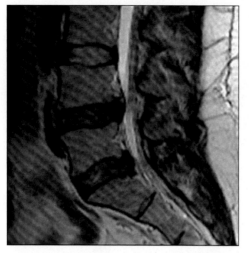

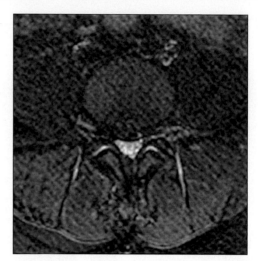

Sagittal T2WI MR shows bulging discs at L4-5 and L5-S1 with associated hypointensities. Minimal height loss is present at L4-5.

Axial T2WI MR with fat suppression shows broad-based disc bulge at L4-5, indenting ventral thecal sac.

TERMINOLOGY

Abbreviations and Synonyms
- Anular bulge

Definitions
- Generalized extension of disc beyond edges of vertebral ring apophyses

IMAGING FINDINGS

General Features
- Best diagnostic clue: Circumferential disc "expansion" beyond confines of vertebral endplates
- Location
  ○ Cervical: C5-6 and C6-7 most common
  ○ Lumbar: L4-5 and L5-S1 most common
- Size: Short radius of extension: ≤ 3 mm
- Morphology
  ○ Broad-based
    ▪ > 50% of disc circumference

Radiographic Findings
- Radiography
  ○ Disc height loss
  ○ Endplate sclerosis and spurring
  ○ Facet arthropathy
  ○ Degenerative spondylolisthesis

- Myelography
  ○ Smooth indentation on anterior thecal sac
    ▪ Central canal and subarticular recesses usually not compromised
    ▪ Unless short pedicles also present
  ○ Bulging disc accentuated by upright myelography
    ▪ Especially at L4-5

CT Findings
- NECT
  ○ Smooth broad-based radial disc bulge
  ○ Vacuum disc phenomenon
- Bone CT
  ○ Better osseous detail with sagittal and coronal reformation

MR Findings
- T1WI: Hypointense bulging disc
- T2WI
  ○ Hypointense bulging disc
    ▪ Dessication and fibrosis
    ▪ Initially seen as linear hypointensity
    ▪ Mild hypointensity likely related to normal aging
- T1 C+
  ○ Enhancing anular tears
  ○ Enhancing fibrovascular marrow in adjacent vertebral endplates
- Disc height loss
- Anular tear

DDx: Disc-Endplate Abnormalities

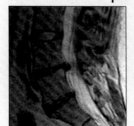

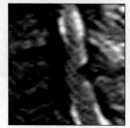

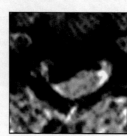

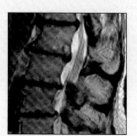

Disc Protrusion   *OPLL*   *OPLL*   *Endplate Spurs*

VERTEBRAL DISC BULGE

Key Facts

Terminology
- Anular bulge
- Generalized extension of disc beyond edges of vertebral ring apophyses

Imaging Findings
- Best diagnostic clue: Circumferential disc "expansion" beyond confines of vertebral endplates
- Size: Short radius of extension: ≤ 3 mm
- > 50% of disc circumference
- Smooth indentation on anterior thecal sac
- Central canal and subarticular recesses usually not compromised
- Bulging disc accentuated by upright myelography
- Hypointense bulging disc
- Disc height loss

- Anular tear
- Extension of contrast into anulus
- T1WI and T2WI MRI with sagittal and axial planes

Top Differential Diagnoses
- Disc protrusion
- Ossification of posterior longitudinal ligament

Pathology
- Genetics: Genetic predisposition to disc degeneration
- Epidemiology: Up to 39% of asymptomatic adults have bulging discs

Clinical Issues
- 82% without progression after one year
- > 80-90% success rate with conservative treatment

- Endplate spurs
- Ligamentum flavum hypertrophy
- Facet arthropathy

Nuclear Medicine Findings
- Bone Scan
  - Uptake of radiotracer in endplates and posterior elements
    - Degenerative changes

Other Modality Findings
- Discography
  - Indications
    - Failed conservative therapy
    - Normal or equivocal MRI findings
    - To correlate disc pathology with symptoms
    - In absence of disc herniation
  - Pain responses
    - No pain, dissimilar pain, similar pain, exact pain
    - Concordant response: Absent painful response in control disc
    - Exact pain in symptomatic disc
  - Extension of contrast into anulus
    - Concentric or circumferential tear
    - Radial tear
  - Dallas discogram description
    - Grade 0: Contrast confined within nucleus pulposus
    - Grade 1: Inner third of anulus
    - Grade 2: Middle third
    - Grade 3: Outer third
    - Focal or < 30° of disc circumference
    - Grade 4 (April and Bogduk): Outer third of anulus
    - > 30° of disc circumference
  - Extension of contrast beyond anulus
    - Grade 5 (Schellhas)
    - Full thickness tear
    - Focal or diffuse

Imaging Recommendations
- Best imaging tool
  - T1WI and T2WI MRI with sagittal and axial planes
  - Only discography can identify symptomatic disc

DIFFERENTIAL DIAGNOSIS

Disc protrusion
- < 50% of disc circumference
- May exceed 3 mm in radius
- Associated central canal, subarticular or foraminal narrowing

Ossification of posterior longitudinal ligament
- Most common in cervical spine (70%)
- Continuous, segmental, mixed or retrodiscal
- Hypointense on T1WI and T2WI
- Vertical extension
- Radiolucent line between ossified ligament and posterior margin of vertebral body on CT

Vertebral endplate spur
- Often associated with bulging disc
- Continuous with vertebral endplate
- Focal or diffuse
- Marrow signal may be present

PATHOLOGY

General Features
- Genetics: Genetic predisposition to disc degeneration
- Etiology
  - Environmental factors
    - Heavy lifting
    - Twisting
    - Flexion and extension
    - Acute trauma
  - Age
  - Poor posture
  - Repetitive micro trauma
    - Endplate injury
    - Rim lesion: Horizontal tear in outer anulus at its attachment to ring apophysis
  - Interruption of nutritional supply to disc
  - Decreasing water content in nucleus pulposus

VERTEBRAL DISC BULGE

II

2

20

- Proteoglycans replaced by fibrocartilage and fibrosis
  - Increasing disc stiffness
- Ineffective cushioning
  - Decreasing intra-disc pressure
- Unequal force distribution to anulus
  - Increasing pressure on anulus posteriorly and posterolaterally
  - Concentric tear ± radial tear → disc bulge and herniation
- Epidemiology: Up to 39% of asymptomatic adults have bulging discs
- Associated abnormalities
  - Osteoporosis
  - Scoliosis
    - Asymmetric lateral bulge
  - Spondylolisthesis
    - Posterior bulge
- Anatomy
  - Central nucleus pulposus
    - Shock absorbing
    - Proteoglycans and glycosaminoglycans
    - High water content (70-90%)
    - Few collagen fibers
  - Transition zone
  - Peripheral anulus fibrosus
    - Tensile strength
    - Outer zone: Dense collagen fibers in concentric lamellae
    - Inner zone: Fibrocartilage
    - Avascular
    - Receives nutrients through diffusion from adjacent vertebral endplates
    - Outer third innervated by sinuvertebral nerve

Microscopic Features

- Myxomatous degeneration of anulus fibrosus
- A combination of anulus, nucleus, fibrocartilage or apophyseal bone

CLINICAL ISSUES

Presentation

- Most common signs/symptoms
  - Low back pain
  - Other signs/symptoms
    - Radiculopathy
    - Neurogenic claudication
- Clinical profile
  - Worsening pain with flexion and increased intra-abdominal pressure
    - Increasing intra-disc pressure
  - Pain relieved by lying flat with flexed hips and knees

Demographics

- Age: 30-70

Natural History & Prognosis

- 82% without progression after one year
- > 80-90% success rate with conservative treatment

Treatment

- Conservative
  - NSAIDs

- Physical therapy
- Epidural injection
  - Cortisone ± lidocaine
- Surgical
  - Discectomy with stabilization if intractable pain
    - About 75% success rate

DIAGNOSTIC CHECKLIST

Image Interpretation Pearls

- Axial and sagittal CT or MRI differentiates disc bulge from disc herniation

SELECTED REFERENCES

1. Lebkowski WJ et al: Degenerated lumbar intervertebral disc. A morphological study. Pol J Pathol. 53(2):83-6, 2002
2. Ido K et al: The validity of upright myelography for diagnosing lumbar disc herniation. Clin Neurol Neurosurg. 104(1):30-5, 2002
3. Fredericson M et al: Changes in posterior disc bulging and intervertebral foraminal size associated with flexion-extension movement: a comparison between L4-5 and L5-S1 levels in normal subjects. Spine J. 1(1):10-7, 2001
4. Botwin KP et al: Role of weight-bearing flexion and extension myelography in evaluating the intervertebral disc. Am J Phys Med Rehabil. 80(4):289-95, 2001
5. Luoma K et al: Low back pain in relation to lumbar disc degeneration. Spine. 25(4):487-92, 2000
6. Adams MA et al: Mechanical initiation of intervertebral disc degeneration. Spine. 25(13):1625-36, 2000
7. Milette PC et al: Differentiating lumbar disc protrusions, disc bulges, and discs with normal contour but abnormal signal intensity. Magnetic resonance imaging with discographic correlations. Spine. 24(1):44-53, 1999
8. Sambrook PN et al: Genetic influences on cervical and lumbar disc degeneration: a magnetic resonance imaging study in twins. Arthritis Rheum. 42(2):366-72, 1999
9. Harada A et al: Correlation between bone mineral density and intervertebral disc degeneration. Spine. 23(8):857-61; discussion 862, 1998
10. Maezawa S et al: Pain provocation at lumbar discography as analyzed by computed tomography/discography. Spine. 17(11):1309-15, 1992
11. Cowan NC et al: The natural history of sciatica: a prospective radiological study. Clin Radiol. 46(1):7-12, 1992
12. Ito S et al: An observation of ruptured annulus fibrosus in lumbar discs. J Spinal Disord. 4(4):462-6, 1991
13. Bernard TN Jr: Lumbar discography followed by computed tomography. Refining the diagnosis of low-back pain. Spine. 15(7):690-707, 1990
14. Tervonen O et al: Lumbar disc degeneration. Correlation between CT and CT/discography. Acta Radiol. 31(6):551-4, 1990
15. Kambin P et al: Annular protrusion: pathophysiology and roentgenographic appearance. Spine. 13(6):671-5, 1988
16. Sachs BL et al: Dallas discogram description. A new classification of CT/discography in low-back disorders. Spine. 12(3):287-94, 1987

VERTEBRAL DISC BULGE

IMAGE GALLERY

Typical

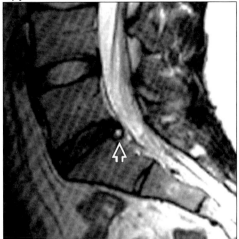
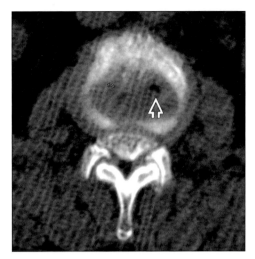

(Left) Sagittal T2WI MR shows a disc bulge at L5-S1 with associated anular fissure (arrow). Disc dessication is also present. *(Right)* Axial NECT after myelography shows mild circumferential disc bulge with associated vacuum disc phenomenon (arrow). There is mild central canal narrowing.

Typical

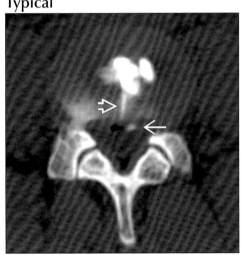
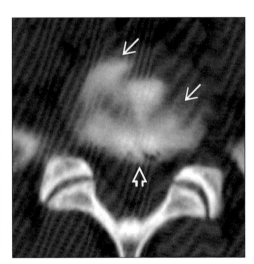

(Left) Axial NECT after discography shows a full thickness radial tear (open arrow) through anulus. There is a broad-based anular bulge with a small amount of extravasated contrast (arrow). *(Right)* Axial NECT after discography shows multiple circumferential anular tears (arrows). These coalesce into a large dorsal anular defect, allowing contrast extending beyond anulus (open arrow).

Typical

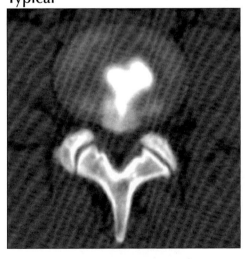
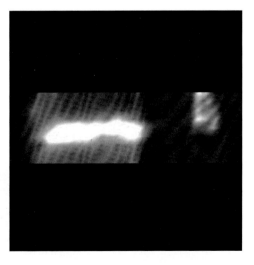

(Left) Axial NECT after discography shows a radial tear extending into middle third of dorsal anulus with associated focal anular bulge. *(Right)* Axial NECT after discography with sagittal reformation shows a full thickness tear in dorsal anulus with contrast extending slightly beyond confines of vertebral endplates.

VERTEBRAL DISC ANULAR TEAR

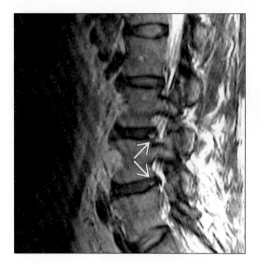

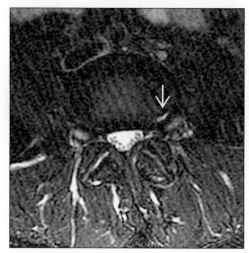

Sagittal T2WI MR shows small foci of high intensity (arrows) in the far left lateral disc margins of L3-4 and L4-5 levels. Note signal loss of parent discs.

Axial T2WI MR shows crescentic, focal high signal in L3-4 disc (arrow), in anulus within foraminal zone. Sagittal T2WI showed an identical focus cross-referenced to this site.

TERMINOLOGY

Abbreviations and Synonyms
- Anular fissure; anular defect; high intensity zone (HIZ) in posterior anulus
  - Term "tear" inaccurately implies acute traumatic etiology, rather than the typical cause of repetitive stress

Definitions
- Disruption of concentric collagenous fibers comprising the anulus fibrosus

IMAGING FINDINGS

General Features
- Best diagnostic clue: Abnormal signal focus (HIZ) at posterior disc margin on MRI
- Location: Posterior margin of lumbar, thoracic, or cervical disc
- Size: Typically a 1-2 mm focus
- Morphology: Well-circumscribed
- Typically seen with degenerating disc
- Classic imaging appearance
  - Focal HIZ in the anulus on T2WI with low signal of parent disc
  - Contrast-enhancement on T1WI

CT Findings
- CECT
  - CECT can show enhancement of disc margin
  - CT post discography shows intradiscal dye at posterior margin of or leaking through anulus

MR Findings
- T1WI: Contrast-enhancing nidus in disc margin
- T2WI: High signal zone at edge of disc which has low intrinsic signal
- T1 C+: Focally enhancing nidus in posterior disc margin

Other Modality Findings
- Discography demonstrates contrast leak from central site of injection through anulus
- Discography is more a provocative test (symptom simulation), rather than a diagnostic imaging modality
  - Separates symptomatic tears (internal disc disruption syndrome-IDD) from incidental ones
  - If typical pain reproduced
  - No double-blind prospective studies exist to verify IDD theory
  - Several studies show poor correlation between presence of tear and concordant symptoms at discography

---

DDx: Abnormal Disc Signal

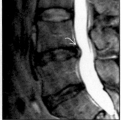

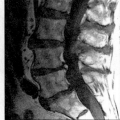

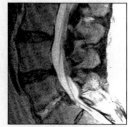

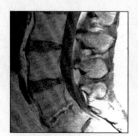

| *Disc Protrusion* | *Disc Fat: Marrow* | *Discitis, T2WI* | *Discitis, T1C+* |

VERTEBRAL DISC ANULAR TEAR

Key Facts

Terminology
- Anular fissure; anular defect; high intensity zone (HIZ) in posterior anulus

Imaging Findings
- Focal HIZ in the anulus on T2WI with low signal of parent disc
- Contrast-enhancement on T1WI
- T1 C+: Focally enhancing nidus in posterior disc margin
- Discography is more a provocative test (symptom simulation), rather than a diagnostic imaging modality

Pathology
- Autopsy demonstrates high prevalence of tears
- Direct association with disc degeneration

- MRI shows anular tears in majority of asymptomatic individuals
- Associated abnormalities: Disc protrusion or extrusion (herniation)

Clinical Issues
- Chronic back pain or sciatica in absence of mechanical nerve root compromise
- Controversial role of anular tear

Diagnostic Checklist
- Other sources of low back pain or disc pathology; e.g., disc infection
- Incidentally seen focal high intensity zone in anulus of otherwise normal disc is essentially a normal finding

Imaging Recommendations
- Sagittal heavily T2WI with thin-sections
- Contrast-enhanced T1WI

DIFFERENTIAL DIAGNOSIS

Discitis
- Diffuse signal alteration of disc
- Enhancement throughout disc and/or paralleling endplate(s)
- Abnormal marrow adjacent to interspace
- Epidural abscess may be present

Focal disc protrusion
- High signal zone represents both the anular defect and disc material extending beyond normal margin of interspace
- Often accompanies anular defect when a complete anular radial tear occurs

Focal fat or ossification with fatty marrow
- HIZ on T1WI in disc margin
- HIZ fades on T2WI, or with fat-saturation pulse
- CT (or plain x-ray) shows ossification of posterior disc

PATHOLOGY

General Features
- General path comments
  - Anulus composed of dense, concentric, crescentically ordered collagen layers
    - Vertically oriented
    - Attach to hyaline cartilage endplate at rim (Sharpey fibers)
    - Contains small blood vessels and nociceptive nerve fibers in outer lateral edge
    - Blood vessels and nerve fibers diminish with age
    - With age inner anulus expands at expense of nucleus
  - Anulus in cervical discs of adults differs from lumbar
    - Absence or attrition of thick posterior anulus

    - Only a thin layer of vertical collagen fibers exists
    - Posterior longitudinal ligament contains the disc within interspace
- Genetics
  - Genetic predisposition to "weak" collagen has been demonstrated in electron microscopic studies
  - Anular defects associated with certain familial conditions such as Scheuermann syndrome
- Etiology
  - With age anulus demonstrates focal lamellar thickening
  - Concentric tear
    - Repetitive stress on spinal motion element leads to lamellar separation, defect parallels lamellar orientation
  - Transverse tear
    - Micro trauma produces defects in anular attachment at endplate rim
  - Radial fissure or tear
    - Various factors including loss of nutrient vessels can lead to total lamellar disruption through outer margin
- Epidemiology
  - Autopsy demonstrates high prevalence of tears
    - Increase with age
  - Direct association with disc degeneration
  - Discography shows presence of anular tears in up to 80% of degenerated discs
  - MRI shows anular tears in majority of asymptomatic individuals
    - Some tears seen only on CE T1WI
    - 96% of all tears enhance
    - Most annular tears persist for months on follow-up MRI
- Associated abnormalities: Disc protrusion or extrusion (herniation)

Gross Pathologic & Surgical Features
- Separation of lamellar structure in concentric tears
- Transverse disruption of fibers in rim or radial fissures

Microscopic Features
- Granulation tissue with microvascularity invades tears

○ Source of enhancement

Staging, Grading or Classification Criteria
- Concentric tears are essentially an aging variant
- Rim tears and radial tears may have clinical consequences in some cases
- Dallas discogram description
  - ○ Grade 0: Contrast confined within nucleus pulposus
  - ○ Grade 1: Inner third of anulus
  - ○ Grade 2: Middle third
  - ○ Grade 3: Outer third
  - ○ Focal or < 30° of disc circumference
  - ○ Grade 4: (April and Bogduk): Outer third anulus
  - ○ > 30° of disc circumference
- Extension of contrast beyond anulus
  - ○ Grade 5 (Schellhas)
  - ○ Full thickness tear
  - ○ Focal or diffuse

CLINICAL ISSUES

Presentation
- Most common signs/symptoms
  - ○ Back or radicular pain
    - Recurrent meningeal nerve and ventral ramus of somatic spinal nerve are sources of innervation
    - Pain may be radicular in distribution
    - Anular disruption may allow inflammatory substances to leak from nucleus
    - Most anular tears are asymptomatic
  - ○ Other signs/symptoms
    - Reproducibility of pain with discography
- Clinical profile
  - ○ Chronic back pain or sciatica in absence of mechanical nerve root compromise
  - ○ Controversial role of anular tear
    - Most tears are incidental findings

Demographics
- Age
  - ○ Up to 25% of normal individuals under 20 show anular defects
  - ○ Majority of adult individuals harbor anular defects
- Gender: No gender differences

Natural History & Prognosis
- Most are asymptomatic or self-limited
  - ○ Scar endpoint of inflammation
- Some felt to be cause of chronic back pain and sciatica
- Good in most symptomatic cases
- Up to 1/3 of chronic pain sufferers have recurrent symptoms despite any therapy

Treatment
- Symptomatic pain relief with NSAIDs
- Chronic pain may prompt patients to undergo fusion as last resort

DIAGNOSTIC CHECKLIST

Consider
- Other sources of low back pain or disc pathology; e.g., disc infection

Image Interpretation Pearls
- Incidentally seen focal high intensity zone in anulus of otherwise normal disc is essentially a normal finding

SELECTED REFERENCES

1. Munter FM et al: Serial MR Imaging of Annular Tears in Lumbar Intervertebral Disks. AJNR Am J Neuroradiol. 23(7):1105-9, 2002
2. Slipman CW et al: Side of symptomatic annular tear and site of low back pain: is there a correlation? Spine. 26(8):E165-9, 2001
3. Weishaupt D et al: Painful Lumbar Disk Derangement: Relevance of Endplate Abnormalities at MR Imaging. Radiology. 218(2):420-7, 2001
4. Schollmeier G et al: Observations on fiber-forming collagens in the anulus fibrosus. Spine. 25(21): 2736-41, 2000
5. Mercer S et al: The ligaments and annulus fibrosus of human adult cervical intervertebral discs. Spine. 24(7): 619-26; discussion 627-8, 1999
6. Ahn JM et al: Peripheral focal low signal intensity areas in the degenerated annulus fibrosus on T2-weighted fast spin echo MR images: correlation with macroscopic and microscopic findings in elderly cadavers. Skeletal Radiol. 28(4):209-14, 1999
7. Saifuddin A et al: The value of lumbar spine magnetic resonance imaging in the demonstration of anular tears. Spine. 23(4):453-7, 1998
8. Ito M et al: Predictive signs of discogenic lumbar pain on magnetic resonance imaging with discography correlation. Spine. 23(11):1252-8; discussion 1259-60, 1998
9. Stadnik TW et al: Annular tears and disk herniation: prevalence and contrast enhancement on MR images in the absence of low back pain or sciatica. Radiology. 206(1):49-55, 1998
10. Vernon-Roberts B et al: Pathogenesis of tears of the anulus investigated by multiple-level transaxial analysis of the T12-L1 disc. Spine 22(22): 2641-6, 1997
11. Wood KB et al: Magnetic resonance imaging of the thoracic spine. Evaluation of asymptomatic individuals. J Bone Joint Surg Am. 77(11):1631-8, 1995
12. Bogduk N et al: The innervation of the cervical intervertebral discs. Spine. 13(1): 2-8, 1988
13. Yu SW et al: Tears of the anulus fibrosus: correlation between MR and pathologic findings in cadavers. AJNR Am J Neuroradiol. 9(2):367-70, 1988
14. Pooni JS et al: Comparison of the structure of human intervertebral discs in the cervical, thoracic and lumbar regions of the spine. Surg Radiol Anat. 8(3): 175-82, 1986
15. Johnson EF et al: The distribution and arrangement of elastic fibres in the intervertebral disc of the adult human. J Anat. 135 (Pt 2): 301-9, 1982

VERTEBRAL DISC ANULAR TEAR

IMAGE GALLERY

Typical

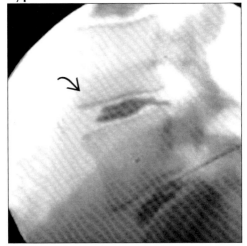 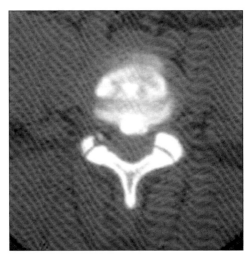

(Left) Lateral radiography during discography shows leakage of intradiscal contrast at L4-5 (arrow); fissured degenerated parent & L5-S1 disc. Symptoms were reproduced with injection of L5-S1 disc, not L4-5. *(Right)* Axial bone CT after the discogram (left) shows the leakage of contrast into the ventral epidural space at L4-5, verifying the presence of the anular defect.

Typical

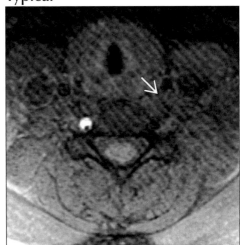 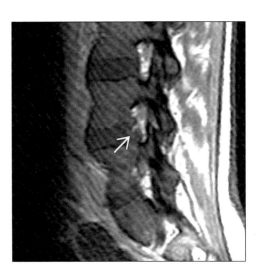

(Left) Axial T2WI MR shows semilunar high signal in the posterolateral anulus within the L4-5 foramen (arrow), the low signal of the disc indicative of its degeneration. *(Right)* Sagittal T1 C+ MR shows enhancing high signal focus (arrow) in the foraminal margin of the L4-5 disc.

Typical

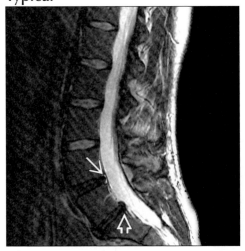 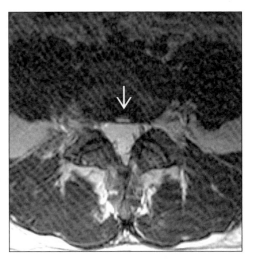

(Left) Sagittal T2WI MR demonstrates difference between anular tear in L4-5 disc (arrow), and disc protrusion at L5-S1, with absence of focal high signal due to chronic fibrosis (open arrow). *(Right)* Axial T2WI MR shows high signal zone in anulus at midline of L4-5 disc (arrow), which cross-referenced to mid-sagittal slice of T2WI.

INTERVERTEBRAL DISC HERNIATION, CERVICAL

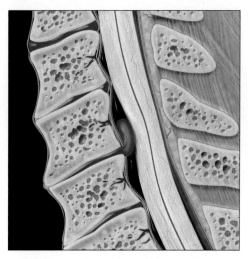

Sagittal graphic shows disc extrusion, with base of herniation smaller than epidural component, effaces thecal sac and causes cord compression.

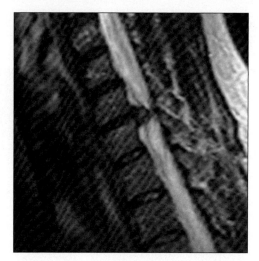

Sagittal T2WI MR shows C5-6 disc extrusion with base of herniation smaller than component extending into epidural space.

TERMINOLOGY

Abbreviations and Synonyms

- Abbreviation: Cervical disc herniation (CDH)
- Synonyms: Protruded disc, extruded disc, free fragment, sequestered disc
- Nonstandard: Prolapse, herniated nucleus pulposus (HNP), rupture

Definitions

- Localized (< 50% of disc circumference) displacement of disc material beyond edges of vertebral ring apophyses

IMAGING FINDINGS

General Features

- Best diagnostic clue: Small mass in spinal canal, contiguous with intervertebral disc
- Location
  - Ventral epidural
  - C6-7 level most common, with compression of C7 root
  - C5-6 second most common location, compressing C6 root
- Size: Variable
- Morphology

  - Protrusion
    - Protrusion is herniated disc with broad-base at parent disc
    - Greatest diameter of protrusion in any plane < distance between edges of base in same plane
    - Focal: < 25% of disc circumference
    - Broad-based: > 25%, but < 50% of disc circumference (greater than 50% is defined as bulge)
  - Extrusion
    - Extrusion is herniated disc with narrow or no base at parent disc
    - Greatest diameter of extrusion in any plane > distance between edges of base in same plane
    - Sequestered or free fragment: Extruded disc without contiguity to parent disc
    - Migrated: Disc material displaced away from site of herniation, regardless of continuity to parent disc
  - Intravertebral herniation (Schmorl node)

Radiographic Findings

- Myelography
  - Extradural defect at intervertebral disc level
  - Effacement or cut-off of root sleeves

CT Findings

- NECT

DDx: Cervical Extradural Disease

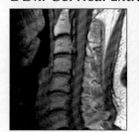

OPLL

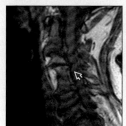

Osteophyte

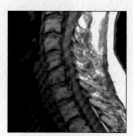

Spondylosis

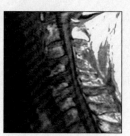

Post-operative

INTERVERTEBRAL DISC HERNIATION, CERVICAL

Key Facts

Terminology
- Abbreviation: Cervical disc herniation (CDH)
- Synonyms: Protruded disc, extruded disc, free fragment, sequestered disc
- Nonstandard: Prolapse, herniated nucleus pulposus (HNP), rupture

Imaging Findings
- Best diagnostic clue: Small mass in spinal canal, contiguous with intervertebral disc
- Protrusion is herniated disc with broad-base at parent disc
- Greatest diameter of protrusion in any plane < distance between edges of base in same plane
- Extrusion is herniated disc with narrow or no base at parent disc

- Greatest diameter of extrusion in any plane > distance between edges of base in same plane
- Sequestered or free fragment: Extruded disc without contiguity to parent disc

Top Differential Diagnoses
- OPLL
- Osteophyte
- Tumor
- Abscess

Clinical Issues
- Clinical symptoms affected by level, location and size of herniation
- Neck pain and stiffness, with radiating pain to shoulder and upper extremity

---

- Ventral epidural soft tissue density extending dorsally into spinal canal contiguous with disc
- Displaces exiting nerve roots and distorts thecal sac

MR Findings
- T1WI
  - Isointense to parent disc
  - May show low signal if calcified or associated with vacuum phenomenon
- T2WI: Isointense to hyperintense
- T2* GRE: Variable in signal reflecting hydration of disc material (hyperintense) or calcification (hypointense)
- T1 C+
  - No enhancement of disc material
  - May enhance peripherally after intravenous contrast material due to granulation tissue or dilated epidural plexus
  - May rarely diffusely enhance if associated with granulation tissue, or post-contrast imaging delayed due to diffusion
- Variable amount of exiting root and thecal sac impingement
- Variable amount of degenerative changes at same or other disc levels

Imaging Recommendations
- Best imaging tool: MR
- Protocol advice: Sagittal, axial T1WI and T2WI; intravenous contrast if question of tumor, infection

DIFFERENTIAL DIAGNOSIS

OPLL
- Flowing low signal epidural space on all sequences
- May show increased signal on T1WI due to fatty marrow content

Osteophyte
- Sharp margins not arising directly from intervertebral disc level
- May show increased signal on T1WI due to fatty marrow content

Tumor
- Homogeneous enhancement, irregular and infiltrative
- Not arising out of intervertebral disc

Hemorrhage
- Elongated within the epidural space
- Tends to be posterior
- Isointense in hyperacute phase, increased signal in subacute stage on T1WI

Abscess
- May mimic large herniation with peripheral enhancement
- Increased signal on T2WI, endplate destruction

PATHOLOGY

General Features
- General path comments: Composed of combination of nucleus pulposus, fragmented anulus, cartilage, and fragmented apophyseal bone
- Genetics
  - Congenitally weak collagen predisposes to degenerative disc disease
  - Increased incidence of spondylosis in Marfan syndrome
- Etiology
  - Degenerative breach in anulus
  - May be post-traumatic
  - Disc material extends through defect
  - Protrusions may be contained by thin annuloligamentous complex
- Epidemiology: 10% of people under age 40 have cervical herniation
- Associated abnormalities: 20% of people over age 40 have cervical foraminal stenosis

Gross Pathologic & Surgical Features
- Nucleus pulposus
  - Gelatinous material with high water content and few collagen fibers
  - Water content decreases with age

- Anulus fibrosus
  - Fibrocartilage, with collagen fibers in concentric lamellae

Microscopic Features
- Degeneration shows cracks, fissures within nucleus; endplate fragmentation; granulation tissue; thickening endplate trabeculae

CLINICAL ISSUES

Presentation
- Most common signs/symptoms
  - Clinical symptoms affected by level, location and size of herniation
  - Neck pain and stiffness, with radiating pain to shoulder and upper extremity
  - May include paresthesia, hyperesthesia and weakness
    - Neck pain (90%)
    - Paresthesia (89%)
    - Radicular pain (65%)
    - Weakness (15%)
  - Central herniations produce cord compression; paracentrals compress ipsilateral hemicord
  - Lateral herniations compress anterior cervical root giving weakness without pain
  - Lateral herniations compress root and dorsal root ganglion causing pain
- Clinical profile
  - 4th-5th decades
  - Risk factors include increasing age; heavy physical work; work dissatisfaction; depression; history of headache

Demographics
- Age: Adult population
- Gender: M > F

Natural History & Prognosis
- Acute radiculopathy usually self-limited disorder with full recovery expected
- Chronic nonspecific pain much more variable
  - 90% back to work by 3 months
  - Continuous or recurrent pain affects 30-40%

Treatment
- Options, risks, complications
  - Conservative treatment
    - Exercise and physical conditioning
    - Nonsteroidal anti-inflammatory drugs
    - Transcutaneous electrical stimulation
    - Epidural steroid injection
    - Opioids
    - Atypical analgesics such as antidepressants, antiepileptic drugs, neuroleptics
  - Multiple surgical approaches without clear consensus
    - Anterior discectomy with fusion (with or without anterior plating and screw fixation)
    - Anterior discectomy without fusion
    - Hemilaminectomy and foraminotomy
  - Compressive cervical myelopathy with herniation and spondylosis treated by corpectomy with strut graft or with multilevel laminectomy

DIAGNOSTIC CHECKLIST

Consider
- OPLL if extradural disease low in signal on all sequences

Image Interpretation Pearls
- Define herniation by level, size, location (central, paracentral, lateral), effect on thecal sac and cord, migration away from disc level
- Combination of axial T1WI and gradient echo T2* better define disc contour due to variable disc signal
- FLAIR insensitive in the spine for intrinsic cord signal abnormality such as contusion, myelomalacia
  - Use fast STIR as additional sequence for cord disease combined with standard fast spin echo T2WI

SELECTED REFERENCES

1. Furusawa N et al: Herniation of cervical intervertebral disc: immunohistochemical examination and measurement of nitric oxide production. Spine. 26(10): 1110-6, 2001
2. Fardon DF et al: Nomenclature and classification of lumbar disc pathology. Recommendations of the Combined task Forces of the North American Spine Society, American Society of Spine Radiology, and American Society of Neuroradiology. Spine. 26(5): E93-E113, 2001
3. Campi A et al: Comparison of MRI pulse sequences for investigation of lesions of the cervical spinal cord. Neuroradiology. 42(9): 669-75, 2000
4. Grob D: Surgery in the degenerative cervical spine. Spine. 23(24): 2674-83, 1998
5. Ahlgren BD et al: Cervical Radiculopathy. Orthop Clin North Am. 27(2): 253-63, 1996
6. Jensen MC et al: Magnetic resonance imaging of the lumbar spine in people without back pain. N Engl J Med. 331(2): 69-73, 1994
7. Radhakrishnan K et al: Epidemiology of cervical radiculopathy. A population-based study from Rochester, Minnesota, 1976 through 1990. Brain. 117 (Pt 2): 325-35, 1994
8. Sze G et al: Fast spin-echo MR imaging of the cervical spine: influence of echo train length and echo spacing on image contrast and quality. AJNR Am J Neuroradiol. 14(5): 1203-13, 1993
9. Jahnke RW et al: Cervical stenosis, spondylosis, and herniated disc disease. Radiol Clin North Am. 29(4): 777-91, 1991
10. Boden SD et al: Abnormal magnetic-resonance scans of the cervical spine in asymptomatic subjects. A prospective investigation. J Bone Joint Surg Am. 72(8): 1178-84, 1990
11. Modic MT et al: Imaging of degenerative disease of the cervical spine. Clin Orthop. (239): 109-20, 1989
12. Brown BM et al: Preoperative evaluation of cervical radiculopathy and myelopathy by surface-coil MR imaging. AJR Am J Roentgenol. 151(6): 1205-12, 1988
13. Simon JE et al: Diskogenic disease of the cervical spine. Semin Roentgenol. 23(2): 118-24, 1988
14. Crandall PH et al: Cervical spondylotic myelopathy. J Neurosurg. 25(1): 57-66, 1966

INTERVERTEBRAL DISC HERNIATION, CERVICAL

IMAGE GALLERY

Typical

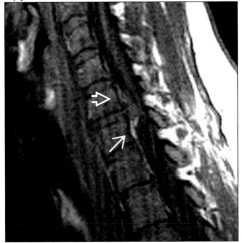
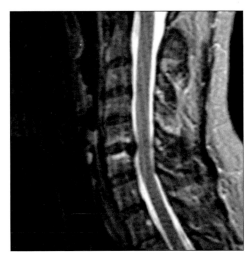

(Left) Sagittal T1WI MR shows extrusion displacing cervical cord. High signal inferior to CDH is epidural fat (arrow). Isointense signal superior to herniation is epidural plexus (open arrow). (Right) Sagittal T2WI MR shows small central protrusion as low signal effacing ventral thecal sac but not distorting the cord. Type I degenerative endplate changes are present as high signal at C5-6.

Typical

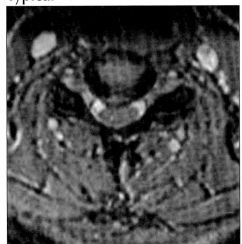
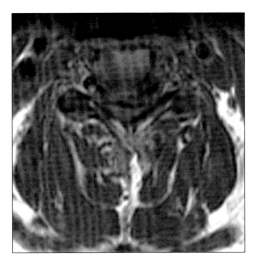

(Left) Axial T2* GRE MR shows small focal protrusion touching ventral cord. Herniation is < 25% of the disc margin. (Right) Axial T1WI MR shows broad-based extrusion severely impinging upon cord. Herniation is > 25% and < 50% of disc circumference.

Typical

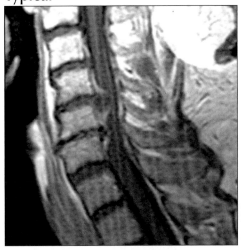
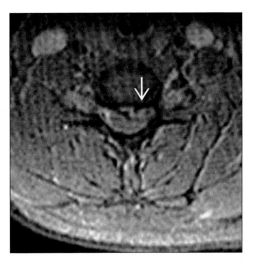

(Left) Sagittal T1 C+ MR shows C4-5 extrusion impinging upon cord. Smaller C5-6 protrusion also effaces ventral cord. Peripheral enhancement related to epidural plexus and granulation tissue. (Right) Axial T2* GRE MR shows left sided extrusion (arrow) effacing left side of thecal sac and cord, and extending towards left neural foramen.

INTERVERTEBRAL DISC HERNIATION, THORACIC

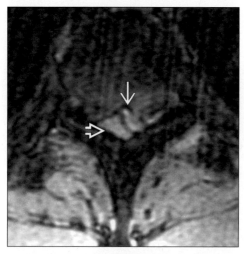

Axial T2* GRE MR through the upper thoracic spine shows large left sided extrusion (arrow) compressing the left side of thoracic cord (open arrow).

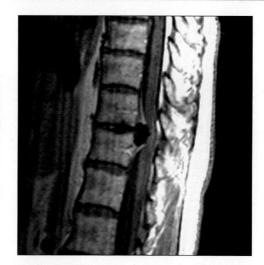

Sagittal T1WI MR with contrast shows large hypointense mass contiguous with disc space reflecting calcified disc extrusion. Prominent distended epidural veins "tent" around herniation.

TERMINOLOGY

Abbreviations and Synonyms

- Thoracic disc herniation (TDH); dorsal spinal herniation
- Protruded disc, extruded disc, free fragment, sequestered disc
- Nonstandard: Prolapse, herniated nucleus pulposus (HNP), rupture

Definitions

- Localized (< 50% of disc circumference) displacement of disc material beyond edges of vertebral ring apophyses

IMAGING FINDINGS

General Features

- Best diagnostic clue: Small mass in spinal canal contiguous with intervertebral disc
- Location
  - Ventral epidural
  - T6 ⇒ T11 most common
  - Rare in upper thoracic spine (T1-T3)
- Size: Variable
- Morphology
  - Protrusion
    - Herniated disc with broad base at parent disc
    - Greatest diameter of herniated disc in any plane < distance between edges of base in same plane
    - Focal: < 25% of disc circumference
    - Broad-based: > 25%, but < 50% of disc circumference (greater than 50% is defined as bulge)
  - Extrusion
    - Herniated disc with narrow or no base at parent disc
    - Greatest diameter of herniated disc in any plane > distance between edges of base in same plane
    - Sequestered or free fragment: Extruded disc without contiguity to parent disc
    - Migrated: Disc material displaced away from site of herniation, regardless of continuity to parent disc
  - Intravertebral herniation (Schmorl node)

Radiographic Findings

- Myelography
  - Extradural defect at intervertebral disc level
  - Effacement or cut-off of root sleeves
  - Displacement or compression of cord

CT Findings

- NECT
  - Ventral epidural soft tissue density extending dorsally into spinal canal contiguous with disc

DDx: Thoracic Extramedullary Lesions

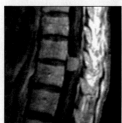

Meningioma

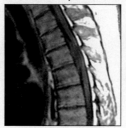

Chondroid Tumor

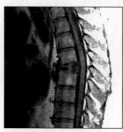

Multiple Myeloma

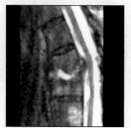

Infection

INTERVERTEBRAL DISC HERNIATION, THORACIC

Key Facts

Terminology
- Thoracic disc herniation (TDH); dorsal spinal herniation
- Protruded disc, extruded disc, free fragment, sequestered disc

Imaging Findings
- T6 ⇒ T11 most common
- Rare in upper thoracic spine (T1-T3)

Top Differential Diagnoses
- Osteophyte
- Tumor
- Hemorrhage
- Abscess

Clinical Issues
- Protean symptomatology
- Pain: Axial, localized or radicular (76%)
- Myelopathy
- As in cervical and lumbar spine, high percentage of herniations remain without major neurologic compromise
- 20-30% may require surgery
- Thoracic disc surgery uncommon, represents 1-2% of all disc surgery
- Surgery for intractable pain, neurologic dysfunction

Diagnostic Checklist
- Calcification (65%)
- Multiple herniation (14%)
- Intradural herniations (7%)

○ Displaces cord and thecal sac
○ May be completely or partially calcified

MR Findings
- T1WI
  ○ Isointense to hypointense to parent disc
  ○ May show low signal if calcified or associated with vacuum phenomenon
  ○ Herniation may only be inferred by mass effect upon the cord if lesion very low in signal
- T2WI: Variable signal reflecting hydration state and presence or absence of calcification
- STIR: Variable signal reflecting hydration state and presence or absence of calcification
- T2* GRE: Variable signal reflecting hydration of disc material (hyperintense) or calcification (hypointense)
- T1 C+
  ○ No enhancement of disc material
  ○ May enhance peripherally after intravenous contrast material due to granulation tissue or dilated epidural plexus
  ○ Peripheral enhancement may give "lifted band" or "tent" configuration

Imaging Recommendations
- Best imaging tool: MR
- Protocol advice: Sagittal, axial T1WI and T2WI; intravenous contrast if question of tumor, infection

DIFFERENTIAL DIAGNOSIS

Osteophyte
- Sharp margins not arising directly from intervertebral disc level
- May show increased signal on T1WI due to fatty marrow content

Tumor
- Homogeneous enhancement
- Not arising out of intervertebral disc
- Irregular and infiltrative

Hemorrhage
- Elongated within epidural space, tends to be posterior
- Isointense in hyperacute phase; increased signal in subacute stage on T1WI

Abscess
- May mimic large herniation with peripheral enhancement
- Increased signal on T2WI
- Associated with endplate destruction of disc space infection and adjacent osteomyelitis

PATHOLOGY

General Features
- General path comments: Composed of combination of nucleus pulposus, fragmented anulus, cartilage, and fragmented apophyseal bone
- Genetics: Congenitally weak collagen predisposes to degenerative disc disease
- Etiology
  ○ Degenerative breach in the anulus
  ○ Prior history of trauma (37%)
  ○ Disc material extends through defect
  ○ Protrusions may be contained by thin annuloligamentous complex
- Epidemiology
  ○ Uncommon entity
  ○ Estimated 2-3 cases per 1,000 patients with disc protrusions
  ○ One patient per million population per annum
- Associated abnormalities
  ○ Signs of disc degeneration elsewhere in spine
    ▪ Loss of disc space height
    ▪ Loss of disc signal on T2WI
    ▪ Vacuum disc
    ▪ Scheuermann endplate irregularity
    ▪ Linear remodeling of endplate directed to herniation
  ○ Disc bulge or tear at other thoracic levels

INTERVERTEBRAL DISC HERNIATION, THORACIC

Gross Pathologic & Surgical Features
- Nucleus pulposus
  - Gelatinous material with high water content and few collagen fibers
  - Water content decreases with age
- Anulus fibrosus
  - Fibrocartilage, with collagen fibers in concentric lamellae

Microscopic Features
- Degeneration shows cracks, fissures within nucleus; endplate fragmentation; granulation tissue; thickening endplate trabeculae

CLINICAL ISSUES

Presentation
- Most common signs/symptoms
  - Protean symptomatology
  - Pain: Axial, localized or radicular (76%)
  - Myelopathy
    - Motor impairment (60%)
    - Hyperreflexia, spasticity (58%)
    - Sensory impairment (61%)
    - Bladder dysfunction (24%)
  - Other signs/symptoms
    - May rarely present as abdominal pain
- Clinical profile
  - 5th decade
  - Prior trauma history
  - History of Scheuermann

Demographics
- Age: Adult population
- Gender: M = F

Natural History & Prognosis
- Asymptomatic population
  - Thoracic disc herniation (37%)
  - Disc bulge (53%)
  - Anular tear (58%)
- Thoracic disc herniations
  - As in cervical and lumbar spine, high percentage of herniations remain without major neurologic compromise
  - 20-30% may require surgery
  - Small herniations (0-10% canal compromise) tend to remain stable in size, and remain asymptomatic
  - Large herniations (> 20% canal compromise) tend to decrease in size

Treatment
- Options, risks, complications
  - Thoracic disc surgery uncommon, represents 1-2% of all disc surgery
  - Surgery for intractable pain, neurologic dysfunction
  - Variety of surgical approaches
    - Transthoracic
    - Transfacet pedicle sparing
    - Lateral extracavitary
    - Transpedicular
  - Causes of surgical failure for thoracic herniations
    - Misidentified level

- Cord injury/vascular injury
- Migrated disc fragment missed
- Intradural disc extension missed
- Lack of adequate visualization during surgery

DIAGNOSTIC CHECKLIST

Consider
- Calcification (65%)
- Multiple herniation (14%)
- Intradural herniations (7%)

Image Interpretation Pearls
- T2WI critical since herniation may not be visible on T1WI due to calcification
- Check and recheck herniation level, counting from C2 and L5 levels
- Combination of axial T1WI and gradient echo T2* better define disc contour due to variable disc signal

SELECTED REFERENCES

1. Dickman CA et al: Reoperation for herniated thoracic discs. J Neurosurg. 91(2 Suppl): 157-62, 1999
2. Levi N et al: Thoracic disc herniation. Unilateral transpedicular approach in 35 consecutive patients. J Neurosurg Sci. 43(1): 37-42; discussion 42-3, 1999
3. Stillerman CB et al: Experience in the surgical management of 82 symptomatic herniated thoracic discs and review of the literature. J Neurosurg. 88(4): 623-33, 1998
4. Korovessis PG et al: Three-level thoracic disc herniation: case report and review of the literature. Eur Spine J. 6(1): 74-6, 1997
5. Wood KB et al: The natural history of asymptomatic thoracic disc herniations. Spine. 22(5): 525-9; discussion 529-30, 1997
6. Wood KB et al: Magnetic resonance imaging of the thoracic spine. Evaluation of asymptomatic individuals. J Bone Joint Surg Am. 77(11): 1631-8, 1995
7. Whitcomb DC et al: Chronic abdominal pain caused by thoracic disc herniation. Am J Gastroenterol. 90(5): 835-7, 1995
8. Boukobza M et al: Thoracic disc herniation and spinal cord compression. MRI and gadolinium-enhancement. J Neuroradiol. 20(4): 272-9, 1993
9. Dietze DD Jr et al: Thoracic disc herniations. Neurosurg Clin N Am. 4(1): 75-90, 1993
10. Brown CW et al: The natural history of thoracic disc herniation. Spine. 17(6 Suppl): S97-102, 1992
11. Parizel PM et al: Gd-DTPA-enhanced MR in thoracic disc herniations. Neuroradiology. 31(1): 75-9, 1989
12. Blumenkopf B: Thoracic intervertebral disc herniations: diagnostic value of magnetic resonance imaging. Neurosurgery. 23(1): 36-40, 1988
13. Ross JS et al: Thoracic disk herniation: MR imaging. Radiology. 165(2): 511-5, 1987
14. Benson MK et al: The clinical syndromes and surgical treatment of thoracic intervertebral disc prolapse. J Bone Joint Surg Br. 57(4): 471-7, 1975
15. Carson J et al: Diagnosis and treatment of thoracic intervertebral disc protrusions. J Neurol Neurosurg Psychiatry. 34(1): 68-77, 1971

INTERVERTEBRAL DISC HERNIATION, THORACIC

IMAGE GALLERY

Typical

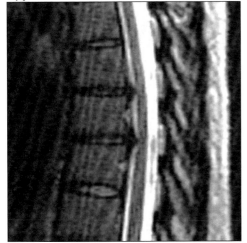
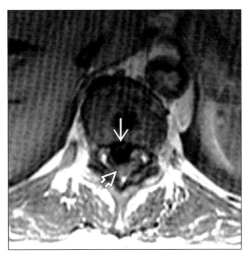

(Left) Sagittal T2WI MR shows small focal midthoracic disc protrusions, effacing thecal sac but not deforming thoracic cord. *(Right)* Axial T1 C+ MR shows large thoracic calcified extrusion as low signal ventral epidural mass (arrow) effacing cord (open arrow).

Typical

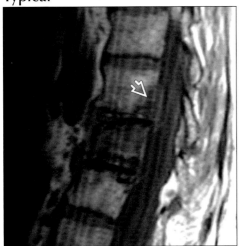
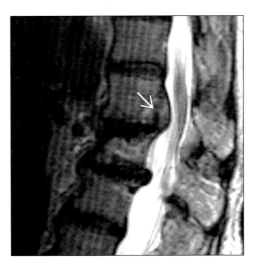

(Left) Sagittal T1WI MR shows large thoracic disc extrusion at T10-11 (open arrow) migrating superiorly behind T10 vertebral body. There is severe disc degeneration at T10-11 and T11-12 with vacuum disc. *(Right)* Sagittal T2WI MR shows the large disc extrusion as intermediate signal intensity, migrating superiorly behind T10 body reflecting free fragment (arrow).

Typical

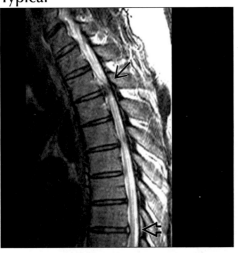
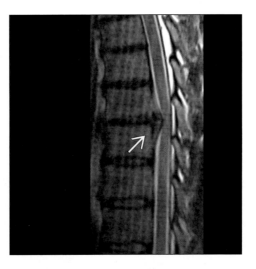

(Left) Sagittal T1WI MR shows large extrusion at T2-3 level (arrow) effacing thecal sac. Second smaller disc protrusion present at T7-8 (open arrow). *(Right)* Sagittal T2WI MR shows large thoracic disc extrusion compressing anterior cord (arrow). There are sloping margins to lesion related to displaced posterior longitudinal ligament and veins.

INTERVERTEBRAL DISC HERNIATION, LUMBAR

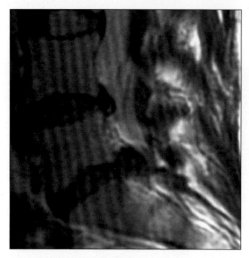

Sagittal T2WI MR shows a disc extrusion at L5-S1. A disc protrusion is present at L4-5. Note the "mushroom" appearance of extrusion.

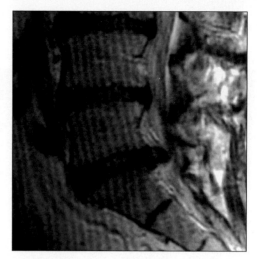

Sagittal T2WI MR shows a "tongue-like" disc protrusion at L5-S1. The greatest cranial-caudal dimension of protruded disc is the same as that of its base.

TERMINOLOGY

Abbreviations and Synonyms
- Nonstandard: "Slipped" or prolapsed disc
- Nonstandard: Herniated nucleus pulposus

Definitions
- Localized (< 50% of disc circumference) displacement of disc material beyond confines of disc space
- Protrusion
  - Herniated disc with broad-base at parent disc
    - Greatest dimension of disc herniation in any plane ≤ distance between edges of the base in same plane
- Extrusion
  - Herniated disc with narrow or no base at parent disc
    - Greatest dimension of disc herniation in any plane > distance between edges of the base in same plane
- Sequestered: Free fragment
  - Extruded disc without continuity to parent disc
- Migrated
  - Disc material displaced away from site of herniation
  - Regardless of continuity
- Intravertebral herniation: Schmorl node

IMAGING FINDINGS

General Features
- Best diagnostic clue: Anterior extradural mass contiguous with disc space extending into spinal canal
- Location
  - Most common: L4-5 or L5-S1
    - 90% of lumbar disc herniation
  - Axial plane
    - Central, subarticular (lateral recess), foraminal, extraforaminal (far lateral)
  - Sagittal plane
    - Disc level, infrapedicle, pedicle, suprapedicle
- Size: Variable
- Morphology
  - Focal: < 25% of disc circumference
  - Broad-based: > 25% but < 50% of disc circumference

Radiographic Findings
- Radiography
  - Disc height loss
  - Degenerative changes
    - Endplate spurring and sclerosis
    - Facet arthropathy
- Myelography: Extradural mass indenting thecal sac and nerve root sleeves

DDx: Intraspinal Extradural Masses

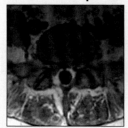

Peridural Fibrosis

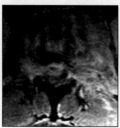

Epidural Abscess

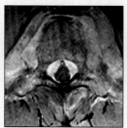

Epidural Lymphoma

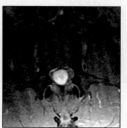

Nerve Sheath Tumor

INTERVERTEBRAL DISC HERNIATION, LUMBAR

Key Facts

Terminology
- Nonstandard: Herniated nucleus pulposus
- Localized (< 50% of disc circumference) displacement of disc material beyond confines of disc space

Imaging Findings
- Best diagnostic clue: Anterior extradural mass contiguous with disc space extending into spinal canal
- Most common: L4-5 or L5-S1
- 90% of lumbar disc herniation
- Myelography: Extradural mass indenting thecal sac and nerve root sleeves
- T1WI: Isointense to parent disc
- Peripheral enhancement

- Variable extent of nerve impingement and central stenosis
- Intravenous gadolinium in post-operative patients

Top Differential Diagnoses
- Peridural fibrosis
- Epidural abscess
- Epidural metastasis

Pathology
- Epidemiology: Up to one-third of asymptomatic adults have disc herniation

Clinical Issues
- Back pain ± radiculopathy resolves within 6-8 weeks
- Conservative treatment alone

CT Findings
- NECT
  - Anterior extradural soft tissue mass
    - Displacing nerve root and distorting thecal sac
- CECT: Mild peripheral enhancement
- Bone CT
  - Degenerative endplate and facet changes

MR Findings
- T1WI: Isointense to parent disc
- T2WI
  - Iso- to hyperintense
    - Depending on degree of disc hydration
- T1 C+
  - Peripheral enhancement
    - Diffuse enhancement if imaged > 30 minutes after injection
- Variable extent of nerve impingement and central stenosis
  - Enhancing nerve root likely due to venous congestion ± inflammation
- Disc hypointensity and height loss

Other Modality Findings
- Discography
  - Pain responses
    - No pain, dissimilar pain, similar pain, exact pain
    - Concordant response: Lack of painful response in control disc
    - Exact pain in symptomatic disc
  - Extension of contrast beyond anulus fibrosus
    - Grade 5 (Schellhas)
    - Full thickness tear
    - Focal or diffuse

Imaging Recommendations
- Best imaging tool: MRI: T2WI and T1WI in sagittal and axial planes
- Protocol advice
  - Intravenous gadolinium in post-operative patients
    - Distinguishes scar tissue from recurrent disc herniation

DIFFERENTIAL DIAGNOSIS

Peridural fibrosis
- Early and homogeneous enhancement
- More infiltrative and less discrete
- Surrounding thecal sac and nerve root

Epidural abscess
- Discitis
- Osteomyelitis
- Peripheral enhancement

Epidural metastasis
- Osseous involvement
- Epidural component elongated in cranial-caudal dimension
- Paravertebral extension

Nerve sheath tumor
- Avid enhancement
- 15% "dumbbell" configuration

PATHOLOGY

General Features
- Genetics
  - Gene variations associated with lumbar disc degeneration
    - Collagen IX and XI genes
    - Vitamin D receptor gene
    - Aggrecan gene
- Etiology
  - Environmental factors
    - Heavy lifting
    - Twisting
    - Flexion and extension
    - Acute trauma
  - Repetitive micro trauma
    - Rim lesion: Horizontal tear in outer anulus at its attachment to ring apophysis
    - Endplate separation → interrupted nutritional supply to disc

- ○ Decreased water content in nucleus pulposus
  - ▪ Proteoglycans replaced by fibrocartilage and fibrosis
  - ○ Ineffective cushioning
  - ○ Unequal force distribution to anulus
    - ▪ Coalescing concentric tears → radial tear → disc herniation
- Epidemiology: Up to one-third of asymptomatic adults have disc herniation
- Associated abnormalities
  - ○ Transitional vertebra below the level of herniation
  - ○ Scoliosis
- Anatomy
  - ○ Central nucleus pulposus
    - ▪ Shock absorbing
    - ▪ Proteoglycans and glycosaminoglycans
    - ▪ High water content
    - ▪ Few collagen fibers
  - ○ Transition zone
  - ○ Peripheral anulus fibrosus
    - ▪ Tensile strength
    - ▪ Outer zone: Dense collagen fibers in concentric lamellae
    - ▪ Inner zone: Fibrocartilage

Microscopic Features

- Combination of nucleus pulposus, anulus, cartilage, fragmented apophyseal bone

CLINICAL ISSUES

Presentation

- Most common signs/symptoms
  - ○ Radiculopathy: Posterolateral radiating pain down lower extremity
  - ○ Other signs/symptoms
    - ▪ Low back pain
    - ▪ Positive straight-leg raising test (Lasegues sign)
    - ▪ Cauda equina syndrome
- Clinical profile
  - ○ Worsening symptoms during lumbar flexion
    - ▪ Sitting, bending
    - ▪ Increased pressure on nucleus pulposus
  - ○ Worsening pain with increased intraabdominal pressure
    - ▪ Coughing, sneezing
  - ○ Pain relieved by lying flat

Demographics

- Age
  - ○ 30 to 60
    - ▪ Mean: 40s
  - ○ Increasing age correlates with more cephalad level of herniation
- Gender: Slight male predominance

Natural History & Prognosis

- Back pain ± radiculopathy resolves within 6-8 weeks
  - ○ Conservative treatment alone
  - ○ 90% of patients
    - ▪ 70% within first four weeks
- 5% recurrent disc herniation

Treatment

- Conservative
  - ○ NSAIDs
  - ○ Bed rest
    - ▪ 2 to 7 days
  - ○ Physical therapy
  - ○ Epidural injection
    - ▪ Cortisone ± lidocaine
- Chymopapain chemonucleolysis
  - ○ Less invasive
  - ○ 70-80% long term success rate
  - ○ 3.7% complication rate
    - ▪ Predominantly discitis
  - ○ 0.45% severe complication
    - ▪ Anaphylaxis, paraplegia, death
  - ○ Not indicated in large herniation and free fragment
- Indications of surgery
  - ○ Intractable pain
  - ○ Cauda equina syndrome
  - ○ Progressive neurologic deficits
- Surgical
  - ○ Laminotomy and discectomy
    - ▪ ≥ 90% success rate
    - ▪ 5% "failed back" syndrome

DIAGNOSTIC CHECKLIST

Image Interpretation Pearls

- Sagittal imaging best at discriminating extrusion from protrusion
  - ○ "Mushroom" appearance of extrusion due to focal expansion

SELECTED REFERENCES

1. Dammers R et al: Lumbar disc herniation: level increases with age. Surg Neurol. 58(3-4):209-12; discussion 212-3, 2002
2. Ito T et al: Types of lumbar herniated disc and clinical course. Spine. 26(6):648-51, 2001
3. Consensus statement on nomenclature and classification of lumbar disc pathology by NASS, ASSR, and ASNR, 2001
4. Carragee EJ et al: Provocative discography in patients after limited lumbar discectomy: A controlled, randomized study of pain response in symptomatic and asymptomatic subjects. Spine. 25(23):3065-71, 2000
5. Kawaguchi Y et al: Association between an aggrecan gene polymorphism and lumbar disc degeneration. Spine. 24(23):2456-60, 1999
6. Videman T et al: Magnetic resonance imaging findings and their relationships in the thoracic and lumbar spine. Insights into the etiopathogenesis of spinal degeneration. Spine. 20(8):928-35, 1995
7. Weber H: The natural history of disc herniation and the influence of intervention. Spine. 19(19):2234-8; discussion 2233, 1994
8. Brock M et al: The form and structure of the extruded disc. Spine. 17(12):1457-61, 1992
9. Muralikuttan KP et al: A prospective randomized trial of chemonucleolysis and conventional disc surgery in single level lumbar disc herniation. Spine. 17(4):381-7, 1992
10. Hashimoto K et al: Magnetic resonance imaging of lumbar disc herniation. Comparison with myelography. Spine. 15(11):1166-9, 1990

INTERVERTEBRAL DISC HERNIATION, LUMBAR

IMAGE GALLERY

Typical

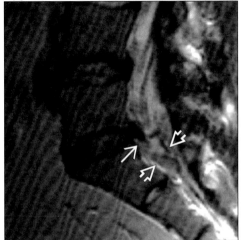
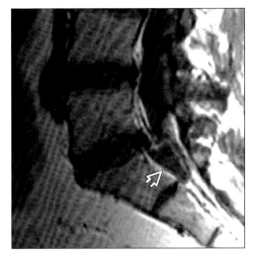

(Left) Sagittal T2WI MR shows a disc fragment (open arrows) migrated caudally from its parent disc at L5-S1, with a thin attachment (arrow). *(Right)* Sagittal T1 C+ MR shows migrated disc fragment (arrow) posterior to S1 segment demonstrating mild peripheral enhancement.

Typical

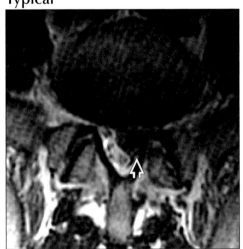
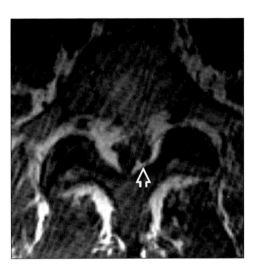

(Left) Axial T2WI MR shows a left subarticular disc protrusion (arrow) at L5-S1 distorting thecal sac and obliterating subarticular recess. The traversing left S1 nerve root is impinged. *(Right)* Axial T1WI MR shows a free disc fragment (arrow) to the left of thecal sac at L5-S1.

Typical

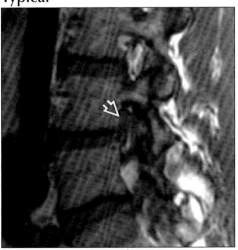
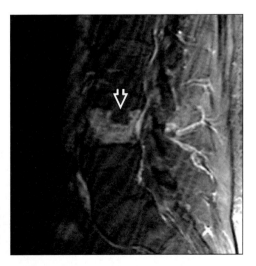

(Left) Sagittal T1WI MR shows a foraminal disc extrusion (arrow) at L4-5 obliterating perineural fat. The exiting L4 nerve root is impinged. *(Right)* Sagittal T1 C+ MR with fat suppression shows intravertebral disc herniation (arrow) at superior endplate of L4 with surrounding marrow enhancement.

FORAMINAL DISC EXTRUSION

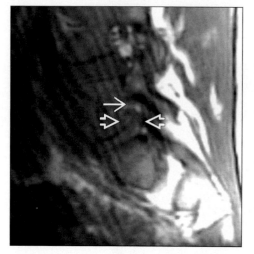

Sagittal T1WI MR shows L5-S1 foraminal disc extrusion (open arrows), displacing exiting L5 nerve root (arrow).

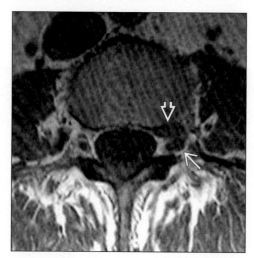

Axial T1WI MR shows a left L4-5 foraminal disc extrusion (open arrow), contacting exiting left L4 nerve root (arrow).

TERMINOLOGY

Abbreviations and Synonyms
- Nonstandard: Lateral herniated nucleus pulposus (HNP)

Definitions
- Extruded disc material within neural foramen

IMAGING FINDINGS

General Features
- Best diagnostic clue
  - Obliterated perineural fat in neural foramen on sagittal images
    - Soft tissue mass contiguous with parent disc
- Location
  - Lumbar: L3-4 and L4-5 most common
  - Cervical: C5-6 and C6-7 most common
  - Thoracic: Rare
    - Herniation: 3 in 1,000 incidence
- Size: Restricted by neural foramen
- Morphology
  - Typical "mushroom" appearance of central or subarticular disc extrusion absent
    - Conforms to neural foramen on sagittal images

Radiographic Findings
- Radiography
  - Nonspecific degenerative changes
    - Disc height loss
    - Endplate sclerosis and spurs
    - Spondylolisthesis
    - Facet arthropathy
- Myelography
  - Often missed on myelography
  - Sensitivity < 13%
  - Post-myelography CT improves sensitivity

CT Findings
- NECT
  - Foraminal soft tissue mass
    - Same density as disc
  - Neural foramen not enlarged
- CECT: May show peripheral enhancement
- Bone CT
  - Same as radiography
  - Vacuum disc phenomenon

MR Findings
- T1WI: Isointense to parent disc
- T2WI
  - Iso-, hypo-, or hyperintense to parent disc
    - Depending on hydration status
- T1 C+

DDx: Foraminal Masses

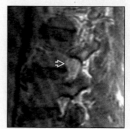

Schwannoma

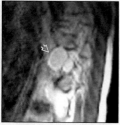

N. Sheath Diverticulum

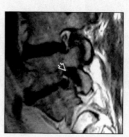

Facet Arthropathy

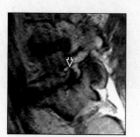

Endplate Spur

FORAMINAL DISC EXTRUSION

Key Facts

Terminology
- Nonstandard: Lateral herniated nucleus pulposus (HNP)
- Extruded disc material within neural foramen

Imaging Findings
- Obliterated perineural fat in neural foramen on sagittal images
- Often missed on myelography
- T1WI: Isointense to parent disc
- May enhance peripherally
- Variable extent of impingement on exiting nerve root
- Contacted, displaced, flattened
- Nerve root may show postgadolinium enhancement
- Extraforaminal component best seen on axial imaging

- Disc height loss
- Degenerative endplate changes
- Contrast extravasation into neural foramen and extraforaminal space

Top Differential Diagnoses
- Schwannoma
- Spinal nerve root diverticulum
- Large facet osteophyte

Pathology
- Uncommon
- 5-10% of all disc herniations

Clinical Issues
- Severe radicular pain
- Favorable outcome with conservative measures

  - ○ May enhance peripherally
  - ○ Enhancing anular tear
- Variable extent of impingement on exiting nerve root
  - ○ Contacted, displaced, flattened
  - ○ Nerve root may show postgadolinium enhancement
    - Venous congestion ± inflammation
- Extraforaminal component best seen on axial imaging
  - ○ May involve adjacent nerve root
- Disc height loss
- Degenerative endplate changes

Nuclear Medicine Findings
- Bone Scan
  - ○ Limited role
    - Radiotracer uptake in endplates and facet joints

Other Modality Findings
- Discography
  - ○ Contrast extravasation into neural foramen and extraforaminal space
    - Most sensitive and specific
    - Invasive

Imaging Recommendations
- Best imaging tool: T1WI and T2WI MRI in sagittal and axial planes

DIFFERENTIAL DIAGNOSIS

Schwannoma
- Enlarged neural foramen due to chronic remodeling
- "Dumbbell" appearance on axial imaging
  - ○ 15% of schwannomas
- Diffuse post-contrast-enhancement
  - ○ Unless necrosis present

Spinal nerve root diverticulum
- Cerebral spinal fluid intensity on all sequences
- No enhancement
- May opacify with contrast on myelography
- Enlarged neural foramen

Large facet osteophyte
- Hypointense on T1WI and T2WI
- Contiguous with facet joint
- Cephalad and posterior portion of neural foramen
  - ○ Best seen on sagittal images
- Osseous density on CT

Endplate osteophyte
- Often associated with herniation
- Contiguous with endplate
- Hypointense on T1WI and T2WI
- Marrow intensity may be present

PATHOLOGY

General Features
- General path comments
  - ○ Anatomy
    - Central nucleus pulposus
    - Peripheral anulus fibrosus
    - Avascular
    - Nutrition and waste removal through diffusion from adjacent endplates
    - Outer anulus innervated by sinuvertebral nerve
- Genetics
  - ○ Genetic predisposition to herniation
    - 5x risk of developing herniation in adults < 21years
    - If positive family history of herniation
- Etiology
  - ○ Environmental factors
    - Heavy lifting
    - Twisting
    - Flexion and extension
    - Lateral bending
    - Acute trauma
  - ○ Age
  - ○ Poor posture
  - ○ Repetitive microtrauma
    - Endplate injury

FORAMINAL DISC EXTRUSION

- Rim lesion: Horizontal tear in outer anulus at its attachment to ring apophysis
  - ○ Interruption of nutritional supply to disc
  - ○ Decreasing water content in nucleus pulposus
    - Proteoglycans replaced by fibrocartilage and fibrosis
    - Increasing stiffness
    - Decreasing intra-disc pressure
  - ○ Ineffective cushioning
  - ○ Unequal force distribution to anulus
    - Concentric tear ± radial tear → disc herniation
- Epidemiology
  - ○ Uncommon
    - 5-10% of all disc herniations
- Associated abnormalities
  - ○ Spondylolisthesis
  - ○ Scoliosis

Microscopic Features
- Myxomatous degeneration of anulus fibrosus
- Composed of a combination of nucleus pulposus, fragmented anulus, cartilage, and fragmented apophyseal bone

CLINICAL ISSUES

Presentation
- Most common signs/symptoms
  - ○ Severe radicular pain
    - More symptomatic compared to other disc herniations
    - Mass effect on exiting nerve root in narrow confines of neural foramen
    - Chemical irritation of nerve root
    - Lumbar: 25% sciatic and 75% femoral distribution
  - ○ Other signs/symptoms
    - Muscle weakness
    - Positive femoral stretch test
- Clinical profile
  - ○ Lateral bending, sitting, and increased intraabdominal pressure worsen pain
  - ○ Pain relieved by rest with hip and knee in flexion

Demographics
- Age
  - ○ 50s to 70s
    - Older than those with posterolateral herniation
- Gender: M = F
- Ethnicity: No racial predilection

Natural History & Prognosis
- May stabilize or resolve spontaneously
- Favorable outcome with conservative measures
- Mild residual radicular pain may be present after lumbar surgery

Treatment
- Conservative
  - ○ Indicated if no or minor neurologic impairment
  - ○ NSAIDs
  - ○ Bed rest
    - 2 to 7 days
  - ○ Physical therapy
  - ○ Selective nerve root block

- Cortisone ± lidocaine
- 60-80% asymptomatic after 1 year
- Surgery
  - ○ Indications
    - Failed conservative therapy after 6-8 weeks
    - Progressive neurologic deficits
  - ○ Lumbar
    - Inter-laminal approach with partial medial facetectomy
    - Pars interarticularis fenestration preserves facet integrity
  - ○ Cervical
    - Anterior or posterior approach
    - Laminotomy-foraminotomy
    - Discectomy
    - Stabilization

DIAGNOSTIC CHECKLIST

Image Interpretation Pearls
- Look for foraminal mass contiguous with disc on sagittal plane
- Look for lateral or far lateral mass at disc level on axial plane

SELECTED REFERENCES

1. Narozny M et al: Therapeutic efficacy of selective nerve root blocks in the treatment of lumbar radicular leg pain. Swiss Med Wkly. 131(5-6):75-80, 2001
2. Consensus statement on nomenclature and classification of lumbar disc pathology by NASS, ASSR, and ASNR, 2001
3. Shao KN et al: Far lateral lumbar disc herniation.. Zhonghua Yi Xue Za Zhi (Taipei). 63(5):391-8, 2000
4. Hsieh MS et al: Diagnosis of herniated intervertebral disc assisted by 3-dimensional, multiaxial, magnetic resonance imaging. J Formos Med Assoc. 98(5):347-55, 1999
5. Di Lorenzo N et al: Pars interarticularis fenestration in the treatment of foraminal lumbar disc herniation: a further surgical approach. Neurosurgery. 42(1):87-9; discussion 89-90, 1998
6. Matsui H et al: Familial predisposition for lumbar degenerative disc disease. A case-control study. Spine. 23(9):1029-34, 1998
7. Weiner BK et al: Foraminal injection for lateral lumbar disc herniation. J Bone Joint Surg Br. 79(5):804-7, 1997
8. Ashkenazi E et al: Foraminal herniation of a lumbar disc mimicking neurinoma on CT and MR imaging. J Spinal Disord. 10(5):448-50, 1997
9. Segnarbieux F et al: Disco-computed tomography in extraforaminal and foraminal lumbar disc herniation: influence on surgical approaches. Neurosurgery. 34(4):643-7; discussion 648, 1994
10. Varlotta GP et al: Familial predisposition for herniation of a lumbar disc in patients who are less than twenty-one years old. J Bone Joint Surg Am. 73(1):124-8, 1991
11. Kunogi J et al: Diagnosis and operative treatment of intraforaminal and extraforaminal nerve root compression. Spine. 16(11):1312-20, 1991
12. An HS et al: Herniated lumbar disc in patients over the age of fifty. J Spinal Disord. 3(2):143-6, 1990
13. Osborn AG et al: CT/MR spectrum of far lateral and anterior lumbosacral disc herniations. AJNR 9:775-8, 1988
14. Jackson RP et al: Foraminal and extraforaminal lumbar disc herniation: diagnosis and treatment. Spine. 12(6):577-85, 1987

FORAMINAL DISC EXTRUSION

IMAGE GALLERY

Typical

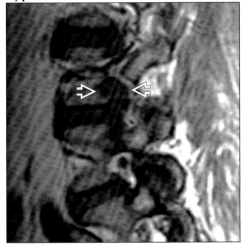
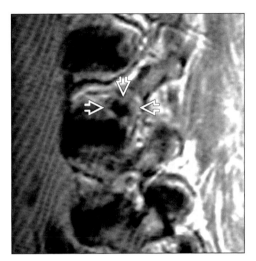

(Left) Sagittal T1WI MR shows large L4-5 disc extrusion *(arrows)*, completely filling neural foramen and obliterating perineural fat. Exiting L4 nerve root cannot be identified *(Courtesy J. Ross, MD)*. *(Right)* Sagittal T1 C+ MR shows L4-5 foraminal disc extrusion with peripheral enhancement *(arrows)*.

Typical

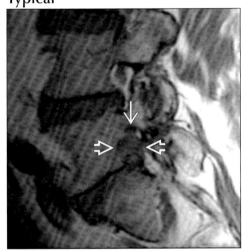
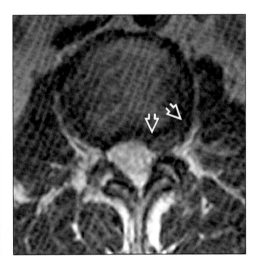

(Left) Sagittal T1WI MR shows L5-S1 foraminal extrusion *(open arrows)*, displacing and flattening exiting L5 nerve root *(arrow)*. *(Right)* Axial T2WI MR shows a left foraminal disc herniation *(arrows)*, also distorting thecal sac.

Typical

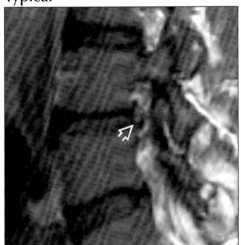
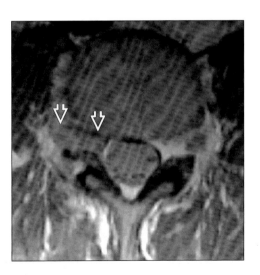

(Left) Sagittal T2WI MR shows L4-5 disc foraminal disc herniation with associated anular tear *(arrow)*. *(Right)* Axial PD/Intermediate MR shows a large right foraminal disc herniation *(arrows)*, effacing perineural fat. The exiting nerve root cannot be visualized.

SPONDYLOLISTHESIS

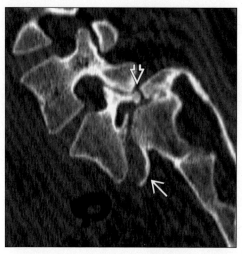

Sagittal bone CT shows grade 4 spondylolisthesis due to spondylolysis (open arrow). Chronicity of displacement is evident by bony remodeling (arrow).

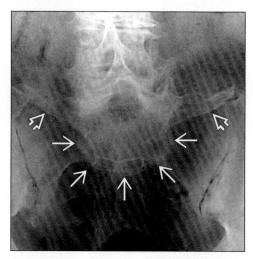

Anteroposterior radiography shows "Napoleon's hat" sign. Hat is inverted; crown (arrows) is anterior cortex of vertebral body, and brim (open arrows) is transverse process.

TERMINOLOGY

Definitions
- Displacement of vertebral body, described relative to inferior vertebra
- Anterolisthesis: Anterior displacement of vertebral body relative to one below
- Retrolisthesis: Posterior displacement of vertebral body relative to one below
- Spondyloptosis: Vertebral body displaced completely anteriorly, with inferior displacement to level of vertebral body below

IMAGING FINDINGS

General Features
- Best diagnostic clue: Displacement of posterior cortex of vertebral body on lateral radiograph
- Location: Most common in lower lumbar spine

Radiographic Findings
- Radiography
  - Evaluate percentage or grade of listhesis on neutral, flexion and extension lateral
  - Lateral flexion and extension to evaluate for instability
    - Instability rarely seen in degenerative listhesis

- Instability sometimes present with spondylolysis
- Instability almost always seen with traumatic spondylolisthesis
  - "Napoleon's hat" sign
    - Severe spondylolisthesis results in focal kyphosis
    - Kyphotic, subluxed vertebra resembles an upside down curved hat on AP radiographs
  - Evaluate for fracture, spondylolysis
  - Degenerative: Degenerative disc disease and facet osteoarthritis present

CT Findings
- Bone CT
  - Evaluate for pars interarticularis defects, fractures, spinal stenosis

MR Findings
- Spondylolysis notoriously difficult to see on MRI
- Obtain stack axial images as well as axials angled through intervertebral disc
- Sagittal, axial T1WI and T2WI to evaluate spinal stenosis and neural foraminal encroachment
- Look for hematoma as sign of acute traumatic spondylolysis

Nuclear Medicine Findings
- Bone Scan
  - Increased uptake at acute or subacute pars defects
  - Chronic pars defects photopenic

DDx: Causes of Spondylolisthesis

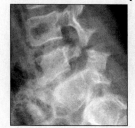
Spondylolysis

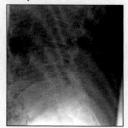
Degenerative

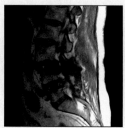
Above Fusion

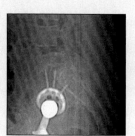
Neuropathic

SPONDYLOLISTHESIS

Key Facts

Terminology
- Displacement of vertebral body, described relative to inferior vertebra

Imaging Findings
- Evaluate percentage or grade of listhesis on neutral, flexion and extension lateral
- Protocol advice: Thin-slice CT with sagittal reformations

Top Differential Diagnoses
- Physiologic motion
- Displaced vertebral body fracture

Pathology
- Spondylolysis
- Trauma at sites other than pars interarticularis
- Degenerative
- Postsurgical

  ○ Increased uptake at degenerated facet joints and discs

Imaging Recommendations
- Best imaging tool: CT scan
- Protocol advice: Thin-slice CT with sagittal reformations

DIFFERENTIAL DIAGNOSIS

Physiologic motion
- Slight subluxations normal in young patients

Displaced vertebral body fracture
- Fracture often best seen on CT

PATHOLOGY

General Features
- Etiology
  - Spondylolysis
    - Acute trauma or fatigue fracture
  - Trauma at sites other than pars interarticularis
    - Shear injury
    - Fractures of posterior elements
  - Degenerative
    - May be related to alignment of facet joints
  - Postsurgical
    - Destabilization of spine at wide laminectomy
    - Late complication above or below fusion
  - Tumor
  - Infection
  - Neuropathic arthropathy
- Associated abnormalities: Scoliosis may develop

Staging, Grading or Classification Criteria
- Grade I: < 25% displacement vertebral body
- Grade II: 25-50% displacement vertebral body
- Grade III: 50-75% displacement vertebral body
- Grade IV: 75-100% displacement vertebral body
- Grade V: Spondyloptosis

CLINICAL ISSUES

Presentation
- Most common signs/symptoms: Back pain, radiculopathy, neurogenic claudication

Demographics
- Gender: More common in women

Treatment
- Options, risks, complications
  - Listhesis usually fused in situ, or with slight correction of deformity
  - Correction of spondylolisthesis may result in neurologic compromise

SELECTED REFERENCES

1. Lamm M et al: Acute traumatic L5-S1 spondylolisthesis. J Spinal Disord Tech. 16(6):524-7, 2003
2. Pneumaticos SG et al: Scoliosis associated with lumbar spondylolisthesis: a case presentation and review of the literature. Spine J. 3(4):321-4, 2003
3. Bassewitz H et al: Lumbar stenosis with spondylolisthesis: current concepts of surgical treatment. Clin Orthop. (384):54-60, 2001
4. Nizard RS et al: Radiologic assessment of lumbar intervertebral instability and degenerative spondylolisthesis. Radiol Clin North Am. 39(1):55-71, v-vi, 2001
5. Cinotti G et al: Predisposing factors in degenerative spondylolisthesis. A radiographic and CT study. Int Orthop. 21(5):337-42, 1997
6. Herkowitz HN: Spine update. Degenerative lumbar spondylolisthesis. Spine. 20(9):1084-90, 1995

IMAGE GALLERY

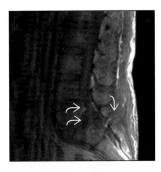 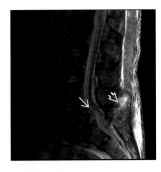

(Left) Sagittal T1WI MR shows L5/S1 spondylolisthesis in patient run over by a truck. Mixed low and high signal hematoma is present behind L5 vertebral body and between posterior elements L5 and S1 (arrows). (Right) Sagittal STIR MR shows traumatic L5-S1 spondylolisthesis with large hematoma (arrow) deviating nerve roots posteriorly. Posterior ligamentous disruption also evident (open arrow).

SPONDYLOLYSIS

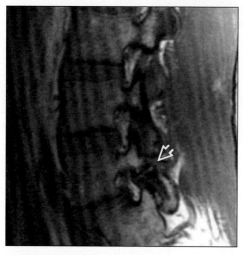

Sagittal T2WI MR shows a well corticated linear defect in L5 pars interarticularis (arrow).

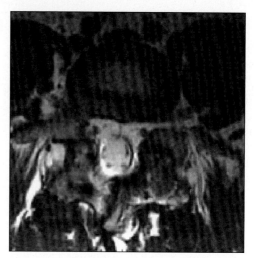

Axial T2WI MR shows bilateral L5 pars defects with elongated anterior-posterior dimension of the spinal canal.

TERMINOLOGY

Abbreviations and Synonyms
- Isthmic spondylolysis

Definitions
- Defects in pars interarticularis (PI) thought to result from repetitive stress injury

IMAGING FINDINGS

General Features
- Best diagnostic clue: Elongation of spinal canal at the level of pars defects on axial imaging
- Location
  - Most common at L5: 82%
  - L4 second most common: 11%
  - 10-15% unilateral defects
    - Unilateral healing or union of fractures that were initially bilateral
- Morphology: Horizontal orientation on axial imaging

Radiographic Findings
- Radiography
  - Radiolucent band in PI on oblique views of lumbar spine
    - Discontinuity in the neck of "Scotty dog"
  - Oblique lucency at base of laminae on lateral view
  - Variable degree of spondylolisthesis
    - "Inverted Napoleon hat" sign on frontal view: Spondylolisthesis at L5
  - Disc height loss at the level below spondylolysis
  - Sclerotic endplate changes and spurring
  - Contralateral pedicle and lamina hypertrophy and sclerosis
    - Unilateral spondylolysis
    - Best seen on frontal lumbar spine
- Myelography: Neural foraminal narrowing with anterolisthesis and disc height loss

CT Findings
- Bone CT
  - "Incomplete ring" sign on axial imaging
    - Disruption of ring formed by vertebral body and arch
  - May simulate facet joints
    - "Extra facet" sign
    - Horizontal vs. oblique orientation
    - Irregular vs. smooth bony cortex
  - Pars defects well seen on oblique reformation
  - Variable spondylolisthesis and foraminal narrowing on sagittal reformation
    - Disc space loss
    - Degenerative endplate changes

MR Findings
- T1WI

DDx: Spondylolisthesis

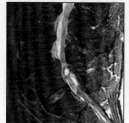

Degenerative

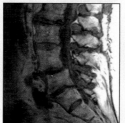

Degenerative

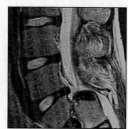

Post-traumatic

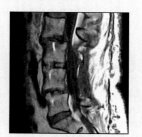

Iatrogenic

SPONDYLOLYSIS

Key Facts

Terminology
- Isthmic spondylolysis
- Defects in pars interarticularis (PI) thought to result from repetitive stress injury

Imaging Findings
- Best diagnostic clue: Elongation of spinal canal at the level of pars defects on axial imaging
- Most common at L5: 82%
- 10-15% unilateral defects
- Radiolucent band in PI on oblique views of lumbar spine
- Oblique lucency at base of laminae on lateral view
- "Incomplete ring" sign on axial imaging
- May simulate facet joints

- Focally decreased signal in PI on sagittal and axial imaging
- STIR: Marrow edema adjacent to pars defects
- SPECT increases sensitivity

Top Differential Diagnoses
- Degenerative spondylolisthesis
- Traumatic spondylolisthesis

Pathology
- General path comments: Thought to result from a combination of "weak" bone and repetitive trauma during growth spurt

Diagnostic Checklist
- Look for integrity of pars interarticular on sagittal MRI

- Focally decreased signal in PI on sagittal and axial imaging
  - Similar appearance on T2WI
- T2WI: Hyperintensity may be present within pars defects
- STIR: Marrow edema adjacent to pars defects
- Elongation of spinal canal
- Horizontal configuration of affected neural foramina on sagittal imaging
  - Anterolisthesis
  - Disc height loss
  - Loss of fat surrounding exiting nerve roots
- Sensitivity of MRI: 57-86%
- Specificity: 81-82%

Nuclear Medicine Findings
- Bone Scan
  - Foci of increased radiotracer uptake in posterior elements
    - Suggests bone healing
    - SPECT increases sensitivity

Imaging Recommendations
- Best imaging tool
  - Axial thin-section CT with bone algorithm
    - Sagittal and oblique reformation

DIFFERENTIAL DIAGNOSIS

Degenerative spondylolisthesis
- Most common at L4-5
- Secondary to bilateral facet arthropathy
- Older patients
- Most common grade I

Traumatic spondylolisthesis
- Acute fracture through PI or other posterior elements
- Multiple fractures and dislocations present

Pathologic spondylolisthesis
- Underlying bony abnormality affecting posterior elements
  - Metabolic, neoplastic, dysplastic

Dysplastic spondylolisthesis
- Congenital insufficiency of L5-S1 articulation allowing listhesis
- No pars defects or elongation

Iatrogenic spondylolisthesis
- Post-surgical
- Instability from excessive removal of posterior elements

Mimickers of spondylolysis on sagittal MR
- Sclerosis of neck of PI
- Partial volume averaging of superior facet spur lateral to PI
- Partial facetectomy
- Blastic metastasis to PI

PATHOLOGY

General Features
- General path comments: Thought to result from a combination of "weak" bone and repetitive trauma during growth spurt
- Genetics
  - Predisposing familial conditions to spondylolysis
    - Marfan syndrome
    - Osteogenesis imperfecta
    - Osteopetrosis
    - Other inherited traits
- Etiology
  - Participation in gymnastics, weight lifting, wrestling, football, etc.
    - Starting at a young age
    - Training more than 15 hours per week
    - Repetitive exposure to rotation, flexion-extension, and hyperextension
  - Repeated micro-fractures of PI lead to fatigue fracture
    - Usually occurs during growth spurt
- Epidemiology
  - Prevalence of 4.4% at age 6
    - Incidence of 3.3%

SPONDYLOLYSIS

- ○ 5-7% in general population
  - ■ 22-44% in competitive athletes in diving, weight lifting, wrestling
- Associated abnormalities
  - ○ Scoliosis
  - ○ 50% with spondylolisthesis
  - ○ Spina bifida occulta
  - ○ Scheuermann disease

Microscopic Features
- New bone and cartilaginous matrix if healing present
- Fibrocartilaginous tissue within pars defects if not healed

CLINICAL ISSUES

Presentation
- Most common signs/symptoms
  - ○ Chronic low back pain
    - ■ Usually presents during adolescent growth spurt
  - ○ Other symptoms
    - ■ Back spasm
    - ■ Hamstring tightness
    - ■ Radiculopathy and cauda equina syndrome
    - ■ Gait disturbance
- Clinical profile: Pain exacerbated by rigorous activities
- 80% without symptoms

Demographics
- Age: 10-20 years
- Gender: M:F = 2-3:1
- Ethnicity
  - ○ In 30-40% of Eskimos
  - ○ Higher incidence in Caucasian males: 6.4%

Natural History & Prognosis
- Progressive spondylolisthesis occurs during skeletal immaturity
  - ○ More common in females
  - ○ Risk of progression: 3-28%
- Little slippage with horizontal sacrum
  - ○ Lumbosacral angle ≥ 100°
- Progressive spondylolisthesis with vertical sacrum
  - ○ Lumbosacral angle < 100°
- Progression from grade 1 spondylolisthesis: Superior vertebral body subluxed by one-fourth of a vertebral body
- To grade 2: Subluxation by half a vertebral body
- To grade 3: Subluxation by three-fourths of a vertebral body
- To grade 4: Subluxation by whole width of a vertebral body

Treatment
- Conservative measures in patients with grade 1 and 2 spondylolisthesis
  - ○ Modification of activity
  - ○ Anti-inflammatory medications
  - ○ Epidural steroid injection
  - ○ Back brace
  - ○ Physical therapy
  - ○ Two-thirds success rate of symptomatic relief
- Surgical interventions in patients who
  - ○ Fail conservative treatment

- ○ Have worsening slippage
- ○ To preserve neural function and prevent instability
  - ■ Posterior or posterolateral fusion
  - ■ Stabilization with fusion or cast immobilization
  - ■ Possible decompression

DIAGNOSTIC CHECKLIST

Image Interpretation Pearls
- Look for integrity of pars interarticular on sagittal MRI
  - ○ At the level of facet joints

SELECTED REFERENCES

1. McTimoney CA et al: Current evaluation and management of spondylolysis and spondylolisthesis. Curr Sports Med Rep. 2(1):41-6, 2003
2. Merbs CF: Asymmetrical spondylolysis. Am J Phys Anthropol. 119(2):156-74, 2002
3. Logroscino G et al: Spondylolysis and spondylolisthesis in the pediatric and adolescent population. Childs Nerv Syst. 17(11):644-55, 2001
4. Standaert CJ et al: Spondylolysis. Phys Med Rehabil Clin N Am. 11(4):785-803, 2000
5. Saifuddin A et al: The value of lumbar spine MRI in the assessment of the pars interarticularis. Clin Radiol. 52(9):666-71, 1997
6. Ulmer J et al: MR Imaging of Lumbar Spondylolysis: The Importance of Ancillary Observations. AJR. 169:233-9, 1997
7. Ohmori K et al: Vertebral slip in lumbar spondylolysis and spondylolisthesis. Long-term follow-up of 22 adult patients. J Bone Joint Surg Br. 77(5):771-3, 1995
8. Ulmer JL et al: Distinction between degenerative and isthmic spondylolisthesis on sagittal MR images: importance of increased anteroposterior diameter of the spinal canal ("wide canal sign"). AJR Am J Roentgenol. 163(2):411-6, 1994
9. Jinkins JR et al: Spondylolysis, spondylolisthesis, and associated nerve root entrapment in the lumbosacral spine: MR evaluation. AJR Am J Roentgenol. 159(4):799-803, 1992
10. Reynolds R: Spondylolysis and Spondylolisthesis. Seminars in Spine Surgery. 4:235-47, 1992
11. Danielson BI et al: Radiologic progression of isthmic lumbar spondylolisthesis in young patients. Spine. 16(4):422-5, 1991
12. Frennered AK et al: Natural history of symptomatic isthmic low-grade spondylolisthesis in children and adolescents: a seven-year follow-up study. J Pediatr Orthop. 11(2):209-13, 1991
13. Rossi F et al: Lumbar spondylolysis: occurrence in competitive athletes. Updated achievements in a series of 390 cases. J Sports Med Phys Fitness. 30(4):450-2, 1990
14. Johnson D et al: MR Imaging of the Pars Interarticularis. AJR. 152:327-32, 1989
15. Rossi F: Spondylolysis, spondylolisthesis and sports. J Sports Med Phys Fitness. 18(4):317-40, 1978
16. Wiltse LL et al: Classification of spondylolisis and spondylolisthesis. Clin Orthop. (117):23-9, 1976
17. Wiltse LL: Spondylolisthesis. West J Med. 122(2):152-3, 1975

SPONDYLOLYSIS

IMAGE GALLERY

Typical

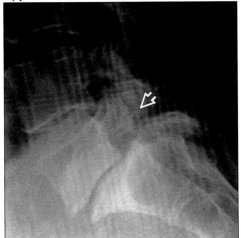

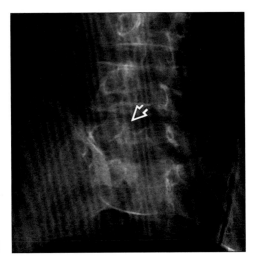

(Left) Lateral radiography shows a defect and mild angulation in L5 pars interarticularis (arrow). There is disc height loss at L5-S1 with associated sclerotic endplate changes. (Right) Coronal oblique radiography shows a thin lucency (arrow) in right L5 pars interarticularis with adjacent bony sclerosis.

Typical

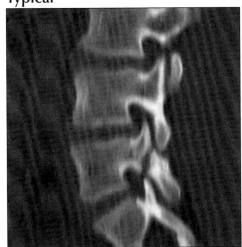

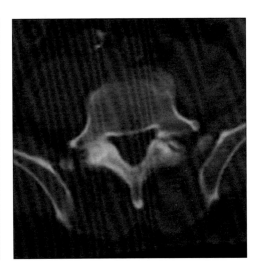

(Left) Sagittal bone CT with sagittal reformation shows a L5 pars defect without anterolisthesis. (Right) Axial bone CT at L5 shows a left-sided pars defect. Right-sided pars fracture has healed.

Typical

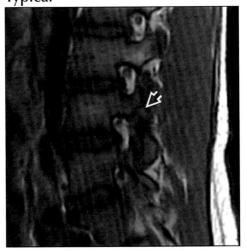

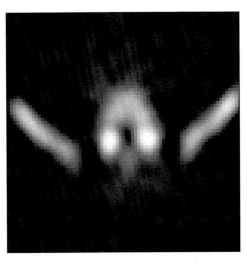

(Left) Sagittal T1WI MR shows a defect in L4 pars interarticularis (arrow). Fractures at this level are much less common than those at L5. (Right) Axial bone scan with SPECT shows increased radiotracer uptake in bilateral L5 pars interarticularis.

FACET ARTHROPATHY, CERVICAL

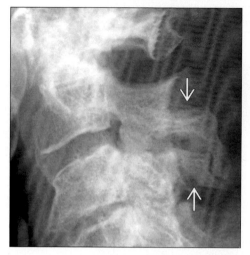

Lateral radiography shows severe facet hypertrophic degenerative arthropathy at C2-3 (arrows).

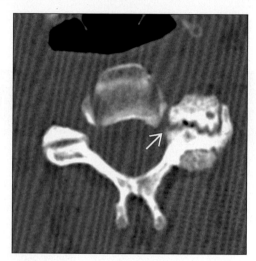

Axial NECT shows severe left facet degenerative arthropathy with foraminal stenosis (arrow). "Vacuum phenomenon" present in left facet joint.

TERMINOLOGY

Abbreviations and Synonyms
- Facet arthrosis, degenerative facet disease, degenerative joint disease

Definitions
- Osteoarthritis of synovially-lined apophyseal joints

IMAGING FINDINGS

General Features
- Best diagnostic clue: Osseous facet overgrowth impinging on neural foramina in conjunction with articular joint space narrowing
- Location
  - Normal anatomy
    - C2 ⇒ C7 levels have two sets of paired joints
    - Facet or zygapophyseal joints posteriorly, with oblique orientation
    - Uncovertebral joints (joints of Luschka, neurocentral joints) formed by curved edges of vertebral bodies at lateral margins
  - Arthropathy most common in mid/lower cervical spine
- Size: Facets may show minimal abnormality or large osteophytes approximating size of facet themselves

- Morphology: Osseous facet overgrowth and cartilage erosion with joint space narrowing

Radiographic Findings
- Radiography
  - Poor for demonstrating early facet degeneration
  - Later changes well-demonstrated
  - Plain films demonstrate facet arthrosis well, not soft tissues
  - Oblique views demonstrate facet joints best
    - Facet joint osteophytes producing foraminal narrowing
    - Associated with degenerative disc disease
    - "Mushroom cap" facet appearance
    - Joint space narrowing with sclerosis and bone eburnation
    - Intra-articular gas ("vacuum phenomenon")
    - Anterolisthesis, retrolisthesis not uncommon
- Fluoroscopy: Same as plain radiography; can observe motion abnormalities on flexion-extension
- Myelography: CT myelography portrays facet relationship to adjacent contrast-opacified thecal sac and nerve root sleeves

CT Findings
- NECT
  - CT more sensitive than plain films for detecting presence and degree of arthrosis

DDx: Facet Arthropathy, Cervical

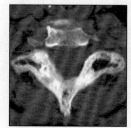

Paget Disease

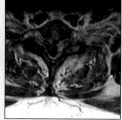

Septic Facet

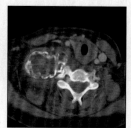

Myositis Ossif

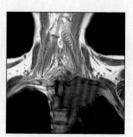

Metastasis

FACET ARTHROPATHY, CERVICAL

Key Facts

Terminology
- Facet arthrosis, degenerative facet disease, degenerative joint disease
- Osteoarthritis of synovially-lined apophyseal joints

Imaging Findings
- Best diagnostic clue: Osseous facet overgrowth impinging on neural foramina in conjunction with articular joint space narrowing
- Size: Facets may show minimal abnormality or large osteophytes approximating size of facet themselves
- CT more sensitive than plain films for detecting presence and degree of arthrosis

Top Differential Diagnoses
- Septic facet
- Healing facet fracture

- Inflammatory arthritides
- Paget disease
- Myositis ossificans
- Tumor

Pathology
- Epidemiology: Facet joint degeneration begins in first two decades of life
- Associated abnormalities: Frequently seen in conjunction with spondylosis

Clinical Issues
- Mechanical neck pain (facet arthrosis syndrome)
- Radiculopathy
- Facet disease may be asymptomatic incidental finding on imaging

○ Facet joint osteophytes producing foraminal narrowing
○ "Mushroom cap" facet appearance
○ Joint space narrowing with sclerosis and bone eburnation
○ Intra-articular gas ("vacuum phenomenon")
○ CT myelography shows facet relationship to adjacent contrast-opacified thecal sac and nerve root sleeves
- CECT
  ○ Inflammatory soft tissue changes surrounding facet joint are common
    ■ May appear aggressive even in absence of infection

MR Findings
- T1WI
  ○ Enhancing inflammatory soft tissue changes surrounding facet joint are common
    ■ May appear aggressive even in absence of infection
  ○ Conversely, some patients show variable synovial thickening
    ■ Irritation of the synovium can produce synovial hyperplasia with paradoxical joint space widening
    ■ Frequently see motion at affected levels on flexion-extension plain films
- T2WI
  ○ Osteophyte proliferation limiting neural foramina
  ○ Joint space narrowing, thinning of articular cartilage
  ○ Facet effusions as linear hyperintensity
- T2* GRE
  ○ Shows osseous changes well
  ○ Tends to overemphasize the degree of foraminal or central canal narrowing
- T1 C+: Enhancement of synovium, epidural and foraminal venous plexus

Nuclear Medicine Findings
- Bone Scan: Increased uptake with degenerative disc disease, facet arthropathy

Imaging Recommendations
- Plain films useful to demonstrate presence and severity of facet degenerative changes
- Sagittal and axial T1WI and T2WI best demonstrate degenerative facet compression of adjacent thecal sac
  ○ 3D gradient echo T2* for foraminal detail
- Consider CT myelography if MRI contraindications or when MRI does not adequately demonstrate facet relationship to neural foramina

DIFFERENTIAL DIAGNOSIS

Septic facet
- T2 hyperintensity extending into adjacent soft tissues

Healing facet fracture
- Trauma history and search for fracture line

Inflammatory arthritides
- Look for ankylosis or erosions, cranial settling, atlanto-axial subluxation (rheumatoid arthritis)

Paget disease
- Thickened cortex, trabeculae, bony expansion

Myositis ossificans
- Trauma history, circumscribed calcification

Tumor
- Metastasis, lymphoma, sarcoma

PATHOLOGY

General Features
- General path comments
  ○ Degenerative (hypertrophic) inflammatory changes in synovial joints
    ■ Progression similar to that in other joints except for early focal full-thickness cartilage necrosis
  ○ Normal bone mineralization (in contrast to rheumatoid arthritis)

○ Joint traction during subluxation may produce gas in joint ("vacuum phenomenon")
○ Associated with synovial cysts, degenerative disc disease
○ Biomechanical stress is exacerbated in facets that are more horizontal in the sagittal plane and more angled in the axial plane
• Genetics: Genetic predisposition pondered but not proven
• Etiology
○ Frequently seen in elderly population
  ▪ Probably related to minor repetitive trauma coupled with abnormal biomechanics
○ May see earlier presentation after trauma, with kyphosis/scoliosis, or following surgical fusion at adjacent level
• Epidemiology: Facet joint degeneration begins in first two decades of life
• Associated abnormalities: Frequently seen in conjunction with spondylosis

Gross Pathologic & Surgical Features
• Most common locations
○ Mid/lower cervical spine
○ Thoracic spine uncommon
• Joint space narrowing, capsular laxity may permit subluxation of the superior facet on the inferior facet (degenerative spondylolisthesis)
• Subsequently see ulceration, fibrillation, loss of joint space, eburnation, and osteophyte formation

Microscopic Features
• Findings are similar to those seen in synovial joints at other locations
○ Osseous proliferation
○ Fibrillation and erosion of articular joint cartilage
○ Preservation of bone density

Staging, Grading or Classification Criteria
• Grading scale (Pathria et al) - based on imaging studies
○ Grade 0: Normal
○ Grade I: Mild narrowing and joint irregularity
○ Grade II: Moderate narrowing and joint irregularity, sclerosis, and osteophyte formation
○ Grade III: Severe narrowing and almost total loss of joint space, sclerosis, and osteophyte formation

CLINICAL ISSUES

Presentation
• Most common signs/symptoms
○ Mechanical neck pain (facet arthrosis syndrome)
  ▪ Pain is related to irritation of nervous innervation of the joint from medial branch(es) of the dorsal primary ramus, capsular distension, inflammatory synovitis, entrapment of synovial villi between two articular processes, or actual nerve impingement by osteophytes
  ▪ Aggravated by rest, worse in the morning, and relieved by repeated gentle motion
○ Radiculopathy
○ Other signs/symptoms

  ▪ Facet disease may be asymptomatic incidental finding on imaging
  ▪ Myelopathy (rarely)
• Clinical profile
○ Clinical pain syndrome produces symptoms that frequently are aggravated by rest and alleviated by movement
○ Poor correlation between duration and severity of pain and extent of facet degeneration

Demographics
• Age: Universal after age 60 years
• Gender: No gender preference

Natural History & Prognosis
• Can show progressive symptoms/signs
• Variable (depending on severity)

Treatment
• Mechanical pain - conservative medical therapy
• Foraminal narrowing with radiculopathy - foraminotomy
• Subluxation
○ Cervical - transarticular fusion with lateral mass screws or anterior cervical discectomy and fusion

DIAGNOSTIC CHECKLIST

Consider
• Best detail of foraminal bony narrowing with thin-section CT with oblique reformats

Image Interpretation Pearls
• 3D gradient echo T2* images overemphasize degree of foraminal or central canal narrowing

SELECTED REFERENCES

1. Roberts CC et al: Oblique reformation in cervical spine computed tomography: a new look at an old friend. Spine. 28(2):167-70, 2003
2. Birchall D et al: Evaluation of magnetic resonance myelography in the investigation of cervical spondylotic radiculopathy. Br J Radiol. 76(908):525-31, 2003
3. Truumees E et al: Cervical spondylotic myelopathy and radiculopathy. Instr Course Lect. 49:339-60, 2000
4. Ross JS: Magnetic resonance imaging of the postoperative spine. Semin Musculoskelet Radiol. 4(3):281-91, 2000
5. Kaiser JA et al: Imaging of the cervical spine. Spine. 23(24):2701-12, 1998
6. Grob D: Surgery in the degenerative cervical spine. Spine 23(24): 2674-83, 1998
7. Czervionke LF et al: Imaging of the spine. Techniques of MR imaging. Orthop Clin North Am. 28(4):583-616, 1997
8. Yousem DM et al: Degenerative narrowing of the cervical spine neural foramina: evaluation with high-resolution 3DFT gradient-echo MR imaging. AJNR Am J Neuroradiol. 12(2):229-36, 1991
9. Oegema TR Jr et al: The inter-relationship of facet joint osteoarthritis and degenerative disc disease. Br J Rheumatol 30(Suppl 1): 16-20, 1991
10. Pathria M et al: Osteoarthritis of the facet joints: accuracy of oblique radiographic assessment. Radiology. 164(1):227-30, 1987

FACET ARTHROPATHY, CERVICAL

IMAGE GALLERY

Typical

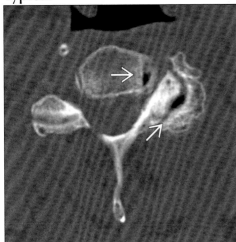 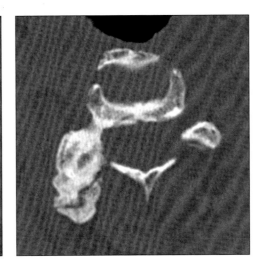

(Left) Axial NECT shows severe left facet degenerative arthropathy and foraminal stenosis. "Vacuum phenomenon" present in facet joint and uncovertebral joint (arrows). *(Right)* Axial NECT shows severe, exuberant right facet degenerative arthropathy.

Typical

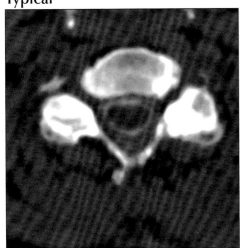 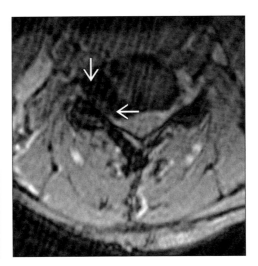

(Left) Axial CECT following myelography shows bilateral foraminal degenerative change, stenosis with relatively mild impingement upon thecal sac. *(Right)* Axial T2* GRE MR shows severe right uncovertebral hypertrophic degenerative arthropathy with severe foraminal stenosis (arrows).

Typical

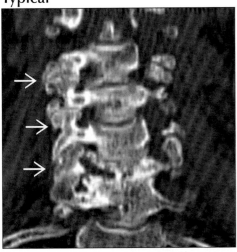 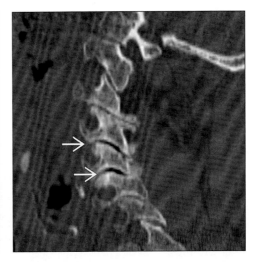

(Left) Coronal NECT shows multilevel severe facet hypertrophic degenerative arthropathy with foraminal stenosis (arrows). *(Right)* Sagittal NECT shows hypertrophic facet degenerative arthropathy with "vacuum phenomenon" (arrows).

FACET ARTHROPATHY, LUMBAR

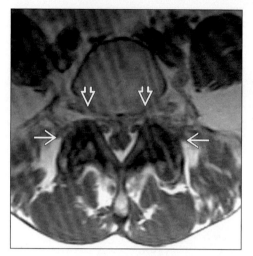

Axial T1WI MR shows marked facet hypertrophic degenerative arthropathy with enlarged facets (arrows), producing foraminal stenosis (open arrows).

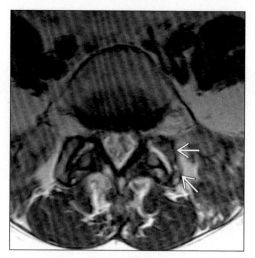

Axial T2WI MR shows bilateral facet hypertrophy and small bilateral facet effusions (arrows).

TERMINOLOGY

Abbreviations and Synonyms
- Facet arthrosis, degenerative facet disease, degenerative joint disease

Definitions
- Osteoarthritis of synovially-lined lumbar apophyseal joints

IMAGING FINDINGS

General Features
- Best diagnostic clue: Osseous facet overgrowth impinging on the neural foramina in conjunction with articular joint space narrowing
- Location: Facet joints of lumbar spine
- Size: May be minimal abnormality or large osteophytes approximating size of facet themselves
- Morphology: Osseous facet overgrowth and cartilage erosion with joint space narrowing

Radiographic Findings
- Radiography
  - Plain films poor for demonstrating early facet degeneration
  - Later changes well demonstrated
  - Oblique views demonstrate facet joints best

- Facet joint osteophytes producing foraminal narrowing
- Associated with degenerative disc disease
- "Mushroom cap" facet appearance
- Joint space narrowing with sclerosis and bone eburnation
- Intra-articular gas ("vacuum phenomenon")
- Spondylolisthesis not uncommon
- Fluoroscopy: Same as plain radiography; can observe motion abnormalities on flexion-extension
- Myelography: CT myelography shows facet relationship to adjacent contrast-opacified thecal sac and nerve root sleeves

CT Findings
- NECT
  - CT more sensitive than plain films for detecting presence and degree of arthrosis
  - Facet joint osteophytes producing foraminal narrowing
  - "Mushroom cap" facet appearance
  - Joint space narrowing with sclerosis and bone eburnation
  - Intra-articular gas ("vacuum phenomenon")
  - CT myelography shows facet relationship to adjacent contrast-opacified thecal sac and nerve root sleeves
- CECT

DDx: Facet Arthropathy, Lumbar

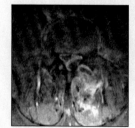

Septic Facet

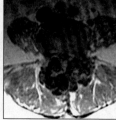

Tumoral Calcinosis

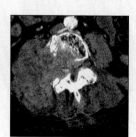

Tumor

FACET ARTHROPATHY, LUMBAR

Key Facts

Terminology
- Facet arthrosis, degenerative facet disease, degenerative joint disease
- Osteoarthritis of synovially-lined lumbar apophyseal joints

Imaging Findings
- Best diagnostic clue: Osseous facet overgrowth impinging on the neural foramina in conjunction with articular joint space narrowing
- Size: May be minimal abnormality or large osteophytes approximating size of facet themselves
- CT more sensitive than plain films for detecting presence and degree of arthrosis

Top Differential Diagnoses
- Septic facet

- Inflammatory arthritides
- Paget disease
- Tumor
- Tumoral calcinosis

Pathology
- Epidemiology: Facet joint degeneration begins in first two decades of life
- Findings similar to those seen in synovial joints at other locations
- Osseous proliferation
- Fibrillation and erosion of articular joint cartilage
- Preservation of bone density

Clinical Issues
- Mechanical back pain (facet arthrosis syndrome) most common symptom

---

- ○ Inflammatory soft tissue changes surrounding facet joint are common
  - ■ May appear aggressive even in absence of infection

MR Findings
- T1WI
  - ○ Joint space narrowing, thinning of articular cartilage
    - ■ Conversely, some patients show variable synovial thickening
    - ■ Irritation of the synovium can produce synovial hyperplasia with paradoxical joint space widening
- T2WI
  - ○ Osteophyte proliferation narrowing neural foramina
  - ○ Foraminal compromise often combination of disease
    - ■ Facet hypertrophic degenerative arthropathy, particularly superior articular facet extending into lumbar foramen
    - ■ Ligamentous buckling/thickening
    - ■ Disc bulge/osteophyte extending into inferior portion of lumbar foramen
- STIR: May show marrow hyperintensity due to edema, type I endplate-like changes
- T2* GRE
  - ○ Shows osseous changes well
  - ○ Tends to overemphasize the degree of foraminal or central canal narrowing
- T1 C+
  - ○ Enhancing inflammatory soft tissue changes surrounding facet joint not uncommon
    - ■ May appear aggressive even in absence of infection

Nuclear Medicine Findings
- Bone Scan: Increased uptake with degenerative disc disease, facet arthrosis

Imaging Recommendations
- Plain films useful to demonstrate presence and severity of facet degenerative changes
- Sagittal and axial T1WI and T2WI best demonstrate degenerative facet compression of adjacent thecal sac and fat-filled neural foramina

- Consider CT myelography if MRI contraindications or MRI does not adequately demonstrate facet relationship to neural foramina

DIFFERENTIAL DIAGNOSIS

Septic facet
- T2 hyperintensity extending into soft tissues, epidural abscess/phlegmon

Inflammatory arthritides
- Look for ankylosis/erosions involving facet and SI joints

Paget disease
- Thickened cortex, trabeculae, bony expansion

Tumor
- Metastasis, lymphoma
- Soft tissue enhancing mass, bone destruction

Tumoral calcinosis
- Large, lobulated calcific mass, no enhancing soft tissue component (rare)

PATHOLOGY

General Features
- General path comments
  - ○ Normal bone mineralization (in contrast to rheumatoid arthritis)
  - ○ Degenerative (hypertrophic) inflammatory changes in synovial joints
    - ■ Progression is similar to that seen in other joints except for early focal full-thickness cartilage necrosis
  - ○ Joint traction during subluxation may produce gas in joint ("vacuum phenomenon")
  - ○ Associated with synovial cysts, degenerative disc disease, canal stenosis

FACET ARTHROPATHY, LUMBAR

- Biomechanical stress is exacerbated in facets that are more horizontal in the sagittal plane and more angled in the axial plane
- Genetics: No genetic basis proven
- Etiology
  - Elderly population
    - Probably related to minor repetitive trauma coupled with abnormal biomechanics
  - May see earlier presentation after trauma, with kyphosis/scoliosis, or following surgical fusion at adjacent level
- Epidemiology: Facet joint degeneration begins in first two decades of life
- Associated abnormalities
  - Foraminal stenosis, central canal stenosis
  - Synovial cyst, extending dorsal or ventral to facet joint

Gross Pathologic & Surgical Features
- Joint space narrowing, capsular laxity may permit subluxation of the superior facet on the inferior facet (degenerative spondylolisthesis)
- Subsequently see ulceration, fibrillation, loss of joint space, eburnation, and osteophyte formation

Microscopic Features
- Findings similar to those seen in synovial joints at other locations
  - Osseous proliferation
  - Fibrillation and erosion of articular joint cartilage
  - Preservation of bone density

Staging, Grading or Classification Criteria
- Grading scale (Pathria et al) - based on imaging studies
  - Grade 0: Normal
  - Grade I: Mild narrowing and joint irregularity
  - Grade II: Moderate narrowing and joint irregularity, sclerosis, and osteophyte formation
  - Grade III: Severe narrowing and almost total loss of joint space, sclerosis, and osteophyte formation

CLINICAL ISSUES

Presentation
- Most common signs/symptoms
  - Mechanical back pain (facet arthrosis syndrome) most common symptom
    - Low back stiffness
    - Pain is related to irritation of nervous innervation of the joint from medial branch(es) of the dorsal primary ramus, capsular distension, inflammatory synovitis, entrapment of synovial villi between two articular processes, or actual nerve impingement by osteophytes
    - Aggravated by rest, worse in the morning, and relieved by repeated gentle motion
    - Pain is centered in the hips, buttocks or thighs, does not extend below knees, has no radicular pattern, and is aggravated by hyperextension
    - Straight leg raise usually negative
  - Other signs/symptoms
    - Facet disease may be asymptomatic incidental finding on imaging

- Clinical profile
  - Clinical pain syndrome produces symptoms that frequently are aggravated by rest and alleviated by movement
  - Poor correlation between duration and severity of pain and extent of facet degeneration

Demographics
- Age
  - Virtually universal after age 60 years
  - Identifiable to varying degrees in majority of adults
- Gender: No gender preference

Natural History & Prognosis
- Can show progressive symptoms/signs
- Variable (depending on severity)

Treatment
- Mechanical pain - conservative medical therapy
- Foraminal narrowing with radiculopathy - nerve root blocks, foraminotomy
- Subluxation
  - Lumbar - posterior fusion with pedicle screws and rods (rarely in conjunction with anterior interbody fusion)

DIAGNOSTIC CHECKLIST

Consider
- Best bony detail with thin-section CT with reformats

Image Interpretation Pearls
- Important to recognize multifactorial nature of foraminal narrowing: Bony facet, ligament, disc, osteophyte

SELECTED REFERENCES

1. Cinotti G et al: Stenosis of lumbar intervertebral foramen: anatomic study on predisposing factors. Spine. 27(3):223-9, 2002
2. Narozny M et al: Therapeutic efficacy of selective nerve root blocks in the treatment of lumbar radicular leg pain. Swiss Med Wkly. 131(5-6):75-80, 2001
3. Jenis LG et al: Foraminal stenosis of the lumbar spine: a review of 65 surgical cases. Am J Orthop. 30(3):205-11, 2001
4. Jenis LG et al: Spine update. Lumbar foraminal stenosis. Spine. 25(3):389-94, 2000
5. Ross JS: Magnetic resonance imaging of the postoperative spine. Semin Musculoskelet Radiol. 4(3):281-91, 2000
6. Postacchini F: Surgical management of lumbar spinal stenosis. Spine. 24(10):1043-7, 1999
7. Czervionke LF et al: Imaging of the spine. Techniques of MR imaging. Orthop Clin North Am. 28(4):583-616, 1997
8. Mehta M et al: Mechanical back pain and the facet joint syndrome. Disabil Rehabil 16(1): 2-12, 1994
9. Griffiths HJ et al: Disease of the lumbosacral facet joints. Neuroimaging Clinics of North America 3(3):567-75, 1993
10. Oegema TR Jr et al: The inter-relationship of facet joint osteoarthritis and degenerative disc disease. Br J Rheumatol 30(Suppl 1): 16-20, 1991
11. Pathria M et al: Osteoarthritis of the facet joints: accuracy of oblique radiographic assessment. Radiology. 164(1):227-30, 1987

FACET ARTHROPATHY, LUMBAR

IMAGE GALLERY

Typical

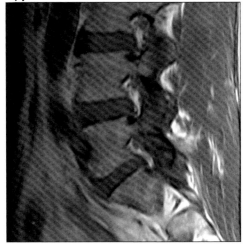
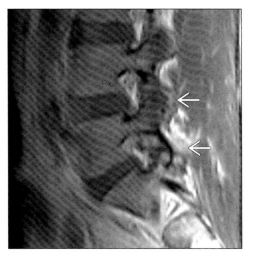

(Left) Sagittal T1WI MR shows L4-5, L5-S1 facet degenerative arthropathy with hypertrophy and low signal. (Right) Sagittal T1 C+ MR shows enhancement of the L4-5, L5-S1 facets (arrows) due to degenerative arthropathy.

Typical

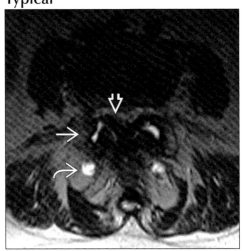
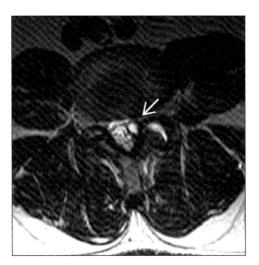

(Left) Axial T2WI MR shows degenerative facet hypertrophy, with bilateral effusions (arrow), thickened ligamentum flavum (open arrow), and posteriorly directed synovial cysts (curved arrow). (Right) Axial T2WI MR shows degenerated left facet with effusion and synovial cyst compressing the left dorsal aspect of thecal sac (arrow).

Typical

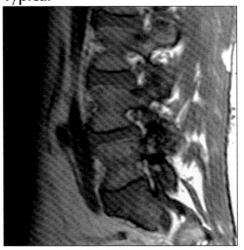
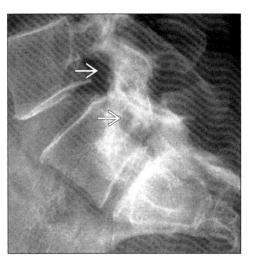

(Left) Sagittal T1WI MR shows degenerated facets spanning L3-4 through L5-S1 levels, narrowing the neural foramina. (Right) Lateral radiography shows facet hypertrophy and bony eburnation of the L4-5 and L5-S1 facets (arrows).

FACET JOINT SYNOVIAL CYST

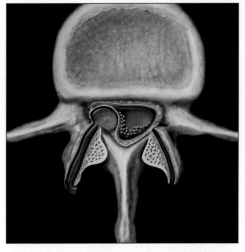

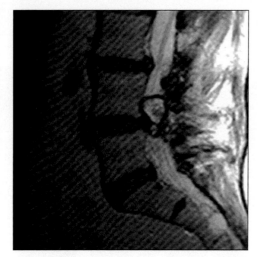

Axial graphic depicts right facet joint synovial cyst. Fluid expands right facet joint, extending into subarticular recess in a loculated collection, there is mass effect on the thecal sac.

Sagittal T2WI MR shows a slightly lobulated predominantly hyperintense mass in the spinal canal at L4-5.

TERMINOLOGY

Abbreviations and Synonyms
- Facet joint ganglion cyst

Definitions
- Synovial cyst formed from degenerative facet joint

IMAGING FINDINGS

General Features
- Best diagnostic clue: Posterolateral extradural cystic mass communicating with facet joint
- Location
  - Posterolateral to thecal sac
  - Adjacent to facet joint
  - Lumbar spine: 90%
    - 70-80% at L4-5
    - L3-4 and L5-S1: Less common
  - Uncommon
    - Cervical and thoracic spine
    - Foraminal
    - Far lateral extra-foraminal
    - Bilateral
- Size: 1-2 cm
- Morphology
  - Round
  - Lobulated
  - Sharply marginated

Radiographic Findings
- Radiography
  - Degenerative changes
    - Disc space loss
    - Vacuum disc phenomenon
    - Endplate sclerosis and spurring
    - Facet arthropathy
    - Spondylolisthesis without spondylolysis
    - Lateral listhesis
    - Scoliosis
    - Worst at the level of synovial cyst
- Myelography
  - Circumscribed posterolateral extradural mass
  - Central canal and subarticular narrowing
  - High sensitivity
  - Low specificity

CT Findings
- NECT
  - Difficult to detect because of fluid density
  - Increased density from hemorrhage
  - Mural calcifications
  - Intra-cystic gas
  - Facet joint gas
- CECT: Mild rim-enhancement
- Bone CT

DDx: Intraspinal Extradural Masses

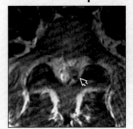

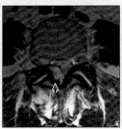

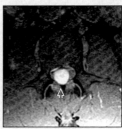

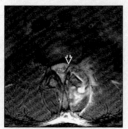

Free Disc Fragment *Ganglion Cyst* *Schwannoma* *Periarticular Abscess*

FACET JOINT SYNOVIAL CYST

Key Facts

Terminology
- Synovial cyst formed from degenerative facet joint

Imaging Findings
- Best diagnostic clue: Posterolateral extradural cystic mass communicating with facet joint
- Lumbar spine: 90%
- 70-80% at L4-5
- Increased density from hemorrhage
- Mural calcifications
- Hyperintense
- Low intensity rim
- T1 C+: Enhancing wall
- Well circumscribed
- Variable central canal, subarticular, or lateral recess narrowing

Top Differential Diagnoses
- Extruded disc fragment
- Ganglion cyst
- Nerve sheath tumor

Pathology
- Invariably associated with degenerative disc and facet disease

Clinical Issues
- Chronic low back pain
- Acute pain from hemorrhage
- May spontaneously regress
- High post-surgical success rate in symptomatic patients
- Laminectomy with cyst excision

- ○ Same as radiographic findings
- ○ Better osseous detail with sagittal and coronal reformation
- ○ Erosion of vertebral arch uncommon

MR Findings
- T1WI
  - ○ Hypointense
    - ▪ Similar to CSF
  - ○ Hyperintense
    - ▪ Hemorrhagic or proteinaceous content
- T2WI
  - ○ Hyperintense
    - ▪ If direct communication with facet joint present
    - ▪ Best seen on sagittal T2WI
  - ○ Hypointense
    - ▪ Hemorrhage
  - ○ Low intensity rim
- STIR: Hyperintense
- T1 C+: Enhancing wall
- Well circumscribed
- Ligamentum flavum hypertrophy
- Facet arthropathy
- Variable central canal, subarticular, or lateral recess narrowing
  - ○ Impingement of traversing nerve root
- High sensitivity and specificity

Nuclear Medicine Findings
- Bone Scan
  - ○ Radiotracer uptake in vertebral endplates and posterior elements
    - ▪ Degenerative changes

Other Modality Findings
- Facet joint arthrogram
  - ○ Contrast extending from facet joint into synovial cyst
    - ▪ Not a consistent finding

Imaging Recommendations
- Best imaging tool
  - ○ MRI of lumbar spine
    - ▪ Axial and sagittal T2WI

DIFFERENTIAL DIAGNOSIS

Extruded disc fragment
- Not contiguous with facet joint
- Usually anterior epidural
- Posterolateral uncommon
- Not as hyperintense on T2WI

Ganglion cyst
- Likely from ligamentum flavum
- Difficult to distinguish by imaging
- Different pathologically
- Contains myxoid material
- Lined by fibrous connective tissue capsule

Nerve sheath tumor
- Intradural extramedullary most common
- "Dumbbell" lesion less common
- Intense post-contrast-enhancement

Septic facet arthritis
- Abscess extending out from facet joint
  - ○ Simulating synovial cyst
- Surrounding soft tissue edema and enhancement
- Adjacent marrow edema

Asymmetric ligamentum flavum hypertrophy
- Hypointense on T2WI
- More broad-based contour
- Diffuse ligamentum flavum thickening

PATHOLOGY

General Features
- General path comments
  - ○ Thickened connective tissue and synovium
  - ○ Invariably associated with degenerative disc and facet disease
- Etiology
  - ○ Stress loading on lumbar spine
  - ○ Facet osteoarthropathy
  - ○ Joint fluid accumulation
  - ○ Facet instability and hypermobility

FACET JOINT SYNOVIAL CYST

- ▪ Greatest mobility at L4-5
  - ○ Synovial proliferation
  - ○ Cyst formation
- Associated abnormalities
  - ○ Degenerative spondylolisthesis
  - ○ Rheumatoid arthritis
  - ○ Calcium pyrophosphate deposition disease

Gross Pathologic & Surgical Features
- Encapsulated
- Serous, mucinous, ± hemorrhagic fluid
- White myxoid material

Microscopic Features
- Fibrous connective tissue
- Inflammatory cell infiltration
- Calcific deposits
- Lined with hypervascular synovium

CLINICAL ISSUES

Presentation
- Most common signs/symptoms
  - ○ Chronic low back pain
  - ○ Other signs/symptoms
    - ▪ Acute pain from hemorrhage
    - ▪ Radicular symptoms
    - ▪ Neurogenic claudication
    - ▪ Cauda equina syndrome
    - ▪ Myelopathy if cervical or thoracic

Demographics
- Age: ≥ 60
- Gender: More common in females
- Ethnicity: No racial predilection

Natural History & Prognosis
- May spontaneously regress
- High post-surgical success rate in symptomatic patients

Treatment
- Conservative
  - ○ Bed rest
  - ○ Analgesics
  - ○ Epidural and facet injection
  - ○ Bracing
- Laminectomy with cyst excision
  - ○ In setting of intractable pain
  - ○ To relieve nerve compression and central stenosis
  - ○ Hemilaminectomy and flavectomy also performed
- Less permanent
  - ○ Percutaneous cyst aspiration
    - ▪ Under CT guidance
  - ○ Steroid injection into cyst
    - ▪ Half to two-thirds of patients have excellent symptomatic relief after 6 months

DIAGNOSTIC CHECKLIST

Consider
- Thin-section sagittal T2WI may show communication between facet joint and adjacent synovial cyst

Image Interpretation Pearls
- Well-circumscribed T2 hyperintense mass
- Thin hypointense rim
- Posterolateral to thecal sac
- Abutting facet joint

SELECTED REFERENCES

1. Houten JK et al: Spontaneous regression of symptomatic lumbar synovial cysts. Report of three cases. J Neurosurg. 99(2 Suppl):235-8, 2003
2. Swartz PG et al: Spontaneous resolution of an intraspinal synovial cyst. AJNR Am J Neuroradiol. 24(6):1261-3, 2003
3. Gadgil AA et al: Bilateral symptomatic synovial cysts of the lumbar spine caused by calcium pyrophosphate deposition disease: a case report. Spine. 27(19):E428-31, 2002
4. Phuong LK et al: Far lateral extraforaminal lumbar synovial cyst: report of two cases. Neurosurgery. 51(2):505-7; discussion 507-8, 2002
5. Metellus P et al: An unusual presentation of a lumbar synovial cyst: case report. Spine. 27(11):E278-80, 2002
6. Gishen P et al: Percutaneous excision of a facet joint cyst under CT guidance. Cardiovasc Intervent Radiol. 24(5):351-53, 2001
7. Tillich M et al: Symptomatic intraspinal synovial cysts of the lumbar spine: correlation of MR and surgical findings. Neuroradiology. 43(12):1070-5, 2001
8. Bureau NJ et al: Lumbar facet joint synovial cyst: percutaneous treatment with steroid injections and distention--clinical and imaging follow-up in 12 patients. Radiology. 221(1):179-85, 2001
9. Banning CS et al: Patient outcome after resection of lumbar juxtafacet cysts. Spine. 26(8):969-72, 2001
10. Trummer M et al: Diagnosis and surgical management of intraspinal synovial cysts: report of 19 cases. J Neurol Neurosurg Psychiatry. 70(1):74-7, 2001
11. Apostolaki E et al: MR imaging of lumbar facet joint synovial cysts. Eur Radiol. 10(4):615-23, 2000
12. Bandiera S et al: Hemorrhagic synovial lumbar cyst: a case report and review of the literature. Chir Organi Mov. 84(2):197-203, 1999
13. Howington JU et al: Intraspinal synovial cysts: 10-year experience at the Ochsner Clinic. J Neurosurg. 91(2 Suppl):193-9, 1999
14. Jonsson B et al: Lumbar nerve root compression by intraspinal synovial cysts. Report of 8 cases. Acta Orthop Scand. 70(2):203-6, 1999
15. Parlier-Cuau C et al: Symptomatic lumbar facet joint synovial cysts: clinical assessment of facet joint steroid injection after 1 and 6 months and long-term follow-up in 30 patients. Radiology. 210(2):509-13, 1999
16. Sampson MA et al: Acute extradural compression due to an intraspinal synovial cyst: CT and myelogram appearances. Clin Radiol. 41(6):433-4, 1990
17. Liu SS et al: Synovial cysts of the lumbosacral spine: diagnosis by MR imaging. AJR Am J Roentgenol. 154(1):163-6, 1990
18. Jackson DE et al: Intraspinal Synovial Cysts: MR Imaging. Radiology 170 (2): 527-30, 1989
19. Onofrio BM et al: Synovial cysts of the spine. Neurosurgery. 22(4):642-7, 1988
20. Wang AM et al: Synovial cysts of the lumbar spine: CT evaluation. Comput Radiol. 11(5-6):253-7, 1987

FACET JOINT SYNOVIAL CYST

IMAGE GALLERY

Typical

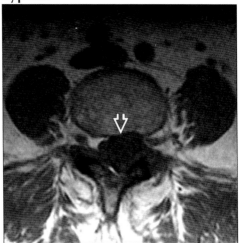 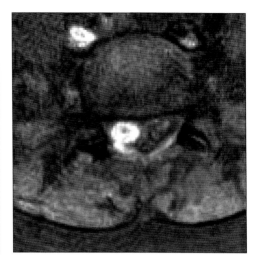

(Left) Axial T1WI MR shows a large fluid intensity mass (arrow) within left lateral aspect of spinal canal with significant mass effect. *(Right)* Axial T1WI MR with fat suppression shows a hyperintense extradural mass within right subarticular/lateral recess, compatible with a hemorrhagic synovial cyst.

Typical

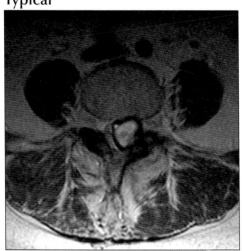 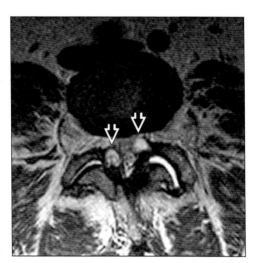

(Left) Axial T2WI MR shows a well-circumscribed hyperintense mass with a hypointense rim abutting left L4-5 facet joint, narrowing the central canal. *(Right)* Axial T2WI MR shows bilateral subarticular hyperintense masses (arrows) at L4-5, consistent with bilateral facet synovial cysts.

Typical

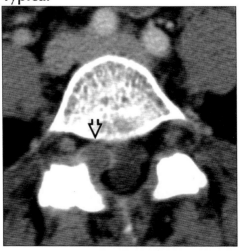 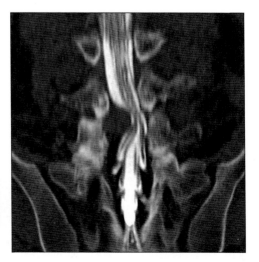

(Left) Axial CECT shows a right-sided circumscribed juxta-articular mass (arrow), slightly hyperdense than CSF, with a thin rim of mild enhancement, causing subarticular stenosis. *(Right)* Axial bone CT after myelography with coronal reformation shows an extradural mass abutting right L4-5 facet joint, distorting thecal sac.

ACQUIRED SPINAL STENOSIS, LUMBAR

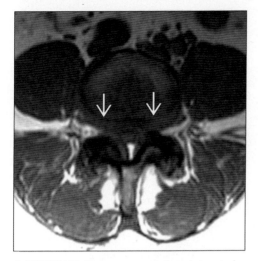

Axial T1WI MR shows severe central canal stenosis due to bulging anulus (arrows) and posterior facet hypertrophic degenerative arthopathy combining to compress the thecal sac.

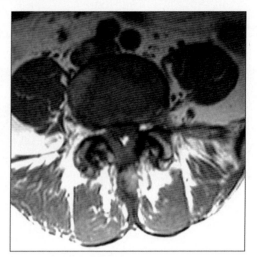

Axial T1WI MR shows central canal stenosis primarily related to facet and ligamentous hypertrophy/thickening with little ventral epidural disease.

TERMINOLOGY

Abbreviations and Synonyms
- Spondylosis, central canal stenosis, lumbar canal stenosis

Definitions
- Spinal canal narrowing in lumbar spine
- Secondary to multifactorial degenerative changes, being progressive and dynamic process

IMAGING FINDINGS

General Features
- Best diagnostic clue: Trefoil appearance of lumbar spinal canal on axial imaging
- Location: Most common in lower lumber spine where there is most mobility (L4-5)
- Size
  - Sagittal diameter of lumbar canal less than 12 mm relative stenosis
  - Sagittal diameter of lumbar canal less than 10 mm absolute stenosis
- Morphology
  - Obliterated perineural fat in lumbar neural foramina on sagittal imaging
  - Narrowed lumbar lateral recess on axial imaging

Radiographic Findings
- Radiography
  - Disc space narrowing, osteophytes
  - Facet osteoarthritis, spondylosis, spondylolisthesis
  - Interpedicular distance narrowing if combined with congenital stenosis
- Myelography
  - 93% accurate for spinal stenosis
  - Hourglass constriction at single or multiple levels
  - Patient positioning in extension accentuates stenosis
    - Dynamic changes: If block at stenotic level, forward flexion often allows contrast past stenotic level

CT Findings
- NECT
  - Direct visualization of compressing disc disease (bulge), facet arthopathy, and ligamentous thickening
  - Trefoil pattern of canal, with compression of thecal sac
  - Reformats allow visualization of foraminal stenosis
    - Rostrocaudal subluxation of facets associated with loss of disc space height
    - Osteophyte impinging upon neural foramen

MR Findings
- T1WI

DDx: Extradural Disease

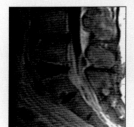

Epidural Abscess

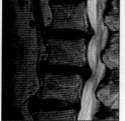

Herniation

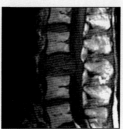

Metastatic

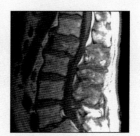

Paget Disease

ACQUIRED SPINAL STENOSIS, LUMBAR

Key Facts

Terminology

- Spondylosis, central canal stenosis, lumbar canal stenosis
- Spinal canal narrowing in lumbar spine
- Secondary to multifactorial degenerative changes, being progressive and dynamic process

Imaging Findings

- Best diagnostic clue: Trefoil appearance of lumbar spinal canal on axial imaging
- Location: Most common in lower lumber spine where there is most mobility (L4-5)
- Sagittal diameter of lumbar canal less than 12 mm relative stenosis

Clinical Issues

- Chronic low back pain

- Bilateral lower extremity pain, paresthesia, and weakness
- Exacerbation by prolonged standing and walking
- Relieve of pain by squatting or sitting (flexion) in 80%
- Degree of spinal stenosis on imaging may not correlate with symptomatology
- Majority of symptomatic patients stable over months to years (40-70%)
- History of back pain < 5 years and leg pain < 6 months have success with nonoperative treatment
- Operative treatment primarily surgical decompression with laminectomies and fusion
- > 70% complete relief of preoperative symptoms
- Other surgery: Expansive laminoplasty or fenestration procedure

- MRI equivalent to CT myelogram in diagnosing lumbar spinal stenosis, but provides additional information on the spinal cord
- Degenerative disc disease with variable degree of herniation
- Trefoil appearance of spinal canal on axial imaging
- Thickened ligamentum flavum
- Vertebral endplate osteophytes
- Facet joint hypertrophy
- Obliterated perineural fat in neural foramina on sagittal imaging
- Short pedicles
- T2WI
  - Trefoil appearance of spinal canal on axial imaging
  - Hourglass appearance of central canal on sagittal T2WI
  - Elongated and redundant nerve roots above and below level of stenosis
  - Narrowed lateral recess on axial imaging
- T1 C+: Enhancing and crowded nerve roots

Imaging Recommendations

- Best imaging tool
  - MRI
  - Conventional T1W and T2W sagittal and axial images with 4-5 mm slice thickness

DIFFERENTIAL DIAGNOSIS

Infection

- Disc space and vertebral body hyperintensity on T2WI, with endplate irregularity
- Enhancement of epidural phlegmon, peripheral enhancement of abscess

Disc herniation

- Focal lesion arising from intervertebral disc

Metastatic disease

- Diffuse or focal hypointensity on T1WI, ventral epidural soft tissue from contiguous extension

Paget disease

- Expansion of vertebral body
- Patchy hyperintensity of vertebral body on T1WI

Epidural hemorrhage

- Variable signal intensity depending on evolving hemoglobin
- Acute onset of symptoms

PATHOLOGY

General Features

- General path comments: Age related degenerative disease involving disc and facets
- Genetics: None for acquired stenosis
- Etiology
  - Degenerative changes involving discs, vertebral endplates, facet joints, and ligamentum flavum
  - Congenitally short pedicles often contribute to acquired spinal stenosis
- Epidemiology: Fifth decade and later
- Associated abnormalities: Congenitally short pedicles often present

Gross Pathologic & Surgical Features

- Disc degeneration
  - Loss of nuclear definition, fibrosis and fissuring
  - Osteophyte formation
  - Anular disruption
  - Loss of facet joint space and cartilage, subchondral sclerosis, osteophytosis

Microscopic Features

- Fissuring of disc, loss of cartilaginous endplate, granulation tissue, bony sclerosis

Staging, Grading or Classification Criteria

- Normal lumbar canal
  - > 12 mm AP diameter
  - Cross-section area > 77 mm square
- 50% reduction in cross section area of bony canal motor and sensory deficits occur (animal model)

ACQUIRED SPINAL STENOSIS, LUMBAR

CLINICAL ISSUES

Presentation
- Most common signs/symptoms
  - Symptoms include
    - Chronic low back pain
    - Bilateral lower extremity pain, paresthesia, and weakness
    - Exacerbation by prolonged standing and walking
    - Relieve of pain by squatting or sitting (flexion) in 80%
  - Neurogenic claudication
    - Leg pain (80%)
    - Numbness, tingling (60%)
    - Cramping, weakness (50%)
  - Other signs/symptoms
    - Bladder dysfunction and sexual difficulty (10%)
    - Radicular pain (10%)
    - Negative straight leg raise
  - Degree of spinal stenosis on imaging may not correlate with symptomatology
- Clinical profile: Insidious onset of low back pain, paresthesia, difficulty walking

Demographics
- Age: > 50
- Gender
  - M = F
  - Associated degenerative spondylolisthesis 4x more common in women

Natural History & Prognosis
- Majority of symptomatic patients stable over months to years (40-70%)
- 1/3 improve with non-operative treatment
- 1/3 deteriorate
- History of back pain < 5 years and leg pain < 6 months have success with non-operative treatment

Treatment
- Nonoperative
  - Analgesic medications: Salicylates, NSAIDs
  - Antidepressants (manage chronic pain and associated depression)
  - Exercise
  - Injection therapy (epidural steroids)
  - Other: TENS, thermal therapy
- Operative
  - Operative treatment primarily surgical decompression with laminectomies and fusion
    - > 70% complete relief of pre-operative symptoms
  - Other surgery: Expansive laminoplasty or fenestration procedure
  - Post-operative complications
    - Mortality 0.09%; increases to 0.6% in patients > 75
    - Radicular deficit (5%)
    - CSF fistula/pseudomeningocele (5%)
    - Infection (0.5-8%)

DIAGNOSTIC CHECKLIST

Consider
- MR myelography using bright CSF echo planar sequence or thin-section fast T2 weighted images

Image Interpretation Pearls
- Border of thecal sac and ligamentum flavum indistinct on axial T1WI
- Axial T2WI mandatory for stenosis identification

SELECTED REFERENCES

1. Binder DK et al: Lumbar spinal stenosis. Semin Neurol. 22(2): 157-66, 2002
2. Yukawa Y et al: A comprehensive study of patients with surgically treated lumbar spinal stenosis with neurogenic claudication. J Bone Joint Surg Am. 84-A(11): 1954-9, 2002
3. Speciale AC et al: Observer variability in assessing lumbar spinal stenosis severity on magnetic resonance imaging and its relation to cross-sectional spinal canal area. Spine. 27(10): 1082-6, 2002
4. Cinotti G et al: Stenosis of lumbar intervertebral foramen: anatomic study on predisposing factors. Spine. 27(3): 223-9, 2002
5. Cirak B et al: Surgical therapy for lumbar spinal stenosis: evaluation of 300 cases. Neurosurg Rev. 24(2-3): 80-2, 2001
6. Sheehan JM et al: Degenerative lumbar stenosis: the neurosurgical perspective. Clin Orthop. (384): 61-74, 2001
7. Borenstein DG et al: The value of magnetic resonance imaging of the lumbar spine to predict low-back pain in asymptomatic subjects : a seven-year follow-up study. J Bone Joint Surg Am. 83-A(9): 1306-11, 2001
8. Schonstrom N et al: Imaging lumbar spinal stenosis. Radiol Clin North Am. 39(1): 31-53, v, 2001
9. Pui MH et al: Value of magnetic resonance myelography in the diagnosis of disc herniation and spinal stenosis. Australas Radiol. 44(3): 281-4, 2000
10. Mariconda M et al: Factors influencing the outcome of degenerative lumbar spinal stenosis. J Spinal Disord. 13(2): 131-7, 2000
11. Beattie PF et al: Associations between patient report of symptoms and anatomic impairment visible on lumbar magnetic resonance imaging. Spine. 25(7): 819-28, 2000
12. Ross JS: Magnetic resonance imaging of the postoperative spine. Semin Musculoskelet Radiol. 4(3):281-91, 2000
13. Jinkins JR: MR evaluation of stenosis involving the neural foramina, lateral recesses, and central canal of the lumbosacral spine. Magn Reson Imaging Clin N Am. 7(3): 493-511, viii, 1999
14. Herno A et al: Long-term clinical and magnetic resonance imaging follow-up assessment of patients with lumbar spinal stenosis after laminectomy. Spine. 24(15): 1533-7, 1999
15. Hilibrand AS et al: Degenerative lumbar stenosis: diagnosis and management. J Am Acad Orthop Surg. 7(4): 239-49, 1999
16. Postacchini F: Surgical management of lumbar spinal stenosis. Spine. 24(10): 1043-7, 1999
17. Alfieri KM et al: MR imaging of spinal stenosis. Applied Radiology. August:18-26, 1997
18. Amunosen T et al: Lumbar spinal stenosis: clinical and radiologic features. Spine. 20:1178-86, 1995
19. Modic MT et al: Imaging of degenerative disease of the cervical spine. Clin Orthop. 239:109-20, 1989

ACQUIRED SPINAL STENOSIS, LUMBAR

IMAGE GALLERY

Typical

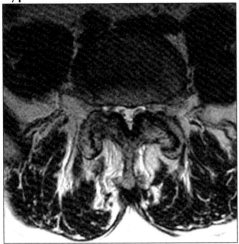
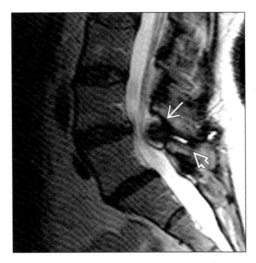

(Left) Axial T2WI MR shows severe central canal stenosis with marked facet arthopathy. The thecal sac has assumed a trefoil appearance. *(Right)* Sagittal T2WI MR shows severe central stenosis L4-5 due to marked posterior ligamentum flavum thickening (arrow). Hyperintensity within interspinous ligament denotes degeneration (open arrow).

Typical

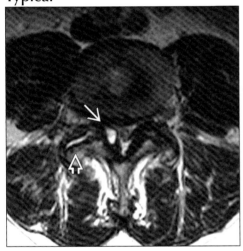
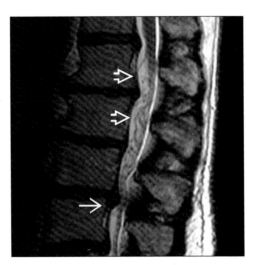

(Left) Axial T2WI MR shows severe central stenosis with disc bulge, facet arthropathy, ligamentous thickening. Right synovial cyst further compresses thecal sac (arrow). Right facet effusion (open arrow). *(Right)* Sagittal T2WI MR shows canal stenosis at L3-4 with bulging disc, ligamentous thickening (arrow). Serpentine areas of low signal within cephalad thecal sac due to redundant nerve roots (open arrows).

Typical

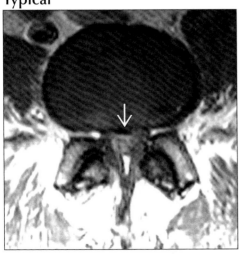
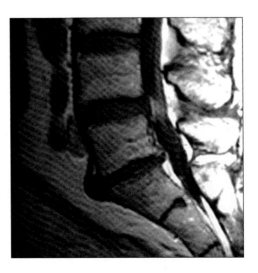

(Left) Axial T1 C+ MR shows central canal stenosis with facet arthropathy and ligamentous thickening. There is diffuse enhancement of the intrathecal roots (arrow). *(Right)* Sagittal T1 C+ MR shows focal enhancement of the roots at the stenotic L4-5 level.

ACQUIRED SPINAL STENOSIS, CERVICAL

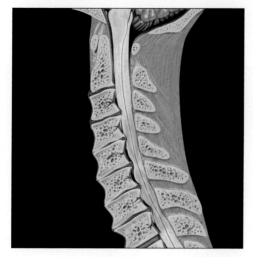

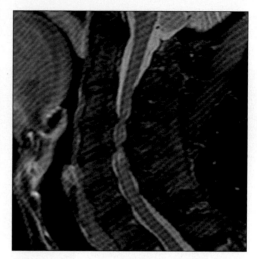

Sagittal graphic shows disc degeneration with osteophyte formation causing central stenosis and cord compression at multiple levels (cervical spondylosis).

Sagittal STIR MR shows severe central canal stenosis at C3-4, C4-5 with marked narrowing of subarachnoid space. Hyperintensity within cord at C4-5 reflects contusion/myelomalacia.

TERMINOLOGY

Abbreviations and Synonyms
- Acquired spinal stenosis, cervical (ASSC)
- Cervical spondylosis; cervical spondylotic myelopathy

Definitions
- Spinal canal and neural foraminal narrowing in cervical spine secondary to multifactorial degenerative changes

IMAGING FINDINGS

General Features
- Best diagnostic clue: Completely effaced cerebral spinal fluid in cervical spine at disc levels
- Location: Cervical spine, ventral epidural, centered at disc levels
- Size: Sagittal diameter of cervical canal < 13 mm
- Morphology
  - Extradural degenerative change compressing thecal sac and cord
  - Congenitally short pedicles often contribute to acquired spinal stenosis

Radiographic Findings
- Radiography: Disc space height loss, osteophyte extending into canal, multilevel degenerative change

- Myelography
  - Obliterated subarachnoid space at disc levels
  - Multiple horizontal "bars" or ridges on AP view due to subarachnoid space narrowing
  - Cord widened on AP view due to compression
  - Multiple levels of root cutoff

CT Findings
- NECT
  - Disc-osteophyte complex protruding into the canal and compressing thecal sac and cord
  - Uncovertebral and facet joint hypertrophy
  - Narrowing of the neural foramina

MR Findings
- T1WI
  - Completely effaced subarachnoid space at disc levels in cervical spine ⇒ "washboard spine"
  - Variable degree of cord compression
  - Disc disease: Disc herniations, osteophytes, disc bulges
- T2WI
  - Intramedullary T2 hyperintensity represents myelomalacia, demyelination, or edema
  - Narrowing of subarachnoid space due to ventral and dorsal epidural disease
    - Ventral low T2 signal due to disc/osteophyte complex

DDx: Myelopathy

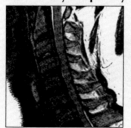

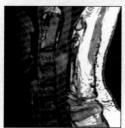

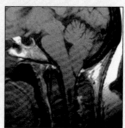

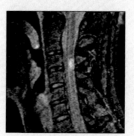

OPLL *Astrocytoma* *Syrinx* *MS*

ACQUIRED SPINAL STENOSIS, CERVICAL

Key Facts

Terminology
- Acquired spinal stenosis, cervical (ASSC)
- Cervical spondylosis; cervical spondylotic myelopathy
- Spinal canal and neural foraminal narrowing in cervical spine secondary to multifactorial degenerative changes

Imaging Findings
- Best diagnostic clue: Completely effaced cerebral spinal fluid in cervical spine at disc levels
- Intramedullary T2 hyperintensity represents myelomalacia, demyelination, or edema
- Narrowing of subarachnoid space due to ventral and dorsal epidural disease
- Ventral low T2 signal due to disc/osteophyte complex

(continued)
- Dorsal low T2 signal due to ligamentous thickening
- T1 C+: Cord myelomalacia, contusion may enhance after gadolinium

Clinical Issues
- ASSC has no pathognomic symptoms or signs
- Spastic paraparesis commonly seen
- Natural history of insidious onset, periods of static disability, and episodic worsening
- New signs and symptoms (75%)
- Slow steady progression of disability (20%)
- Rapid onset with long period of stability (5%)

Diagnostic Checklist
- OPLL if confluent anterior epidural disease
- MRI of cervical spine may overestimate neural foraminal stenosis

---

      - Dorsal low T2 signal due to ligamentous thickening
- T2* GRE
  - Narrowing of neural foramina
  - Uncovertebral and facet joint hypertrophy
- T1 C+: Cord myelomalacia, contusion may enhance after gadolinium

Imaging Recommendations
- Sagittal and axial T1WI, sagittal T2WI, axial T2* imaging (2-3 mm thickness, 3D preferred)

DIFFERENTIAL DIAGNOSIS

Ossification of posterior longitudinal ligament
- A cause of cervical spinal stenosis
- Thick band of hypointensity along posterior vertebral margin
- Central hyperintensity within band represents fatty marrow

Cord tumor
- Intramedullary mass with enhancement

Syrinx
- Linear hyperintensity on T2WI, with or without cord expansion, multiple septations

Multiple sclerosis
- Focal cord hyperintensity on T2WI
- Brain periventricular lesions

Motor neuron disease
- Distinguished on clinical grounds, diagnosis of exclusion

PATHOLOGY

General Features
- General path comments: Age related degenerative disease

- Etiology
  - Degenerative changes involving discs, vertebral endplates, uncovertebral joints, facet joints, and ligamentum flavum
  - Congenitally short pedicles often present
- Epidemiology: Fifth decade and later
- Associated abnormalities: Lumbar canal stenosis (> 5%)

Gross Pathologic & Surgical Features
- Multilevel disc degeneration with decreased disc hydration and fissures
- Disc herniation, bulge with associated broad osteophytes
- Uncovertebral joint osteoarthritic change with foraminal stenosis

Microscopic Features
- Cord destruction of gray and white matter, with demyelination above and below compression levels

Staging, Grading or Classification Criteria
- Sagittal diameter of spinal canal < 13 mm stenotic
- Torg ratio
  - Spinal canal: Vertebral body ratio < 0.8 on plain radiographs = cervical stenosis
  - Poor correlation of Torg ratio and sagittal diameter of spinal canal on CT
  - Not absolute, multiple factors involved in producing neurapraxia with trauma
- AP compression ratio (AP diameter cord/transverse diameter)
  - < 0.40 have worse outcome after surgical decompression
- Cord T2 hyperintensity
  - More clinically symptomatic
  - Less postoperative improvement

CLINICAL ISSUES

Presentation
- Most common signs/symptoms
  - ASSC has no pathognomic symptoms or signs

ACQUIRED SPINAL STENOSIS, CERVICAL

- Spastic paraparesis commonly seen
- Upper extremity numbness, weakness ("myelopathic hand")
- Gait disturbance, loss of position and vibration sense
- Chronic neck pain radiating to occiput and upper extremities
  - Cord syndromes
    - Transverse: Severe spasticity, sphincter involvement, Lhermitte
    - Motor system: Spasticity but minimal sensory disturbance
    - Central cord: Severe motor and sensory disturbance, worse for upper extremities
    - Brown-Sequard: Contralateral sensory and ipsilateral motor deficits
    - Brachialgia cord syndrome: Lower motor neuron ⇒ upper extremity involvement, upper motor neuron ⇒ lower extremity involvement, radicular pain
- Clinical profile: Neck pain, "heaviness" in arms, ataxic gait, hyperreflexia, extensor plantar reflex

Demographics
- Age: > 50
- Gender: M > F

Natural History & Prognosis
- Natural history of insidious onset, periods of static disability, and episodic worsening
  - New signs and symptoms (75%)
  - Slow steady progression of disability (20%)
  - Rapid onset with long period of stability (5%)
- Continued pain, disability and poor outcomes (30-50%)
- More favorable outcome if treated early
- Severity and duration of pre-operative neurologic deficits predictive of the degree of neurologic recovery

Treatment
- Cervical spine
  - Medications
    - Anti-inflammatories, narcotics, antidepressants, muscle relaxants
  - Soft collar immobilization and traction
  - Physical therapy
    - Isometrics
    - Aerobic conditioning
    - Flexibility exercises
  - Depending on site of compression
    - Anterior corpectomy or interbody arthrodesis
    - Posterior decompression with laminectomies
    - Open-door laminaplasties with or without foraminotomies
- Prognostic factors for good surgical outcome
  - Young age
  - < 1 year of symptoms
  - Unilateral motor deficit
  - Presence of Lhermitte sign
- Post-operative complications
  - Neurologic deterioration (5%)
  - Vertebral artery injury
  - Graft extrusion or fracture
  - Instrumentation failure or migration

- Airway obstruction
- Adjacent level degeneration
- Reduced mobility

DIAGNOSTIC CHECKLIST

Consider
- OPLL if confluent anterior epidural disease

Image Interpretation Pearls
- MRI of cervical spine may overestimate neural foraminal stenosis
  - Short TE on axial T2* images decreases this artifact

SELECTED REFERENCES

1. Mayr MT et al: Cervical spinal stenosis: outcome after anterior corpectomy, allograft reconstruction, and instrumentation. J Neurosurg. 96(1 Suppl): 10-6, 2002
2. Tani S et al: Laminoplasty with preservation of posterior cervical elements: surgical technique. Neurosurgery. 50(1): 97-101; discussion 101-2, 2002
3. Edwards CC 2nd et al: Corpectomy versus laminoplasty for multilevel cervical myelopathy: an independent matched-cohort analysis. Spine. 27(11): 1168-75, 2002
4. Geck MJ et al: Surgical options for the treatment of cervical spondylotic myelopathy. Orthop Clin North Am. 33(2): 329-48, 2002
5. Handa Y et al: Evaluation of prognostic factors and clinical outcome in elderly patients in whom expansive laminoplasty is performed for cervical myelopathy due to multisegmental spondylotic canal stenosis. A retrospective comparison with younger patients. J Neurosurg. 96(2 Suppl): 173-9, 2002
6. Epstein N: Posterior approaches in the management of cervical spondylosis and ossification of the posterior longitudinal ligament. Surg Neurol. 58(3-4): 194-207; discussion 207-8, 2002
7. Yue WM et al: The Torg--Pavlov ratio in cervical spondylotic myelopathy: a comparative study between patients with cervical spondylotic myelopathy and a nonspondylotic, nonmyelopathic population. Spine. 26(16): 1760-4, 2001
8. Emery SE: Cervical spondylotic myelopathy: diagnosis and treatment. J Am Acad Orthop Surg. 9(6): 376-88, 2001
9. Fouyas IP et al: Surgery for cervical radiculomyelopathy. Cochrane Database Syst Rev. (3): CD001466, 2001
10. Satomi K et al: Short-term complications and long-term results of expansive open-door laminoplasty for cervical stenotic myelopathy. Spine J. 1(1): 26-30, 2001
11. Kawakami M et al: A comparative study of surgical approaches for cervical compressive myelopathy. Clin Orthop. (381): 129-36, 2000
12. Alfieri KM et al: MR imaging of spinal stenosis. Applied Radiology. August:18-26, 1997
13. Amunosen T et al: Lumbar spinal stenosis: clinical and radiologic features. Spine 20:1178-86, 1995
14. Modic MT et al: Imaging of degenerative disease of the cervical spine. Clin Orthop 239:109-20, 1989

ACQUIRED SPINAL STENOSIS, CERVICAL

IMAGE GALLERY

Typical

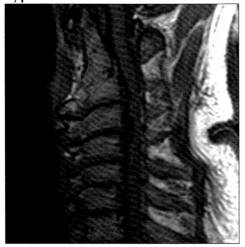
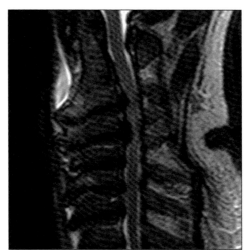

(Left) Sagittal T1WI MR shows severe multilevel disc degeneration with severe central canal stenosis at C3-4, C4-5 with cord compression. Note calcification/ossification of C2-3 disc. (Right) Sagittal T2WI MR shows severe central stenosis with obliteration of subarachnoid space at C3-5, C4-5 with ventral disc/osteophyte complexes.

Typical

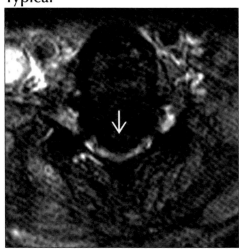
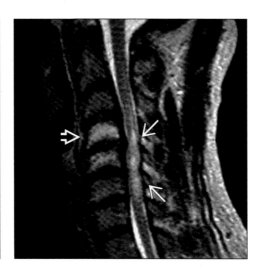

(Left) Axial T2* GRE MR shows marked central stenosis with large ventral disc/osteophyte (arrow). There is bilateral foraminal stenosis. (Right) Sagittal T2WI MR shows narrowing at C3-4 through C5-6 with disc/osteophyte complex and hyperintense cord contusion/myelomalacia (arrows). Type I degenerative endplate change at C4-5 (open arrow).

Typical

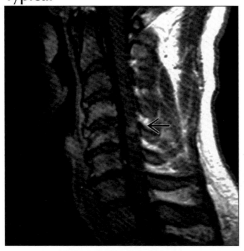
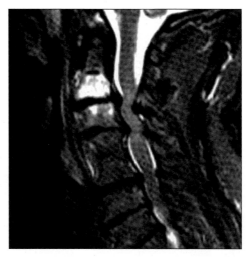

(Left) Sagittal T1 C+ MR shows enhancement of cord contusion (arrow). Extradural disease is of low signal and not well defined on T1W sequence. (Right) Sagittal STIR MR shows severe multilevel stenosis, worst at C2-3, C3-4. Cord hyperintensity present at both levels. Congenital fusion of C4 and C5 bodies accelerates degenerative process.

DEGENERATIVE SCOLIOSIS

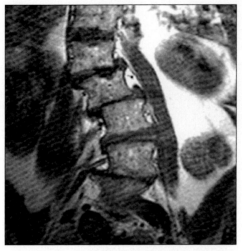

Coronal T1WI MR shows moderate levoscoliosis centered at L3-4. There is right lateral listhesis of L1 on L2, and L2 on L3. Disc height loss and degenerative endplate changes are present.

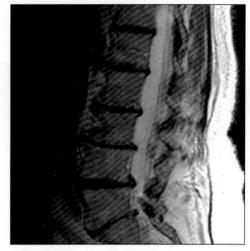

Sagittal T2WI MR in the same patient shows loss of lumbar lordosis with multi-level disc space narrowing and degenerative endplate changes.

TERMINOLOGY

Abbreviations and Synonyms
- "De novo" scoliosis

Definitions
- Lateral curvature in spine due to degenerative disc and facet disease in older patients

IMAGING FINDINGS

General Features
- Best diagnostic clue: Lateral curvature in spine with associated degenerative changes
- Location
  - T12 to L5
    - Most common from L1 to L4
  - Apex of curvature most common at L2-3 interspace
- Size
  - Curvature ranging from 14-80 degrees
    - Mean: 24-43 degrees
  - Average curvature per segment less than 10 degrees
- Morphology
  - Moderate curvature over a short spinal segment
  - Levo or dextroscoliosis
    - 57-68% levoscoliosis

Radiographic Findings
- Radiography
  - Lateral listhesis
    - In > ¾ of patients
    - Average translation: < 10 mm
  - Vertebral rotation
    - Most common grade 2
  - Disc space loss
    - Worse on concave side
    - Vacuum disc phenomenon
  - Endplate sclerosis
  - Circumferential endplate spurring
    - Most significant on concave side
  - Facet arthropathy
    - Concave > convex side
  - Spondylolisthesis
    - In > 50% of patients
    - L4-5 most common
    - Usually not beyond grade 1
  - Loss of lumbar lordosis
  - Flexion-extension views
    - Vertebral body subluxation
- Myelography
  - Post-myelographic CT improves sensitivity and specificity
    - Especially with multi-detector row helical CT
  - Variable central stenosis

DDx: Scoliosis

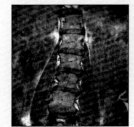

Idiopathic

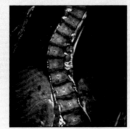

Neuromuscular

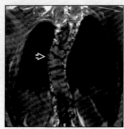

Congenital

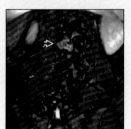

Osteoblastoma

DEGENERATIVE SCOLIOSIS

Key Facts

Terminology
- Lateral curvature in spine due to degenerative disc and facet disease in older patients

Imaging Findings
- Most common from L1 to L4
- Apex of curvature most common at L2-3 interspace
- Moderate curvature over a short spinal segment
- Lateral listhesis
- Vertebral rotation
- Disc space loss
- Endplate sclerosis
- Circumferential endplate spurring
- Facet arthropathy
- Spondylolisthesis
- Loss of lumbar lordosis

- Variable central stenosis
- Subarticular recess stenosis
- Neural foraminal stenosis

Top Differential Diagnoses
- Adult idiopathic scoliosis

Pathology
- Epidemiology: Prevalence around 6%

Clinical Issues
- Risk factors for curve progression
- Cobb angle > 30 degrees
- Lateral listhesis > 6 mm
- Grade 2 or 3 vertebral rotation
- Inter-crest line through L5 or L4-5 disc space
- 3 degrees per year

- Disc herniation, endplate spurring, spondylolisthesis, ligamentum flavum hypertrophy
  - Subarticular recess stenosis
    - May be asymmetric
    - Concave side of curvature
    - Ligamentum flavum hypertrophy and facet arthropathy
  - Neural foraminal stenosis
    - Worse at concave side
    - Foraminal disc herniation, endplate spurring, or disc space loss

CT Findings
- Bone CT
  - Same findings as radiography
  - Better osseous detail
    - Sagittal and coronal reformation
    - Facet arthropathy well-delineated
  - Similar accuracy compared to CT-myelography and MRI

MR Findings
- Same findings as CT-myelography
- Underestimates nerve root compression in lateral recess compared to conventional myelography
  - 28-29% vs. 5-7%
- Disc herniation well visualized
  - Anterior, posterior, foraminal, far lateral
- Excellent characterization of central canal and neural foramina

Nuclear Medicine Findings
- Bone Scan
  - Spinal curvature
  - Asymmetric uptake of radiotracer at endplates and facets

Other Modality Findings
- Axial loading during CT myelography or MRI may provide additional information
  - Worsening disc herniation
  - Worsening central canal, lateral recess, or neural foraminal narrowing

Imaging Recommendations
- Best imaging tool
  - Noncontrast-enhanced MRI
    - Similar sensitivity and specificity as CT-myelography
    - Non-invasive
- Protocol advice
  - Include coronal T1 on lumbar MRI
    - Characterization of scoliosis
    - Additional information on lateral endplate spurring, disc bulge, and far lateral nerve root

DIFFERENTIAL DIAGNOSIS

Adult idiopathic scoliosis
- Juvenile idiopathic scoliosis present in adults
- Most common
  - 85% of all scoliosis
- Strongly familial: 80%
  - Female predilection: 7-9:1
- Long, smooth S-shaped spinal curvature
  - Thoracic and lumbar component

Neuromuscular
- Cerebral palsy, poliomyelitis, muscular dystrophy, syringohydromyelia, cord neoplasm
- Single long smooth curve

Congenital scoliosis
- Failure of vertebral formation or segmentation
  - Wedge vertebra, hemivertebra, pedicle bar, block vertebra
- Acute curvature
- Associated with spinal dysraphic, genitourinary, or cardiac anomalies

Post-traumatic, inflammatory, or neoplastic
- Juvenile rheumatoid arthritis, tuberculosis, radiation therapy, osteoid osteoma, osteoblastoma
- Vertebral deformities present

DEGENERATIVE SCOLIOSIS

Dysplasias
- Neurofibromatosis type 1 (NF1), Marfan syndrome, Ehlers-Danlos syndrome
- Posterior vertebral scalloping
  - Dural ectasia
- High thoracic acute curvature in NF1
  - Associated with wedge-shaped vertebra, block vertebra, spina bifida occulta

PATHOLOGY

General Features
- General path comments: Degenerative disease of spine
- Etiology
  - Degenerative disc at L3-4 and L4-5
  - Facet arthropathy
  - Loss of lordosis
  - Instability in sagittal and coronal plane
    - Leading to spondylolisthesis and scoliosis
- Epidemiology: Prevalence around 6%
- Associated abnormalities
  - Osteoarthritis
    - Hip and knee
    - May be unilateral
  - Spondylosis
    - Cervical and thoracic
  - No association with osteoporosis

CLINICAL ISSUES

Presentation
- Most common signs/symptoms
  - Low back pain
  - Other signs/symptoms
    - Radiculopathy
    - Neurogenic claudication
    - Deformity and waist asymmetry
    - Gait disturbance
- Clinical profile
  - Pain worse with prolonged spinal extension
  - Radiculopathy not reliably relieved by flexion
    - In contrast to spinal stenosis without scoliosis

Demographics
- Age: Sixth decade
- Gender: M < F
- Ethnicity: More common in Caucasians

Natural History & Prognosis
- Curvature may regress
  - Especially in early course of disease
- Risk factors for curve progression
  - Cobb angle > 30 degrees
  - Lateral listhesis > 6 mm
  - Grade 2 or 3 vertebral rotation
  - Inter-crest line through L5 or L4-5 disc space
- 3 degrees per year
- 73% of patients
- Biochemical changes in cross-link profile of intervertebral discs
  - Tissue remodeling
  - Increased tissue turnover

- May have implications on disease progression

Treatment
- Non-operative
  - Physical therapy
  - NSAIDs
  - Epidural injection
  - Brace
- Surgery
  - Preserves neural function and prevents instability
  - Decompression
    - Alone or with fusion
    - Posterior or in combination with anterior fusion
    - With instrumentation

DIAGNOSTIC CHECKLIST

Image Interpretation Pearls
- Presence of extensive degenerative disc disease and facet arthropathy indicates degenerative scoliosis

SELECTED REFERENCES

1. Tsuchiya K et al: Application of multi-detector row helical scanning to postmyelographic CT. Eur Radiol. 13(6):1438-43, 2003
2. Bartynski WS et al: Lumbar root compression in the lateral recess: MR imaging, conventional myelography, and CT myelography comparison with surgical confirmation. AJNR Am J Neuroradiol. 24(3):348-60, 2003
3. Gupta MC: Degenerative scoliosis. Options for surgical management. Orthop Clin North Am. 34(2):269-79, 2003
4. Daffner SD et al: Adult degenerative lumbar scoliosis. Am J Orthop. 32(2):77-82; discussion 82, 2003
5. Murata Y et al: Changes in scoliotic curvature and lordotic angle during the early phase of degenerative lumbar scoliosis. Spine. 27(20):2268-73, 2002
6. Willen J et al: The diagnostic effect from axial loading of the lumbar spine during computed tomography and magnetic resonance imaging in patients with degenerative disorders. Spine. 26(23):2607-14, 2001
7. McPhee IB et al: The surgical management of degenerative lumbar scoliosis. Posterior instrumentation alone versus two stage surgery. Bull Hosp Jt Dis. 57(1):16-22, 1998
8. Duance VC et al: Changes in collagen cross-linking in degenerative disc disease and scoliosis. Spine. 23(23):2545-51, 1998
9. Pritchett JW et al: Degenerative symptomatic lumbar scoliosis. Spine. 18(6):700-3, 1993
10. Thornbury JR et al: Disk-caused nerve compression in patients with acute low-back pain: diagnosis with MR, CT myelography, and plain CT. Radiology. 186(3):731-8, 1993
11. Ogilvie JW: Adult scoliosis: evaluation and nonsurgical treatment. Instr Course Lect. 41:251-5, 1992
12. Aebi M: Correction of degenerative scoliosis of the lumbar spine. A preliminary report. Clin Orthop. (232):80-6, 1988
13. Grubb SA et al: Degenerative adult onset scoliosis. Spine. 13(3):241-5, 1988
14. Gillespie T 3rd et al: Progressive senile scoliosis: seven cases of increasing spinal curves in elderly patients. Skeletal Radiol. 13(4):280-6, 1985
15. Robin GC et al: Scoliosis in the elderly: a follow-up study. Spine. 7(4):355-9, 1982

DEGENERATIVE SCOLIOSIS

IMAGE GALLERY

Typical

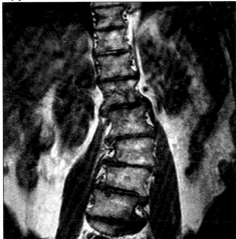 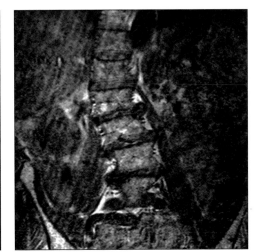

(Left) Coronal T1WI MR shows mild levoscoliosis centered at L2-3. There is left lateral listhesis of L4 on L5 with multi-level degenerative disc and endplate disease. *(Right)* Coronal T1WI MR shows dextroscoliosis centered at L2-3. Asymmetric disc space narrowing and degenerative endplate changes are evident.

Typical

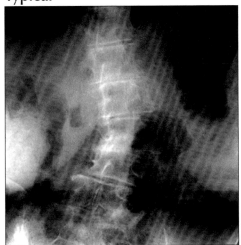 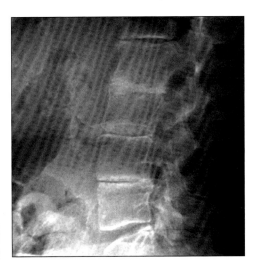

(Left) Anteroposterior radiography shows lumbar rotatory levoscoliosis with associated disc height loss and endplate sclerosis. There is left lateral listhesis of L4 on 5. *(Right)* Lateral radiography shows loss of lumbar lordosis with multi-level disc space loss and degenerative endplate changes, worst at L2-3.

Typical

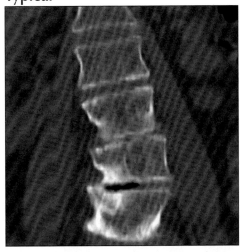 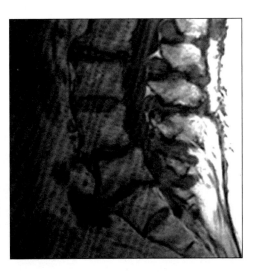

(Left) Axial bone CT with coronal reformation shows mild levoscoliosis at L4-5 with vacuum disc phenomenon and right-sided endplate sclerosis. There is disc height loss at L3-4 and L4-5. *(Right)* Sagittal T1WI MR shows grade 1 anterolisthesis of L4 on 5. Degenerative disc and endplate disease is present at L2-3, L4-5, and L5-S1.

NEUROGENIC (CHARCOT) ARTHROPATHY

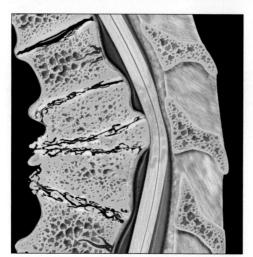

Sagittal graphic shows arthropathy centered at 3 adjacent discs with endplate erosions, bony debris, and deformity.

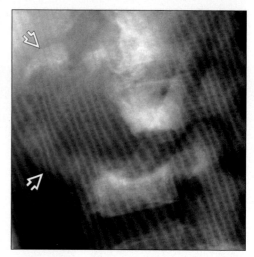

Lateral radiography shows neuropathic spine secondary to traumatic paraplegia. Note bony debris (arrows) sclerosis, and destructive arthropathy with malalignment.

TERMINOLOGY

Abbreviations and Synonyms
- Neuropathic spine, neuropathic arthropathy

Definitions
- A destructive arthropathy which occurs when pain and proprioception are diminished or lost, while joint mobility is maintained

IMAGING FINDINGS

General Features
- Best diagnostic clue: Florid destruction of discs and facet joints with preserved bone density, involving 1-2 spinal levels
- Location
  - Almost always in lumbar spine
  - Sometimes occurs in lower thoracic spine

Radiographic Findings
- Radiography
  - Early stages mimic severe degenerative disc disease
    - Disc space narrowing
    - Discogenic sclerosis
    - Large osteophytes, often much larger than in degenerative disc disease
  - Vertebral endplate destruction

- Facet joint destructive arthropathy
- Preserved bone density
- Nonunited fractures
- Bony debris around vertebrae
  - Small, nonunited fracture fragments
- Spondylolisthesis
- Often rapidly progressive
- Vacuum phenomenon
- Disorganization

CT Findings
- Bone CT
  - Destruction of vertebral endplates, facet joints
  - Bony debris and nonunited fractures
  - Soft tissue mass, which may be large
    - Enhances with contrast administration

MR Findings
- T1WI
  - Severe discogenic marrow changes
  - Facet arthropathy
  - Low signal intensity soft tissue mass
  - Bone debris best seen on this sequence
- T2WI
  - Bone marrow edema often severe, diffuse
  - Soft tissue mass intermediate to high signal intensity
  - May have high signal intensity in the disc
  - Fluid collections may be present
  - Bone debris may be obscured by inflammatory tissue

DDx: Neurogenic Arthropathy

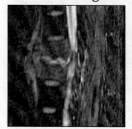

Osteomyelitis

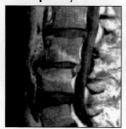

DDD Instability

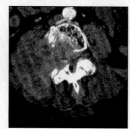

Tumor

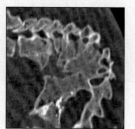

Tuberculosis

NEUROGENIC (CHARCOT) ARTHROPATHY

Key Facts

Terminology
- A destructive arthropathy which occurs when pain and proprioception are diminished or lost, while joint mobility is maintained

Imaging Findings
- Almost always in lumbar spine
- Early stages mimic severe degenerative disc disease
- Vertebral endplate destruction
- Facet joint destructive arthropathy
- Preserved bone density
- Bony debris around vertebrae
- Spondylolisthesis
- Often rapidly progressive
- Vacuum phenomenon

- Enhancement may mimic infection, but often more diffuse
- Best imaging tool: CT: Preserved bone density, bony debris best seen on CT, helps distinguish from infection

Top Differential Diagnoses
- Pyogenic infection
- Atypical infection: Tuberculosis, fungi
- Soft tissue sarcoma: Malignant fibrous histiocytoma or osteosarcoma
- Degenerative disc disease (DDD) with instability

Pathology
- Diabetes Mellitus: Most common cause
- Neurosyphilis: Originally described by Charcot
- Following traumatic paraplegia

- STIR: Similar to T2WI but more pronounced edema
- T1 C+
  - Enhancement may mimic infection, but often more diffuse
  - Enhancement centers on disc, facet joints
  - Fluid collections tend not to enhance as much as an abscess
  - Chronic, inactive neuropathic joint shows little or no enhancement

Nuclear Medicine Findings
- Bone Scan: Positive on all three phases
- PET: Uptake with FDG
- Gallium scan
  - Positive
- WBC scan
  - Positive in active neuropathic joint

Imaging Recommendations
- Best imaging tool: CT: Preserved bone density, bony debris best seen on CT, helps distinguish from infection
- Protocol advice: Thin-section CT with reformatted images in coronal and sagittal planes

DIFFERENTIAL DIAGNOSIS

Pyogenic infection
- Bones usually osteopenic but occasionally see sclerosing variant
- Bone destruction extends across disc space
- May see cloaca, sequestrum in bone
- Paraspinous soft tissue abscess shows rim-enhancement
- Uncommon to destroy both discs and facet joints except in patients with failed fusion
- Fever, elevated ESR and CRP useful
- Cultures negative in 50%

Atypical infection: Tuberculosis, fungi
- Bone density preserved
- Paraspinous soft tissue mass

- Amorphous calcifications in intraosseous and soft tissue cold abscesses
- Cultures often negative
- Pulmonary tuberculosis may be absent
- Rely on histology rather than culture for diagnosis

Soft tissue sarcoma: Malignant fibrous histiocytoma or osteosarcoma
- Reactive spindle cells in soft tissue mass of Charcot joint may be misdiagnosed as sarcoma by unwary pathologists
- Centered in soft tissues
- Soft tissue sarcomas rarely destroy intervertebral discs or facet joints

Bone tumor
- Rare to involve two adjacent vertebrae
- Tends to spare disc space

Degenerative disc disease (DDD) with instability
- Severe DDD may show endplate erosion, especially if instability present
- Erosion similar to very early neuropathic joint however, other signs of neuropathic joint absent
- DDD slowly progressive

PATHOLOGY

General Features
- General path comments
  - Occurs when there is preserved mobility with impaired proprioception and pain
  - Because proprioception is impaired, joint is stressed beyond normal range of motion
  - Because pain is diminished or absent, patient does not self protect following minor injury
  - Abnormal joint motion results in
    - Disruption of joint capsule and stabilizing ligaments
    - Microfractures and/or major fractures
  - Fractures fail to heal because of continued motion

NEUROGENIC (CHARCOT) ARTHROPATHY

- Motion at fracture leads to
  - Exuberant, nonbridging peripheral callus formation
  - Joint subluxation and/or dislocation
  - Soft tissue reparative response
  - Nonunited bone fragments (bone debris)
- Etiology
  - Diabetes Mellitus: Most common cause
    - Diabetic neuropathy in chronic diabetes mellitus
  - Neurosyphilis: Originally described by Charcot
    - More commonly involves hips, knees than spine
  - Following traumatic paraplegia
    - Paraplegic patients who are physically active put stress on insensate spine
    - Seen > 5 years following traumatic paraplegia
    - Below level of loss of sensation
    - Often presents as instability in wheel chair
  - Congenital insensitivity to pain
  - Other causes or neuropathic joint occur in peripheral joints but not in spine

Gross Pathologic & Surgical Features
- Bone sclerosis due to
  - Affected level continues to be stressed, i.e., no disuse osteopenia
  - Callus formation
  - Bone debris

Microscopic Features
- Bone and cartilage fragments
- Histiocytes and lymphoplasmacytic infiltrate
- Fibrosis, granulation tissue without acute inflammation
- Mimics chronic infection

CLINICAL ISSUES

Presentation
- Most common signs/symptoms
  - Instability of spine
  - Spine deformity
  - Some cases are painless
  - Pain may be present
    - Common misconception is that pain must be absent to make diagnosis of neuropathic joint
    - Pain is, however, less severe than expected for severity of joint destruction
- Clinical profile
  - Middle-aged diabetic patient with nonspecific back pain
  - Paraplegic patient complaining of instability while seated

Natural History & Prognosis
- Treated with rigid internal fixation and fusion of affected spinal levels
- Most cases do well following fusion
- May become superinfected

Treatment
- Options, risks, complications
  - Fusion with rigid internal fixation
  - Can also be treated with bracing, but success limited

DIAGNOSTIC CHECKLIST

Consider
- Distinction between neuropathic joint and infection is one of most difficult problems radiographically
- Important differential diagnostic consideration for infection when patient
  - Has predisposing cause for neuropathic joint
  - Has no systemic signs of infection
  - Has negative cultures (percutaneous or open)
  - Has preserved bone density, disorganization and bone debris

Image Interpretation Pearls
- Only two processes can destroy a joint in a month: Infection and neurogenic arthropathy
- Nuclear medicine studies unreliable in differentiation of neuropathic joint from infection

SELECTED REFERENCES

1. Wagner SC et al: Can imaging findings help differentiate spinal neuropathic arthropathy from disk space infection? Initial experience. Radiology. 214(3):693-9, 2000
2. Palestro CJ et al: Radionuclide imaging in orthopedic infections. Semin Nucl Med. 27(4):334-45, 1997
3. Standaert C et al: Charcot spine as a late complication of traumatic spinal cord injury. Arch Phys Med Rehabil. 78(2):221-5, 1997
4. Arnold PM et al: Surgical management of lumbar neuropathic spinal arthropathy (Charcot joint) after traumatic thoracic paraplegia: report of two cases. J Spinal Disord. 8(5):357-62, 1995
5. Park YH et al: Imaging findings in spinal neuroarthropathy. Spine. 19(13):1499-504, 1994
6. Heggeness MH: Charcot arthropathy of the spine with resulting paraparesis developing during pregnancy in a patient with congenital insensitivity to pain. A case report. Spine. 19(1):95-8, 1994
7. Montgomery TJ et al: Traumatic neuropathic arthropathy of the spine. Orthop Rev. 22(10):1153-7, 1993
8. Harrison MJ et al: Spinal Charcot arthropathy. Neurosurgery. 28(2):273-7, 1991
9. Crim JR et al: Spinal neuroarthropathy after traumatic paraplegia. AJNR Am J Neuroradiol. 9(2):359-62, 1988
10. Kalen V et al: Charcot arthropathy of the spine in long-standing paraplegia. Spine. 12(1):42-7, 1987
11. Fishel B et al: Multiple neuropathic arthropathy in a patient with syphilis. Clin Rheumatol. 4(3):348-52, 1985

NEUROGENIC (CHARCOT) ARTHROPATHY

IMAGE GALLERY

Typical

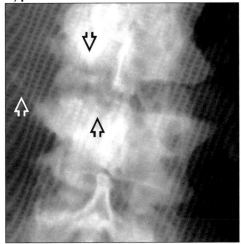
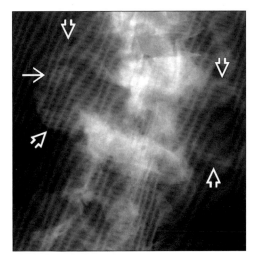

(Left) Anteroposterior radiography shows early neuropathic joint mimicking severe degenerative disc disease. Clues to diagnosis are focal endplate destruction (black arrows) and bony debris (white arrow). *(Right)* Anteroposterior radiography shows neuropathic joint which developed over a two month interval. Note scoliosis, florid osteophytes (open arrows), bone debris (arrow) and peridiscal destruction.

Typical

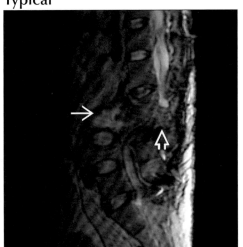
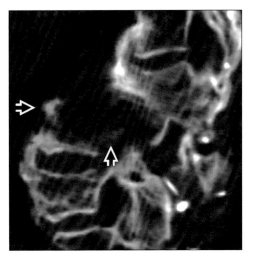

(Left) Sagittal STIR MR shows neuropathic joint at L2-3; paraplegic patient. Chronic fluid collection (arrow) was sterile. Granulation tissue (open arrow) was present posteriorly. *(Right)* Sagittal bone CT shows neuropathic joint in paraplegic patient. Note preserved bone density, bony debris (arrows) and gross instability of all three columns.

Typical

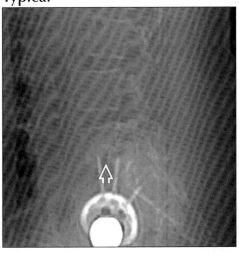
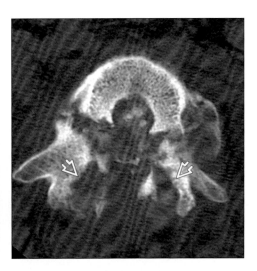

(Left) Lateral radiography shows endplate destruction (arrow), preserved bone density and instability in diabetic patient. Multiple cultures were negative. Patient did well following fusion. *(Right)* Axial bone CT shows nonunited fractures, bone debris, preserved bone density, and destruction of facet joints (arrows) in diabetic patient with L5-S1 neuropathic joint.

DISH

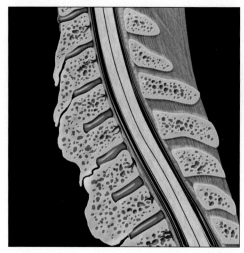

Sagittal graphic shows bulky flowing ossification of the anterior longitudinal ligament extending over more than four contiguous vertebra. Disc spaces are relatively preserved.

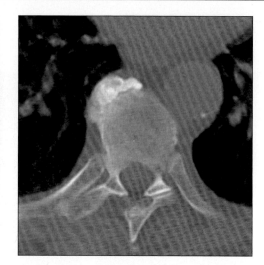

Axial bone CT of the thoracic spine demonstrates characteristic right-sided flowing ALL ossification. The left side adjacent to the aorta is typically spared.

TERMINOLOGY

Abbreviations and Synonyms
- Diffuse idiopathic skeletal hyperostosis (DISH), senile ankylosing hyperostosis, asymmetrical skeletal hyperostosis, Forestier disease

Definitions
- Bulky flowing ossification of anterior longitudinal ligament (ALL)

IMAGING FINDINGS

General Features
- Best diagnostic clue: Flowing anterior vertebral ossification with relatively minimal degenerative disc disease, facet arthropathy, and absent facet ankylosis
- Location: Thoracic spine (100%) > cervical (65-80%), lumbar spine (68-90%); R > L
- Size: Range from small, focal → large, extensive
- Morphology: Bulky flowing multilevel ossification (R > L) anterior to vertebral bodies

Radiographic Findings
- Radiography
  - Flowing anterior vertebral ossification, variably distinguishable from anterior vertebral body cortex
    - Earliest sign = new bone formation adjacent to mid-vertebral body
    - May co-exist with spondylosis
  - Relative preservation of disc spaces, facets
- Fluoroscopy: Lateral flexion-extension imaging assesses dynamic spinal mobility
- Myelography
  - Similar osseous findings to plain radiography
  - No canal stenosis unless concurrent OPLL

CT Findings
- Bone CT
  - Thick ALL ossification, R > L
  - Relatively minimal degenerative disc, facet disease
  - Absent facet, sacroiliac joint erosion or ankylosis
  - DISH changes detectable in-between disc levels
    - Spondylosis centered at disc level

MR Findings
- T1WI
  - Flowing ALL ossification along anterior vertebral bodies; may be difficult to distinguish from anterior vertebral body
    - ALL marrow is not contiguous with vertebral body marrow
    - Hypointense if predominantly calcified
    - Isointense → hyperintense if marrow fat present

DDx: Diffuse Idiopathic Skeletal Hyperostosis (DISH)

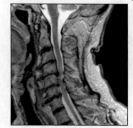
Spondylosis

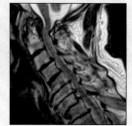
Spondylosis

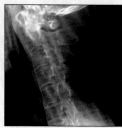
Ankylosing Spondylitis

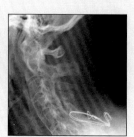
Psoriatic Arthritis

DISH

Key Facts

Terminology
- Diffuse idiopathic skeletal hyperostosis (DISH), senile ankylosing hyperostosis, asymmetrical skeletal hyperostosis, Forestier disease

Imaging Findings
- Best diagnostic clue: Flowing anterior vertebral ossification with relatively minimal degenerative disc disease, facet arthropathy, and absent facet ankylosis
- Location: Thoracic spine (100%) > cervical (65-80%), lumbar spine (68-90%); R > L
- No canal stenosis unless concurrent OPLL

Top Differential Diagnoses
- Spondylosis
- Ankylosing spondylitis
- Psoriatic or reactive (Reiter) arthritis

Pathology
- ↓ Spine mobility 2° ALL ossification; relative protection from degenerative disc disease & facet arthropathy

Clinical Issues
- Frequently incidental finding; patient may complain of intermittent spinal stiffness, restricted mobility
- Pain related to associated enthesitis, tendinitis
- Anterior osteophytes may compress esophagus ⇒ dysphagia

Diagnostic Checklist
- DISH is largely asymptomatic and incidentally detected
- Look carefully for signs of associated OPLL ⇒ myelopathy 2° to central canal stenosis

---

- T2WI: Similar findings to T1WI; ALL ossification may be hypointense unless substantial fatty marrow content
- T2* GRE: Hypointense flowing "mass" within ALL
- T1 C+: +/- Minimal enhancement (similar to vertebral marrow)

Imaging Recommendations
- Best imaging tool: Lateral radiography inexpensive, reliable for detecting DISH
- Protocol advice
  - AP and lateral plain radiographs
  - Axial bone algorithm CT with sagittal and coronal reformats to confirm plain film diagnosis (if necessary)
  - MRI unnecessary for DISH diagnosis
    - Reserve MRI to evaluate for co-existent OPLL or if cord compression or spondylosis are being considered within differential diagnosis

DIFFERENTIAL DIAGNOSIS

Spondylosis
- Rarely contiguous across four or more vertebral levels; usually confined to disc interspace vicinity
- More substantial facet, disc degenerative changes than DISH
- No predisposition to right or left side

Ankylosing spondylitis
- Thin intervertebral syndesmophytes instead of bulky flowing DISH ossification
- Sacroiliac (SI) joint, facet erosion/ankylosis
- Appropriate clinical history; HLA B27 ≥ 90%

Psoriatic or reactive (Reiter) arthritis
- Large bulky osteophytes; often lateral with skips areas
- Erosive or ankylosing changes of SI joints, appropriate clinical history

PATHOLOGY

General Features
- General path comments
  - ↓ Spine mobility 2° ALL ossification; relative protection from degenerative disc disease & facet arthropathy
  - +/- Co-existent exuberant ossification of tendon, ligament, or joint capsule insertions ("enthesitis")
  - Dysphagia 2° DISH probably multifactorial
    - Combination of direct mechanical compression + inflammation/fibrosis of esophageal wall, esophageal denervation
  - R > L predilection; attributed to effect of repetitive aortic pulsations retarding proliferative ossification
- Etiology
  - Exact cause for exaggerated response to new bone formation stimuli unknown
  - Possible associations with diabetes mellitus, dyslipidemia, hyperuricemia, alcohol intake and poor dietary habits postulated but not definitively proven
- Epidemiology
  - Reported incidence varies widely
    - Conservative estimate is 6-12% adults over 40 years manifest some findings of DISH; actual incidence may be substantially higher
    - More common in elderly men
- Associated abnormalities
  - Ossification of posterior longitudinal ligament (OPLL)
  - Exuberant enthesial reaction at tendon, ligament, and joint capsule insertions
    - Iliac crest (66%), ischial tuberosities (53%) ⇒ "pelvic whiskering"
    - Lesser (42%) and greater (36%) femoral trochanters, patellar quadriceps insertion (29%)
    - Osseous bridging of fibula → tibia (10%)
    - Distal metacarpal, phalangeal periarticular capsular hyperostosis (13%)

DISH

Gross Pathologic & Surgical Features
- Bulky anterior vertebral ossification with normal cortical bone, marrow appearance

Microscopic Features
- Normal-appearing Haversian bone, marrow within ossified ligament

Staging, Grading or Classification Criteria
- Three primary diagnostic criteria for DISH
  - Flowing anterior ossification extending over at least 4 contiguous vertebral bodies
  - No apophyseal or SI joint ankylosis
  - Relatively minimal degenerative disc changes, no facet ankylosis

CLINICAL ISSUES

Presentation
- Most common signs/symptoms
  - Frequently incidental finding; patient may complain of intermittent spinal stiffness, restricted mobility
    - Often worse in morning, after prolonged sitting, or during cold winter weather
    - May be relieved by mild activity
  - Pain related to associated enthesitis, tendinitis
  - Other signs/symptoms
    - Anterior osteophytes may compress esophagus ⇒ dysphagia
    - Stridor (extremely rare) requiring tracheostomy
- Clinical profile: Usually incidental observation in asymptomatic Caucasian patient imaged for unrelated reasons

Demographics
- Age: Middle-age ⇒ older adults; uncommon before age 50, common in elderly
- Gender: M:F = 2:1
- Ethnicity
  - Caucasian > > African-American, Native-American or Asian populations
  - ↓ Incidence in osteoporotic Caucasian populations

Natural History & Prognosis
- Nearly always incidental finding without additive morbidity or mortality
  - Severe cases may rarely produce dysphagia
  - May be mildly increased predisposition to fracture 2° decreased flexibility
  - ↑ Risk of heterotopic ossification after total hip arthroplasty

Treatment
- Vast majority of cases incidental ⇒ merit conservative (observational) management
- Consider osteophyte resection if severe symptoms directly referable to DISH

DIAGNOSTIC CHECKLIST

Consider
- DISH is largely asymptomatic and incidentally detected
  - Look carefully for signs of associated OPLL ⇒ myelopathy 2° to central canal stenosis

Image Interpretation Pearls
- Flowing ossification classically R > L
- Discs/facet joints relatively preserved, no SI joint erosion or ankylosis
- May co-exist with degenerative spondylosis

SELECTED REFERENCES

1. Mader R: Diffuse idiopathic skeletal hyperostosis: a distinct clinical entity. Isr Med Assoc J. 5(7):506-8, 2003
2. Belanger TA et al: Diffuse idiopathic skeletal hyperostosis: musculoskeletal manifestations. J Am Acad Orthop Surg. 9(4):258-67, 2001
3. Le Hir PX et al: Hyperextension vertebral body fractures in diffuse idiopathic skeletal hyperostosis: a cause of intravertebral fluidlike collections on MR imaging. AJR Am J Roentgenol. 173(6):1679-83, 1999
4. Papakostas K et al: An unusual case of stridor due to osteophytes of the cervical spine: (Forestier's disease). J Laryngol Otol. 113(1):65-7, 1999
5. Ehara S et al: Paravertebral ligamentous ossification: DISH, OPLL and OLF. Eur J Radiol. 27(3):196-205, 1998
6. Cammisa M et al: Diffuse idiopathic skeletal hyperostosis. Eur J Radiol. 27 Suppl 1:S7-11, 1998
7. Weinfeld RM et al: The prevalence of diffuse idiopathic skeletal hyperostosis (DISH) in two large American Midwest metropolitan hospital populations. Skeletal Radiol. 26(4):222-5, 1997
8. Mata S et al: A controlled study of diffuse idiopathic skeletal hyperostosis. Clinical features and functional status. Medicine (Baltimore). 76(2):104-17, 1997
9. Van Dooren-Greebe RJ et al: Prolonged treatment with oral retinoids in adults: no influence on the frequency and severity of spinal abnormalities. Br J Dermatol. 134(1):71-6, 1996
10. McCafferty RR et al: Ossification of the anterior longitudinal ligament and Forestier's disease: an analysis of seven cases. J Neurosurg. 83(1):13-7, 1995
11. Nesher G et al: Rheumatologic complications of vitamin A and retinoids. Semin Arthritis Rheum. 24(4):291-6, 1995
12. Burkus JK et al: Hyperextension injuries of the thoracic spine in diffuse idiopathic skeletal hyperostosis. Report of four cases. J Bone Joint Surg Am. 76(2):237-43, 1994
13. Mata S et al: Chest radiographs as a screening test for diffuse idiopathic skeletal hyperostosis. J Rheumatol. 20(11):1905-10, 1993
14. Ramos-Remus C et al: Radiologic features of DISH may mimic ankylosing spondylitis. Clin Exp Rheumatol. 11(6):603-8, 1993
15. Schlapbach P et al: Diffuse idiopathic skeletal hyperostosis (DISH) of the spine: a cause of back pain? A controlled study. Br J Rheumatol. 28(4):299-303, 1989
16. Resnick D et al: Association of diffuse idiopathic skeletal hyperostosis (DISH) and calcification and ossification of the posterior longitudinal ligament. AJR Am J Roentgenol. 131(6):1049-53, 1978

DISH

IMAGE GALLERY

Typical

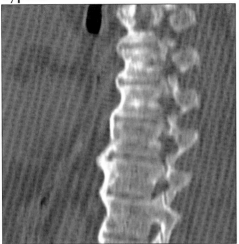 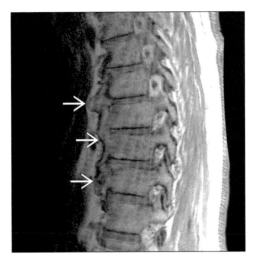

(Left) Sagittal bone CT to the right of midline reveals flowing ALL ossification over more than 4 contiguous levels, typical of DISH. *(Right)* Sagittal T1WI MR right parasagittal slice shows bulky flowing ALL ossification (arrows) spanning more than four vertebral levels, but minimal disc abnormality typical of DISH.

Variant

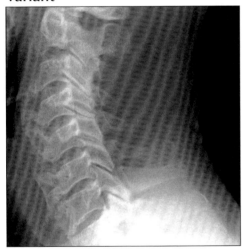 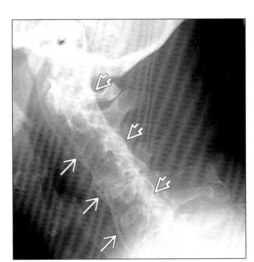

(Left) Lateral radiography shows a large anterior ossified mass that is discontinuous at several disc spaces, a variation implying some degree of continued cervical spine mobility. *(Right)* Lateral radiography depicts typical ALL ossification (DISH, arrows) as well as concurrent PLL ossification (OPLL, open arrows).

Variant

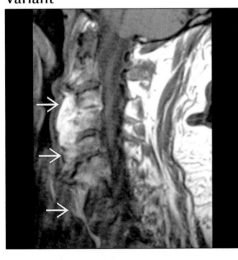 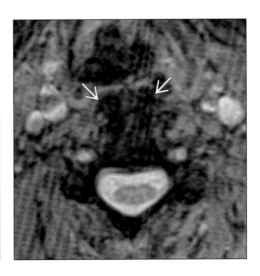

(Left) Sagittal T1WI MR shows bulky anterior flowing ossification (arrows) consistent with DISH. Fatty marrow is responsible for high T1 signal intensity. *(Right)* Axial T2* GRE MR demonstrates large bulky ossification (arrows) of ALL, displacing the aerodigestive tract anteriorly.

OPLL

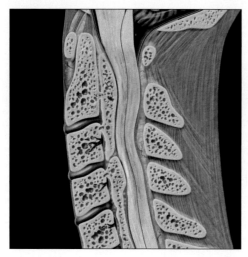

Sagittal graphic shows flowing multilevel ossification within the posterior longitudinal ligament (PLL) producing canal narrowing, cord compression.

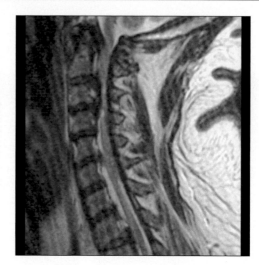

Sagittal T2WI MR demonstrates bulky multifocal PLL ossification producing severe central canal stenosis and cord compression at upper cervical, cervicothoracic junction.

TERMINOLOGY

Abbreviations and Synonyms
- Ossification of posterior longitudinal ligament

Definitions
- Ossification within spinal posterior longitudinal ligament (PLL)

IMAGING FINDINGS

General Features
- Best diagnostic clue: Flowing multilevel ossification posterior to vertebral bodies, with relatively minimal degenerative disc disease, absent facet ankylosis
- Location: Midcervical (C3-C5) > mid-thoracic (T4-T7)
- Size: Mild focal thickening → extensive flowing ossification (≈ 2-5 mm thickness)
- Morphology: PLL ossification narrows AP spinal canal dimension → spinal stenosis, cord compression

Radiographic Findings
- Radiography
  - Flowing posterior ossification behind vertebral bodies
    - Often superimposed over facet complex on lateral projection
    - Requires high index of suspicion to diagnose; subtle finding, easy to overlook
- Fluoroscopy: Flex-extend imaging determines dynamic range
- Myelography
  - Flowing PLL ossification narrows ventral spinal canal
    - Spinal stenosis → cord compression
    - +/- Spinal block (severe cases)

CT Findings
- NECT: Characteristic "upside down T" or "bowtie" PLL configuration on axial images
- Bone CT
  - PLL ossification appearance similar to NECT findings
    - Cortical bone surrounding central marrow space
    - May appear contiguous with adjacent vertebral cortex or distinct from posterior vertebral body
    - PLL, vertebral marrow spaces discrete

MR Findings
- T1WI
  - Posterior flowing ossification extending over multiple levels on sagittal images
  - Characteristic "upside down T" or "bowtie" configuration on axial images
  - Usually low signal intensity on all pulse sequences

DDx: Ossification of Posterior Longitudinal Ligament (OPLL)

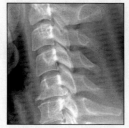

Spondylosis

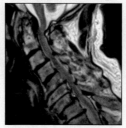

Spondylosis

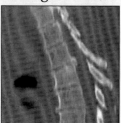

Ca++ HNP

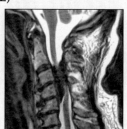

Meningioma

OPLL

Key Facts

Terminology
- Ossification of posterior longitudinal ligament

Imaging Findings
- Best diagnostic clue: Flowing multilevel ossification posterior to vertebral bodies, with relatively minimal degenerative disc disease, absent facet ankylosis
- Location: Midcervical (C3-C5) > mid-thoracic (T4-T7)
- Characteristic "upside down T" or "bowtie" configuration on axial images

Top Differential Diagnoses
- Spondylosis
- Calcified herniated disc
- Meningioma
- Cervical peridural calcification of hemodialysis

Pathology
- Epidemiology: 2-4% prevalence in Japan; much less common elsewhere
- Bulky posterior ligamentous ossification with normal cortical bone, marrow

Clinical Issues
- Symptomatic myelopathy almost universal if canal diameter < 6 mm; rare if > 14 mm
- ↑ Risk for developing progressive myelopathy if > 60% canal stenosis, ↑ cervical range of motion

Diagnostic Checklist
- Overly "thick" hypointense PLL on MRI strongly suggestive of OPLL
- Requires high index of suspicion, careful observation to diagnose on plain radiographs

---

    ■ May show high signal intensity if significant marrow fat content
- T2WI
  - PLL findings similar to T1WI
  - +/- Cord hyperintensity 2° myelomalacia, edema
- T2* GRE
  - Hypointense signal intensity within PLL ossification
  - Caveat: Exaggerates severity of stenosis 2° to magnetic susceptibility effects

Imaging Recommendations
- Best imaging tool: Multiplanar MR imaging
- Protocol advice
  - Sagittal T1WI, T2WI to evaluate spinal cord compression, extent of ligamentous ossification
  - Axial T2WI images to determine stenosis severity, confirm cord signal abnormality
  - CT with sagittal reformats to confirm MR diagnosis, clarify extent of ossification for surgical planning

DIFFERENTIAL DIAGNOSIS

Spondylosis
- Usually centered at disc interspace; rarely contiguous across 4 or more vertebral levels
- More substantial facet, disc degenerative changes than OPLL
- Absence of characteristic "T-shaped" PLL ossification

Calcified herniated disc
- Focal calcified "mass" centered at a single disc space level
- Lacks characteristic "T-shaped" PLL ossification

Meningioma
- Avidly enhancing dural based mass + dural "tail", smooth margins
- Often T2 hypointense 2° to calcification
- Lacks characteristic "T-shaped" PLL ossification

Cervical peridural calcification of hemodialysis
- Curvilinear dural calcification; may be circumferential

- Hemodialysis patient +/- myelopathy, sensory abnormalities
- Requires dural resection in addition to laminectomy/laminoplasty

PATHOLOGY

General Features
- General path comments
  - Idiopathic PLL ossification predominately described in Japanese > other Asian populations, less common in Caucasians
  - More recently described early-stage "OPLL in evolution" noted in both Asian, Caucasian populations
    - Hypertrophied PLL with punctate calcifications rather than smooth, flowing ossific mass
    - Difficult to distinguish from more common spondylosis at this early stage
  - OPLL patients have higher bone mineral density (BMD) than age-matched controls
    - Possible predisposition for excessive bone deposition
- Genetics: Chromosome 6 XI collagen (alpha) 2 gene (COL11A2) ⇒ abnormal N-propeptide, OPLL susceptibility
- Etiology
  - Not conclusively determined
  - Postulated etiologies include infectious agents, autoimmune disorders, or trauma
- Epidemiology: 2-4% prevalence in Japan; much less common elsewhere
- Associated abnormalities
  - Diffuse idiopathic skeletal hyperostosis (DISH)
  - Enthesial, tendinous, and ligamentous ossifications (if concurrent DISH)

Gross Pathologic & Surgical Features
- Bulky posterior ligamentous ossification with normal cortical bone, marrow
- OPLL may transgress dura

Microscopic Features
- Histologically normal Haversian bone, marrow within ossified ligament

CLINICAL ISSUES

Presentation
- Most common signs/symptoms
  - Incidental observation in asymptomatic patient
  - Symptomatic patients present with myelopathy referable to stenosis level
    - Symptomatic myelopathy almost universal if canal diameter < 6 mm; rare if > 14 mm
    - Canal diameter 6-14 mm variable presentation; greater cervical mobility → more likely to be symptomatic
- Clinical profile: Classic presentation is Japanese patient with progressive quadriparesis or paraparesis

Demographics
- Age: Usually age > 50 years; rare < 30 years
- Gender: M:F = 2:1
- Ethnicity: ↑ Prevalence in Japanese population

Natural History & Prognosis
- Mild cases asymptomatic → incidental discovery
- Spastic paresis → paralysis (17-22%)
  - Patients with mild OPLL at diagnosis rarely develop severe canal stenosis on follow-up
  - Patients presenting with myelopathy very likely to clinically progress
  - Mild trauma may exacerbate myelopathy
- ↑ Risk for developing progressive myelopathy if > 60% canal stenosis, ↑ cervical range of motion
  - ↓ Spinal mobility appears to protect spinal cord from injury

Treatment
- Asymptomatic patients: Careful observation, non-operative management
- Symptomatic or high grade stenosis patients: Anterior (corpectomy) or posterior (laminectomy or laminoplasty) decompression

DIAGNOSTIC CHECKLIST

Consider
- Look carefully for OPLL on lateral plain films; confirm with multiplanar CT or MRI

Image Interpretation Pearls
- Search for flowing multilevel ossification behind vertebral bodies
- Overly "thick" hypointense PLL on MRI strongly suggestive of OPLL
- Requires high index of suspicion, careful observation to diagnose on plain radiographs

SELECTED REFERENCES

1. Matsunaga S et al: Clinical course of patients with ossification of the posterior longitudinal ligament: a minimum 10-year cohort study. J Neurosurg. 100(3 Suppl):245-8, 2004
2. Shiraishi T et al: Cervical peridural calcification in patients undergoing long-term hemodialysis. Report of two cases. 100(3 Suppl): 284-6, 2004
3. Kamizono J et al: Occupational recovery after open-door type laminoplasty for patients with ossification of the posterior longitudinal ligament. Spine. 28(16):1889-92, 2003
4. Epstein NE et al: In vitro characteristics of cultured posterior longitudinal ligament tissue. Spine. 27(1):56-8, 2002
5. Epstein N: Diagnosis and surgical management of cervical ossification of the posterior longitudinal ligament. Spine J. 2(6):436-49, 2002
6. Matsunaga S et al: Trauma-induced myelopathy in patients with ossification of the posterior longitudinal ligament. J Neurosurg. 97(2 Suppl):172-5, 2002
7. Matsunaga S et al: J Neurosurg. 96(2 Suppl):168-72, 2002
8. Epstein NE: Identification of ossification of the posterior longitudinal ligament extending through the dura on preoperative computed tomographic examinations of the cervical spine. Spine. 26(2):182-6, 2001
9. Matsunaga S et al: Quality of life in elderly patients with ossification of the posterior longitudinal ligament. Spine. 26(5):494-8, 2001
10. Sakou T et al: Recent progress in the study of pathogenesis of ossification of the posterior longitudinal ligament. J Orthop Sci. 5(3):310-5, 2000
11. Yamauchi T et al: Bone mineral density in patients with ossification of the posterior longitudinal ligament in the cervical spine. J Bone Miner Metab. 17(4):296-300, 1999
12. Koga H et al: Genetic mapping of ossification of the posterior longitudinal ligament of the spine. Am J Hum Genet. 62(6):1460-7, 1998
13. Ehara S et al: Paravertebral ligamentous ossification: DISH, OPLL and OLF. Eur J Radiol. 27(3):196-205, 1998
14. Matsunaga S et al: The natural course of myelopathy caused by ossification of the posterior longitudinal ligament in the cervical spine. Clin Orthop. (305):168-77, 1994
15. Epstein NE: The surgical management of ossification of the posterior longitudinal ligament in 43 north americans. Spine. 19(6):664-72, 1994
16. Epstein NE: Ossification of the posterior longitudinal ligament in evolution in 12 patients. Spine. 19(6):673-01, 1994
17. Epstein N: The surgical management of ossification of the posterior longitudinal ligament in 51 patients. J Spinal Disord. 6(5):432-54; discussion 454-5, 1993

OPLL

IMAGE GALLERY

Typical

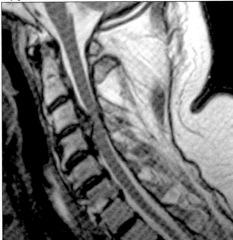 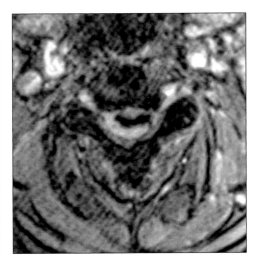

(Left) Sagittal T2WI MR reveals a large focal PLL ossification with marrow signal intensity causing severe cord compression. Intramedullary high signal intensity corresponds to clinical myelopathy. *(Right)* Axial T2* GRE MR depicts hypointense "bowtie" PLL ossification producing severe central canal stenosis.

Typical

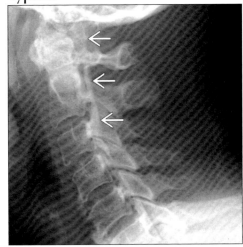 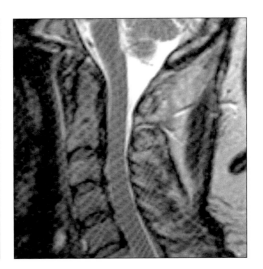

(Left) Lateral radiography shows bulky flowing PLL ossification (arrows). Diagnosis is more difficult in mid and lower cervical spine because of overlapping facet density that partially obscures OPLL. *(Right)* Sagittal T2WI MR shows moderate flowing PLL ossification that mildly narrows the central canal but does not produce significant cord compression.

Variant

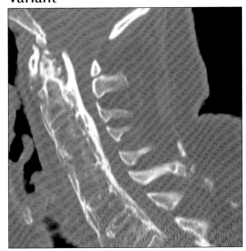 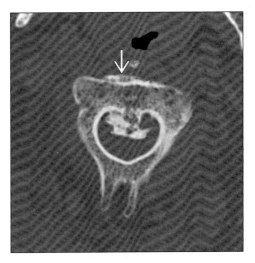

(Left) Sagittal bone CT shows extensive flowing PLL ossification that severely narrows the central canal. Also noted is concurrent ALL ossification (DISH). *(Right)* Axial bone CT reveals bulky "upside-down T" PLL ossification that severely narrows the central canal at C2. Mild concurrent ALL ossification (arrow) is typical of DISH.

OSSIFICATION LIGAMENTUM FLAVUM

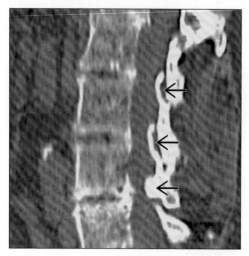

Sagittal NECT shows dorsal curvilinear ossification within ligamentum flavum (arrows) producing mild central canal narrowing.

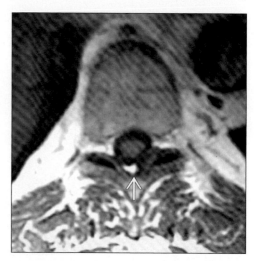

Axial T1WI MR reveals focal ossification within the ligamentum flavum (arrow). Hyperintense signal intensity similar to regional fat indicates fatty marrow.

TERMINOLOGY

Abbreviations and Synonyms
- Ossification of ligamentum flavum (OLF), ossification of the vertebral arch ligaments (OVAL), ligamentum flavum "pseudogout"

Definitions
- Ossification of spinal ligamentum flavum

IMAGING FINDINGS

General Features
- Best diagnostic clue: Linear thickening of ligamentum flavum with imaging characteristics similar to adjacent vertebral marrow ossification
- Location
  - Ligamentum flavum (ventromedial to facets and lamina, dorsal to thecal sac)
  - Lower thoracic > cervical, upper thoracic, lumbar
- Size: Multi- or single level, small or large
- Morphology
  - Linear ossification localized within ligamentum flavum
  - Symmetric, bilateral > unilateral

Radiographic Findings
- Radiography: Thin curvilinear "calcification" ventral to lamina; difficult to appreciate on plain radiography
- Myelography
  - Thin curvilinear "calcification" ventral to lamina
  - +/- Dorsal thecal sac impression
    - Usually minimal; rare cases show significant compression → myelographic block

CT Findings
- NECT
  - Curvilinear hyperdense thickening of ligamentum flavum
  - CT best shows ossification, but poor for determining cord status
- Bone CT
  - Hyperdense nodular or linear ossification within ligamentum flavum
  - "V-shape" on axial images

MR Findings
- T1WI
  - Hypo- to hyperintense linear "mass" within ligamentum flavum +/- cord compression
    - "V-shape" on axial images
    - Thinner lesions usually hypointense 2° to minimal marrow relative to cortical bone

---

DDx: OLF, Spine

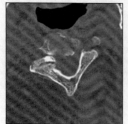

Cervical Facet Arth.

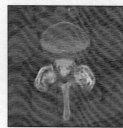

Lumbar Facet Arth.

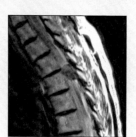

Meningioma

OSSIFICATION LIGAMENTUM FLAVUM

Key Facts

Terminology
- Ossification of ligamentum flavum (OLF), ossification of the vertebral arch ligaments (OVAL), ligamentum flavum "pseudogout"

Imaging Findings
- Best diagnostic clue: Linear thickening of ligamentum flavum with imaging characteristics similar to adjacent vertebral marrow ossification
- Symmetric, bilateral > unilateral
- Thin curvilinear "calcification" ventral to lamina
- +/- Dorsal thecal sac impression
- "V-shape" on axial images

Top Differential Diagnoses
- Facet arthrosis
- Meningioma

Pathology
- Pathogenesis probably related to hydroxyapatite (HAD) or calcium pyrophosphate deposition (CPPD) in ligament → calcification, ossification

Clinical Issues
- Incidental observation on imaging study ordered for other reasons
- Chronic thoracic myelopathy
- Duration of pre-operative symptoms = most important predictor of long term post-operative outcome

Diagnostic Checklist
- Consider OLF in a patient presenting with progressive myelopathy, particularly if Japanese or North African descent

---

- Thicker lesions more likely to mimic marrow signal intensity (isointense → hyperintense) of adjacent vertebral body
- T2WI
  - Hypointense linear "mass" within ligamentum flavum +/- cord myelomalacia, ↑ signal intensity 2° to compression
  - Large lesions may mimic marrow signal intensity of adjacent vertebra, but usually hypointense
- T2* GRE
  - Hypointense ligamentum flavum thickening
  - GRE always overemphasizes degree of canal narrowing 2° to susceptibility artifact

Imaging Recommendations
- CT imaging best modality for primary diagnosis, "lesion conspicuity"
  - Sagittal reformats excellent for determining longitudinal extent
- Multiplanar MR imaging to determine relationship to and effect on regional soft tissues
  - Sagittal T1WI, T2WI evaluate longitudinal extent of ligamentous ossification, degree of cord compression
  - Axial T1WI, T2WI evaluate canal caliber

DIFFERENTIAL DIAGNOSIS

Facet arthrosis
- Substantially more common than OLF
- Facet joint space shows characteristic degenerative changes
  - Centered in joint space rather than ligamentum flavum
- Commonly co-exists with OLF as unrelated finding

Meningioma
- "En plaque" calcified meningioma mimics OLF when small
  - Arises from dural surface; centered in spinal canal, not ligamentum flavum
  - Almost always enhance; look for dural "tail"

PATHOLOGY

General Features
- General path comments
  - Calcium pyrophosphate dihydrate crystal deposition disease (CPPD/CDD) noted in variety of vertebral structures other than ligamentum flavum
    - Intervertebral disc, anterior longitudinal ligament (ALL), posterior longitudinal ligament (PLL), interspinous/supraspinous ligaments, apophyseal and SI joints
  - Debated whether ossified ligamentum flavum is different than "calcification" of ligamentum flavum 2° to crystal deposition
- Etiology
  - In majority of patients (idiopathic presentation), mechanism is unclear
    - Some cases clearly associated with metabolic or endocrine disease
  - Pathogenesis probably related to hydroxyapatite (HAD) or calcium pyrophosphate deposition (CPPD) in ligament → calcification, ossification
- Epidemiology
  - Probably more common than currently appreciated
    - Most cases incidental, asymptomatic, and unrecognized on imaging
- Associated abnormalities
  - Variably co-exists with DISH, OPLL
  - Rare association with Bartter syndrome, hypomagnesemia

Gross Pathologic & Surgical Features
- Ectopic bone formation within ligamentum flavum

Microscopic Features
- Ligamentous tissue hyperplasia, cell proliferation ⇒ endochondral ossification of ligamentum flavum
- Polarized-light microscopy: Characteristic rod-shaped, birefringent crystals

OSSIFICATION LIGAMENTUM FLAVUM

CLINICAL ISSUES

Presentation
- Most common signs/symptoms
  - Incidental observation on imaging study ordered for other reasons
  - Chronic thoracic myelopathy
    - Ambulation difficulty, weakness, back pain, and lower extremity paresthesias
    - Posterior column findings usually first followed by progressive spastic paraparesis
  - Back pain +/- radicular symptoms
- Clinical profile: Symptomatic patients present similarly to other cause of myelopathy

Demographics
- Age: 4th → 6th decade
- Gender: M > F
- Ethnicity: Symptomatic presentation more common in Japanese, North African descent > > Caucasian > African-American

Natural History & Prognosis
- Most patients remain asymptomatic
- Minority of patients manifest progressive myelopathy; symptoms may improve or stabilize following surgery
  - Persistent post-operative spasticity suggests irreversible cord injury
- Duration of pre-operative symptoms = most important predictor of long term post-operative outcome

Treatment
- Conservative observation in asymptomatic, mild cases
- Posterior decompression (laminectomy or laminoplasty), ligamentum flavum resection in symptomatic cases

DIAGNOSTIC CHECKLIST

Consider
- Consider OLF in a patient presenting with progressive myelopathy, particularly if Japanese or North African descent
- Important to exclude co-existent OPLL, other myelopathic lesions

Image Interpretation Pearls
- Distinguish from facet arthropathy by location in ligamentum flavum, observation above or below facet joint level

SELECTED REFERENCES

1. Takeuchi A et al: Thoracic paraplegia due to missed thoracic compressive lesions after lumbar spinal decompression surgery. Report of three cases. J Neurosurg. 100(1 Suppl):71-4, 2004
2. Miyakoshi N et al: Factors related to long-term outcome after decompressive surgery for ossification of the ligamentum flavum of the thoracic spine. J Neurosurg. 99(3 Suppl):251-6, 2003
3. Ben Hamouda K et al: Thoracic myelopathy caused by ossification of the ligamentum flavum: a report of 18 cases. J Neurosurg. 99(2 Suppl):157-61, 2003
4. Seichi A et al: Image-guided resection for thoracic ossification of the ligamentum flavum. J Neurosurg. 99(1 Suppl):60-3, 2003
5. Muthukumar N et al: Tumoral calcium pyrophosphate dihydrate deposition disease of the ligamentum flavum. Neurosurgery. 53(1):103-8; discussion 108-9, 2003
6. Mizuno J et al: Unilateral ossification of the ligamentum flavum in the cervical spine with atypical radiological appearance. J Clin Neurosci. 9(4):462-4, 2002
7. Akhaddar A et al: Thoracic spinal cord compression by ligamentum flavum ossifications. Joint Bone Spine. 69(3):319-23, 2002
8. Li KK et al: Myelopathy caused by ossification of ligamentum flavum. Spine. 27(12):E308-12, 2002
9. Vasudevan A et al: Ossification of the ligamentum flavum. J Clin Neurosci. 9(3):311-3, 2002
10. Hirai T et al: Ossification of the posterior longitudinal ligament and ligamentum flavum: imaging features. Semin Musculoskelet Radiol. 5(2):83-8, 2001
11. Trivedi P et al: Thoracic myelopathy secondary to ossified ligamentum flavum. Acta Neurochir (Wien). 143(8):775-82, 2001
12. Xiong L et al: CT and MRI characteristics of ossification of the ligamenta flava in the thoracic spine. Eur Radiol. 11(9):1798-802, 2001
13. Muthukumar N et al: Calcium pyrophosphate dihydrate deposition disease causing thoracic cord compression: case report. Neurosurgery. 46(1):222-5, 2000
14. Yamagami T et al: Calcification of the cervical ligamentum flavum--case report. Neurol Med Chir (Tokyo). 40(4):234-8, 2000
15. Ono K et al: Pathology of ossification of the posterior longitudinal ligament and ligamentum flavum. Clin Orthop. (359):18-26, 1999
16. Wang PN et al: Ossification of the posterior longitudinal ligament of the spine. A case-control risk factor study. Spine. 24(2):142-4; discussion 145, 1999
17. Ehara S et al: Paravertebral ligamentous ossification: DISH, OPLL and OLF. Eur J Radiol 27(3): 196-205, 1998
18. al-Orainy IA et al: Ossification of the ligament flavum. Eur J Radiol. 29(1):76-82, 1998
19. Ido K et al: Surgical treatment for ossification of the posterior longitudinal ligament and the yellow ligament in the thoracic and cervico-thoracic spine. Spinal Cord. 36(8):561-6, 1998
20. Fam AG: Calcium pyrophosphate crystal deposition disease and other crystal deposition diseases. Curr Opin Rheumatol. 7(4):364-8, 1995
21. Imai S et al: Cervical radiculomyelopathy due to deposition of calcium pyrophosphate dihydrate crystals in the ligamentum flavum: historical and histological evaluation of attendant inflammation. J Spinal Disord. 7(6):513-7, 1994
22. Delamarter RB et al: Lumbar spinal stenosis secondary to calcium pyrophosphate crystal deposition (pseudogout). Clin Orthop. (289):127-30, 1993
23. Gomez H et al: Myeloradiculopathy secondary to pseudogout in the cervical ligamentum flavum: case report. Neurosurgery. 25(2):298-302, 1989
24. Kawano N et al: Calcium pyrophosphate dihydrate crystal deposition disease in the cervical ligamentum flavum. J Neurosurg. 68(4):613-20, 1988
25. Berghausen EJ et al: Cervical myelopathy attributable to pseudogout. Case report with radiologic, histologic, and crystallographic observations. Clin Orthop. (214):217-21, 1987
26. Resnick D et al: Vertebral involvement in calcium pyrophosphate dihydrate crystal deposition disease. Radiographic-pathological correlation. Radiology. 153(1):55-60, 1984

OSSIFICATION LIGAMENTUM FLAVUM

IMAGE GALLERY

Typical

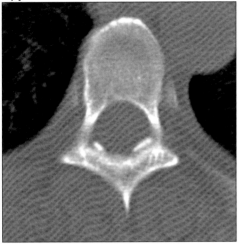
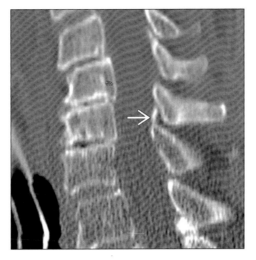

(Left) Axial bone CT shows bilateral linear ligamentum flavum ossification in an asymptomatic patient imaged for lumbar trauma. *(Right)* Sagittal bone CT in a patient with severe degenerative disc disease demonstrates fine linear OLF *(arrow)* incidentally noted during work-up for chronic neck pain.

Typical

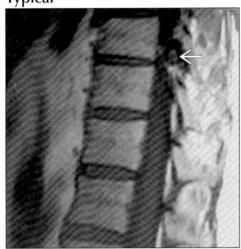
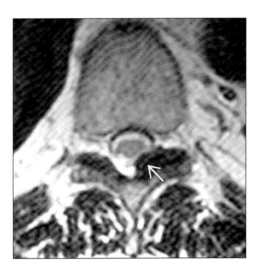

(Left) Sagittal T1WI MR reveals focal nodular OLF in the thoracic ligamentum flavum *(arrow)*, mildly narrowing the central canal. *(Right)* Axial T2WI MR depicts unilateral hypointense ossification *(arrow)* within the left ligamentum flavum producing mild narrowing of the lateral spinal canal and neural foramen.

Typical

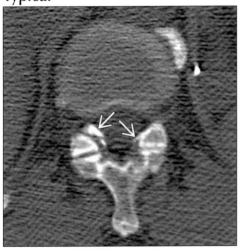
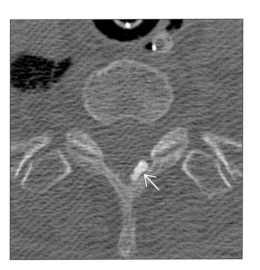

(Left) Axial bone CT reveals asymmetric bilateral OLF *(arrows)* co-existing with mild facet arthropathy. *(Right)* Axial bone CT obtained for trauma shows focal nodular ossification *(arrow)* in the OLF, an incidental asymptomatic finding.

ADULT RHEUMATOID ARTHRITIS

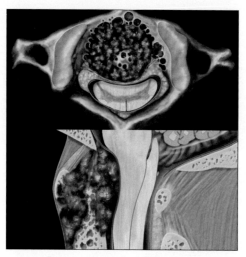

Axial and sagittal graphics show erosion of dens by pannus. Rupture of transverse ligament of dens is evident on axial graphic. Note mass effect on spinal cord.

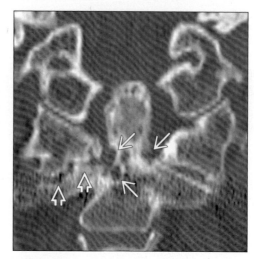

Coronal bone CT shows severe erosions at base of dens (arrows) and right C1-C2 facet joint (open arrows). Early erosion seen at left C1-C2 facet joint.

TERMINOLOGY

Abbreviations and Synonyms
- Rheumatoid arthritis (RA)

Definitions
- Most common inflammatory arthritis involving synovium
- Inflamed and thickened synovium is called pannus

IMAGING FINDINGS

General Features
- Best diagnostic clue: C1/2 subluxation in patient with peripheral rheumatoid arthritis
- Location
  - Involves synovial joints (facet and uncovertebral joints)
  - Involves synovium of bursae (e.g., odontoid process bursa) and tendon sheaths
  - Most often involves hands, feet
  - Never involves spine without hands and/or feet
  - Cervical spine: Approximately 60% of RA patients
  - Rarely involves sacroiliac joints and lumbar spine
- Morphology: Erosive arthropathy

Radiographic Findings
- Radiography

- Abnormal alignment often overshadows erosions in cervical spine
- Neutral, flexion and extension lateral radiographs performed for evaluation
  - Motion should be maximal which is comfortable for patient without technologist assistance
  - Subluxations primarily seen in flexion
  - Extension views useful to assess reducibility of subluxations
- C1-C2 instability in 33% of all RA patients
  - Normal: 4 mm between inferior margin anterior ring of C1 and dens
  - High correlation to neurologic symptoms with distance 9 mm or more
  - Extension view useful to determine if pannus precludes full reduction
  - Odontoid erosions may lead to complete destruction of odontoid
- Atlanto-axial subluxation in 5% of patients with cervical RA
  - Associated with high mortality rate
- Instability may also be present at lower levels of cervical spine
- Often multilevel subluxations ("stepladder subluxations")
- Facet and uncovertebral joint erosions
  - Ankylosis of spine not seen in adult RA
- Osteopenia: Interpret with care

DDx: Cervical Spine Inflammatory Arthritis

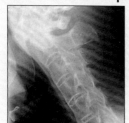

Ankylosing Spondylitis

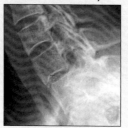

Psoriatic

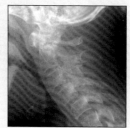

Juvenile

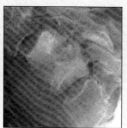

Hemodialysis

ADULT RHEUMATOID ARTHRITIS

Key Facts

Terminology
- Inflamed and thickened synovium is called pannus

Imaging Findings
- Never involves spine without hands and/or feet
- Cervical spine: Approximately 60% of RA patients
- Rarely involves sacroiliac joints and lumbar spine
- C1-C2 instability in 33% of all RA patients
- Atlanto-axial subluxation in 5% of patients with cervical RA
- Instability may also be present at lower levels of cervical spine
- Cervical spine radiographs in flexion/extension to assess for instability
- MR imaging in patients with cord symptoms

Top Differential Diagnoses
- Seronegative spondyloarthropathy
- Juvenile chronic arthritis
- Degenerative disc disease

Pathology
- Rheumatoid factor may be negative initially
- Epidemiology: 1% of population has rheumatoid arthritis

Clinical Issues
- Morning pain and stiffness
- Radiculopathy common with cervical spine involvement

- ■ Not radiographically evident unless severe
- ■ Can be masked by or mistaken for senile osteoporosis
- ■ Can be absent ("robust RA")
- ○ Disc and adjacent vertebral body destruction (extremely rare)
  - ■ Synovitis extends from apophyseal joint
  - ■ Difficult to distinguish from infection - may require biopsy
- ○ AP, odontoid radiographs useful for erosions, rotary subluxations

CT Findings
- Bone CT
  - ○ Erosion of odontoid more apparent than on radiographs
  - ○ May see pannus around dens
  - ○ Erosions of uncovertebral and facet joints well seen
  - ○ Pre-operative planning and post-operative follow-up

MR Findings
- T1WI
  - ○ Pannus is low signal intensity, mass-like
  - ○ Erosions well seen
- T2WI
  - ○ Pannus is heterogeneous signal intensity
    - ■ low signal areas may mimic pigmented villonodular synovitis (PVNS)
  - ○ Bone marrow edema, facet joint effusions common
  - ○ Cord may be compressed by pannus
- T1 C+
  - ○ Increases sensitivity in early diagnosis of RA
  - ○ Pannus enhances avidly
  - ○ Gadolinium excreted rapidly into joint
    - ■ To evaluate synovium must perform imaging in first 5 minutes post injection

Nuclear Medicine Findings
- 3-phase technetium bone scan, Gallium scan, WBC scan all positive
  - ○ Due to hyperemia, white blood cells present in RA
  - ○ Can usually distinguish from infection by distribution, time course

Imaging Recommendations
- Cervical spine radiographs in flexion/extension to assess for instability
- Plain radiographs of hands and/or feet to confirm diagnosis
- Thin-section bone algorithm CT with sagittal and coronal reformats for surgical planning
- MR imaging in patients with cord symptoms

DIFFERENTIAL DIAGNOSIS

Seronegative spondyloarthropathy
- Psoriatic arthritis, Reiter disease, ankylosing spondylitis
- Sacroiliac joints always involved if cervical spine disease present
- Corner erosions of anterior cortex vertebral bodies
- Bony ankylosis

Juvenile chronic arthritis
- Growth disturbance common
- Fusion of vertebral bodies, facet joints

Degenerative disc disease
- Disc space narrowing, discogenic sclerosis
- Osteophyte formation

Gout
- Rare in spine
- Usually centered on disc

Infection
- Usually lumbar or thoracic spine
- Usually centered on disc

Hemodialysis arthropathy
- Rare in spine
- Centered on intervertebral disc

ADULT RHEUMATOID ARTHRITIS

PATHOLOGY

General Features
- General path comments
  - Erythrocyte sedimentation rate, C-reactive protein elevated
  - Rheumatoid factor may be negative initially
    - Eventually positive in up to 95% of RA patients
    - False positive RF seen in elderly patients, systemic lupus erythematosus, sarcoid, cryoglobulinemia, cirrhosis, endocarditis
  - Polyarticular synovial inflammation leads to articular destruction
- Genetics: Strong hereditary component
- Etiology: Common arthritis of unknown etiology
- Epidemiology: 1% of population has rheumatoid arthritis
- Associated abnormalities
  - Lungs: Interstitial lung disease, rheumatoid lung nodules, pleural effusions
  - Soft tissues: Rheumatoid nodules

Gross Pathologic & Surgical Features
- Upper cervical abnormalities are most common manifestation of cervical spine RA
  - Pannus erodes transverse atlantoaxial ligament
    - Permits subluxation of the anterior C1 ring relative to the dens
    - Often asymptomatic but can result in cord compression when neck flexed
  - Cranial settling, atlantoaxial subluxation
    - Due to erosion of occipital condylar-C1 facet joints and occiput-C1 ligaments

Microscopic Features
- Thickened synovium containing plasma cells, multinucleated giant cells, polymorphonuclear leukocytes, lymphocytes

Staging, Grading or Classification Criteria
- 1987 American Rheumatology Association Criteria
  - Morning stiffness at least 1 hr, 6 weeks
  - Swelling 3 or more joints, 6 weeks
  - Swelling wrist, MCP or PIP joints, 6 weeks
  - Symmetrical swelling
  - Hand x-ray changes
  - Subcutaneous nodules
- Presence of any four of the seven criteria yields 93% sensitivity, 90% specificity

CLINICAL ISSUES

Presentation
- Most common signs/symptoms
  - Morning pain and stiffness
  - Radiculopathy common with cervical spine involvement
  - Other signs/symptoms
    - Pathologic fracture
    - Cervical myelopathy
    - Peripheral nerve compression, especially in carpal tunnel

Demographics
- Age: Occurs at all ages, most common in middle-age
- Gender: M:F = 2-3:1

Natural History & Prognosis
- May develop radiculopathy, myelopathy
- Increased morbidity, mortality with craniocervical junction instability

Treatment
- Medical treatment
  - Disease modifying agents (DMARDS) are anti tumor necrosis factor
    - Can dramatically slow disease progression
  - Corticosteroids, methotrexate
- Surgical treatment
  - C1/2 transarticular surgical fusion for atlantoaxial subluxation
  - Transoral odontoid resection for dens/pannus cord compression

DIAGNOSTIC CHECKLIST

Image Interpretation Pearls
- Flexion-extension views often technically inadequate due to lack of patient motion
  - Do not misinterpret as stability

SELECTED REFERENCES

1. Neva MH et al: Early and extensive erosiveness in peripheral joints predicts atlantoaxial subluxations in patients with rheumatoid arthritis. Arthritis Rheum. 48(7):1808-13, 2003
2. Emery P et al: Role of biologics in early arthritis. Clin Exp Rheumatol. 21(5 Suppl 31):S191-4, 2003
3. Casey AT et al: Rheumatoid arthritis of the cervical spine: current techniques for management. Orthop Clin North Am. 33(2):291-309, 2002
4. Roche CJ et al: The rheumatoid cervical spine: signs of instability on plain cervical radiographs. Clin Radiol. 57(4):241-9, 2002
5. Riew KD et al: Diagnosing basilar invagination in the rheumatoid patient. The reliability of radiographic criteria. J Bone Joint Surg Am. 83-A(2):194-200, 2001
6. Reijnierse M et al: Neurologic dysfunction in patients with rheumatoid arthritis of the cervical spine. Predictive value of clinical, radiographic and MR imaging parameters. Eur Radiol 11(3): 467-73, 2001
7. Riise T et al: High mortality in patients with rheumatoid arthritis and atlantoaxial subluxation. J Rheumatol. 28(11):2425-9, 2001
8. Neva MH et al: Prevalence of radiological changes in the cervical spine-a cross sectional study after 20 years from presentation of rheumatoid arthritis. J Rheumatol 27(1): 90-3, 2000
9. Zoli A et al: Craniocervical junction involvement in rheumatoid arthritis: a clinical and radiological study. J Rheumatol. 27(5):1178-82, 2000
10. Janssen H et al: MR imaging of arthritides of the cervical spine. Magn Reson Imaging Clin N Am. 8(3):491-512, 2000

ADULT RHEUMATOID ARTHRITIS

IMAGE GALLERY

Typical

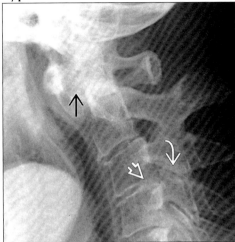 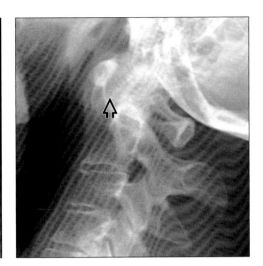

(Left) Lateral radiography shows C1-2 subluxation (arrow) in flexed position. Subaxial disease also evident, causing C3-4 uncovertebral (open arrow) and facet (curved arrow) erosions. *(Right)* Lateral radiography shows that C1-2 subluxation (arrow) improves but does not resolve when neck is extended. This indicates amount of space-occupying pannus between C1 and C2 preventing reduction.

Typical

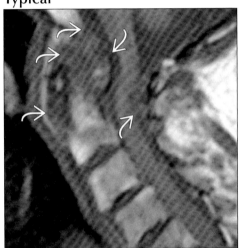 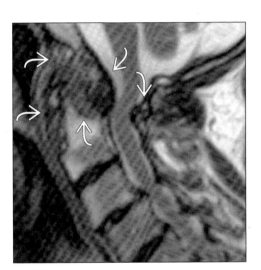

(Left) Sagittal T1WI MR shows heterogeneous signal intensity pannus (arrows) surrounding dens, eroding clivus and compressing cord both anteriorly and posteriorly. Dens is severely eroded. *(Right)* Sagittal T2WI MR shows heterogeneous signal intensity pannus (arrows). There is spinal cord compression at C1-2 and C3-4. C3-4 subluxation is from uncovertebral, facet erosions (not shown).

Variant

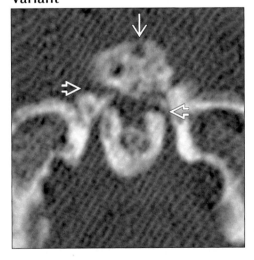 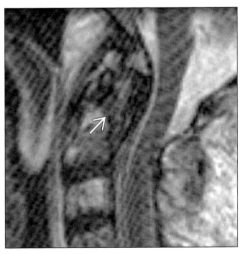

(Left) Axial bone CT shows pathologic oblique fracture of dens (open arrows) in longstanding RA. Note odontoid erosions (arrow). *(Right)* Sagittal T2WI MR shows pathologic oblique fracture of dens (arrow). Pannus formation and hematoma are seen surrounding dens, and there is prevertebral hematoma.

JUVENILE CHRONIC ARTHRITIS

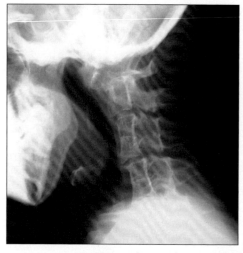 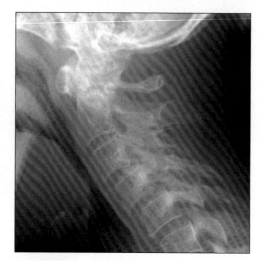

Lateral radiography shows multiple vertebral fusions in adult patient with history of JCA. Fused vertebrae are tall and narrow. Odontoid process is eroded, and there is C1-2 subluxation.

Lateral radiography shows adult-type juvenile onset RA, with odontoid erosion and multilevel facet erosions resulting in "stepladder" subluxations of cervical spine.

TERMINOLOGY

Abbreviations and Synonyms
- Juvenile chronic arthritis (JCA)
- Juvenile rheumatoid arthritis (JRA)
- Juvenile idiopathic arthritis (JIA)

Definitions
- A spectrum of idiopathic inflammatory arthropathies occurring in childhood

IMAGING FINDINGS

General Features
- Best diagnostic clue: Cervical spine subluxations and growth disturbance
- Location
  - Cervical spine
  - Occasionally thoracic spine
  - Juvenile onset ankylosing spondylitis (AS) involves sacroiliac joints, uncommonly progresses to remainder of spine
  - Peripheral arthropathy: Oligoarticular in large joints, or mimicking adult RA in small joints

Radiographic Findings
- Radiography
  - Cervical vertebral fusions

- Involve discs and/or facet joints
- Most commonly involves C4 vertebra
- May involve multiple levels
- Accelerated degenerative disc disease at unfused levels
  - Growth disturbances
    - Fused vertebrae small in anteroposterior dimension if fused early in childhood
    - Bony overgrowth due to hyperemia may also be seen
    - Cranial settling, basilar invagination common
    - Temporomandibular joint involvement, mandibular hypoplasia often visible on c-spine radiographs
  - Multilevel vertebral subluxations
    - Craniocervical
    - Atlanto-axial
    - Subaxial
    - May be rotary as well as anteroposterior
  - Erosions
    - Odontoid process characteristically involved
    - Facet, uncovertebral, costovertebral, costotransverse joints
    - Erosions in facet joints proceed to ankylosis
    - May involve thoracic as well as cervical spine
    - Often difficult to see on radiographs
  - Juvenile (AS)
    - Sacroiliac joint (SIJ) erosions

DDx: Juvenile Chronic Arthritis

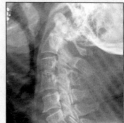 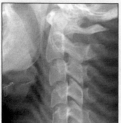 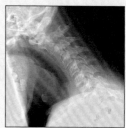 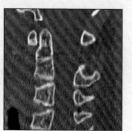

Congenital Fusion   *Physiologic Sublux.*   *Down Syndrome*   *Osteogen. Imperf.*

JUVENILE CHRONIC ARTHRITIS

Key Facts

Terminology
- Juvenile chronic arthritis (JCA)
- A spectrum of idiopathic inflammatory arthropathies occurring in childhood

Imaging Findings
- Best diagnostic clue: Cervical spine subluxations and growth disturbance
- Cervical vertebral fusions
- Growth disturbances
- Multilevel vertebral subluxations
- Erosions
- Visualization of bone erosions
- Pannus low signal intensity
- Cartilage erosions visible much earlier than bony erosions

- Pannus intermediate to high signal intensity

Top Differential Diagnoses
- Congenital spinal fusion
- Physiologic subluxations
- Down syndrome
- Osteogenesis imperfecta

Pathology
- JCA is divided into 5 categories
- Oligoarticular JRA
- Still disease
- Seronegative polyarticular JRA
- Juvenile onset adult RA
- Juvenile onset AS

- Do not diagnose juvenile AS based on SIJ widening without erosions; SIJs normally wide in children
- Usually spares remainder of spine
- Periostitis at entheses
- Oligoarticular involvement of lower extremities
- Peripheral involvement
  - Erosions occur later than in adult RA because of thicker cartilage
  - Overgrowth of epiphyses due to periarticular hyperemia
  - Shortening of bones because of premature physeal closure
  - Thin, gracile bones
  - Periarticular periostitis
  - Bony ankylosis

CT Findings
- Bone CT
  - Can be used for early diagnosis of erosions
  - Radiation considerations have led to preference for MRI

MR Findings
- T1WI
  - Visualization of bone erosions
  - Pannus low signal intensity
- T2WI
  - Cartilage erosions visible much earlier than bony erosions
  - Pannus intermediate to high signal intensity
  - Joint effusions: Facet and sacroiliac joints
- STIR
  - Pannus intermediate to high signal intensity
  - Joint effusions: Facet and sacroiliac joints
- T1 C+
  - Avid enhancement at erosions, in pannus
  - Contrast excreted into synovial joints by 10 minutes post injection
    - Evaluation of pannus must be performed immediately post injection

Nuclear Medicine Findings
- Bone Scan

- Positive 3-phase bone scan
- Oligoarticular disease easily misdiagnosed as infection on bone scan
- Gallium Scan
  - Positive
- WBC Scan
  - Positive
  - High concentration of WBC in joints affected by JCA

Imaging Recommendations
- Best imaging tool: Earliest diagnosis by MRI
- Protocol advice
  - Sagittal T1WI, STIR, axial T2WI FSE
  - Gadolinium increases sensitivity in early diagnosis, but usually not needed

DIFFERENTIAL DIAGNOSIS

Congenital spinal fusion
- Isolated anomaly or in association with syndromes such as VACTERL
- No systemic symptoms
- Often have kyphosis, scoliosis
- May have Sprengel deformity

Physiologic subluxations
- Normal vertebral morphology
- Subluxations usually less than 2 mm

Down syndrome
- Vertebral subluxations
- Normal vertebral morphology

Osteogenesis imperfecta
- Subluxations
- Diffuse osteopenia
- Vertebra plana and fractures
- No systemic symptoms

JUVENILE CHRONIC ARTHRITIS

PATHOLOGY

General Features
- Etiology: Unknown
- Epidemiology: Patients with severe hand JCA usually also have cervical spine involvement
- Associated abnormalities
  - Young children may have fever, anemia, hepatosplenomegaly
  - Secondary amyloidosis may be present
    - Causes nephropathy

Gross Pathologic & Surgical Features
- Because cartilage thicker in children, bone erosions are less commonly seen than in adults
- Growth disturbance is often the most outstanding feature
- Fusion of joints common in appendicular skeleton as well as spine
- Periostitis may be seen around joints

Microscopic Features
- Thickened synovium containing plasma cells, multinucleated giant cells, PMNs, lymphocytes

Staging, Grading or Classification Criteria
- JCA is divided into 5 categories →
- Oligoarticular JRA
  - 40% of patients
  - RF negative
  - Involves 1 to several large joints (e.g., knee, hip, shoulder, elbow)
- Still disease
  - 20% of patients
  - RF negative
  - Under 5 years old
  - Systemic disease, growth disturbance
  - Fever, anemia, hepatosplenomegaly
- Seronegative polyarticular JRA
  - 25% of patients
  - Adult distribution, but seronegative
- Juvenile onset adult RA
  - 5% of patients
  - RF positive
- Juvenile onset AS
  - 10% of patients
  - Almost all HLA-B27 positive
  - Usually adolescent males
  - Primarily involves SIJs, lower extremity joints
  - Enthesopathy a prominent feature

CLINICAL ISSUES

Presentation
- Most common signs/symptoms
  - Vague, pauciarticular pain
  - Limited neck movement
  - Peripheral tenosynovitis may be presenting complaint
  - Other signs/symptoms
    - Still disease: Fever, anemia, hepatosplenomegaly
    - Juvenile onset AS: Chronic low back pain, limited motion

Demographics
- Age
  - Younger children often have systemic disease (Still)
  - Older children and adolescents present with joint pain
- Gender: Females more common than males except for juvenile onset AS

Natural History & Prognosis
- Growth disturbances lead to premature osteoarthritis
- Often "burns out" as children approach adulthood
  - Duration of symptoms in childhood correlated to risk of continued disease in adulthood
- Psychosocial issues from chronic disease in childhood

Treatment
- Options, risks, complications: NSAIDs, steroids, methotrexate, anti tumor necrosis factor (TNF) medications

DIAGNOSTIC CHECKLIST

Consider
- Underdiagnosed; consider in child with vague, chronic articular or neck pain

SELECTED REFERENCES

1. Kekilli E et al: Cervical involvement in juvenile-onset ankylosing spondylitis with bone scintigraphy. Rheumatol Int. 24(3):164-5, 2004
2. Laiho K et al: The cervical spine in juvenile chronic arthritis. Spine J. 2(2):89-94, 2002
3. Burgos-Vargas R et al: A short-term follow-up of enthesitis and arthritis in the active phase of juvenile onset spondyloarthropathies. Clin Exp Rheumatol. 20(5):727-31, 2002
4. Haapasaari J et al: MRI diagnosis and successful treatment of upper cervical spine synovitis in a patient with juvenile chronic arthritis. Clin Exp Rheumatol. 20(2):256-7, 2002
5. Roche CJ et al: The rheumatoid cervical spine: signs of instability on plain cervical radiographs. Clin Radiol. 57(4):241-9, 2002
6. Laiho K et al: The cervical spine in mutilant juvenile chronic arthritis. Joint Bone Spine. 68(5):425-9, 2001
7. Prieur AM et al: Prognostic factors in juvenile idiopathic arthritis. Curr Rheumatol Rep. 3(5):371-8, 2001
8. Cunnane G: Amyloid precursors and amyloidosis in inflammatory arthritis. Curr Opin Rheumatol. 13(1):67-73, 2001
9. Janssen H et al: MR imaging of arthritides of the cervical spine. Magn Reson Imaging Clin N Am. 8(3):491-512, 2000
10. Zoli A et al: Craniocervical junction involvement in rheumatoid arthritis: a clinical and radiological study. J Rheumatol. 27(5):1178-82, 2000
11. Ansell BM: Prognosis in juvenile arthritis. Adv Exp Med Biol. 455:27-33, 1999
12. Husby G: Treatment of amyloidosis and the rheumatologist. State of the art and perspectives for the future. Scand J Rheumatol. 27(3):161-5, 1998
13. Schneider R et al: Systemic onset juvenile rheumatoid arthritis. Baillieres Clin Rheumatol. 12(2):245-71, 1998
14. Tucker LB: Juvenile rheumatoid arthritis. Curr Opin Rheumatol. 5(5):619-28, 1993

JUVENILE CHRONIC ARTHRITIS

IMAGE GALLERY

Typical

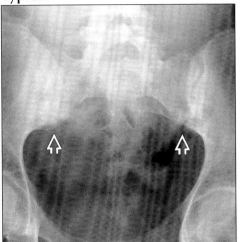
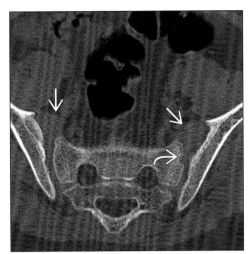

(Left) Anteroposterior radiography shows sclerosis and poor definition of SI joints (arrows) indicating sacroiliitis in 17 yo male with low back and left knee pain. Knee MRI showed inflammatory arthropathy. *(Right)* Axial bone CT shows left SI joints erosions (curved arrow) and bilateral effusions (arrows) in child with inflammatory arthropathy.

Typical

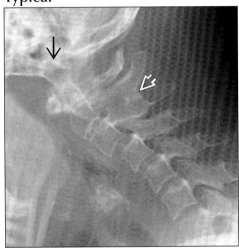
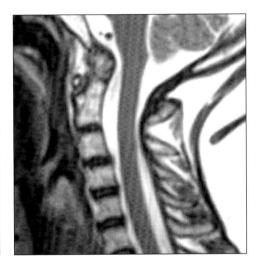

(Left) Lateral radiography shows posterior fusion at C2-3 (open arrow) due to JRA. Dens is large and appears fused to clivus (arrow). Subluxations are seen at C3-4 and C4-5. *(Right)* Sagittal T2WI MR shows enlargement of dens, which abuts clivus. Lateral images showed fused facet joints at C2-3.

Typical

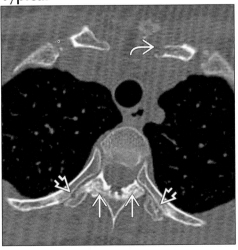
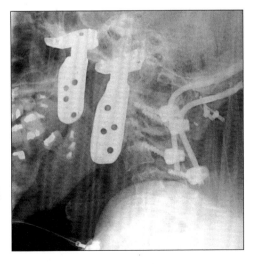

(Left) Axial bone CT shows erosions due to JCA, involving facet joints (arrows), costotransverse joints (open arrows) and left sternoclavicular joint (curved arrow). *(Right)* Lateral radiography shows surgical fusion from occiput to C4 for instability from JCA. Note mandibular hypoplasia and temporomandibular joint prostheses.

SERONEGATIVE SPONDYLOARTHROPATHY

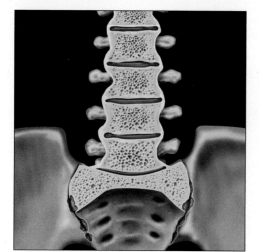

Coronal graphic shows bilateral sacroiliac erosions and flowing syndesmophytes along lateral margins of lumbar vertebrae.

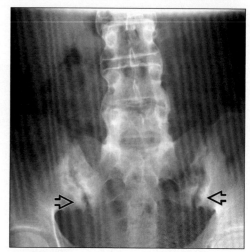

Anteroposterior radiography shows bilateral sacroiliitis (arrows), with joint widening and multiple small erosions, as well as reactive sclerosis. Diffuse ankylosis lumbar spine also seen.

TERMINOLOGY

Abbreviations and Synonyms
- Ankylosing spondylitis (AS)
- Reactive arthropathy: Previously called Reiter syndrome
- Undifferentiated spondyloarthropathy (USpA)

Definitions
- RF (rheumatoid factor) negative inflammatory arthritis and enthesopathy affecting the spine and sacroiliac joints
- Syndesmophyte: Paraspinous ligamentous or disc ossification bridging two adjacent vertebral bodies
- Enthesopathy: Inflammation at attachments of ligaments and tendons (entheses)

IMAGING FINDINGS

General Features
- Best diagnostic clue: SI joint erosion or ankylosis
- Location
  - First involves sacroiliac joints
  - Second involves thoracolumbar junction
  - May involve entire spine

Radiographic Findings
- Radiography

- Sacroiliac joint (SIJ) erosive arthritis
  - Affects lower third of joint (synovial portion)
  - Erosions seen first on iliac side of joint
  - Erosions best seen on PA or Ferguson rather than AP view
  - Oblique views often not contributory because of difficulty positioning
  - Earliest sign: Loss of definition of subchondral bone plate
  - Erosions small, multiple, "serrated steak knife"
  - Progresses to joint space widening
  - Fusion a late phenomenon
  - Bilaterally symmetric: Ankylosing spondylitis, arthritis of inflammatory bowel disease
  - Bilateral but asymmetric: Reactive arthropathy, psoriatic arthritis
- Corner erosions vertebral bodies
  - "Squaring" anterior vertebral margin
  - Progresses to corner erosions
  - Sclerotic repair leads to "shiny corner" sign (Romanus lesion)
- Ossification of outer fibers anulus fibrosis
  - Thin ossification at vertebral margins
  - When multilevel results in "bamboo spine" appearance; more common in AS
  - Susceptible to fracture
- Ossification of paraspinous ligaments

DDx: Spectrum of Sacroiliitis

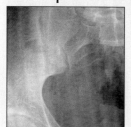

Early Erosions

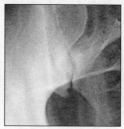

Erosions, Sclerosis

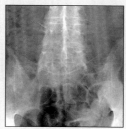

Joint Fusion

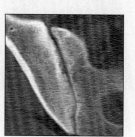

CT of Erosions

SERONEGATIVE SPONDYLOARTHROPATHY

Key Facts

Terminology
- RF (rheumatoid factor) negative inflammatory arthritis and enthesopathy affecting the spine and sacroiliac joints

Imaging Findings
- Best diagnostic clue: SI joint erosion or ankylosis
- Sacroiliac joint (SIJ) erosive arthritis
- Corner erosions vertebral bodies
- Ossification of outer fibers anulus fibrosis
- Ossification of paraspinous ligaments
- Kyphotic deformity thoracic and lumbar spine
- Fractures through syndesmophytes and/or vertebral bodies
- Start with plain films; use CT if plain films are negative

- MR/CT in combination to evaluate bone and cord status following trauma

Top Differential Diagnoses
- Rheumatoid arthritis
- Juvenile chronic arthritis
- Infectious sacroiliitis
- Diffuse idiopathic skeletal hyperostosis (DISH)
- Retinoid therapy

Clinical Issues
- Low back pain, greatest in morning
- Pathologic fracture
- Most cases mild, limited to SIJs
- Some progress to extensive spine ankylosis over period of years

---

- May be bulky; more common in psoriatic and reactive arthropathy
- Distinguished from osteophytes by origin from mid vertebral body rather than endplate
○ Kyphotic deformity thoracic and lumbar spine
○ Facet joint arthritis
  - Erosions progress to fusion
○ Atlantoaxial subluxation
○ Fractures through syndesmophytes and/or vertebral bodies
  - Often difficult to see because of osteopenia, spinal deformity
  - Unstable; involve all spinal columns
○ Accelerated degenerative disc disease in unfused regions due to increased stress
  - May mimic discitis or neuropathic disease
○ Other joints of axial skeleton may show erosions progressing to fusion
  - Costotransverse, costovertebral joints
  - Sternoclavicular, acromioclavicular joints
  - Pubic symphysis
○ Peripheral arthritis
  - Erosions
  - Periosteal new bone at entheses; "whiskered" appearance
  - Psoriatic: Affects hands > feet
  - Reactive, AS: Affects feet more than hands
○ Bone mineral density
  - Normal early in course of disease
  - Diffuse osteopenia in areas of ankylosis

CT Findings
- Bone CT
○ Highly sensitive to early sacroiliac erosions
○ Commonly shows involvement of costotransverse and costovertebral joints
○ Useful to evaluate fractures

MR Findings
- T1WI
○ Low signal intensity bone marrow at corner and SIJ erosions
○ Joint erosions and ankylosis

- T2WI: High signal intensity bone marrow at early corner and SIJ erosions
- STIR: High signal intensity bone marrow at early corner and SIJ erosions
- T1 C+: Avid enhancement in active disease
- Marrow in disc spaces (later stages), preservation of central canal

Nuclear Medicine Findings
- Bone Scan: Positive 3-phase bone scan in active disease

Imaging Recommendations
- Start with plain films; use CT if plain films are negative
- MR/CT in combination to evaluate bone and cord status following trauma

DIFFERENTIAL DIAGNOSIS

Rheumatoid arthritis
- Rarely involves SIJs
- Primarily involves cervical spine
- Bony ankylosis not a feature

Juvenile chronic arthritis
- Onset less than age 18
- Growth disturbances of vertebrae
- Bony fusions
- Juvenile onset ankylosing spondylitis usually limited to SIJs, peripheral enthesopathy

Infectious sacroiliitis
- Unilateral

Diffuse idiopathic skeletal hyperostosis (DISH)
- Flowing ossification paraspinous ligaments
- Sacroiliac joints normal

Retinoid therapy
- Flowing ossification paraspinous ligaments
- Sacroiliac joints normal

SERONEGATIVE SPONDYLOARTHROPATHY

PATHOLOGY

General Features
- General path comments: RF negative, elevated ESR
- Genetics
  - Strong association with HLA - B27 haplotype
    - 95% AS, 80% Reiter, 50% psoriatic patients are positive
    - 6-8% of normal population is HLA - B27 positive
    - Psoriatic arthritis in HLA-B27 negative patients spares the spine
    - 1-2% people with HLA-B27 develop spondyloarthropathy
- Etiology
  - Psoriatic arthritis: Associated with psoriasis but may precede psoriatic rash
  - Reactive arthritis: Follows prior bacterial infection - venereal or dysentery
- Epidemiology
  - Approximately 0.1-1% of population
    - Lowest incidence in Sub-Saharan Africa
  - Often mild, undiagnosed
- Associated abnormalities
  - Uveitis, iritis, conjunctivitis seen with all forms
  - AS: Inflammatory bowel disease, aortitis, upper lobe pulmonary fibrosis, rash
  - Reactive: Urethritis/cervicitis, balanitis, heel pain
  - Peripheral arthritis
    - AS, reactive: Predilection for lower extremity, especially hips, knees, plantar aponeurosis
    - Psoriatic: Predilection for hands hands
  - Secondary amyloid leading to nephropathy

Gross Pathologic & Surgical Features
- AS: Extensive ankylosis creates high risk for spinal fractures

Microscopic Features
- Enchondral ossification discs
- Inflammation synovium, subchondral bone, less severe than RA

Staging, Grading or Classification Criteria
- Ankylosing spondylitis
- Reactive spondyloarthropathy
- Psoriatic spondyloarthropathy
- Spondyloarthropathy associated with inflammatory bowel disease
- Undifferentiated spondyloarthropathy (uSpA)
  - Most cases of uSpA can be categorized later in course of disease

CLINICAL ISSUES

Presentation
- Most common signs/symptoms
  - Low back pain, greatest in morning
  - Pathologic fracture
    - Increased fracture risk with multilevel spine ankylosis
    - Often due to minor injury
    - Unstable
    - Most common at cervicothoracic or thoracolumbar junction
  - Other signs/symptoms
    - Fatigue, low grade fever
    - Rarely, cauda equina syndrome (due to synovial cysts)

Demographics
- Age: Early to mid adulthood
- Gender: All types more common in men than women

Natural History & Prognosis
- Most cases mild, limited to SIJs
- Some progress to extensive spine ankylosis over period of years
- Often see exacerbations and remissions

Treatment
- NSAIDs, sulfasalazine, methotrexate

DIAGNOSTIC CHECKLIST

Image Interpretation Pearls
- Look for loss of definition of subchondral bone plate at SIJs as earliest sign

SELECTED REFERENCES

1. Vinson EN et al: MR imaging of ankylosing spondylitis. Semin Musculoskelet Radiol. 7(2):103-13, 2003
2. Queiro R et al: Clinically asymptomatic axial disease in psoriatic spondyloarthropathy. A retrospective study. Clin Rheumatol. 21(1):10-3, 2002
3. Hitchon PW et al: Fractures of the thoracolumbar spine complicating ankylosing spondylitis. J Neurosurg. 97(2 Suppl):218-22, 2002
4. Bollow M et al: Use of contrast enhanced magnetic resonance imaging to detect spinal inflammation in patients with spondyloarthritides. Clin Exp Rheumatol. 20(6 Suppl 28):S167-74, 2002
5. Shih TT et al: Spinal fractures and pseudoarthrosis complicating ankylosing spondylitis: MRI manifestation and clinical significance. J Comput Assist Tomogr. 25(2):164-70, 2001
6. Cunnane G: Amyloid precursors and amyloidosis in inflammatory arthritis. Curr Opin Rheumatol. 13(1):67-73, 2001
7. Sampaio-Barros PD et al: Undifferentiated spondyloarthropathies: a 2-year follow-up study. Clin Rheumatol. 20(3):201-6, 2001
8. Janssen H et al: MR imaging of arthritides of the cervical spine. Magn Reson Imaging Clin N Am. 8(3):491-512, 2000
9. Luong AA et al: Imaging of the seronegative spondylo-arthropathies. Curr Rheumatol Rep 2(4): 288-96, 2000
10. Mitra D et al: The prevalence of vertebral fractures in mild ankylosing spondylitis and their relationship to bone mineral density. Rheumatology (Oxford). 39(1):85-9, 2000
11. Braun JM et al: Radiologic diagnosis and pathology of the spondyloarthropathies. Rheum Dis Clin North Am 24(4): 697-735, 1998
12. Deesomchok U et al: Clinical comparison of patients with ankylosing spondylitis, Reiter's syndrome and psoriatic arthritis. J Med Assoc Thai 76(2): 61-70, 1993
13. Rosenkranz W: Ankylosing spondylitis: cauda equina syndrome with multiple spinal arachnoid cysts. Case report. J Neurosurg. 34(2 Pt 1):241-3, 1971

SERONEGATIVE SPONDYLOARTHROPATHY

IMAGE GALLERY

Typical

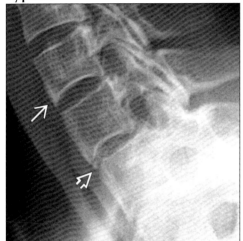
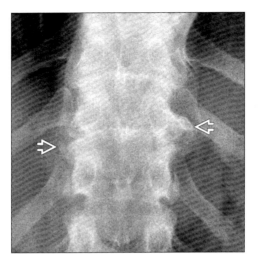

(Left) Lateral radiography shows shiny corner (arrow), vertebral squaring, ossification of outer fibers of anulus fibrosus (open arrow), and anterior longitudinal ligament in psoriatic arthritis. (Right) Anteroposterior radiography shows bulky lateral paraspinous ligamentous ossifications (arrows) in psoriatic arthritis.

Typical

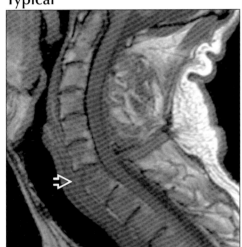
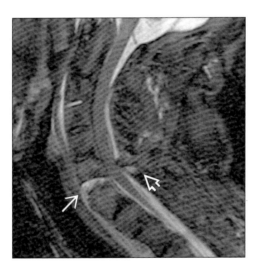

(Left) Sagittal T1WI MR shows C6-7 fracture-dislocation (arrow) through syndesmophytes and posterior ligaments in AS. Thin, low signal intensity syndesmophytes are visible in remainder of visualized spine. (Right) Sagittal STIR MR shows C6-7 fracture (arrow) through syndesmophyte in AS. Hematoma posteriorly (open arrow) indicates interspinous ligament rupture.

Typical

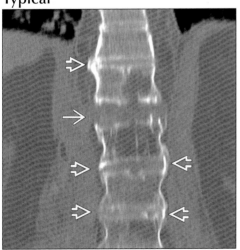
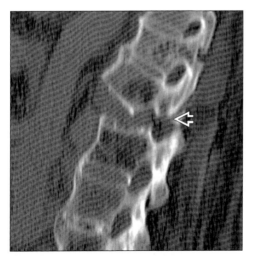

(Left) Coronal bone CT shows thoracolumbar fracture-dislocation (arrow) due to AS. Note thin syndesmophytes creating "bamboo spine" appearance (open arrows). Severe osteopenia is present. (Right) Sagittal bone CT shows fracture-dislocation in AS. Anteriorly, fracture extends through fused disc space; posteriorly, it extends through pars interarticularis (arrow) and interspinous ligaments.

GOUT

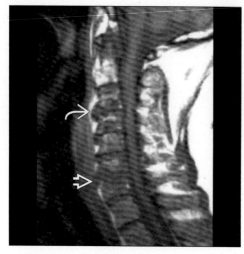

Sagittal PD/Intermediate MR shows punched out vertebral body erosions at multiple levels. There is endplate destruction at C6-7 (open arrow). Curved arrow points to prevertebral tophus.

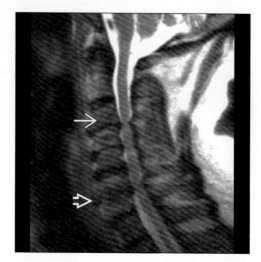

Sagittal T2WI MR shows endplate destruction at C6-7 (open arrow). Intraosseous tophus (arrow) is low signal intensity and almost indistinguishable from the surrounding marrow.

TERMINOLOGY

Definitions
- Arthropathy secondary to urate crystal deposition
- Tophus: Focal mass consisting of crystals and host reaction

IMAGING FINDINGS

General Features
- Best diagnostic clue: Erosive arthritis centered on disc in patient with known gout
- Location
  ○ Generally involves only 1-2 levels
  ○ Disc or facet joints
  ○ Sacroiliac joints
  ○ Usually have peripheral disease also

Radiographic Findings
- Radiography
  ○ Bone mineral density preserved
  ○ Disc space narrowing
  ○ Endplate erosion
  ○ Prevertebral soft tissue mass

CT Findings
- Bone CT
  ○ Endplate destruction
  ○ Soft tissue mass
    ▪ May contain faint calcifications
  ○ Facet joint erosions may be seen

MR Findings
- T1WI: Low signal intensity tophi
- T2WI: Heterogeneous signal intensity tophi
- STIR: Heterogeneous signal intensity tophi
- T1 C+: Variable enhancement
- Endplate destruction seen on all sequences
- Small foci low signal intensity seen on all sequences
- Tophi may compress cord or nerve roots

Nuclear Medicine Findings
- Bone Scan: Increased activity all three phases
- WBC Scan
  ○ Increased activity

Imaging Recommendations
- Best imaging tool: MRI to show tophi, impingement on cord and nerve roots
- Protocol advice: Sagittal T1WI, STIR, axial T2WI

DIFFERENTIAL DIAGNOSIS

Osteomyelitis
- Focal osteopenia on radiographs
- May appear identical on CT, MRI

DDx: Vertebral Endplate Destruction

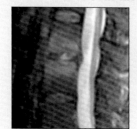

Osteomyelitis

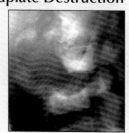

Neuropathic

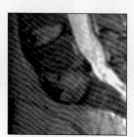

Amyloid

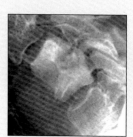

Hemodialysis

GOUT

Key Facts

Terminology
- Arthropathy secondary to urate crystal deposition

Imaging Findings
- Best diagnostic clue: Erosive arthritis centered on disc in patient with known gout
- Best imaging tool: MRI to show tophi, impingement on cord and nerve roots

Top Differential Diagnoses
- Osteomyelitis
- Hemodialysis arthropathy
- Neuropathic arthropathy
- Seronegative spondyloarthropathy

Pathology
- General path comments: Specimens must be sent to pathology in alcohol; formalin dissolves crystals

---

Hemodialysis arthropathy
- Patient history is key
- Imaging findings identical

Neuropathic arthropathy
- Extensive bone destruction
- Bony debris

Seronegative spondyloarthropathy
- Vertebral body corner erosions
- Ligament ossification, vertebral fusion

PATHOLOGY

General Features
- General path comments: Specimens must be sent to pathology in alcohol; formalin dissolves crystals
- Etiology
  - High levels of serum uric acid lead to soft tissue crystal deposition
  - May be secondary to chronic diseases
    - Renal disease, myeloproliferative disorders
- Epidemiology: Spine involvement rare

Gross Pathologic & Surgical Features
- Chalky white tophi

Microscopic Features
- Polarized light: Negatively birefringent crystals
- Tophi: Deposits of crystals surrounded by fibrous tissue, rimmed by mononuclear cells and giant cells

CLINICAL ISSUES

Presentation
- Most common signs/symptoms
  - Back pain, often acute and severe
  - Other signs/symptoms
    - Fever
    - Neurologic symptoms
- Clinical profile: Associated with obesity, rich diet

Demographics
- Gender
  - M:F = 20:1
    - Female patients almost always post menopausal

Natural History & Prognosis
- Most cases respond to medical therapy

Treatment
- Medical
  - Nonsteroidal anti-inflammatory medications
  - Colchicine
  - Uric acid production inhibitors (e.g., Allopurinol)
  - Uricosuric medications (e.g., probenecid)
- Surgical decompression for neurologic symptoms

SELECTED REFERENCES

1. Hsu CY et al: Tophaceous gout of the spine: MR imaging features. Clin Radiol. 57(10):919-25, 2002
2. Barrett K et al: Tophaceous gout of the spine mimicking epidural infection: case report and review of the literature. Neurosurgery. 48(5):1170-2; discussion 1172-3, 2001
3. King JC et al: Gouty arthropathy of the lumbar spine: a case report and review of the literature. Spine. 22(19):2309-12, 1997
4. Bonaldi VM et al: Tophaceous gout of the lumbar spine mimicking an epidural abscess: MR features. AJNR Am J Neuroradiol. 17(10):1949-52, 1996
5. Duprez TP et al: Gout in the cervical spine: MR pattern mimicking diskovertebral infection. AJNR Am J Neuroradiol. 17(1):151-3, 1996
6. Varga J et al: Tophaceous gout of the spine in a patient with no peripheral tophi: case report and review of the literature. Arthritis Rheum. 28(11):1312-5, 1985
7. Bullough PG et al: Atlas of Orthopaedic Pathology. Philadelphia, University Park Press. pp.5.4-5.5, 1984
8. Jajic I: Gout in the spine and sacro-iliac joints: radiological manifestations. Skeletal Radiol. 8(3):209-12, 1982

IMAGE GALLERY

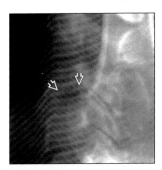 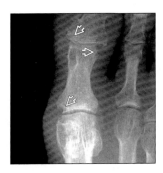

(Left) Lateral radiography shows severe disc space narrowing at C7-T1, with a punched-out erosion (arrows) at C7. (Right) Anteroposterior radiography of toe shows classic sharply marginated erosions with overhanging edges (arrows), and soft tissue masses. Almost all patients with spinal gout have peripheral disease.

CPPD

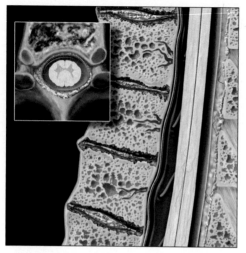

Sagittal graphic shows crystal deposition and degeneration of the intervertebral disc. Calcification of the ligamentum flavum is also evident, best seen on axial inset graphic.

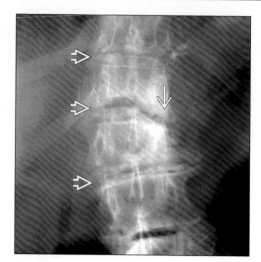

Anteroposterior radiography shows linear disc calcifications (open arrows) due to CPPD. Endplate erosions (arrow) may mimic infection or neuropathic arthropathy.

TERMINOLOGY

Abbreviations and Synonyms
- Calcium pyrophosphate dihydrate deposition disease

Definitions
- Pseudogout: Acute painful episode due to CPPD

IMAGING FINDINGS

General Features
- Best diagnostic clue: Linear disc or ligament calcific deposits
- Location: Cervical, thoracic or lumbar spine

Radiographic Findings
- Radiography
  - Linear disc calcifications
  - Majority of cases show calcification pubic symphysis and/or triangular fibrocartilage of wrist

CT Findings
- Bone CT
  - Linear disc calcifications
  - Calcification ligamentum flavum
  - Calcification facet joints
  - Globular perivertebral calcific deposits

MR Findings
- T1WI: Low to intermediate signal
- T2WI: Heterogeneous signal
- Not easily seen unless globular, tumoral configuration

Nuclear Medicine Findings
- Bone Scan
  - Positive on delayed images
  - Positive 3-phase scan in acute pseudogout attack

Imaging Recommendations
- Best imaging tool: CT scan
- Protocol advice: Thin-section CT with sagittal, coronal reformats

DIFFERENTIAL DIAGNOSIS

Degenerative disc disease
- Disc bulges and herniations may calcify when chronic

Seronegative spondyloarthropathy
- Calcification outer fibers anulus, paraspinous ligaments
- Progresses to ossification

Hemodialysis arthropathy
- Endplate erosions
- Calcifications due to hydroxyapatite deposition

DDx: Spine Arthritis with Calcification

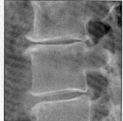

Calcified Disc Bulges

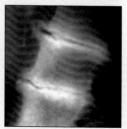

Ochronosis

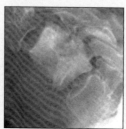

Hemodialysis

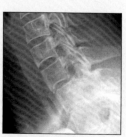

Psoriatic

CPPD

Key Facts

Terminology
- Calcium pyrophosphate dihydrate deposition disease
- Pseudogout: Acute painful episode due to CPPD

Imaging Findings
- Linear disc calcifications
- Calcification ligamentum flavum
- Calcification facet joints
- Globular perivertebral calcific deposits

Top Differential Diagnoses
- Degenerative disc disease
- Seronegative spondyloarthropathy
- Hemodialysis arthropathy
- Ochronosis

Ochronosis
- Diffuse disc calcifications and degeneration

Gout
- Endplate erosions
- Calcification usually minimal

PATHOLOGY

General Features
- General path comments
  - Crystals deposited in hyaline and fibrocartilage, joint capsules, ligaments
  - Occasionally tumoral deposits of calcification develop
    - Less common, usually hydroxyapatite crystals in addition to CPPD
  - Specimens must be sent to pathology in alcohol; crystals dissolve in formalin
- Etiology: Idiopathic or associated with: Hyperparathyroidism, hemochromatosis, gout, hypophosphatasia
- Epidemiology: At least 5% of elderly have CPPD at some location in autopsy series
- Associated abnormalities: May coexist with gout, hydroxyapatite deposition

Gross Pathologic & Surgical Features
- Chalky white deposits of crystals

Microscopic Features
- Rhomboidal crystals with weak positive birefringence

CLINICAL ISSUES

Presentation
- Most common signs/symptoms
  - Back pain indistinguishable from degenerative disc disease
  - Other signs/symptoms
    - Acute episode of pain, sometimes with fever
    - Neurologic symptoms due to tumoral calcific deposits

Demographics
- Age: Older patients, generally over 50 years old

Treatment
- Options, risks, complications: Tumoral deposits may require surgical decompression

SELECTED REFERENCES

1. Finckh A et al: The cervical spine in calcium pyrophosphate dihydrate deposition disease. A prevalent case-control study. J Rheumatol. 31(3):545-9, 2004
2. Muthukumar N et al: Tumoral calcium pyrophosphate dihydrate deposition disease of the ligamentum flavum. Neurosurgery. 53(1):103-8; discussion 108-9, 2003
3. Chen CF et al: Calcium pyrophosphate dihydrate crystal deposition disease in cervical radiculomyelopathy. J Chin Med Assoc. 66(4):256-9, 2003
4. Fujishiro T et al: Pseudogout attack of the lumbar facet joint: a case report. Spine. 27(17):E396-8, 2002
5. Steinbach LS et al: Calcium pyrophosphate dihydrate crystal deposition disease: imaging perspectives. Curr Probl Diagn Radiol. 29(6):209-29, 2000
6. Berlemann U et al: Calcium pyrophosphate dihydrate deposition in degenerate lumbar discs. Eur Spine J. 7(1):45-9, 1998
7. Markiewitz AD et al: Calcium pyrophosphate dihydrate crystal deposition disease as a cause of lumbar canal stenosis. Spine. 21(4):506-11, 1996
8. Brown TR et al: Deposition of calcium pyrophosphate dihydrate crystals in the ligamentum flavum: evaluation with MR imaging and CT. Radiology. 178(3):871-3, 1991
9. el-Khoury GY et al: Massive calcium pyrophosphate crystal deposition at the craniovertebral junction. AJR Am J Roentgenol. 145(4):777-8, 1985

IMAGE GALLERY

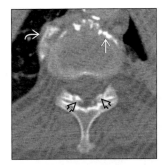 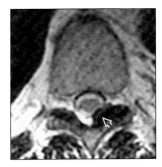

(Left) Axial bone CT shows calcification of ligamentum flavum (open arrows) and disc (arrow) in CPPD. Paraspinous ossification due to DISH (curved arrow) also present. *(Right)* Axial T2WI MR shows mild impression on thecal sac due to calcification of ligamentum flavum (arrow) in CPPD.

HEMODIALYSIS SPONDYLOARTHROPATHY

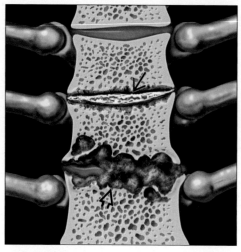

Coronal graphic shows 2 types of hemodialysis arthropathy: Crystal deposition (arrow) and amyloid deposition (open arrow) both cause endplate erosions.

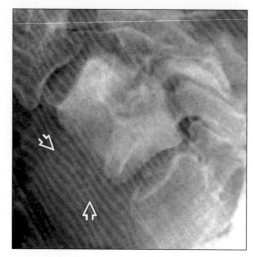

Lateral radiography shows severe endplate destruction at C5-6, resulting in kyphosis. Faint calcifications are visible in anterior soft tissues (arrows) and are due to hydroxyapatite.

IMAGING FINDINGS

General Features
- Best diagnostic clue: Peridiscal destructive arthritis in patient on long term hemodialysis
- Location: Cervical, thoracic or lumbar spine

Radiographic Findings
- Radiography
  - Centered on intervertebral disc
  - Endplate destruction
  - Soft tissue mass
    - May contain amyloid
    - May contain crystals with visible calcification

CT Findings
- Bone CT
  - Sharply marginated erosions
  - Soft tissue mass

MR Findings
- T1WI: Low signal intensity
- T2WI: Low to intermediate signal intensity
- STIR: Low to intermediate signal intensity

Nuclear Medicine Findings
- Bone Scan: Positive 3 phase bone scan

Imaging Recommendations
- Best imaging tool: MRI
- Protocol advice: T2WI, STIR to differentiate from infection

DIFFERENTIAL DIAGNOSIS

Infection
- Calcifications usually absent
- Osteoporosis usually present
- High signal intensity on T2WI, STIR

Neuropathic joint
- Lumbar spine
- Imaging appearance may be identical

Gout
- Imaging appearance may be identical

Longus coli tendonitis
- Due to hydroxyapatite deposition
- Seen in older patients in absence of hemodialysis
- Disc spaces not affected

Calcium pyrophosphate deposition disease
- Disc, ligamentum flavum calcifications

DDx: Hemodialysis Arthropathy

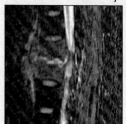

Osteomyelitis

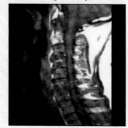

Gout

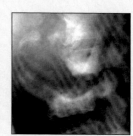

Neuropathic

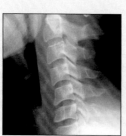

Tendinopathy

HEMODIALYSIS SPONDYLOARTHROPATHY

Key Facts

Imaging Findings
- Best diagnostic clue: Peridiscal destructive arthritis in patient on long term hemodialysis
- Location: Cervical, thoracic or lumbar spine
- Soft tissue mass
- May contain amyloid
- May contain crystals with visible calcification

Top Differential Diagnoses
- Infection
- Neuropathic joint
- Gout
- Longus coli tendonitis
- Calcium pyrophosphate deposition disease

Diagnostic Checklist
- History is key to making diagnosis

PATHOLOGY

General Features
- General path comments
  - Two types of arthropathy associated with hemodialysis
    - Amyloid deposition: Beta-2 microglobulin
    - Crystal deposition: Hydroxyapatite
- Etiology: Beta-2 microglobulin not efficiently removed by dialysis, accumulates in soft tissues
- Epidemiology
  - Rare
  - Incidence increases with length of time on dialysis
- Associated abnormalities: Amyloid deposition may lead to carpal tunnel syndrome, destructive arthropathy peripheral joints

Gross Pathologic & Surgical Features
- Amyloid: Waxy, tan tissue
- Crystal: Chalky, semiliquid material

Microscopic Features
- Amyloid: Apple-green birefringence under polarized light
- Hydroxyapatite: Electron microscopy for definitive diagnosis of crystal type

CLINICAL ISSUES

Presentation
- Most common signs/symptoms
  - Asymptomatic unless severe
  - Other signs/symptoms
    - Back pain
    - Radiculopathy
    - Rarely cord compression

Natural History & Prognosis
- Indolent
- May result in spinal instability

Treatment
- Options, risks, complications: Fusion for stabilization

DIAGNOSTIC CHECKLIST

Image Interpretation Pearls
- History is key to making diagnosis

SELECTED REFERENCES

1. Theodorou DJ et al: Imaging in dialysis spondyloarthropathy. Semin Dial. 15(4):290-6, 2002
2. Leone A et al: Destructive spondyloarthropathy of the cervical spine in long-term hemodialyzed patients: a five-year clinical radiological prospective study. Skeletal Radiol. 30(8):431-41, 2001
3. Mikawa Y et al: Compression of the spinal cord due to destructive spondyloarthropathy of the atlanto-axial joints. J Bone Joint Surg Am. 78(12):1911-4, 1996
4. Maruyama H et al: A magnetic resonance imaging study of destructive spondyloarthropathy in long-term hemodialysis patients. Nephron. 59(1):71-4, 1991
5. Sethi D et al: Dialysis arthropathy: a clinical, biochemical, radiological and histological study of 36 patients. Q J Med. 77(282):1061-82, 1990
6. Rafto SE et al: Spondyloarthropathy of the cervical spine in long-term hemodialysis. Radiology. 166(1 Pt 1):201-4, 1988
7. Naidich JB et al: Spondyloarthropathy from long-term hemodialysis. Radiology. 167(3):761-4, 1988

IMAGE GALLERY

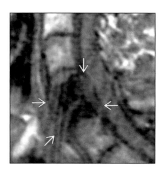 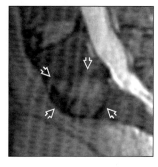

(Left) Sagittal T1WI MR shows soft tissue mass *(arrows)* due to crystal deposition anterior and posterior to sclerotic C5 and C6 vertebrae. Spinal cord is mildly compressed. *(Right)* Sagittal T2WI MR shows amyloid deposit *(arrows)* at L5-S1 causing extensive erosion of the adjacent vertebral bodies.

CALCIFIC TENDINITIS, LONGUS COLI

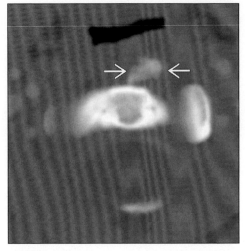

Axial bone CT shows amorphous focal calcification anterior to C2 (arrows) and prevertebral soft tissue swelling.

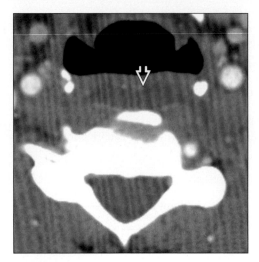

Axial CECT shows prevertebral fluid collection (arrow) dissecting along fascial planes, at level below longus coli calcifications.

TERMINOLOGY

Abbreviations and Synonyms
- Calcific tendinopathy, longus coli

Definitions
- Longus coli muscle is a deep flexor of the neck, located anterior to anterior longitudinal ligament

IMAGING FINDINGS

General Features
- Best diagnostic clue: Focal calcification and soft tissue swelling in prevertebral space
- Location: Upper cervical spine
- Morphology: Amorphous calcification

Radiographic Findings
- Radiography
  - Retropharyngeal soft tissue swelling
  - Retropharyngeal calcification
    - Fluffy, amorphous
    - Anterior to anterior longitudinal ligament

CT Findings
- Bone CT
  - Fluffy, amorphous calcification longus coli
  - Decreased attenuation in longus coli muscle
  - Elongated fluid collection extending along fascial planes
  - No enhancement of fluid with contrast administration

MR Findings
- T1WI
  - Prevertebral soft tissue swelling
  - Low signal intensity calcific deposits
- T2WI
  - High signal intensity along longus coli
  - Fluid extending along fascial planes
  - Low signal intensity calcific deposits
- T1 C+
  - Heterogeneous enhancement around calcific deposit
  - Fluid collection does not enhance

Imaging Recommendations
- Best imaging tool: CT scan
- Protocol advice: Bone and soft tissue algorithm

DIFFERENTIAL DIAGNOSIS

Retropharyngeal abscess
- Rounded fluid collection on CT, MR
- Rim-enhancement of fluid
- This morphology differs from elongated collection along fascial planes due to tendinitis longus coli

DDx: Calcific Tendonitis, Longus Coli

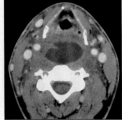

Abscess

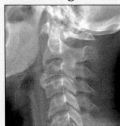

Ligament Ossification

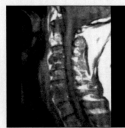

Gout

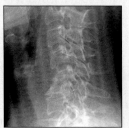

Osteomyelitis

CALCIFIC TENDINITIS, LONGUS COLI

Key Facts

Imaging Findings
- Best diagnostic clue: Focal calcification and soft tissue swelling in prevertebral space
- Retropharyngeal calcification

Top Differential Diagnoses
- Retropharyngeal abscess
- Cervical osteomyelitis
- Paraspinal ligament ossification

Pathology
- Etiology: Deposition of hydroxyapatite (HADD) crystals in longus coli muscle

Clinical Issues
- Clinical profile: Patient with sudden onset of neck pain and stiffness
- Resolves in 1-2 weeks

Cervical osteomyelitis
- Centered on disc
- Endplate erosions
- Soft tissue mass

Paraspinal ligament ossification
- Juxtaposed to vertebrae
- Forms well-defined bone, not amorphous calcification
- Seen in seronegative arthropathies, DISH, retinoid therapy

Gout
- Peridiscal erosions
- Soft tissue mass
- Faint calcifications

Hemodialysis arthropathy
- Centered on disc
- Amorphous calcifications
- Focal soft tissue mass

PATHOLOGY

General Features
- Etiology: Deposition of hydroxyapatite (HADD) crystals in longus coli muscle

Gross Pathologic & Surgical Features
- Chalky, semiliquid calcific deposits

Microscopic Features
- Crystals amorphous on light microscopy
- Electron microscopy for definitive diagnosis of crystal type

CLINICAL ISSUES

Presentation
- Most common signs/symptoms
  - Neck pain and stiffness
  - Odynophagia
  - Other signs/symptoms
    - Mild leukocytosis and fever
- Clinical profile: Patient with sudden onset of neck pain and stiffness

Demographics
- Age: Middle-aged and older patients

Natural History & Prognosis
- Resolves in 1-2 weeks

Treatment
- Options, risks, complications: Nonsteroidal anti-inflammatory medications

SELECTED REFERENCES

1. Diaw AM et al: Calcium hydroxyapatite deposition disease of the neck: finding in three patients. J Belge Radiol. 81(2):73-4, 1998
2. Claudepierre P et al: Misleading clinical aspects of hydroxyapatite deposits: a series of 15 cases. J Rheumatol. 24(3):531-5, 1997
3. De Maeseneer M et al: Calcific tendinitis of the longus colli muscle. Head Neck. 19(6):545-8, 1997
4. Smith RV et al: Hydroxyapatite deposition disease: an uncommon cause of acute odynophagia. Otolaryngol Head Neck Surg. 114(2):321-3, 1996
5. Ring D et al: Acute calcific retropharyngeal tendinitis. Clinical presentation and pathological characterization. J Bone Joint Surg Am. 76(11):1636-42, 1994
6. Hall FM et al: Calcific tendinitis of the longus coli: diagnosis by CT. AJR Am J Roentgenol. 147(4):742-3, 1986

IMAGE GALLERY

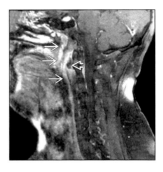 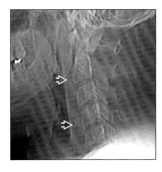

(Left) Sagittal T1 C+ MR shows thickening of prevertebral soft tissues (arrows) and enhancement around focal calcification (open arrow). (Right) Lateral radiography shows diffuse prevertebral soft tissue swelling, with calcification at C2 and C4 levels (arrows).

PART III

Infection and Inflammatory Disorders

Infections   1

Inflammatory & Autoimmune   2

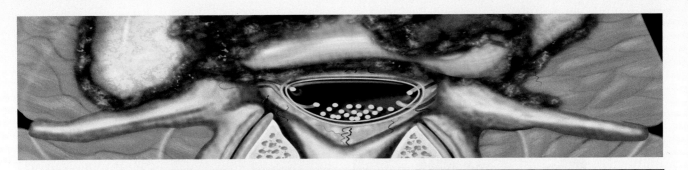

SECTION 1: Infections

INFECTIONS, PATHWAYS OF SPREAD

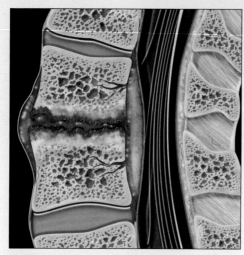

Sagittal graphic shows lumbar disc space infection, vertebral body osteomyelitis with endplate destruction and marrow edema. There are ventral and dorsal abscess collections.

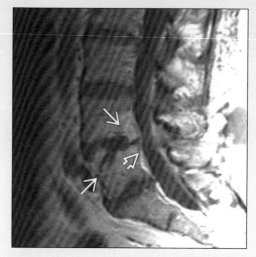

Sagittal T1 C+ MR shows pyogenic disc space infection at L4-5 with endplate destruction (arrows), irregular enhancement of bodies and disc, and epidural phlegmon (open arrow).

TERMINOLOGY

Abbreviations and Synonyms
- Osteomyelitis spread, infection extension; infection spread; metastatic infection
- Disc space infection (DSI)

Definitions
- Dissemination or extension of infection by direct, hematogenous, lymphatic and other routes

PATHOLOGY ISSUES

General Considerations
- Routes of spread
  - Tissue (interstitial) spaces
  - Lymphatic system
  - Hematogenous
  - Coelomic spaces
  - Cerebrospinal fluid space
- Types of spinal infection
  - Disc space infection/vertebral osteomyelitis
    - Extension into epidural space, paravertebral region, psoas muscles
  - Isolated epidural abscess without DSI
    - Hematogenous spread, or direct extension following instrumentation/catheter placement
  - Subdural empyema
  - Meningitis
  - Intramedullary spinal cord abscess
  - Septic arthritis/facet joint
- Pyogenic infection pathoanatomy different for adults and children
  - Adults: Vertebral endplates infected first with spread to adjacent disc space ⇒ spread to adjacent vertebral body, paravertebral tissues, epidural space
  - Children: Vascular channels cross growth plate allowing primary infection of intervertebral disc, with secondary infection of vertebral body
- Disc space infection

- Lumbar (45%) > thoracic (35%) > cervical (20%)
- DSI ⇒ epidural abscess
  - Cervical spine > thoracic > lumbar
- Risk factors
  - Age > 50
  - Diabetes
  - Rheumatoid arthritis
  - AIDS
  - Chronic steroid administration
  - Paraplegia
  - Urinary tract instrumentation
  - Prior spinal fracture
- Staph aureus most common organism (> 50%)
  - Pseudomonas may occur with drug abuse
  - Salmonella classic infection of sickle cell patients (S. aureus most common in this population)

Classification
- Waldvogel classification of bone infection
  - Hematogenous or secondary to contiguous infection
  - Contiguous infection either without or with vascular insufficiency
  - Acute or chronic phase
    - Acute phase shows suppurative infection with edema, vascular congestion, vessel thrombosis
    - Chronic infection shows infected dead bone (sequestra), ischemic tissue, refractory clinical course
- Cierny & Mader classification of bone infection
  - 4 anatomic disease types and 3 host categories
    - ⇒ 12 clinical stages
  - Anatomic disease types
    - Early hematogenous or medullary osteomyelitis
    - Superficial osteomyelitis (contiguous spread type)
    - Localized; full thickness sequestration
    - Diffuse osteomyelitis
  - Host classification
    - A: Normal physiologic response
    - B: Locally or systemically compromised response
    - C: Treatment of osteomyelitis would be worse than infection itself

DIFFERENTIAL DIAGNOSIS

Disc space irregularity
- Pyogenic disc space infection
- TB, fungal disc space infection
- Type I degenerative endplate changes
- Hemodialysis spondyloarthropathy
- Gout
- Seronegative spondyloarthropathy

Epidural mass
- Metastatic disease
- Abscess/phlegmon
- Disc herniation/osteophyte
- Primary bone tumor
- Hemorrhage

Subdural mass
- Postoperative benign effusion

- Hemorrhage
- Empyema

Meningeal/leptomeningeal
- Bacteria infection
- Viral infection (CMV)
- Autoimmune (AIDP, CIDP)
- Leptomeningeal metastatic disease
- Arachnoiditis

Cord
- Primary tumor (astrocytoma, ependymoma with ring-enhancement)
- Demyelinating disease may give ring-enhancement, cord edema
- Bacterial or parasitic infection (rare)

- Spinal tuberculosis classification (Mehta 2001)
  - Stable anterior lesions without kyphotic deformity
    - Treated with anterior debridement and strut grafting
  - Global lesions, kyphosis, instability
    - Treated with posterior instrumentation, anterior strut grafting
  - High risk for transthoracic surgery (medical or anesthetic complications)
    - Treated with posterior decompression, instrumentation
  - Isolated posterior lesions
    - Treated with posterior decompression

ANATOMY-BASED IMAGING ISSUES

Key Concepts or Questions
- Direct extension
  - Bone in contact with adjacent infection giving osteomyelitis
  - Typical route for intramedullary spinal cord abscess
    - Infection through congenital dysraphism/dermal sinus mechanism of infection → 40% of intramedullary abscesses
- Lymphatic spread
  - Limited in importance relative to hematogenous spread
- Hematogenous spread
  - Major pathway of infection spread to axial skeleton
    - Major pathway of intramedullary spinal cord abscess in adults
  - Arterial or venous route (controversial as to relative importance)
  - Arterial route important in spine infection spread
    - Metaphyseal bone near anterior longitudinal ligament has end arteriole network making it susceptible to bacterial seeding
    - Distal nonanastomosing vessels have slow flow, and occlusion leads to avascular necrosis
    - Segmental arteries usually supply two adjacent vertebral bodies and intervening disc, giving typical disc space infection pattern

- Venous route classically through Batson plexus
  - Longitudinal network of valveless veins running parallel to spinal column
  - Lie outside of thoracoabdominal cavity
  - Communicate with multiple venous systems: Spine, vena cava, portal, azygos, intercostal, pulmonary and renal
  - Flow direction in Batson plexus variable due to variable intrathoracic or intraabdominal pressure
  - Pharyngovertebral plexus serves same purpose
- CSF spread
  - Cranial ⇔ spinal
- Extension
  - Spine ⇒ psoas muscle
  - Extension to mediastinum
  - Extension through dura ⇒ meningitis

Other Imaging Issues
- Grisel syndrome ⇒ unilateral or bilateral subluxation C1 on C2, associated with an infectious condition in the head or neck
  - Associated with head/neck infection

CLINICAL IMPLICATIONS

Clinical Importance
- Spine = 2-5% of all osteomyelitis sites
- Axial spine pain most common presentation
- Progressive, although may have insidious onset
- Pain may be constant, without relief from rest
- Fever variable, and present in < 50% of cases
  - High grade fever in < 5%
- Motor/sensory deficits in 10-15%
  - Rare intramedullary abscess always present with motor and/or sensory neurological deficits
- Delay in diagnosis common
  - Intramedullary abscess fatal 8%, persistent neurologic deficit 70%
- Lab abnormalities
  - Erythrocyte sedimentation rate positive in > 90%
  - C reactive protein also elevated

INFECTIONS, PATHWAYS OF SPREAD

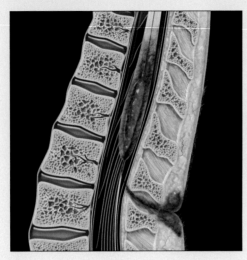

Sagittal graphic shows dermal sinus extending from skin surface to conus, with conus abscess, edema.

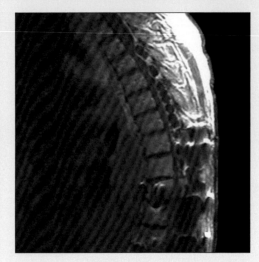

Sagittal T1W C+ MR shows extensive dorsal epidural abscess throughout thoracic spine with cord compression. Note extensive metal artifact from prior anterior/posterior fixation.

- ○ WBC elevation variable, average 12,000 (range 4,000-24,000)
- Blood cultures positive 25-60% cases
- Operative treatment
  - ○ May be necessary to obtain diagnosis
  - ○ Abscess drainage
  - ○ Presence of neurologic deficit
  - ○ Spine instability
  - ○ Spinal deformity
  - ○ Failure of medical treatment
    - No clinical/laboratory improvement with appropriate parenteral antibiotics in 2-3 weeks
  - ○ Medical treatment (I.V. antibiotics) first line of therapy if no acute or evolving neurologic deficit
    - 6 week course of I.V. antibiotics (culture specific) ± oral antibiotics with completion of I.V. regimen
    - External spine immobilization/bracing
    - Recurrent bacteremia, paravertebral abscesses, chronically draining sinuses associated with relapse
- Autofusion of infected level with successful non-operative treatment common (50-100%)

CUSTOM DIFFERENTIAL DIAGNOSIS

Hematogenous spread of infection
- Presumed typical route for pyogenic DSI
  - ○ Decreased T1 signal with loss of disc margin, endplate irregularity
  - ○ Increased T2 signal from intervertebral disc, adjacent vertebral bodies
  - ○ Enhancement of vertebral bodies, endplates, anulus (variable)

CSF spread of infection
- Hematogenous seeding
- Meningitis extension from cranial infection
- Associated with dermal sinus, CSF leak

Direct extension of infection
- Typical iatrogenic route
  - ○ Operative seeding
  - ○ Anesthetic catheter placement
  - ○ Lumbar puncture, discography
- Extension from adjacent soft tissue infection
  - ○ Mycotic infection extension from aorta

Lymphatic spread
- Uncommon route

SELECTED REFERENCES

1. Weinberg J et al: Infections of the spine: what the orthopedist needs to know. Am J Orthop. 33(1):13-7, 2004
2. Ledermann HP et al: MR imaging findings in spinal infections: rules or myths? Radiology. 228(2):506-14, 2003
3. McHenry MC et al: Vertebral osteomyelitis: long-term outcome for 253 patients from 7 Cleveland-area hospitals. Clin Infect Dis. 34(10):1342-50, 2002
4. Mehta JS et al: Tuberculosis of the thoracic spine. A classification based on the selection of surgical strategies. J Bone Joint Surg Br. 83(6):859-63, 2001
5. Gouliamos AD et al: MR imaging of tuberculous vertebral osteomyelitis: pictorial review. Eur Radiol. 11(4):575-9, 2001
6. Hadjipavlou AG et al: Hematogenous pyogenic spinal infections and their surgical management. Spine. 25(13):1668-79, 2000
7. Mader JT et al: Antimicrobial treatment of chronic osteomyelitis. Clin Orthop. (360):47-65, 1999
8. Mader JT et al: Staging and staging application in osteomyelitis. Clin Infect Dis. 25(6):1303-9, 1997
9. Mader JT et al: A practical guide to the diagnosis and management of bone and joint infections. Drugs. 54(2):253-64, 1997

INFECTIONS, PATHWAYS OF SPREAD

IMAGE GALLERY

Typical

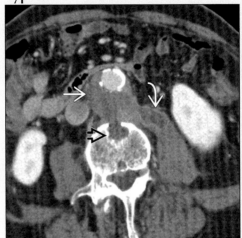
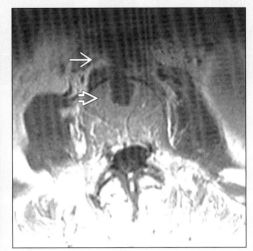

(Left) Axial CECT shows direct extension of infection from mycotic aortic aneurysm (arrow) into vertebral body (open arrow), and left psoas muscle (curved arrow). *(Right)* Axial T1 C+ MR shows direct extension of infection from mycotic aortic aneurysm (arrow), erosion of ventral vertebral body and osteomyelitis (open arrow). There is also direct extension into psoas.

Typical

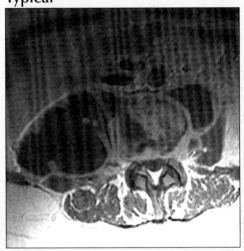
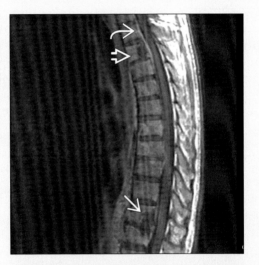

(Left) Axial T1 C+ MR shows extension of tuberculous spondylitis from vertebral body into psoas muscles bilaterally, forming large abscesses. Enhancing phlegmon also present in ventral epidural space. *(Right)* Sagittal T1 C+ MR shows multifaceted appearance of TB, with areas mimicking pyogenic infection (arrow), focal lesions like metastatic disease (open arrow), and dural enhancement (curved arrow).

Typical

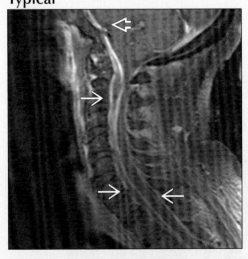
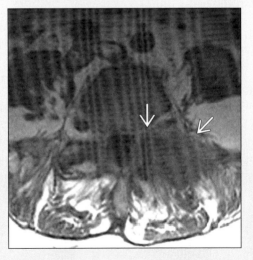

(Left) Sagittal T1 C+ MR with fat suppression shows extensive subdural empyema with peripheral enhancement (arrows) throughout the cervical spine, and extending along clivus (open arrow). *(Right)* Axial T1WI MR of lumbar spine shows left septic facet (arrows) with left facet bone destruction and infection extending into adjacent soft tissues.

PYOGENIC OSTEOMYELITIS

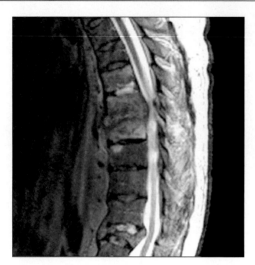

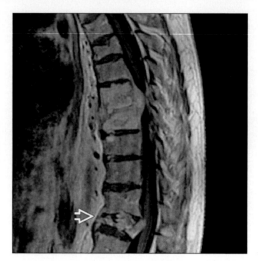

Sagittal T2WI MR shows hyperintense marrow in three consecutive thoracic vertebrae with loss of endplate definition. Intervertebral discs appear hyperintense and narrowed.

Sagittal T1 C+ MR shows enhancing vertebrae, disc, and epidural phlegmon, compatible with spondylodiscitis. Another infectious focus is present more caudally (arrow).

TERMINOLOGY

Abbreviations and Synonyms
- Pyogenic spondylodiscitis

Definitions
- Bacterial suppurative infection of vertebrae and intervertebral disc

IMAGING FINDINGS

General Features
- Best diagnostic clue: Ill-defined hypointense vertebral marrow on T1WI with loss of endplate definition on both sides of the disc
- Location
  - All spinal segments involved
    - Lumbar (48%) > thoracic (35%) > cervical spine (6.5%)
- Size
  - 2 adjacent vertebrae with intervening disc
    - 2/3 of pyogenic vertebral osteomyelitis
- Morphology
  - Disc space narrowing
  - Loss of vertebral endplate cortex
  - Ill-defined marrow signal alteration
  - Vertebral collapse

- Paraspinal ± epidural infiltrative soft tissue ± loculated fluid collection
  - In 75% of pyogenic vertebral osteomyelitis
- Variable central canal narrowing

Radiographic Findings
- Radiography
  - Negative up to 2-8 weeks after onset of symptoms
  - Initial endplate and vertebral osteolysis followed by increased bone density
  - Paraspinal soft tissue density
  - Fusion across disc space late in disease course

CT Findings
- NECT
  - Iso- to hypodense paraspinal soft tissue enlargement
    - ± Soft tissue gas
- CECT: Enhancing disc, marrow, and paravertebral soft tissue
- Bone CT
  - Endplate osteolytic/osteosclerotic changes
  - Bony sequestra
  - Spinal deformity best seen on coronal and sagittal reformation

MR Findings
- Disc space narrowing
  - Hypointense on T1WI
  - Variable, typically hyperintense on T2WI

DDx: Focal Vertebral Marrow Abnormality Adjacent to Endplate

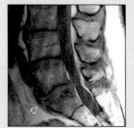

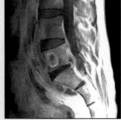

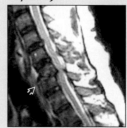

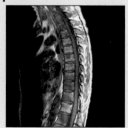

Type I Endplate   *TB Spondylitis*   *Hemodia. Spondylo.*   *Metastases*

PYOGENIC OSTEOMYELITIS

Key Facts

Terminology
- Pyogenic spondylodiscitis
- Bacterial suppurative infection of vertebrae and intervertebral disc

Imaging Findings
- Best diagnostic clue: Ill-defined hypointense vertebral marrow on T1WI with loss of endplate definition on both sides of the disc
- Lumbar (48%) > thoracic (35%) > cervical spine (6.5%)
- 2 adjacent vertebrae with intervening disc
- Disc space narrowing
- Loss of vertebral endplate cortex
- Ill-defined marrow signal alteration
- Vertebral collapse

- Paraspinal ± epidural infiltrative soft tissue ± loculated fluid collection
- Variable central canal narrowing
- CECT: Enhancing disc, marrow, and paravertebral soft tissue
- Cord compression with ill-defined T2 hyperintensity

Top Differential Diagnoses
- Degenerative endplate changes
- Tuberculous vertebral osteomyelitis
- Spinal neuropathic arthropathy
- Chronic hemodialysis spondyloarthropathy

Clinical Issues
- Acute or chronic back pain
- Focal spinal tenderness
- Fever

- ○ Diffuse post-gadolinium enhancement
- Vertebral marrow signal abnormality abutting disc
  - ○ Hypointense on T1WI
  - ○ Hyperintense on fat-saturated T2WI or STIR
  - ○ Avid enhancement with gadolinium
- Paraspinal and epidural phlegmon or abscess
  - ○ Isointense to muscle on T1WI
  - ○ Hyperintense on T2WI
  - ○ Diffuse or rim-enhancement
- Cord compression with ill-defined T2 hyperintensity

Ultrasonographic Findings
- Real Time: Anechoic or hypoechoic paraspinal abscess
- Color Doppler: Hyperemia and increased vascularity surrounding abscess

Nuclear Medicine Findings
- Bone Scan: 3 phase technetium Tc 99m diphosphonate scan shows arterial hyperemia and progressive skeletal radionuclide uptake
- Gallium Scan
  - ○ Increased uptake of gallium citrate (Ga 67)
    - ▪ Increased sensitivity with SPECT
  - ○ May be used in combination with bone scan
- WBC Scan
  - ○ Often false negative in patients with chronic vertebral osteomyelitis

Imaging Recommendations
- Best imaging tool
  - ○ Sagittal and axial T2WI and T1WI MRI
    - ▪ Sensitivity 96%, specificity 92%, accuracy 94%
  - ○ SPECT Ga 67 scan good alternative
    - ▪ Sensitivity and specificity in low 90%
- Protocol advice
  - ○ STIR or FSE T2 with fat suppression most sensitive for marrow edema and epidural involvement
  - ○ Post-gadolinium T1WI with fat suppression also improves MR sensitivity

DIFFERENTIAL DIAGNOSIS

Degenerative endplate changes
- Most common mimic
- Disc desiccation
  - ○ Hypointense on T1WI and T2WI
  - ○ Mild post-gadolinium enhancement, often linear
- Vertebral endplates preserved
- Degenerative marrow pattern
- Disc aspiration in difficult cases
  - ○ Hyperintense disc space on T2WI, endplate irregularity

Tuberculous vertebral osteomyelitis
- Mid-thoracic or thoracolumbar > lumbar, cervical
- Vertebral collapse and gibbus deformity
- ± Endplate destructive changes
- Subligamentous spread of infection
- Large dissecting paraspinal abscesses out of proportion to vertebral involvement

Spinal neuropathic arthropathy
- Sequela of spinal cord injury
- Disc space loss/T2 hyperintensity, endplate erosion/sclerosis, osteophytosis, soft tissue mass
  - ○ Present in both spondylodiscitis and neuropathic spine
- Vacuum disc/rim-enhancement, facet involvement, spondylolisthesis, debris, disorganization
  - ○ More common in neuropathic spine

Chronic hemodialysis spondyloarthropathy
- Cervical spine most common
- Disc space loss, endplate erosion, vertebral destruction
- Vertebral marrow hypointense on both T1WI and T2WI
- Low to intermediate disc signal intensity on T2WI
- ± Soft tissue component
- Clinical history of renal disease and hemodialysis
- Presence of amyloid on biopsy

Spinal metastases
- Discrete or ill-defined vertebral lesions
  - ○ Hypointense on T1WI

PYOGENIC OSTEOMYELITIS

- ○ Hyperintense on T2WI
- ○ Post-gadolinium enhancement
- Non-contiguous vertebral involvement
- Posterior elements commonly effected
- Disc space preserved

PATHOLOGY

General Features

- General path comments: Along a spectrum of suppurative infection involving disc, vertebrae, and adjacent soft tissue
- Etiology
  - ○ Predisposing factors
    - Intravenous drug use
    - Immunocompromised state
    - Chronic medical illnesses such as renal failure, cirrhosis, cancer, diabetes
  - ○ Staphylococcus aureus is the most common pathogen
    - Escherichia coli most common within gram-negative bacilli
    - Salmonella more common in patients with sickle cell disease
  - ○ Bacteremia from an extraspinal primary source
    - Most common route of infection
    - GU or GI tract, lungs, cardiac, mucous/cutaneous sources
    - Vascularized subchondral bone adjacent to endplate seeded primarily
    - Secondary infection of intervertebral disc and adjacent vertebra
    - Intervertebral disc first site of infection in children due to presence of vascularity
  - ○ Direct inoculation from penetrating trauma, surgical intervention, or diagnostic procedures
    - Epidural injection/catheter
  - ○ Extension from adjacent infection in paraspinal soft tissues
    - Diverticulitis, appendicitis, inflammatory bowel disease
    - Pyelonephritis
- Epidemiology: 2-7% of osteomyelitis in US
- Associated abnormalities
  - ○ Spinal meningitis
  - ○ Myelitis

Gross Pathologic & Surgical Features

- Necrotic bone
- Suppurative soft tissue

Microscopic Features

- Bone/disc fragments
- Leukocytes, micro-organisms, cellular debris
- Vascular proliferation

CLINICAL ISSUES

Presentation

- Most common signs/symptoms
  - ○ Acute or chronic back pain
  - ○ Focal spinal tenderness

- ○ Fever
- ○ Other signs/symptoms
  - Myelopathy if cord compromised
  - Elevated erythrocyte sedimentation rate, C-reactive protein, and white cell count
- Clinical profile: Average duration of symptoms for 7 weeks before diagnosis

Demographics

- Age
  - ○ Bimodal distribution
    - Pediatric patients
    - 60-70s
- Gender: Slight male predominance

Natural History & Prognosis

- Vertebral collapse
- Irreversible neurological deficits
- Mortality rate of 2-12%
- Favorable outcome with resolution of symptoms if prompt diagnosis and treatment
  - ○ Residual functional deficits may be present in 15% of patients
- Recurrence due to incomplete treatment: 2-8%

Treatment

- Early empiric antibiotics with broad spectrum coverage until causative pathogen isolated
  - ○ Coverage should be effective against staphylococci, gram negatives, and anaerobes
- Organism specific parenteral antibiotics for 6-8 weeks
- Spinal immobilization with bracing for 6-12 weeks
- Surgical treatment
  - ○ Laminectomy, debridement, ± stabilization
  - ○ Especially if epidural abscess, instability present

DIAGNOSTIC CHECKLIST

Image Interpretation Pearls

- Diffusely enhancing disc, adjacent vertebral marrow, and soft tissue with endplate erosion highly suggestive of vertebral osteomyelitis

SELECTED REFERENCES

1. Ledermann HP et al: MR imaging findings in spinal infections: rules or myths? Radiology. 228(2):506-14, 2003
2. Love C et al: Diagnosing spinal osteomyelitis: a comparison of bone and Ga-67 scintigraphy and magnetic resonance imaging. Clin Nucl Med. 25(12):963-77, 2000
3. Wagner SC et al: Can imaging findings help differentiate spinal neuropathic arthropathy from disk space infection? Initial experience. Radiology. 214(3):693-9, 2000
4. Carragee EJ: The clinical use of magnetic resonance imaging in pyogenic vertebral osteomyelitis. Spine. 22(7):780-5, 1997
5. Dagirmanjian A et al: MR Imaging of Vertebral Osteomyelitis Revisited. AJR. 167:1539-43, 1996
6. Thrush A et al: MR Imaging of Infectious Spondylitis. AJNR. 11:1171-80, 1990
7. Modic MT et al: Vertebral osteomyelitis: assessment using MR. Radiology. 157(1):157-66, 1985

IMAGE GALLERY

Typical

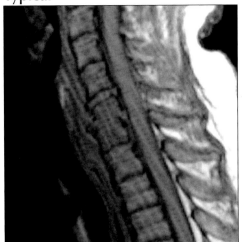
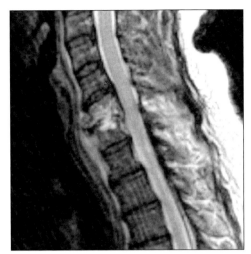

(Left) Sagittal T1WI MR shows C6 and C7 vertebral endplate erosion with associated hypointense marrow and intervertebral disc space narrowing. (Right) Sagittal T2WI MR demonstrates hyperintensity in C6 vertebra, extending into disc space and C7 vertebra. Prevertebral phlegmon is also present.

Typical

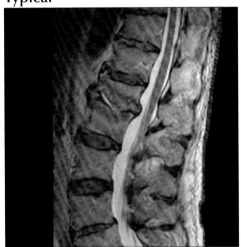
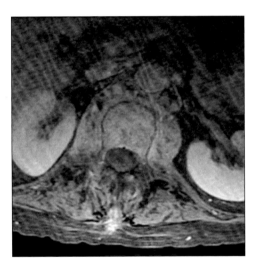

(Left) Sagittal T2WI MR shows vertebral collapse, endplate erosion, and hyperintense narrowed disc space at L1-2, compatible with discitis and vertebral osteomyelitis. (Right) Axial T1 C+ MR with fat suppression reveals enhancing paravertebral phlegmon at L1-2.

Typical

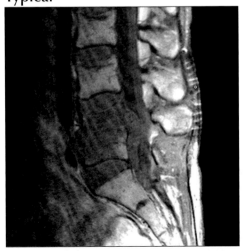
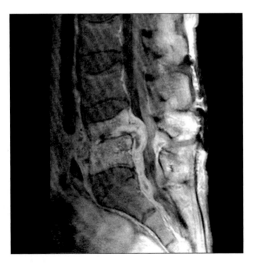

(Left) Sagittal T1WI MR in a patient with history of lumbar surgery shows hypointense marrow, vertebral collapse, endplate erosion, disc space loss, and epidural soft tissue at L4-5. (Right) Sagittal T1 C+ MR demonstrates enhancing vertebrae, disc, & epidural abscess extending from L4-5 to S1. Consistent with pyogenic vertebral osteomyelitis. Central canal narrowing is present at L4-5.

GRANULOMATOUS OSTEOMYELITIS

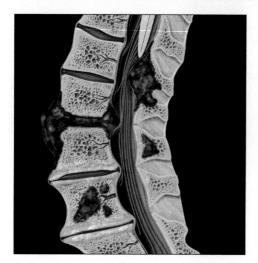

Sagittal graphic through lumbar spine depicts multifocal granulomatous osteomyelitis. Frank abscesses are present at L3-4 disc space and between spinous process of L2 and L3.

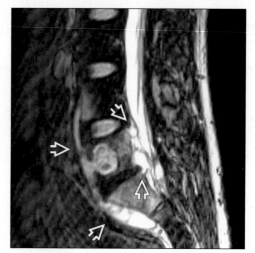

Sagittal STIR MR shows classic TS. There is an anterior intraosseous abscess in L5 with ventral extension. Subligamentous spread of infection is present (arrows), reaching anterior L4.

TERMINOLOGY

Abbreviations and Synonyms
- Tuberculous spondylitis (TS): Pott disease

Definitions
- Granulomatous infection of spine and adjacent soft tissue typically caused by tuberculosis or brucellosis

IMAGING FINDINGS

General Features
- Best diagnostic clue
  - Gibbus vertebrae with relatively intact intervertebral discs and large paraspinal abscesses in TS
  - Anterosuperior epiphysitis at L4 with associated sacroiliitis in brucellar spondylitis (BS)
- Location
  - TS
    - Mid-thoracic or thoracolumbar > lumbar, cervical
    - Anterior vertebral body
    - Isolated posterior element involvement possible
    - Laminae > pedicles > spinous process > transverse process
  - BS
    - Lower lumbar spine (L4) > cervical = thoracic
    - Sacroiliac joints

- Posterior elements not effected
- Anterior endplate at diskovertebral junction involved in focal BS
- Entire vertebral body effected in diffuse BS
- Size: Multiple (non)contiguous vertebrae
- Morphology
  - TS
    - Vertebral collapse and gibbus deformity
    - ± Destruction of intervertebral discs
    - Epidural soft tissue mass
    - Large dissecting paraspinal abscesses over considerable distance
    - Out of proportion relative to degree of vertebral destruction
  - BS
    - Vertebrae morphologically intact despite osteomyelitis
    - Spinal deformity rare
    - Destruction of intervertebral discs
    - Epidural soft tissue mass
    - Paraspinal soft tissues rarely effected

Radiographic Findings
- Radiography
  - Findings may not be present until weeks after onset of infection
  - Endplate irregularity and osteolysis
  - Vertebral sclerosis
    - Focal in BS vs. diffuse in TS

DDx: Vertebral Disc and Marrow Abnormalities

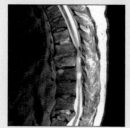

Pyogenic Spondylitis

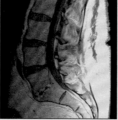

Pyogenic Spondylitis

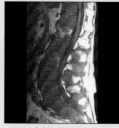

Metastases

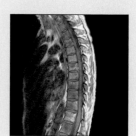

Metastases

GRANULOMATOUS OSTEOMYELITIS

Key Facts

Terminology
- Tuberculous spondylitis (TS): Pott disease
- Granulomatous infection of spine and adjacent soft tissue typically caused by tuberculosis or brucellosis

Imaging Findings
- Gibbus vertebrae with relatively intact intervertebral discs and large paraspinal abscesses in TS
- Size: Multiple (non)contiguous vertebrae
- Endplate irregularity and osteolysis
- Vertebral sclerosis
- Fusion across disc space in late TS and BS
- NECT: Calcifications of chronic paravertebral abscesses: TS > BS
- Osseous destruction

- T2WI: Hyperintense marrow, disc, soft tissue infection
- Marrow, subligamentous, discal, dural enhancement
- Diffuse or peripherally enhancing soft tissue
- Increased radionuclide uptake in spine and paraspinal soft tissue

Top Differential Diagnoses
- Pyogenic spondylitis (PS)
- Fungal spondylitis
- Spinal metastases

Clinical Issues
- Chronic back pain
- Focal tenderness
- Fever

- Fusion across disc space in late TS and BS
- Disc gas and endplate osteophytes in BS

CT Findings
- NECT: Calcifications of chronic paravertebral abscesses: TS > BS
- CECT: Diffuse or peripherally enhancing epidural and paraspinal soft tissue
- Bone CT
  - Osseous destruction
    - Focal in BS vs. diffuse in TS
  - Bony sequestra

MR Findings
- T1WI
  - Hypointense marrow in adjacent vertebrae
  - Hypointense intraosseous, extradural, paraspinal abscesses
- T2WI: Hyperintense marrow, disc, soft tissue infection
- STIR: Hyperintense marrow, disc, phlegmon/abscess
- T1 C+
  - Marrow, subligamentous, discal, dural enhancement
  - Diffuse or peripherally enhancing soft tissue
- Cord displacement or compression from epidural abscess
- 39% with extradural infection without bone destruction
- Atypical findings in TS
  - Isolated vertebral body or posterior element involvement
    - Hypointense on T1WI
    - Hyperintense on T2WI
    - Diffuse enhancement
  - Sacral involvement

Nuclear Medicine Findings
- Bone Scan: Increased spinal radionuclide uptake
- Gallium Scan
  - Increased radionuclide uptake in spine and paraspinal soft tissue
    - 100% sensitive and specific for vertebral osteomyelitis

Imaging Recommendations
- Best imaging tool
  - Sagittal and axial T1WI, T2WI and T1 C+ MR
    - Evaluate extent of disease and assess response to treatment
- Protocol advice: Sagittal STIR or FSE T2 with fat-saturation most sensitive for bone marrow edema and epidural involvement

DIFFERENTIAL DIAGNOSIS

Pyogenic spondylitis (PS)
- Peak incidence in older patients
- Predilection for lower lumbar spine
- Initial infection in subchondral bone adjacent to endplate
  - Intervertebral discs typically effected
- Posterior element involvement less common
- Soft tissue calcifications and spinal deformity infrequent

Fungal spondylitis
- May be indistinguishable from TS
  - ± Posterior element involvement
  - Disc space may be spared
- Vertebral deformity less common than TS
- Paraspinal involvement not as extensive as TS

Spinal metastases
- Hypointense on T1WI and hyperintense on T2WI
  - Post-gadolinium enhancement
  - Posterior elements typically involved
- Extraosseous epidural or paraspinal extension
- Pathologic compression fractures
- Disc space preserved
- May be difficult to distinguish from isolated tuberculous, fungal, or brucellar spondylitis

GRANULOMATOUS OSTEOMYELITIS

PATHOLOGY

General Features
- General path comments: Granulomatous destruction of spinal column with adjacent soft tissue infection
- Etiology
  - TS
    - Hematogenous spread or through lymphatics from pulmonary origin
    - Initial inoculum in anterior vertebral body
    - Spread to (non)adjacent vertebral bodies beneath longitudinal ligaments
    - Sparing of intervertebral disc due to lack of proteolytic enzymes
    - Paraspinal, subarachnoid dissemination of disease
  - BS
    - Access to spine via hematogenous dissemination
    - Direct extension to adjacent discs and vertebrae
  - Other pathogens causing granulomatous osteomyelitis (Streptomycis, Madurella) uncommon
- Epidemiology
  - Rising incidence of tuberculosis in past two decades
  - TS in less than 1% of patients with tuberculosis
  - Concomitant pulmonary tuberculosis in about 10% of patients
  - TS more aggressive in children
    - Kyphosis and cord compression more common
  - Brucellosis uncommon in US: 100-200 cases per year
    - Prevalent in Mediterranean, South and Central America, Middle East with reported incidence between 6-58%
- Associated abnormalities
  - Intramedullary abscess
  - Arachnoiditis

Microscopic Features
- Both TS and BS show caseating granulomas and nonspecific inflammatory reaction
- Acid fast bacilli isolated < 50% of time
- Brucellar species very difficult to culture

CLINICAL ISSUES

Presentation
- Most common signs/symptoms
  - Chronic back pain
  - Focal tenderness
  - Fever
  - Other signs/symptoms
    - Paraparesis
    - Kyphosis
    - Sensory disturbance
    - Bladder and bowel dysfunction
- Clinical profile
  - Gradual, insidious onset of symptoms results in diagnostic delay
    - Mean delay of 14 weeks
  - Fever relatively infrequent in TS compared to PS
  - Neurologic deficits more common with TS compared to BS and PS

Demographics
- Age

- TS: Most prevalent in 50s
- BS: More common in 60s
- Gender
  - M = F in TS
  - M:F = 2.4:1 in BS

Natural History & Prognosis
- Prognosis depends on early diagnosis and institution of appropriate therapy
- If untreated
  - Progressive vertebral collapse
  - Irreversible neurologic deficits
  - Death
- With proper treatment
  - Favorable outcome with resolution of symptoms
    - Especially with early presentation and lack of neurologic deficits or spinal deformity

Treatment
- Antibrucellar medications highly effective
  - Surgical debridement rarely indicated
- Long term antituberculous medication for at least one year
- Surgical decompression in setting of neurologic deficits ± spinal deformity
  - Indicated in 10-25% of TS
  - Laminectomy and debridement in absence of vertebral destruction
  - Debridement and fusion if spinal deformity present

DIAGNOSTIC CHECKLIST

Image Interpretation Pearls
- Thoracic spondylitis with posterior element involvement and large paraspinal abscesses suggestive of TS
- BS should be in differential diagnosis of lumbar spondylitis at L4 with associated bilateral sacroiliitis

SELECTED REFERENCES
1. Akman S et al: Magnetic resonance imaging of tuberculous spondylitis. Orthopedics. 26(1):69-73, 2003
2. Narlawar RS et al: Isolated tuberculosis of posterior elements of spine: magnetic resonance imaging findings in 33 patients. Spine. 27(3):275-81, 2002
3. Gouliamos AD et al: MR imaging of tuberculous vertebral osteomyelitis: pictorial review. Eur Radiol. 11(4):575-9, 2001
4. Hadjipavlou AG et al: The effectiveness of gallium citrate Ga 67 radionuclide imaging in vertebral osteomyelitis revisited. Am J Orthop. 27(3):179-83, 1998
5. Sharif HS et al: Granulomatous spinal infections: MR imaging. Radiology. 177(1):101-7, 1990
6. Sharif HS et al: Brucellar and tuberculous spondylitis: comparative imaging features. Radiology. 171(2):419-25, 1989
7. Smith AS et al: MR imaging characteristics of tuberculous spondylitis vs vertebral osteomyelitis. AJNR. 10:619-25, 1989

GRANULOMATOUS OSTEOMYELITIS

IMAGE GALLERY

Typical

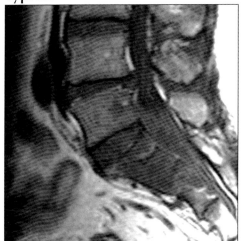 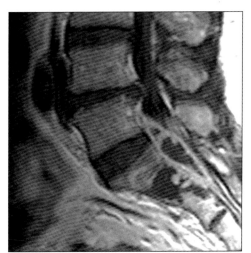

(Left) Sagittal T1WI MR shows hypointense S1 & S2 bodies from TB osteomyelitis with epidural extension (incidental herniation L4-5). (Right) Sagittal T1 C+ MR shows irregular peripheral enhancement of sacral TB osteomyelitis and epidural abscess. Note sparring of L5 disc space.

Typical

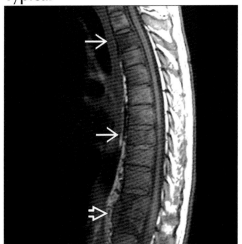 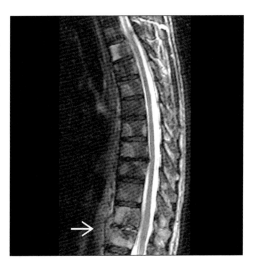

(Left) Sagittal T1WI MR shows diffuse TB involvement of thoracic spine with focal bone (arrows) and paravertebral (open arrow) patterns. (Right) Sagittal T2WI MR shows multiple foci of hyperintensity within vertebral bosies form TB osteomyelitis. Note prevertebral extension (arrow).

Typical

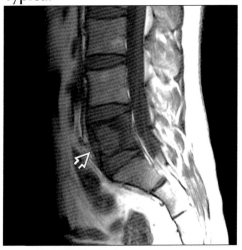 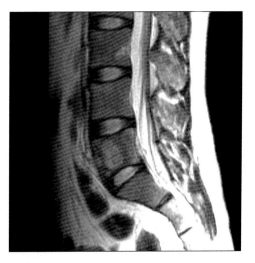

(Left) Sagittal T1WI MR of a patient with TS shows a well-defined intraosseous lesion in L5, slightly hypointense compared to marrow, with surrounding edema. There is ventral subligamentous spread (arrow). (Right) Sagittal T2WI MR shows L5 intraosseous lesion, which is hyperintense. Anterior vertebral cortex of L5 appears eroded.

OSTEOMYELITIS, C1-C2

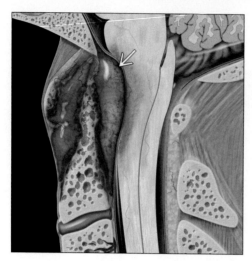

Sagittal graphic shows osteomyelitis involving odontoid with bone destruction, extension to anterior arch of C1, epidural abscess formation (open arrow).

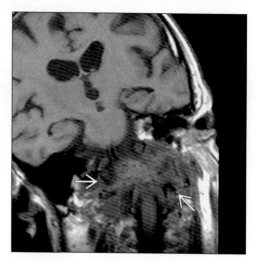

Coronal T1WI MR shows craniocervical osteomyelitis with extensive soft tissue destruction involving C0-C1, C1-C2 articulations (arrows) with lateral subluxation of cranium.

TERMINOLOGY

Abbreviations and Synonyms
- Atlanto-axial osteomyelitis

Definitions
- Infection of C1-2 articulation (pyogenic or tuberculous)

IMAGING FINDINGS

General Features
- Best diagnostic clue: Soft tissue mass and bone destruction at C1-2 level
- Location: C1 anterior arch, atlanto-axial joint, dens, C2 body
- Size: Variable, may have large epidural abscess
- Morphology: Irregular soft tissue mass involving multiple spaces/vertebral bodies

Radiographic Findings
- Radiography
  - Gross bone destruction manifested late in course
    - Sensitivity 80%, specificity 50-60%
  - Early changes with indistinct anterior margin of C1, prevertebral soft tissue swelling
- Fluoroscopy: Useful in assessing C1-2 subluxation

- Myelography: May show nonspecific extradural defect in contrast column at C1-2 related to epidural extension of infection

CT Findings
- NECT
  - Variable bone destruction involving anterior arch C1, odontoid and body of C2
  - Soft tissue mass adjacent to bone lesions within prevertebral space, variable extension into epidural space
- CECT: Enhancement of soft tissue component; may show nonenhancing abscess focus
- CTA: Useful if question of skull base, C1-2 instability with vertebral artery compromise

MR Findings
- T1WI
  - Low signal mass centered at C1-2 with variable involvement of odontoid and lateral masses C2
  - May show enlarged atlanto-dental interval
  - Prevertebral increased soft tissue/edema
  - Epidural mass with thecal sac/cord compression
- T2WI: Diffuse increased signal from vertebral bodies, soft tissue mass
- STIR: Diffuse increased signal from vertebral bodies, soft tissue mass
- DWI
  - May show restricted diffusion of abscess component

DDx: Cranio-Cervical Junction Abnormality

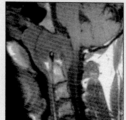

Chordoma

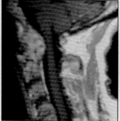

Rheumatoid Arthritis

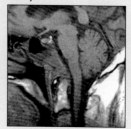

Metastasis

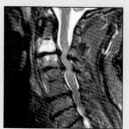

Type I Endplate

Key Facts

Imaging Findings
- Best imaging tool: MRI with contrast ± MRA; shows bone involvement, prevertebral soft tissues, epidural space, vertebral arteries

Top Differential Diagnoses
- C1-C2 osteoarthritis
- Rheumatoid arthritis
- Chordoma
- Primary bone tumor
- Nasopharyngeal carcinoma
- Extension of skull base osteomyelitis
- Degenerative endplate changes
- Odontoid fracture
- Hemodialysis spondyloarthropathy
- Gout

Pathology
- Staph aureus most common organism in USA

Clinical Issues
- IV antibiotics, followed by prolonged oral antibiotic administration
- Surgical decompression/stabilization

Diagnostic Checklist
- Grisel syndrome: Inflammatory, non-traumatic subluxation of C1-C2 following peripharyngeal infection
- Attributed to laxity of transverse/alar ligaments by hyperemia
- Associated with otitis media, pharyngitis, retropharyngeal abscess, upper respiratory infections

---

- o Brain diffusion shows posterior circulation infarcts if vertebral artery compromise
- T1 C+
  - o Diffuse enhancement of vertebral bodies, soft tissue mass within prevertebral region/epidural space
    - Phlegmon shows diffuse enhancement
    - Abscess shows peripheral enhancement, central nonenhancing pus
- MRA: Useful if question of skull base, C1-2 instability with vertebral artery compromise

Nuclear Medicine Findings
- Bone Scan
  - o Technetium-99m methylene diphosphonate SPECT
    - Arterial hyperemia with progressive increased uptake in osteomyelitis
  - o High sensitivity (90%), low specificity (75%)
    - Three phase bone scanning overall accuracy 90%
    - Specificity increased by combining indium-labeled WBC scan or gallium-67 scan
    - Unreliable for diagnosis of active TB (scans cold in 35-40%)
- PET
  - o FDG PET shows nonspecific increased uptake with infection, tumor
    - No uptake with degenerative endplate changes
- Gallium Scan
  - o Increased uptake, nonspecific
- WBC Scan
  - o Increased uptake in acute phase
  - o High specificity, low sensitivity

Imaging Recommendations
- Best imaging tool: MRI with contrast ± MRA; shows bone involvement, prevertebral soft tissues, epidural space, vertebral arteries
- Protocol advice: T1WI, T2WI axial, sagittal images; post-contrast axial, sagittal with fat suppression; 3D TOF MRA

DIFFERENTIAL DIAGNOSIS

C1-C2 osteoarthritis
- May show pseudo pannus from osteoarthritic degenerative change
- Bone irregularity, low signal, and soft tissue mass dorsal to odontoid

Rheumatoid arthritis
- Erosion of odontoid, soft tissue pannus, C1-2 subluxation, subaxial subluxations

Chordoma
- Soft tissue mass, increased T2W signal

Metastatic disease
- Focal low signal on T1WI, with bone destruction, epidural extension
- Multiple lesions

Primary bone tumor
- Enhancing soft tissue mass destroying vertebral body/posterior elements
- Center of lesion in C2 body, not at C1-2 articulation

Nasopharyngeal carcinoma
- Center of soft tissue at nasopharynx, with clival involvement

Extension of skull base osteomyelitis
- Sphenoid, petrous apex inflammatory change with secondary inferior extension

Degenerative endplate changes
- Parallel signal alteration of vertebral endplates, associated with evidence of disc degeneration
- PET hypometabolic

Odontoid fracture
- Fracture line defined by GRE, T1W images, STIR shows marrow/prevertebral edema

Hemodialysis spondyloarthropathy
- Low signal on T1WI involving endplates similar to pyogenic disc space infection

OSTEOMYELITIS, C1-C2

- May be indistinguishable from pyogenic disc space infection

Gout

- Rarely vertebral involvement with low signal involving endplates, similar to disc space infection

PATHOLOGY

General Features

- General path comments
  - Staph aureus most common organism in USA
  - Mycobacterium tuberculosis most common worldwide
  - Brucella, Pseudomonas, Serratia & Candida organisms common in IV drug addicts, immunocompromised patients
  - Infection starts as septic arthritis of C1-2
- Etiology
  - Hematogenous seeding to capillary ends/end arterioles in subchondral regions
  - Many vascular anastomoses
    - Pharyngovertebral plexus drains posterosuperior nasopharynx inferiorly to basiocciput penetrating atlanto-occipital membrane
    - Pharyngovertebral plexus ⇔ lymphatics
    - Periodontoidal venous plexus ⇔ pharyngovertebral veins
    - Batson plexus allows seeding from viscera
- Epidemiology
  - Uncommon; most cervical infections C5 & C6 region
  - Risk factors include diabetes, drug abuse, endocarditis, immunocompromise
- Associated abnormalities: C1-C2 subluxation, cervicomedullary junction compression; vertebral artery compression

CLINICAL ISSUES

Presentation

- Most common signs/symptoms
  - Neck pain, stiffness, limited range of motion, dysphagia
  - Other signs/symptoms
    - Triad of fever, pain, neurologic deficit in minority of cases
    - C1-2 subluxation, medulla compression and motor/sensory deficit
    - Vertebral artery compression with posterior circulation infarction

Demographics

- Age: Adult > child
- Gender: No gender preference

Treatment

- I.V. antibiotics, followed by prolonged oral antibiotic administration
- Surgical decompression/stabilization
  - Variable approaches; anterior debridement and posterior cervical-occipital arthrodesis

DIAGNOSTIC CHECKLIST

Consider

- Grisel syndrome: Inflammatory, non-traumatic subluxation of C1-C2 following peripharyngeal infection
  - Attributed to laxity of transverse/alar ligaments by hyperemia
  - Associated with otitis media, pharyngitis, retropharyngeal abscess, upper respiratory infections
  - Present with pain, head tilt, restricted neck movement
  - Head position classically 20° tilt, 20° rotation giving "cock-robin" position

Image Interpretation Pearls

- Severe C1-2 subluxation: Check posterior circulation for infarcts due to vertebral compression, check for medullary compression

SELECTED REFERENCES

1. Krishnan A et al: Craniovertebral junction tuberculosis: a review of 29 cases. J Comput Assist Tomogr. 25(2): 171-6, 2001
2. Magliulo G et al: Osteomyelitis of the skull base with atypical onset and evolution. Ann Otol Rhinol Laryngol. 109(3): 326-30, 2000
3. Chan LL et al: Imaging of mucormycosis skull base osteomyelitis. AJNR Am J Neuroradiol. 21(5): 828-31, 2000
4. Subburaman N et al: Skull base osteomyelitis interpreted as malignancy. J Laryngol Otol. 113(8): 775-8, 1999
5. Chong VF et al: The retropharyngeal space: route of tumour spread. Clin Radiol. 53(1): 64-7, 1998
6. Swift AC et al: Skull base osteitis following fungal sinusitis. J Laryngol Otol. 112(1): 92-7, 1998
7. Jones DC et al: Oropharyngeal morbidity following transoral approaches to the upper cervical spine. Int J Oral Maxillofac Surg. 27(4): 295-8, 1998
8. Baker LL et al: Atlanto-axial subluxation and cervical osteomyelitis: two unusual complications of adenoidectomy. Ann Otol Rhinol Laryngol. 105(4):295-9, 1996
9. Lam CH et al: Conservative therapy of atlantoaxial osteomyelitis. A case report. Spine. 21(15):1820-3, 1996
10. Gormley W et al: Spontaneous atlantoaxial osteomyelitis: no longer a rare case? Case report. Neurosurgery. 35(1):132-5; discussion 135-6, 1994
11. Wetzel FT et al: Grisel's syndrome. Clin Orthop. (240):141-52, 1989
12. Wilson BC et al: Nontraumatic subluxation of the atlantoaxial joint: Grisel's syndrome. Ann Otol Rhinol Laryngol. 96(6):705-8, 1987
13. Zigler JE et al: Pyogenic osteomyelitis of the occiput, the atlas, and the axis. A report of five cases. J Bone Joint Surg Am. 69(7):1069-73, 1987

IMAGE GALLERY

Typical

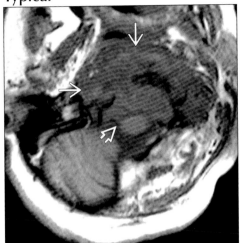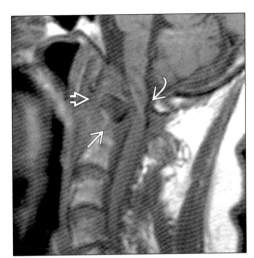

(Left) Axial T1WI MR shows large destructive mass engulfing C0-C1 articulation (arrows) with destruction of anterior arch C1, prevertebral extension, epidural extension effacing cord (open arrow). (Right) Sagittal T1WI MR shows C1-2 infection involving odontoid (arrow), with atlanto-axial joint extension (open arrow), C1-2 subluxation, cord compression (curved arrow).

Typical

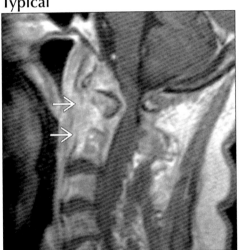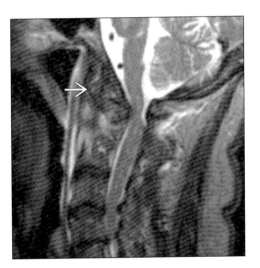

(Left) Sagittal T1 C+ MR shows C1-2 osteomyelitis with extensive enhancement of C2 body, odontoid with extensive prevertebral phlegmon (arrows). There is atlanto-axial subluxation and cord compression. (Right) Sagittal T2WI MR shows increased signal from odontoid/body of C2 in this case of C1-2 osteomyelitis. Anterior arch of C1 is involved by phlegmon (arrow), with C1-2 subluxation and cord compression.

Variant

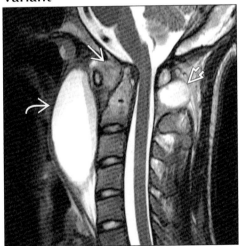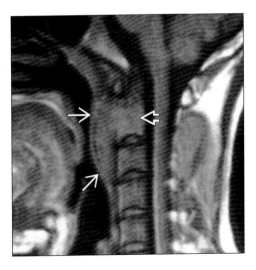

(Left) Sagittal T2WI MR shows tuberculous spondylitis involving C1-2 articulation, with C1-2 subluxation (arrow), dorsal (open arrow) and ventral (curved arrow) abscesses (Courtesy R. Harnsberger, MD). (Right) Sagittal T1WI MR shows tuberculous osteomyelitis involving C2 body (open arrow), extending ventral to C1-2 articulation into prevertebral soft tissues (arrows).

SEPTIC FACET JOINT ARTHRITIS

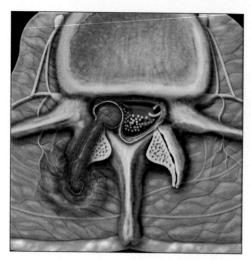

Axial graphic through lumbar vertebra demonstrates right facet joint osteomyelitis and abscess, extending into subarticular recess and posterior paraspinal muscle.

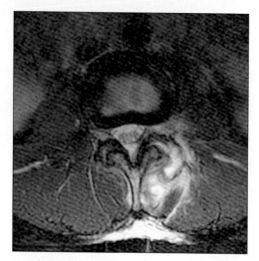

Axial T2WI MR with fat suppression through lumbar vertebra shows fluid intensity expanding left facet joint & extending posteriorly. There is hyperintense edema in surrounding soft tissue.

TERMINOLOGY

Abbreviations and Synonyms
- Pyogenic facet joint infection

Definitions
- Suppurative bacterial infection of facet joint, adjacent soft tissue

IMAGING FINDINGS

General Features
- Best diagnostic clue: Abnormal enhancement within facet joint with associated facet marrow, adjacent soft tissue edema
- Location: Lumbar spine most common: 97%
- Size
  - Typically single level involvement
    - Unilateral
- Morphology
  - Facet joint widening
  - Eroded facet cortex
  - Ill-defined facet marrow signal alteration

Radiographic Findings
- Radiography
  - May be negative up to 2-8 weeks after onset of infection

  - Osteolytic/sclerotic facet joint
  - Periarticular soft tissue density
- Fluoroscopy
  - ± Instability on flexion/extension views
    - ≥ 4 mm of translation
    - > 10° of angular motion between adjacent vertebrae
    - Up to 3 mm of translation considered normal

CT Findings
- NECT
  - Low density within expanded facet joint
  - ± Juxtaarticular, epidural, and paraspinal phlegmon or abscess
- CECT
  - Diffuse or rim-enhancement within facet joint
    - ± Extraarticular extension
  - Diffuse or peripherally enhancing epidural and paraspinal soft tissue
- Bone CT
  - Mixed lytic/sclerotic facet changes
  - Bony debris
  - Spondylolisthesis best seen on sagittal reformation

MR Findings
- T1WI
  - Hypointensity within facet joint
  - Ill-defined hypointense facet marrow
- T2WI

DDx: Facet Joint Lesions

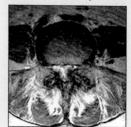
Facet Osteoarthritis

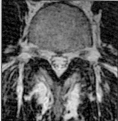
Facet Osteoarthritis

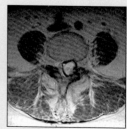
Synovial Cyst

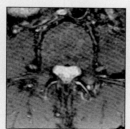
Metastasis

SEPTIC FACET JOINT ARTHRITIS

Key Facts

Terminology
- Pyogenic facet joint infection

Imaging Findings
- Best diagnostic clue: Abnormal enhancement within facet joint with associated facet marrow, adjacent soft tissue edema
- Location: Lumbar spine most common: 97%
- Typically single level involvement
- Facet joint widening
- Eroded facet cortex
- Low density within expanded facet joint
- Diffuse or rim-enhancement within facet joint
- Diffuse or peripherally enhancing epidural and paraspinal soft tissue

- Uptake of technetium 99m diphosphonate in posterior elements

Top Differential Diagnoses
- Facet joint osteoarthritis
- Rheumatoid arthritis
- Metastases

Pathology
- Staphylococcus aureus most common
- Bacteremia from an extraspinal primary source
- Uncommon entity

Clinical Issues
- Difficult to distinguish from spondylodiscitis clinically

- ○ Hyperintensity within facet joint
- ○ Periarticular soft tissue edema
- STIR: Hyperintense facet marrow
- T1 C+
  - ○ Diffuse or rim-enhancement within joint
  - ○ Enhancing marrow abutting facet joint
  - ○ Enhancing soft tissue or peripherally enhancing fluid collection
    - Contiguous with facet joint
    - Epidural or paraspinal extension
- ± Central canal or neural foraminal narrowing

Ultrasonographic Findings
- Real Time: Anechoic or hypoechoic extraarticular abscess
- Power Doppler: Hyperemia and increased vascularity surrounding abscess

Nuclear Medicine Findings
- Bone Scan
  - ○ Uptake of technetium 99m diphosphonate in posterior elements
    - More laterally located and vertically oriented
    - Improved lesion localization with SPECT
- Gallium Scan
  - ○ Increased uptake of gallium citrate (Ga 67)
    - Increased sensitivity with SPECT

Imaging Recommendations
- Best imaging tool: Sagittal and axial T1WI and T2WI MRI
- Protocol advice
  - ○ Sagittal STIR or FSE T2 with fat-saturation most sensitive for bone marrow edema and epidural involvement
  - ○ Post-gadolinium T1WI with fat-saturation better delineates extent of facet, epidural, and paraspinal involvement

DIFFERENTIAL DIAGNOSIS

Facet joint osteoarthritis
- Joint space narrowing

- Vacuum phenomenon
- Cortical eburnation
  - ○ Subcortical cystic change
- Osteophytosis
- Typically without marrow signal changes
  - ○ Marrow edema may represent stress reaction
- ± Fluid within facet joint
- Symmetric bilaterally
  - ○ Unless scoliosis present
- Associated ligamentum flavum thickening
- ± Spondylolisthesis
- No soft tissue edema or abscess
- Normal erythrocyte sedimentation rate, C-reactive protein

Facet synovial cyst
- L4-5 most common
- Juxtaarticular thin walled, well-defined mass
  - ○ Hypointense on T1WI
  - ○ Hyperintense on T2WI
  - ○ ± Mild peripheral enhancement
- No marrow signal abnormality or cortical erosion
- No soft tissue edema or enhancement
- Associated facet arthropathy and ligamentum flavum thickening

Rheumatoid arthritis
- Cervical spine most commonly effected
- Atlantoaxial subluxation & dens erosion most common findings
- Facet joint erosion
  - ○ Widened joint space
  - ○ Enhancing synovium
  - ○ ± Ankylosis
- Enhancing soft tissue pannus

Metastases
- Multi-focal discrete or ill-defined lesion in posterior elements
  - ○ Hypointense on T1WI
  - ○ Hyperintense on T2WI
  - ○ Post-gadolinium enhancement
  - ○ ± Surrounding marrow edema
- Osseous destruction

SEPTIC FACET JOINT ARTHRITIS

- Facet joint may be preserved

PATHOLOGY

General Features
- General path comments: Hematogenous infection of facet joint and adjacent soft tissue
- Genetics: No genetic predisposition
- Etiology
  - Predisposing factors
    - Intravenous drug abuse
    - Immunocompromised state
    - Diabetes, cirrhosis, renal failure, cancer, other chronic medical illnesses
  - Staphylococcus aureus most common
  - Bacteremia from an extraspinal primary source
    - Most common route of infection
    - GU or GI tract, lungs, or cutaneous source
  - Direct inoculation from penetrating trauma, surgical intervention, or diagnostic procedures
    - Facet joint injection
  - Extension from adjacent infection in paraspinal soft tissues
    - Diverticulitis, appendicitis, inflammatory bowel disease
    - Renal abscess
- Epidemiology
  - Uncommon entity
    - < 50 reported cases in literature
    - 4-5% of infectious spondylitis in one series
- Associated abnormalities
  - Spondylodiscitis
  - Epidural abscess: 25%
    - Cord compression
    - Foraminal narrowing
  - Paraspinal abscess
  - Spinal meningitis

Gross Pathologic & Surgical Features
- Necrotic bone
- Suppurative soft tissue

Microscopic Features
- Bone/synovial fragments
- Leukocytes, micro-organisms, cellular debris
- Granulation tissue

CLINICAL ISSUES

Presentation
- Most common signs/symptoms
  - Acute or chronic back pain
  - Focal tenderness
  - Fever
  - Other signs/symptoms
    - Neurological impairment in 38% of cases
    - Radiculopathy
    - Paraparesis
    - Sensory disturbance
    - Sphincter dysfunction
    - Elevated erythrocyte sedimentation rate, C-reactive protein, white count

- Clinical profile
  - Acute back pain mimics disc herniation
  - Difficult to distinguish from spondylodiscitis clinically

Demographics
- Age: 50-60s
- Gender: Slight male predominance
- Ethnicity: No racial predilection

Natural History & Prognosis
- Osseous destruction
- Spinal instability
- Progressive neurologic deterioration
- Sepsis and death
- Favorable outcome with intravenous antibiotics alone: 71%
- Success rate improved if combined with percutaneous drainage: 85%

Treatment
- Intravenous antibiotics
- Percutaneous drainage
- Surgery
  - Decompressive laminectomy
  - Indicated when epidural abscess and neurological deficits present

DIAGNOSTIC CHECKLIST

Consider
- Imaging guided facet joint aspiration if blood culture negative

Image Interpretation Pearls
- Enhancing facet joint with juxtaarticular, paraspinal, or epidural phlegmon or abscess characteristic of septic facet joint arthritis

SELECTED REFERENCES

1. Coscia MF et al: Pyogenic lumbar facet joint arthritis with intradural extension: a case report. J Spinal Disord Tech. 15(6):526-8, 2002
2. Muffoletto AJ et al: Hematogenous pyogenic facet joint infection. Spine. 26:1570-6, 2001
3. Muffolerro AJ et al: Hematogenous pyogenic facet joint infection of the subaxial cervical spine. A report of two cases and review of the literature. J Neurosurg. 95(1 Suppl):135-8, 2001
4. Rombauts PA et al: Septic arthritis of a lumbar facet joint caused by Staphylococcus aureus. Spine. 25:1736-8, 2000
5. Fujiwara A et al: Septic arthritis of a lumbar facet joint: report of a case with early MRI findings. J Spinal Disord. 11(5):452-3, 1998
6. Ergan M et al: Septic arthritis of lumbar facet joint. A review of six cases. Rev Rhum Engl Ed. 64:386-95, 1997
7. Baltz MS et al: Lumbar facet joint infection associated with epidural and paraspinal abscess. Clin Orthop. (339):109-12, 1997
8. Swayne LC et al: Septic arthritis of a lumbar facet joint: detection with bone SPECT imaging. J Nucl Med. 30(8):1408-11, 1989

SEPTIC FACET JOINT ARTHRITIS

IMAGE GALLERY

Typical

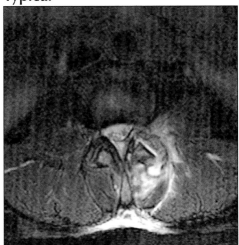 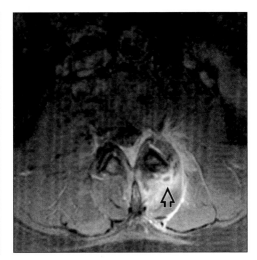

(Left) Axial T2WI MR with fat suppression through a lumbar vertebra shows fluid in left facet joint with posterior extension and loculation. Edema is present in surrounding soft tissue. *(Right)* Axial T1 C+ MR with fat suppression shows enhancement in left facet joint with posterior abscess (arrow). Enhancement also present in epidural and paraspinal soft tissue.

Typical

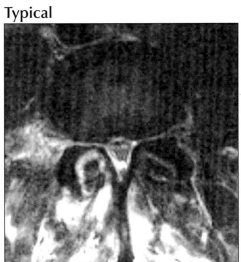 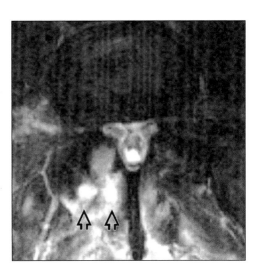

(Left) Axial T2WI MR through lumbar vertebra shows asymmetric hyperintensity in right facet joint. *(Right)* Axial T2WI MR demonstrates a phlegmon expanding right facet joint with extension (arrows) into posterior paraspinal muscle.

Typical

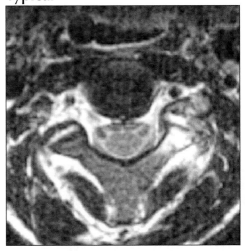 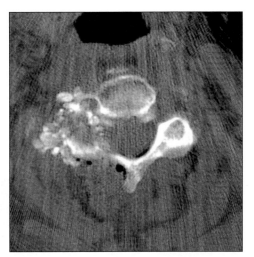

(Left) Axial PD/Intermediate MR through a cervical vertebra shows hyperintensity in left facet joint with adjacent marrow edema. Blood culture was positive for E. coli. *(Right)* Axial bone CT through a cervical vertebra shows osseous destruction in right facet joint with low density, surrounding bony debris, compatible with septic facet arthritis.

EPIDURAL ABSCESS

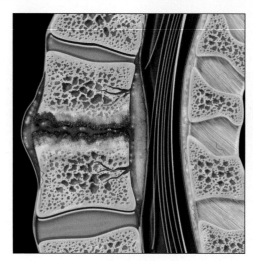

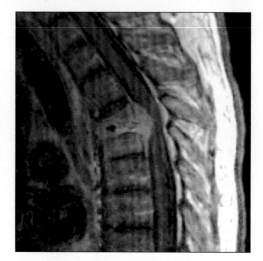

Sagittal graphic through lumbar spine demonstrates vertebral osteomyelitis with intervertebral abscess extending ventrally and dorsally, narrowing central canal.

Sagittal T1 C+ MR through thoracic spine shows discitis and osteomyelitis with contiguous enhancing ventral epidural phlegmon, narrowing central canal.

TERMINOLOGY

Abbreviations and Synonyms
- Spinal epidural abscess (SEA)
- Spinal dural empyema

Definitions
- Extradural spinal infection with abscess formation

IMAGING FINDINGS

General Features
- Best diagnostic clue: Findings of spondylodiscitis, with adjacent enhancing epidural phlegmon ± peripherally enhancing fluid collection
- Location
  - Posterior epidural space (80%) > anterior (20%) > circumferential (caudal to S2)
  - Lower thoracic and lumbar > cervical and upper thoracic
- Size: Multi-segmental
- Morphology: Focal or diffuse elongated epidural soft tissue

Radiographic Findings
- Radiography
  - Endplate erosion
  - Vertebral height loss

- Myelography: Epidural mass impeding cerebral spinal fluid flow

CT Findings
- CECT: Enhancing epidural mass narrowing central canal
- Bone CT
  - Cortical destruction
  - Vertebral collapse

MR Findings
- T1WI: Iso- to hypointense to cord
- T2WI: Hyperintense
- STIR: Hyperintense
- T2* GRE: Iso- to hyperintense
- DWI: Hyperintense
- T1 C+
  - Homogeneously or heterogeneously enhancing phlegmon
  - Peripherally enhancing necrotic abscess
  - Diffuse dural enhancement in extensive SEA
  - Enhancing prominent anterior epidural veins or basivertebral venous plexus above or below abscess
- Various degree of encroachment on central canal and intervertebral foramina
- Signal alteration in spinal cord from
  - Cord compression
  - Cord ischemia
  - Direct infection

DDx: Epidural Masses

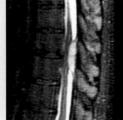

Metastasis

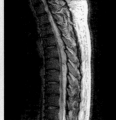

Hematoma

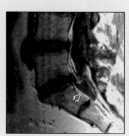

Disc Fragment

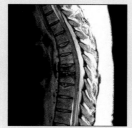

Epi. Lipomatosis

EPIDURAL ABSCESS

Key Facts

Terminology
- Extradural spinal infection with abscess formation

Imaging Findings
- Best diagnostic clue: Findings of spondylodiscitis, with adjacent enhancing epidural phlegmon ± peripherally enhancing fluid collection
- Posterior epidural space (80%) > anterior (20%) > circumferential (caudal to S2)
- Lower thoracic and lumbar > cervical and upper thoracic
- Size: Multi-segmental
- T1WI: Iso- to hypointense to cord
- T2WI: Hyperintense
- Homogeneously or heterogeneously enhancing phlegmon
- Peripherally enhancing necrotic abscess

Top Differential Diagnoses
- Extradural metastasis
- Epidural hematoma
- Extruded/migrated disc

Pathology
- Staphylococcus aureus is most common pathogen
- Mycobacterium tuberculosis is next most frequent cause: 25%
- Cord symptoms likely from combination of compressive & ischemic effects

Clinical Issues
- Acute or subacute spinal pain and tenderness
- Fever

- Persistent epidural enhancement without mass effect on follow-up MR imaging
  - Probable sterile granulation tissue or fibrosis
  - Correlation with erythrocyte sedimentation rate for disease activity

Nuclear Medicine Findings
- Gallium Scan
  - Increased uptake in spinal or epidural area

Imaging Recommendations
- Best imaging tool: Sagittal and axial T1WI and T2WI MR with gadolinium
- Protocol advice: Sagittal STIR or T2WI with fat-saturation increases lesion conspicuity by suppressing signal from epidural fat and vertebral marrow

DIFFERENTIAL DIAGNOSIS

Extradural metastasis
- Well circumscribed extra-osseous soft tissue mass
  - Hypointense on T1WI and hyperintense on T2WI
  - Diffuse enhancement
  - Often contiguous with vertebral lesion
    - Destruction of posterior vertebra/pedicle
  - ± Expansion of involved vertebral body
  - Intervertebral discs uneffected
- Pathologic compression fractures
- Sparing of spinal column in some cases
  - Spinal epidural lymphoma

Epidural hematoma
- Heterogeneously hyperintense on T2WI
- Acute hemorrhage isointense on T1WI
  - Subacute and chronic hemorrhage hyperintense
- No significant post-gadolinium enhancement
- Intact vertebrae in absence of trauma

Extruded/migrated disc
- Associated parent disc height loss, protrusion, degeneration
  - Iso/hypointense on T2WI
- More focal appearance
- ± Mild peripheral post-gadolinium enhancement
- Vertebral endplates intact
  - ± Enhancing fibrovascular marrow

Epidural lipomatosis
- Excessive epidural fat in thoracic and lumbar canal
- Homogenous and hyperintense on T1WI and T2WI
- Signal loss with fat suppression
- Mass effect on spinal cord

PATHOLOGY

General Features
- General path comments: Suppuration of epidural space from adjacent infection or bacteremia
- Genetics: No genetic predilection
- Etiology
  - Staphylococcus aureus is most common pathogen
    - 57-73% of reported cases
  - Mycobacterium tuberculosis is next most frequent cause: 25%
  - Fungal infection less common
    - More common in immunocompromised host
    - May be chronic and indolent
  - Predisposing factors
    - Intravenous drug abuse
    - Immunocompromised state
    - Diabetes mellitus, chronic renal failure, alcoholism, cancer, or other chronic illnesses
  - Anterior SEA arises from adjacent discitis & vertebral osteomyelitis
  - Posterior SEA from GU or GI tract, lungs, cardiac, mucous/cutaneous sources through hematogenous dissemination
    - Mucous/cutaneous source most common
  - Direct inoculation from penetrating trauma, surgical intervention, or diagnostic procedures
    - Risk of SEA in epidural anesthesia: 5.5%
    - Extradural hematoma may become infected in blunt trauma

EPIDURAL ABSCESS

- ○ Extension from adjacent infection in paraspinal soft tissues
  - ▪ Diverticulitis, appendicitis, pyelonephritis
- ○ Anterior cranial-caudal epidural extension by tracking beneath posterior longitudinal ligament
- ○ Tuberculous infection tends to spread beneath anterior longitudinal ligament
  - ▪ Intervertebral discs spared
- ○ Cord symptoms likely from combination of compressive & ischemic effects
  - ▪ Cord ischemia from compromised epidural venous plexuses
- Epidemiology: 0.2 to 2.8 cases per 10,000
- Associated abnormalities
  - ○ Discitis
  - ○ Osteomyelitis
  - ○ Paraspinal abscess
  - ○ Septic facet arthritis
  - ○ Spinal instability

Microscopic Features
- Leukocytes, micro-organisms, cellular debris
- Granulation tissue
- Increased vascularity

CLINICAL ISSUES

Presentation
- Most common signs/symptoms
  - ○ Acute or subacute spinal pain and tenderness
  - ○ Fever
  - ○ Other signs/symptoms
    - ▪ Radiculopathy
    - ▪ Paraparesis
    - ▪ Paresthesia
    - ▪ Loss of bladder and bowel control
    - ▪ Paralysis
- Clinical profile
  - ○ In patients with septicemia or chronic illness neurologic symptoms may be obscured by systemic complaints
  - ○ Lumbar SEA mimics disc herniation
  - ○ Abscess from hematogenous spread progresses rapidly
    - ▪ Abscess from discitis/osteomyelitis tends to smolder

Demographics
- Age
  - ○ All ages reported
  - ○ Peak incidence in 60s and 70s
- Gender: M:F = 1:0.56
- Ethnicity: No racial predilection

Natural History & Prognosis
- Irreversible neurologic deficit and death if untreated or delay in treatment
- Prognosis influenced by
  - ○ Age
    - ▪ Children with better prognosis than adults
  - ○ Severity of initial neurologic deficits
    - ▪ Thecal compression > 50% associated with poor prognosis

- ○ Co-morbidities
- ○ Duration between onset of neurologic deficits and time of surgical intervention
  - ▪ Early diagnosis & institution of treatment improve prognosis
- Mortality rate 12-30%

Treatment
- Emergent surgical decompression with drainage of abscess
  - ○ Even in absence of initial neurologic compromise
    - ▪ Rapid progression of neurologic deficits can occur despite appropriate medical therapy
- Early empiric antibiotics with broad spectrum coverage until causative pathogen isolated
  - ○ Coverage should be effective against staphylococci, gram negatives, and anaerobes
- Organism specific intravenous antibiotics followed by long term parenteral antibiotics for 6-8 weeks
- Medical therapy alone if
  - ○ Substantial operative risks
  - ○ Extensive cranial-caudal involvement of spinal canal
  - ○ Paralysis > 3 days

DIAGNOSTIC CHECKLIST

Image Interpretation Pearls
- Epidural soft tissue with homogeneous or peripheral enhancement plus adjacent spondylodiscitis characteristic of SEA

SELECTED REFERENCES

1. Eastwood JD et al: Diffusion-weighted imaging in a patient with vertebral and epidural abscesses. AJNR Am J Neuroradiol. 23(3):496-8, 2002
2. Varma R et al: Imaging of pyogenic infectious spondylodiskitis. Radiol Clin North Am. 39(2):203-13, 2001
3. Reihsaus E et al: Spinal epidural abscess: a meta-analysis of 915 patients. Neurosurg Rev. 23(4):175-204; discussion 205, 2000
4. Ruiz A et al: MR imaging of infections of the cervical spine. Magn Reson Imaging Clin N Am. 8(3):561-80, 2000
5. Tung GA et al: Spinal epidural abscess: correlation between MRI findings and outcome. Neuroradiology. 41(12):904-9, 1999
6. Sampath P et al: Spinal epidural abscess: a review of epidemiology, diagnosis, and treatment. J Spinal Disord. 12(2):89-93, 1999
7. Mackenzie AR et al: Spinal epidural abscess: the importance of early diagnosis and treatment. J Neurol Neurosurg Psychiatry. 65:209-12, 1998
8. Khanna RK et al: Spinal epidural abscess: evaluation of factors influencing outcome. Neurosurgery. 39(5):958-64, 1996
9. Numaguchi Y et al: Spinal epidural abscess: evaluation with gadolinium-enhanced MR imaging. Radiographics. 13(3):545-59; discussion 559-60, 1993
10. Nussbaum ES et al: Spinal Epidural Abscess: A Report of 40 Cases and Review. Surg Neurol. 38:225-31, 1992
11. Sandhu FS et al: Spinal epidural abscess: evaluation with contrast-enhanced MR imaging. AJNR Am J Neuroradiol. 12(6):1087-93, 1991

EPIDURAL ABSCESS

IMAGE GALLERY

Typical

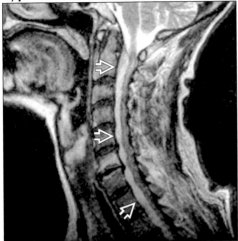 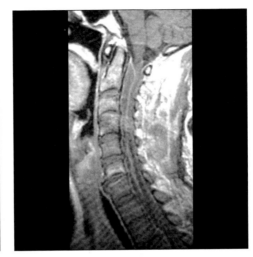

(Left) Sagittal T2WI MR through cervical spine shows an extensive ventral epidural hyperintense collection (arrows) from C2 to upper thoracic spine, with significant mass effect on cervical cord. *(Right)* Sagittal T1 C+ MR shows the same collection with peripheral enhancement, compatible with an epidural abscess.

Typical

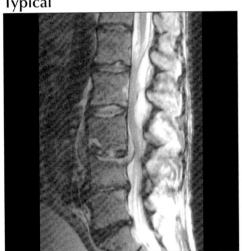 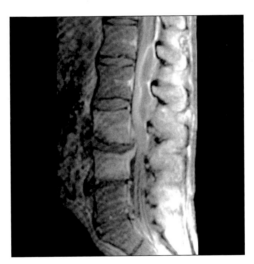

(Left) Sagittal T2WI MR through lumbar spine demonstrates discitis and osteomyelitis at L3-4 with associated hyperintense epidural abscess. A second epidural abscess is present dorsally from L1-3. *(Right)* Sagittal T1 C+ MR with fat suppression shows abscesses with peripheral enhancement. There is significant mass effect on cauda equina.

Typical

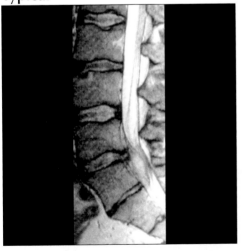 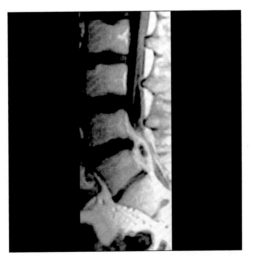

(Left) Sagittal T2WI MR through lumbar spine demonstrates ventral epidural hyperintense collection from L5 to S1, narrowing central canal. *(Right)* Sagittal T1 C+ MR shows thick peripheral enhancement in this collection, consistent with an epidural abscess.

SUBDURAL ABSCESS

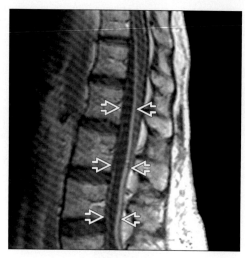

Sagittal T1 C+ MR through thoracolumbar spine shows an extensive ventral intraspinal rim-enhancing fluid collection (arrows).

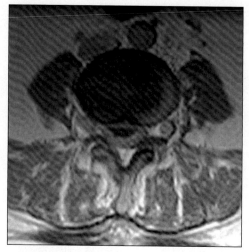

Axial T1 C+ MR confirms subdural location of this collection, compatible with subdural abscess. Enhancing nerve roots are also present, due to spinal meningitis.

TERMINOLOGY

Abbreviations and Synonyms
- Spinal subdural empyema
- Spinal subdural abscess (SSA)

Definitions
- Collection of pus in "potential" space between dura and arachnoid

IMAGING FINDINGS

General Features
- Best diagnostic clue: Intradural extramedullary ring-enhancing fluid collection on axial imaging
- Location: Thoracolumbar region most common
- Size
  - Focal abscess
  - Multifocal phlegmon or abscesses extending over multiple spinal levels
- Morphology
  - Thin, elongated fluid collection
  - Diffuse subdural thickening

Radiographic Findings
- Radiography: Typically noncontributory unless spondylodiscitis also present
- Myelography

  - Block of cerebral spinal fluid (CSF)
  - Intradural irregularities
  - Cord swelling

CT Findings
- NECT
  - Increased subdural density
  - ± Intradural extramedullary gas
- CECT
  - Homogeneous subdural enhancement
  - Peripherally enhancing fluid collection

MR Findings
- T1WI
  - Intermediate signal intensity (SI)
  - Effaced CSF
- T2WI
  - Hyperintense
    - Presence suggested by mass effect on cord
  - Obliterated subarachnoid space
- PD/Intermediate: Hyperintense
- STIR: Hyperintense
- T2* GRE: Hyperintense
- T1 C+
  - Heterogeneous, diffuse subdural enhancement
  - Rim-enhancing fluid collection
  - Intraspinal contents from outer to inner on axial imaging

DDx: Intraspinal Collections and Abnormal Enhancement

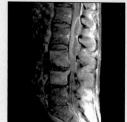

Epidural Abscess

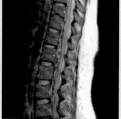

Subdural Hematoma

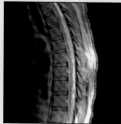

Spinal Meningitis

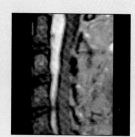

CSF Leakage Syndrome

SUBDURAL ABSCESS

Key Facts

Terminology
- Spinal subdural empyema
- Collection of pus in "potential" space between dura and arachnoid

Imaging Findings
- Best diagnostic clue: Intradural extramedullary ring-enhancing fluid collection on axial imaging
- Intermediate signal intensity (SI)
- Effaced CSF
- Heterogeneous, diffuse subdural enhancement
- Rim-enhancing fluid collection

Top Differential Diagnoses
- Spinal epidural abscess
- Subdural hematoma
- Spinal meningitis

Pathology
- Staphylococcus aureus most common

Clinical Issues
- Fever
- Neck or back pain
- Paraparesis, quadriparesis
- Paresthesia, sensory level
- Laminectomy and durotomy for abscess drainage and irrigation

Diagnostic Checklist
- (Rim)-enhancing intradural extramedullary collection suspicious for SSA
- Especially if outlined by epidural fat and CSF on axial imaging

---

        ▪ Epidural fat, enhancing dura and subdural abscess, CSF, cord
- Cord displacement
  ○ ± Impingement
  ○ ± Edema

Nuclear Medicine Findings
- Gallium Scan
  ○ Increased intraspinal uptake of gallium citrate (Ga 67)
    ▪ Improved sensitivity with SPECT

Imaging Recommendations
- Best imaging tool: Sagittal and axial T1WI and T2WI MR
- Protocol advice
  ○ Intravenous gadolinium increases sensitivity in detecting SSA
    ▪ Axial imaging confirms subdural location

DIFFERENTIAL DIAGNOSIS

Spinal epidural abscess
- Difficult to distinguish clinically
- Lower thoracic and lumbar spine
- Typically associated with spondylodiscitis
- Intermediate SI on T1WI, hyperintense on T2WI
  ○ Diffuse or rim-enhancement
- Variable mass effect on spinal cord

Subdural hematoma
- Other than trauma, lumbar puncture in patients with coagulopathy is the most common cause
- More common in lumbar or thoracolumbar region
- Predominantly hypointense on T2WI or gradient echo
  ○ Isointense on T1WI
- No post-gadolinium enhancement

Spinal meningitis
- Hematogenous dissemination of bacteria from extraspinal source
- Increased CSF intensity on T1WI
- Diffuse CSF enhancement

- Smooth or nodular leptomeningeal or nerve root enhancement
- ± Cord edema

CSF leakage syndrome
- From prior spinal trauma, diagnostic or interventional procedure, or spontaneous
- Low opening pressure on lumbar puncture
- Diffuse smooth dural thickening and enhancement
  ○ Likely from dural venous engorgement
- May see cerebellar tonsillar descent and effaced pre-pontine space in posterior fossa

Idiopathic hypertrophic spinal pachymeningitis
- Unknown etiology
- Diagnosis of exclusion
- Fibrous inflammatory thickening of dura mater
- Thickened dura iso- to hypointense on T1WI and T2WI
  ○ Marked post-contrast-enhancement

PATHOLOGY

General Features
- General path comments: Suppuration of spinal subdural space
- Genetics: No genetic predilection
- Etiology
  ○ Predisposing factors
    ▪ Intravenous drug abuse
    ▪ Immunocompromised state
    ▪ Alcoholism
    ▪ Diabetes, cirrhosis, renal failure, or other chronic medical illnesses
  ○ Mechanism of inoculation
    ▪ Hematogenous dissemination from extraspinal focus of infection
    ▪ Mucous/cutaneous source most common
    ▪ Contiguous spread from adjacent abscess
    ▪ Direct inoculation through trauma or interventional procedures

SUBDURAL ABSCESS

- Lumbar puncture, cervical/lumbar discogram
- Unexplained source of infection
  ○ Common pathogens
  - Staphylococcus aureus most common
  - Gram negative bacilli
  ○ Cord symptoms likely from a combination of compressive and ischemic effects
- Epidemiology
  ○ Rare
  ○ About 50 reported cases of SSA in the literature
- Associated abnormalities
  ○ Spinal meningitis
  ○ Spinal epidural abscess
  ○ Usually not associated with vertebral osteomyelitis
- Anatomy
  ○ Subdural space
  - "Potential" space between dura mater and arachnoid membrane
  ○ Factors contributing to low incidence of SSA compared cranial subdural abscess
  - Lack of venous sinuses
  - Epidural space may act as a filter
  - Centripetal blood flow in the spine vs. centrifugal blood flow in the brain

Gross Pathologic & Surgical Features

- Turbid CSF
- Frank pus

CLINICAL ISSUES

Presentation

- Most common signs/symptoms
  ○ Fever
  ○ Neck or back pain
  ○ Tenderness
  ○ Other signs/symptoms
  - Paraparesis, quadriparesis
  - Paresthesia, sensory level
  - Gait disturbance
  - Meningismus
  - Hyporeflexia
  - Bladder or bowl dysfunction
- Clinical profile
  ○ Triad of fever, neck or back pain, and cord compression
  - 38% of reported cases
  ○ Source of infections such as cellulitis, furuncles, dental abscess may be present
  ○ Difficult to distinguish from spinal epidural abscess clinically

Demographics

- Age: All ages reported
- Gender: M:F = 1:2
- Ethnicity: No racial predilection

Natural History & Prognosis

- If left untreated, progressive neurologic deterioration
  ○ Sepsis, death
- 20% survival rate if intravenous antibiotics only
- 82% survival rate if surgical treatment

Treatment

- Supportive care with hydration and pain management
- Intravenous dexamethasone to decrease inflammatory reaction and brain/cord edema
- Percutaneous imaging guided catheter drainage
- Surgery
  ○ Laminectomy and durotomy for abscess drainage and irrigation
  ○ Recommended in all surgical candidates
- Empiric intravenous antibiotics with Gram-positive cocci coverage until positive culture results

DIAGNOSTIC CHECKLIST

Image Interpretation Pearls

- (Rim)-enhancing intradural extramedullary collection suspicious for SSA
  ○ Especially if outlined by epidural fat and CSF on axial imaging

SELECTED REFERENCES

1. Ozates M et al: Spinal subdural tuberculous abscess. Spinal Cord. 38(1):56-8, 2000
2. Schneider P et al: Spinal subdural abscess in a pediatric patient: a case report and review of the literature. Pediatr Emerg Care. 14(1):22-3, 1998
3. Martin RJ et al: Neurosurgical care of spinal epidural, subdural, and intramedullary abscesses and arachnoiditis. Orthop Clin North Am. 27(1):125-36, 1996
4. Sathi S et al: Spinal subdural abscess: successful treatment with limited drainage and antibiotics in a patient with AIDS. Surg Neurol. 42(5):424-7, 1994
5. Levy ML et al: Subdural empyema of the cervical spine: clinicopathological correlates and magnetic resonance imaging. Report of three cases. J Neurosurg. 81(1):160, 1994
6. Krauss WE et al: Infections of the dural spaces. Neurosurg Clin N Am. 3(2):421-33, 1992
7. Bartels RH et al: Spinal subdural abscess. Case report. J Neurosurg. 76(2):307-11, 1992
8. Harries-Jones R et al: Meningitis and spinal subdural empyema as a complication of sinusitis. J Neurol Neurosurg Psychiatry. 53(5):441, 1990
9. Hershkowitz S et al: Spinal empyema in Crohn's disease. J Clin Gastroenterol. 12(1):67-9, 1990
10. Lownie SP et al: Spinal subdural empyema complicating cervical discography. Spine. 14(12):1415-7, 1989
11. Butler EG et al: Spinal subdural abscess. Clin Exp Neurol. 25:67-70, 1988
12. Knudsen LL et al: Computed tomographic myelography in spinal subdural empyema. Neuroradiology. 29(1):99, 1987
13. Harris LF et al: Subdural empyema and epidural abscess: recent experience in a community hospital. South Med J. 80(10):1254-8, 1987
14. Theodotou B et al: Spinal subdural empyema: diagnosis by spinal computed tomography. Surg Neurol. 21(6):610-2, 1984
15. Reddy DR et al: Pneumococcal spinal subdural abscess (a case report). J Postgrad Med. 19(4):190-2, 1973
16. Hirson C: Spinal subdural abscess. Lancet. 2(7424):1215-7, 1965

SUBDURAL ABSCESS

IMAGE GALLERY

Typical

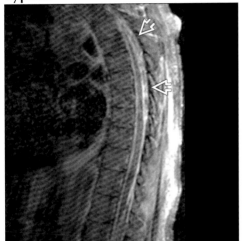 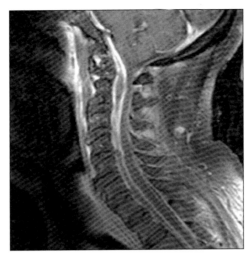

(Left) Sagittal T1 C+ MR with fat suppression through thoracic spine shows dorsal subdural heterogeneously enhancing collection (arrows), consistent with abscess. *(Right)* Sagittal T1 C+ MR with fat suppression through cervical spine demonstrates diffuse ventral subdural abscess with intracranial extension.

Typical

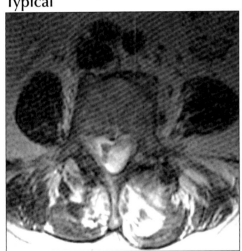 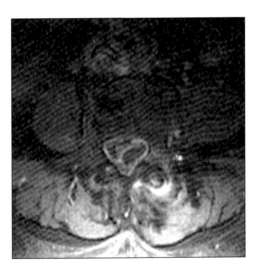

(Left) Axial T2WI MR through lumbar spine shows a left-sided intraspinal hyperintense collection compressing cauda equina. *(Right)* Axial T1 C+ MR with fat suppression shows the same fluid collection with peripheral enhancement, proven to be a subdural abscess at surgery.

Typical

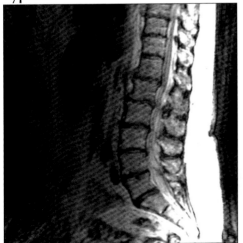 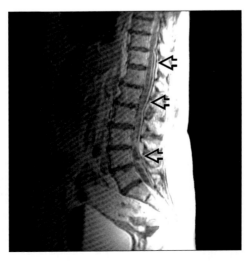

(Left) Sagittal T2WI MR through thoracolumbar spine shows diffuse and heterogeneous extramedullary hyperintense collection. *(Right)* Sagittal T1 C+ MR in same patient shows an extensive rim-enhancing subdural empyema (arrows), corresponding to hyperintense collection on T2WI.

PARASPINAL ABSCESS

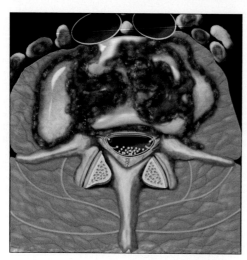

Axial graphic through a lumbar disc space demonstrates an extensive abscess infiltrating bilateral psoas muscles and epidural space. Abnormal retroperitoneal lymph nodes are also present.

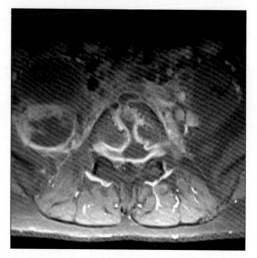

Axial T1 C+ MR with fat suppression in patient with tuberculous spondylitis shows intraosseous & right psoas abscesses, plus prevertebral phlegmon, abscess.

TERMINOLOGY

Abbreviations and Synonyms
- Paraspinal abscess (PA)

Definitions
- Infection of soft tissues surrounding spine

IMAGING FINDINGS

General Features
- Best diagnostic clue: Paravertebral enhancing phlegmon or peripherally enhancing liquified collection
- Location
  - Prevertebral space
  - Paravertebral soft tissue
    - Psoas
    - Iliacus
    - Posterior paraspinous muscles
- Size
  - Variable
  - Craniocaudal extension
    - Subligamentous
    - Along muscle plane
- Morphology
  - Ill-defined infiltrative paraspinal soft tissue

  - Focal or diffuse muscle enlargement
    - Intramuscular fluid collection
    - Thick or thin, smooth or irregular wall
  - Obliterated soft tissue fascial plane

Radiographic Findings
- Radiography
  - Paraspinal soft tissue density
  - Enlarged psoas shadow
  - Endplate osteolysis
  - Disc space narrowing
  - Vertebral collapse

CT Findings
- NECT
  - Amorphous soft tissue density
  - Low density intra-muscular collection
    - Intra-abscess gas
  - Calcified psoas abscesses characteristic of tuberculous paraspinal abscess
- CECT
  - Diffuse or peripheral enhancement
  - Enhancing disc space
- Bone CT
  - Endplate destruction
  - Bony sequestra
  - Spinal deformity

DDx: Paraspinal Soft Tissue Mass

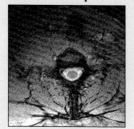

Lymphoma

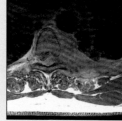

Lymphoma

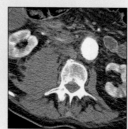

Hematoma

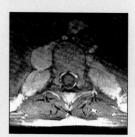

Extra. Hematopoiesis

PARASPINAL ABSCESS

Key Facts

Terminology
- Infection of soft tissues surrounding spine

Imaging Findings
- Best diagnostic clue: Paravertebral enhancing phlegmon or peripherally enhancing liquified collection
- Ill-defined infiltrative paraspinal soft tissue
- Focal or diffuse muscle enlargement
- Obliterated soft tissue fascial plane
- Low density intra-muscular collection
- Intra-abscess gas
- Calcified psoas abscesses characteristic of tuberculous paraspinal abscess
- T2WI: Hyperintense
- T1 C+: Diffuse or peripheral enhancement

- Real Time: Anechoic or hypoechoic intramuscular collection
- Power Doppler: Hyperemia and increased vascularity surrounding abscess
- Increased uptake on In-111 WBC scan

Top Differential Diagnoses
- Neoplasm, primary or metastatic
- Retroperitoneal hematoma
- Extramedullary hematopoiesis

Pathology
- General path comments: Suppuration of paraspinal soft tissue from direct extension or hematogenous dissemination of pathogens

MR Findings
- T1WI
  - Iso- to hypointense
    - Difficult to distinguish from normal musculature
- T2WI: Hyperintense
- PD/Intermediate: Hyperintense
- STIR: Hyperintense
- T2* GRE: Iso- to hyperintense
- T1 C+: Diffuse or peripheral enhancement
- Features of spondylitis
  - Hyperintense disc on T2WI
  - Endplate erosion
  - Marrow edema
  - Enhancing disc and marrow
- Intraspinal extension with cord compression

Ultrasonographic Findings
- Real Time: Anechoic or hypoechoic intramuscular collection
- Power Doppler: Hyperemia and increased vascularity surrounding abscess

Nuclear Medicine Findings
- Gallium Scan
  - Increased radionuclide uptake
- WBC Scan
  - Increased uptake on In-111 WBC scan

Imaging Recommendations
- Best imaging tool: Sagittal and axial T1WI and T2WI MRI with gadolinium
- Protocol advice
  - T2WI with fat suppression or STIR improves detection of early paraspinal inflammation
  - Post-gadolinium T1WI with fat suppression also improves lesion conspicuity

DIFFERENTIAL DIAGNOSIS

Neoplasm, primary or metastatic
- Discrete or infiltrative soft tissue mass
  - Isointense to muscle on T1WI

  - Hyperintense on T2WI
    - Lymphoma with intermediate signal intensity (SI)
    - Desmoid, calcifications with low SI
  - Post-gadolinium enhancement
    - Necrotic component mimics abscess
- Variable vertebral involvement
  - Intervertebral discs typically spared

Retroperitoneal hematoma
- Infiltrative soft tissue
  - Hyperdense on CT
  - Hypointense on T1WI and T2WI in acute stage
  - Hyperintense on T1WI in later stage
  - ± Mild enhancement
- Diffuse muscular enlargement
  - Fluid-fluid level present if anti-coagulated

Extramedullary hematopoiesis
- Along thoracic and lumbar spine
- Paravertebral mass
  - Homogeneous and well-defined
  - Iso- to hypointense on T1WI
  - Iso- to hyperintense on T2WI
  - ± Mild enhancement
- Diffuse vertebral marrow hypointensity
  - Relatively hyperintense intervertebral discs spared

PATHOLOGY

General Features
- General path comments: Suppuration of paraspinal soft tissue from direct extension or hematogenous dissemination of pathogens
- Genetics: No genetic predisposition
- Etiology
  - Most common pathogens
    - Staphylococcus aureus
    - Mycobacterium tuberculosis
    - Escherichia coli
  - Fungal infection rare
    - More common in immunocompromised host
  - Predisposing factors

PARASPINAL ABSCESS

- Intravenous drug abuse
- Immunocompromised state
- Diabetes mellitus, alcoholism, cirrhosis, chronic renal failure, and other chronic medical illnesses
  - Direct extension from adjacent infection
    - Spondylodiscitis
    - Septic facet arthritis
    - Appendicitis
    - Diverticulitis
    - Inflammatory bowel disease
    - Perinephric abscess
  - Transcutaneous infection of deep tissue
    - Trauma
    - Epidural injection or catheter placement
    - Facet joint injection
    - Spine or GI surgery
  - Hematogenous spread from distant sites
  - Primary PA uncommon
- Epidemiology: > 90% cases of tuberculous spondylitis associated with intra- or paraspinal abscess
- Associated abnormalities: Epidural abscess

Gross Pathologic & Surgical Features
- Necrotic soft tissue with thick green brown fluid

Microscopic Features
- Leukocytes, micro-organisms, cellular debris
- Granulation tissue, increase vascularity

CLINICAL ISSUES

Presentation
- Most common signs/symptoms
  - Fever
  - Back pain and tenderness
  - Other signs/symptoms
    - Lower extremity pain
    - Paraspinal muscle spasm
  - If epidural component present
    - Weakness
    - Paresthesia
    - Sphincter dysfunction
- Clinical profile: Diagnosis may be delayed due to chronic and insidious symptomatology

Demographics
- Age: 50-60s
- Gender: M:F = 3:1
- Ethnicity: No racial predilection

Natural History & Prognosis
- Depends on host immune response
  - May be contained with early treatment
  - Overwhelming sepsis leading to death in debilitated host
- Progressive neurological impairment if spondylitis ± epidural abscess present
- Dependent on
  - Co-morbidities
  - Extent of spinal involvement
  - Degree of neurologic compromise

Treatment
- Long term intravenous antibiotics

- Analgesic medications
- Percutaneous catheter drainage
- Surgical debridement
  - Spinal stabilization may be required if instability present

DIAGNOSTIC CHECKLIST

Image Interpretation Pearls
- Peripherally enhancing collection in paravertebral soft tissue with associated spondylitis characteristic of PA

SELECTED REFERENCES

1. Martinez V et al: Tuberculous paravertebral abscess. Lancet. 363(9409):615, 2004
2. Ledermann HP et al: MR imaging findings in spinal infections: rules or myths? Radiology. 228(2):506-14, 2003
3. Gouliamos AD et al: MR imaging of tuberculous vertebral osteomyelitis: pictorial review. Eur Radiol. 11(4):575-9, 2001
4. Hill JS et al: A Staphylococcus aureus paraspinal abscess associated with epidural analgesia in labour. Anaesthesia. 56(9):873-8, 2001
5. Veillard E et al: Prompt regression of paravertebral and epidural abscesses in patients with pyogenic discitis. Sixteen cases evaluated using magnetic resonance imaging. Joint Bone Spine. 67(3):219-27, 2000
6. Tzen KY et al: The role of 67Ga in the early detection of spinal epidural abscesses. Nucl Med Commun. 21(2):165-70, 2000
7. Cook NJ et al: Paraspinal abscess following facet joint injection. Clin Rheumatol. 18(1):52-3, 1999
8. Raj V et al: Paraspinal abscess associated with epidural in labour. Anaesth Intensive Care. 26(4):424-6, 1998
9. Staatz G et al: Spondylodiskitic abscesses: CT-guided percutaneous catheter drainage. Radiology. 208(2):363-7, 1998
10. Pascaretti C et al: Epidural involvement in nontuberculous disk space infections. Incidence by magnetic resonance imaging, impact and prognosis. Rev Rhum Engl Ed. 64(10):556-61, 1997
11. Cecil M et al: Paraspinal pyomyositis, a rare cause of severe back pain: case report and review of the literature. Am J Orthop. 26(11):785-7, 1997
12. Bertol V et al: Neurologic complications of lumbar epidural analgesia: spinal and paraspinal abscess. Neurology. 48(6):1732-3, 1997
13. Baltz MS et al: Lumbar facet joint infection associated with epidural and paraspinal abscess. Clin Orthop. (339):109-12, 1997
14. Dagirmanjian A et al: MR imaging of vertebral osteomyelitis revisited. AJR. 167:1539-43, 1996
15. Nussbaum ES et al: Spinal tuberculosis: a diagnostic and management challenge. J Neurosurg. 83:243-7, 1995
16. Shanley DJ: Tuberculosis of the spine: imaging features. AJR Am J Roentgenol. 164(3):659-64, 1995
17. Pegues DA et al: Infectious complications associated with temporary epidural catheters. Clin Infect Dis. 19(5):970-2, 1994
18. Post MJ et al: Magnetic resonance imaging of spinal infection. Rheum Dis Clin North Am. 17(3):773-94, 1991
19. Smevik B et al: Computed tomography of a tuberculous paravertebral abscess. Z Kinderchir. 43(6):430-2, 1988
20. Lee JK et al: Psoas muscle disorders: MR imaging. Radiology. 160(3):683-7, 1986

IMAGE GALLERY

Typical

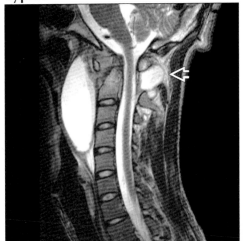
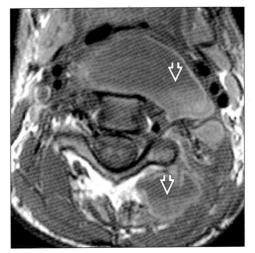

(Left) Sagittal T2WI MR in a patient with chronic neck pain shows a large prevertebral fluid collection from skull base to C5 without vertebral involvement. A posterior collection is also present (arrow). *(Right)* Axial T1WI MR shows fluid collections with fluid debris levels (arrows). Acid fast bacilli were cultured from these abscesses.

Typical

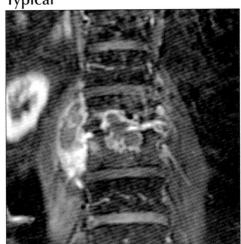
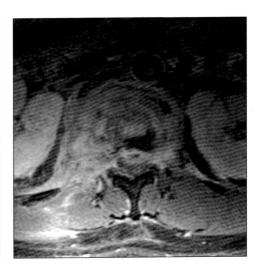

(Left) Coronal T1 C+ MR with fat suppression in patient with tuberculous spondylitis demonstrates intraosseous abscess spanning two vertebrae and right psoas abscess. *(Right)* Axial T1 C+ MR with fat suppression in patient with pyogenic spondylitis shows circumferential enhancing paravertebral phlegmon with epidural extension, narrowing spinal canal.

Typical

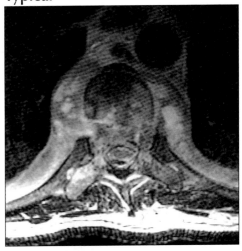
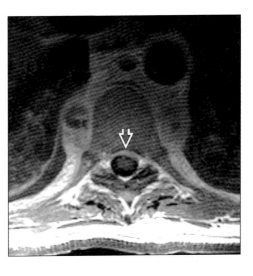

(Left) Axial T2WI MR through thoracic spine shows enlarged bilateral paravertebral soft tissues with multiple hyperintense collections. *(Right)* Axial T1WI MR shows centrally nonenhancing abscesses within bilateral enhancing phlegmon. Epidural extension is present (arrow).

VIRAL MYELITIS

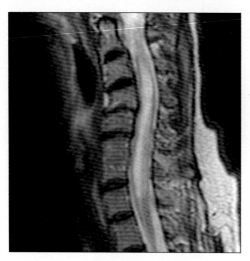

Sagittal T2WI MR shows long, edematous cervical cord segment in patient with onset of progressive weakness and radiculopathy over two days. Consitent with ATM.

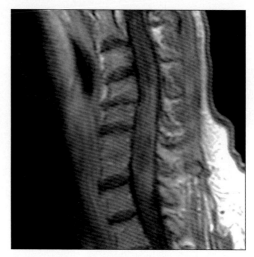

Sagittal T1 C+ MR shows ill-defined enhancement of enlarged cord in patient with two day history of progressive weakness and radiculopathy. Consitent with ATM.

TERMINOLOGY

Abbreviations and Synonyms
- Acute transverse myelitis, viral, ATM

Definitions
- Acute inflammatory insult of spinal cord due to direct viral infection or post-viral immunologic attack

IMAGING FINDINGS

General Features
- Best diagnostic clue: Swollen, edematous cord with segmental contiguous involvement
- Location: Cervical, thoracic segments; isolated conus involvement rare
- Size: From one segment to extensive cord involvement
- Morphology: Fusiform expansion of cord

Radiographic Findings
- Myelography: Focal or diffuse cord enlargement

CT Findings
- CECT
  - May see vague contrast-enhancement
  - Intrathecal contrast (post-myelogram) outlines symmetrically swollen cord

MR Findings
- T1WI
  - Expanded cord, fills canal
  - May see central low signal simulating syrinx, but intensity higher than CSF
- T2WI: Diffuse increase in signal intensity through involved segment
- T1 C+: Variable, non-focal enhancement of involved cord segment

Imaging Recommendations
- Best imaging tool: MRI
- Protocol advice: T2WI with thin (3 mm) sagittal sections; T1 C+ to exclude focal lesion as cause of cord edema

DIFFERENTIAL DIAGNOSIS

"Idiopathic" transverse myelitis
- Identical clinical picture
- No etiology found
- Up to 40% of cases preceded by upper respiratory tract infection
- Presence of CSF lymphocytes and neutrophils indicative of some type of inflammation in most cases
- Typically long segment of cord involvement by swelling, edema, vague diffuse enhancement

DDx: Acute Myelopathy

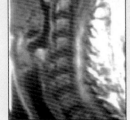

Transverse Myelitis

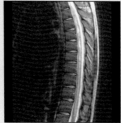

ADEM

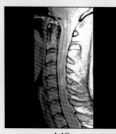

MS

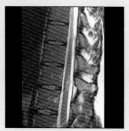

MS

Key Facts

Terminology
- Acute inflammatory insult of spinal cord due to direct viral infection or post-viral immunologic attack

Imaging Findings
- Best diagnostic clue: Swollen, edematous cord with segmental contiguous involvement
- Expanded cord, fills canal
- May see central low signal simulating syrinx, but intensity higher than CSF
- T2WI: Diffuse increase in signal intensity through involved segment
- T1 C+: Variable, non-focal enhancement of involved cord segment

Top Differential Diagnoses
- "Idiopathic" transverse myelitis

- Multiple sclerosis (MS)
- Acute disseminated encephalomyelitis (ADEM)
- Neuromyelitis optica
- Spinal arteriovenous malformation (AVM)
- Arteritis
- Acute cord infarct

Pathology
- Since eradication of polio, other enteroviruses most common etiology
- Herpes

Diagnostic Checklist
- Long, segmental cord enlargement and edema without focal lesions strong diagnostic clue in patients with acute onset of myelopathy

---

- "Idiopathic" likely because of incomplete evaluation and/or follow-up
- May represent collateral damage of immune attack following an infection already mopped up by host's defenses

Multiple sclerosis (MS)
- Up to 33% may have isolated cord lesions (no brain lesions)
- Most lesions are focal (1-2 segments), may be multiple
- 20% demonstrate monosegmental involvement
- Acute lesions exhibit focal enhancement with short segment edema
- No peripheral nervous system involvement
- 90% of cases show oligoclonal bands

Acute disseminated encephalomyelitis (ADEM)
- Mimic of multiple sclerosis
- Related to vaccination or immune insult
- Monophasic illness

Neuromyelitis optica
- Myelitis and optic neuritis
- Often a manifestation of ADEM, or systemic lupus erythematosus

Spinal arteriovenous malformation (AVM)
- High-flow AVM may cause acute myelopathy due to bleed or venous thrombosis
- Subacute onset of myelopathy, including edema, cord swelling may be due to "steal" & resulting ischemia
- Dural AVM may cause stuttering symptoms or acute myelopathy (due to venous thrombosis ⇒ Foix-Alajouanine syndrome)

Arteritis
- Small vessel vasculitis may have no imaging abnormality

Acute cord infarct
- Acute stroke-like presentation
- Motor signs predominate

- May be related to recent aortic aneurysm surgery or aortic dissection (vertebral artery dissection if cervical)
- More often due to atherosclerotic occlusion of ventral spinal artery (of Adamkiewicz)
- Conus involvement common (due to single ventral spinal artery)

Mycoplasma myelitis
- Coincident with a mycoplasma pneumonitis

PATHOLOGY

General Features
- General path comments: Swollen, soft cord
- Etiology
  - Since eradication of polio, other enteroviruses most common etiology
    - Coxsackie, echovirus, hepatitis, rubella, measles, mumps
  - Herpes
    - Ebstein-Barr, varicella zoster, cytomegalus virus, herpes simplex, herpes virus 6, herpes B (monkey virus)
  - Retrovirus
    - HTLV I and II, HIV
    - In immunocompromised hosts
  - Other
    - Influenza, rabies, West Nile
- Epidemiology
  - 1/100,000 per year
  - More common in immunocompromised
- Associated abnormalities
  - Peripheral neuropathy
  - Encephalitis

Gross Pathologic & Surgical Features
- Edematous, boggy cord
- May have necrosis

Microscopic Features
- Lymphocytic infiltrate
- Vascular thickening
- Demyelination

VIRAL MYELITIS

CLINICAL ISSUES

Presentation
- Most common signs/symptoms
  - Limb weakness
  - Areflexia
  - Other signs/symptoms
    - Sensory dysesthesia
    - Pain
- Clinical profile
  - Acute onset of weakness following febrile illness or upper respiratory tract infection
  - Reaches nadir at 1 week
  - CSF shows elevated mononuclear counts, protein level
  - Specific diagnosis through viral titers or polymerase chain reaction on CSF samples

Demographics
- Age: Typically younger patients
- Gender: No preference
- Ethnicity: All

Natural History & Prognosis
- Most cases leave lasting residual; significant minority resolve
- Disease course one to twelve weeks

Treatment
- Supportive; steroids and antiviral agents often used, variable efficacy

DIAGNOSTIC CHECKLIST

Consider
- Obtaining brain MRI to exclude multiple sclerosis, ADEM

Image Interpretation Pearls
- Long, segmental cord enlargement and edema without focal lesions strong diagnostic clue in patients with acute onset of myelopathy

SELECTED REFERENCES

1. Jeha LE et al: West Nile virus infection: a new acute paralytic illness. Neurology. 61(1):55-9, 2003
2. Zandman-Goddard G et al: Transverse myelitis associated with chronic hepatitis C. Clin Exp Rheumatol. 21(1):111-3, 2003
3. Fujimoto H et al: Epstein-Barr virus infections of the central nervous system. Intern Med. 42(1):33-40, 2003
4. Karacostas D et al: Cytomegalovirus-associated transverse myelitis in a non-immunocompromised patient. Spinal Cord. 40(3):145-9, 2002
5. Gorson KC et al: Nonpoliovirus poliomyelitis simulating Guillain-Barre syndrome. Arch Neurol. 58(9):1460-4, 2001
6. McMinn P et al: Neurological manifestations of enterovirus 71 infection in children during an outbreak of hand, foot, and mouth disease in Western Australia. Clin Infect Dis. 32(2):236-42, 2001
7. Andersen O: Myelitis. Curr Opin Neurol. 13(3):311-6, 2000
8. Gruhn B et al: Successful treatment of Epstein-Barr virus-induced transverse myelitis with ganciclovir and cytomegalovirus hyperimmune globulin following unrelated bone marrow transplantation. Bone Marrow Transplant. 24(12):1355-8, 1999
9. Nakajima H et al: Herpes simplex virus myelitis: clinical manifestations and diagnosis by the polymerase chain reaction method. Eur Neurol. 39(3):163-7, 1998
10. Haanpaa M et al: CSF and MRI findings in patients with acute herpes zoster. Neurology. 51(5):1405-11, 1998
11. Ku B et al: Acute transverse myelitis caused by Coxsackie virus B4 infection: a case report. J Korean Med Sci. 13(4):449-53, 1998
12. Salonen O et al: Myelitis associated with influenza A virus infection. J Neurovirol. 3(1):83-5, 1997
13. de Silva SM et al: Zoster myelitis: improvement with antiviral therapy in two cases. Neurology. 47(4):929-31, 1996
14. Moulignier A et al: AIDS-associated cytomegalovirus infection mimicking central nervous system tumors: a diagnostic challenge. Clin Infect Dis. 22(4):626-31, 1996
15. Ebo DG et al: Herpes zoster myelitis occurring during treatment for systemic lupus erythematosus. J Rheumatol. 23(3):548-50, 1996
16. Breningstall GN et al: Acute transverse myelitis and brainstem encephalitis associated with hepatitis A infection. Pediatr Neurol. 12(2):169-71, 1995
17. Campi A et al: Acute transverse myelopathy: spinal and cranial MR study with clinical follow-up. AJNR Am J Neuroradiol. 16(1):115-23, 1995
18. Gilden DH et al: Varicella-zoster virus myelitis: an expanding spectrum. Neurology. 44(10):1818-23, 1994
19. Caldas C et al: Case report: transverse myelitis associated with Epstein-Barr virus infection. Am J Med Sci. 307(1):45-8, 1994
20. Kyllerman MG et al: PCR diagnosis of primary herpesvirus type I in poliomyelitis-like paralysis and respiratory tract disease. Pediatr Neurol. 9(3):227-9, 1993
21. Chang CM et al: Postinfectious myelitis, encephalitis and encephalomyelitis. Clin Exp Neurol. 29:250-62, 1992
22. Cumming WJ: Myelitis and toxic, inflammatory and infectious disorders. Curr Opin Neurol Neurosurg. 5(4):549-53, 1992
23. Hwang YM et al: A case of herpes zoster myelitis: positive magnetic resonance imaging finding. Eur Neurol. 31(3):164-7, 1991
24. Iwamasa T et al: Acute ascending necrotizing myelitis in Okinawa caused by herpes simplex virus type 2. Virchows Arch A Pathol Anat Histopathol. 418(1):71-5, 1991
25. Dawson DM et al: Acute nontraumatic myelopathies. Neurol Clin. 9(3):585-603, 1991
26. Power C et al: Pathological and molecular biological features of a myelopathy associated with HTLV-1 infection. Can J Neurol Sci. 18(3):352-5, 1991
27. Wiley CA et al: Acute ascending necrotizing myelopathy caused by herpes simplex virus type 2. Neurology. 37(11):1791-4, 1987
28. Awerbuch G et al: Demonstration of acute post-viral myelitis with magnetic resonance imaging. Pediatr Neurol. 3(6):367-9, 1987

IMAGE GALLERY

Typical

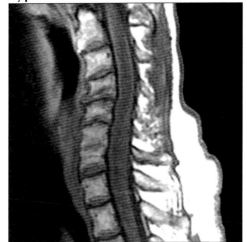 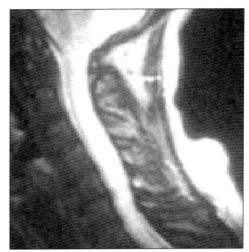

(Left) Sagittal T1WI MR shows enlarged cord with central tubular low signal simulating syrinx, though central signal not that of free fluid. Patient had 2 day history of weakness and radiculopathy. (Right) Sagittal T2WI MR shows diffuse edema and swelling of cervical cord in ER patient complaining of severe neck, arm pain and weakness.

Typical

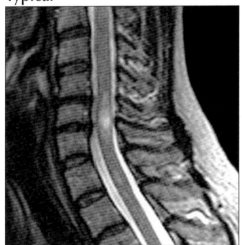 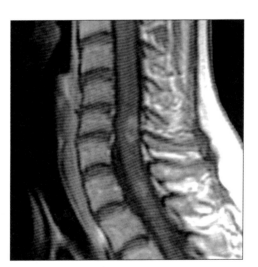

(Left) Sagittal T2WI MR shows focal lesion in lower cervical cord which demonstrates mild expansion. Patient had onset of weakness shortly after viral illness. (Right) Sagittal T1 C+ MR demonstrates ill-defined focus of enhancement in region of cord which showed high signal on T2WI: Patient developed weakness shortly after onset of viral illness.

Typical

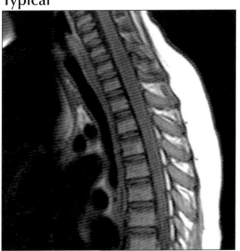 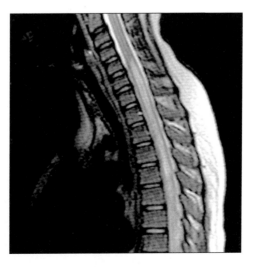

(Left) Sagittal T1WI MR shows large cervicothoracic cord filling canal, central low signal. Patient with leg weakness, peripheral neuropathy. (Right) Sagittal T2WI MR depicts expanded, edematous cervico-thoracic cord in patient with weakness, peripheral neuropathy.

HIV

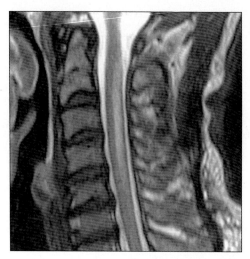

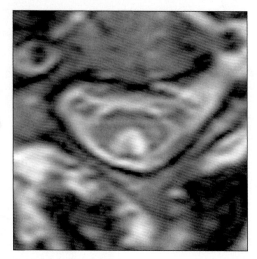

Sagittal T2WI MR demonstrates intramedullary hyperintensity within posterior cervical cord in patient with HIV myelopathy (Courtesy Florian P. Thomas, MD, PhD).

Axial T2WI MR shows hyperintensity within posterior cervical cord in patient with HIV myelopathy (Courtesy Florian P. Thomas, MD, PhD).

TERMINOLOGY

Abbreviations and Synonyms
- Synonyms: AIDS or HIV → myelopathy or myelitis

Definitions
- Myelopathy resulting from primary HIV infection

IMAGING FINDINGS

General Features
- Best diagnostic clue: Spinal cord T2 hyperintensity which may show patchy enhancement
- Location: Thoracic > cervical; mid to low thoracic cord with ↑ rostral involvement as disease progresses
- Morphology
  - Most common: Atrophy (72%)
  - Common
    - Diffuse nonspecific T2 hyperintensity of spinal cord with no definite pattern (29%)
    - Atrophy + diffuse intrinsic abnormality (14%)
  - Classic: T2 hyperintensity involving white matter (WM) tracts laterally & symmetrically

MR Findings
- T1WI
  - May be normal
  - Cord atrophy

- T2WI
  - May be normal
  - Hyperintensity either diffusely or involving WM tracts laterally & symmetrically
  - Cord atrophy
- STIR: Foci of hyperintensity
- T1 C+: Visible lesions may enhance

Imaging Recommendations
- Best imaging tool: MRI C+

DIFFERENTIAL DIAGNOSIS

B12 deficiency
- May appear identical to HIV myelopathy
- Negative HIV test

Varicella Zoster virus
- Intrinsic myelopathy
- PCR-positive for virus in CSF

CMV myelitis
- Cause of HIV-related polyradiculopathy
- MRI may show nerve root & conus leptomeningeal thickening, enhancement
- Characteristic intranuclear inclusions

Multiple sclerosis
- Similar appearance

DDx: HIV Myelopathy Mimics

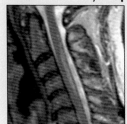

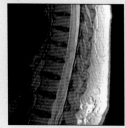

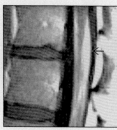

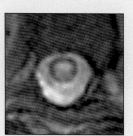

B12 Deficiency

Varicella Zoster

CMV

Transverse Myelitis

HIV

Key Facts

Terminology
- Synonyms: AIDS or HIV → myelopathy or myelitis
- Myelopathy resulting from primary HIV infection

Imaging Findings
- Best diagnostic clue: Spinal cord T2 hyperintensity which may show patchy enhancement
- Location: Thoracic > cervical; mid to low thoracic cord with ↑ rostral involvement as disease progresses
- Best imaging tool: MRI C+

Top Differential Diagnoses
- B12 deficiency
- Varicella Zoster virus
- CMV myelitis
- Multiple sclerosis
- Transverse myelitis

- HTLV1 (human T-cell leukemia/lymphoma virus)
- Lymphoma

Pathology
- General path comments: Diagnosis is one of exclusion based on clinical, laboratory, & radiologic findings
- Most common cause of spinal cord disease in AIDS patients is AIDS-associated myelopathy with prevalence of 20-55%

Clinical Issues
- Insidious onset of progressive spastic paraparesis with ataxia, urinary problems & sensory loss

Diagnostic Checklist
- Need to exclude other treatable causes of myelopathy

- Waxing & waning symptoms
- Negative HIV test

Transverse myelitis
- Indistinguishable by imaging from HIV myelitis
- Inflammation across the width of enlarged spinal cord
- Uncertain etiology
- Will have normal CD4 count & negative HIV test

HTLV1 (human T-cell leukemia/lymphoma virus)
- Intrinsic myelopathy
- HTLV myelopathy may respond to corticosteroids or interferon

Lymphoma
- Destructive lesion with enhancing paraspinal and/or intradural component
- Neoplastic cells in CSF

PATHOLOGY

General Features
- General path comments: Diagnosis is one of exclusion based on clinical, laboratory, & radiologic findings
- Genetics
  - Neurotropism is property specific to certain HIV strains & may be related to monocyte tropism
    - Would explain why HIV expression occurs in CNS of certain AIDS patients but not others
  - May relate to polymorphism of genes encoding for enzymes of transmethyl cycle
    - Methylation is essential for myelin formation, stabilization, & repair → interference with transmethyl pathway at any level can cause WM vacuolization in spinal cord
    - Usually mild or asymptomatic in normal individuals
    - ↑ Demand for methyl donors or inhibition of methylation (as may occur in HIV infection) may induce metabolic stress & hypomethylation

- Result is genetic predisposition to cord disease in these susceptible & HIV infected individuals
- Etiology
  - Primary HIV infection = DNA lentivirus/retrovirus that attacks spine monocytes & macrophages
  - Possible mechanisms
    - Infection by HIV-1 may stimulate macrophages to phagocytize myelin
    - HIV-1-infected macrophages may secrete factors that directly damage neural tissue
    - Macrophages are likely to ingest myelin that has been damaged by any mechanism
    - Associated with abnormal B12 utilization
  - Disease of cord & brain often occur separately suggesting different pathogenetic mechanisms
- Epidemiology
  - Most common cause of spinal cord disease in AIDS patients is AIDS-associated myelopathy with prevalence of 20-55%
  - Although frequent, often non-diagnosed → ≈ 10% have symptoms
  - Up to 20% in clinical & 55% in histologic studies
- Associated abnormalities
  - Opportunistic CNS & PNS infections (e.g., CMV, PML)
  - Opportunistic malignancies (e.g., lymphoma)

Microscopic Features
- Vacuolar myelopathy (VM)
  - Direct injury of neurons by HIV
  - Intramyelin & periaxonal vacuolation of WM with posterior & lateral column demyelination
- Electron microscopy
  - Intramyelinic or periaxonal vacuoles, rarely disrupted axons
  - Myelin within macrophages
  - HIV-1 budding from macrophages
- RNA analysis demonstrates
  - HIV-1 expression in mononuclear & multinucleated macrophages in areas of myelopathy
  - HIV RNA detected in 100% of cords with VM
  - Level of RNA expression correlates directly with extent of spinal cord pathology & clinical findings

- In children, spinal cord WM is also effected
  - Diffuse demyelination with axonal loss & a more prominent inflammatory infiltrate
  - Typical VM is rarely observed
  - Difference may be from different myelin structure or alternative pathologic mechanisms in children
- In rare cases there is evidence of partial remyelination
- Pathology changes observed in brains of patients with AIDS are morphologically different with myelin pallor, microglial infiltrates, & reactive astrocytosis

Staging, Grading or Classification Criteria
- Criteria for diagnosis of AIDS-associated myelopathy
- (1) Male or female > 18 yrs with HIV-1 infection
- (2) AIDS-associated myelopathy, with or without neuropathy & dementia
  - (A) At least two of the following symptoms
    - Paresthesia &/or numbness in lower extremities or all four limbs
    - Weakness of limbs
    - Unsteady, stiff, or uncoordinated gait
    - Sensation of electric shock through back and legs on neck flexion
    - Urinary frequency, urgency, incontinence, or retention
    - Fecal incontinence or retention
    - Sexual dysfunction with male erectile impairment
  - (B) At least two of the following signs
    - Reduction in vibratory and/or position sensation
    - Brisk deep tendon reflexes
    - Abnormal plantar response
    - Lhermitte sign
    - Spastic, ataxic, or ataxospastic gait
- (3) Signs & symptoms of AIDS-associated myelopathy for at least 6 weeks
- (4) Abnormal somatosensory evoked potentials
- (5) No other determinable cause for spinal cord disease by serologic & CSF studies

CLINICAL ISSUES

Presentation
- Most common signs/symptoms
  - Insidious onset of progressive spastic paraparesis with ataxia, urinary problems & sensory loss
    - Occurs in later stages of disease
    - May need to urinate every 2-3 hours
    - Difficulty in obtaining or maintaining an erection
    - Stiffness in legs develops, often accompanied by cramps & spasms → walking becomes difficult
    - Weakness with degrees of paralysis develops
    - In final stages, there may be severe paralysis of legs & loss of urinary control with incontinence
    - Loss of anal sphincter control → incontinence
    - Painless initially, in later stages cramps & spasms may cause serious discomfort or pain
    - Arms & hands generally not effected
  - May have acute myelitic syndrome occurring shortly after seroconversion
- Clinical profile
  - Very low CD4 + lymphocyte counts
  - Often have vitamin B12 deficiency
    - Relationship to pathogenesis not yet understood

- May be related to polymorphism of transmethyl cycle enzyme genes

Natural History & Prognosis
- Prognosis is poor

Treatment
- MRI is essential in exclusion of other extrinsic or intrinsic processes, but there are caveats
  - Normal-appearing spinal cord is often seen in patients with mild & severe myelopathy
  - Cord atrophy & signal abnormality are found in both mildly & severely myelopathic patients
- Historically no known treatment
  - Treatment studies are underway using highly active antiretroviral therapy (HAART)
    - Now less common with HAART
    - Estimated < 10% of patients with AIDS now develop spinal cord pathology
  - Improvement with L-methionine has been reported

DIAGNOSTIC CHECKLIST

Consider
- Need to exclude other treatable causes of myelopathy

Image Interpretation Pearls
- MRI is often noncontributory but may reveal unsuspected coexisting conditions or other explanation for patient symptoms
- Spinal cord atrophy is the most common abnormal MR finding typically involving the thoracic cord with or without cervical cord involvement

SELECTED REFERENCES

1. Portegies P et al: Guidelines for the diagnosis and management of neurological complications of HIV infection. Eur J Neurol. 11(5):297-304, 2004
2. Di Rocco A: HIV-associated Myelopathy. Curr Treatment Options Infect Dis. 5:457-465, 2003
3. Di Rocco A: Diseases of the spinal cord in human immunodeficiency virus infection. Semin Neurol. 19(2):151-5, 1999
4. Chong J et al: MR findings in AIDS-associated myelopathy. AJNR Am J Neuroradiol. 20(8):1412-6, 1999
5. Quencer RM: AIDS-associated myelopathy: clinical severity, MR findings, and underlying etiologies. AJNR Am J Neuroradiol. 20(8):1387-8, 1999
6. Weiser B et al: Human immunodeficiency virus type 1 expression in the central nervous system correlates directly with extent of disease. Proc Natl Acad Sci U S A. 87(10):3997-4001, 1990
7. Eilbott DJ et al: Human immunodeficiency virus type 1 in spinal cords of acquired immunodeficiency syndrome patients with myelopathy: expression and replication in macrophages. Proc Natl Acad Sci U S A. 86(9):3337-41, 1989

HIV

III 1 41

IMAGE GALLERY

Typical

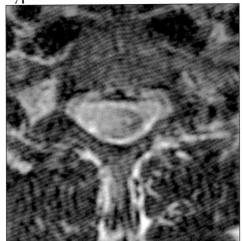 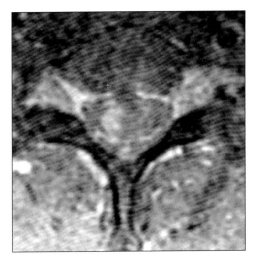

(Left) Axial T2WI MR shows diffuse hyperintensity within the right hemicord from HIV myelopathy. *(Right)* Axial T1 C+ MR with fat suppression reveals enhancement within right hemicord consistent with HIV myelopathy.

Typical

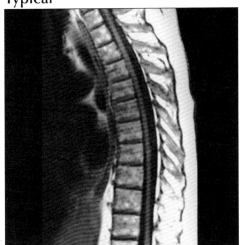 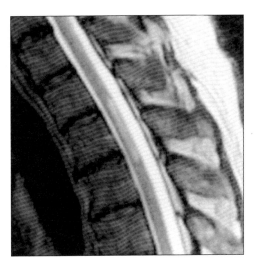

(Left) Sagittal T1WI MR shows diffuse cord atrophy from HIV myelopathy. Not shown is diffuse T2WI intramedullary hyperintensity without enhancement (Courtesy Scott W. Atlas, MD, with permission from AJNR). *(Right)* Sagittal T2WI MR shows intramedullary hyperintensity, primarily posteriorly, in a patient with HIV myelopathy (Courtesy Scott W. Atlas, MD, with permission from AJNR).

Typical

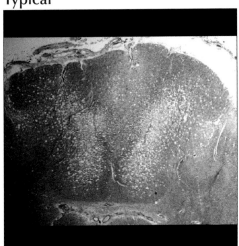 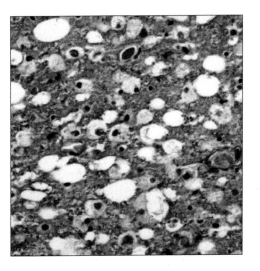

(Left) Micropathology, low power with Luxol fast blue stain, shows extensive spongiform changes within white matter from vacuolar myelopathy (Courtesy Robert E. Schmidt, MD). *(Right)* Micropathology, high power with Luxol fast blue stain, shows marked vacuolation within white matter from HIV myelopathy (Courtesy Robert E. Schmidt, MD).

MYELITIS-CORD ABSCESS

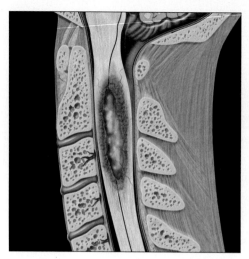

Sagittal graphic shows irregular abscess cavity in cervical cord, with cord expansion and edema.

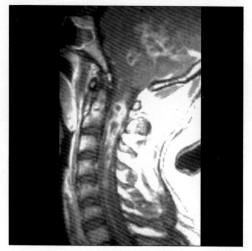

Sagittal T1 C+ MR shows extensive irregular enhancement involving cerebellum, cervical cord reflecting Streptococcal abscesses (Courtesy J. Illes, MD).

TERMINOLOGY

Abbreviations and Synonyms
- Intramedullary spinal cord abscess (ISCA)

Definitions
- Infection of spinal cord with necrosis
  - Pyogenic infection most common

IMAGING FINDINGS

General Features
- Best diagnostic clue: Ring-enhancing mass within cord, with appropriate clinical history of inflammation/infection
- Location: Intramedullary
- Size: Variable, usually less than 2 cm
- Morphology: Round or oblong irregular area of ring-enhancement, with associated edema

Radiographic Findings
- Myelography: Nonspecific findings of symmetrical cord enlargement, or myelographic block from intramedullary lesion

CT Findings
- NECT: Normal, or ill-defined cord irregularity and expansion

MR Findings
- T1WI
  - Ill-defined low signal from expanded cord
  - Abscess cord may show focal low signal
- T2WI: Increased T2W signal from abscess core and surrounding edema; cord expansion
- PD/Intermediate: Increased signal from abscess and surrounding edema
- STIR: Good definition of cord edema
- DWI
  - May show positive diffusion (reduced ADC) similar to brain abscess
    - Lack of diffusion restriction does not exclude abscess
- T1 C+: Irregular ring-enhancing lesion with cord expansion

Imaging Recommendations
- Best imaging tool: MRI with contrast defines cord abnormality, edema, enhancing abscess
- Protocol advice: Sagittal, axial T1W, T2W images, post-contrast sagittal, axial T1W

DDx: Cord T2 Hyperintensity

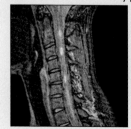

Multiple Sclerosis

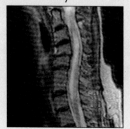

Viral Myelitis

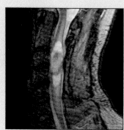

Astrocytoma

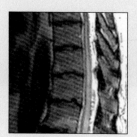

Type I Fistula

MYELITIS-CORD ABSCESS

Key Facts

Terminology
- Intramedullary spinal cord abscess (ISCA)

Imaging Findings
- Best diagnostic clue: Ring-enhancing mass within cord, with appropriate clinical history of inflammation/infection

Top Differential Diagnoses
- Acute transverse/viral myelitis
- Hypervascular cord neoplasms
- Multiple sclerosis
- Type I dural fistula
- Cavernous malformation
- Cord infarction
- Intradural/extramedullary tumors

Pathology
- Routes of infection: Majority of cases idiopathic/cryptogenic
- Hematogenous spread (10%)
- Contiguous spread from adjacent infection (25% of these cases from dermal sinus tract)
- Direct implantation such as trauma, or surgical
- Multiple organisms involved

Clinical Issues
- Often present with signs/symptoms of structural cord lesion, rather than infection
- Mixed neurologic deficits including fever, pain, motor deficit, sensory disturbance, and sphincter dysfunction

DIFFERENTIAL DIAGNOSIS

Acute transverse/viral myelitis
- Rapid onset of paraplegia with or without sensory symptoms, bladder dysfunction
- Multiple viral agents implicated, either immune mediated or direct viral invasion of cord
  - Echovirus, Coxsackie, cytomegalovirus, varicella-zoster, herpes simplex, Epstein-Barr, mumps, hepatitis, rubella, measles
- 1/3 improve, 1/3 partial improvement, 1/3 fail to improve
- Nonspecific T2 hyperintensity in cord, with variable enhancement (no ring-enhancement)

Hypervascular cord neoplasms
- Ependymoma (mass centrally located; no syrinx)
- Hemangioblastoma (focal pial based mass ± cyst
- Astrocytoma (usually not hypervascular; peritumoral edema common)
- Vascular metastasis (known primary, e.g., renal cell carcinoma)

Multiple sclerosis
- Peripheral in location
- Less than two vertebral segments in length
- 90% incidence of associated intracranial lesions
- May show ring-enhancement

Type I dural fistula
- May rarely show only cord expansion and edema on T2WI, without prominent vessels
- No cord ring-enhancement

Cavernous malformation
- Mottled or speckled pattern of prior hemorrhage, hemosiderin rim

Cord infarction
- Focal hyperintensity on T2WI in slightly expanded cord
- May show patchy ill-defined enhancement in subacute phase
- Abrupt onset of weakness and loss of sensation

Intradural/extramedullary tumors
- Enhancing schwannoma/meningioma with demarcation between lesion and cord margin

PATHOLOGY

General Features
- General path comments
  - Rare, < 100 cases described
  - Routes of infection: Majority of cases idiopathic/cryptogenic
    - Hematogenous spread (10%)
    - Contiguous spread from adjacent infection (25% of these cases from dermal sinus tract)
    - Direct implantation such as trauma, or surgical
  - Microbiology
    - Multiple organisms involved
    - Staph aureus
    - Staph epidermidis
    - Bacteroides
    - Haemophilus species
    - Listeria monocytogenes
- Etiology
  - Two major etiologies
    - Adult ISCA either hematogenous seeding from cardiopulmonary source, or idiopathic
    - Children often have spinal dysraphism allowing direct extension of infection (40%)
- Epidemiology
  - Intramedullary infection rare
  - 0.2-2.2 cases per 10,000 tertiary care hospital admissions
- Associated abnormalities: Dermal sinus tract or dysraphism commonly present in children presenting with cord abscess

CLINICAL ISSUES

Presentation
- Most common signs/symptoms

MYELITIS-CORD ABSCESS

- ○ Often present with signs/symptoms of structural cord lesion, rather than infection
- ○ Mixed neurologic deficits including fever, pain, motor deficit, sensory disturbance, and sphincter dysfunction
- ○ Other signs/symptoms
  - ▪ Incontinence, meningismus
  - ▪ Triad of fever, pain, neurologic deficit in 25%
- ○ Delay in diagnosis common (time from symptom onset to diagnosis > 30 days)
  - ▪ Fever < 50%
- ○ Children
  - ▪ Paralysis (60%)
  - ▪ Fever (> 50%)
  - ▪ Urinary retention (30%)
  - ▪ Back pain (28%)
  - ▪ Nausea/vomiting (10%)
  - ▪ 20% recover without neurologic sequelae

Demographics
- Age: Adults and children (mean age 34 years)
- Gender: M:F = 3:1
- Ethnicity: None known

Natural History & Prognosis
- Associated with high mortality and morbidity
- Mortality of 24% reported from years 1944-1977
  - ○ Mortality of 8% in antibiotic era (1977-1997)
- Quick surgical drainage and aggressive intravenous antibiotics required
- Persistent neurologic deficit with successful treatment > 70%

Treatment
- Early surgical drainage followed by antibiotic therapy
  - ○ Laminectomy with myelotomy and drainage
  - ○ I.V. antibiotic coverage 4-6 weeks, with 2-3 additional months oral antibiotics
- Surgically treated mortality approximately 14%

DIAGNOSTIC CHECKLIST

Consider
- Ampicillin empiric coverage in idiopathic cases for L. monocytogenes
- Serial WBC count, ESR, enhanced MRI, important for post-operative follow-up, detection of recurrence

Image Interpretation Pearls
- MR brain to exclude concomitant brain abscess

SELECTED REFERENCES

1. Berger JR et al: Infectious myelopathies. Semin Neurol. 22(2): 133-42, 2002
2. Krishnan A et al: Craniovertebral junction tuberculosis: a review of 29 cases. J Comput Assist Tomogr. 25(2): 171-6, 2001
3. Chidambaram B et al: Intramedullary abscess of the spinal cord. Pediatr Neurosurg. 34(1): 43-4, 2001
4. Durmaz R et al: Multiple nocardial abscesses of cerebrum, cerebellum and spinal cord, causing quadriplegia. Clin Neurol Neurosurg. 103(1): 59-62, 2001
5. Rossi FH et al: Listeria spinal cord abscess responsive to trimethoprim-sulfamethoxazole monotherapy. Can J Neurol Sci. 28(4): 354-6, 2001
6. Elmac I et al: Cervical spinal cord intramedullary abscess. Case report. J Neurosurg Sci. 45(4): 213-5; discussion 215, 2001
7. Ruiz A et al: MR imaging of infections of the cervical spine. Magn Reson Imaging Clin N Am. 8(3): 561-80, 2000
8. Desai KI et al: Holocord intramedullary abscess: an unusual case with review of literature. Spinal Cord. 37(12): 866-70, 1999
9. Mukunda BN et al: Solitary spinal intramedullary abscess caused by Nocardia asteroides. South Med J. 92(12): 1223-4, 1999
10. Murphy KJ et al: Spinal cord infection: myelitis and abscess formation. AJNR Am J Neuroradiol. 19(2): 341-8, 1998
11. Sverzut JM et al: Spinal cord abscess in a heroin addict: case report. Neuroradiology. 40(7): 455-8, 1998
12. Chan CT et al: Intramedullary abscess of the spinal cord in the antibiotic era: clinical features, microbial etiologies, trends in pathogenesis, and outcomes. Clin Infect Dis. 27(3): 619-26, 1998
13. Derkinderen P et al: Intramedullary spinal cord abscess associated with cervical spondylodiskitis and epidural abscess. Scand J Infect Dis. 30(6): 618-9, 1998
14. Friess HM et al: MR of staphylococcal myelitis of the cervical spinal cord. AJNR Am J Neuroradiol. 18(3): 455-8, 1997
15. Martin RJ et al: Neurosurgical care of spinal epidural, subdural, and intramedullary abscesses and arachnoiditis. Orthop Clin North Am. 27(1): 125-36, 1996
16. Banuelos AF et al: Central nervous system abscesses due to Coccidioides species. Clin Infect Dis. 22(2): 240-50, 1996
17. Chu JY et al: Listeria spinal cord abscess--clinical and MRI findings. Can J Neurol Sci. 23(3): 220-3, 1996
18. Lindner A et al: Magnetic resonance image findings of spinal intramedullary abscess caused by Candida albicans: case report. Neurosurgery. 36(2): 411-2, 1995
19. Pfadenhauer K et al: Spinal manifestation of neurolisteriosis. J Neurol. 242(3): 153-6, 1995
20. Bartels RH et al: Intramedullary spinal cord abscess. A case report. Spine. 20(10): 1199-204, 1995
21. King SJ et al: MRI of an abscess of the cervical spinal cord in a case of Listeria meningoencephalomyelitis. Neuroradiology. 35(7): 495-6, 1993

IMAGE GALLERY

Typical

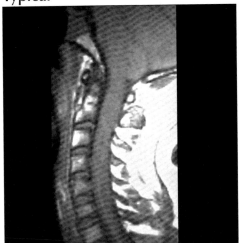
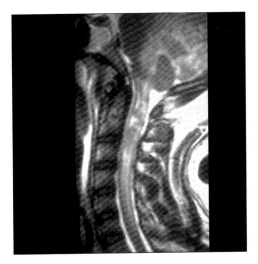

(Left) Sagittal T1WI MR with extensive cerebellar, cervical cord Strep abscesses shows diffuse cord expansion, loss of CSF signal, and poor definition of 4th ventricle due to edema (Courtesy J. Illes, MD). *(Right)* Sagittal T2WI MR shows diffuse T2 hyperintensity involving cerebellum, brain stem, cervical cord from diffuse Strep abscesses (Courtesy J. Illes, MD).

Typical

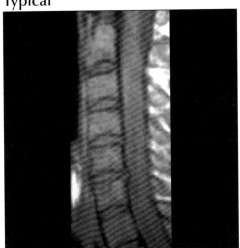
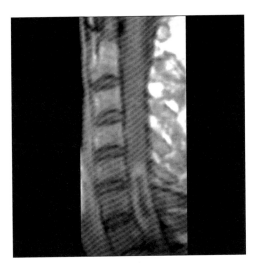

(Left) Sagittal T1WI MR shows diffuse cord enlargement filling the thecal sac from C1 to C7 level. Abscess cavity at C6-7 level is not defined without contrast (Courtesy J. Illes, MD). *(Right)* Sagittal T1 C+ MR shows irregular ring-enhancement of cord at C6 & C7 levels reflecting focal cord abscess (Courtesy J. Illes, MD).

Typical

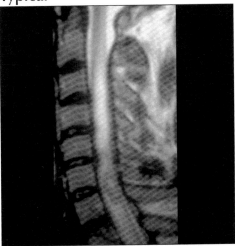
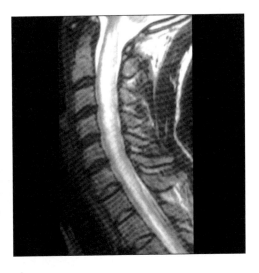

(Left) Sagittal T2WI MR shows cord abscess as irregular low signal within cord at C6-7. There is extensive T2 hyperintense cord edema extending to C2 level (Courtesy J. Illes, MD). *(Right)* Sagittal T2WI MR shows extensive cord T2 hyperintensity, diffuse cord expansion extending from C1 to T2 level due to cord herpes myelitis.

SPINAL MENINGITIS

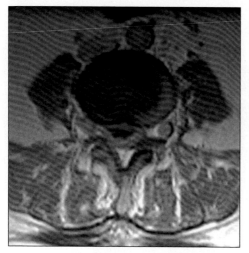

Axial T1 C+ MR shows clumped, diffusely enhancing nerve roots in patient with Staph. aureus meningitis.

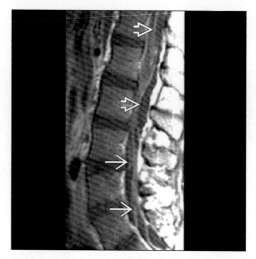

Sagittal T1 C+ MR shows diffuse enhancement of multiple nerve roots (arrows) in patient with meningitis, dorsal subdural empyema (open arrows).

TERMINOLOGY

Abbreviations and Synonyms
- Infectious arachnoiditis

Definitions
- Infection of spinal cord leptomeninges and subarachnoid space

IMAGING FINDINGS

General Features
- Best diagnostic clue: Diffuse, extensive subarachnoid enhancement
- Location: All spinal segments involved
- Size: Diffuse or focal
- Morphology
  - Smooth or irregular meningeal enhancement
  - Diffuse cerebral spinal fluid (CSF) enhancement

Radiographic Findings
- Myelography
  - Block of CSF
  - Irregular contour of thecal sac
  - Nodular or band-like filling defects adherent to cord surface
  - Thickened nerve roots
  - Focal or diffuse cord swelling

CT Findings
- NECT: Increased CSF density
- CECT: Enhancing CSF ± meninges

MR Findings
- T1WI
  - Increased CSF intensity
  - Indistinct cord-CSF interface
  - Irregular cord outline
  - Clumped nerve roots
- T2WI
  - Obliterated subarachnoid space
  - Nodular or band-like filling defects in subarachnoid space
  - Hyperintense cord signal intensity (SI)
    - ± Focal or diffuse cord swelling
- T1 C+
  - Smooth or nodular meningeal enhancement
  - Homogenously enhancing CSF
  - Smooth or nodular nerve root enhancement
  - ± Segmental or focal intramedullary enhancement

Imaging Recommendations
- Best imaging tool
  - Axial and sagittal T1WI and T2WI MRI
    - Positive in advanced bacterial meningitis or granulomatous infection

DDx: Leptomeningeal/Nerve Root Enhancement

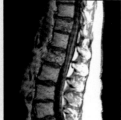

Metastasis

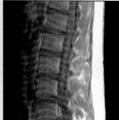

Sarcoidosis

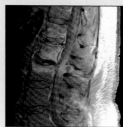

Arachnoiditis

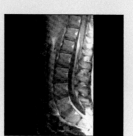

Guillain-Barré

SPINAL MENINGITIS

Key Facts

Terminology
- Infectious arachnoiditis
- Infection of spinal cord leptomeninges and subarachnoid space

Imaging Findings
- Location: All spinal segments involved
- NECT: Increased CSF density
- Increased CSF intensity
- Indistinct cord-CSF interface
- Irregular cord outline
- Clumped nerve roots
- Smooth or nodular meningeal enhancement
- Homogenously enhancing CSF
- Smooth or nodular nerve root enhancement
- ± Segmental or focal intramedullary enhancement

Top Differential Diagnoses
- Carcinomatous meningitis
- Sarcoidosis
- Lumbar arachnoiditis
- Guillain-Barré syndrome
- Intracranial hypotension

Clinical Issues
- Acute onset of fever, chills, headache, + altered level of consciousness

---

- Protocol advice: Intravenous gadolinium increases sensitivity in detecting meningeal disease

DIFFERENTIAL DIAGNOSIS

Carcinomatous meningitis
- Primary CNS neoplasm
- Metastatic lung, breast carcinoma, melanoma, lymphoma
- Thickened blurred nerve roots on T1WI and T2WI
  ○ Obliterated CSF
- Focal or diffuse, "sheet-like" or nodular enhancement along cord or nerve roots

Sarcoidosis
- Noncaseating granulomatous inflammation of spinal cord & its coverings
- Protean imaging findings
  ○ Leptomeningeal + nerve root enhancement mimics spinal meningitis
  ○ Cord edema with focal intramedullary enhancement simulates myelitis
- Concurrent systemic manifestations & elevated angiotensin converting enzyme level help make diagnosis
  ○ Clinical CNS involvement in 5% of patients with sarcoidosis

Lumbar arachnoiditis
- Commonly associated with prior surgery
  ○ ± Exposure to myelographic agents
- Cauda equina typically involved
- Clumped nerve roots forming central mass or multiple cords
- "Empty sac sign" with nerve roots adherent to periphery of thecal sac
- ± Nerve root enhancement
- Loculated CSF

Guillain-Barré syndrome
- Inflammatory demyelination typically following recent viral illness
  ○ Autoimmune response suspected

- Ascending paralysis
- Diffuse enhancement of conus and cauda equina
  ○ ± Nerve root thickening

Intracranial hypotension
- From prior spinal trauma, diagnostic or interventional procedure, or spontaneous
- Increased dural venous engorgement
- Low opening pressure on lumbar puncture
- Diffuse smooth meningeal thickening & enhancement
- May see cerebellar tonsillar descent + effaced pre-pontine space in posterior fossa

Idiopathic hypertrophic spinal pachymeningitis
- Diagnosis of exclusion
- Unknown etiology
- Fibrous inflammatory thickening of dura mater
- Thickened dura iso- to hypointense on T1WI and T2WI
  ○ Marked post-contrast-enhancement

Subdural hematoma
- Other than trauma, lumbar puncture in patients with coagulopathy is most common cause
- More common in lumbar or thoracolumbar region
- Predominantly hypointense on T2WI or gradient echo
  ○ Isointense on T1WI
- No post-gadolinium enhancement

PATHOLOGY

General Features
- General path comments: Infection of CSF and meningeal coverings surrounding spinal cord
- Etiology
  ○ Acute meningitis: Onset of symptoms < 24 hr
    ▪ Almost always bacterial
    ▪ Newborn: Group B Streptococcus, gram negative bacilli, Listeria monocytogenes

SPINAL MENINGITIS

- 2 months to 12 years: Haemophilus influenzae, Streptococcus pneumoniae, & Neisseria meningitides
  - Adults: Above, plus streptococci + staphylococci
  ○ Subacute meningitis: Symptoms develop in 1-7 days
    - Mostly viral (e.g., HIV-related CMV radiculomyelitis), some bacterial (e.g., Lyme disease)
  ○ Chronic meningitis: Fluctuating symptoms for > 7 days
    - Tuberculosis
    - Syphilis
    - Fungal: Coccidioidomycosis, cryptococcosis, and aspergillosis
  ○ Mechanism of inoculation
    - Hematogenous dissemination from extraspinal focus of infection
    - Contiguous spread from adjacent spondylodiscitis, spinal epidural abscess
    - Direct inoculation through trauma or interventional procedures
    - Unexplained source of infection: Probably bacteria colonized in nasopharynx
  ○ Pathophysiology of bacterial meningitis
    - Initial acute inflammatory exudate in subarachnoid space
    - Toxic mediators potentiate inflammatory response
    - Increased permeability of blood-cord barrier
    - Influx of inflammatory cells
    - Spinal cord swelling and edema likely due to ischemia from vasculitis, venous congestion; and/or direct infection
- Epidemiology: Incidence of bacterial meningitis: 2-3 per 100,000
- Associated abnormalities
  ○ Spondylodiscitis
  ○ Spinal epidural abscess
  ○ Subdural empyema
  ○ Subarachnoid cysts
    - Fibrin deposition results in loculation of subarachnoid space
  ○ Myelitis
  ○ Cord abscess
  ○ Syringomyelia
    - Blocked CSF flow results in increased pressure within cord and subsequent central canal expansion

Microscopic Features
- Cellular debris, inflammatory cells, and micro-organisms
- Tuberculous meningitis
  ○ Small tubercles consist of epithelioid cells, Langerhan giant cells, & foci of caseation

CLINICAL ISSUES

Presentation
- Most common signs/symptoms
  ○ Acute onset of fever, chills, headache, + altered level of consciousness
  ○ Other signs/symptoms
    - Generalized convulsions

- Neck stiffness
- Paraparesis
- Paresthesia
- Gait disturbance
- Urinary bladder dysfunction
- Clinical profile: Milder symptoms with protracted course in tuberculous or fungal meningitis

Demographics
- Age
  ○ Newborns
  ○ Infants: Peak age 3-8 months
  ○ Adults: 20s; 60s
- Gender
  ○ No gender preference among adults
  ○ M:F = 3:1 in neonates

Natural History & Prognosis
- Prognosis depends on severity of disease, causative pathogen, patient age + co-morbidities
  ○ Mortality of bacterial meningitis: 20-90%
    - Depending on initial neurologic impairment & rate of progression
    - Chronic disabilities include paralysis, seizures, deafness, etc.
  ○ Viral meningitis generally less severe
    - Full recovery expected within 2 weeks in most cases

Treatment
- Supportive care with hydration and pain management
- Intravenous dexamethasone to decrease inflammatory reaction and brain/cord edema
- Empiric intravenous antibiotics based on suspected organisms in each age group
- Organism specific intravenous antibiotics
- Preventive oral antibiotics for close contacts of patients with Neisseria meningitides

DIAGNOSTIC CHECKLIST

Image Interpretation Pearls
- Imaging often negative in early spinal meningitis
- Increased CSF SI on T1WI with diffuse post-gadolinium enhancement suggestive of spinal meningitis

SELECTED REFERENCES

1. Hunter JV et al: Neuroimaging of central nervous system infections. Semin Pediatr Infect Dis. 14(2):140-64, 2003
2. Kaplan SL: Clinical presentations, diagnosis, and prognostic factors of bacterial meningitis. Infect Dis Clin North Am. 13(3):579-94, vi-vii, 1999
3. Meltzer CC et al: MR imaging of the meninges. Part I. Normal anatomic features and nonneoplastic disease. Radiology. 201(2):297-308, 1996
4. Post MD et al: Magnetic resonance imaging of spinal infection. Rheum Dis Clin North Am. 17:773-94, 1991
5. Chang KH et al: Tuberculous arachnoiditis of the spine: Findings on Myelography, CT, and MR imaging. AJNR. 10:1255-62, 1989

SPINAL MENINGITIS

IMAGE GALLERY

Typical

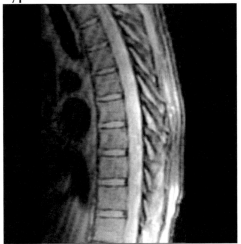
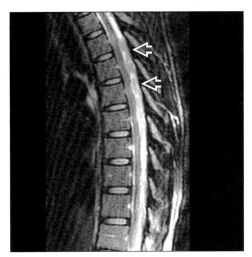

(Left) Sagittal T1WI MR through thoracic spine shows diffusely increased CSF signal intensity, obscuring cord-CSF interface. *(Right)* Sagittal T2WI MR with fat suppression demonstrates hyperintense CSF with areas of subtle low intensities (arrows) due to bacterial meningitis. Mild mass effect on thoracic cord is suggested.

Typical

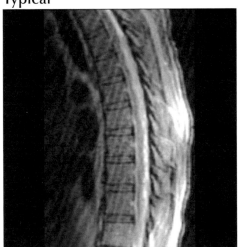
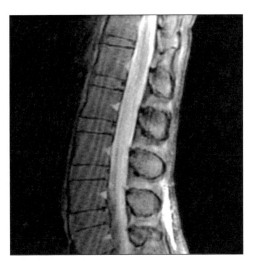

(Left) Sagittal T1 C+ MR with fat suppression demonstrates diffusely enhancing CSF, with mild heterogeneity. CSF culture confirmed bacterial meningitis. *(Right)* Sagittal T1 C+ MR with fat suppression through lumbar spine shows enhancing CSF with indistinct, enhancing nerve roots.

Typical

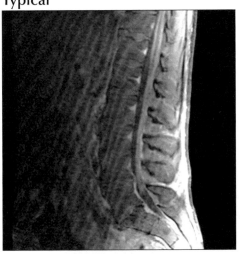
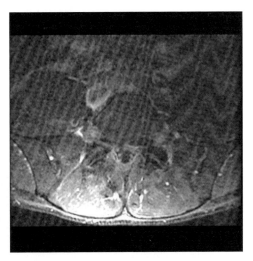

(Left) Sagittal T1 C+ MR with fat suppression through lumbar spine with spinal meningitis shows leptomeningeal and nerve root enhancement. *(Right)* Axial T1 C+ MR with fat suppression in same patient demonstrates enhancing nerve roots with mildly enhancing dura.

ECHINOCOCCUS

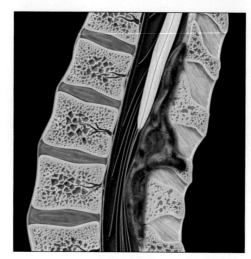

Sagittal graphic of lumbar spine shows cystic mass involving posterior elements with extension into dorsal epidural space, thecal sac & cauda equina compression.

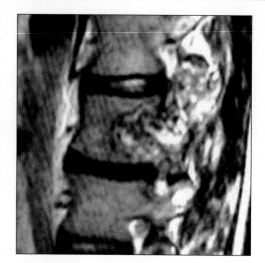

Sagittal T2WI MR shows lobulated extradural heterogeneous T2 hyperintense mass (with permission Athanassopoulou et al, MRI in spinal hydatid disease, {online case 1855}, Euromultimedia).

TERMINOLOGY

Abbreviations and Synonyms
- Synonyms: Hydatidosis, hydatid disease, hydatid cyst disease

Definitions
- Disease caused by cyst stage of infestation by tapeworm of genus echinococcus
- Liver, lung involvement most common, bone involvement rare
- Multiple Echinococcal species produce disease; complex life cycle
  - E. granulosus = causative agent of Hydatid disease in man/other mammals
    - Dog as definite host; parasitized by adult tapeworm
    - Gravid proglottids shed by tapeworm, disintegrate in dog intestine
    - Eggs passed in feces
    - Mammals act as intermediate host after ingestion of eggs (typically sheep, cattle)
    - Eggs hatch in intestine, penetrates gut wall, travel via lymphatic/blood vessels throughout body
    - Development of cysts to produce infective protoscolices takes 1 to 2 years
    - Dogs then ingest protoscolices on death of intermediate host (predation/scavenging)

- Cyst wall digested in gut, allowing development of adult worms
  - E. multilocularis = causative agent of alveolar hydatid disease in man/other mammals
    - Fox is most important definitive host
    - Cyst grows invasively by external budding, diffuse growth through infected organ
  - E. vogeli = polycystic form in Central & South America
    - Bush dogs as definitive hosts

IMAGING FINDINGS

General Features
- Best diagnostic clue: Multiloculated, multiseptated T2 hyperintense vertebral body/posterior element mass without significant enhancement in endemic area for echinococcus
- Location: Thoracic spine most common
- Size: Variable, up to several centimeters
- Morphology: Round, multiseptated, multiloculated cysts, bone expansion

Radiographic Findings
- Radiography
  - Multiloculated osteolytic lesions give "bunch of grapes" morphology
  - Nonspecific bone destruction

DDx: Heterogeneous T2 Hyperintense Masses

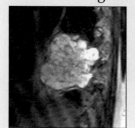

Chondrosarcoma

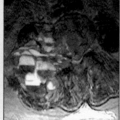

Osteosarcoma

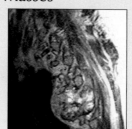

Renal Cell Met

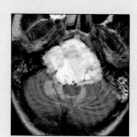

Chordoma

Key Facts

Terminology
- Synonyms: Hydatidosis, hydatid disease, hydatid cyst disease
- Disease caused by cyst stage of infestation by tapeworm of genus echinococcus
- Liver, lung involvement most common, bone involvement rare
- E. granulosus = causative agent of Hydatid disease in man/other mammals
- Dog as definite host; parasitized by adult tapeworm
- E. multilocularis = causative agent of alveolar hydatid disease in man/other mammals
- E. vogeli = polycystic form in Central & South America

Imaging Findings
- Best diagnostic clue: Multiloculated, multiseptated T2 hyperintense vertebral body/posterior element mass without significant enhancement in endemic area for echinococcus
- Location: Thoracic spine most common

Pathology
- Intramedullary cyst
- Intradural/extramedullary
- Extradural intraspinal
- Vertebral disease
- Paravertebral

Diagnostic Checklist
- Hydatid cyst fluid highly allergenic, cyst rupture may cause anaphylaxis

---

- Myelography: May show block with significant epidural extension of cysts

CT Findings
- NECT
  - Multiloculated osteolytic lesions in vertebral body, posterior elements
  - Paraspinal mass associated with vertebral body lesions
- CECT: Minimal/no enhancement of paraspinal/vertebral body cysts

MR Findings
- T1WI
  - CSF signal multiseptated/multicystic lesions
  - Degenerated cysts may be isointense to muscle
- T2WI
  - CSF signal multiseptated/multicystic lesions
  - Epidural extension of soft tissue with cord compression
  - Degenerated cysts may show low signal relative to CSF
- STIR: CSF signal multiseptated/multicystic lesions
- T1 C+: Minimal or no enhancement of large cystic lesions

Imaging Recommendations
- Best imaging tool
  - MR shows bone, epidural, paravertebral extension and degree of neural compromise
  - CT shows bone morphology, degree of bone destruction
- Protocol advice: Sagittal, axial T1WI + T2WI, post-contrast sagittal, axial T1WI

DIFFERENTIAL DIAGNOSIS

Primary bone neoplasm
- Osteosarcoma, chondrosarcoma, ABC, giant cell, chordoma

Metastatic disease
- Cystic metastases; such as renal cell, thyroid

Tuberculosis
- Vertebral body, posterior element and epidural space involvement
- Diffuse + peripheral enhancement of phlegmon, cold abscesses

Other parasitic diseases
- Cord inflammatory myelopathy with schistosomiasis
- Complex cystic intramedullary enhancing mass with cysticercosis

PATHOLOGY

General Features
- General path comments
  - Bone involvement rare: Incidence ranges from 0.5-2% of all cases of echinococcosis
    - Vertebrae most common bone involved
    - Vertebrae > long bone epiphyses > ilium > skull > ribs
  - No pericyst formation in bone involvement
    - Parasite expands by exogenous proliferation with irregular pattern
    - Bone resorption due to pressure erosion & necrosis
  - Typical involvement of vertebral bodies, contiguous ribs & paravertebral tissue
    - Disc space generally spared
- Etiology
  - Usual cause is accidental ingestion of dog feces containing echinococcal eggs
  - Cysts slowly grow in vertebral body/posterior elements with subsequent extension into pre/paravertebral region, ribs, epidural space with cord compression
- Epidemiology
  - Echinococcus common in Southern South America, Mediterranean, Middle East, Central Asia, Africa
  - US: California, Arizona, New Mexico, Utah

Gross Pathologic & Surgical Features
- Spherical, fluid filled hollow cyst, containing multiple protoscolices, brood capsules, daughter cysts

ECHINOCOCCUS

Microscopic Features
- Outer laminated hyaline wall
- Inner nucleated germinal layer, studded with developing brood capsules
  - Protoscolices formed within brood capsules

Staging, Grading or Classification Criteria
- Five categories of spine involvement
  - Intramedullary cyst
  - Intradural/extramedullary
  - Extradural intraspinal
  - Vertebral disease
  - Paravertebral

CLINICAL ISSUES

Presentation
- Most common signs/symptoms
  - Back pain, myelopathy, radiculopathy depending upon anatomic location of infestation
  - Other signs/symptoms
    - Progressive weakness, numbness of extremities

Demographics
- Age: Any age
- Gender: No gender predilection
- Ethnicity: Related to endemic geographic locations

Natural History & Prognosis
- Indolent, progressive course without treatment

Treatment
- Oral treatment with albendazole or mebendazole
- Surgical resection for neural compression
- Recurrence rate of spinal hydatid cysts after surgery 18%

DIAGNOSTIC CHECKLIST

Consider
- Hydatid cyst fluid highly allergenic, cyst rupture may cause anaphylaxis
- Disease is indolent with latent period of multiple years before cysts reach symptomatic size

Image Interpretation Pearls
- Lack of significant enhancement is critical differential feature of echinococcal cysts

SELECTED REFERENCES

1. Hadjipavlou AG et al: Effectiveness and pitfalls of percutaneous transpedicle biopsy of the spine. Clin Orthop. (411):54-60, 2003
2. El Kohen A et al: Multiple hydatid cysts of the neck, the nasopharynx and the skull base revealing cervical vertebral hydatid disease. Int J Pediatr Otorhinolaryngol. 67(6):655-62, 2003
3. Karadereler S et al: Primary spinal extradural hydatid cyst in a child: case report and review of the literature. Eur Spine J. 11(5):500-3, 2002
4. Sener RN et al: Multiple, primary spinal-paraspinal hydatid cysts. Eur Radiol. 11(11):2314-6, 2001
5. Stabler A et al: Imaging of spinal infection. Radiol Clin North Am. 39(1):115-35, 2001
6. Hassan FO et al: Primary pelvic hydatid cyst: an unusual cause of sciatica and foot drop. Spine. 26(2):230-232, 2001
7. Bruschi F et al: Immunochemical and molecular characterization of vertebral hydatid fluid. Scand J Infect Dis. 31(3):322-3, 1999
8. Savas R et al: Spinal cord compression due to costal Echinococcus multilocularis. Comput Med Imaging Graph. 23(2):85-8, 1999
9. Normelli HC et al: Vertebral hydatid cyst infection (Echinococcus granulosus): a case report. Eur Spine J. 7(2):158-61, 1998
10. Mazyad MA et al: Spinal cord hydatid cysts in Egypt. J Egypt Soc Parasitol. 28(3):655-8, 1998
11. von Sinner WN et al: Case report 833: Primary spinal echinococcosis (Echinococcus granulosus) of lumbosacral spine with destruction of the left pedicles of L3-5 and extension of a large paraspinal cystic mass into the spinal canal. Skeletal Radiol. 23(3):220-3, 1994
12. Sharif HS: Role of MR imaging in the management of spinal infections. AJR Am J Roentgenol. 158(6):1333-45, 1992
13. Dernevik L et al: Management of dumbbell tumours. Reports of seven cases. Scand J Thorac Cardiovasc Surg. 24(1):47-51, 1990
14. Richards KS et al: Effect of albendazole on human hydatid cysts: an ultrastructural study. HPB Surg. 2(2):105-12; discussion 112-3, 1990
15. Charles RW et al: Echinococcal infection of the spine with neural involvement. Spine. 13(1):47-9, 1988
16. Bhargava S: Radiology--including computed tomography--of parasitic diseases of the central nervous system. Neurosurg Rev. 6(3):129-37, 1983
17. Braithwaite PA et al: Vertebral hydatid disease: radiological assessment. Radiology. 140(3):763-6, 1981
18. Kaufman DM et al: Infectious agents in spinal epidural abscesses. Neurology. 30(8):844-50, 1980
19. Karvounis PC et al: Intradural spinal echinococcus simulating lumbar disc protrusion. Neurochirurgia (Stuttg). 20(2):58-60, 1977

IMAGE GALLERY

Typical

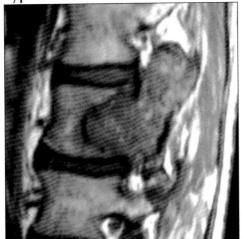
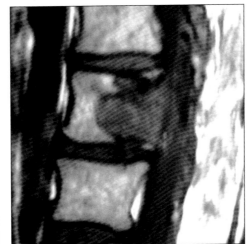

(Left) Sagittal T1WI MR shows nonspecific lobulated vertebral mass involving posterior elements (with permission Athanassopoulou et al, MRI in spinal hydatid disease, {online case 1855}, Euromultimedia). *(Right)* Sagittal T1WI MR shows intermediate signal mass involving thoracic vertebral body (with permission Athanassopoulou et al, MRI in spinal hydatid disease, {online case 1855}, Euromultimedia).

Typical

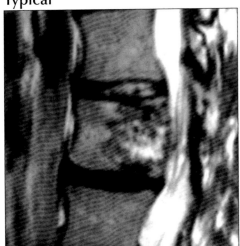
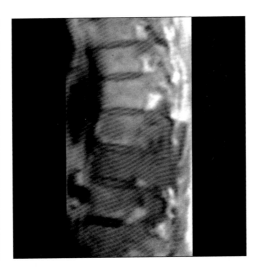

(Left) Sagittal T2WI MR shows heterogeneous signal vertebral mass (with permission Athanassopoulou et al, MRI in spinal hydatid disease, {online case 1855}, Euromultimedia). *(Right)* Sagittal T1WI MR shows complex echinococcal mass involving multiple vertebral bodies & posterior elements, epidural extension, sparing of disc spaces (Courtesy J. Beltran, MD).

Typical

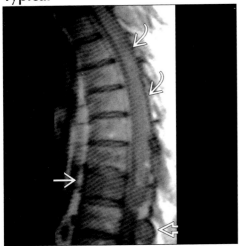
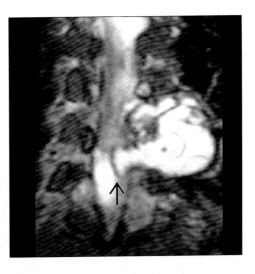

(Left) Sagittal T1WI MR shows complex echinococcal mass involving vertebral body (arrow), posterior elements (open arrow) and diffuse epidural extension (curved arrows) (Courtesy J. Beltran, MD). *(Right)* Coronal T2WI MR shows complex T2 hyperintense mass in paravertebral region with multiple septa, with epidural extension (arrow) (Courtesy J. Beltran, MD).

SCHISTOSOMIASIS

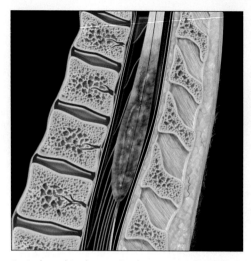

Sagittal graphic shows schistosomiasis involving conus medullaris with granulomatous inflammatory response.

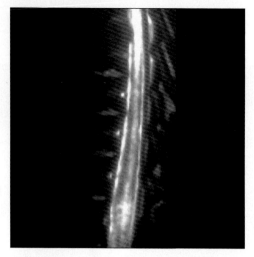

Sagittal T2WI MR shows diffuse cord T2 hyperintensity centered on conus medullaris, with moderate cord expansion in patient with schistosomiasis (Courtesy R. Mendonca, MD).

TERMINOLOGY

Abbreviations and Synonyms
- Synonym: Bilharziasis
- Katayama fever = acute schistosomiasis

Definitions
- CNS infection from parasitic trematodes (blood flukes) of genus Schistosoma
- Complex life cycle
  - Infect particular species fresh water snails within endemic areas
  - Infected snails release free swimming larvae (cercariae) which attach to host mammal
  - Cercariae migrate through skin to dermal veins ⇒ pulmonary vasculature
  - Cercariae metamorphose to "schistosomula" ⇒ loosing forked tails, developing lipid teguments, incorporating host proteins (major histocompatibility complexes & blood group antigens)
  - Migrate through lung capillaries ⇒ portal veins where they mature
  - Male and female pair off & migrate together, produce eggs
    - S. mansoni, S. japonicum ⇒ mesenteric veins
    - S. hematobium ⇒ vesicular (bladder) veins
  - Eggs are antigenic & induce inflammatory response

  - Migrate through bowel or bladder wall & shed in feces, urine
  - Shed eggs mature into free swimming "miracidia" ⇒ infect freshwater snail
    - Two generations of "sporocysts" multiple in snail intermediate host

IMAGING FINDINGS

General Features
- Best diagnostic clue: Myelopathy, cord enhancement, edema in patient from endemic area
- Location: Thoracic cord, conus
- Size: Variable, up to few centimeters
- Morphology: Variable, generally ill-defined cord enlargement

Radiographic Findings
- Myelography
  - Enlarged cord/intramedullary mass
  - Block with marked cord expansion/pseudotumoral form

CT Findings
- CECT: Diffuse cord enlargement & patchy enhancement

DDx: Myelopathy & Increased Cord T2 Signal

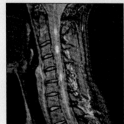

Multiple Sclerosis

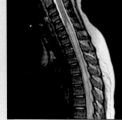

Trans. Myelitis

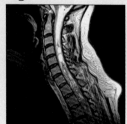

Astrocytoma

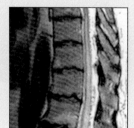

Dural Fistula

SCHISTOSOMIASIS

Key Facts

Terminology
- Synonym: Bilharziasis
- CNS infection from parasitic trematodes (blood flukes) of genus Schistosoma
- Infect particular species fresh water snails within endemic areas

Imaging Findings
- Best diagnostic clue: Myelopathy, cord enhancement, edema in patient from endemic area

Top Differential Diagnoses
- Multiple sclerosis
- ADEM
- Intramedullary neoplasm
- Infarction
- Tuberculosis
- Pyogenic abscess
- Viral or idiopathic transverse myelitis
- Spinal dural fistula
- Sarcoidosis

Pathology
- Vascular obstruction secondary to granuloma formation with intense inflammatory reaction, ischemic necrosis

Clinical Issues
- 3 Clinical patterns of cord involvement
- Myelitic
- Granulomatous/pseudotumoral
- Radicular/myeloradicular
- Oral treatment with antihelmintics: Praziquantel and oxamniquine

MR Findings
- T1WI: Enlarged cord/conus medullaris
- T2WI: Diffuse increased signal within cord over several segments
- T2* GRE: No gross hemorrhage
- T1 C+
  - Heterogeneous cord enhancement
  - May extend over several segments

Imaging Recommendations
- Best imaging tool: MR with contrast
- Protocol advice: Sagittal, axial T1WI + T2WI, sagittal + axial post-contrast

DIFFERENTIAL DIAGNOSIS

Multiple sclerosis
- Central enhancement of peripheral cord lesions
- May show ring-enhancement
- Presence of typical intracranial periventricular, subcallosal, brainstem, cerebellar white matter lesions

ADEM
- Diffuse cord enlargement, patchy multisegmental enhancement

Intramedullary neoplasm
- No leptomeningeal enhancement
- Peri-tumoral edema
- Cystic & hemorrhagic components

Infarction
- Immediate onset of neurologic deficit
- Initial findings of T2 hyperintensity, without enhancement or mass effect

Tuberculosis
- Vertebral body, epidural, leptomeningeal abnormalities

Pyogenic abscess
- Focal, irregular focus of ring-enhancement with edema

Viral or idiopathic transverse myelitis
- Usually single lesion
- May be mono- or multisegmental

Spinal dural fistula
- Cord enlargement, T2 hyperintensity
- Prominent vessels on cord surface
- Stuttering course of myelopathic progression

Sarcoidosis
- Cord and leptomeningeal enhancement
- Intracranial leptomeningeal enhancement, particularly midline about optic chiasm

PATHOLOGY

General Features
- General path comments
  - Presence of eggs in CNS induces cell-mediated periovular granulomatous reaction
  - Human schistosomiasis most often caused by Schistosoma haematobium, Schistosoma mansoni, Schistosoma japonicum
  - Vascular obstruction secondary to granuloma formation with intense inflammatory reaction, ischemic necrosis
- Etiology
  - Early stage of disease more often produce CNS symptoms
    - Anomalous migration of adult worms causes CNS infestation, with subsequent in-situ egg deposition
  - Chronic hepatosplenic, cardiopulmonary, urinary schistosomiasis usually asymptomatic
    - Random, occasional embolization of eggs from portal mesenteric system to brain & cord
- Epidemiology
  - Infection effects 200 million individuals in 74 countries of Latin America, Africa and Asia
    - Second to malaria worldwide socioeconomic impact
  - Man, other mammals as definitive hosts; aquatic & amphibious snails as intermediate hosts

SCHISTOSOMIASIS

- ○ Prevalence of CNS involvement varies from 1-30% of infected individuals
- ○ Spinal cord schistosomiasis one of most common causes of non-traumatic myelopathies in endemic areas
- Associated abnormalities
  - ○ Egg retention & granuloma formation in bowel causes bloody diarrhea, cramping, inflammatory colon polyps
  - ○ Urinary tract involvement leads to dysuria, hematuria, bladder polyps, ulcers, obstructive uropathy, increased risk of bladder squamous carcinoma
  - ○ Unshed eggs ⇒ portal circulation ⇒ hepatic perisinusoidal obstruction, portal hypertension, splenomegaly, ascites

Microscopic Features
- Large necrotic-exudative granulomas

Staging, Grading or Classification Criteria
- CSF bilharzia enzyme-linked immunosorbent assay (ELISA) test
  - ○ Antibody testing cannot distinguish active infection from inactive infection
- Urine, stool analysis
- Colon biopsy

CLINICAL ISSUES

Presentation
- Most common signs/symptoms
  - ○ CNS involvement frequently asymptomatic
  - ○ Fever, malaise, arthralgias, diarrhea
  - ○ 3 Clinical patterns of cord involvement
    - Myelitic
    - Granulomatous/pseudotumoral
    - Radicular/myeloradicular
  - ○ Spine involvement generally as transverse myelitis pattern, or spinal cord infarction
    - Transverse myelitis
    - Tetraparesis, paraparesis
    - Anterior spinal artery occlusion
    - Radiculopathy
  - ○ Other signs/symptoms
    - Bowel, bladder dysfunction
- Clinical profile
  - ○ CSF pleocytosis, elevated protein content, oligoclonal IgG bands
  - ○ Stool smear examination with quantitative Kato-Katz oogram if suspected schistosomiasis

Demographics
- Age: Any age (peak in 2nd decade)
- Gender: M > F
- Ethnicity: No ethnic predisposition, infection related to location of endemic schistosomiasis

Natural History & Prognosis
- Most patients improve with appropriate antihelmintic drug treatment
- Acute schistosomiasis up to 25% mortality

- End-stage hepatosplenic disease, varices, pulmonary hypertension, CNS disease associated with high mortality

Treatment
- Oral treatment with antihelmintics: Praziquantel and oxamniquine
- Steroids to decrease inflammatory response

DIAGNOSTIC CHECKLIST

Consider
- Patients with spinal involvement may have no other clinical evidence of schistosomiasis

SELECTED REFERENCES

1. Cohen-Gadol AA et al: Spinal cord biopsy: a review of 38 cases. Neurosurgery. 52(4): 806-15; discussion 815-6, 2003
2. Samandouras G et al: Schistosoma haematobium presenting as an intrinsic conus tumour. Br J Neurosurg. 16(3): 296-300, 2002
3. Olson S et al: Spinal schistosomiasis. J Clin Neurosci. 9(3): 317-20, 2002
4. Junker J et al: Cervical intramedullar schistosomiasis as a rare cause of acute tetraparesis. Clin Neurol Neurosurg. 103(1): 39-42, 2001
5. Leite CC et al: Clinics in diagnostic imaging (52). Spinal cord schistosomiasis. Singapore Med J. 41(8): 417-9, 2000
6. Mazyad MA et al: Spinal cord schistosomiasis and neurologic complications. J Egypt Soc Parasitol. 29(1): 179-82, 1999
7. Bennett G et al: Schistosomal myelitis: findings at MR imaging. Eur J Radiol. 27(3): 268-70, 1998
8. Murphy KJ et al: Spinal cord infection: myelitis and abscess formation. AJNR Am J Neuroradiol. 19(2): 341-8, 1998
9. Pittella JE: Neuroschistosomiasis. Brain Pathol. 7(1): 649-62, 1997
10. Ueki K et al: Schistosoma mansoni infection involving the spinal cord. Case report. J Neurosurg. 82(6): 1065-7, 1995
11. Haribhai HC et al: Spinal cord schistosomiasis. A clinical, laboratory and radiological study, with a note on therapeutic aspects. Brain. 114 (Pt 2): 709-26, 1991
12. Bloom K et al: Paraplegia from schistosomiasis. Paraplegia. 28(7): 455-9, 1990
13. Bac DJ et al: Schistosomiasis in ectopic or unusual sites. A report of 5 cases. S Afr Med J. 72(10): 717-8, 1987
14. Scrimgeour EM et al: Involvement of the central nervous system in Schistosoma mansoni and S. haematobium infection. Brain. 108 (Pt 4):1023-38, 1985
15. Queiroz LS et al: Massive spinal cord necrosis in schistosomiasis. Arch Neurol. 36(8): 517-9, 1979
16. Siddorn JA: Schistosomiasis and anterior spinal artery occlusion. Am J Trop Med Hyg. 27(3): 532-4, 1978
17. Norfray JF et al: Schistosomiasis of the spinal cord. Surg Neurol. 9(1): 68-71, 1978
18. Lechtenberg R et al: Schistosomiasis of the spinal cord. Neurology. 27(1): 55-9, 1977

IMAGE GALLERY

Typical

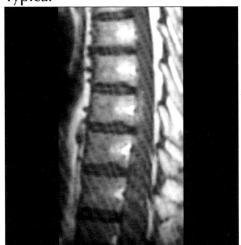 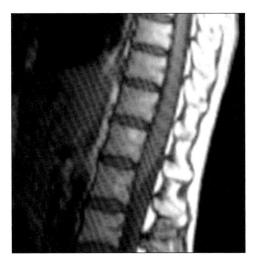

(Left) Sagittal T1 C+ MR shows patchy enhancement of distal thoracic cord & conus due to schistosomiasis (Courtesy R. Mendonca, MD). *(Right)* Sagittal T1WI MR shows mild diffuse cord/conus enlargement with schistosomiasis infection (Courtesy A. Aul, MD).

Typical

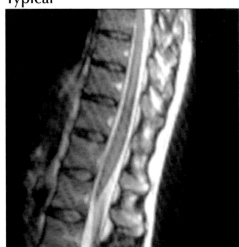 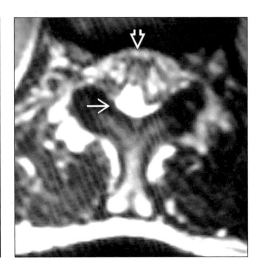

(Left) Sagittal T2WI MR shows diffuse patchy T2 hyperintensity throughout distal thoracic cord & conus in patient with schistosomiasis (Courtesy A. Aul, MD). *(Right)* Axial T2WI MR shows T2 hyperintensity involving distal conus (open arrow) & dorsal hyperintense mass (arrow) presumed to be schistosomiasis granulomatous inflammatory change (Courtesy A. Aul, MD).

Typical

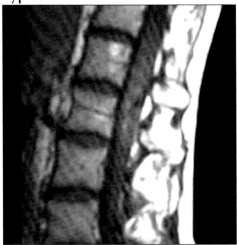 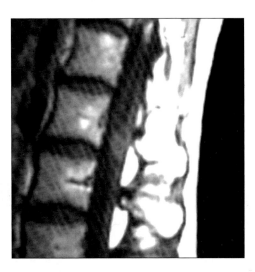

(Left) Sagittal T1 C+ MR shows patchy conus enhancement due to schistosomiasis infection. Ovoid intradural lesion below conus presumed granuloma (Courtesy A. Aul, MD). *(Right)* Sagittal T1 C+ MR shows shows ovoid intradural lesion below conus level presumed to be schistosomiasis granulomatous inflammatory mass (Courtesy A. Aul, MD).

CYSTICERCOSIS

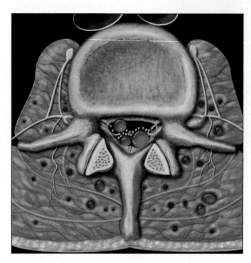

Axial graphic shows multiple subarachnoid cysts (cysticerci) distorting nerve roots, with multiple additional lesion within muscles.

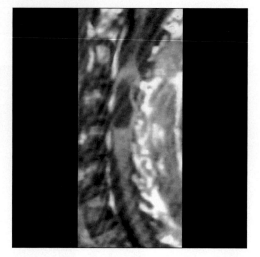

Sagittal T1 C+ MR of cervical spine shows complex multicystic/solid mass with cord enhancement in this patient with intramedullary cysticercosis (Courtesy R. Mendonca, MD).

TERMINOLOGY

Abbreviations and Synonyms
- Neurocysticercosis (NCC); intramedullary spinal cord cysticercosis

Definitions
- CNS parasitic infection caused by pork tapeworm, Taenia solium
- Classified as extraspinal (vertebral body) or intraspinal (extradural, subarachnoid, intramedullary)

IMAGING FINDINGS

General Features
- Best diagnostic clue: Intradural cyst with evidence of similar lesions in brain (cyst with "dot" appearance)
- Location
  - Parenchymal, leptomeningeal, intraventricular, spinal
    - Spinal NCC rare
    - Spinal involvement is thoracic 60-75%
- Size
  - Cyst size variable, 5-20 mm
    - Cysts contain scolex which is 1-4 mm
- Morphology
  - Round or ovoid cyst

- Imaging varies with developmental stage of infection, host response
- Inflammatory response may give edema

Radiographic Findings
- Radiography: May show soft tissue calcifications
- Myelography
  - Variety of appearances depending upon region involved
    - Intradural-extramedullary lesions with subarachnoid cysts
    - Enlarged cord ± myelographic block with intramedullary disease

CT Findings
- CECT: Focal cystic low attenuation, subarachnoid or intramedullary, cord enlargement ± enhancement

MR Findings
- T1WI
  - Subarachnoid: CSF signal cystic lesions, variable mass effect on adjacent cord/cauda equina
  - Intramedullary: Focal cystic lesion(s), ± syrinx cavitation
- T2WI
  - Subarachnoid: CSF signal cystic lesions
  - Intramedullary: Focal cystic lesion showing ↑ T2 signal, cord edema extending over several segments
- T1 C+

DDx: Cystic Intradural Lesions

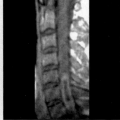
Abscess

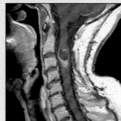
Ependymoma

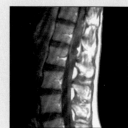
Hemangioblastoma

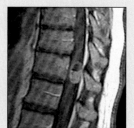
Schwannoma

CYSTICERCOSIS

Key Facts

Terminology
- CNS parasitic infection caused by pork tapeworm, Taenia solium
- Classified as extraspinal (vertebral body) or intraspinal (extradural, subarachnoid, intramedullary)

Top Differential Diagnoses
- Pyogenic abscess
- Granulomatous disease
- Neoplasm
- Arachnoid cyst
- Other parasitic infections
- Syrinx
- Schwannoma

Pathology
- Cysticercosis most common worldwide parasitic infection
- CNS infection in 60-90% of cases
- Thickened, opaque arachnoid, pachymeningitis
- Subarachnoid or intramedullary cysts with cleavage plane from normal tissue; surrounding soft yellowish granulation tissue

Clinical Issues
- Spastic paraparesis, quadriparesis, flaccid paralysis
- Sensory level
- Bladder dysfunction
- Enzyme-linked immunoelectrotransfer blot (EITB) reportedly > 90% sensitivity

---

- ○ Subarachnoid: Peripheral cyst enhancement
- ○ Intramedullary: Peripheral enhancement of cyst
  - ■ May show only nonspecific sheet-like enhancement of subarachnoid space, cord pial surface

Imaging Recommendations
- Best imaging tool: MR imaging with contrast defines intradural extramedullary, intramedullary cysts, associated edema
- Protocol advice: Sagittal, axial T1WI, T2WI, T1 C+, include brain imaging in addition to spine imaging

DIFFERENTIAL DIAGNOSIS

Pyogenic abscess
- Irregular ring-enhancement with cord edema, expansion

Granulomatous disease
- Tuberculosis, sarcoidosis
- Not cystic
- Generally leptomeningeal pattern of intradural involvement

Neoplasm
- Primary or metastatic
- Irregular solid or ring-enhancement
- Associated cysts with astrocytoma, ependymoma, hemangioblastoma

Arachnoid cyst
- CSF signal/attenuation
- No enhancement

Other parasitic infections
- May have cystic component (echinococcus)
- May show myelitis pattern without focal cyst (schistosomiasis)

Syrinx
- Central cord linear CSF signal intensity associated with Chiari I

- Loculation or beaded appearance over several segments
- No enhancement

Schwannoma
- Intradural extramedullary mass
- May show cystic degeneration with thin rim-enhancement

PATHOLOGY

General Features
- General path comments
  - ○ Spinal involvement uncommon (5% of cases of NCC)
  - ○ Approximately 50 cases of spinal involvement reported
  - ○ Subarachnoid form most common spinal type
- Etiology
  - ○ Caused by larval form of pig tapeworm, T. solium
  - ○ Man intermediate parasitic host in tapeworm lifecycle
    - ■ Fecal-oral route of infection
    - ■ Contaminated water, food ⇒ ingestion of eggs
    - ■ GI tract ⇒ hematogenous dissemination to CNS and muscle
    - ■ After cysticerci lodged in tissue, do not move to other sites
  - ○ Downward migration of larvae from cerebral to spinal subarachnoid space ⇒ leptomeningeal form
  - ○ Hematogenous dissemination, spread through ventriculo-ependymal pathways ⇒ intramedullary form
  - ○ Predilection of cysticerci for thoracic cord related to higher percentage blood flow to thoracic segment
  - ○ Subarachnoid cysticercosis caused by two different larval types
    - ■ Cysticercus cellulosae ⇒ larval worm with simple bladder and scolex
    - ■ Cysticercus racemosus ⇒ "grape-like" cluster of larvae (without scolex) ⇒ chronic granulomatous meningitis

CYSTICERCOSIS

- Epidemiology
  - Cysticercosis most common worldwide parasitic infection
  - CNS infection in 60-90% of cases
  - Endemic in Mexico, Central & South America, eastern Europe, Asia, India, Africa

Gross Pathologic & Surgical Features

- Thickened, opaque arachnoid, pachymeningitis
- Subarachnoid or intramedullary cysts with cleavage plane from normal tissue; surrounding soft yellowish granulation tissue

Microscopic Features

- Cyst wall has 3 layers: Outer (cuticular layer), middle cellular (pseudoepithelial) layer, inner reticular (fibrillary) layer
- Inflammatory reaction with edema, adjacent gliosis
- Cyst wall degeneration with calcification
- Adjacent acute, chronic inflammatory cell infiltrate giving "cysticercal abscess", arachnoiditis

CLINICAL ISSUES

Presentation

- Most common signs/symptoms
  - Commonly asymptomatic
  - Spine symptoms
    - Spastic paraparesis, quadriparesis, flaccid paralysis
    - Sensory level
    - Bladder dysfunction
    - Neck, low back pain
  - Other signs/symptoms: Brain involvement
    - Seizure, headache, hydrocephalus, focal neurologic deficit, stroke
- Clinical profile
  - Diagnosed confirmed by ELISA of serum or CSF
    - > 70% sensitivity, highly specific for cysticercal antigens; sensitivity ↑ if assay performed on CSF
    - Increased sensitivity as number of lesion increase, if assay performed on CSF
    - 2/3 spinal NCC reported with negative ELISA
    - Enzyme-linked immunoelectrotransfer blot (EITB) reportedly > 90% sensitivity
  - Peripheral blood eosinophilia 25%
  - CSF: Nonspecific protein elevation, lymphocytosis

Demographics

- Age: Any age
- Gender: M = F
- Ethnicity: In US, Hispanic & Asian patients common ⇒ endemic area immigration

Natural History & Prognosis

- Satisfactory surgical outcome with intramedullary disease in 60-75%
  - Parenchymal gliosis, pachyleptomeningitis may cause cord vascular compromise
- Various degree of post-operative motor, sensory, urologic deficits

Treatment

- Options, risks, complications
  - Surgical resection of intramedullary lesion
  - Steroids to decrease inflammation
  - Oral treatment with praziquantel or albendazole
  - Postoperative course of anticysticercal necessary since generalized disease with focal spinal manifestation

DIAGNOSTIC CHECKLIST

Consider

- Spinal cysticercosis often accompanied by intracranial disease

Image Interpretation Pearls

- Only spinal findings may be chronic inflammatory arachnoiditis ⇒ altered CSF flow dynamics ⇒ syringomyelia

SELECTED REFERENCES

1. Parmar H et al: MR imaging in intramedullary cysticercosis. Neuroradiology. 43(11): 961-7, 2001
2. Del Brutto OH et al: Proposed diagnostic criteria for neurocysticercosis. Neurology. 57(2): 177-83, 2001
3. Mathuriya SN et al: Intramedullary cysticercosis : MRI diagnosis. Neurol India. 49(1): 71-4, 2001
4. Rahalkar MD et al: The many faces of cysticercosis. Clin Radiol. 55(9): 668-74, 2000
5. Zee CS et al: Imaging of neurocysticercosis. Neuroimaging Clin N Am. 10(2): 391-407, 2000
6. Garg RK: Neurocysticercosis. Postgrad Med J. 74(872): 321-6, 1998
7. Sawhney IM et al: Uncommon presentations of neurocysticercosis. J Neurol Sci. 154(1): 94-100, 1998
8. Leite CC et al: MR imaging of intramedullary and intradural-extramedullary spinal cysticercosis. AJR Am J Roentgenol. 169(6): 1713-7, 1997
9. Mohanty A et al: Spinal intramedullary cysticercosis. Neurosurgery. 40(1): 82-7, 1997
10. Corral I et al: Intramedullary cysticercosis cured with drug treatment. A case report. Spine. 21(19): 2284-7, 1996
11. Creasy JL et al: Magnetic resonance imaging of neurocysticercosis. Top Magn Reson Imaging. 6(1): 59-68, 1994
12. Isidro-Llorens A et al: Spinal cysticercosis. Case report and review. Paraplegia. 31(2): 128-30, 1993
13. Zee CS et al: CT myelography in spinal cysticercosis. J Comput Assist Tomogr. 10(2): 195-8, 1986
14. Akiguchi I et al: Intramedullary spinal cysticercosis. Neurology. 29(11): 1531-4, 1979
15. Firemark HM: Spinal cysticercosis. Arch Neurol. 35(4): 250-1, 1978
16. Kurrein F et al: Cysticercosis of the spine. Ann Trop Med Parasitol. 71(2): 213-7, 1977

CYSTICERCOSIS

IMAGE GALLERY

Typical

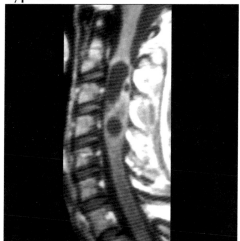
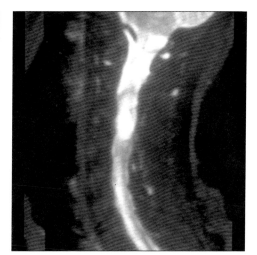

(Left) Sagittal T1 C+ MR of cervical spine shows complex intramedullary multicystic mass with patchy peripheral enhancement in cysticercosis (Courtesy R. Mendonca, MD). *(Right)* Sagittal T2WI MR of cervical spine shows heterogeneous T2 signal from expanded upper cervical cord in intramedullary cysticercosis (Courtesy R. Mendonca, MD).

Typical

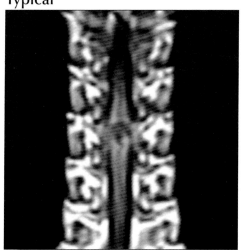
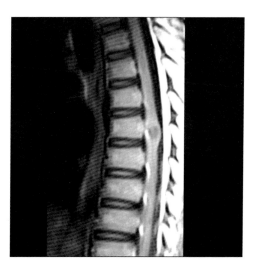

(Left) Coronal T1WI MR shows focal, well-defined cyst in mid-thoracic cord with mild focal cord expansion in this patient with intramedullary cysticercosis (Courtesy H. Shah, MD). *(Right)* Sagittal T1 C+ MR shows focal, well-defined cyst in midthoracic cord with mild focal dorsal cord expansion in this patient with intramedullary cysticercosis (Courtesy H. Shah, MD).

Typical

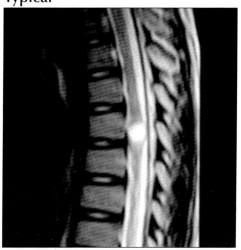
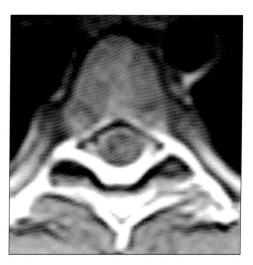

(Left) Sagittal T2WI MR shows well-defined T2 hyperintense cyst in thoracic cord with mild focal cord expansion but no adjacent edema in this patient with intramedullary cysticercosis (Courtesy H. Shah, MD). *(Right)* Axial T1 C+ MR shows focal, well-defined nonenhancing cyst in thoracic cord with mild focal cord expansion in this patient with intramedullary cysticercosis (Courtesy H. Shah, MD).

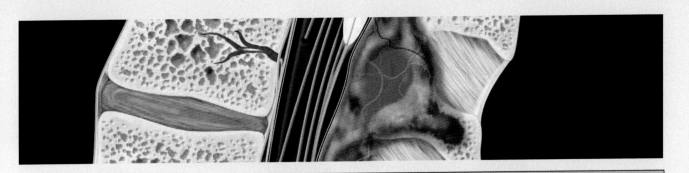

SECTION 2: Inflammatory & Autoimmune

GUILLAIN-BARRE SYNDROME

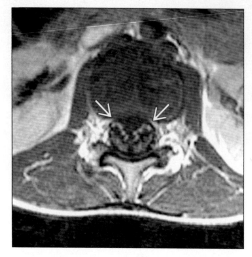

Axial T1 C+ MR in patient with ascending paralysis demonstrates preferential enhancement of ventral cauda equina (arrows).

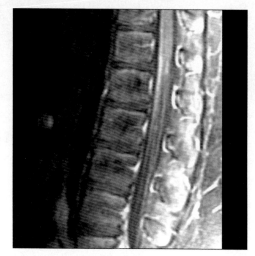

Sagittal T1 C+ MR (with fat-saturation) of an 8 year old shows diffuse pial enhancement of conus, and thickened, enhancing cauda equina roots. Note normal conus size.

TERMINOLOGY

Abbreviations and Synonyms
- Guillain-Barre syndrome (GBS)
- Acute inflammatory demyelinating polyradiculoneuropathy (AIDP)
- Ascending paralysis

Definitions
- Autoimmune post-infectious or post-vaccinial acute inflammatory demyelination of peripheral nerves, nerve roots, cranial nerves

IMAGING FINDINGS

General Features
- Best diagnostic clue: Smooth pial enhancement of the cauda equina and conus medullaris
- Location: On imaging, typically the cauda equina, especially ventral roots
- Size: Nerve roots may be slightly enlarged
- Morphology: Symmetric, smooth appearance of roots

Radiographic Findings
- Myelography
  - May see symmetric enlargement of cauda roots

- Lumbar puncture typically done in early stages to assess spinal fluid chemistry, protein levels, bacteriology

CT Findings
- CECT
  - Rare: May see symmetric enhancement of lumbar roots
  - Difficult to diagnose with CT

MR Findings
- T2WI
  - Should see normal conus
  - May see slight prominence of root size
- T1 C+
  - Avid enhancement of cauda equina
    - Roots may be slightly thickened, not nodular
  - Axial images show preferential contrast accentuation of ventral roots in cauda
  - Pial surface of distal cord and conus enhances variably
    - Conus not enlarged

Imaging Recommendations
- Sagittal and axial T1WI without and with gadolinium contrast

DDx: Causes of Enhancing Conus and Cauda

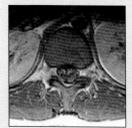

CIDP

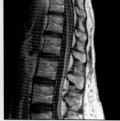

Meningitis

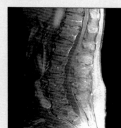

Blood Induced

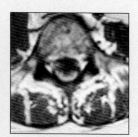

Metastases

GUILLAIN-BARRE SYNDROME

Key Facts

Terminology
- Autoimmune post-infectious or post-vaccinial acute inflammatory demyelination of peripheral nerves, nerve roots, cranial nerves

Imaging Findings
- Avid enhancement of cauda equina
- Roots may be slightly thickened, not nodular
- Axial images show preferential contrast accentuation of ventral roots in cauda

Top Differential Diagnoses
- Miller-Fischer syndrome (MFS)
- Chronic polyneuropathies
- Vasculitic neuropathy
- Carcinomatous or lymphomatous meningitis
- Chemical or post-surgical arachnoiditis

- Physiological nerve root enhancement

Pathology
- Inflammatory (postulated autoimmune or viral) demyelination
- Usually follows recent viral illness

Clinical Issues
- Acute flaccid paralysis or
- Distal paraesthesia followed by rapid ascending paralysis
- Most patients somewhat better by 2-3 months
- Mortality up to 8%

Diagnostic Checklist
- Clinical setting of nerve root enhancement in cauda critical in differential diagnosis

DIFFERENTIAL DIAGNOSIS

Miller-Fischer syndrome (MFS)
- Ataxia, areflexia, ophthalmoplegia
- May have similar trigger

Chronic polyneuropathies
- Subacute inflammatory demyelinating polyradiculoneuropathy (SIDP)
- Chronic inflammatory demyelinating polyradiculoneuropathy (CIDP)
  - Both show slower onset, more protracted course
- Hereditary polyneuropathies
  - Charcot-Marie-Tooth
  - Dejerine-Sottas

Vasculitic neuropathy
- Polyarteritis nodosa or Churg-Strauss most commonly
- Cranial nerves and respiratory nerves frequently spared

Acute transverse myelitis
- Cranial nerves always spared

Bacterial or granulomatous meningitis
- Acute onset
- Fever, headache, + LP

Carcinomatous or lymphomatous meningitis
- Enhancement is frequently more nodular than GBS
- Conus deposits frequently cause T2 signal abnormality

Chemical or post-surgical arachnoiditis
- Hemorrhage-induced arachnoidal inflammation
- Chemotherapy; systemic (vincristine neuropathy), or intrathecal

Physiological nerve root enhancement
- Much more subtle enhancement of normal roots
- Absent clinical syndrome
- Post-operative up to 6 weeks

PATHOLOGY

General Features
- General path comments
  - Lesions are scattered throughout peripheral nerves, nerve roots, cranial nerves
  - Both cell-mediated and humoral mechanisms involved in pathogenesis
- Genetics
  - May be first presentation of genetic or hereditary disorders
    - 17p12 mutation
    - Reported association with HLA typing and Guillain-Barre subtypes
- Etiology
  - Inflammatory (postulated autoimmune or viral) demyelination
    - Antecedent event or "trigger" in 70% GBS cases
    - Usually follows recent viral illness
    - Campylobacter (C.) jejuni infection can be trigger
    - 1/3 have antibodies against nerve gangliosides which cross-react with C. jejuni liposaccharide constituents
    - Vaccination (influenza, others) can be a trigger in rare cases
  - More tenuous association with prior recent surgery or systemic illness
- Epidemiology
  - Incidence: 0.6-2.73 cases per 100,000 population per year
  - Affects all ages, races, socioeconomic status
  - Most common cause of paralysis in Western countries

Gross Pathologic & Surgical Features
- Thickened nerve roots

Microscopic Features
- Focal segmental demyelination
- Perivascular and endoneural lymphocytic/monocytic (macrophages) infiltrates
- Axonal degeneration in conjunction with segmental demyelination in severe cases

GUILLAIN-BARRE SYNDROME

Staging, Grading or Classification Criteria
- Spectrum of disease extends to subacute inflammatory demyelinating polyradiculoneuropathy (SIDP)
- SIDP a bridge to chronic inflammatory demyelinating polyradiculopathy (CIDP)
  - Both entities exhibit slower onset, protracted course, exacerbations, lesser cranial nerve involvement

CLINICAL ISSUES

Presentation
- Most common signs/symptoms
  - Classically presents with "ascending paralysis"
  - Ascent up to brainstem may involve cranial nerves
    - Respiratory paralysis requiring ventilator in severe cases
  - Other signs/symptoms
    - Sensory loss common but less severe
    - Numbness tingling
- Distal paraesthesias rapidly followed by "ascending paralysis"
  - Frequently bilateral and symmetric
  - May require prolonged respiratory support in severe cases
- Autonomic disturbances
- Cranial nerve involvement common
  - Facial nerve involved in up to 50% of cases
  - Ophthalmoparesis in 10-20% of cases

Demographics
- Age: Typically children, young adults
- Gender: No preference
- Ethnicity: All

Natural History & Prognosis
- Acute flaccid paralysis or
- Distal paraesthesia followed by rapid ascending paralysis
  - Most often bilateral, symmetric
- Cranial nerve involvement common
  - Facial nerve in 50%
  - Ophthalmoparesis in < 10%
- Clinical nadir at 4 weeks
- Most patients somewhat better by 2-3 months
  - 30-50% have persistent symptoms at 1 year
  - Permanent deficits in 5-10%
- 2-10% relapse
  - 6% develop chronic course resembling CIDP
  - Earliest stages of SIDP, CIDP may be indistinguishable clinically from Guillain-Barre
- Mortality up to 8%

Treatment
- Medical management with plasma exchange or intravenous gamma globulin
- No proven benefit from corticosteroid administration
- Intensive care management in severe cases

DIAGNOSTIC CHECKLIST

Consider
- Clinical setting of nerve root enhancement in cauda critical in differential diagnosis

Image Interpretation Pearls
- Anterior cauda nerve root and pial conus enhancement without significant enlargement or nodularity is strong clue

SELECTED REFERENCES

1. Cheng BC et al: Guillain-Barre syndrome in southern Taiwan: clinical features, prognostic factors and therapeutic outcomes. Eur J Neurol. 10(6):655-62, 2003
2. Chang YW et al: Spinal MRI of vincristine neuropathy mimicking Guillain-Barre syndrome. Pediatr Radiol. 33(11):791-3, 2003
3. Molinero MR et al: Epidemiology of childhood Guillain-Barre syndrome as a cause of acute flaccid paralysis in Honduras: 1989-1999. J Child Neurol. 18(11):741-7, 2003
4. Oh SJ et al: Subacute inflammatory demyelinating polyneuropathy. Neurology. 61(11):1507-12, 2003
5. Haber P et al: Influenza vaccination and Guillain Barre syndrome. Clin Immunol. 109(3):359; author reply 360-1, 2003
6. Wilmshurst JM et al: Lower limb and back pain in Guillain-Barre syndrome and associated contrast enhancement in MRI of the cauda equina. Acta Paediatr. 90(6):691-4, 2001
7. Kehoe M: Guillain-Barre syndrome--a patient guide and nursing resource. Axone. 22(4):16-24, 2001
8. Duarte J et al: Hypertrophy of multiple cranial nerves and spinal roots in chronic inflammatory demyelinating neuropathy. J Neurol Neurosurg Psychiatry. 67(5):685-7, 1999
9. Berciano J: MR imaging in Guillain-Barre syndrome. Radiology. 211(1):290-1, 1999
10. Vroomen PC et al: The clinical significance of gadolinium enhancement of lumbar disc herniations and nerve roots on preoperative MRI. Neuroradiology. 40(12):800-6, 1998
11. Byun WM et al: Guillain-Barre syndrome: MR imaging findings of the spine in eight patients. Radiology. 208(1):137-41, 1998
12. Iwata F et al: MR imaging in Guillain-Barre syndrome. Pediatr Radiol. 27(1):36-8, 1997
13. Gorson KC et al: Prospective evaluation of MRI lumbosacral nerve root enhancement in acute Guillain-Barre syndrome. Neurology. 47(3):813-7, 1996
14. Perry JR: MRI in Guillain-Barre syndrome. Neurology. 45(5):1024-5, 1995
15. Bertorini T et al: Contrast-enhanced magnetic resonance imaging of the lumbosacral roots in the dysimmune inflammatory polyneuropathies. J Neuroimaging. 5(1):9-15, 1995
16. Georgy BA et al: MR of the spine in Guillain-Barre syndrome. AJNR Am J Neuroradiol. 15(2):300-1, 1994
17. Crino PB et al: Magnetic resonance imaging of the cauda equina in Guillain-Barre syndrome. Neurology 44(7): 1334-6, 1994
18. Patel H et al: MRI of Guillain-Barre syndrome. J Comput Assist Tomogr. 17(4):651-2, 1993
19. Jinkins JR et al: MRI of benign lumbosacral nerve root enhancement. Semin Ultrasound CT MR. 14(6):446-54, 1993

GUILLAIN-BARRE SYNDROME

IMAGE GALLERY

Typical

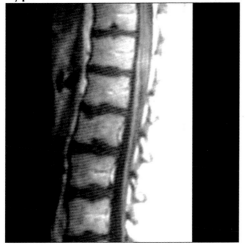
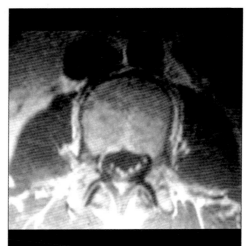

(Left) Sagittal T1 C+ MR in 32 year old woman recuperating from ascending lower extremity paralysis shows enhancement of conus pial surface, and thickened, enhancing cauda equina. *(Right)* Axial T1 C+ MR in the same case shows enhancement and slight thickening of ventral cauda equina roots.

Typical

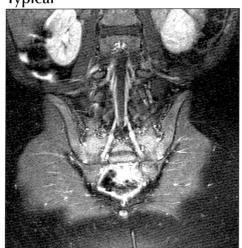
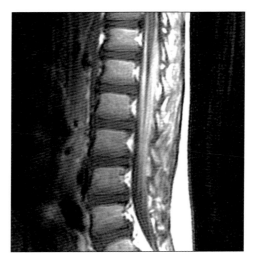

(Left) Coronal T1 C+ MR with fat-saturation shows enhancement of spinal nerves and lumbar plexus roots in child with GBS (Courtesy S. Blaser, MD). *(Right)* Sagittal T1 C+ MR shows striking enhancement of cauda equina and surface of conus simulating carcinomatous meningitis in patient with GBS (Courtesy S. Blaser, MD).

Variant

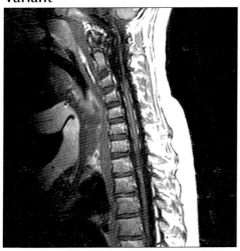
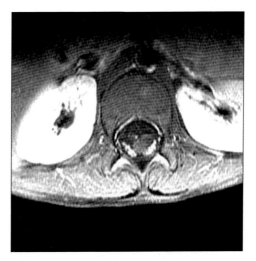

(Left) Sagittal T1 C+ MR off midline shows enhancing cervical roots in child with GBS (Courtesy S. Blaser, MD). *(Right)* Axial T1 C+ MR in patient with GBS demonstrates preferential enhancement of dorsal roots-an atypical finding (Courtesy S. Blaser, MD).

CIDP

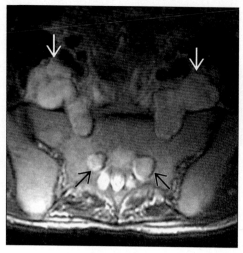

Axial T2WI MR shows marked enlargement of the lumbar/sacral nerve roots (black arrows) and lumbosacral trunk (arrows).

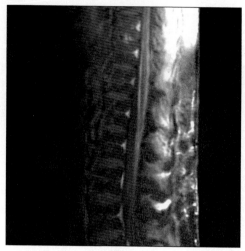

Sagittal T1 C+ MR demonstrates diffuse pial thickening and enhancement extending into the cauda equina nerve roots. Clinical course distinguished from Guillain-Barre (AIDP).

TERMINOLOGY

Abbreviations and Synonyms
- Chronic inflammatory demyelinating polyneuropathy (CIPD), chronic inflammatory demyelinating polyradiculoneuropathy

Definitions
- Chronic acquired, immune-mediated demyelinating neuropathy characterized by relapsing or progressive muscle weakness +/- sensory loss

IMAGING FINDINGS

General Features
- Best diagnostic clue: Enlargement and abnormal T2 hyperintensity of nerve roots, plexi, or peripheral nerves
- Location
  - Spinal nerve roots and peripheral nerves (extraforaminal > intradural)
  - Lumbar > cervical, brachial plexus, thoracic/intercostal > cranial nerve
- Size: Nerve size varies small → very large
- Morphology: Focal or diffuse fusiform enlargement of cauda equina, nerve roots/plexi, and peripheral nerves

CT Findings
- NECT: Isodense nerve enlargement
- CECT: Mild to moderate nerve enhancement

MR Findings
- T1WI: Isointense enlargement of cauda equina and proximal peripheral nerves
- T2WI: Enlargement, abnormal hyperintensity of intradural and extradural spinal nerves/branches
- FLAIR
  - No utility for spine imaging
  - Sagittal FLAIR may reveal hyperintense brain lesions similar to multiple sclerosis (MS)
- T1 C+: Mild to moderate nerve enhancement

Ultrasonographic Findings
- Real Time: Hypoechoic, hypertrophic nerves

Imaging Recommendations
- T2WI, enhanced coronal and axial T1WI sequences with fat suppression best delineate nerve lesions
- Brain MRI to detect subclinical CNS demyelination

DIFFERENTIAL DIAGNOSIS

Guillain-Barre (AIDP)
- Pial, nerve root enhancement similar to CIDP

DDx: Chronic Immune Demyelinating Polyneuropathy

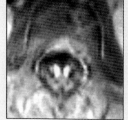

Guillan-Barre (AIDP)

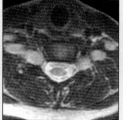

Charcot-Marie-Tooth

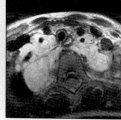

Neurofibromatosis 1

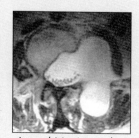

Lateral Meningocele

CIDP

Key Facts

Terminology
- Chronic inflammatory demyelinating polyneuropathy (CIPD), chronic inflammatory demyelinating polyradiculoneuropathy
- Chronic acquired, immune-mediated demyelinating neuropathy characterized by relapsing or progressive muscle weakness +/- sensory loss

Imaging Findings
- Best diagnostic clue: Enlargement and abnormal T2 hyperintensity of nerve roots, plexi, or peripheral nerves
- Sagittal FLAIR may reveal hyperintense brain lesions similar to multiple sclerosis (MS)

Top Differential Diagnoses
- Guillain-Barre (AIDP)

- Inherited demyelinating neuropathy
- Neurofibromatosis type 1
- Lateral meningocele

Pathology
- Hallmarks of CIDP: Enlarged nerves with "onion bulb" formations, demyelination

Clinical Issues
- Mixed sensorimotor neuropathy
- Symmetric proximal and distal weakness, sensory loss
- Clinical course: Chronic progressive, step-wise progressive, or recurrent behavior

Diagnostic Checklist
- Consider CIDP in differential of nerve root/peripheral nerve enlargement

- Distinguish from CIDP by onset duration, clinical course
  - Acute onset of ascending paralysis with relative sensory preservation

Inherited demyelinating neuropathy
- Charcot-Marie-Tooth, Dejerine-Sottas neuropathies
- Genetic testing, clinical phenotype help distinguish from CIDP

Neurofibromatosis type 1
- Diffuse nerve root enlargement, enhancement
- Genetic testing, distinctive clinical stigmata distinguish from CIDP

Lateral meningocele
- CSF density/signal intensity (not solid) +/- foraminal enlargement, dural ectasia
- Usually co-existing NF1 or connective tissue disorder (Marfan syndrome)

PATHOLOGY

General Features
- General path comments
  - Acquired, immune-mediated multifocal demyelinating neuropathy affecting primarily spinal nerves, plexi, and proximal nerve trunks
    - Putative pathogenic mechanisms broadly resemble MS; considered by some to be peripheral counterpart of MS
- Etiology
  - Exact pathogenesis of CIDP unclear; involves both cellular and humoral immune factors
    - Chemokines released into CSF from inflamed spinal nerve roots ⇒ attract T cells, monocytes, and macrophages to PNS and precipitate release of proinflammatory enzymes
    - Activated CD4 T cells, antimyelin antibodies/complement cross-react with myelin and PNS antigens
  - Idiopathic or secondary (CIDP with concurrent disease)

    - Connective tissue disease, diabetes mellitus, IgG or IgA monoclonal gammopathy, hepatitis C infection, Sjögren syndrome, inflammatory bowel disease, human immunodeficiency virus (HIV), and lymphoma
    - Although precise relationship of secondary diseases to CIDP is unclear, neuropathy frequently responds to therapy-like idiopathic CIDP
- Epidemiology: Prevalence 2-7.7/100,000 U.S. population
- Associated abnormalities: +/- Concurrent CNS demyelination

Gross Pathologic & Surgical Features
- Extensive fusiform nerve enlargement +/- gross onion bulb formations

Microscopic Features
- Hallmarks of CIDP: Enlarged nerves with "onion bulb" formations, demyelination
  - Macrophage, T cell infiltration ⇒ perivascular inflammatory infiltrates, nerve demyelination and remyelination
  - "Onion bulb" formation 2° to excessive Schwann cell process proliferation ⇒ segmental repetitive demyelination/remyelination

CLINICAL ISSUES

Presentation
- Most common signs/symptoms
  - Mixed sensorimotor neuropathy
  - Symmetric proximal and distal weakness, sensory loss
  - Other signs/symptoms
    - Occasional pure motor neuropathy
    - Symptomatic lumbar stenosis 2° to nerve root hypertrophy
- Clinical profile
  - CIDP is usually a clinical diagnosis based on presence of progressive weakness/sensory loss and response to corticosteroid therapy

- +/- Concurrent CNS demyelination (frequently subclinical)
- Laboratory abnormalities
  - Abnormal EMG/NCV: Key electrophysiologic features ⇒ nerve conduction block, slowed conduction velocities suggestive of demyelination
  - ↑ CSF protein
- Diagnosis relies primarily on clinical, electrophysiologic examination supplemented by nerve biopsy
- ≥ 50% of CIDP patients have atypical features; asymmetry, distal weakness, sensory loss only

Demographics

- Age: Adult > childhood
- Gender: M = F

Natural History & Prognosis

- Clinical course: Chronic progressive, step-wise progressive, or recurrent behavior
  - Mildly affected patients tend to recover; severely affected patients more likely to have chronic symptoms or mortality related to CIDP
  - Prolonged remission/cure is exception, not rule
  - Atypical and secondary CIDP respond similarly to classic CIDP
- Average disease duration = 7.5 years

Treatment

- Immunomodulation or immunosuppression therapy
  - Prednisolone therapy, plasmapheresis, or intravenous immunoglobulin (IVIG)

DIAGNOSTIC CHECKLIST

Consider

- Consider CIDP in differential of nerve root/peripheral nerve enlargement

Image Interpretation Pearls

- MRI findings imperfectly correlate with clinical disease activity/severity, laboratory findings

SELECTED REFERENCES

1. Saperstein DS et al: Current concepts and controversy in chronic inflammatory demyelinating polyneuropathy. Curr Neurol Neurosci Rep. 3(1):57-63, 2003
2. Rodriguez-Casero MV et al: Childhood chronic inflammatory demyelinating polyneuropathy with central nervous system demyelination resembling multiple sclerosis. Neuromuscul Disord. 13(2):158-61, 2003
3. Ropper AH: Current treatments for CIDP. Neurology. 60(8 Suppl 3):S16-22, 2003
4. Toyka KV et al: The pathogenesis of CIDP: rationale for treatment with immunomodulatory agents. Neurology. 60(8 Suppl 3):S2-7, 2003
5. Haq RU et al: Chronic inflammatory demyelinating polyradiculoneuropathy in diabetic patients. Muscle Nerve. 27(4):465-70, 2003
6. Press R et al: Aberrated levels of cerebrospinal fluid chemokines in Guillain-Barre syndrome and chronic inflammatory demyelinating polyradiculoneuropathy. J Clin Immunol. 23(4):259-67, 2003
7. Odaka M et al: Patients with chronic inflammatory demyelinating polyneuropathy initially diagnosed as Guillain-Barre syndrome. J Neurol. 250(8):913-6, 2003
8. Fee DB et al: Resolution of chronic inflammatory demyelinating polyneuropathy-associated central nervous system lesions after treatment with intravenous immunoglobulin. J Peripher Nerv Syst. 8(3):155-8, 2003
9. Cocito D et al: Different clinical, electrophysiological and immunological features of CIDP associated with paraproteinaemia. Acta Neurol Scand. 108(4):274-80, 2003
10. Oguz B et al: Diffuse spinal and intercostal nerve involvement in chronic inflammatory demyelinating polyradiculoneuropathy: MRI findings. Eur Radiol. 13 Suppl 4:L230-4, 2003
11. Magda P et al: Comparison of electrodiagnostic abnormalities and criteria in a cohort of patients with chronic inflammatory demyelinating polyneuropathy. Arch Neurol. 60(12):1755-9, 2003
12. Costello F et al: Childhood-onset chronic inflammatory demyelinating polyradiculoneuropathy with cranial nerve involvement. J Child Neurol. 17(11):819-23, 2002
13. Saperstein DS et al: Clinical spectrum of chronic acquired demyelinating polyneuropathies. Muscle Nerve. 24(3):311-24, 2001
14. Cros D: Peripheral Neuropathy. First ed. Philadelphia: Lippincott Williams & Wilkins: 432, 2001
15. Sabatelli M et al: Pure motor chronic inflammatory demyelinating polyneuropathy. J Neurol. 248(9):772-7, 2001
16. Taniguchi N et al: Sonographic detection of diffuse peripheral nerve hypertrophy in chronic inflammatory demyelinating polyradiculoneuropathy. J Clin Ultrasound. 28(9):488-91, 2000
17. Van den Bergh PY et al: Chronic demyelinating hypertrophic brachial plexus neuropathy. Muscle nerve 23(2): 283-8, 2000
18. Duarte J et al: Hypertrophy of multiple cranial nerves and spinal roots in chronic inflammatory demyelinating neuropathy. J Neurol Neurosurg Psychiatry. 67(5):685-7, 1999
19. Midroni G et al: MRI of the cauda equina in CIDP: clinical correlations. J Neurol Sci. 170(1):36-44, 1999
20. Mizuno K et al: Chronic inflammatory demyelinating polyradiculoneuropathy with diffuse and massive peripheral nerve hypertrophy: distinctive clinical and magnetic resonance imaging features. Muscle Nerve. 21(6):805-8, 1998
21. Kuwabara S et al: Magnetic resonance imaging at the demyelinative foci in chronic inflammatory demyelinating polyneuropathy. Neurology. 48(4):874-7, 1997
22. Simmons Z et al: Chronic inflammatory demyelinating polyradiculoneuropathy in children: I. Presentation, electrodiagnostic studies, and initial clinical course, with comparison to adults. 20(12):1569-75, 1997
23. Van Es HW et al: Magnetic resonance imaging of the brachial plexus in patients with multifocal motor neuropathy. Neurology. 48(5):1218-24, 1997
24. Goldstein JM et al: Nerve root hypertrophy as the cause of lumbar stenosis in chronic inflammatory demyelinating polyradiculoneuropathy. Muscle Nerve. 19(7):892-6, 1996
25. Schady W et al: Massive nerve root enlargement in chronic inflammatory demyelinating polyneuropathy. J Neurol Neurosurg Psychiatry. 61(6):636-40, 1996

CIDP

IMAGE GALLERY

Typical

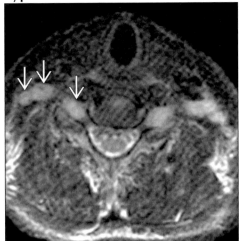
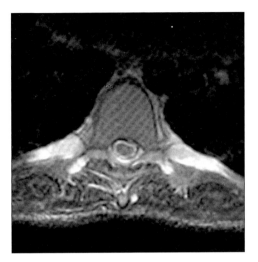

(Left) Axial T2WI MR reveals bilateral symmetric enlargement, hyperintensity of cervical nerve roots and brachial plexus (arrows). *(Right)* Axial T2WI MR shows diffuse thickening and hyperintensity of thoracic nerve roots and paraspinal intercostal nerves.

Typical

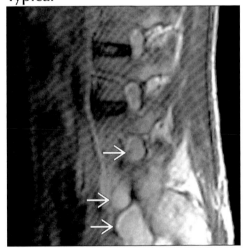
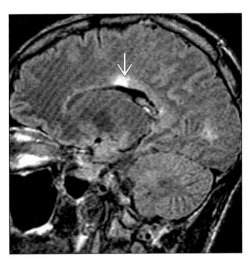

(Left) Sagittal T2WI MR depicts enlarged lumbar nerve roots extending into extraforaminal ventral primary rami (arrows). *(Right)* Sagittal FLAIR MR of the brain in a CIDP patient shows a typical paraventricular demyelinating lesion (arrow) similar to those seen in multiple sclerosis patients.

Typical

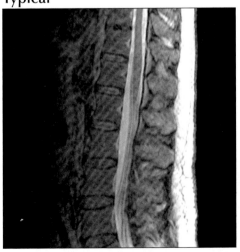
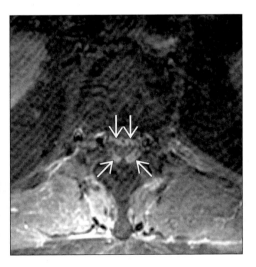

(Left) Sagittal T2WI MR demonstrates diffuse thickening of the intradural cauda equina nerve roots. *(Right)* Axial T1 C+ MR shows thickening and enhancement of ventral and dorsal cauda equina nerve roots (arrows).

ARACHNOIDITIS, LUMBAR

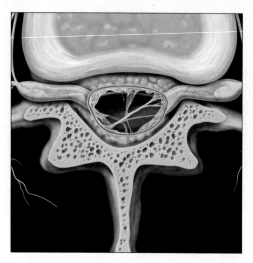

Axial graphic of a lumbar vertebra demonstrates nerve roots plastered against the periphery of thecal sac, with multiple adhesions compartmentalizing arachnoid space.

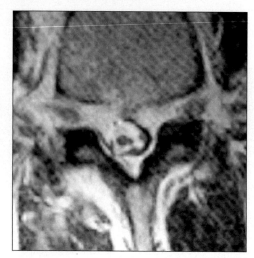

Axial T2WI MR shows centrally and peripherally clumped nerve roots.

TERMINOLOGY

Abbreviations and Synonyms
- Chronic adhesive arachnoiditis

Definitions
- Post-inflammatory adhesion and clumping of nerve roots

IMAGING FINDINGS

General Features
- Best diagnostic clue: Absence of discrete nerve roots in thecal sac
- Location
  - Lumbar spine
    - Cauda equina
- Morphology
  - Intrathecal cords
  - "Empty sac"
  - Soft tissue mass

Radiographic Findings
- Radiography: Evidence of prior lumbar surgery
- Myelography
  - Type I
    - "Featureless sac sign"
    - Homogeneous filling of thecal sac
    - Absent or blunted nerve root sleeve filling
  - Type II
    - Localized or diffuse intrathecal filling defects
    - Flow of myelographic contrast may be obstructed
    - "Candle-guttering sign"
    - Loculated, clumped contrast: Must be distinguished from epidural or subdural injection
  - Two types form continuum of findings

CT Findings
- NECT
  - Post-myelography
    - "Empty thecal sac sign"
    - Absent nerve root sleeve filling
    - Nerve roots adherent to thecal sac
    - Clumped nerve roots forming soft tissue mass(es)
    - Irregular contrast collections
  - Thickened retracted dura
  - Distorted thecal sac
- CECT: Enhancing nerve roots and dura
- Bone CT
  - Rare calcifications of nerve roots or soft tissue mass
    - Arachnoiditis ossificans

MR Findings
- T1WI
  - ± Residual Pantopaque (high signal droplets)
  - Indistinct cord due to increased cerebral spinal fluid (CSF) intensity

DDx: Entities Simulating Lumbar Arachnoiditis

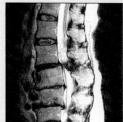

Spinal Stenosis

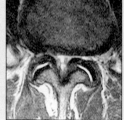

Spinal Stenosis

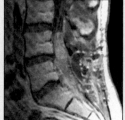

Ependymoma

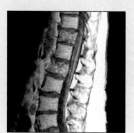

Intradural Mets

ARACHNOIDITIS, LUMBAR

Key Facts

Terminology
- Chronic adhesive arachnoiditis
- Post-inflammatory adhesion and clumping of nerve roots

Imaging Findings
- Best diagnostic clue: Absence of discrete nerve roots in thecal sac
- Absent or blunted nerve root sleeve filling
- Flow of myelographic contrast may be obstructed
- Clumped nerve roots forming cords
- Nerve roots adhering to walls of thecal sac
- "Empty thecal sac sign"
- Soft tissue mass filling most of thecal sac (type III)
- Intradural cysts

- Minimal to mild cord, nerve root, and dural enhancement
- Findings extend over at least two lumber vertebrae

Top Differential Diagnoses
- Spinal stenosis
- Cauda equina neoplasms
- Intradural metastases

Pathology
- Now more commonly associated with prior lumbar surgery
- 6-16% of postoperative patients

Clinical Issues
- Chronic low back pain

- T2WI
  - Discrete nerve roots absent
  - Clumped nerve roots forming cords
    - Centrally = type I
    - Peripheral = type II
    - May involve only 2-3 nerve roots
  - Nerve roots adhering to walls of thecal sac
    - "Empty thecal sac sign"
    - Central CSF without nerve roots
    - Thickened thecal sac wall
  - Soft tissue mass filling most of thecal sac (type III)
    - Clumped nerve roots
    - Decreased sac diameter
    - Obliterated subarachnoid space
  - Intradural cysts
    - Loculated CSF
    - Formed by adhesions
    - Mass effect present
    - May be septated
- T1 C+
  - Minimal to mild cord, nerve root, and dural enhancement
    - Smooth, linear
    - Nodular
    - Mass-like intradural enhancement
    - Also in postoperative patients without myelographic evidence of arachnoiditis
    - No correlation between degree of enhancement and severity of symptoms
- Findings extend over at least two lumber vertebrae

Imaging Recommendations
- Best imaging tool: Spine T1WI and T2WI MRI in sagittal and axial planes with gadolinium

DIFFERENTIAL DIAGNOSIS

Spinal stenosis
- Clumped nerve roots at site of stenosis
- Tortuous, elongated roots cephalad to stenosis
- Degenerative changes prominent
  - Disc herniation

  - Endplate spur
  - LAX, thickened ligamentum flavum
  - Facet arthropathy

Cauda equina neoplasms
- Myxopapillary ependymoma most common
  - Cysts and hemorrhage present
- Large nerve sheath tumor
- Paraganglioma rare
- All with avid post-gadolinium enhancement
- Displacement of conus

Carcinomatous meningitis
- Smooth or nodular nerve root enhancement
- Clumping of nerve roots usually absent

Intradural metastases
- Nodules or masses within cauda equina
- Significant post-gadolinium enhancement

PATHOLOGY

General Features
- General path comments: Inflammation of all three meningeal layers and nerve roots
- Genetics: No familial predilection
- Etiology
  - Historically more commonly related to trauma or spinal meningitis
    - Tuberculosis
    - Syphilis
    - Fungal
    - Parasitic
    - Cord and nerve roots involved in infectious meningitis
  - Now more commonly associated with prior lumbar surgery
    - Especially when multi-level or complicated
    - In combination with antecedent myelography
    - Ionic water or oil-based agents
    - Nonionic water-soluble contrast less likely to cause arachnoiditis

- Myelography alone elicits an intrathecal inflammatory response
- Intrathecal hemorrhage
  - Shown to irritate meninges in animal models
  - Dorsal thoracic arachnoiditis more common in subarachnoid hemorrhage
- Other causes
  - Spinal anesthesia
  - Degenerative disc disease
- Pathophysiology
  - Infectious meningitis: Vascular congestion, inflammatory exudate
  - Fibrin deposition
  - Fibrocytes proliferate
  - Perineural and leptomeningeal fibrosis
  - Nerve roots adhere to one another, thecal sac
  - CSF loculation
- Epidemiology
  - Uncommon
    - < 1,000 cases reported in literature over 50 years
  - Clinical syndrome more common
    - 6-16% of post-operative patients
- Associated abnormalities
  - Syringomyelia
    - Not lined by ependyma
    - Alteration in CSF circulation
    - Increased amount of CSF entering cord
    - Symptoms higher in cord

Gross Pathologic & Surgical Features
- Inflammatory, collagenous mass
- Maybe calcified
- Posterior nerve roots involved more commonly

Microscopic Features
- Collagen formation
- Chronic lymphocytic infiltration
- Small foci of calcifications

CLINICAL ISSUES

Presentation
- Most common signs/symptoms
  - Chronic low back pain
  - Radicular or non-radicular leg pain
    - Simulates spinal stenosis and polyneuropathy
  - Other signs/symptoms
    - Paraparesis
    - Hypoesthesia
    - Gait disorder
    - Bladder and bowel dysfunction
- Clinical profile
  - No defining clinical symptomatology
  - Radiological findings may be present without clinical symptoms

Demographics
- Gender: No gender predilection
- Ethnicity: No racial predilection

Natural History & Prognosis
- Symptoms usually static
  - Fluctuate in severity
- Small percentage with progressive neurologic deficits

- 1.8% in one series

Treatment
- Intrathecal steroid injection
- Spinal cord stimulation
  - Treatment of choice when pain is the predominant symptom
  - Immediate success rate (pain relief): > 70%
  - Intermediate success rate: > 50%
  - Long term success rate: > 30%
- Pain rehabilitation
- Laminectomy with microlysis of adhesions
  - Reserved for patients with progressive neurologic deficits
  - 50% initial success rate
  - Effectiveness decreases over time

DIAGNOSTIC CHECKLIST

Image Interpretation Pearls
- Absent discrete nerve roots in thecal sac with clumping or "empty sac sign" highly suggestive of lumbar arachnoiditis

SELECTED REFERENCES

1. Ross JS: Magnetic resonance imaging of the postoperative spine. Semin Musculoskelet Radiol. 4(3):281-91, 2000
2. Petty PG et al: Symptomatic lumbar spinal arachnoiditis: fact or fallacy? J Clin Neurosci. 7(5):395-9, 2000
3. Long DM: Chronic adhesive spinal arachnoiditis: pathogenesis, prognosis, and treatment. Neurosurgery Quarterly. 2:296-318, 1992
4. Sklar EM et al: Complications of epidural anesthesia: MR appearance of abnormalities. Radiology. 181(2):549-54, 1991
5. Johnson CE et al: Benign lumbar arachnoiditis: MR imaging with gadopentetate dimeglumine. AJR Am J Roentgenol. 155(4):873-80, 1990
6. Delamarter RB et al: Diagnosis of lumbar arachnoiditis by magnetic resonance imaging. Spine. 15:304-10, 1990
7. Caplan LR et al: Syringomyelia and arachnoiditis. J Neurol Neurosurg Psychiatry. 53(2):106-13, 1990
8. Augustijn P et al: Chronic spinal arachnoiditis following intracranial subarachnoid haemorrhage. Clin Neurol Neurosurg. 91(4):347-50, 1989
9. Sklar E et al: Acquired spinal subarachnoid cysts: evaluation with MR, CT myelography, and intraoperative sonography. AJNR Am J Neuroradiol. 10(5):1097-104, 1989
10. Ross JS et al: MR imaging of lumbar arachnoiditis. AJR. 149:1025-32, 1987
11. Burton CV et al: Causes of failure of surgery on the lumbar spine. Clin Orthop. (157):191-9, 1981
12. Quiles M et al: Lumbar adhesive arachnoiditis. Etiologic and pathologic aspects. Spine. 3(1):45-50, 1978
13. Quencer RM et al: The postoperative myelogram. Radiographic evaluation of arachnoiditis and dural/arachnoidal tears. Radiology. 123(3):667-79, 1977
14. Jorgensen J et al: A clinical and radiological study of chronic lower spinal arachnoiditis. Neuroradiology. 9(3):139-44, 1975

ARACHNOIDITIS, LUMBAR

IMAGE GALLERY

Typical

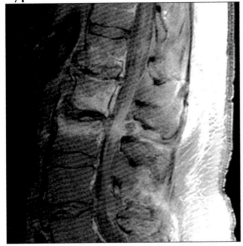
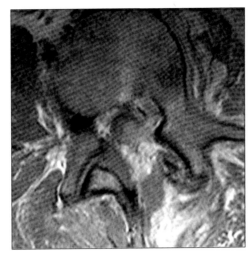

(Left) Sagittal T1 C+ MR with fat suppression shows mass-like enhancement within thecal sac at L2-3, involving adherent nerve roots. *(Right)* Axial T1 C+ MR with fat suppression in same patient shows intradural mass-like enhancement and paradural post-surgical changes.

Typical

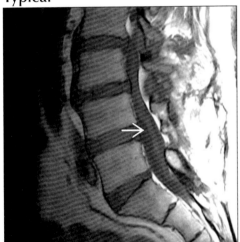
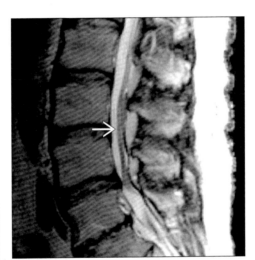

(Left) Sagittal T1WI MR shows a cord-like thickening (arrow) within thecal sac extending from L3 to S1. *(Right)* Sagittal T2WI MR shows an intrathecal conglomerate of nerve roots (arrow).

Typical

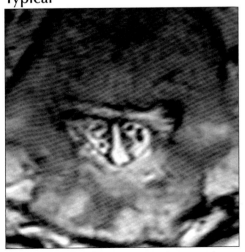
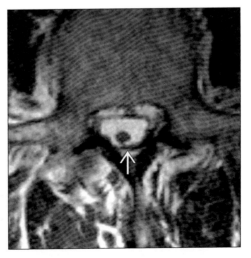

(Left) Axial T2WI MR shows compartmentalized nerve roots and loculated CSF from intrathecal adhesions. Post-surgical changes involve posterior elements. *(Right)* Axial T2WI MR shows centrally clumped nerve roots forming a mass. Posterior thecal sac is thickened (arrow) from adherent nerve roots.

ARACHNOIDITIS OSSIFICANS, LUMBAR

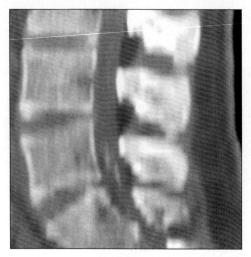

Axial bone CT with sagittal reformation shows two intraspinal thin linear calcifications at L5-S1.

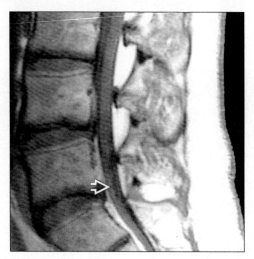

Sagittal T1WI MR shows a conglomerate of lumbar nerve roots consistent with arachnoiditis. A subtle linear intrathecal hypointensity (arrow) corresponds to a calcification on CT.

TERMINOLOGY

Definitions
- Intradural ossification associated with post-inflammatory adhesion and clumping of lumbar nerve roots

IMAGING FINDINGS

General Features
- Best diagnostic clue: Focal calcific density on CT or hyperintensity on T1WI and T2WI within lumbar nerve root aggregate
- Location: Lumbar spine
- Morphology
  ○ Thin, linear
  ○ Mass-like, globular

Radiographic Findings
- Radiography: Intraspinal ossification
- Myelography: Intrathecal contrast may obscure calcifications

CT Findings
- Bone CT
  ○ Calcific densities within clumped nerve roots
  ○ Calcifications may surround conus medullaris, cauda equina

MR Findings
- Clumped nerve roots forming cords and mass(es)
- Focal signal alteration distinct from nerve root conglomerate
  ○ Variable signal intensity
    ▪ Hypo- or hyperintense on T1WI and T2WI
  ○ Hyperintensity represents fatty marrow
  ○ May exert mass effect on conus and cauda equina
  ○ No post-gadolinium enhancement
- Variable nerve root enhancement
- Intraspinal cysts and loculations

Imaging Recommendations
- Best imaging tool: Axial thin-section bone CT with sagittal reformation

DIFFERENTIAL DIAGNOSIS

Retained Pantopaque
- Hyperintense on T1WI
- Iso- to hypointense on T2WI
- Differentiated from calcification by CT

Intrathecal primary neoplasm, metastases
- More vigorous enhancement of mass, nerve roots, or focal nodules

DDx: Entities Simulating Arachnoiditis Ossificans

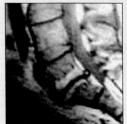

Retained Pantopaque

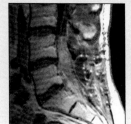

Ependymoma

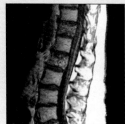

Intradural Mets

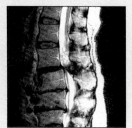

Spinal Stenosis

ARACHNOIDITIS OSSIFICANS, LUMBAR

Key Facts

Terminology
- Intradural ossification associated with post-inflammatory adhesion and clumping of lumbar nerve roots

Imaging Findings
- Best diagnostic clue: Focal calcific density on CT or hyperintensity on T1WI and T2WI within lumbar nerve root aggregate

- Hypo- or hyperintense on T1WI and T2WI
- No post-gadolinium enhancement

Pathology
- Osseous metaplasia from chronic inflammation and fibrosis

Diagnostic Checklist
- Thin-section bone CT when heterogeneous intrathecal signal present in setting of arachnoiditis

---

- Mass or nodules isointense on T1WI and hyperintense on T2WI

Spinal stenosis
- Clumped nerve roots
- Degenerative changes prominent
- No intrathecal calcification

Calcified dural plaques
- Thin, patchy dural calcifications
- Asymptomatic

PATHOLOGY

General Features
- Etiology
  - Prior trauma, lumbar surgery, subarachnoid hemorrhage, myelography, spinal anesthesia
  - Pathophysiology of lumbar arachnoiditis
    - Fibrin deposition
    - Proliferating fibroblasts
    - Perineural and leptomeningeal fibrosis
  - Ossification results from
    - Intrathecal hematoma
    - Incorporated bone fragments
    - Osseous metaplasia from chronic inflammation and fibrosis
    - End-stage chronic arachnoiditis
- Epidemiology: Rare
- Associated abnormalities: Syringomyelia

Gross Pathologic & Surgical Features
- Calcified inflammatory, collagenous mass

Microscopic Features
- Osteoblastic proliferation with osseous metaplasia
- Mature bone with osseous marrow and trabeculae

CLINICAL ISSUES

Presentation
- Most common signs/symptoms
  - Low back pain
  - Other signs/symptoms
    - Radicular or non-radicular leg pain
    - Paraparesis
    - Bladder and bowel dysfunction
- Clinical profile
  - No defining clinical symptomatology

- Simulates spinal stenosis and polyneuropathy

Natural History & Prognosis
- Possible progressive neurologic impairment

Treatment
- Decompressive laminectomy over entire length of ossification with some reported success
- No therapeutic advantage in resecting intradural ossifications

DIAGNOSTIC CHECKLIST

Consider
- Thin-section bone CT when heterogeneous intrathecal signal present in setting of arachnoiditis

SELECTED REFERENCES

1. Faure A et al: Arachnoiditis ossificans of the cauda equina. Case report and review of the literature. J Neurosurg. 97(2 Suppl):239-43, 2002
2. Frizzell B et al: Arachnoiditis ossificans: MR imaging features in five patients. AJR 177:461-4, 2001
3. Long DM: Chronic adhesive spinal arachnoiditis: pathogenesis, prognosis, and treatment. Neurosurgery Quarterly. 2:296-318, 1992

IMAGE GALLERY

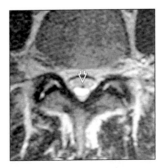 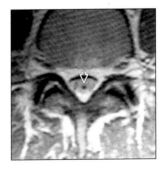

(Left) Axial T2WI MR confirms the focal intrathecal hypointensity (arrow) at dorsal aspect of clumped nerve roots. (Right) Axial PD/Intermediate MR shows the same focal hypointensity (arrow), corresponding to calcification on CT.

SARCOIDOSIS

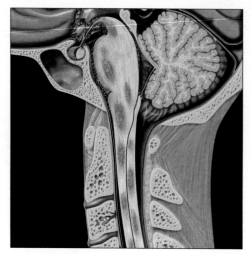

Sagittal graphic depicts multiple intramedullary sarcoid granulomas in brainstem and upper cervical cord.

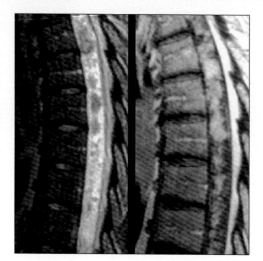

Sagittal T2WI MR (left) shows diffuse IM T2 hyperintensities with nodular isointensities. Sagittal T1 C+ MR (right) shows nodular and mass-like enhancement (Courtesy A. Osborn, MD).

TERMINOLOGY

Abbreviations and Synonyms
- Neurosarcoidosis

Definitions
- Noncaseating granulomatous disease of spine and spinal cord

IMAGING FINDINGS

General Features
- Best diagnostic clue: Combination of leptomeningeal and peripheral intramedullary (IM) mass-like enhancement suggestive of spinal sarcoidosis
- Location
  - Intramedullary
    - Cervical
    - Upper thoracic
  - Extramedullary intradural
    - Cauda equina
    - Dural involvement without segmental predilection
  - Extradural
  - Vertebral
    - Lower thoracic and upper lumbar spine
- Size: Variable
- Morphology: Variable

Radiographic Findings
- Myelography: Nonspecific cord expansion

CT Findings
- NECT: Cord expansion
- Bone CT
  - Multiple lytic lesions in spine
    - Sclerotic margins
  - Sclerotic or mixed lytic and sclerotic lesions also possible

MR Findings
- T1WI
  - Fusiform cord enlargement
  - Cord atrophy in late stages
  - Iso- to hypointense lesions
- T2WI
  - Hyperintensity
    - Focal or diffuse
- STIR: Lesions hyperintense
- T1 C+
  - Enhancing dural masses
    - Variable cord and nerve root compression
  - Leptomeningeal enhancement
    - Smooth or nodular
    - 60% of cord lesions
    - Including cauda equina

DDx: Intramedullary Lesions and Leptomeningeal Enhancement

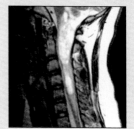

Astrocytoma

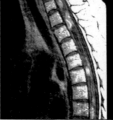

Intramedullary Mets

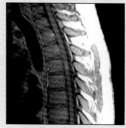

Multiple Sclerosis

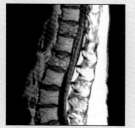

Leptomeningeal Mets

SARCOIDOSIS

Key Facts

Terminology
- Noncaseating granulomatous disease of spine and spinal cord

Imaging Findings
- Best diagnostic clue: Combination of leptomeningeal and peripheral intramedullary (IM) mass-like enhancement suggestive of spinal sarcoidosis
- Multiple lytic lesions in spine
- Fusiform cord enlargement
- Cord atrophy in late stages
- Hyperintensity
- Enhancing dural masses
- Leptomeningeal enhancement
- Peripheral IM enhancement
- Mass-like IM enhancement

Top Differential Diagnoses
- Intramedullary neoplasm
- Multiple sclerosis

Pathology
- General path comments: Noncaseating granulomatous inflammation
- Clinical CNS involvement in patients with sarcoidosis: 5%
- Intraoperative frozen-sections may be misinterpreted for gliomas

Diagnostic Checklist
- Protean imaging manifestations
- Mimicking multiple spinal pathologies
- Invariable presence of systemic disease helps make the diagnosis and avoid spinal cord biopsy

---

- ○ Peripheral IM enhancement
  - ▪ Broad-based contact with cord surface
- ○ Mass-like IM enhancement
  - ▪ Focal or multifocal
- ○ Diffuse or patchy IM enhancement
- ○ Enhancing vertebral lesions
- Regression of findings during steroid therapy
  - ○ Decreased enhancement
  - ○ Poor correlation with clinical response
- Rare: IM calcifications or cysts

Nuclear Medicine Findings
- Bone Scan: Multifocal uptake of radiotracer in vertebral sarcoid lesions
- PET: Increased metabolic activity in cord lesions
- Gallium Scan
  - ○ Increased central nervous system uptake
    - ▪ < 5% of patients

Imaging Recommendations
- Best imaging tool: Sagittal and axial T1WI and T2WI MRI with gadolinium

DIFFERENTIAL DIAGNOSIS

Intramedullary neoplasm
- Lack of leptomeningeal enhancement
- Typically holocord enhancement on axial imaging
- Peri-tumoral edema
- Cystic ± hemorrhagic components
- Degree of enhancement does not regress significantly after corticosteroid treatment

Multiple sclerosis
- Lack of leptomeningeal enhancement
- Central enhancement in peripheral lesions
- < Half cross-sectional area of spinal cord
- Presence of intracranial periventricular, subcallosal, brainstem, and cerebellar white matter lesions in 90% of cases

Cord ischemia and infarct
- Immediate onset

- ○ Minutes, rather than days, weeks
- Ventral location
- No mass effect initially
- No significant enhancement

Idiopathic transverse myelitis
- Peripheral enhancement in central lesions
- 3 to 4 segments in length
- > Two-thirds cross-sectional area of spinal cord
- Diagnosis of exclusion

Lymphoma
- Protean manifestations
- Nodular leptomeningeal enhancement
- Look for vertebral & epidural masses

Intradural metastases
- Smooth enhancement along cord or roots
  - ○ Carcinomatous meningitis
- Multifocal discrete nodules
- Thickening of cauda equina
- Focal masses

PATHOLOGY

General Features
- General path comments: Noncaseating granulomatous inflammation
- Genetics
  - ○ Major histocompatibility complex or complement receptor gene on macrophages may be involved
    - ▪ Exaggerated response to chemotactic factors
- Etiology
  - ○ Exaggerated T-cell mediated immune response suspected
    - ▪ Self antigen or infectious agents
  - ○ Faulty suppression mechanism
- Epidemiology
  - ○ Incidence of sarcoidosis
    - ▪ 10-40 per 100,000 in US and Europe
  - ○ Clinical CNS involvement in patients with sarcoidosis: 5%
    - ▪ Spinal intramedullary sarcoidosis: < 1%

SARCOIDOSIS

- o Imaging evidence of CNS involvement: 10%
- o CNS involvement at autopsy: 15-25%
- o Isolated neurosarcoidosis: 1.5%
- • Associated abnormalities
  - o Intracranial sarcoidosis
  - o Systemic sarcoidosis
- • Pathophysiology of IM involvement
  - o Leptomeningeal granulomatous inflammation
  - o Central intramedullary spread via perivascular space
    - ▪ Cord enlargement and faint enhancement
  - o Focal or multifocal enhancement
    - ▪ Normal cord contour
  - o Resolved inflammation
    - ▪ No enhancement
    - ▪ Normal or atrophic cord

Gross Pathologic & Surgical Features
- • Granuloma resembles neoplasm
- • Intraoperative frozen-sections may be misinterpreted for gliomas

Microscopic Features
- • Epithelioid cell noncaseating granulomas
  - o Surrounded by lymphocytes and mononuclear phagocytes
  - o Negative stains for infectious agents
  - o Granulomas smaller compared to those in systemic disease
    - ▪ Fewer multinucleated giant cells
- • Areas of neural tissue infarction
- • Perivascular lymphocytic infiltrate
  - o Also involving adventitia of vessels

CLINICAL ISSUES

Presentation
- • Most common signs/symptoms
  - o Lower extremity weakness
  - o Other signs/symptoms
    - ▪ Paresthesia
    - ▪ Radiculopathy
    - ▪ Bladder and bowel dysfunction
- • Clinical profile: Acute to subacute onset

Demographics
- • Age: 20-40 years old
- • Gender
  - o Male > female in spinal sarcoidosis
  - o Slight female predominance in systemic sarcoidosis
- • Ethnicity
  - o Sarcoidosis relatively more common in Northern Europeans and African-Americans
  - o Rare in Asians

Natural History & Prognosis
- • Favorable response to corticosteroid therapy
  - o Two-thirds of neurosarcoidosis
- • One-third with remitting relapsing course

Treatment
- • Intravenous ± oral corticosteroids
  - o Chronic steroid therapy may be required
- • Immunosuppressive therapy
  - o Cyclophosphamide

- o Azathioprine
- o Methotrexate
- o Cyclosporine
- • Low dose radiation
  - o 1-3,000 rads over days to weeks

DIAGNOSTIC CHECKLIST

Image Interpretation Pearls
- • Protean imaging manifestations
  - o Mimicking multiple spinal pathologies
  - o Invariable presence of systemic disease helps make the diagnosis and avoid spinal cord biopsy

SELECTED REFERENCES

1. Smith JK et al: Imaging manifestations of neurosarcoidosis. AJR Am J Roentgenol. 182(2):289-95, 2004
2. Bose B: Extramedullary sarcoid lesion mimicking intraspinal tumor. Spine J. 2(5):381-5, 2002
3. Dubey N et al: Role of fluorodeoxyglucose positron emission tomography in the diagnosis of neurosarcoidosis. J Neurol Sci. 205(1):77-81, 2002
4. Gullapalli D et al: Neurologic manifestations of sarcoidosis. Neurol Clin. 20(1):59-83, vi, 2002
5. Bode MK et al: Isolated neurosarcoidosis - MR findings and pathologic correlation. Acta Radiol. 42(6):563-7, 2001
6. Vinas FC et al: Spinal cord sarcoidosis: a diagnostic dilemma. Neurol Res. 23(4):347-52, 2001
7. Maroun FB et al: Sarcoidosis presenting as an intramedullary spinal cord lesion. Can J Neurol Sci. 28(2):163-6, 2001
8. Hayat GR et al: Solitary intramedullary neurosarcoidosis: role of MRI in early detection. J Neuroimaging. 11(1):66-70, 2001
9. Yasui K et al: Correlation of magnetic resonance imaging findings and histopathology of lesion distribution of spinal cord sarcoidosis at post-mortem. Neuropathol Appl Neurobiol. 26(5):481-7, 2000
10. Koike H et al: Differential response to corticosteroid therapy of MRI findings and clinical manifestations in spinal cord sarcoidosis. J Neurol. 247(7):544-9, 2000
11. Dumas JL et al: Central nervous system sarcoidosis: follow-up at MR imaging during steroid therapy. Radiology. 214(2):411-20, 2000
12. Christoforidis GA et al: MR of CNS sarcoidosis: correlation of imaging features to clinical symptoms and response to treatment. AJNR Am J Neuroradiol. 20(4):655-69, 1999
13. Hashmi M et al: Diagnosis and treatment of intramedullary spinal cord sarcoidosis. J Neurol. 245(3):178-80, 1998
14. Jallo GI et al: Intraspinal sarcoidosis: diagnosis and management. Surg Neurol. 48(5):514-20; discussion 521, 1997
15. Lexa FJ et al: MR of sarcoidosis in the head and spine: spectrum of manifestations and radiographic response to steroid therapy. AJNR 5:973-82, 1994
16. Junger SS et al: Intramedullary spinal sarcoidosis: clinical and magnetic resonance imaging characteristics. Neurology. 43(2):333-7, 1993
17. Seltzer S et al: CNS sarcoidosis: evaluation with contrast-enhanced MR imaging. AJNR Am J Neuroradiol. 12(6):1227-33, 1991
18. Nesbit GM et al: Spinal cord sarcoidosis: a new finding at MR imaging with Gd-DTPA enhancement. Radiology. 173(3):839-43, 1989
19. Terunuma H et al: Sarcoidosis presenting as progressive myelopathy. Clin Neuropathol. 7(2):77-80, 1988

SARCOIDOSIS

IMAGE GALLERY

Typical

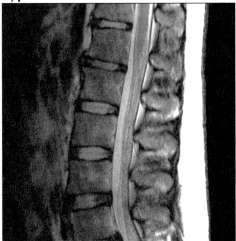 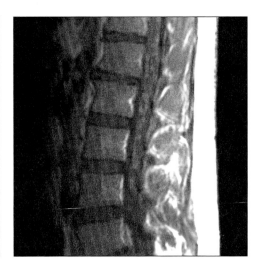

(Left) Sagittal T2WI MR shows subtle isointense nodules interspersed throughout cauda equina. *(Right)* Sagittal T1 C+ MR shows numerous enhancing nodules along surface of nerve roots and conus medullaris.

Typical

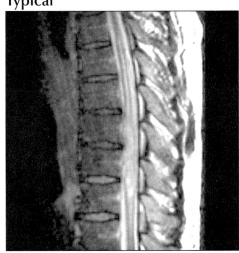 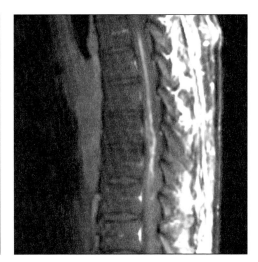

(Left) Sagittal T2WI MR through thoracic spine in a patient with sarcoidosis shows intramedullary hyperintensity cranial and rostral to a mildly expansile lesion in mid-thoracic cord. *(Right)* Sagittal T1 C+ MR with fat suppression in same patient shows heterogeneous intramedullary enhancement corresponding to T2 abnormality. Posterior mediastinal lymphadenopathy is evident.

Typical

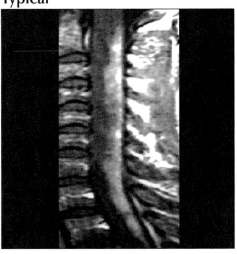 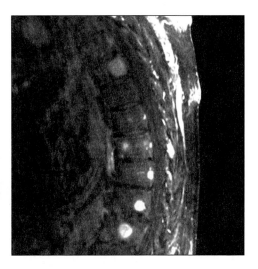

(Left) Sagittal T1 C+ MR shows diffuse mildly heterogenous enhancement involving mid and dorsal aspect of cervical cord from C2 to T2-3. *(Right)* Sagittal T1 C+ MR with fat suppression shows "multiple vertebral sarcoid" lesions with homogeneous enhancement.

MULTIPLE SCLEROSIS, SPINAL CORD

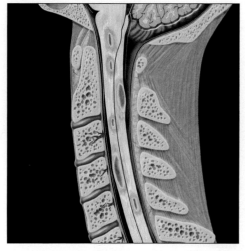

Sagittal graphic depicts multiple demyelinating plaques in cervical cord.

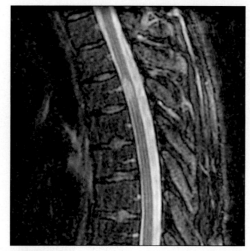

Sagittal STIR MR shows a hyperintense demyelinating plaque within thoracic cord without significant cord expansion.

TERMINOLOGY

Abbreviations and Synonyms
- Spinal cord multiple sclerosis (MS)

Definitions
- Primary demyelinating disease of central nervous system with multiple lesions disseminated over time and space

IMAGING FINDINGS

General Features
- Best diagnostic clue: Concomitant intracranial lesions in periventricular, subcallosal, brain stem, or cerebellar white matter
- Location
  - 10-20% isolated spinal cord disease
  - Cervical is the most commonly affected spinal cord segment
    - Two-thirds of cord lesions
  - Dorsolateral aspect of cord
  - Does not respect gray-white boundary
- Size
  - Less than half cross-sectional area of spinal cord
  - Less than two vertebral segments in length
- Morphology

  - Wedge shaped on axial MRI
    - Apex directed centrally

Radiographic Findings
- Myelography: Nonspecific mild cord expansion

MR Findings
- T1WI
  - Iso- to hypointense lesions
    - In cord (unlike brain) rarely visible as hypointense on T1
- T2WI
  - Well-circumscribed hyperintense lesions
    - Complete demyelination
  - Ill-defined mildly hyperintense areas
    - Partial demyelination
- STIR: Improved lesion detection
- FLAIR: Lower sensitivity compared to STIR in cord imaging
- DWI: Increased mean diffusivity
- T1 C+
  - Variable
    - Homogeneous, nodular, or ring-enhancement during acute or subacute phase
    - Enhancement lasts 1-2 months
    - Does not reflect disease progression
    - No enhancement during chronic phase
- MRS: Decreased N-acetylaspartate level
- Solitary or multifocal lesions

DDx: Cervical Intramedullary Lesions

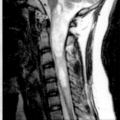

Astrocytoma

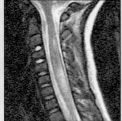

Cord Ischemia

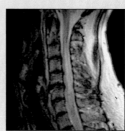

Idiop. Tr. Myelitis

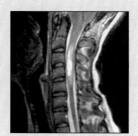

Syringohydromyelia

MULTIPLE SCLEROSIS, SPINAL CORD

Key Facts

Terminology
- Primary demyelinating disease of central nervous system with multiple lesions disseminated over time and space

Imaging Findings
- 10-20% isolated spinal cord disease
- Cervical is the most commonly affected spinal cord segment
- Dorsolateral aspect of cord
- Does not respect gray-white boundary
- Well-circumscribed hyperintense lesions
- Homogeneous, nodular, or ring-enhancement during acute or subacute phase
- MRS: Decreased N-acetylaspartate level
- Cord atrophy

- Useful for monitoring disease progression and therapeutic efficacy

Top Differential Diagnoses
- Intramedullary neoplasm
- Spinal cord ischemia and infarct
- Idiopathic transverse myelitis

Pathology
- Autoimmune, cell-mediated inflammatory process focused on CNS myelin

Diagnostic Checklist
- Imaging findings must be correlated with clinical and laboratory features to confirm diagnosis
- Caution: Acute MS can mimic cord neoplasm!

- ○ Larger lesions formed by coalescence of smaller plaques
- Normal or mild focal cord expansion
  - ○ Cord edema
    - ▪ Resolves after 6-8 weeks
- Cord atrophy
  - ○ Usually in late stage
  - ○ May be seen in early disease course
  - ○ Useful for monitoring disease progression and therapeutic efficacy
  - ○ Correlates with clinical disability

Other Modality Findings
- Magnetization transfer (MT) imaging
  - ○ Reduction in MT ratio in spinal cord
  - ○ Better correlation with disability and axonal loss

Imaging Recommendations
- Best imaging tool: T1WI and T2WI spinal cord MRI in sagittal and axial planes with gadolinium

DIFFERENTIAL DIAGNOSIS

Intramedullary neoplasm
- Cord expansion
- Entire cross-section of spinal cord
- Peritumoral edema
- Diffuse or partial enhancement
- Cystic ± hemorrhagic components

Spinal cord ischemia and infarct
- Sudden onset of symptom
- Posterior columns typically spared in anterior spinal infarct

Idiopathic transverse myelitis
- Lesion centrally located
- 3-4 segments in length
- Occupying more than two thirds of cord's cross-sectional area
- Variable enhancement
- No associated intracranial lesions
- Diagnosis of exclusion

Syringohydromyelia
- Central cystic lesion
- Cerebral spinal fluid intensity on all sequences
- No abnormal enhancement

PATHOLOGY

General Features
- General path comments: Focal regions of demyelination of varying size and age scattered throughout CNS white matter
- Genetics: Low familial incidence
- Etiology
  - ○ Autoimmune, cell-mediated inflammatory process focused on CNS myelin
    - ▪ Infectious agents may play a primary or secondary role
- Epidemiology
  - ○ Increasing prevalence further north from equator
    - ▪ 30-80 per 100,000 in Northern US and Europe
    - ▪ 6-14 per 100,000 in Southern US and Europe
    - ▪ 1 per 100,000 in equatorial regions
- Associated abnormalities
  - ○ 90% incidence of associated intracranial lesions
  - ○ Neurofibromatosis type I

Microscopic Features
- Discrete lesions of myelin destruction
- Active lesions with macrophages and lymphocytes
- Chronic lesions with gliosis and cavitation
- Perivascular cuffs of lymphocytes and mononuclear cells
- Involvement of dorsal horns common

CLINICAL ISSUES

Presentation
- Most common signs/symptoms
  - ○ Paresthesia
  - ○ Other signs/symptoms
    - ▪ Muscle weakness

MULTIPLE SCLEROSIS, SPINAL CORD

III

2

22

- Spasm
- Gait disturbance
- Bladder and bowel dysfunction
- Hyperreflexia
- Clinical profile: Cord lesions may be asymptomatic

Demographics
- Age
  - Onset 30-40
  - Onset < 18 years of age
    - 3-5% of MS cases
- Gender
  - Adult females more susceptible than males (1.7:1)
    - Men more likely to have progressive relapsing and secondary progressive MS
    - Women more likely to have relapsing remitting MS
  - Both sexes are equally affected in primary progressive MS
- Ethnicity: Western Europeans with higher risk

Natural History & Prognosis
- Benign: 20%
  - Complete recovery after 1-2 attacks
  - Some may experience progressive MS after 10-15 years
- Relapsing remitting: 25%
  - Distinct periods of new or worsening symptoms alternating with complete or partial recovery
  - 90% will evolve into progressive MS after 25 years
- Secondary progressive: 40%
  - From relapsing remitting MS
  - Worsening deficits and disabilities
  - Incomplete and infrequent remission
- Primary progressive: 12%
  - Steady progression of symptoms
    - Motor dysfunction common
    - Primary cord involvement
    - No distinct attacks
- Progressive relapsing: 3%
  - Similar to primary progressive MS
  - Includes distinct periods of exacerbation without recovery
  - High mortality rate

Treatment
- IV and oral prednisone
- Plasmapheresis
  - If no response to steroid therapy
- Beta interferon
  - Inhibition of immune cells
- Glatiramer acetate
  - Synthetic protein similar to myelin protein
  - Serves as a substrate for T-cells
- Mitoxantrone
  - Suppression of T lymphocytes and B lymphocytes
- Supportive therapy
  - Anticholinergics
  - Smooth muscle relaxants
- Physical therapy

DIAGNOSTIC CHECKLIST

Consider
- Brain MRI including high-resolution fast spin echo T2 through corpus callosum
  - Presence of periventricular, subcallosal, brain stem, or cerebellar white matter lesions suggests MS

Image Interpretation Pearls
- Imaging findings must be correlated with clinical and laboratory features to confirm diagnosis
- Caution: Acute MS can mimic cord neoplasm!

SELECTED REFERENCES

1. International Working Group for Treatment Optimization in MS: Treatment optimization in multiple sclerosis: report of an international consensus meeting. Eur J Neurol. 11(1):43-7, 2004
2. Pretorius PM et al: The role of MRI in the diagnosis of MS. Clin Radiol. 58(6):434-48, 2003
3. Steiner I et al: Infection and the etiology and pathogenesis of multiple sclerosis. Curr Neurol Neurosci Rep. 1(3):271-6, 2001
4. Filippi M et al: Overview of diffusion-weighted magnetic resonance studies in multiple sclerosis. J Neurol Sci. 186 Suppl 1:S37-43, 2001
5. Poser CM et al: Diagnostic criteria for multiple sclerosis. Clin Neurol Neurosurg. 103(1):1-11, 2001
6. Simon JH: Brain and spinal cord atrophy in multiple sclerosis. Neuroimaging Clin N Am. 10(4):753-70 ,ix, 2000
7. Hickman SJ et al: Imaging of the spine in multiple sclerosis. Neuroimaging Clin N Am. 10(4):689-704 ,viii, 2000
8. Bastianello S et al: MRI of spinal cord in MS. J Neurovirol. 6 Suppl 2:S130-3, 2000
9. Simon JH: The contribution of spinal cord MRI to the diagnosis and differential diagnosis of multiple sclerosis. J Neurol Sci. 172 Suppl 1:S32-5, 2000
10. van Waesberghe JH et al: Magnetization transfer imaging of the spinal cord and the optic nerve in patients with multiple sclerosis. Neurology. 53(5 Suppl 3):S46-8, 1999
11. McFarland HF: The lesion in multiple sclerosis: clinical, pathological, and magnetic resonance imaging considerations. J Neurol Neurosurg Psychiatry. 64 Suppl 1:S26-30, 1998
12. Miller DH: Magnetic resonance imaging and spectroscopy in multiple sclerosis. Curr Opin Neurol. 8(3):210-5, 1995
13. Tartaglino LM et al: Multiple Sclerosis in the Spinal Cord: MR Appearance and Correlation with Clinical Parameters. Radiology. 195:725-32, 1995
14. Campi A et al: Acute Transverse Myelopathy: Spinal and Cranial MR Study with Clinical Follow-up. AJNR. 16:115-23, 1995
15. Jeffery DR et al: Transverse myelitis. Retrospective analysis of 33 cases, with differentiation of cases associated with multiple sclerosis and parainfectious events. Arch Neurol. 50(5):532-5, 1993
16. Thomas DJ et al: Magnetic resonance imaging of spinal cord in multiple sclerosis by fluid-attenuated inversion recovery. Lancet. 341(8845):593-4, 1993
17. Maravilla KR et al: Magnetic Resonance Demonstration of Multiple Sclerosis Plaques in the Cervical Cord. AJNR. 5:685-9, 1984

MULTIPLE SCLEROSIS, SPINAL CORD

IMAGE GALLERY

Typical

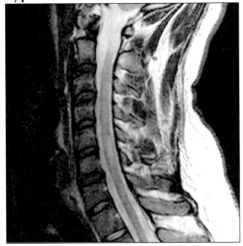
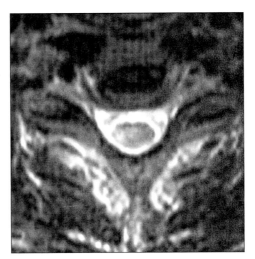

(Left) Sagittal T2WI MR of cervical cord shows an ill-defined intramedullary hyperintense lesion at C5-6. (Right) Axial T2WI MR of cervical cord in another patient shows a poorly defined wedge-shaped mildly hyperintense plaque within right lateral aspect of the cord.

Typical

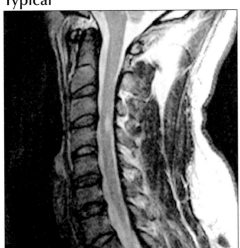
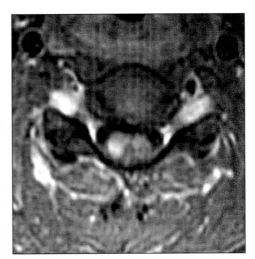

(Left) Sagittal T2WI MR of cervical cord shows a more discrete demyelinating focus at C3-4. (Right) Axial T1 C+ MR with fat suppression of cervical cord in a separate case shows right peripheral nodular enhancement.

Variant

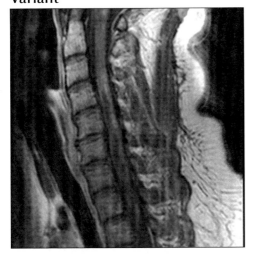
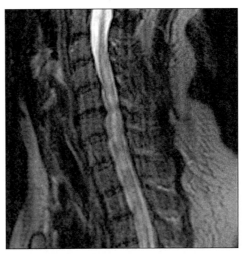

(Left) Sagittal C+ MR shows diffuse cord expansion, extensive multilevel cord enhancement in acute exacerbation of MS. (Right) Sagittal T2W MR shows diffuse cord enlargement & hyperintensity throughout cervical segment into upper thoracic cord in case of acute MS exacerbation.

ADEM, SPINAL CORD

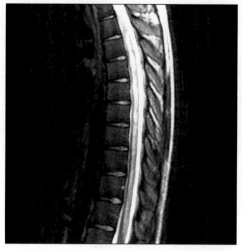

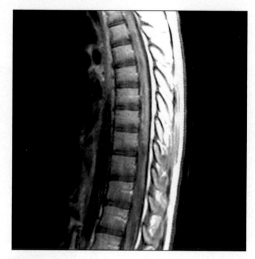

Sagittal T2WI MR shows multiple focal lesions with high signal intensity throughout thoracic cord in patient suffering from lower extremity weakness, paresthesias, after viral illness.

Sagittal T1 C+ MR exhibits patch enhancement throughout thoracic spine (which showed multiple focal high signal lesions on T2WI) in patient with ADEM.

TERMINOLOGY

Abbreviations and Synonyms
- Acute disseminated encephalomyelitis (ADEM)

Definitions
- Para/postinfectious immune mediated inflammatory disorder of the white matter

IMAGING FINDINGS

General Features
- Best diagnostic clue: Multifocal white matter lesions with relatively little mass effect or vasogenic edema
- Location
  - Anywhere in the spinal cord white matter
  - Brain almost always involved
- Size: Punctate to segmental
- Morphology: Plump lesions with feathery edges

Radiographic Findings
- Myelography: May see focal cord swelling

CT Findings
- CECT: May see (multi)focal intramedullary enhancement

MR Findings
- T1WI: Focal low signal and slight cord swelling
- T2WI
  - Multifocal flame shaped white matter lesions with slight cord swelling
  - Dorsal white matter more voluminous
  - May see gray matter involvement
- PD/Intermediate: Sometimes depict the lesions more sensitively
- T2* GRE: Same as T2WI, not as sensitive
- T1 C+
  - Variable enhancement, depending on stage of disease
  - Punctate, ring-shaped, or fluffy enhancement
  - May see nerve enhancement

Imaging Recommendations
- Best imaging tool: Pre- and post-contrast MRI
- Protocol advice: Include brain MRI whenever suspicious cord lesions found

DIFFERENTIAL DIAGNOSIS

Multiple sclerosis
- Indistinguishable on single study
- Brain MRI may help differentiate (cranial nerve involvement indicates ADEM)

DDx: Non-Neoplastic Cord Lesions

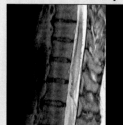

Dural AVM

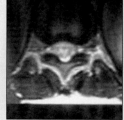

Cord Infarct

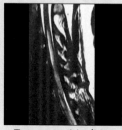

Transverse Myelitis

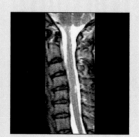

MS

ADEM, SPINAL CORD

Key Facts

Terminology
- Acute disseminated encephalomyelitis (ADEM)
- Para/postinfectious immune mediated inflammatory disorder of the white matter

Imaging Findings
- Best diagnostic clue: Multifocal white matter lesions with relatively little mass effect or vasogenic edema
- Anywhere in the spinal cord white matter
- Brain almost always involved
- Multifocal flame shaped white matter lesions with slight cord swelling
- Variable enhancement, depending on stage of disease

Top Differential Diagnoses
- Multiple sclerosis
- Immune-mediated vasculitis

- Viral or idiopathic transverse myelitis

Pathology
- Autoimmune process producing inflammatory reaction

Clinical Issues
- Paresis
- Cranial nerve palsies
- Abnormal CSF
- Usually no oligoclonal bands
- Age: Typically childhood or young adult
- 50-60% recover completely

Diagnostic Checklist
- Re-scanning if initially negative
- Caution: ADEM can mimic cord neoplasm!

- Clinical course (relapsing-remitting) indicates MS

Immune-mediated vasculitis
- Systemic lupus erythematosus

Viral or idiopathic transverse myelitis
- Usually single lesion
- Mono- to multisegmental

Cord infarct
- Stroke-like, acute presentation
- Focal, segmental lesion in gray matter
- Typically conus involvement

Arteriovenous malformation (AVM)
- High flow AVM demonstrates obvious serpentine structures with flow void at periphery of abnormal cord
- Dural AVF often show distal cord signal increase only, not multi-focal
  - Stuttering course of paresis
  - No cranial nerve findings
  - Signal abnormality spares cord periphery
  - MRA will show abnormal vessels

PATHOLOGY

General Features
- General path comments
  - Tumefactive swelling in some larger, acute lesions
    - Most lesions show no gross features
- Genetics: HLA-DR linkage
- Etiology
  - Autoimmune process producing inflammatory reaction
  - Predisposing infection
    - Mumps
    - Strep
    - Mycoplasma
    - Chickenpox
    - Influenza
    - Epstein-Barr
  - Post-vaccinial association in some reported cases

- Polio vaccine
- Rubella vaccine
- Sporadically reported other post-vaccinial cases
- Following intravenous immunoglobulin administration
- Epidemiology: Unknown
- Increasingly recognized
  - More sensitive imaging tools

Gross Pathologic & Surgical Features
- Slight swelling to tumefactive necrosis

Microscopic Features
- Acute myelin loss
- Lymphocytic infiltrate
- Axonal Preservation
- Astroglial reaction, proliferation

CLINICAL ISSUES

Presentation
- Most common signs/symptoms
  - Paresis
  - Cranial nerve palsies
  - Other signs/symptoms
    - Decreased consciousness
    - Behavioral changes
    - Convulsions
- Clinical profile
  - Usual prodromal phase
    - Fever
    - Malaise
    - Myalgia
  - Abnormal CSF
    - Increased protein
    - Usually no oligoclonal bands
    - Leukocytosis

Demographics
- Age: Typically childhood or young adult
- Gender: Some reports suggest male predominance
- Ethnicity: All

Natural History & Prognosis
• 50-60% recover completely
• Neurologic sequelae in 30-40%
• 10% mortality
• May see striking cord atrophy in chronic phase

Treatment
• Options, risks, complications
  ○ Immunomodulation, supportive
  ○ Plasmapheresis in fulminant case

DIAGNOSTIC CHECKLIST

Consider
• Re-scanning if initially negative
  ○ Typically delay between clinical onset and appearance of imaging findings

Image Interpretation Pearls
• Check thin-section intracranial slices on T1 C+ for cranial nerve enhancement
• Caution: ADEM can mimic cord neoplasm!

SELECTED REFERENCES

1. Garg RK: Acute disseminated encephalomyelitis. Postgrad Med J. 79(927):11-7, 2003
2. Miravalle A et al: Encephalitis complicating smallpox vaccination. Arch Neurol. 60(7):925-8, 2003
3. Dale RC: Acute disseminated encephalomyelitis. Semin Pediatr Infect Dis. 14(2):90-5, 2003
4. Idrissova ZhR et al: Acute disseminated encephalomyelitis in children: clinical features and HLA-DR linkage. Eur J Neurol. 10(5):537-46, 2003
5. Khong PL et al: Childhood acute disseminated encephalomyelitis: the role of brain and spinal cord MRI. Pediatr Radiol. 32(1):59-66, 2002
6. Au WY et al: Acute disseminated encephalomyelitis after para-influenza infection post bone marrow transplantation. Leuk Lymphoma. 43(2):455-7, 2002
7. Murthy SN et al: Acute disseminated encephalomyelitis in children. Pediatrics. 110(2 Pt 1):e21, 2002
8. Khong PL et al: Childhood acute disseminated encephalomyelitis: the role of brain and spinal cord MRI. Pediatr Radiol. 32(1):59-66, 2002
9. Inglese M et al: Magnetization transfer and diffusion tensor MR imaging of acute disseminated encephalomyelitis. AJNR Am J Neuroradiol. 23(2):267-72, 2002
10. Arya SC: Acute disseminated encephalomyelitis associated with poliomyelitis vaccine. Pediatr Neurol. 24(4):325, 2001
11. Lin WC et al: Sequential MR studies of a patient with white matter disease presenting psychotic symptoms: ADEM versus single-episode MS. Kaohsiung J Med Sci. 17(3):161-6, 2001
12. Miyazawa R et al: Plasmapheresis in fulminant acute disseminated encephalomyelitis. Brain Dev. 23(6):424-6, 2001
13. Bastianello S: Magnetic resonance imaging of MS-like disease. Neurol Sci. 22 Suppl 2:S103-7, 2001
14. Tsuru T et al: Acute disseminated encephalomyelitis after live rubella vaccination. Brain Dev. 22(4):259-61, 2000
15. Singh S et al: Acute disseminated encephalomyelitis and multiple sclerosis: magnetic resonance imaging differentiation. Australas Radiol. 44(4):404-11, 2000
16. Pradhan S et al: Intravenous immunoglobulin therapy in acute disseminated encephalomyelitis. J Neurol Sci. 165(1):56-61, 1999
17. Murthy JM et al: Clinical, electrophysiological and magnetic resonance imaging study of acute disseminated encephalomyelitis. J Assoc Physicians India. 47(3):280-3, 1999
18. Murthy JM: MRI in acute disseminated encephalomyelitis following Semple antirabies vaccine. Neuroradiology. 40(7):420-3, 1998
19. Kumada S et al: Encephalomyelitis subsequent to mycoplasma infection with elevated serum anti-Gal C antibody. Pediatr Neurol. 16(3):241-4, 1997
20. Patel SP et al: Neuropsychiatric features of acute disseminated encephalomyelitis: a review. J Neuropsychiatry Clin Neurosci. 9(4):534-40, 1997
21. Kinoshita A et al: Inflammatory demyelinating polyradiculitis in a patient with acute disseminated encephalomyelitis (ADEM). J Neurol Neurosurg Psychiatry. 60(1):87-90, 1996
22. Kleiman M et al: Acute disseminated encephalomyelitis: response to intravenous immunoglobulin. J Child Neurol. 10(6):481-3, 1995
23. Baum PA et al: Deep gray matter involvement in children with acute disseminated encephalomyelitis. AJNR Am J Neuroradiol. 15(7):1275-83, 1994

ADEM, SPINAL CORD

IMAGE GALLERY

Typical

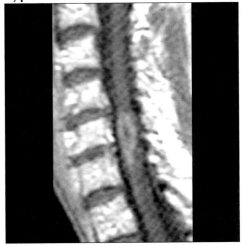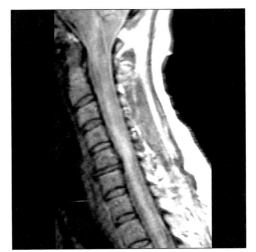

(Left) Sagittal T1 C+ MR shows a vaguely enhancing lesion in cervical cord of patient with ADEM who had numerous cord lesions on T2WI. (Right) Sagittal PD/Intermediate MR exhibits confluent ill-defined intramedullary lesions in patient with ADEM.

Variant

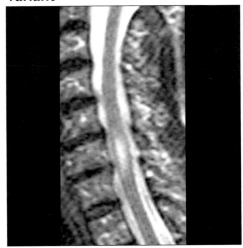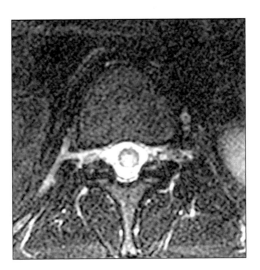

(Left) Sagittal T2WI MR shows focal cord lesion in patient with extremity weakness and cranial nerve findings after a viral illness. (Right) Axial T2WI MR shows lesion in dorsal aspect of cord in patient with ADEM.

Variant

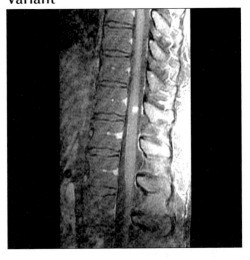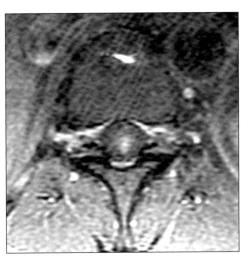

(Left) Sagittal T1 C+ MR shows enhancing focal lesion in distal cord. Patient developed leg weakness and cranial nerve signs after viral illness. (Right) Axial T1 C+ MR shows focal enhancing lesion in distal cord in patient with ADEM.

IDIOPATHIC ACUTE TRANSVERSE MYELITIS

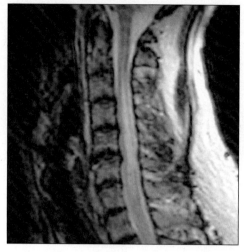

Sagittal T2WI MR shows diffuse intramedullary hyperintensity with mild cord expansion from C2-3 to C7.

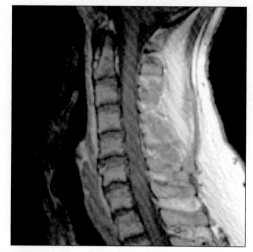

Sagittal T1 C+ MR in the same patient does not show significant post-gadolinium enhancement. Subtle intramedullary hypointensity is present.

TERMINOLOGY

Abbreviations and Synonyms
- Idiopathic acute transverse myelitis (IATM)
- Idiopathic transverse myelopathy

Definitions
- Inflammatory disorder involving both halves of spinal cord resulting in bilateral motor, sensory, and autonomic dysfunction

IMAGING FINDINGS

General Features
- Best diagnostic clue: Central cord lesion more than two vertebral segments in length with eccentric enhancement
- Location
  - Thoracic more common
  - 10% in cervical cord
  - Central cord location on axial imaging
- Size
  - More than two-thirds of cross-sectional area of cord on axial imaging
  - More than two vertebral segments in length
    - Commonly three to four segments
- Morphology: Well-circumscribed

Radiographic Findings
- Myelography
  - To exclude extra-axial compressive etiologies
  - Mild neoplastic cord enlargement
  - Cord swelling may block flow of CSF

MR Findings
- T1WI
  - Smooth cord expansion
    - Less extensive than T2 signal abnormality
  - Cord atrophy in late stage
  - Iso- to hypointense
- T2WI
  - High signal intensity
  - Central dot sign
    - Central gray matter surrounded by edema
- STIR: Hyperintense
- T1 C+
  - Variable post-gadolinium enhancement
    - No enhancement
    - Focal nodular enhancement
    - Subtle diffuse enhancement
    - Patchy enhancement
    - Enhancement at periphery of lesion
    - Meningeal enhancement
    - Preserved cord contour
  - More frequent in subacute than in acute or chronic stage

DDx: Intramedullary T2 Hyperintensity

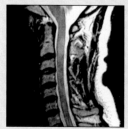

Multiple Sclerosis

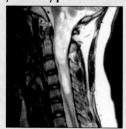

Astrocytoma

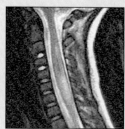

Cord Ischemia

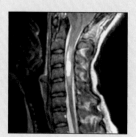

Syringohydromyelia

IDIOPATHIC ACUTE TRANSVERSE MYELITIS

Key Facts

Terminology
- Idiopathic transverse myelopathy
- Inflammatory disorder involving both halves of spinal cord resulting in bilateral motor, sensory, and autonomic dysfunction

Imaging Findings
- Best diagnostic clue: Central cord lesion more than two vertebral segments in length with eccentric enhancement
- Thoracic more common
- Central cord location on axial imaging
- More than two-thirds of cross-sectional area of cord on axial imaging
- More than two vertebral segments in length
- Smooth cord expansion

- High signal intensity
- Variable post-gadolinium enhancement
- Enhancement at periphery of lesion
- Up to 40-50% of cases not demonstrated by MRI

Top Differential Diagnoses
- Multiple sclerosis
- Spinal cord neoplasm

Diagnostic Checklist
- Peripheral enhancement in centrally located T2 hyperintensity more characteristic of IATM
- Central enhancement in peripherally located T2 hyperintensity more characteristic of multiple sclerosis
- Caution: IATM can mimic cord neoplasm!

- ○ Resolves over time
- ○ Not predictive of clinical course
- ○ Enhancement more common when cord enlargement present
- ○ Enhancing area less extensive than T2 hyperintensity
- Solitary or multifocal lesions
- Up to 40-50% of cases not demonstrated by MRI

Imaging Recommendations
- Best imaging tool: Sagittal and axial T2WI and T1WI MRI through spinal cord with gadolinium

DIFFERENTIAL DIAGNOSIS

Multiple sclerosis
- Peripheral in location
- Less than two vertebral segments in length
- Less than half cross-sectional area of cord
- 90% with associated intracranial lesions
- Relapsing and remitting clinical course

Spinal cord neoplasm
- Cord expansion invariably present
- Diffuse or nodular contrast-enhancement
- Extensive peri-tumoral edema
- Cystic ± hemorrhage components
- Slower clinical progression

Cord infarct
- Ventral cord location
- Motor signs greater than sensory
- Immediate onset
  - ○ Minutes, rather than hours, days
- Less mass effect initially

Syringohydromyelia
- Central cystic lesion
- Cerebral spinal fluid intensity on all pulse sequences
- No post-gadolinium enhancement
- Normal cord contour

PATHOLOGY

General Features
- General path comments
  - ○ Perivascular inflammation
  - ○ Demyelination
- Genetics: No familial predisposition
- Etiology
  - ○ Possible association with previous viral infection or vaccination in some cases
  - ○ Autoimmune phenomenon with formation of antigen-antibody complexes
  - ○ Small vessel vasculopathy resulting in cord ischemia
  - ○ Associated demyelinating process
- Epidemiology
  - ○ 4.6 new cases of transverse myelitis per million people per year in US
    - ■ 1,400 new cases per year
  - ○ Majority of cases occurred in late winter through spring in one series
- Associated abnormalities
  - ○ Depression
    - ■ Life time risk > 50%
    - ■ Correlates with severity of sensory symptoms

Microscopic Features
- Necrosis of gray and white matter
- Destruction of neurons, axons, and myelin
- Astrocytic gliosis
- Perivascular lymphocytic infiltrate

CLINICAL ISSUES

Presentation
- Most common signs/symptoms
  - ○ Sensory deficit
    - ■ Loss of pain and temperature sensation
    - ■ Clearly defined upper level
    - ■ Ascending paresthesia in bilateral lower extremities
    - ■ Band-like dysesthesia
  - ○ Other signs/symptoms

- Paraplegia or quadriplegia
- Back ± radicular pain
- Bladder and bowl dysfunction
- Urgency, incontinence, retention
- Hypotonia and hyporeflexia initially
- Spasticity and hyperreflexia over time
  - Acute to subacute onset of symptoms
- Clinical profile
  - Prodrome of generalized body aches
  - Preceding viral-like illness
  - Rapid progression to maximal neurologic deficits within days

Demographics

- Age
  - All ages can be affected
  - Transverse myelitis with two peaks
    - 10-19 and 30-39 years old
- Gender: No gender predilection
- Ethnicity: No racial predilection

Natural History & Prognosis

- One third of patients experience good to complete recovery
  - Symptomatic improvement starting 2-12 weeks after onset
  - Children with slightly better prognosis than adults
- One third fair recovery
  - Residual spasticity and urinary dysfunction
- One third poor recovery
  - Persistent complete deficits
  - Requiring assistance in activities of daily living
- Factors portending poor prognosis
  - Rapid clinical deterioration
  - Back pain
  - Spinal shock: Loss of motor, sensation, sphincter control, and areflexia
  - MRI signal alteration > 10 spinal segments
  - Significant denervation on electromyogram
  - Abnormal somatosensory evoked potential
- Typically monophasic
  - 5-15% recurrence rate
  - If recurrent, must consider
    - Multiple sclerosis: Progression to multiple sclerosis in 2-8% of cases of transverse myelitis
    - SLE
    - Antiphospholipid syndrome
    - Vascular malformation

Treatment

- High dose intravenous steroid pulse therapy
- Physical therapy

DIAGNOSTIC CHECKLIST

Consider

- Brain MRI including high-resolution fast spin echo T2 through corpus callosum
  - To exclude intracranial lesions associated with multiple sclerosis or acute disseminated encephalomyelitis

Image Interpretation Pearls

- Peripheral enhancement in centrally located T2 hyperintensity more characteristic of IATM
- Central enhancement in peripherally located T2 hyperintensity more characteristic of multiple sclerosis
- Caution: IATM can mimic cord neoplasm!

SELECTED REFERENCES

1. Kim KK: Idiopathic recurrent transverse myelitis. Arch Neurol. 60(9):1290-4, 2003
2. Banit DM et al: Recurrent transverse myelitis after lumbar spine surgery: a case report. Spine. 28(9):E165-8, 2003
3. Andronikou S et al: MRI findings in acute idiopathic transverse myelopathy in children. Pediatr Radiol. 33(9):624-9, 2003
4. Transverse Myelitis Consortium Working Group: Proposed diagnostic criteria and nosology of acute transverse myelitis. Neurology. 59(4):499-505, 2002
5. Kerr DA et al: Immunopathogenesis of acute transverse myelitis. Curr Opin Neurol. 15(3):339-47, 2002
6. Scotti G et al: Diagnosis and differential diagnosis of acute transverse myelopathy. The role of neuroradiological investigations and review of the literature. Neurol Sci. 22 Suppl 2:S69-73, 2001
7. Misra UK et al: Role of MRI in acute transverse myelitis. Neurol India. 47(4):253-4, 1999
8. Murthy JM et al: Acute transverse myelitis: MR characteristics. Neurol India. 47(4):290-3, 1999
9. Isoda H et al: MR imaging of acute transverse myelitis (myelopathy). Radiat Med. 16(3):179-86, 1998
10. Tartaglino LM et al: Idiopathic Acute Transverse Myelitis: MR Imaging Findings. Radiology. 201:661-9, 1996
11. Choi KH et al: Idiopathic Transverse Myelitis: MR Characteristics. AJNR. 17:1151-60, 1996
12. Misra UK et al: A clinical, MRI and neurophysiological study of acute transverse myelitis. J Neurol Sci. 138(1-2):150-6, 1996
13. Campi A et al: Acute Transverse Myelopathy: Spinal and Cranial MR Study with Clinical Follow-up. AJNR. 16:115-23, 1995
14. Jeffery DR et al: Transverse myelitis. Retrospective analysis of 33 cases, with differentiation of cases associated with multiple sclerosis and parainfectious events. Arch Neurol. 50(5):532-5, 1993
15. Kelley CE et al: Acute transverse myelitis in the emergency department: a case report and review of the literature. J Emerg Med. 9(6):417-20, 1991
16. Christensen PB et al: Clinical course and long-term prognosis of acute transverse myelopathy. Acta Neurol Scand. 81(5):431-5, 1990
17. Dunne K et al: Acute transverse myelopathy in childhood. Dev Med Child Neurol. 28(2):198-204, 1986
18. Berman M et al: Acute transverse myelitis: incidence and etiologic considerations. Neurology. 31(8):966-71, 1981
19. Lipton HL et al: Acute transverse myelopathy in adults. A follow-up study. Arch Neurol. 28(4):252-7, 1973
20. ALTROCCHI PH: ACUTE TRANSVERSE MYELOPATHY. Arch Neurol. 168:111-9, 1963

IDIOPATHIC ACUTE TRANSVERSE MYELITIS

IMAGE GALLERY

Typical

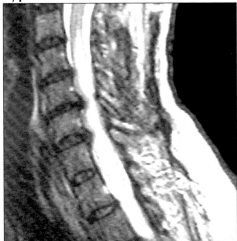
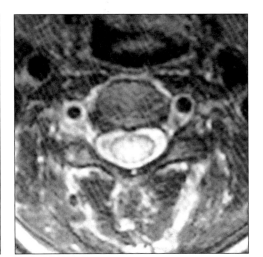

(Left) Sagittal T2WI MR shows diffuse cervical intramedullary hyperintensity. Cervical spondylosis is also evident. (Right) Axial T2WI MR in the same patient shows hyperintensity involving entire cross-sectional area of cervical cord.

Typical

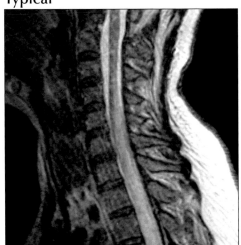
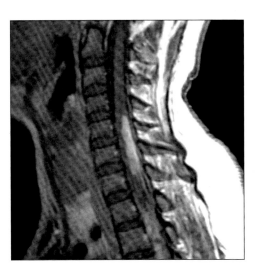

(Left) Sagittal T2WI MR shows diffuse intramedullary hyperintensity involving lower cervical and upper thoracic cord with mild cord expansion. (Right) Sagittal T1 C+ MR shows mass-like enhancement from C5-7 with patchy enhancement in upper thoracic cord.

Typical

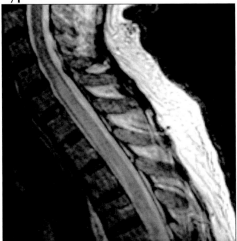
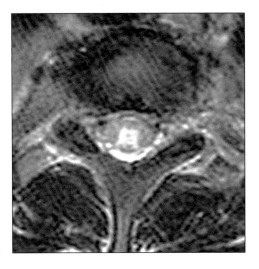

(Left) Sagittal T2WI MR shows patchy intramedullary hyperintensities in cervical and thoracic cord. (Right) Axial T2WI MR in the same patient confirms a well-circumscribed central intramedullary hyperintensity.

VITAMIN B12 DEFICIENCY, SPINAL CORD

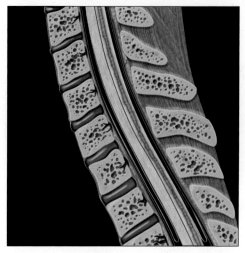

Sagittal graphic shows dorsal column demyelination secondary to Vitamin B12 deficiency. Abnormality is characteristically located in the dorsal spinal columns.

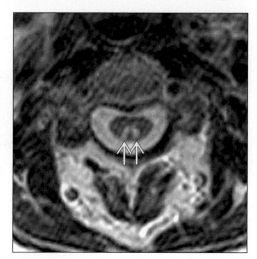

Axial T2WI MR reveals T2 hyperintensity confined to the dorsal columns (arrows) in an "inverted V" configuration characteristic of B12 deficiency.

TERMINOLOGY

Abbreviations and Synonyms
- Subacute combined degeneration, combined system disease

Definitions
- Vitamin B12 deficiency produces selective degeneration of dorsal +/- lateral spinal cord columns

IMAGING FINDINGS

General Features
- Best diagnostic clue: Mild spinal cord enlargement, abnormal T2 hyperintensity within dorsal columns
- Location: Dorsal spinal cord columns +/- lateral columns
- Size: Imaging abnormality confined to abnormal spinal tracts
- Morphology: Mild spinal cord enlargement, abnormal signal intensity within dorsal +/- lateral columns only

CT Findings
- NECT
  - Mild spinal cord enlargement in florid cases
  - Usually normal

MR Findings
- T1WI: Mild spinal cord enlargement, dorsal spinal cord hypointensity
- T2WI
  - Hyperintensity confined to dorsal +/- lateral columns
    - Longitudinal dorsal cord T2 signal abnormality
    - Axial image ⇒ "inverted V" or "inverted rabbit ears" within dorsal spinal cord
- T1 C+: +/- Mild dorsal column enhancement

Other Modality Findings
- Brain MR imaging
  - No specific findings in adults
  - May see severe brain atrophy that improves following parenteral B12 therapy in infants

Imaging Recommendations
- Multiplanar T2WI to confirm localization in dorsal columns, exclude cord infarct or spondylosis

DIFFERENTIAL DIAGNOSIS

Spinal cord infarction
- Hyperacute presentation, motor > sensory symptoms
- Predominantly ventral cord or central gray matter signal changes

DDx: Vitamin B12 Deficiency

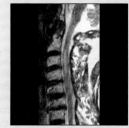

Spinal Cord Infarct

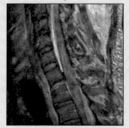

Spinal Cord Contusion

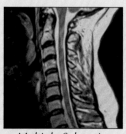

Multiple Sclerosis

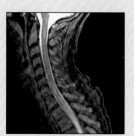

Viral Myelitis

VITAMIN B12 DEFICIENCY, SPINAL CORD

Key Facts

Terminology
- Subacute combined degeneration, combined system disease
- Vitamin B12 deficiency produces selective degeneration of dorsal +/- lateral spinal cord columns

Imaging Findings
- Best diagnostic clue: Mild spinal cord enlargement, abnormal T2 hyperintensity within dorsal columns
- Axial image ⇒ "inverted V" or "inverted rabbit ears" within dorsal spinal cord

Top Differential Diagnoses
- Spinal cord infarction
- Spinal cord contusion
- Inflammatory demyelination
- Infectious myelitis

- Acute transverse myelitis

Pathology
- Methylmalonic acid accumulation believed to cause myelin toxicity ⇒ dorsolateral spinal cord demyelination (myelin sheaths + axons)
- Megaloblastic anemia

Clinical Issues
- Insidious subacute course of clinical symptom onset; functional disturbances increase fairly rapidly → severe disability within weeks to months

Diagnostic Checklist
- Neurologic findings may precede anemia
- Imaging changes may not completely resolve following treatment

Spinal cord contusion
- Cord swelling, T2 hyperintensity +/- hemorrhage
- Associated fracture, soft tissue injury
- History, clinical findings enable diagnosis

Inflammatory demyelination
- Multiple sclerosis or acute disseminated encephalomyelitis (ADEM)
- Lesions more focal, patchy than B12 deficiency, do not show specificity for lateral or dorsal columns
- Characteristic clinical presentation

Infectious myelitis
- HIV vacuolar myelopathy, Varicella-Zoster/Herpes, Lyme disease
- Imaging findings may be identical to B12 deficiency
- Clinical, laboratory findings help distinguish

Acute transverse myelitis
- Acute (non-traumatic) presentation ⇒ diffuse multisegmental cord hyperintensity, swelling
- Idiopathic or known etiology; clinical and laboratory findings may help distinguish cause
- ↑ CSF protein, pleocytosis, +/- oligoclonal bands (28%)

PATHOLOGY

General Features
- General path comments
  - Vitamin B12 (cobalamin) mostly found in meat, lacking in most vegetable
    - Vitamin B12 storage mainly in liver; effects of deficiency may not be appreciated until stores depleted
  - B12 is a coenzyme for two important biochemical enzymatic reactions
    - Homocysteine methylation → methionine
    - Methylmalonyl coenzyme A + succinate → succinyl coenzyme A + methylmalonic acid
  - Methylmalonic acid accumulation believed to cause myelin toxicity ⇒ dorsolateral spinal cord demyelination (myelin sheaths + axons)

- Subsequently, focal myelin swelling progresses to vacuolization → axonal loss, Wallerian degeneration of posterior and lateral columns
- Genetics: Serum Transcobalamin II (TC-II) transporter deficiency in some patients
- Etiology
  - Malabsorption (most common)
    - Pernicious anemia (antibody mediated intrinsic factor disorder) is most common cause of vitamin B12 malabsorption in USA
    - Less common causes include post-gastrectomy, fish tapeworm (D. latum) infestation, Crohn disease, celiac disease, bacterial overgrowth in intestinal blind loops
  - Inadequate B12 intake (rare)
    - Infants of strict vegetarian mothers, Vegans
  - Other metabolic conditions (nitrous oxide anesthesia susceptibility, transcobalamin II deficiency)
    - Nitrous oxide (N2O) inactivates B12 ⇒ accumulation of methylmalonic acid ⇒ myelin toxicity
- Epidemiology: Uncommon
- Associated abnormalities
  - Megaloblastic anemia
  - Extramedullary hematopoiesis (severe anemia)
  - Brain derangements; dementia, psychiatric disorders, optic neuropathy
  - Other (rare) sites of demyelination; peripheral nerves, optic nerves, pyramidal and spinocerebellar tracts, cerebrum/cerebellum

Gross Pathologic & Surgical Features
- Gray discoloration of posterior +/- lateral columns
- +/- Patchy demyelination in cerebral white matter

Microscopic Features
- Early neuropathological findings: Myelin sheath swelling of cervical posterior columns (funiculus gracilis and spinocerebellar tracts), lateral columns
- Late sequelae: Myelin sheath + axonal degeneration/loss → long tract Wallerian degeneration

VITAMIN B12 DEFICIENCY, SPINAL CORD

CLINICAL ISSUES

Presentation

- Most common signs/symptoms
  - Paraesthesias, stiffness, numbness or tingling of limbs (earliest neurological manifestation), mild sensory ataxia, loss of position and vibration sense, spasticity, hyperreflexia and positive Babinski sign
  - Often symmetric, distal → proximal
- Clinical profile
  - Insidious subacute course of clinical symptom onset; functional disturbances increase fairly rapidly → severe disability within weeks to months
    - Spinal cord symptoms appear first with motor (spastic paraparesis, gait unsteadiness) and sensory (paraesthesias, absent reflexes, loss of joint position sense and vibration sense) findings
    - Mental status decline may follow → progressive psychomotor regression (confusion, depression, delusions, mental slowness)
- Laboratory abnormalities
  - Macrocytic anemia (MCV > 100)
  - ↓ Plasma B12 level
  - Abnormal electroneurography, electromyography and evoked potentials

Demographics

- Age: Diagnosis in 5th → 8th decade, uncommonly identified in infants, young adults
- Gender: M ≥ F
- Ethnicity: Pernicious anemia more common in Scandinavian and "English speaking" populations, but found within all racial groups

Natural History & Prognosis

- Spontaneous improvement without treatment uncommon
- Variable clinical improvement following B12 therapy
  - Greatest recovery when treatment is started in early disease stage
- Treatment arrests degenerative process but does not restore destroyed neural fibers

Treatment

- Cornerstones of therapy
  - Life-long parenteral B12 administration
  - Address treatable causes
  - Avoiding N2O anesthesia in vulnerable patients

DIAGNOSTIC CHECKLIST

Consider

- Neurologic findings may precede anemia
- Imaging changes may not completely resolve following treatment

Image Interpretation Pearls

- T2 hyperintensity confined to dorsal columns highly suggestive of diagnosis; confirm with laboratory studies

SELECTED REFERENCES

1. Teplitsky V et al: Hereditary partial transcobalamin II deficiency with neurologic, mental and hematologic abnormalities in children and adults. Isr Med Assoc J. 5(12):868-72, 2003
2. Ilniczky S et al: MR findings in subacute combined degeneration of the spinal cord caused by nitrous oxide anaesthesia--two cases. Eur J Neurol. 9(1):101-4, 2002
3. Srikanth SG et al: MRI in subacute combined degeneration of spinal cord: a case report and review of literature. Neurol India. 50(3):310-2, 2002
4. Ravina B et al: MR findings in subacute combined degeneration of the spinal cord: a case of reversible cervical myelopathy. AJR Am J Roentgenol. 174(3):863-5, 2000
5. Locatelli ER et al: MRI in vitamin B12 deficiency myelopathy. Can J Neurol Sci. 26(1):60-3, 1999
6. Beltramello A et al: Subacute combined degeneration of the spinal cord after nitrous oxide anaesthesia: role of magnetic resonance imaging. J Neurol Neurosurg Psychiatry. 64(4):563-4, 1998
7. Pema PJ et al: Myelopathy caused by nitrous oxide toxicity. AJNR Am J Neuroradiol. 19(5):894-6, 1998
8. Katsaros VK et al: MRI of spinal cord and brain lesions in subacute combined degeneration. Neuroradiology. 40(11):716-9, 1998
9. Hemmer B et al: Subacute combined degeneration: clinical, electrophysiological, and magnetic resonance imaging findings. J Neurol Neurosurg Psychiatry. 65(6):822-7, 1998
10. Yamada K et al: A case of subacute combined degeneration: MRI findings. Neuroradiology. 40(6):398-400, 1998
11. Larner AJ et al: MRI appearances in subacute combined degeneration of the spinal cord due to vitamin B12 deficiency. J Neurol Neurosurg Psychiatry. 62(1):99-100, 1997
12. Weir DG et al: The biochemical basis of the neuropathy in cobalamin deficiency. Baillieres Clin Haematol. 8(3):479-97, 1995
13. Murata S et al: MRI in subacute combined degeneration. Neuroradiology. 36(5):408-9, 1994
14. Timms SR et al: Subacute combined degeneration of the spinal cord: MR findings. AJNR Am J Neuroradiol. 14(5):1224-7, 1993
15. Tracey JP et al: Magnetic resonance imaging in cobalamin deficiency. Lancet. 339(8802):1172-3, 1992
16. Berger JR et al: Reversible myelopathy with pernicious anemia: clinical/MR correlation. Neurology. 41(6):947-8, 1991
17. Healton EB et al: Neurologic aspects of cobalamin deficiency. Medicine (Baltimore). 70(4):229-45, 1991
18. Petito CK et al: Vacuolar myelopathy pathologically resembling subacute combined degeneration in patients with the acquired immunodeficiency syndrome. N Engl J Med. 312(14):874-9, 1985

VITAMIN B12 DEFICIENCY, SPINAL CORD

IMAGE GALLERY

Typical

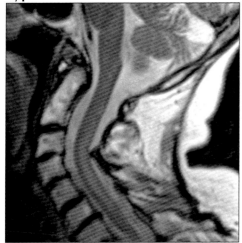
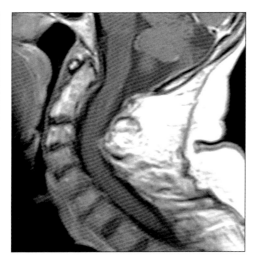

(Left) Sagittal T2WI MR displays characteristic T2 hyperintensity within the dorsal spinal cord. *(Right)* Sagittal T1 C+ MR reveals no abnormal enhancement within dorsal spinal cord.

Typical

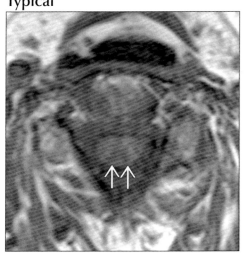
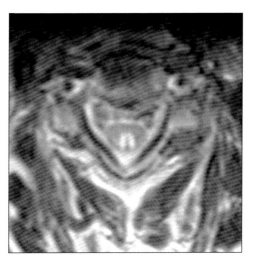

(Left) Axial T1WI MR shows "inverted V" hypointensity confined to dorsal columns (arrows). *(Right)* Axial T2WI MR reveals T2 hyperintensity within dorsal columns typical of B12 deficiency

Typical

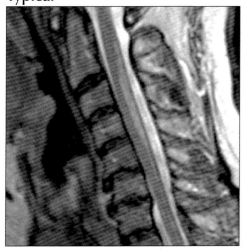
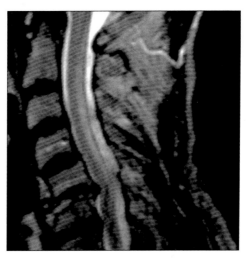

(Left) Sagittal T2WI MR shows characteristic T2 hyperintensity within the dorsal spinal columns. *(Right)* Sagittal T2WI MR demonstrates an incidental large C5/6 herniated disc in addition to typical dorsal cord changes of Vitamin B12 deficiency.

PART IV

Neoplasms, Cysts, and Other Masses

Neoplasms   **1**

Non-Neoplastic Cysts and Tumor Mimics   **2**

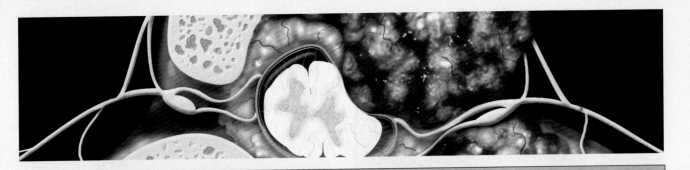

SECTION 1: Neoplasms

NEOPLASMS, PATHWAYS OF SPREAD

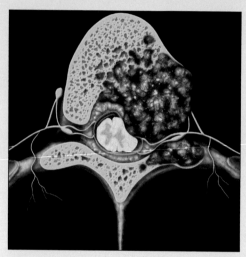

Axial graphic shows hematogenously disseminated lytic metastatic lesion to thoracic vertebral body and pedicle, with subsequent direct epidural tumor extension and cord compression.

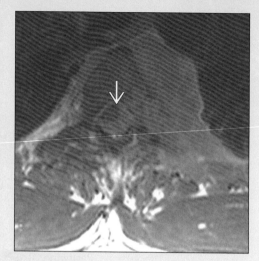

Axial T1WI MR shows large metastatic paravertebral mass lesion involving thoracic body, with extension to posterior elements, chest wall and epidural tumor with cord compression (arrow).

TERMINOLOGY

Abbreviations and Synonyms
- Tumor extension; tumor spread; metastatic spread

Definitions
- Dissemination or extension of tumor by direct, hematogenous or lymphatic and other routes

PATHOLOGY ISSUES

General Considerations
- 40% of patients with cancer develop visceral or bony metastases during illness
- Spinal column most common site of osseous metastases
- Men more commonly affected with vertebral metastases, M:F = 3:2
- Prostate, lung and breast cancer account for vast majority of spine metastases
- Locations: Vertebrae (85%) > paravertebral region > epidural space > intradural
- Locations: Thoracic (70%) > lumbar (20%) > cervical
- Malignant growth defined by 6 changes in cell physiology
  ○ Self-sufficiency in growth signals
  ○ Insensitivity to growth inhibitory signals
  ○ Evasion of programmed cell death
  ○ Unlimited replication potential
  ○ Angiogenesis
  ○ Tissue invasion and metastases
- Routes of spread
  ○ Tissue (interstitial) spaces
  ○ Lymphatic system
    ▪ Lymphatic involvement generally ends with hematogenous dissemination
  ○ Hematogenous
    ▪ Venous invasion more common than arterial
    ▪ Venous tumor emboli go to lungs
    ▪ Portal vein tumor emboli go to liver

- ▪ Lungs to pulmonary veins go to peripheral organs
- ▪ Exceptions include: Paradoxical embolization with patent foramen ovale; retrograde venous embolization
  ○ Coelomic spaces
  ○ Cerebrospinal fluid spaces
- Mechanism of metastatic disease development
  ○ Primary tumor composed of variety of biologically different cells in regards to metastatic potential
  ○ Cells continually shed from primary tumor and gain access to circulation
  ○ Fewer than 0.01-0.1% of tumor cells survive to reach distant site
  ○ Successful tumor spread requires completion of complex pathway including
    ▪ Tumor separation from primary
    ▪ Access to blood, CSF, lymph
    ▪ Survive transport process
    ▪ Attach to endothelium of distant vessel and exit
    ▪ Develop own vascular supply at distant site
  ○ Host environment of distant site is complex and multifactorial
    ▪ Anatomic pathways involved
    ▪ Flow patterns of veins
    ▪ Osteotropism of malignant cells
    ▪ Marrow growth factors
    ▪ Microtrauma
    ▪ Local ischemia
  ○ Basement membrane (BM) is first barrier tumor cells must breach
    ▪ Receptors on on surface of cells recognize glycoprotein (laminin) of BM to which they attach
    ▪ Attachment followed by proteolysis of type IV collagen of BM by tumor specific collagenase
    ▪ Locomotion follows BM lysis, with cells crossing defective BM with access to interstitial space, lymphatics, blood vessels
  ○ Chemokines and neurotransmitters involved in development of metastases

DIFFERENTIAL DIAGNOSIS

Direct extension of tumor
- Primary bone tumor mimic metastasis direct extension: Sarcoma, chordoma, ABC, osteoblastoma
- Infection may show destruction, soft tissue involvement, thecal sac compression

Hematogenous spread of tumor
- Heterogeneous nonmalignant marrow signal may occur with chronic anemia, osteoporosis
- Mottled marrow signal classic sign of multiple myeloma

CSF spread of tumor
- Granulomatous disease (sarcoid, TB) can mimic leptomeningeal mets
- Bacterial meningitis may show irregular leptomeningeal enhancement

Lymphatic spread
- Limited in importance relative to hematogenous spread

CNS tumor types with subarachnoid spread
- Medulloblastoma, PNET
- Ependymoma
- Pineal tumors
- Astrocytoma (glioblastoma)

Spread along CSF pathways from hematogenous dissemination
- Cord and leptomeningeal metastatic disease from lung, breast cancer

---

- Dopamine is activator of migration of breast carcinoma cells
- Catecholamines are chemoattractant for breast carcinoma, and activator of colon carcinoma migration
- Various peptide neurotransmitters increase invasive capacity of prostate carcinoma

ANATOMY-BASED IMAGING ISSUES

Key Concepts or Questions
- Direct extension
  - Primary tumor located in soft tissues extend into vertebral column by direct extension
    - Lung carcinoma extends into chest wall, paravertebral region and spinal column
    - Prostate, bladder, or bowel carcinoma extends into presacral space, and subsequently vertebral column and epidural space
    - Nasopharyngeal carcinoma extends to clivus/skull base or tracks along nerves
    - Rare cases of direct extension of CNS tumor along biopsy, or surgical tract
    - Rare cases of CNS tumor extension through shunt tube giving systemic metastases
  - Hematogenous metastatic vertebral body disease extends into epidural space with neural compression
  - Findings of soft tissue mass with bone destruction, variable neural compromise
  - Direct extension into epidural space more likely from vertebral body through posterior longitudinal ligament (PLL)
    - Anterior longitudinal ligament (ALL) and disc are resistant to tumor invasion
    - ALL stronger than PLL, and has less perforating vessels
    - Dura tough, and is effective barrier to tumor penetration
  - Direct extension from primary cord tumor within substance of cord to infratentorial space
- Lymphatic spread

  - Limited in importance relative to hematogenous spread
  - Local spread of pelvic tumors to lumbar spine without pulmonary metastasis suggest venous or lymphatic route
- Hematogenous spread
  - Major pathway of spread of malignant tumor to axial skeleton
  - Batson plexus
    - Longitudinal network of valveless veins running parallel to spinal column
    - Lie outside of thoracoabdominal cavity
    - Communicate with multiple venous systems: Spine, vena cava, portal, azygos, intercostal, pulmonary and renal
    - Flow direction in Batson plexus variable due to variable intrathoracic or intraabdominal pressure
    - Tumors in multiple sites could deposit metastases along course of venous plexus, without lung or liver involvement
    - Prostate carcinoma cells could seed vertebral bodies via plexus, and not necessarily into vena cava
    - Breast carcinoma might seed vertebral bodies via azygos system into Batson plexus
    - Only 5-10% of portal blood flow might shunt to Batson plexus, giving low frequency of spine mets with GI and GU primaries
    - No clear answer to all metastatic lesions, since review of MR findings in spinal mets shows no consistent pattern
    - Homing properties of tumor cells, and receptive properties of implantation site may be more important than vascular route
- CSF spread
  - Spread along CSF pathway for primary intracranial tumors
    - Tumor emboli which has access to CSF via fragmentation
    - Tumor shedding during surgical manipulation
  - CNS tumor types with subarachnoid spread
    - Medulloblastoma, PNET
    - Ependymoma

NEOPLASMS, PATHWAYS OF SPREAD

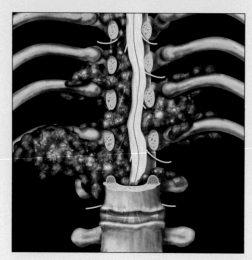

Coronal graphic of thoracolumbar junction shows metastatic neuroblastoma with paravertebral mass, multilevel epidural tumor extension.

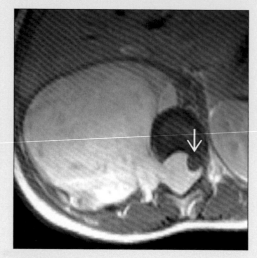

Axial T1WI with contrast shows large paravertebral mass extending into canal and displacing cord (arrow) from neuroblastoma.

- Pineal tumors
- Astrocytoma
- Lymphoma/leukemia
- Choroid plexus papilloma/carcinoma
- Retinoblastoma (poor prognosis with MYCN gene amplification)
  - ○ Spread along CSF pathways from hematogenous dissemination
    - Cord and leptomeningeal metastatic disease from lung, breast cancer

CLINICAL IMPLICATIONS

Clinical Importance
- Spine metastatic involvement present with unrelenting back pain
- Objective signs uncommon, or late in disease (palpable mass, deformity)
- Back pain and weakness sign of epidural tumor extension
- Due to spinothalamic tract crossing pattern, sensory levels may be 1-2 segments below site of compression
- Sensory abnormalities uncommon presenting signs

CUSTOM DIFFERENTIAL DIAGNOSIS

CSF spread of tumor
- Granulomatous disease (sarcoid, TB) can mimic leptomeningeal mets
- Bacterial meningitis may show irregular leptomeningeal enhancement
- Viral infection (CMV) usually shows smooth enhancement of multiple roots
- Parasitic disease may present with subarachnoid seeding (cysticercosis)

Direct extension of tumor
- Primary bone tumor mimic metastasis direct extension: Sarcoma, chordoma, ABC

- Infection may show destruction, soft tissue involvement, thecal sac compression
- Rarely complex aortic aneurysm may show soft tissue mass and vertebral erosion mimicking tumor

Hematogenous spread of tumor
- Heterogeneous nonmalignant marrow signal may occur with chronic anemia, osteoporosis
- Mottled marrow signal classic sign of multiple myeloma
- Disseminated infection (particularly TB) may show tumor metastasis pattern
- TB notorious for presenting with imaging findings typical for neoplasm

SELECTED REFERENCES

1. Demopoulos A: Leptomeningeal metastases. Curr Neurol Neurosci Rep. 4(3):196-204, 2004
2. Entschladen F et al: Tumour-cell migration, invasion, and metastasis: navigation by neurotransmitters. Lancet Oncol. 5(4):254-8, 2004
3. Giordana MT et al: Molecular genetic study of a metastatic oligodendroglioma. J Neurooncol. 66(3):265-71, 2004
4. Tosaka M et al: Spinal epidural metastasis from pineal germinoma. Acta Neurochir (Wien). 145(5):407-10; discussion 410, 2003
5. Matthay KK et al: Central nervous system metastases in neuroblastoma: radiologic, clinical, and biologic features in 23 patients. Cancer. 98(1):155-65, 2003
6. Kesari S et al: Leptomeningeal metastases. Neurol Clin. 21(1):25-66, 2003
7. Demopoulos A et al: Neurologic complications of leukemia. Curr Opin Neurol. 15(6):691-9, 2002
8. Van Roy F et al: Tumour invasion: effects of cell adhesion and motility. Trends Cell Biol. 2(6):163-9, 1992
9. Batson OV: The Function of the vertebral veins and their role in the spread of metastasis. Ann Surg. (312): 49, 1940

IMAGE GALLERY

Typical

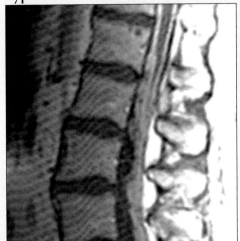
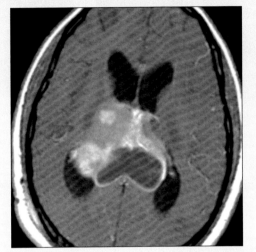

(Left) Sagittal T1 C+ MR shows bulky nodular and linear enhancement of leptomeninges in this patient with CSF spread of supratentorial glioblastoma. *(Right)* Axial T1 C+ MR in same case shows large cystic and solid enhancing mass involving corpus callosum, with intraventricular extension.

Typical

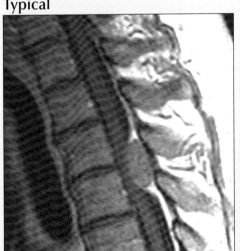
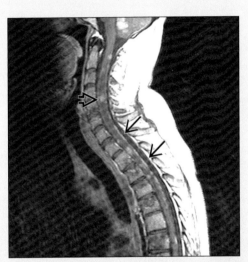

(Left) Sagittal T1 C+ MR shows focal epidural mass with cord compression from metastatic melanoma. Route of dissemination is hematogenous. *(Right)* Sagittal T1 C+ MR in extensive metastatic breast carcinoma shows foci of enhancement from leptomeningeal *(arrows)* and intramedullary *(open arrow)* metastases. Note multiple vertebral body mets.

Typical

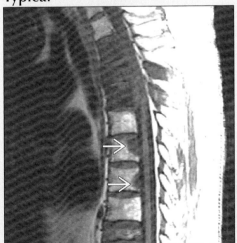
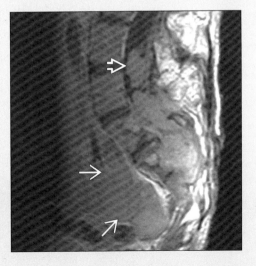

(Left) Sagittal T1WI MR shows foci of low signal throughout thoracic bodies and posterior elements due to prostate metastases. Note the propensity of some lesions to center at basivertebral veins *(arrows)*. *(Right)* Sagittal T1 C+ MR shows large lobulated malignant peripheral nerve sheath tumor (MPNST) extending from pelvis *(arrows)* through sacrum into lumbar nerve roots *(open arrow)*.

BLASTIC OSSEOUS METASTASES

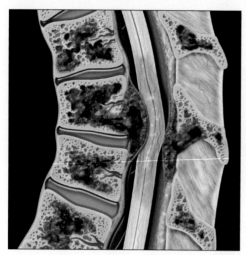

Sagittal graphic of thoracic spine shows multiple metastatic lesions in vertebral bodies, posterior elements with dorsal + ventral epidural extension, cord compression.

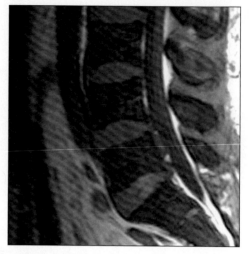

Sagittal T1WI MR in this patient with prostate carcinoma shows diffuse low signal throughout all vertebral bodies and posterior elements from metastatic disease.

TERMINOLOGY

Abbreviations and Synonyms
- Sclerotic metastases, osteosclerotic metastases

Definitions
- Extension of primary tumor to spine, where bone production exceeds bone destruction

IMAGING FINDINGS

General Features
- Best diagnostic clue: Lesion destroys posterior cortex, pedicle
- Location: Vertebral body and posterior elements
- Size: Variable, can be few mm to > 10 cm
- Morphology: Round focus of sclerosis, or mixed lytic/sclerotic

Radiographic Findings
- Radiography
  - Multiple dense foci scattered throughout bodies, posterior elements
    - Sclerosis may occur as discrete nodular appearance, mottled areas, to larger regions of diffuse increased density
- Myelography

  - Myelography, myelo-CT (use only if MR unavailable)
    - Extradural compression
    - "Block" (ill-defined "feathered" edge to contrast column)

CT Findings
- NECT
  - Sclerotic lesion(s), well-defined ⇒ ill-defined margins
    - Posterior vertebral body involved in almost all cases
    - 80% anterior body
    - 60% pedicle
    - 20% spinous, transverse processes and/or laminae
  - Location proportionate to red marrow (L > T > C spine)
  - +/- Paraspinous/epidural soft tissue mass
  - Uncommon patterns
    - Diffuse sclerosis ("ivory" vertebra)
    - Lytic lesion with sclerotic rim
- CECT: Enhancement not detectable due to sclerosis

MR Findings
- T1WI
  - Signal intensity different from uninvolved marrow
  - Hypointense
    - Solitary or multiple focal lesions

DDx: Increased Vertebra Density

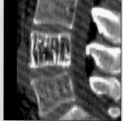

Hemangioma

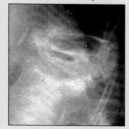

Osteonecrosis

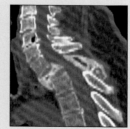

Paget Disease

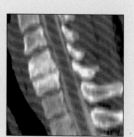

Degenerative Disc

BLASTIC OSSEOUS METASTASES

Key Facts

Terminology
- Extension of primary tumor to spine, where bone production exceeds bone destruction

Imaging Findings
- Sclerosis may occur as discrete nodular appearance, mottled areas, to larger regions of diffuse increased density
- MR image entire spinal axis
- Radionuclide studies for screening of entire skeleton

Top Differential Diagnoses
- Hemangioma
- Renal osteodystrophy
- Paget disease
- Hematopoietic malignancy
- Benign (osteoporotic) compression fracture

- Inhomogeneous marrow

Pathology
- Osteosclerotic primaries include prostate, carcinoid, bladder, nasopharynx, medulloblastoma, neuroblastoma
- Mixed lytic and blastic primaries include lung, breast, cervix, ovarian

Diagnostic Checklist
- Defining response to therapy of sclerotic lesion difficult since osteolytic conversion (tumor progression) and fading (good response) may look identical
- Metastatic "ivory vertebral body" seen with prostate, lymphoma, myeloma, chordoma

---

- Diffuse involvement/replacement of fatty marrow causes generalized vertebral low signal (discs are "brighter" than bone)
  - Cortex (especially posterior), pedicle sclerotic
  - Intervertebral discs generally spared
  - May cause pathologic fracture with paraspinal/epidural mass
    - Usually involves more than one quadrant
    - "Draped curtain" sign = tumor spreads posteriorly into epidural space with relative midline sparing
- T2WI: Sclerotic metastases generally hypointense
- STIR: May show slight hyperintensity
- DWI: Hyperintense, showing restricted diffusion (efficacy controversial)
- T1 C+
  - Lesions show variable enhancement depending upon degree of sclerosis
  - Contrast may mask bone lesions if fat suppression not used

Nuclear Medicine Findings
- Bone Scan
  - SPECT superior to planar imaging
  - Tc99m SPECT has high sensitivity with larger lesions, cortical involvement
  - False negatives most common with myeloma, leukemia, anaplastic carcinomas
  - Diffuse increase uptake ("superscan") most common with prostate carcinoma
  - Diffuse increase uptake excluding calvarium ("headless bone scan") uncommon with prostate carcinoma
- PET
  - FDG-PET has better specificity, but lower sensitivity for detecting malignant bone metastases when compared with bone scan
  - FDG PET/CT has better specificity for detection of malignant involvement of the spine than does FDG PET alone

Other Modality Findings
- Biochemical markers indicate presence/extent of skeletal metastases

Imaging Recommendations
- MR image entire spinal axis
  - Standard MRI + STIR or fat-suppressed T2WI
  - Contrast-enhanced, fat-saturated T1WI
- Radionuclide studies for screening of entire skeleton

DIFFERENTIAL DIAGNOSIS

Hemangioma
- "Corduroy" appearance of thickened trabeculae
- Typical lesion shows T1 hyperintensity

Renal osteodystrophy
- "Rugger-jersey" appearance on radiographs
- vertebral body low T1 signal, no paravertebral or epidural soft tissue component

Paget disease
- Expansion of body with thickened trabeculae ("picture-frame" vertebrae)

Hematopoietic malignancy
- Plasmacytoma, multiple myeloma (MM), lymphoma, leukemia
- Radionuclide studies negative/equivocal in 25% of MM
- Diffuse marrow involvement more common than metastasis

Benign (osteoporotic) compression fracture
- May be difficult to distinguish acute osteoporotic fracture (DWI may be helpful)
  - 1/3 of fracture in patients with known primary tumor are benign
  - 1/4 of fracture in apparently osteopenic patients are from malignant disease
- Marrow signal with late subacute/chronic benign fractures similar to normal marrow (suppresses on STIR)

Inhomogeneous marrow
- Focal/irregular, patchy fatty marrow in older patients
- Intact pedicle, posterior vertebral cortex

BLASTIC OSSEOUS METASTASES

PATHOLOGY

General Features
- General path comments: Marrow initially infiltrated, trabeculae destroyed, then cortex
- Etiology
  - Hematogenous dissemination (arterial or venous via Batson plexus) > perineural, lymphatic, CSF spread
  - Marrow infiltration precedes osseous destruction/sclerosis
    - Posterior vertebral body first, then pedicle
  - Primary tumor
    - Osteosclerotic primaries include prostate, carcinoid, bladder, nasopharynx, medulloblastoma, neuroblastoma
    - Mixed lytic and blastic primaries include lung, breast, cervix, ovarian
- Epidemiology
  - Vertebral metastases
    - 10-40% of patients with systemic cancer
    - Account for 40% of all bone metastases
  - 90% of prostate metastases involve spine, with lumbar 3x more often than cervical
  - Epidural spinal cord compression in 5% of adults with systemic cancers (70% solitary, 30% multiple sites)

Gross Pathologic & Surgical Features
- Softened, eroded bone +/- adjacent soft tissue mass

Microscopic Features
- Varies with histology of primary, osteoclastic/blastic response

Staging, Grading or Classification Criteria
- Surgical stratification (Tomita et al)
  - Grade of malignancy (slow growth, 1 point ⇒ rapid growth, 4 points)
  - Visceral metastases (no metastases, 0 points ⇒ untreatable, 4 points)
  - Bone metastases (solitary, 1 point ⇒ multiple 2 points)
  - Total 2-3 points suggest wide excision for long term control
  - Total 8-10 points indicate nonoperative supportive care

CLINICAL ISSUES

Presentation
- Most common signs/symptoms
  - Progressive axial, referred, or radicular pain
    - Pain associated with cord compression not relieved by recumbent position
  - Epidural tumor extension may cause paralysis, sensory loss, incontinence
  - Compression fracture
  - Other signs/symptoms
    - Hypercalcemia
    - Focal tenderness
    - Soft tissue mass
- Clinical profile: Elderly male with prostate carcinoma, new onset leg weakness, back pain

Demographics
- Age: Children and adults
- Gender: Predilection varies with specific tumor

Natural History & Prognosis
- Relentless, progressive; pathologic fracture, ESCC may ensue
- Varies with histology of primary lesion

Treatment
- Pain relief with opioid medications, steroids for cord edema, pain
- Radiation therapy
- Surgical decompression, stabilization
- Vertebroplasty
- Embolization

DIAGNOSTIC CHECKLIST

Consider
- Defining response to therapy of sclerotic lesion difficult since osteolytic conversion (tumor progression) and fading (good response) may look identical

Image Interpretation Pearls
- Metastatic "ivory vertebral body" seen with prostate, lymphoma, myeloma, chordoma

SELECTED REFERENCES

1. Wahl RL: Current status of PET in breast cancer imaging, staging, and therapy. Semin Roentgenol. 36(3):250-60, 2001
2. Tomita K et al: Surgical strategy for spinal metastases. Spine. 26(3):298-306, 2001
3. Castillo M et al: Diffusion-weighted MR imaging offers no advantage over routine noncontrast MR imaging in the detection of vertebral metastases. AJNR. 21: 948-53, 2000
4. Chamberlain MC et al: Epidural spinal cord compression. Neuro-oncol. 1: 120-3, 1999
5. Vanel D et al: MRI of bone metastases. Eur Radiol. 8: 1345-51, 1998
6. Ontell FK et al: Blastic osseous metastases in ovarian carcinoma. Can Assoc Radiol J. 46(3):231-4, 1995
7. Olson EM et al: Osseous metastasis in medulloblastoma: MRI findings in an unusual case. Clin Imaging. 15(4):286-9, 1991
8. Thrall JH et al: Skeletal metastases. Radiol Clin North Am. 25(6):1155-70, 1987
9. Galasko CS: Mechanisms of lytic and blastic metastatic disease of bone. Clin Orthop. (169):20-7, 1982
10. Kongtawng T et al: Radiographic evaluation of treatment of advanced carcinoma of the prostate. South Med J. 71(3):247-50, 1978
11. Joffe N et al: Osteoblastic bone metastases secondary to adenocarcinoma of the pancreas. Clin Radiol. 29(1):41-6, 1978
12. Lokich JJ: Osseous metastases: radiographic monitoring of therapeutic response. Oncology. 35(6):274-6, 1978

IMAGE GALLERY

Typical

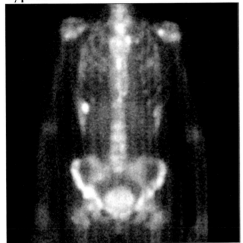
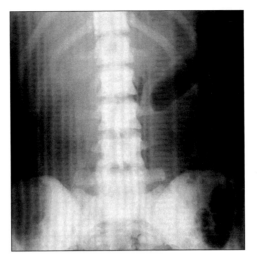

(Left) Anteroposterior bone scan shows multiple foci of increase uptake throughout spine, pelvis, ribs from breast carcinoma. *(Right)* Anteroposterior radiography shows diffuse sclerosis of vertebral bodies, pelvis from breast carcinoma.

Typical

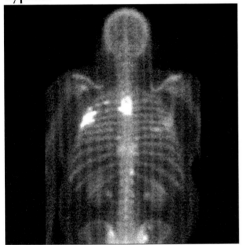
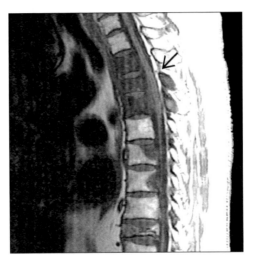

(Left) Anteroposterior bone scan shows marked abnormal uptake in thoracic spine, multiple ribs in this patient with prostate carcinoma. *(Right)* Sagittal T1WI MR shows low signal throughout multiple bodies from prostate carcinoma. There is confluent involvement of upper thoracic spine with epidural extension, cord compression (arrow).

Typical

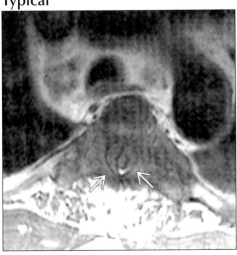
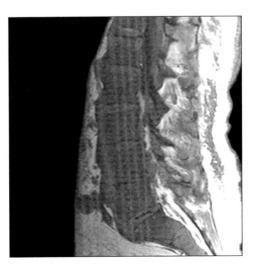

(Left) Axial T1WI MR shows diffuse low signal within thoracic body and posterior elements from prostate carcinoma. Epidural extension severely compresses cord (arrows). *(Right)* Sagittal T1WI MR shows diffuse hypointensity within all lumbar vertebral bodies and posterior element due to blastic metastases.

LYTIC OSSEOUS METASTASES

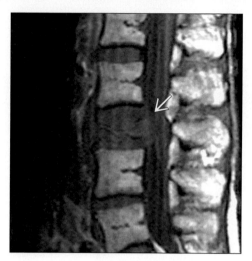

Sagittal T1WI MR shows collapse of L3 with diffuse low signal. There is convex posterior margin to L3, with severe cauda equina compression (arrow) and anterior paravertebral soft tissue.

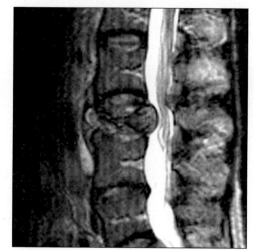

Sagittal T2WI MR shows severe collapse of L3 with slight heterogeneous increased signal. Convex posterior body margin and thecal sac compression are well-defined.

TERMINOLOGY

Abbreviations and Synonyms
- Osteolytic metastases

Definitions
- Extension of primary tumor to spine, where bone destruction exceeds bone production

IMAGING FINDINGS

General Features
- Best diagnostic clue: Lesion destroys posterior cortex, pedicle
- Location: Vertebral body and posterior elements
- Size: Variable, can be few mm to > 10 cm
- Morphology: Round focus with bone destruction

Radiographic Findings
- Radiography
  - Radiography requires 50-70% bone destruction for detection, and > 1 cm
    - AP: Absent ("missing") pedicle, +/- paraspinous soft tissue mass
    - Lateral: Destroyed posterior cortical line
  - Plain films detect level of neural compression < 25%
- Myelography

- Myelography, myelo-CT (use only if MR unavailable)
  - Extradural compression
  - "Block" (ill-defined "feathered" edge to contrast column)

CT Findings
- NECT
  - Lytic, permeative destructive lesion(s)
    - Posterior vertebral body involved in almost all cases
    - 80% anterior body
    - 60% pedicle
    - 20% spinous, transverse processes and/or laminae
  - Location proportionate to red marrow (L > T > C spine)
  - +/- Paraspinous/epidural soft tissue mass
  - Uncommon patterns
    - Lytic lesion with sclerotic rim
- CECT: Enhancement often not detectable

MR Findings
- T1WI
  - Signal intensity different from uninvolved marrow
  - T1 hypointense
    - Solitary or multiple focal lesions
    - Diffuse involvement/replacement of fatty marrow causes generalized vertebral low signal (discs "brighter" than bone)

DDx: Metastatic Disease

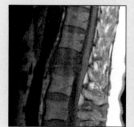
Benign Fracture

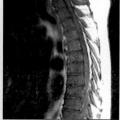
Leukemia

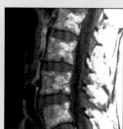
Normal Marrow

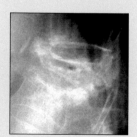
Osteonecrosis

LYTIC OSSEOUS METASTASES

Key Facts

Terminology

- Extension of primary tumor to spine, where bone destruction exceeds bone production

Imaging Findings

- Radiography requires 50-70% bone destruction for detection, and > 1 cm
- Tc99m SPECT has high sensitivity with larger lesions, cortical involvement
- MR scan entire spinal axis

Top Differential Diagnoses

- Hematopoietic malignancy
- Benign (osteoporotic) compression fracture
- Normal heterogeneous marrow
- Avascular necrosis

Pathology

- Lytic metastases include: Breast, lung, kidney, thyroid, oropharyngeal and nasopharyngeal, GI tract, bladder, uterine, ovarian, melanoma, chordoma, paraganglioma
- Expansile osteolytic lesions with kidney, thyroid metastasis
- Spine most frequent site of skeletal metastases

Clinical Issues

- Pain: Progressive axial, referred, or radicular
- Epidural tumor extension may cause paralysis, sensory loss, incontinence

Diagnostic Checklist

- Only accurate investigation to establish presence and site of compressive lesion is MR

- ○ Cortex (especially posterior), pedicle destroyed
- ○ Intervertebral discs generally spared
- ○ May cause pathologic fracture with paraspinal/epidural mass
  - ▪ Usually involves more than one quadrant
  - ▪ "Draped curtain" sign = tumor spreads posteriorly into epidural space with relative midline sparing
- T2WI
  - ○ Hypointense ⇒ hyperintense to normal marrow
  - ○ "Target sign" ⇒ hyperintense rim surrounding hypointense metastasis on T2WI
- STIR: High intensity lesion in posterior vertebra/pedicle
- DWI: Hyperintense (efficacy controversial)
- T1 C+: Lesions diffusely enhance (may mask lesions if no fat suppression used)

Nuclear Medicine Findings

- Bone Scan
  - ○ SPECT superior to planar imaging
  - ○ Tc99m SPECT has high sensitivity with larger lesions, cortical involvement
  - ○ Uptake in regions of bone production, not uptake directly by tumor
  - ○ Predict level of neural compression < 20%
  - ○ Bone scan false negatives most common with myeloma, leukemia, anaplastic carcinomas
- PET
  - ○ FDG-PET has better specificity, but lower sensitivity for detecting malignant bone metastases when compared with bone scan
  - ○ FDG PET/CT has better specificity for detection of malignant involvement of the spine than does FDG PET alone

Other Modality Findings

- Biochemical markers indicate presence/extent of skeletal metastases

Imaging Recommendations

- MR scan entire spinal axis
  - ○ Standard MRI + STIR or fat-suppressed T2WI (scan entire spine)
  - ○ Contrast-enhanced, fat-saturated T1WI

- Radionuclide studies for screening of entire skeleton

DIFFERENTIAL DIAGNOSIS

Hematopoietic malignancy

- Plasmacytoma, multiple myeloma (MM), lymphoma, leukemia
- Radionuclide studies negative/equivocal in 25% of MM
- Diffuse marrow involvement more common than metastasis

Benign (osteoporotic) compression fracture

- May be difficult to distinguish acute osteoporotic Fx (DWI may be helpful)
  - ○ 1/3 of Fxs in patients with known primary tumor are benign
  - ○ 1/4 of Fxs in apparently osteopenic patients are from malignant disease
- Marrow signal with late subacute/chronic benign fractures similar to normal marrow (suppresses on STIR)

Normal heterogeneous marrow

- Focal/irregular, patchy fatty marrow in older patients
- Intact pedicle, posterior vertebral cortex and no epidural soft tissue

Avascular necrosis

- Vacuum cleft below endplate, usually anterior vertebral body

PATHOLOGY

General Features

- General path comments
  - ○ Marrow initially infiltrated, trabeculae destroyed, then cortex
  - ○ May cause pathologic fracture (breast, lung), cord compression
  - ○ Both bone resorption and bone formation often present

LYTIC OSSEOUS METASTASES

- ○ Lytic lesions
  - Lytic metastases include: Breast, lung, kidney, thyroid, oropharyngeal and nasopharyngeal, GI tract, bladder, uterine, ovarian, melanoma, chordoma, paraganglioma
  - Expansile osteolytic lesions with kidney, thyroid metastasis
- Etiology
  - ○ Hematogenous dissemination (arterial or venous via Batson plexus) > perineural, lymphatic, CSF spread
  - ○ Marrow infiltration precedes osseous destruction
    - Posterior vertebral body first, then pedicle
  - ○ Primary tumor (adults)
    - Lung, breast, prostate, lymphoma, renal most common spinal metastases
    - Unknown primary in 15-25%
  - ○ Primary tumor (children): Sarcomas (Ewing, neuroblastoma), hematologic malignancies
- Epidemiology
  - ○ Spine most frequent site of skeletal metastases
  - ○ Vertebral metastases
    - 10-40% of patients with systemic cancer
    - Account for 40% of all bone metastases
  - ○ Epidural spinal cord compression (ESCC) in 5% of adults with systemic cancers (70% solitary, 30% multiple sites)
  - ○ ESCC occurs in 5% of children with malignant solid tumors
    - Invades canal via neural foramen
    - Circumferential cord compression common
  - ○ MRI of entire spine in patients with suspected epidural extension show multiple sites in one-third of patients

Gross Pathologic & Surgical Features
- Softened, eroded bone +/- adjacent soft tissue mass

Microscopic Features
- Varies with histology of primary, osteoclastic/blastic response

Staging, Grading or Classification Criteria
- Surgical stratification (Tokuhashi et al)
  - ○ 6 parameters scored
  - ○ General condition, number of extraspinal bone metastases, number of metastases in vertebral body, metastases to major internal organs, primary site of the cancer, severity of spinal cord palsy
  - ○ Excisional operation > 9 points
  - ○ Palliative operation < 5 points
- Surgical stratification (Tomita et al)
  - ○ Grade of malignancy (slow growth, 1 point ⇒ rapid growth, 4 points)
  - ○ Visceral metastases (no metastasis, 0 points ⇒ untreatable, 4 points)
  - ○ Bone metastases (solitary, 1 point; multiple, 2 points)
  - ○ Total 2-3 points suggest wide excision for long term local control ⇒
  - ○ Total 8-10 points indicated nonoperative supportive care

CLINICAL ISSUES

Presentation
- Most common signs/symptoms
  - ○ Pain: Progressive axial, referred, or radicular
  - ○ Epidural tumor extension may cause paralysis, sensory loss, incontinence
  - ○ Compression fracture
  - ○ Other signs/symptoms
    - Hypercalcemia, focal tenderness, soft tissue mass
- Clinical profile: Back pain, weakness in patient with known primary tumor

Demographics
- Age
  - ○ Children and adults
  - ○ Middle age to elderly most common
- Gender: Varies with specific tumor type

Natural History & Prognosis
- Spine metastases found in 5-10% of cancer patients
- Relentless, progressive; pathologic fracture, ESCC may ensue
- Varies with histology of primary lesion

Treatment
- Radiation therapy
- Surgical decompression, stabilization
- Vertebroplasty, embolization

DIAGNOSTIC CHECKLIST

Consider
- Only accurate investigation to establish presence and site of compressive lesion is MR

Image Interpretation Pearls
- Persistence of marrow low T1 signal after therapy may be either residual active tumor or fibrosis

SELECTED REFERENCES
1. Chang EL, Lo S. Diagnosis and management of central nervous system metastases from breast cancer. Oncologist. 8(5):398-410, 2003
2. Aebi M. Spinal metastasis in the elderly. Eur Spine J. 12 Suppl 2:S202-13, 2003
3. Lipton A. Bone metastases in breast cancer. Curr Treat Options Oncol. 4(2):151-8, 2003
4. Tomita K et al: Surgical strategy for spinal metastases. Spine. 26(3):298-306, 2001
5. Murphy KJ et al: Percutaneous vertebroplasty in benign and malignant disease. Neuroimaging Clin N Am. 10(3):535-45, 2000
6. Wetzel FT et al: Management of metastatic disease of the spine. Orthop Clin North Am. 31(4):611-21, 2000
7. Castillo M et al: Diffusion-weighted MR imaging offers no advantage over routine noncontrast MR imaging in the detection of vertebral metastases. AJNR. 21: 948-53, 2000
8. Chamberlain MC et al: Epidural spinal cord compression. Neuro-oncol. 1: 120-3, 1999
9. Cook AM et al: Magnetic resonance imaging of the whole spine in suspected malignant spinal cord compression: impact on management. Clin Oncol (R Coll Radiol). 10(1):39-43, 1998

IMAGE GALLERY

Typical

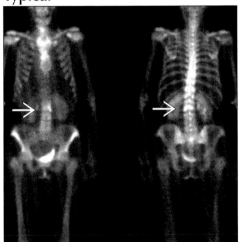
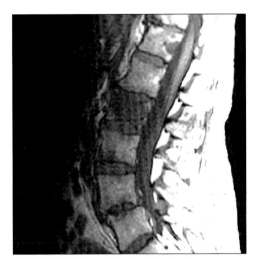

(Left) Bone scan shows increased uptake in L2 body in this patient with squamous vulvar carcinoma, consistent with metastatic disease (arrows). *(Right)* Sagittal T1WI MR shows focal low signal from L2 body reflecting bone metastasis without epidural extension. Additional metastases present in L3, T12 not identified on bone scan.

Typical

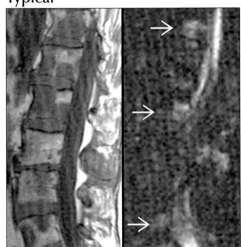
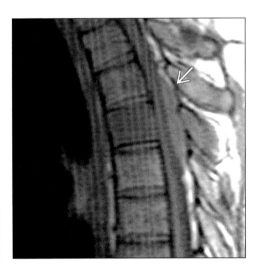

(Left) T1WI MR (left side) shows multiple foci of low signal due to lung metastases. Diffusion MR (b = 600) (right side) shows restricted diffusion from multiple metastatic lesions (arrows). *(Right)* Sagittal T1WI MR shows diffuse metastatic involvement of T5 with low signal, and extensive posterior epidural extension with cord compression (arrow).

Typical

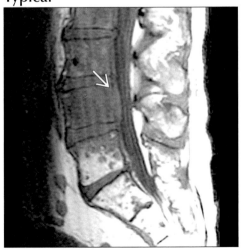
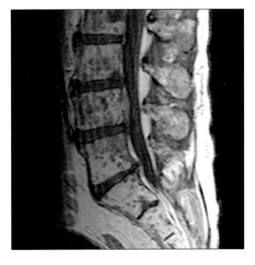

(Left) Sagittal T1WI MR shows recurrent disease in this patient with lung carcinoma and prior radiation therapy to spine. Diffuse low signal present in L2-L4, with epidural extension at L4 (arrow). *(Right)* Sagittal T1 C+ MR shows multiple low signal metastatic lesions which are less conspicuous due to diffuse tumor enhancement matching signal of fatty marrow.

HEMANGIOMA

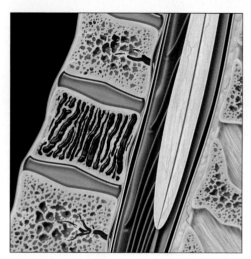

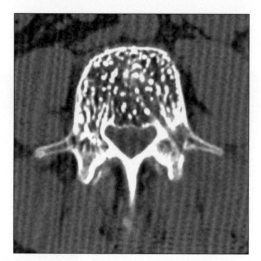

Sagittal graphic of thoracolumbar junction shows the typical striated pattern of hemangioma, with thickened bony trabeculae. There is no extraosseous extension or thecal sac compromise.

Axial NECT shows typical corduroy pattern of thickened trabeculae and intervening low attenuation fat.

TERMINOLOGY

Abbreviations and Synonyms
- Vertebral hemangioma (VH), intraosseous hemangioma, extraosseous hemangioma, compressive hemangioma

Definitions
- Benign vertebral body vascular tumor
- Incidental lesion identified on imaging performed for unrelated reasons
- Radiographic diagnostic criteria are lesion growth, bone destruction, vertebral collapse, absence of fat in lesion, and active vascular component
- Rarer presentation (clinical or radiographic) is "aggressive hemangioma"
- May extend epidurally and cause cord compression

IMAGING FINDINGS

General Features
- Best diagnostic clue: Well-circumscribed, hypodense lesion with coarse vertical trabeculae ("white polka dots") on axial CT
- Location: Vertebral body, posterior elements
- Size: Variable, may encompass whole vertebral body
- Morphology: Well-circumscribed, thickened trabeculae

Radiographic Findings
- Radiography: Vertebral body lesion with coarse vertical trabeculae resembling corduroy or honeycomb

CT Findings
- NECT
  - Hypodense lesion centered in vertebral body
    - Sparse, thickened trabeculae surrounded by hypodense fat
    - "Spotted" appearance on axial images
    - Aggressive lesions show avid contrast-enhancement

MR Findings
- Typical "benign" (fatty stroma) hemangioma
  - T1WI: Hyperintense, with avid contrast-enhancement
  - T2WI: Hyperintense
  - Occasional radiographically benign lesions are isointense or hypointense on T1WI, and difficult to distinguish from metastases
- "Aggressive" ("malignant") hemangioma
  - T1WI: Isointense to hypointense, with avid contrast-enhancement
  - T2WI: Hyperintense
  - Pathologic fracture or epidural extension common
  - Clinically aggressive hemangiomas are usually radiographically aggressive as well

DDx: Vertebral Body T1 Hyperintensity

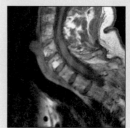

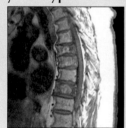

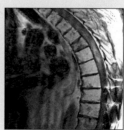

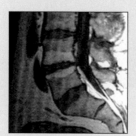

Fatty Marrow

Paget Disease

Radiation Change

Type II Endplate

HEMANGIOMA

Key Facts

Terminology
- Benign vertebral body vascular tumor
- Incidental lesion identified on imaging performed for unrelated reasons
- Radiographic diagnostic criteria are lesion growth, bone destruction, vertebral collapse, absence of fat in lesion, and active vascular component
- Rarer presentation (clinical or radiographic) is "aggressive hemangioma"
- May extend epidurally and cause cord compression

Imaging Findings
- Best diagnostic clue: Well-circumscribed, hypodense lesion with coarse vertical trabeculae ("white polka dots") on axial CT
- Both CT and MR can permit a specific diagnosis

- MR best demonstrates aggressive characteristics
- Sagittal and axial T1WI images most useful to characterize composition
- Axial T2WI and enhanced T1WI best for characterizing epidural extent and cord compromise (aggressive lesions)
- Axial bone algorithm CT is most useful for characteristic features that distinguish hemangioma from metastatic lesion

Pathology
- Slow growing
- Capillary, cavernous, or venous origin
- Most common spinal axis tumor
- 10-12% of adult population
- 25-30% multiple; particularly in thoracic spine

Angiographic Findings
- Conventional: Angiography unnecessary unless embolization is being considered

Nuclear Medicine Findings
- Bone Scan: Studies usually normal, lesions not visualized

Other Modality Findings
- Angiography: Normal to hypervascular stain, aggressive lesions stain vividly

Imaging Recommendations
- Both CT and MR can permit a specific diagnosis
  - MR best demonstrates aggressive characteristics
    - Sagittal and axial T1WI images most useful to characterize composition
    - Axial T2WI and enhanced T1WI best for characterizing epidural extent and cord compromise (aggressive lesions)
  - Axial bone algorithm CT is most useful for characteristic features that distinguish hemangioma from metastatic lesion

DIFFERENTIAL DIAGNOSIS

Vertebral metastasis
- Characteristically extends into pedicles
- Hypointense on T1WI, hypointense to hyperintense (to marrow) on T2WI
- May be difficult to distinguish from "aggressive" hemangioma; consider CT

Focal fatty marrow
- Incidental rounded focus of marrow fat that is conspicuous on MR imaging
- STIR sequence will show marked lesion hypointensity; hemangiomas typically retain some high signal due to vascular components

Paget disease
- Expanded body with thickened low signal cortex, heterogeneous signal containing fat

- No regular pattern of vertically oriented trabeculae
- No epidural soft tissue extension (unless degenerated into sarcoma)

Degenerative endplates, type II
- Abuts intervertebral disc, and parallel involvement of endplate
- Usually severe disc degeneration with loss of disc signal on T2WI and loss of disc space height
- Commonly involves adjacent endplates about degenerated disc level

Spinal radiation treatment
- Fatty marrow replacement throughout vertebral body
- Conforms to radiation port

PATHOLOGY

General Features
- General path comments
  - Slow growing
  - Capillary, cavernous, or venous origin
    - Cavernous hemangiomas most common
- Genetics: Rare: Krev interaction-trapped 1 (KRIT1) gene in families with cerebral cavernous malformations, autosomal dominant
- Etiology: Developmental
- Epidemiology
  - Most common spinal axis tumor
  - 10-12% of adult population
  - 25-30% multiple; particularly in thoracic spine
- Associated abnormalities
  - Rare family associated cerebral cavernous malformations, autosomal dominant
  - Vast majority has no associated findings

Gross Pathologic & Surgical Features
- Vast majority confined to vertebral body proper
  - May be small or occupy entire vertebral body
  - Uncommonly involve posterior elements/pedicles (10-15%)
- Thoracic lesions are more often aggressive than at other locations

HEMANGIOMA

Microscopic Features

- Benign lesions show mature, thin-walled, endothelium-lined capillary and cavernous sinuses interspersed among sparse, osseous trabeculae and fatty stromata
- Aggressive lesions contain less fat and more vascular stroma

Staging, Grading or Classification Criteria

- Aggressive lesion features: Typical location between T-3 and T-9, involvement of the entire vertebral body, extension to neural arch, an expanded cortex with indistinct margins, irregular honeycomb pattern, soft tissue mass

CLINICAL ISSUES

Presentation

- Most common signs/symptoms
  - Benign hemangiomas are incidentally discovered
  - Symptomatic (aggressive) hemangiomas present with intense, localized spinal pain, myelopathy and/or radiculopathy from osseous expansion, pathologic fracture, and/or epidural extension
- Clinical profile: Middle-aged women with new onset thoracic region pain

Demographics

- Age: Peak incidence fourth to sixth decades
- Gender: M = F; aggressive lesions slightly more common in women

Natural History & Prognosis

- Benign (fatty) hemangiomas - incidental lesions, excellent prognosis
- Aggressive vascular hemangiomas - variable depending on size of lesion, degree of epidural extension, and presence/absence of cord compression

Treatment

- Annual neurological and radiological examinations for patients with hemangiomas associated with pain
- Regular monitoring for patients with asymptomatic lesions unnecessary unless pain develops at the appropriate spinal level
- Aggressive hemangiomas
  - Direct intralesional injection of ethanol (post ethanol treatment body collapse reported complication)
  - Vertebroplasty in conjunction with embolization and surgery as needed
  - Post-operative radiation therapy in patients following subtotal tumor resection

DIAGNOSTIC CHECKLIST

Consider

- Paget if vertebral body expansion; should have no epidural soft tissue

Image Interpretation Pearls

- Classic hemangioma: Hypodense lesion (CT) with coarse, vertically-oriented trabeculae; hyperintense (MRI) on both T1WI and T2WI

SELECTED REFERENCES

1. Bandiera S et al: Symptomatic vertebral hemangioma: the treatment of 23 cases and a review of the literature. Chir Organi Mov. 87(1): 1-15, 2002
2. Murugan L et al: Management of symptomatic vertebral hemangiomas: review of 13 patients. Neurol India. 50(3): 300-5, 2002
3. Gabal AM: Percutaneous technique for sclerotherapy of vertebral hemangioma compressing spinal cord. Cardiovasc Intervent Radiol. 25(6): 494-500, 2002
4. Miszczyk L et al: The efficacy of radiotherapy for vertebral hemangiomas. Neoplasma. 48(1): 82-4, 2001
5. Bas T et al: Efficacy and safety of ethanol injections in 18 cases of vertebral hemangioma: a mean follow-up of 2 years. Spine. 26(14): 1577-82, 2001
6. Baudrez V et al: Benign vertebral hemangioma: MR-histological correlation. Skeletal Radiol. 30(8): 442-6, 2001
7. Cross JJ et al: Imaging of compressive vertebral hemangiomas. Eur Radiol. 10(6): 997-1002, 2000
8. Doppman JL et al: Symptomatic vertebral hemangiomas: treatment by means of direct intralesional injection of ethanol. Radiology. 214(2): 341-8, 2000
9. Lee S et al: Extraosseous extension of vertebral hemangioma, a rare cause of spinal cord compression. Spine. 24(20): 2111-4, 1999
10. Pastushyn AI et al: Vertebral hemangiomas: diagnosis, management, natural history and clinicopathological correlates in 86 patients. Surg Neurol. 50(6): 535-47, 1998
11. Sakata K et al: Radiotherapy of vertebral hemangiomas. Acta Oncol. 36(7): 719-24, 1997
12. Griffith JF et al: Clinics in diagnostic imaging (25). Aggressive vertebral haemangioma. Singapore Med J. 38(5): 226-30, 1997
13. Jayakumar PN et al: Symptomatic vertebral haemangioma: endovascular treatment of 12 patients. Spinal Cord. 35(9): 624-8, 1997
14. Ide C et al: Vertebral haemangiomas with spinal cord compression: the place of preoperative percutaneous vertebroplasty with methyl methacrylate. Neuroradiology. 38(6): 585-9, 1996
15. Guedea F et al: The role of radiation therapy in vertebral hemangiomas without neurological signs. Int Orthop. 18(2): 77-9, 1994
16. Fox MW et al: The natural history and management of symptomatic and asymptomatic vertebral hemangiomas. J Neurosurg. 78(1): 36-45, 1993
17. Laredo JD et al: Vertebral hemangiomas: fat content as a sign of aggressiveness. Radiology. 177(2):467-72, 1990
18. Nguyen JP et al: Vertebral hemangiomas presenting with neurologic symptoms. Surg Neurol. 27(4):391-7, 1987
19. Nicola N et al: Vertebral hemangioma: retrograde embolization-stabilization with methyl methacrylate. Surg Neurol. 27(5):481-6, 1987
20. Ross JS et al: Vertebral hemangiomas: MR imaging. Radiology. 165(1):165-9, 1987
21. Laredo JD et al: Vertebral hemangiomas: radiologic evaluation. Radiology. 161(1):183-9, 1986

IMAGE GALLERY

Typical

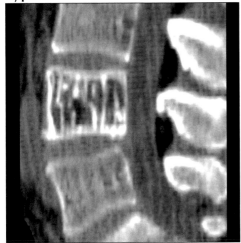
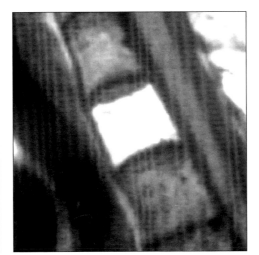

(Left) Sagittal NECT shows thickened vertically oriented trabeculae, with intervening fatty stoma involving L4 body. (Right) Sagittal T1WI MR shows well-defined high signal from the T1 body consistent with hemangioma. There is no epidural soft tissue extension.

Typical

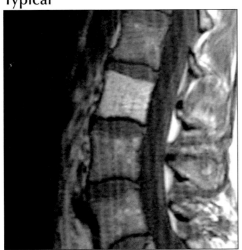
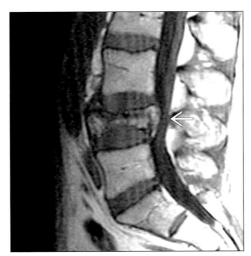

(Left) Sagittal T1WI MR shows fatty signal intensity throughout the L2 body with linear low signal striations due to thickened trabeculae. (Right) Sagittal T1WI MR in patient 6 months following alcohol treatment of L4 hemangioma shows severe L4 collapse, with posterior bony retropulsion and compression of the thecal sac (arrow).

Variant

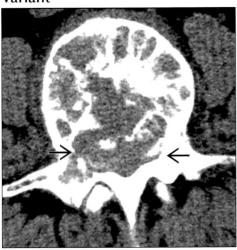
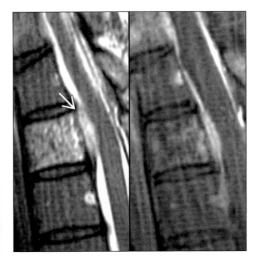

(Left) Axial NECT shows thickened, linear trabeculae within L3 body. There is severe thecal sac compression from soft tissue epidural extension, and bony retropulsion (arrows). (Right) Sagittal T2WI (left side) shows upper thoracic hemangioma with extraosseous extension into epidural space, and cord compression (arrow). Enhanced T1WI (right side) shows enhancing epidural tissue.

OSTEOID OSTEOMA

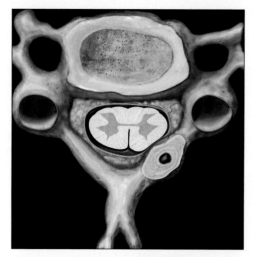

Axial graphic shows small, highly vascular tumor nidus of osteoid osteoma in left lamina, surrounded by dense reactive bone.

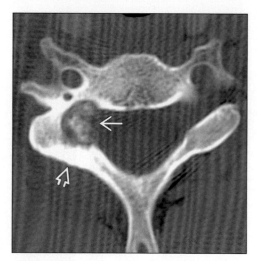

Axial bone CT shows sclerotic C7 OO nidus (arrow). Lesion is sharply demarcated, and surrounded by sclerosis (open arrow). Diagnosis missed on MR, made on radiograph, confirmed on CT.

TERMINOLOGY

Abbreviations and Synonyms
- Osteoid osteoma (OO)

Definitions
- Benign osteoid-producing tumor < 1.5 cm in size
- The tumor is often called a "nidus" to distinguish it from the surrounding sclerotic, reactive bone

IMAGING FINDINGS

General Features
- Best diagnostic clue: Small radiolucent tumor nidus with surrounding sclerosis
- Location
  - 10% of OO occur in spine
  - Almost all involve neural arch
  - Involvement of vertebral body rare
  - 59% lumbar, 27% cervical, 12% thoracic, 2% sacrum
- Size: < 1.5 cm nidus; larger lesions called osteoblastoma
- Morphology: Nidus round or oval

Radiographic Findings
- Radiography
  - Central, lucent tumor nidus often obscured by reactive sclerosis

- Focal scoliosis concave on side of tumor

CT Findings
- CECT
  - Variable enhancement
    - Contrast administration may obscure bony matrix
- Bone CT
  - Central nidus
    - Variable amount of ossification in the nidus
    - Nidus usually predominantly lucent
    - Occasionally nidus is sclerotic
  - Wide peripheral zone of reactive sclerosis surrounds nidus
  - Periosteal reaction variably present, usually unilaminar
  - Soft tissue mass or pleural thickening/effusion often seen
  - Bones adjacent to OO may show sclerosis, periosteal reaction
    - Ribs, adjacent vertebrae affected
  - Ossification of ligamentum flavum has been reported

MR Findings
- T1WI
  - Hypo- or isointense nidus and surrounding reactive zone
  - Cortical thickening
  - Thoracic OO: Pleural thickening and/or effusion

DDx: Osteoid Osteoma

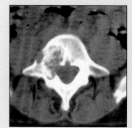
Osteoblastoma

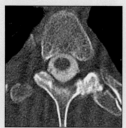
Stress Fracture

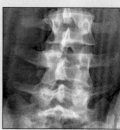
Unilateral Pars Defect

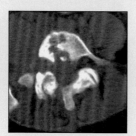
Osteomyelitis

OSTEOID OSTEOMA

Key Facts

Terminology
- Benign osteoid-producing tumor < 1.5 cm in size
- The tumor is often called a "nidus" to distinguish it from the surrounding sclerotic, reactive bone

Imaging Findings
- Best diagnostic clue: Small radiolucent tumor nidus with surrounding sclerosis
- 10% of OO occur in spine
- Central, lucent tumor nidus often obscured by reactive sclerosis
- Focal scoliosis concave on side of tumor

Top Differential Diagnoses
- Osteoblastoma
- Stress fracture of pedicle or lamina
- Unilateral spondylolysis

- Unilateral absent pedicle or pars interarticularis
- Sclerotic metastasis, lymphoma
- Osteomyelitis

Pathology
- Epidemiology: 12% of all benign skeletal neoplasms

Clinical Issues
- Most common signs/symptoms: Night pain relieved by aspirin, NSAIDs
- 70% have scoliosis related to muscle spasm, concave on side of tumor
- Gait disturbance, muscle atrophy, torticollis sometimes seen
- Majority occur in second decade of life

- T2WI
  - Nidus varies from hypointense to hyperintense
  - Surrounding hyperintensity is reactive host response related to prostaglandin release
    - Reactive zone involves much larger area than the tumor
    - Reactive zone may extend to adjacent vertebrae, ribs, and paraspinous soft tissues
    - Severe reactive response may lead to misdiagnosis of malignancy or infection
- T1 C+
  - Contrast-enhancement improves sensitivity of MRI
  - Rapid enhancement pattern typical in nidus: Best seen on dynamic scans
  - Reactive zone enhances more slowly
  - These criteria reportedly result in equal conspicuity of lesion compared to CT
  - However, avid enhancement of reactive zone may obscure nidus relative to marrow fat signal
  - Note that this dedicated protocol centered at a specific level requires a pretest diagnosis of probable OO
- Literature reports high rate of missed MRI diagnosis of OO
  - Lesion may not be seen due to small size of nidus
    - Thin shape, oblique orientation of posterior elements
    - Partial volume averaging with adjacent structures
    - Improve visualization with thin slices, 3-3.5 mm
    - Axial, coronal and sagittal planes
  - Lesion misidentified as reactive zone rather than nidus
    - Misdiagnosis of infection or malignancy common

Nuclear Medicine Findings
- Bone Scan: Positive on all 3 phases of Tc-99m MDP bone scan

Imaging Recommendations
- Bone CT with 1 mm helical sections, IV contrast not needed

DIFFERENTIAL DIAGNOSIS

Osteoblastoma
- Larger (> 1.5 cm)
- Expansile lesion of neural arch/pedicle
- Also a benign tumor of the osteoblast

Stress fracture of pedicle or lamina
- Sclerosis around fracture mimics reactive sclerosis around osteoid osteoma
- CT with MPR or high-resolution MRI will show fracture line
- May occur in patients with pre-existing scoliosis, due to altered stresses
- Pain related to activity, improves at night

Unilateral spondylolysis
- Linear defect pars interarticularis
- Contralateral side is sclerotic
- Painful
- Presents in young patients
- Scoliosis may develop
- May be diagnosed on oblique radiographs, CT

Unilateral absent pedicle or pars interarticularis
- Contralateral side is sclerotic
- Congenital absence of pedicle or pars interarticularis confirmed on CT

Sclerotic metastasis, lymphoma
- Older patients
- Often involves pedicle, destroys posterior body cortex
- Poorly defined, wide zone of transition
- Associated soft tissue mass common
- Often presents with night pain relieved by aspirin, NSAIDs

Osteomyelitis
- Sequestrum or focal abscess can mimic nidus of osteoid osteoma
- Usually involves vertebral bodies
- MR, bone scan may appear very similar

OSTEOID OSTEOMA

- CT usually shows endplate destruction or destructive arthritis of facet joints
- Sequestrum tends to have irregular shape
- Often presents with night pain relieved by aspirin, NSAIDs

Ewing sarcoma
- Diffuse edema may involve adjacent vertebral bodies and ribs
- Pleural thickening, effusion
- Centered in vertebral body
- No nidus on CT scan

PATHOLOGY

General Features
- Etiology: Benign tumor of osteoblastic origin
- Epidemiology: 12% of all benign skeletal neoplasms

Gross Pathologic & Surgical Features
- Sharply-demarcated, round, pink-red mass (nidus)
- Nidus can be shelled out from surrounding, sclerotic reactive bone which does not contain tumor

Microscopic Features
- Web of osteoid trabeculae showing variable amounts of mineralization
- Vascular, fibrous connective tissue
- Similar histologically to osteoblastoma
- No malignant potential
- Reactive zone may contain lymphocytes and plasmocytes

CLINICAL ISSUES

Presentation
- Most common signs/symptoms: Night pain relieved by aspirin, NSAIDs
- Clinical profile
  - 70% have scoliosis related to muscle spasm, concave on side of tumor
  - Gait disturbance, muscle atrophy, torticollis sometimes seen

Demographics
- Age
  - Majority occur in second decade of life
  - Has been reported as late as seventh decade, but very rare
- Gender: M:F = 2-3:1

Natural History & Prognosis
- Resection is curative in most cases
  - Entire nidus must be removed or recurrence is probable
  - Radionuclide labeling can be used to localize intraoperatively
- Spontaneous healing has been reported

Treatment
- Open excision
  - Proximity to vertebral artery should be noted in cervical OO

- CT-guided percutaneous excision
- Thermo/photocoagulation
- Conservative observation (patients with well controlled symptoms)

DIAGNOSTIC CHECKLIST

Consider
- Important cause of painful scoliosis in a child or young adult

Image Interpretation Pearls
- Thin-section CT most accurate in visualizing nidus
- Edema of adjacent bones on MRI mimics extension of infection across discs and joints

SELECTED REFERENCES

1. Liu PT et al: Imaging of osteoid osteoma with dynamic gadolinium-enhanced MR imaging. Radiology. 227(3):691-700, 2003
2. Scuotto A et al: Unusual manifestation of vertebral osteoid osteoma: case report. Eur Radiol. 12(1):109-12, 2002
3. Davies M et al: The diagnostic accuracy of MR imaging in osteoid osteoma. Skeletal Radiol. 31(10):559-69, 2002
4. Lefton DR et al: Vertebral osteoid osteoma masquerading as a malignant bone or soft-tissue tumor on MRI. Pediatr Radiol. 31(2):72-5, 2001
5. Cove JA et al: Osteoid osteoma of the spine treated with percutaneous computed tomography-guided thermocoagulation. Spine. 25(10):1283-6, 2000
6. Radcliffe SN et al: Osteoid osteoma: the difficult diagnosis. Eur J Radiol. 28(1):67-79, 1998
7. Gangi A et al: Percutaneous laser photocoagulation of spinal osteoid osteomas under CT guidance. AJNR Am J Neuroradiol. 19(10):1955-8, 1998
8. Assoun J et al: Osteoid osteoma: MR imaging versus CT. Radiology. 191(1):217-23, 1994
9. Zambelli PY et al: Osteoid osteoma or osteoblastoma of the cervical spine in relation to the vertebral artery. J Pediatr Orthop. 14(6):788-92, 1994
10. Greenspan A: Benign bone-forming lesions: osteoma, osteoid osteoma, and osteoblastoma. Clinical, imaging, pathologic, and differential considerations. Skeletal Radiol. 22(7):485-500, 1993
11. Woods ER et al: Reactive soft-tissue mass associated with osteoid osteoma: correlation of MR imaging features with pathologic findings. Radiology. 186(1):221-5, 1993
12. Klein MH et al: Osteoid osteoma: radiologic and pathologic correlation. Skeletal Radiol. 21(1):23-31, 1992
13. Raskas DS et al: Osteoid osteoma and osteoblastoma of the spine. J Spinal Disord. 5(2): 204-11, 1992
14. Afshani E et al: Common causes of low back pain in children. Radiographics. 11(2): 269-91, 1991
15. Kransdorf MJ et al: Osteoid osteoma. Radiographics. 11(4):671-96, 1991
16. Crim JR et al: Widespread inflammatory response to osteoblastoma: the flare phenomenon. Radiology. 177(3):835-6, 1990

OSTEOID OSTEOMA

IMAGE GALLERY

Typical

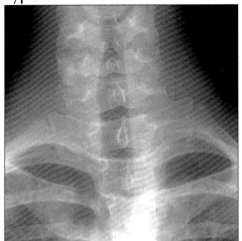 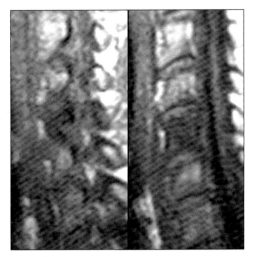

(Left) Anteroposterior radiography shows focal, short-curve levoscoliosis in young man with neck pain. Sclerosis at C6 on right suggested possible diagnosis of OO. (Right) Sagittal T1WI MR images of cervical spine show focal low signal from C5 vertebral body & pedicle from marrow reactive edema is this patient with osteoid osteoma.

Typical

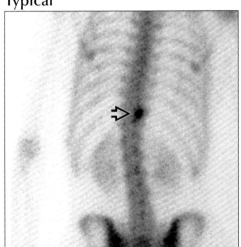 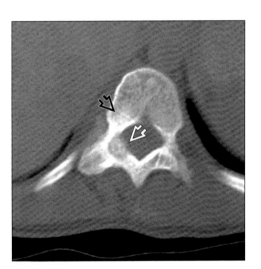

(Left) Posteroanterior bone scan (3 hour image) shows intense, focal uptake on right at T11 (arrow) and scoliosis with concavity on side of OO. (Right) Axial bone CT shows OO nidus centered in lamina (white arrow). Reactive sclerosis extends into vertebral body (black arrow).

Typical

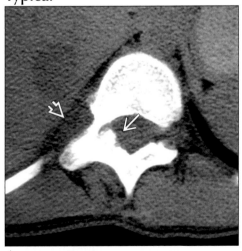 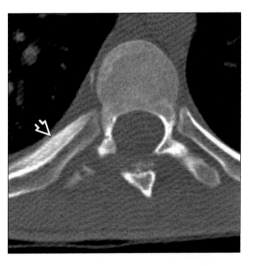

(Left) Axial NECT shows pleural thickening (open arrow) adjacent to OO nidus (arrow). Patient had pleuritic chest pain. (Right) Axial bone CT shows thick, uniform reactive periosteal reaction (arrow) in rib adjacent to OO of adjacent lamina (not shown). Mild pleural thickening is also visible adjacent to rib.

OSTEOBLASTOMA

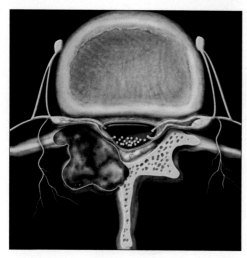

Axial graphic shows expansile, highly vascular osteoblastoma arising in right lamina, and impinging on exiting nerve root.

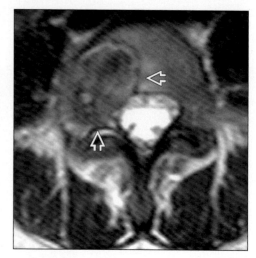

Axial T2WI MR shows OB (arrows) of L5 with characteristic heterogeneous signal intensity. Bony matrix is low signal. There is edema in the adjacent vertebral body.

TERMINOLOGY

Abbreviations and Synonyms
- Osteoblastoma (OB); giant osteoid osteoma

Definitions
- Benign tumor forming osteoid
- Differentiated grossly from osteoid osteoma by larger size (> 1.5 cm)

IMAGING FINDINGS

General Features
- Best diagnostic clue: Expansile mass occurring in posterior elements
- Location
  - 40% of osteoblastomas occur in the spine
    - 40% cervical, 25% lumbar, 20% thoracic, 15-20% sacrum
  - Originate in neural arch
  - May be centered in pedicle, lamina, transverse or spinous process, articular pillar, or pars interarticularis
  - Often extend into vertebral body
- Size: > 1.5 cm
- Morphology: Ovoid lytic lesion, often markedly expansile

Radiographic Findings
- Radiography
  - Geographic lesion
  - Expansile
  - Matrix often not visible on spine radiographs, better seen on CT
  - Usually radiolucent, occasionally sclerotic
  - AP radiograph
    - Lucent or sclerotic pedicle
    - Expansion lateral process
    - Scoliosis in 50-60% of cases
    - Scoliosis concave on side of tumor
  - Lateral radiograph
    - Expanded pedicle, lamina, or spinous process
    - Sharply demarcated lucency posterior portion vertebral body
  - May be occult on radiographs; obtain CT in every case of young patient with painful scoliosis

CT Findings
- CECT: Heterogeneous enhancement obscures bone matrix
- Bone CT
  - Most common appearance
    - Well-circumscribed, expansile lesion of neural arch
    - Often extends into vertebral body
    - Narrow zone of transition, sclerotic rim

DDx: Osteoblastoma

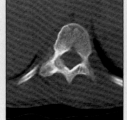

Osteoid Osteoma

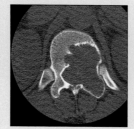

ABC

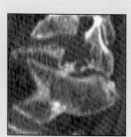

Metastasis

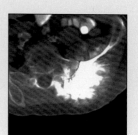

Osteosarcoma

OSTEOBLASTOMA

Key Facts

Terminology
- Osteoblastoma (OB); giant osteoid osteoma
- Benign tumor forming osteoid

Imaging Findings
- 40% of osteoblastomas occur in the spine
- Originate in neural arch
- Matrix often not visible on spine radiographs, better seen on CT
- Scoliosis in 50-60% of cases
- May be occult on radiographs; obtain CT in every case of young patient with painful scoliosis
- Well-circumscribed, expansile lesion of neural arch
- Often extends into vertebral body
- Narrow zone of transition, sclerotic rim
- Variable amount of mineralization

- Inflammatory response may spread far beyond lesion
- May have aneurysmal bone cyst component
- Peritumoral edema may obscure lesion, mimic malignancy or infection on MRI

Top Differential Diagnoses
- Osteoid osteoma (OO)
- Aneurysmal bone cyst (ABC)
- Osteogenic sarcoma (OGS)

Clinical Issues
- 90% in 2nd-3rd decades of life
- 10-15% recurrence for typical OB
- 50% recurrence for aggressive OB

- ○ Aggressive osteoblastoma
  - ■ Cortical breakthrough, wide zone of transition
- ○ Matrix mineralization
  - ■ Variable amount of mineralization
  - ■ May see small, irregular trabeculae
  - ■ Can be difficult to distinguish from calcified cartilage of chondrosarcoma, enchondroma
- ○ Inflammatory response may spread far beyond lesion
  - ■ Widespread, ill-defined sclerotic bone around lesion
  - ■ Periosteal reaction adjacent ribs
  - ■ Pleural thickening effusion
  - ■ Ossification of ligamentum flavum

MR Findings
- T1WI: Low/intermediate signal
- T2WI
  - ○ Intermediate/high signal intensity
  - ○ Low signal areas of bone matrix
  - ○ May have aneurysmal bone cyst component
    - ■ Fluid-fluid levels
  - ○ Extensive peritumoral edema common ("flare phenomenon")
  - ○ Peritumoral edema may involve adjacent bones and soft tissues
  - ○ Peritumoral edema may obscure lesion, mimic malignancy or infection on MRI
  - ○ Pleural effusions common with thoracic OB
- T1 C+
  - ○ Variable enhancement
  - ○ Peritumoral edema may enhance

Angiographic Findings
- Intense tumor blush

Nuclear Medicine Findings
- Bone Scan: Positive 3 phase bone scan

Imaging Recommendations
- CT with sagittal, coronal reformations

DIFFERENTIAL DIAGNOSIS

Osteoid osteoma (OO)
- Smaller (< 1.5 cm)
- Round nidus with surrounding sclerotic bone
- Same age group
- Pain usually more intense
- Scoliosis common

Aneurysmal bone cyst (ABC)
- Expansile lesion of posterior elements
- ABC component present in 10-15% of OB
- ABC may also be isolated, or associated with other tumors
- Multiple blood-filled cavities with fluid-fluid levels
- Matrix absent in ABC without OB

Metastasis
- Older patients
- Usually destroys cortex rather than expanding
- May be expansile, especially in renal cell carcinoma
- Involves posterior elements and/or vertebral body

Osteogenic sarcoma (OGS)
- Sarcoma containing bone matrix
- Rare in spine
- More aggressive appearance on radiographs, CT
- Wider zone of transition
- Cortical breakthrough rather than cortical expansion
- Involves neural arch and/or vertebral body

Chordoma
- Involves vertebral body rather than posterior elements
- Common in sacrum, rare in vertebrae
- No matrix: Purely lytic tumor

Infection
- MRI appearance of OB may mimic infection because of inflammatory change in adjacent bones
- Distinction between OB & infection easily made on CT

Fibrous dysplasia
- Rare in spine
- Expansile lesion of posterior elements

OSTEOBLASTOMA

- May be lytic, or contain "ground glass" matrix or tiny trabeculae of bone

Chondrosarcoma
- Rare in spine
- Involves vertebral body and/or posterior elements
- May have fairly unaggressive features on imaging studies
- Cartilage calcification in arcs and rings

PATHOLOGY

General Features
- General path comments
  ○ Prostaglandins released by tumor cause extensive peritumoral edema
  ○ Pain usually less intense than with OO

Gross Pathologic & Surgical Features
- Friable, highly vascular tumor
- Red color due to vascularity
- Well demarcated from surrounding host bone

Microscopic Features
- Prominent osteoblasts
- Rims of osteoblasts along trabeculae
- Vascular fibrous stroma
- Woven bone matrix of variable quantity
- Cartilage absent
- ABC component found in 10-15%
- "Aggressive" OB
  ○ Same features as above, plus
  ○ More nuclear pleomorphism
  ○ Epithelioid osteoblasts

Staging, Grading or Classification Criteria
- Classic osteoblastoma
- Aggressive osteoblastoma
  ○ Borderline lesion with osteosarcoma
  ○ Locally aggressive but does not metastasize
  ○ Sometimes called pseudomalignant OB

CLINICAL ISSUES

Presentation
- Most common signs/symptoms
  ○ Dull, localized pain
  ○ Scoliosis concave on side of tumor
  ○ Neurologic symptoms due to compression of cord, nerve roots
- Painful scoliosis
  ○ Possible causes in addition to OB include
  ○ Trauma
  ○ OO, other tumors
  ○ Infection
  ○ Spondylolysis
  ○ Renal or retroperitoneal abnormality

Demographics
- Age
  ○ 90% in 2nd-3rd decades of life
  ○ Have been diagnosed in patients up to 7th decade of life

- Gender: M:F = 2-2.5:1

Natural History & Prognosis
- Grow slowly
- 10-15% recurrence for typical OB
- 50% recurrence for aggressive OB

Treatment
- Curettage with bone graft or methylmethacrylate placement
- Pre-operative embolization may be useful

DIAGNOSTIC CHECKLIST

Image Interpretation Pearls
- Aggressive OB is difficult on imaging and histology to distinguish from osteogenic sarcoma
  ○ Wide zone of transition suspicious for osteogenic sarcoma
- OB is important cause of painful scoliosis

SELECTED REFERENCES

1. Biagini R et al: Osteoid osteoma and osteoblastoma of the sacrum. Orthopedics. 24(11):1061-4, 2001
2. Okuda S et al: Ossification of the ligamentum flavum associated with osteoblastoma: a report of three cases. Skeletal Radiol. 30(7):402-6, 2001
3. Shaikh MI et al: Spinal osteoblastoma: CT and MR imaging with pathological correlation. Skeletal Radiol. 28(1):33-40, 1999
4. Saifuddin A et al: Osteoid osteoma and osteoblastoma of the spine. Factors associated with the presence of scoliosis. Spine. 23(1):47-53, 1998
5. Cheung FM et al: Diagnostic criteria for pseudomalignant osteoblastoma. Histopathology. 31(2):196-200, 1997
6. Murphey MD et al: Primary tumors of the spine: Radiologic-pathologic correlation. RadioGraphics. 16: 1131-58, 1996
7. Greenspan A: Benign bone-forming lesions: osteoma, osteoid osteoma, and osteoblastoma. Skeletal Radiol. 22(7):485-500, 1993
8. Boriani S et al: Osteoblastoma of the spine. Clin Ortho Rel Res. 278: 37-45, 1992
9. Nemoto O et al: Osteoblastoma of the spine. Spine. 15: 1272-80, 1990
10. Crim JR et al: Widespread inflammatory response to osteoblastoma: the flare phenomenon. Radiology. 177(3):835-6, 1990
11. Mirra JM et al: Bone tumors: Clinical, radiologic and pathologic correlations. vol. 1. 2nd ed. Philadelphia, Lea & Feibiger. 399-430, 1989

IMAGE GALLERY

Typical

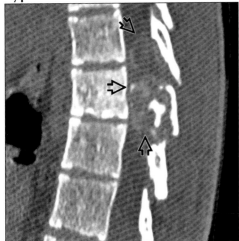 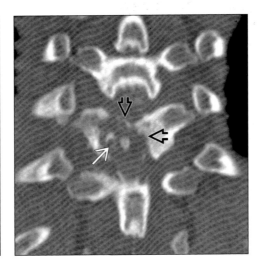

(Left) Sagittal bone CT shows expansile lower thoracic osteoblastoma (arrows) extending from lamina into spinal canal. Lesion is sharply circumscribed, and bilobed, involving 2 adjacent levels. *(Right)* Coronal bone CT shows expansile OB (open arrows) of right lamina. Matrix (arrow) mimics chondroid matrix. Small areas of cortical breakthrough are evident at inferior tumor margin.

Typical

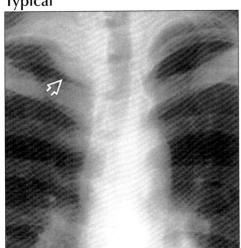 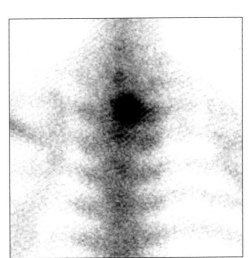

(Left) Anteroposterior radiography shows focal levoscoliosis secondary to upper thoracic OB. Tumor is not visible. Note focal pleural thickening (arrow), a secondary sign of OB. *(Right)* Posteroanterior bone scan shows intense uptake at OB of thoracic spine, with surrounding "flare" of less intense uptake in multiple adjacent bones. Flare reflects inflammatory response around tumor.

Variant

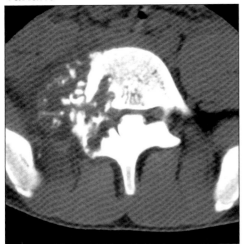 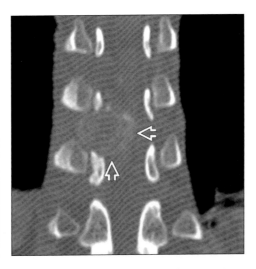

(Left) Axial bone CT shows aggressive OB of L5 centered in pedicle, with extensive cortical breakthrough and soft tissue ossification. Low grade OGS could also have this appearance. *(Right)* Coronal bone CT shows OB with soft tissue mass in spinal canal. Mass originated in lamina. It contains immature ossification (arrows) and is poorly marginated, mimicking OGS.

ANEURYSMAL BONE CYST

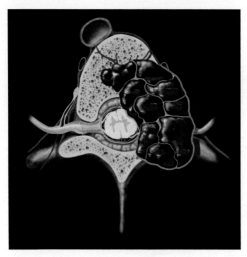

Axial graphic shows aneurysmal bone cyst with expansile, multicystic mass in posterior vertebral body & pedicle extending into epidural space. Fluid-fluid levels are characteristic.

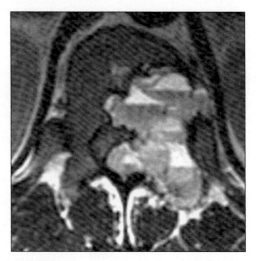

Axial T2WI MR shows ABC with multiple fluid-fluid levels due to layering blood products. Lesion is sharply demarcated, with a narrow zone of transition.

TERMINOLOGY

Abbreviations and Synonyms

- Aneurysmal bone cyst (ABC)

Definitions

- Expansile benign neoplasm containing thin-walled, blood-filled cavities

IMAGING FINDINGS

General Features

- Best diagnostic clue: Expansile multiloculated neural arch mass with fluid-fluid levels
- Location
  ○ 10-30% of ABC occur in spine/sacrum
  ○ Arise in neural arch
  ○ 75-90% extend into vertebral body

Radiographic Findings

- Radiography
  ○ Balloon-like expansile remodeling of bone
    ▪ Centered in neural arch, extends into vertebral body
  ○ Absent pedicle sign: Expansion of pedicle results in loss of pedicle contour on AP radiographs
  ○ Cortical thinning
  ○ Focal cortical destruction common

○ Rare: Vertebral body collapse ("vertebra plana")
○ Rare: Extends to more than 1 vertebral level
○ Rare: Involves adjacent ribs

CT Findings

- NECT
  ○ Balloon-like expansile remodeling of bone
  ○ Thinned, "eggshell" cortex
  ○ Focal cortical destruction common
  ○ Narrow, nonsclerotic zone of transition
  ○ Fluid-fluid levels caused by hemorrhage, blood product sedimentation
  ○ Tumor matrix absent
  ○ Thin bony septa may be present
  ○ Commonly extends into epidural space, may severely narrow spinal canal
- CECT
  ○ Periphery and septa enhance
  ○ Solid ABC variant enhances diffusely

MR Findings

- T1WI
  ○ Lobulated neural arch mass +/- extension into vertebral body
  ○ Cystic spaces of varying sizes within mass
    ▪ Contain fluid-fluid levels due to blood products
    ▪ Cysts separated by septae of varying thickness
  ○ Part or all of mass may be solid
  ○ Hypointense rim around mass

DDx: Aneurysmal Bone Cyst

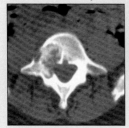
Osteoblastoma

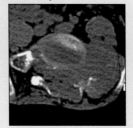
Telangiectatic OGS

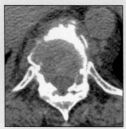
Metastasis

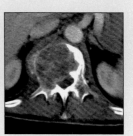
Giant Cell Tumor

ANEURYSMAL BONE CYST

Key Facts

Terminology
- Aneurysmal bone cyst (ABC)
- Expansile benign neoplasm containing thin-walled, blood-filled cavities

Imaging Findings
- 10-30% of ABC occur in spine/sacrum
- Arise in neural arch
- 75-90% extend into vertebral body
- Balloon-like expansile remodeling of bone
- Centered in neural arch, extends into vertebral body
- Absent pedicle sign: Expansion of pedicle results in loss of pedicle contour on AP radiographs
- Cortical thinning
- Focal cortical destruction common

- Fluid-fluid levels caused by hemorrhage, blood product sedimentation
- Tumor matrix absent
- Commonly extends into epidural space, may severely narrow spinal canal

Top Differential Diagnoses
- Osteoblastoma
- Telangiectatic osteogenic sarcoma (OGS)
- Metastases
- Giant cell tumor (GCT)

Clinical Issues
- Back pain, most severe at night
- Scoliosis
- Neurologic signs and symptoms from root and/or cord compression

---

  - Rim of periosteum visible on MR even when no cortex visible on CT
  - Epidural extension well seen
- T2WI
  - Cystic spaces of varying sizes
  - Fluid-fluid levels due to blood products
  - Intensities vary with stage of blood degradation
  - Hypointense rim around mass
  - Epidural extension well seen
- STIR: Similar to T2WI
- T1 C+
  - Enhancement at periphery, septae between cysts
  - Diffuse enhancement in solid ABC variant

Angiographic Findings
- Conventional
  - Hypervascular
  - Vessels more prominent at periphery, drape around lesion

Nuclear Medicine Findings
- Bone Scan
  - Positive 3 phase bone scan
    - May have rim of activity around photopenic region ("donut sign")

Imaging Recommendations
- CT best for diagnosis based on specific imaging features
- CT best to differentiate from telangiectatic OGS
  - Narrow zone of transition in ABC
  - Absence of infiltration into surrounding soft tissues
- MRI shows epidural extent, cord compromise

DIFFERENTIAL DIAGNOSIS

Osteoblastoma
- Same age range
- Expansile lesion of neural arch
- Bone matrix is visible on plain films or CT
- May be associated with ABC

Telangiectatic osteogenic sarcoma (OGS)
- Same age range or older
- Involves vertebral body and/or neural arch
- Also shows fluid-fluid levels
- Has more permeative bone destruction
- Wider zone of transition
- Infiltrates into surrounding soft tissues

Metastases
- Older patients (usually 6th, 7th decades)
- Involves vertebral body +/- neural arch
- Destructive lesion with associated soft tissue mass
- Rare: Vascular metastasis can have fluid levels
- Less expansile, more permeative
- Renal cell carcinoma can have "soap bubble" expansile appearance

Giant cell tumor (GCT)
- Slightly older patients
- Involves vertebral body rather than neural arch
- Expansile, lytic lesion +/- soft tissue mass
- May be associated with ABC

Plasmacytoma
- Older patients, usually over 40 years old
- Solitary plasmacytoma can have expansile appearance
- Involves vertebral body, usually spares neural arch

Tarlov cyst
- Perineural cyst occurring in sacrum, arising in neural foramina
- Causes bone expansion, cortical breakthrough
- No enhancement
- Simple fluid on all pulse sequences

PATHOLOGY

General Features
- General path comments
  - Bone cannot truly expand
  - "Expansile" appearance reflects containment of tumor by appositional periosteal new bone

ANEURYSMAL BONE CYST

- Etiology
  - 3 theories
  - 1: Results from trauma + local circulatory disturbance
  - 2: Underlying tumor induces vascular process (venous obstruction or AV fistulae)
    - 5-35% of ABC associated with other tumor, most commonly GCT or OB
  - 3: Neoplasm with cytogenetic abnormalities
    - More than 1/2 cases show abnormality in chromosomes 17p or 16
- Epidemiology: 1-2% of primary bone tumors are ABC

Gross Pathologic & Surgical Features
- Spongy, red mass
- Multiple blood-filled spaces

Microscopic Features
- Typical
  - Cystic component predominates
    - Cavernous blood-filled cysts of variable sizes
    - Lined by fibroblasts, giant cells, histiocytes, hemosiderin
  - Solid components
    - Septations interposed between blood-filled spaces
    - Contain bland stroma with fibrous tissue, reactive bone, giant cells
- Solid ABC is rare variant
  - 5-8% of all ABCs
  - Solid component predominates
  - Propensity for spine

CLINICAL ISSUES

Presentation
- Most common signs/symptoms
  - Back pain, most severe at night
  - Other signs/symptoms
    - Scoliosis
    - Neurologic signs and symptoms from root and/or cord compression
    - Pathologic fracture
- Clinical profile: Young patient with back pain of insidious onset

Demographics
- Age: 80% less than 20 years old
- Gender: Slightly more common in females
- Familial incidence has been reported

Natural History & Prognosis
- Long term history of untreated ABC variable
  - Grows initially, then usually stabilizes
  - No malignant degeneration
- Recurrence rate 20-30% (increased if incomplete excision)

Treatment
- Embolization
  - Curative as sole therapy in some cases
  - Can also be used pre-operatively
- Surgical excision
- May require instrumentation for stabilization of spine

- Radiation therapy may predispose to radiation-induced sarcoma

DIAGNOSTIC CHECKLIST

Consider
- "Absent pedicle" sign caused by: ABC, osteoblastoma, lytic OGS, metastasis, trauma, congenital absence of pedicle

Image Interpretation Pearls
- Evaluation of pedicles on AP radiograph should be part of routine on every patient

SELECTED REFERENCES

1. Lomasney LM et al: Fibrous dysplasia complicated by aneurysmal bone cyst formation affecting multiple cervical vertebrae. Skeletal Radiol. 32(9):533-6, 2003
2. Pogoda P et al: Aneurysmal bone cysts of the sacrum. Clinical report and review of the literature. Arch Orthop Trauma Surg. 123(5):247-51, 2003
3. Garneti N et al: Cervical spondyloptosis caused by an aneurysmal bone cyst: a case report. Spine. 28(4):E68-70, 2003
4. Chan MS et al: Spinal aneurysmal bone cyst causing acute cord compression without vertebral collapse: CT and MRI findings. Pediatr Radiol. 32(8):601-4, 2002
5. Lam CH et al: Nonteratomatous tumors in the pediatric sacral region. Spine. 27(11):E284-7, 2002
6. Papagelopoulos PJ et al: Treatment of aneurysmal bone cysts of the pelvis and sacrum. J Bone Joint Surg Am. 83-A(11):1674-81, 2001
7. Boriani S et al: Aneurysmal bone cyst of the mobile spine: report on 41 cases. Spine. 26(1):27-35, 2001
8. DiCaprio MR et al: Aneurysmal bone cyst of the spine with familial incidence. Spine. 25(12):1589-92, 2000
9. Bush CH et al: Treatment of an aneurysmal bone cyst of the spine by radionuclide ablation. AJNR Am J Neuroradiol. 21(3):592-4, 2000
10. Ozaki T et al: Aneurysmal bone cysts of the spine. Arch Orthop Trauma Surg. 119(3-4):159-62, 1999
11. Papagelopoulos PJ et al: Aneurysmal bone cyst of the spine. Management and outcome. Spine. 23(5):621-8, 1998
12. de Kleuver M et al: Aneurysmal bone cyst of the spine: 31 cases and the importance of the surgical approach. J Pediatr Orthop B. 7(4):286-92, 1998
13. Murphey MD et al: Primary tumors of the spine: Radiologic-pathologic correlation. RadioGraphics. 16:1131-58, 1996
14. Koci TM et al: Aneurysmal bone cyst of the thoracic spine: evolution after particulate embolization. AJNR Am J Neuroradiol. 16(4 Suppl):857-60, 1995
15. Kransdorf MJ et al: Aneurysmal bone cyst: Concept, controversy, clinical presentation, and imaging. AJR. 164: 573-80, 1995

ANEURYSMAL BONE CYST

IMAGE GALLERY

Typical

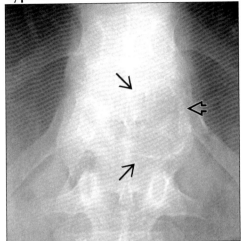
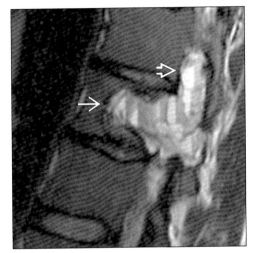

(Left) Anteroposterior radiography shows ABC of T12 with "absent pedicle" sign (open arrow). Arrows show superior and inferior extent of tumor, which involved vertebral body as well as neural arch. *(Right)* Sagittal T2WI MR shows ABC of T12, with vertebral body involvement (arrow) and extension into spinal canal (open arrow). Lesion was centered on pedicle (not shown).

Typical

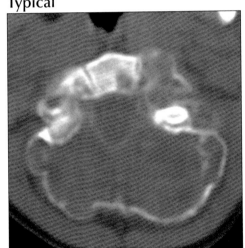
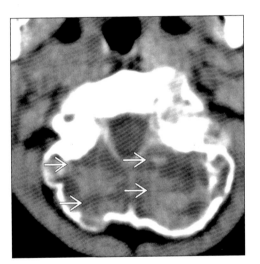

(Left) Axial bone CT shows ABC of C2, causing ballooning of posterior elements and sharply demarcated lytic region in vertebral body. *(Right)* Axial NECT shows ABC of C2, with multiple fluid-fluid levels (arrows) due to layering of blood products.

Typical

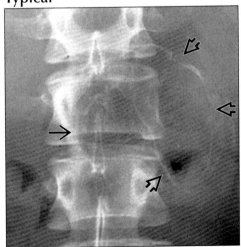
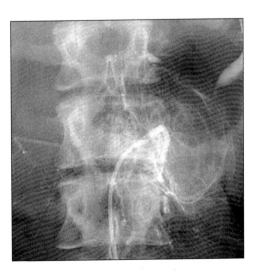

(Left) Anteroposterior radiography shows ABC causing balloon-like expansion of L2 transverse process (open arrows) and pedicle. Sharply-demarcated lytic lesion extends into vertebral body (arrow). *(Right)* Anteroposterior angiography shows ABC of L2 with draping of vessels around lesion periphery, as well as regions of neovascularity centrally.

GIANT CELL TUMOR

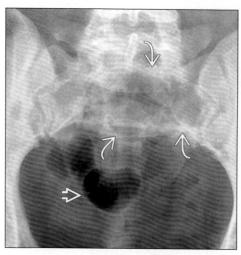

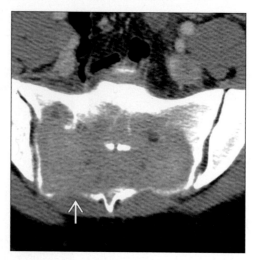

Anteroposterior radiography shows sacral GCT (curved arrows). Recognition of lytic sacral lesions is more difficult because of similar appearance of overlying bowel gas (open arrow).

Axial bone CT shows sacral GCT involving S1 and S2 neural foramina. There is focal cortical destruction (arrow). Zone of transition is narrow.

TERMINOLOGY

Abbreviations and Synonyms
• Giant cell tumor (GCT)

Definitions
• Locally aggressive neoplasm composed of osteoclast-like giant cells

IMAGING FINDINGS

General Features
• Best diagnostic clue: Lytic lesion in vertebral body or sacrum
• Location
  ○ Spine: 3% of all GCT
  ○ Centered in vertebral body
  ○ Sacrum: 4% of all GCT
  ○ Rarely involves multiple sites

Radiographic Findings
• Radiography
  ○ Lytic, expansile lesion
  ○ Narrow zone of transition
  ○ Margin usually not sclerotic
  ○ Matrix absent, but may have residual bone trabeculae
  ○ May have cortical breakthrough

CT Findings
• Bone CT
  ○ Features described for radiography more clearly seen
  ○ May contain fluid attenuation regions due to necrosis or focal aneurysmal bone cyst (ABC) component
  ○ Absence of matrix best seen on noncontrast CT

MR Findings
• T1WI: Low-intermediate signal intensity
• T2WI
  ○ Intermediate-high signal intensity
  ○ Fluid-fluid levels if ABC present
  ○ Use to evaluate extraosseous component of tumor
• STIR: Intermediate-high signal intensity
• T1 C+
  ○ Heterogeneous enhancement
  ○ Areas of necrosis common
• Hemosiderin may be seen, low signal on T1WI and T2WI

Nuclear Medicine Findings
• Bone Scan: Positive all three phases

Imaging Recommendations
• Best imaging tool
  ○ CT scan for diagnosis
  ○ MR for evaluation of spinal canal, nerve roots

DDx: Lytic Lesion Vertebral Body

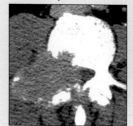

Metastasis

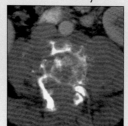

Chordoma

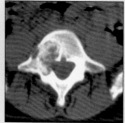

Osteoblastoma

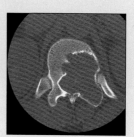

ABC

GIANT CELL TUMOR

Key Facts

Terminology
- Locally aggressive neoplasm composed of osteoclast-like giant cells

Imaging Findings
- Best diagnostic clue: Lytic lesion in vertebral body or sacrum
- Lytic, expansile lesion
- Narrow zone of transition
- Margin usually not sclerotic
- Matrix absent, but may have residual bone trabeculae
- May have cortical breakthrough

Top Differential Diagnoses
- Metastasis
- Aneurysmal bone cyst (ABC)
- Chordoma

- Osteogenic sarcoma (OGS)
- Osteoblastoma
- Myeloma

Pathology
- 5% of all primary bone tumors
- 6th most common primary bone tumor

Clinical Issues
- Most common signs/symptoms: Back pain of insidious onset, greatest at night
- Pathologic fracture in 30%
- Locally aggressive: 12-50% recurrence rate
- Can undergo sarcomatous transformation, spontaneously or in response to radiation therapy

- Protocol advice: Thin-section CT with sagittal, coronal reformations

DIFFERENTIAL DIAGNOSIS

Metastasis
- Usually appears more aggressive, but can be expansile
- Involves vertebral body and neural arch
- Often multiple
- Usually in older patients

Aneurysmal bone cyst (ABC)
- Markedly expansile
- Arises in neural arch, can extend into vertebral body
- Can coexist with GCT

Chordoma
- Lytic, expansile lesion
- Most common in sacrum but can involve vertebral body
- Arises in midline
- No matrix
- Can have large soft tissue component

Osteogenic sarcoma (OGS)
- Wide zone of transition, permeative appearance
- Vertebral body or neural arch
- Soft tissue mass
- Osseous matrix visible in 80%
- May contain large numbers of giant cells

Osteoblastoma
- Lytic, expansile lesion neural arch
- May extend into vertebral body
- Bone matrix visible on CT scan

Myeloma
- Lytic lesion, often expansile
- Vertebral body or sacrum
- Can have sharp zone of transition, geographic appearance
- Usually in older patients
- Look for lesions elsewhere

Brown tumor of hyperparathyroidism
- Radiologically and histologically identical to GCT
- Due to osteoclast stimulation in hyperparathyroidism
- Regresses with successful treatment of hyperparathyroidism

PATHOLOGY

General Features
- Epidemiology
  - 5% of all primary bone tumors
  - 6th most common primary bone tumor

Gross Pathologic & Surgical Features
- Soft, tan tumor
- Tumor tissue well-demarcated
- 10-15% have ABC component
- Surrounding bone is "expanded" with thinning of the cortex
  - This actually represents containment of tumor by deposition of periosteal new bone
- Periphery shows thin layer of fibrous and reactive bone tissue
- Apparent soft tissue extension usually covered by periosteum

Microscopic Features
- Multinucleated osteoclastic giant cells
  - Giant cells have average of 15 nuclei
  - Mitoses are absent
  - Nuclei round or oval, not pleomorphic
  - Abundant cytoplasm
  - No bone or cartilage matrix production by giant cells
- Spindle cell stroma
  - Each cell has single nucleus similar in appearance to the giant cells
- Reactive osteoid may be present
  - Periosteal reaction, not made by tumor cells
- Hemorrhage, necrosis, hemosiderin may be present
- Malignant giant cell tumor
  - Rare tumor

GIANT CELL TUMOR

- ○ Difficult histologic diagnosis
- ○ Anaplasia and pleomorphism of giant cells
- ○ Distinguished from giant cell rich OGS by lack of osteoid formation by tumor cells

Staging, Grading or Classification Criteria

- Typical GCT
  - ○ Grading systems have been proposed, but not predictive of behavior
- Malignant GCT
  - ○ High risk of local recurrence and metastasis to bone, lung, liver

CLINICAL ISSUES

Presentation

- Most common signs/symptoms: Back pain of insidious onset, greatest at night
- Clinical profile
  - ○ Pathologic fracture in 30%
  - ○ Limited range of motion of joint adjacent to affected area

Demographics

- Age
  - ○ 80% 3rd to 5th decade of life
  - ○ In spine, peak incidence 2nd and 3rd decades
  - ○ Rare before skeletal maturity
- Gender: M:F = 1-2.5 in spine (more marked female preponderance than in appendicular skeleton)

Natural History & Prognosis

- Locally aggressive: 12-50% recurrence rate
- Can undergo sarcomatous transformation, spontaneously or in response to radiation therapy
- Pulmonary implants: 1-2%
  - ○ Occurs in patients with stage 3 disease
  - ○ Within 3 years after removal of primary GCT
  - ○ Histologically identical to primary GCT
  - ○ Self limited growth potential
  - ○ May regress spontaneously
  - ○ Resection is curative
- Primary malignant GCT (rare)
  - ○ Poor prognosis
  - ○ Metastasis to lung, liver, bone

Treatment

- Curettage alone associated with high rate of recurrence
- Cryotherapy or thermocoagulation used to reduce recurrence
- Curettage defect filled with methylmethacrylate or bone graft
- Radiation only for cases of unresectable tumor
  - ○ Risk of sarcoma years after treatment
- Arterial embolization
  - ○ Used pre-operatively
  - ○ Used for therapy for unresectable tumor
- Surgical resection of pulmonary implants
  - ○ Good prognosis following resection
- Malignant GCT treated with wide resection, chemotherapy, radiation

DIAGNOSTIC CHECKLIST

Image Interpretation Pearls

- Sacral GCT may be occult on radiographs; have low threshold for CT in patients with atypical sacral pain
- Patients treated with radiation must be followed with MRI because of risk of recurrence, sarcomatous degeneration

SELECTED REFERENCES

1. Bertoni F et al: Malignancy in giant cell tumor of bone. Cancer. 97(10):2520-9, 2003
2. Lackman RD et al: The treatment of sacral giant-cell tumours by serial arterial embolization. J Bone Joint Surg. 84(B):873-7, 2002
3. Garcia-Bravo A et al: Secondary tetraplegia due to giant-cell tumors of the cervical spine. Neurochirurgie. 48(6):527-32, 2002
4. Murphey MD et al: From the archives of AFIP. Imaging of giant cell tumor and giant cell reparative granuloma of bone: radiologic-pathologic correlation. Radiographics. 21(5):1283-309, 2001
5. Meis JM et al: Primary malignant giant cell tumor of bone: "Dedifferentiated" giant cell tumor. Mod Pathol. 2:541-6, 1995
6. Schutte HE et al: Giant cell tumor in children and adolescents. Skeletal Radiol. 22:173-6, 1993
7. Manaster BJ et al: Giant cell tumor of bone. Radiol Clin North Am. 31:299-323, 1993
8. Tubbs WS et al: Benign giant-cell tumor of bone with pulmonary metastases: Clinical findings and radiologic appearance of metastases in 13 cases. Am J Roentgenol. 158:331-4, 1992
9. Aoki J et al: Giant cell tumors of bone containing large amounts of hemosiderin: MR-pathologic correlation. J Comput Assist Tomogr. 15:1024-7, 1991
10. Bridge JA et al: Cytogenetic findings and biologic behavior of giant cell tumors of bone. Cancer. 65:2697-703, 1990
11. Mirra JM et al: Bone tumors: Clinical, radiologic and pathologic correlations. vol. 1. 2nd ed. Philadelphia, Lea &Feibiger. 942-1019, 1989, 1989
12. Carrasco CH et al: Giant cell tumors. Orthop Clin North Am. 20:395-405, 1989

IMAGE GALLERY

Typical

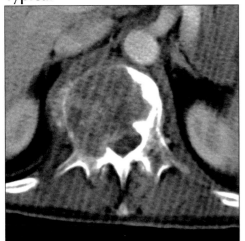
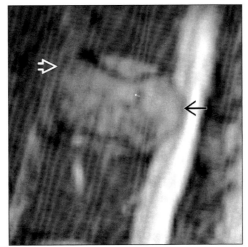

(Left) Axial CECT shows lytic, mildly expansile L1 GCT, centered in vertebral body. Majority of tumor is surrounded by thin rim of reactive bone. There is heterogeneous enhancement with contrast. *(Right)* Sagittal STIR MR shows expansile, heterogeneous L1 GCT. There is encroachment on the spinal canal (arrow) and small area of cortical breakthrough anteriorly (open arrow).

Typical

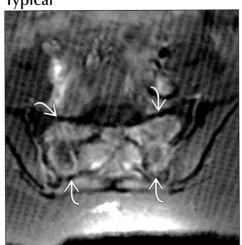
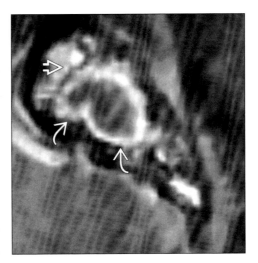

(Left) Axial T1 C+ MR shows treated sacral GCT (arrows) stable for 3 years. Fluid filled areas are surrounded by enhancing fibrosis due to radiation therapy. *(Right)* Sagittal T1 C+ MR shows stable, treated sacral GCT. There is central cyst formation (curved arrows). Insufficiency fracture is seen in superior portion of sacrum (open arrow).

Variant

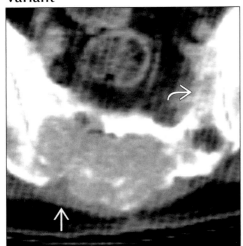
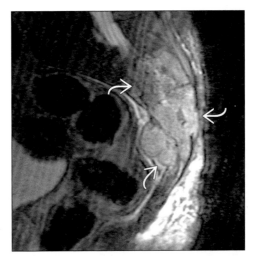

(Left) Axial NECT shows malignant sacral GCT later metastasizing to bone, liver and lung. Note extensive cortical breakthrough, ST mass (arrow), and permeative appearance in left sacral ala (curved arrow). *(Right)* Sagittal STIR MR shows malignant sacral GCT (arrows). Clues indicating tumor is more aggressive than most GCT include larger ST mass and more extensive cortical destruction

OSTEOCHONDROMA

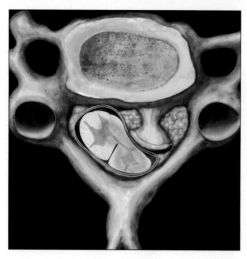

Axial graphic shows a typical osteochondroma (exostosis) protruding into the central canal, producing spinal cord compression.

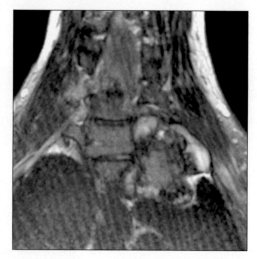

Coronal T2WI MR shows a large left T1 transverse process osteochondroma. Hyperintense cartilage cap thickness > 1.5 cm suggests chondrosarcoma, but benign pathology found at surgery.

TERMINOLOGY

Abbreviations and Synonyms
- Synonyms: OC, osteocartilaginous exostosis, exostosis
- Hereditary multiple exostoses (HME) = familial osteochondromatosis, diaphyseal aclasis

Definitions
- Cartilage-covered osseous excrescence contiguous with parent bone

IMAGING FINDINGS

General Features
- Best diagnostic clue: Sessile or pedunculated osseous "cauliflower" lesion with marrow/cortical continuity with parent vertebra
- Location
  - Bones forming through endochondral ossification
    - Metaphysis of long tubular bones (85%) common, particularly knee
  - < 5% occur in spine
    - Cervical (50%, C2 predilection) > thoracic (T8 > T4 > other levels) > lumbar > > sacrum
    - Spinous/transverse processes > vertebral body
- Size: Vary dramatically; 1-10 cm

Radiographic Findings
- Radiography
  - Sessile/pedunculated osseous protuberance with flaring of parent bone cortex at OC attachment
  - Cartilage cap visible only if extensively mineralized

CT Findings
- CECT: Sessile or pedunculated osseous projection +/- heterogeneous enhancement, cartilaginous cap Ca++
- Bone CT
  - Marrow/cortex continuity with parent bone
  - +/- Chondroid matrix ⇒ "arcs and rings", flocculent Ca++

MR Findings
- T1WI
  - Central hyperintensity surrounded by hypointense cortex
  - Hypo/isointense hyaline cartilage cap
- T2WI
  - Central iso- to hyperintense signal surrounded by hypointense cortex
  - Hyperintense hyaline cartilage cap
- T1 C+: +/- Septal and peripheral cartilage cap enhancement

Ultrasonographic Findings
- Real Time

DDx: Spinal Osteochondroma

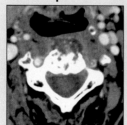

Chondrosarcoma

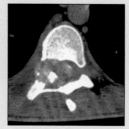

Osteoblastoma

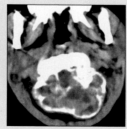

ABC

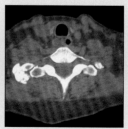

Scleroderma

OSTEOCHONDROMA

Key Facts

Terminology
- Synonyms: OC, osteocartilaginous exostosis, exostosis
- Hereditary multiple exostoses (HME) = familial osteochondromatosis, diaphyseal aclasis

Imaging Findings
- Best diagnostic clue: Sessile or pedunculated osseous "cauliflower" lesion with marrow/cortical continuity with parent vertebra
- Cervical (50%, C2 predilection) > thoracic (T8 > T4 > other levels) > lumbar > > sacrum
- Spinous/transverse processes > vertebral body

Top Differential Diagnoses
- Chondrosarcoma
- Osteoblastoma
- Aneurysmal bone cyst (ABC)

- Metabolic and connective tissue diseases

Pathology
- Narrow stalk (pedunculated) or broad attachment base (sessile) contiguous with vertebral cortex, medullary space

Clinical Issues
- Asymptomatic incidental diagnosis on radiography
- Palpable mass
- Myelopathy; onset often follows trauma

Diagnostic Checklist
- Multiplicity → consider HME
- Interpret cartilage thickness in context of patient age
- Cartilage cap > 1.5 cm in adults raises concern for malignant transformation (chondrosarcoma)

- Hypoechoic nonmineralized cartilage cap easily distinguished from hyperechoic surrounding fat, muscle
- Cartilage cap mineralization and osseous stalk → posterior acoustic shadowing

Nuclear Medicine Findings
- Bone Scan
  - Variable; direct correlation with enchondral bone formation
    - ↑ Radionuclide uptake = metabolically active osteochondroma
    - No ↑ radionuclide uptake = quiescent osteochondroma

Imaging Recommendations
- Best imaging tool: MR imaging
- Protocol advice
  - MRI to measure cartilage cap, determine status of regional neural and musculoskeletal tissue
  - Bone CT to assess mineralization, confirm continuity with vertebral marrow space

DIFFERENTIAL DIAGNOSIS

Chondrosarcoma
- Isolated or 2° malignant OC degeneration
- Lytic destructive lesion with sclerotic margins, soft tissue mass
- Chondroid matrix ("rings and arcs", 50%)

Osteoblastoma
- Expansile lesion of neural arch/pedicle

Aneurysmal bone cyst (ABC)
- Expansile, multicystic; fluid-fluid levels

Metabolic and connective tissue diseases
- E.g., calcium metabolism disorders (hyperparathyroidism), dermatomyositis, scleroderma
- Sheet or tumoral calcification, abnormal lab studies

PATHOLOGY

General Features
- General path comments
  - Benign cartilaginous bone tumor
    - 9% of all bone tumors, most common benign bone tumor (30-45%)
    - Rapid growth, new pain, continued growth of cartilage cap > 1.5 cm thickness after skeletal maturity imply malignant transformation to chondrosarcoma
    - OC complications include deformity, fracture, vascular compromise, neurologic sequelae, overlying bursa formation, and malignant transformation
  - Vertebral OC rare; 1-5% of sporadic OC, 1-9% OC in HME
    - Narrow stalk (pedunculated) or broad attachment base (sessile) contiguous with vertebral cortex, medullary space
    - Hyaline cartilage cap thickness proportional to patient age
  - Many spinal OC are neurologically asymptomatic, produce mechanical impingement symptoms
    - Symptomatic OC arising from posterior vertebral body protrude into canal → cord compression, myelopathy
- Genetics
  - Hereditary multiple exostoses
    - Autosomal dominant, EXT gene locus chromosomes 8, 11, and 19 (tumor suppressor sites)
    - Inactivation of one EXT gene → exostosis; subsequent inactivation of 2nd EXT gene → malignant transformation
- Etiology
  - Idiopathic, trauma, perichondral ring deficiency, radiation induced (dose-dependent)
    - Peripheral portion of epiphyseal cartilage herniates out of growth plate
    - Metaplastic cartilage is stimulated; enchondral bone formation → bony stalk

OSTEOCHONDROMA

- ○ Radiation-induced OC
  - ▪ Most common benign radiation-induced tumor; prevalence 6-24%
  - ▪ Radiation dose 1,500–5,500 cGy; occur at treatment field periphery, latent period 3-17 y, patients generally < 2 yo at time of XRT
  - ▪ Pathologically and radiographically identical to other exostoses
- • Epidemiology
  - ○ Prevalence of solitary OC unknown since many asymptomatic
  - ○ Prevalence of HME 1:50,000 to 1:100,000 in Western populations; up to 1:1,000 in ethnic Chamorros

Gross Pathologic & Surgical Features

- • Osseous excrescence with cortex, medullary cavity contiguous with parent bone
- • Cartilage cap ranges from thick bosselated glistening blue-gray surface (young patients) to several millimeters thick or entirely absent (adults)

Microscopic Features

- • Mature cartilaginous, cancellous, and cortical bone
- • Cartilage cap histology reflects classic growth plate zones

CLINICAL ISSUES

Presentation

- • Most common signs/symptoms
  - ○ Asymptomatic incidental diagnosis on radiography
  - ○ Palpable mass
  - ○ Myelopathy; onset often follows trauma
  - ○ Other signs/symptoms
    - ▪ Cranial nerve deficits (dysphagia, hoarseness), pharyngeal mass, scoliosis, radiculopathy
- • Clinical profile
  - ○ Many solitary OC patients present with painless slowly growing mass, but may manifest identical symptoms to HME patients
  - ○ HME patients more often symptomatic; many exostoses produce impingement, other symptoms referable to OC location
    - ▪ Mechanical pain → 2° to bursitis over exostosis, surrounding tendon/muscle/neural irritation, OC stalk fracture, or infarct/ischemic necrosis

Demographics

- • Age
  - ○ Peak age = 10-30 y
  - ○ Most HME patients diagnosed by age 5 y, virtually all by 12 y
- • Gender: M:F = 3:1

Natural History & Prognosis

- • Post-surgical local recurrence rate < 2%
- • Benign lesions; no propensity for metastasis
- • Malignant transformation < 1% solitary lesions; 3-5% HME
  - ○ Markers for possible malignant degeneration
    - ▪ Growth or new pain after skeletal maturity, ↑ cartilage cap thickness (> 1.5 cm in adults)

Treatment

- • Conservative management in asymptomatic patients
- • Surgical excision, deformity correction in symptomatic patients

DIAGNOSTIC CHECKLIST

Consider

- • Multiplicity → consider HME
- • Interpret cartilage thickness in context of patient age

Image Interpretation Pearls

- • Cartilage cap > 1.5 cm in adults raises concern for malignant transformation (chondrosarcoma)
- • Radiologic features pathognomonic, reflect pathologic appearance

SELECTED REFERENCES

1. Taitz J et al: Osteochondroma after total body irradiation: an age-related complication. Pediatr Blood Cancer. 42(3):225-9, 2004
2. Fiechtl JF et al: Spinal osteochondroma presenting as atypical spinal curvature: a case report. Spine. 28(13):E252-5, 2003
3. Jones KB et al: Of hedgehogs and hereditary bone tumors: re-examination of the pathogenesis of osteochondromas. Iowa Orthop J. 23:87-95, 2003
4. Sharma MC et al: Osteochondroma of the spine: an enigmatic tumor of the spinal cord. A series of 10 cases. J Neurosurg Sci. 46(2):66-70; discussion 70, 2002
5. Pierz KA et al: Hereditary multiple exostoses: one center's experience and review of etiology. Clin Orthop. (401):49-59, 2002
6. Jose Alcaraz Mexia M et al: Osteochondroma of the thoracic spine and scoliosis. Spine. 26(9):1082-5, 2001
7. Wuyts W et al: Molecular basis of multiple exostoses: mutations in the EXT1 and EXT2 genes. Hum Mutat. 15(3):220-7, 2000
8. Ratliff J et al: Osteochondroma of the C5 lamina with cord compression: case report and review of the literature. Spine. 25(10):1293-5, 2000
9. Murphey MD et al: Imaging of osteochondroma: variants and complications with radiologic-pathologic correlation. Radiographics. 20(5):1407-34, 2000
10. Silber JS et al: A solitary osteochondroma of the pediatric thoracic spine: a case report and review of the literature. Am J Orthop. 29(9):711-4, 2000
11. Govender S et al: Osteochondroma with compression of the spinal cord. A report of two cases. J Bone Joint Surg Br. 81(4):667-9, 1999
12. Okuyama K et al: Huge solitary osteochondroma at T11 level causing myelopathy: case report. Spinal Cord. 35(11):773-6, 1997
13. Mikawa Y et al: Cervical spinal cord compression in hereditary multiple exostoses. Report of a case and a review of the literature. Arch Orthop Trauma Surg. 116(1-2):112-5, 1997
14. Murphey MD et al: From the archives of the AFIP. Primary tumors of the spine: radiologic pathologic correlation. Radiographics. 16(5):1131-58, 1996
15. Morikawa M et al: Osteochondroma of the cervical spine: MR findings. Clin Imaging. 19: 275-8, 1995

Typical

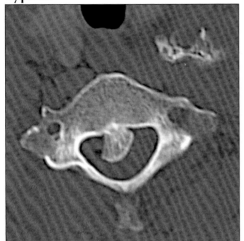
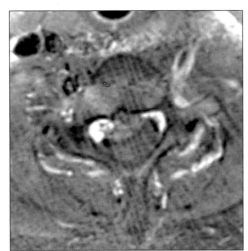

(Left) Axial bone CT shows a typical exostosis protruding into central spinal canal. Marrow contiguity with vertebral body is typical. *(Right)* Axial T1 C+ MR shows a typical exostosis protruding into central spinal canal, producing cord compression. Marrow enhances minimally, similar to parent vertebral body.

Typical

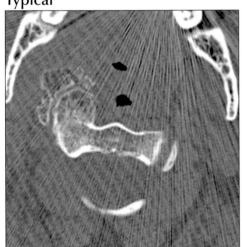
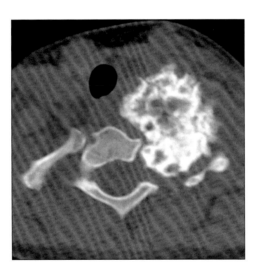

(Left) Axial bone CT shows a mature C2 osteochondroma with ossification of cartilaginous cap (adult patient with soft tissue impingement symptoms). *(Right)* Axial bone CT shows large left T1 exostosis with typical "cauliflower" ossification. Patient presented with brachial plexopathy secondary to regional neural compression.

Typical

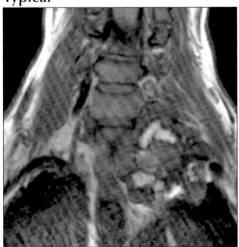
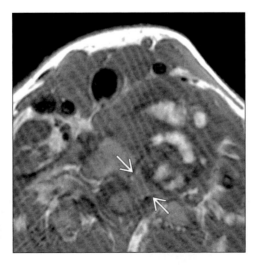

(Left) Coronal T1WI MR demonstrates a large left T1 osteochondroma, with internal marrow high signal and hypointense cartilaginous cap. *(Right)* Axial T1WI MR shows a large left T1 osteochondroma presenting with brachial plexopathy in an HME patient. Tumor fills left C7/T1 foramen (arrows).

CHONDROSARCOMA

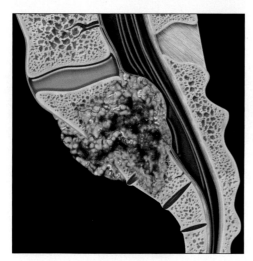

Sagittal graphic of lumbosacral junction shows large soft tissue mass destroying bone, with presacral and epidural extension.

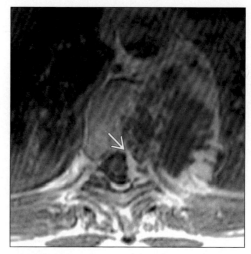

Axial T1 C+ MR shows large mass with peripheral irregular enhancement arising from left side of thoracic vertebral body. There is extension of tumor to left epidural space (arrow).

TERMINOLOGY

Abbreviations and Synonyms
- Conventional chondrosarcoma, dedifferentiated chondrosarcoma, mesenchymal chondrosarcoma

Definitions
- Malignant tumor of connective tissue, characterized by formation of cartilage matrix by tumor cells

IMAGING FINDINGS

General Features
- Best diagnostic clue: Lytic mass with or without chondroid matrix, cortical disruption and extension into soft tissues
- Location
  - Flat bones
    - Pelvis: 25%
    - Ilium: 15%
    - Pubis and ischium: 9%
    - Scapula: 5%
  - Ribs and sternum: 12%
  - Metaphysis/diaphysis of long bones, may extend into epiphysis
    - Femur: 15%
    - Tibia: 5%
    - Humerus: 10%
  - Craniofacial bones: 2%, can arise from laryngeal cartilage
  - Spine and sacrum: 5%
  - Soft tissues (extraskeletal chondrosarcoma)
- Size: 1-40 cm, mean: 10 cm
- Morphology: Ill-defined lytic lesion with or without chondroid matrix

Radiographic Findings
- Radiography
  - Lytic mass with or without chondroid matrix
  - Medullary (central) chondrosarcoma: 85%
    - Expansion of medullary cavity
    - Thickening of cortex with endosteal scalloping
    - Popcorn-like ring and arc calcification
    - Cortical disruption with extension into soft tissue in advanced stages
  - Exostotic (peripheral) chondrosarcoma
    - Thickening of cortex and soft tissue mass at site of attachment to bone
    - Chondroid matrix
    - Late destruction of bone
  - Dedifferentiated chondrosarcoma: 10%
    - Ill-defined, lytic lesion in continuity with cartilaginous tumor
    - Abrupt transition between cartilaginous tumor and dedifferentiated lytic component
  - Mesenchymal chondrosarcoma: < 1%

DDx: Masses with Heterogeneous MR Signal

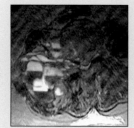
Osteosarcoma

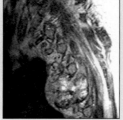
Renal Cell Met

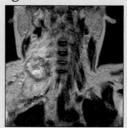
Myositis Ossificans

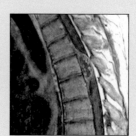
Chondromyxoid Fib

CHONDROSARCOMA

Key Facts

Imaging Findings
- Best diagnostic clue: Lytic mass with or without chondroid matrix, cortical disruption and extension into soft tissues
- Chondroid matrix mineralization of "rings and arcs" (characteristic)

Top Differential Diagnoses
- Lymphoma/metastatic disease
- Chondroblastoma/low grade chondroid lesion
- Osteogenic sarcoma (OGS)
- Malignant fibrous histiocytoma (MFH)
- Myositis ossificans

Pathology
- Can occur as primary chondrosarcoma or as malignant degeneration of osteochondroma or enchondroma
- Third most common primary malignant bone tumor
- 10-25% of all primary bone sarcomas
- Extraskeletal chondrosarcoma: 2% of all soft tissue sarcomas

Clinical Issues
- Dull aching pain at rest, may be severe at night
- Soft tissue swelling, mass
- Prognosis depends on location, size, and histologic grade
- Overall 5 year survival: 48-60%
- Wide surgical excision

- ■ Aggressive lytic bone destruction
- ■ Predilection for mandible, femur, ribs
- ○ Clear cell chondrosarcoma: 5%
  - ■ Round, sharply-marginated, lytic lesion
  - ■ Involves epiphysis of long bones
  - ■ May contain calcifications
  - ■ Surrounding sclerosis
  - ■ Indistinguishable from chondroblastoma (slow growth over years)
- ○ Extraskeletal chondrosarcoma
  - ■ Lobulated soft tissue mass with and without calcification
  - ■ Extremities (thigh) most common

CT Findings
- NECT
  - ○ Chondroid matrix mineralization of "rings and arcs" (characteristic)
  - ○ Nonmineralized portions of tumor hypodense to muscle
    - ■ High water content of hyaline cartilage

MR Findings
- T1WI
  - ○ To determine intramedullary extent and soft tissue invasion
  - ○ Low to intermediate signal intensity
- T2WI: High signal (hyaline cartilage), areas of low signal intensity (mineralization)
- T1 C+
  - ○ Enhancement of septa with ring and arc pattern
  - ○ Nonenhancing areas represent hyaline cartilage, cystic mucoid tissue, necrosis

Nuclear Medicine Findings
- Bone Scan
  - ○ Increased uptake of radiotracer
  - ○ Overestimates extent of lesion due to surrounding hyperemia and edema

Imaging Recommendations
- Best imaging tool: CT shows bone destruction, calcification, extent
- Protocol advice

- ○ CT to evaluate for chondroid matrix, cortical destruction, intra- and extraosseous extension
- ○ MRI to evaluate intramedullary extent and relationship to neurovascular bundle

DIFFERENTIAL DIAGNOSIS

Lymphoma/metastatic disease
- Soft tissue mass
- Irregular margins, multiple sites involved

Chondroblastoma/low grade chondroid lesion
- May be indistinguishable from clear cell chondrosarcoma

Osteogenic sarcoma (OGS)
- Osteoid matrix
- No chondroid matrix
- Usually younger patients

Malignant fibrous histiocytoma (MFH)
- Often purely lytic
- Can have areas of sclerosis, no chondroid matrix
- No significant periosteal reaction

Myositis ossificans
- History of trauma
- Mass has large soft tissue component

PATHOLOGY

General Features
- General path comments: Malignant tumor in which neoplastic cells form cartilage
- Genetics
  - ○ Grade 1 chondrosarcomas: Diploid
  - ○ Grade 2 and 3 chondrosarcomas: Aneuploid, correlate with aggressive behavior
  - ○ High grade lesions: Complex chromosomal aberration with nonreciprocal translocations and deletions

CHONDROSARCOMA

- Accumulation of p53 protein, may be indicator of poor prognosis
- Etiology
  - Can occur as primary chondrosarcoma or as malignant degeneration of osteochondroma or enchondroma
  - Exostotic (peripheral) chondrosarcoma
    - Malignant degeneration of hereditary multiple exostoses, Ollier disease
    - Can arise in cartilage cap of a previously benign osteochondroma
- Epidemiology
  - Third most common primary malignant bone tumor
  - 10-25% of all primary bone sarcomas
  - Extraskeletal chondrosarcoma: 2% of all soft tissue sarcomas

Gross Pathologic & Surgical Features

- Lobulated tumor composed of translucent hyaline nodules (resemble normal cartilage)
  - Mineralization at periphery of nodules
- Focal ivory-like areas represent extensive enchondral ossification
- Hemorrhagic necrosis, especially in high grade tumors
- Central lesions erode and destroy cortex with extension into surrounding soft tissue
  - Cortical disruption earlier in flat bones due to narrow medullary cavity
- Extraosseous component grows on outer bone surface
  - Encircles affected bone

Microscopic Features

- Irregular-shaped lobules of cartilage
- May be separated by narrow, fibrous bands
- Chondrocytes arranged in clusters, can be mononuclear or multinucleated
- Matrix: Mature hyaline cartilage or myxoid stroma
- Immunohistochemistry: Positive for S-100 protein and vimentin
- Dedifferentiated chondrosarcoma: Two components that coexist in one tumor
  - High grade sarcoma +/- heterologous elements (MFH, OGS)
  - Low grade cartilaginous lesion

Staging, Grading or Classification Criteria

- Grade 1 chondrosarcoma: Slowly growing, locally aggressive, indolent course
  - Recurrent growth potential, no metastatic spread
  - Diagnosis requires supportive evidence from clinical and radiographic data
- Grade 2 chondrosarcoma: Locally aggressive tumor with great potential for local recurrence
  - Metastases in 10-15%
- Grade 3 chondrosarcoma: Highly aggressive, rapidly growing
  - Metastases > 50%

CLINICAL ISSUES

Presentation
- Most common signs/symptoms
  - Dull aching pain at rest, may be severe at night

- Duration of symptoms - several months to years
- Clinical profile
  - Soft tissue swelling, mass
  - If lesion is close to joint, restricted range of motion

Demographics
- Age: 20-90 years, peak: 40-60 years
- Gender: M:F = 2:1

Natural History & Prognosis
- Prognosis depends on location, size, and histologic grade
  - Overall 5 year survival: 48-60%
  - 5 year survival 90% for grade 1, 81% for grade 2, 29% for grade 3 tumors
- Recurrence 5-10 years after surgery
  - Recurrence can be associated with increased histologic grade and more aggressive behavior
- Metastases (lung, lymph nodes, liver, kidneys, brain): 66% (grade 3 chondrosarcomas)
- Degeneration into fibrosarcoma, malignant fibrous histiocytoma, osteosarcoma in 10%
- Pelvic chondrosarcoma may invade bladder or colon
- Pathologic fractures rare

Treatment
- Wide surgical excision
- Limited role for chemotherapy or radiation therapy
  - For high grade chondrosarcomas
- Biopsies must be planned with future tumor excision in mind

DIAGNOSTIC CHECKLIST

Consider
- Enlarging or painful enchondroma or osteochondroma suspicious for sarcomatous transformation
- Clear cell chondrosarcoma may be indistinguishable from benign chondroid lesions (chondroblastoma, enchondroma)
- Always consult orthopedic surgeon before biopsy of possible chondrosarcoma

SELECTED REFERENCES
1. Greenspan A et al: Differential diagnosis of tumors and tumor-like lesions of bones and joints. 1st ed. Philadelphia PA, Lippincott-Raven. 169-98, 1998
2. Dorfman HD et al: Bone tumors. 1st ed. St. Louis MO, Mosby. 353-440, 1998
3. Bjornsson J et al: Primary chondrosarcoma of long bones and limb girdles. Cancer. 83:2105-19, 1998
4. Swarts SJ et al: Chromosomal abnormalities in low grade chondrosarcoma and a review of the literature. Cancer Genet Cytogenet .98:126-30, 1997
5. Mercuri M et al: Dedifferentiated chondrosarcoma. Skeletal Radiol. 24:409-16, 1995
6. Aoki J et al: MR of enchondroma and chondrosarcoma: Rings and arcs of Gd-DTPA enhancement. J Comput Assist Tomogr.15:1011-6, 1991

CHONDROSARCOMA

IMAGE GALLERY

Typical

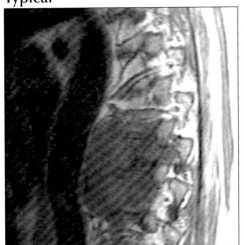 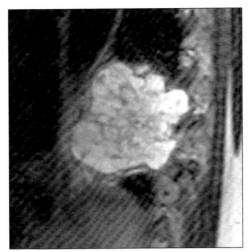

(Left) Sagittal T1WI MR shows large soft tissue mass involving left paravertebral region, extending over multiple levels. *(Right)* Sagittal T2WI MR in same patient shows lobulated mass of increased signal. There is typical linear striations within the mass consistent with chondroid lesion.

Typical

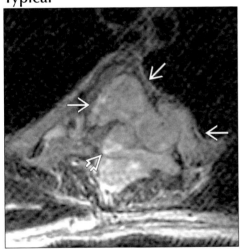 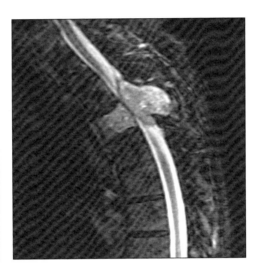

(Left) Axial T2WI MR shows a large, lobulated hyperintense mass involving thoracic body (arrows) with epidural extension (open arrow). *(Right)* Sagittal STIR MR shows hyperintense mass involving upper thoracic body and posterior elements. There is a large amount of dorsal epidural extension with cord compression.

Typical

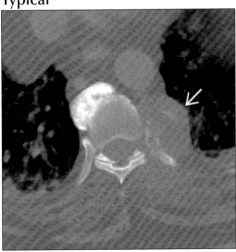 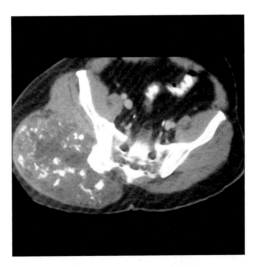

(Left) Axial NECT shows destruction of medial rib, and calcific matrix (arrow) within left paravertebral soft tissue mass. *(Right)* Axial NECT shows a large, partially calcified mass adjacent to the right sacrum, consistent with a soft tissue chondrosarcoma (Courtesy D. Stoller, MD).

OSTEOSARCOMA

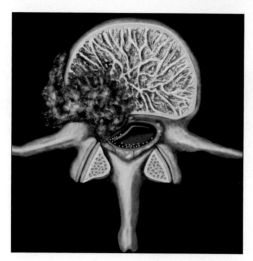

Axial graphic shows secondary osteosarcoma arising in Pagetic vertebral body, destroying cortex & invading adjacent soft tissues. Tumor has wide zone of transition.

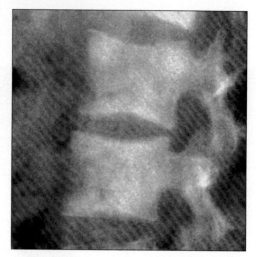

Lateral radiography shows metastatic OGS to lumbar spine. Multiple deposits of amorphous bone matrix are visible in vertebral bodies and pedicles.

TERMINOLOGY

Abbreviations and Synonyms
- Osteogenic sarcoma (OGS)

Definitions
- Sarcoma containing osteoid produced directly by the malignant cells
- Matrix (material produced by tumor cells) is immature, woven osteoid

IMAGING FINDINGS

General Features
- Best diagnostic clue: Aggressive lesion forming immature bone
- Location
  - 4% of all primary OGS occur in spine and sacrum
  - 79% arise in posterior elements
  - 17% involve 2 adjacent spinal levels
  - 84% invade spinal canal
- Size: Several centimeters

Radiographic Findings
- Radiography
  - Wide zone of transition
  - Permeative appearance
  - Cortical breakthrough and soft tissue mass
  - 80% have bone matrix seen on radiographs and/or CT scan
  - 20% have lytic appearance without visible bone matrix

CT Findings
- CECT: Contrast administration tends to obscure bone matrix and is not recommended
- Bone CT
  - Best visualization of bone matrix, wide zone of transition, soft tissue mass
  - Moth eaten bone destruction

MR Findings
- T1WI
  - Low signal intensity: Mineralized tumor
  - Low-intermediate signal intensity: Solid, nonmineralized tumor
- T2WI
  - Low signal intensity: Mineralized tumor
  - High signal intensity: Nonmineralized tumor, soft tissue mass
  - Fluid/fluid levels seen in telangiectatic OGS
- Appearance similar to other sarcomas; use CT for matrix visualization

Nuclear Medicine Findings
- Bone Scan
  - Increased uptake on all three phases

DDx: Osteogenic Sarcoma

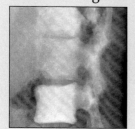

Metastasis

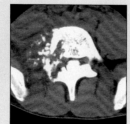

Osteoblastoma

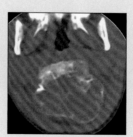

ABC

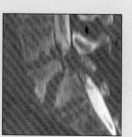

Osteomyelitis

OSTEOSARCOMA

Key Facts

Terminology
- Sarcoma containing osteoid produced directly by the malignant cells

Imaging Findings
- 4% of all primary OGS occur in spine and sacrum
- 79% arise in posterior elements
- 17% involve 2 adjacent spinal levels
- 84% invade spinal canal
- Wide zone of transition
- Permeative appearance
- Cortical breakthrough and soft tissue mass
- 80% have bone matrix seen on radiographs and/or CT scan
- 20% have lytic appearance without visible bone matrix

- Best imaging tool: CT scan

Top Differential Diagnoses
- Sclerotic metastasis
- Osteoblastoma (OB)
- Aneurysmal bone cyst (ABC)
- Osteomyelitis
- Ewing sarcoma
- Chondrosarcoma
- Lymphoma

Clinical Issues
- Insidious onset of back pain
- Median survival 23 months in recent series
- Lower survival rate in sacral tumors

- o For staging, detection of skip lesions, metastases
- PET: Useful in evaluating tumor recurrence

Imaging Recommendations
- Best imaging tool: CT scan
- Protocol advice
  - o MDCT 1-3 mm with reformatted images
  - o MR useful to evaluate for cord, nerve root impingement
  - o Staging should also include bone scan and chest CT scan

DIFFERENTIAL DIAGNOSIS

Sclerotic metastasis
- Most commonly prostate, breast, gastrointestinal
- Sclerosis reactive; doesn't extend beyond borders of bone
- Often multiple

Osteoblastoma (OB)
- Expansile, bone forming lesion in posterior elements
- Can extend into vertebral body
- Aggressive osteoblastoma mimics OGS on imaging studies
- A difficult histologic differential diagnosis

Aneurysmal bone cyst (ABC)
- Fluid-fluid levels similar to telangiectatic OGS
- Expansile lesion centered in posterior elements
- Can have cortical breakthrough
- Zone of transition is narrow, unlike telangiectatic OGS

Osteomyelitis
- Occasionally sclerotic
- Usually involves 2 contiguous vertebrae and intervening disc space

Ewing sarcoma
- Can rarely be sclerotic
- Tends to permeate through cortex rather than cause a large visible area of destruction

Chondrosarcoma
- Ring and arc calcifications

Lymphoma
- Moth-eaten lytic bone destruction
- Can rarely be sclerotic

Malignant giant cell tumor
- Rare entity, most common in sacrum
- Lytic, aggressive mass without bone matrix formation
- Histologically similar to giant-cell rich OGS

Giant bone island
- Sclerotic focus in medullary bone
- Mature cortical bone
- Shows "brush border": Trabeculae merge with adjacent bone

PATHOLOGY

General Features
- General path comments
  - o Malignant tumor which produces osteoid directly from neoplastic cells
  - o Secondary osteosarcoma occurs in Paget disease, irradiated bone, bone infarct
  - o Other malignant tumors (e.g., chondrosarcoma) may contain bone but osteoid is not produced by the malignant cells
- Genetics: Alterations of Rb genes in OGS that develops in association with retinoblastoma
- Etiology
  - o Majority of OGS of unknown etiology = primary OGS
  - o Secondary to predisposing factors (Paget disease, bone infarct, radiation) = secondary OGS
  - o Associated with retinoblastoma
- Epidemiology: OGS is second most common primary bone malignancy (after multiple myeloma)

OSTEOSARCOMA

Gross Pathologic & Surgical Features
- Heterogeneous mass with ossified and non-ossified components
- Ossified areas: Yellow-white, firm, may be as hard as cortical bone
- Less ossified areas: Soft, tan, with foci of hemorrhage and necrosis
- Cortical breakthrough with often large extraosseous tumor mass
- Necrosis common

Microscopic Features
- Pluripotential neoplasm
- Malignant cells produce some osteoid in all subtypes, but it may be difficult to find
- Classic: High degree anaplasia, high mitotic rate
- Tumor cells may be spindle or round, size varies from small to giant
- Telangiectatic OGS
  - Dilated vascular channels lined by multinucleated giant cells
  - Stroma forms osteoid, which may not be a prominent feature

Staging, Grading or Classification Criteria
- Classified by predominant cell type histologically
  - Osteoblastic (conventional), chondroblastic, fibroblastic, telangiectatic, small cell, giant cell, epithelioid
  - Surface OGS not reported in spine
- Surgical staging for malignant musculoskeletal tumors
  - Stage Ia: Low grade, intracompartmental
  - Stage Ib: Low grade, extracompartmental
  - Stage IIa: High grade, intracompartmental
  - Stage IIb: High grade, extracompartmental
  - Stage IIIa: Low or high grade, intracompartmental, metastases
  - Stage IIIb: Low or high grade, extracompartmental, metastases

CLINICAL ISSUES

Presentation
- Most common signs/symptoms
  - Insidious onset of back pain
  - Pain greatest at night
  - Radicular pain
  - Paraplegia
- Clinical profile
  - Pathologic fracture
  - Pulmonary metastases common, can cause pneumothorax (calcifying)
  - Increased serum alkaline phosphatase

Demographics
- Age
  - Spine OGS has peak incidence in 4th decade
  - Later peak incidence than for appendicular OGS
  - Age range 8-80 years in one large series
- Gender: M = F

Natural History & Prognosis
- Median survival 23 months in recent series
- Lower survival rate in sacral tumors
- Survival rate lower than for peripheral OGS due to difficulty of surgical resection
- Metastases: Bone, lung, liver
- 3% of 10 year survivors of all OGS develop a second malignancy

Treatment
- Surgical resection with wide margins
- Adjuvant and neoadjuvant chemotherapy
- Biopsies must be planned with future tumor excision in mind

DIAGNOSTIC CHECKLIST

Image Interpretation Pearls
- All telangiectatic OGS are lytic on radiographs and CT, but not all lytic OGS are telangiectatic

SELECTED REFERENCES

1. Ilaslan H et al: Primary vertebral osteosarcoma: imaging findings. Radiology. 230(3):697-702, 2004
2. Brenner W et al: PET imaging of osteosarcoma. J Nucl Med. 44(6):930-42, 2003
3. Ozaki T et al: Osteosarcoma of the spine: experience of the Cooperative Osteosarcoma Study Group. Cancer. 94(4):1069-77, 2002
4. Bredella MA et al: Value of FDG PET in conjunction with MR imaging for evaluating therapy response in patients with musculoskeletal sarcomas. AJR Am J Roentgenol. 179(5):1145-50, 2002
5. Aung L et al: Second malignant neoplasms in long-term survivors of osteosarcoma: Memorial Sloan-Kettering Cancer Center Experience. Cancer. 95(8):1728-34, 2002
6. Yamamoto T et al: Sacral radiculopathy secondary to multicentric osteosarcoma. Spine. 26(15):1729-32, 2001
7. Iwata A et al: Osteosarcoma as a second malignancy after treatment for neuroblastoma. Pediatr Hematol Oncol. 18(7):465-9, 2001
8. Bramwell VH: Osteosarcomas and other cancers of bone. Curr Opin Oncol. 12(4):330-6, 2000
9. Vuillemin-Bodaghi V et al: Multifocal osteogenic sarcoma in Paget's disease. Skeletal Radiol. 29(6):349-53, 2000
10. Unni KK: Osteosarcoma of bone. J Orthop Sci. 3(5):287-94, 1998
11. Rosenberg ZS et al: Osteosarcoma: Subtle, rare, and misleading plain film features. Am J Roentgenol. 165:1209-14, 1995
12. Tigani D et al: Vertebral osteosarcoma. Ital J Orthop Traumatol. 14(1):5-13, 1988
13. Barwick KW et al: Primary osteogenic sarcoma of the vertebral column: a clinicopathologic correlation of ten patients. Cancer. 46(3):595-604, 1980

IMAGE GALLERY

Typical

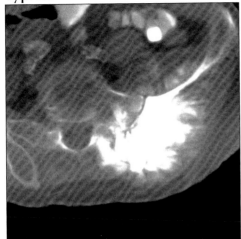
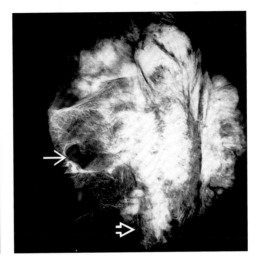

(Left) Axial bone CT shows amorphous ossification in sacrum and left ilium, crossing sacroiliac joint. ST mass is also densely ossified, a distinguishing feature of OGS. (Right) Anteroposterior specimen radiography shows resection of OGS involving sacrum and ilium. Left S1 neural foramen (arrow) lies medial to tumor, which crosses SI joint (open arrow).

Typical

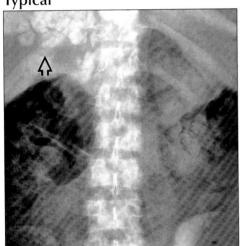
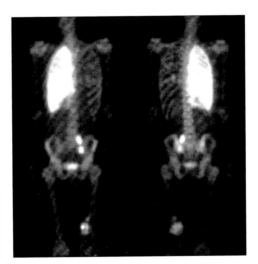

(Left) Anteroposterior radiography shows OGS metastatic to spine, with extensive blastic lesions. Ossified metastatic foci are also seen in the liver (arrow). (Right) Bone scan shows metastatic OGS to spine, ribs, pleural space, and pelvic lymph nodes from femoral primary.

Variant

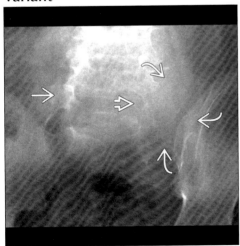
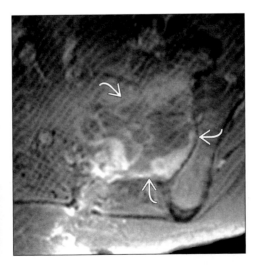

(Left) Anteroposterior radiography shows lytic OGS at left transitional vertebra (curved arrows). Right pedicle is normal (arrow), left pedicle is absent (open arrow). (Right) Axial T1 C+ MR shows telangiectatic OGS of sacrum (arrows). Fluid filled nonenhancing regions are present, as well as enhancing nodules.

CHORDOMA

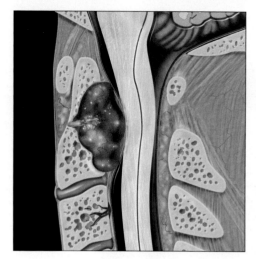

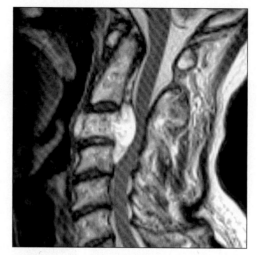

Sagittal graphic of cervical spine shows extradural soft tissue mass with epicenter in posterior aspect of C2 body, causing bone destruction and epidural extension with cord compression.

Sagittal T2WI MR shows hyperintense mass involving C3 body with extensive epidural extension and cord compression.

TERMINOLOGY

Definitions
- Malignant tumor arising from notochord remnants

IMAGING FINDINGS

General Features
- Best diagnostic clue
  - Mass is hyperintense to discs on T2WI, with multiple septa
  - Histologic identification of physaliphorous cell confirms diagnosis
- Location: Sacrococcygeal > spheno-occipital >> vertebral body
- Size: Several cm at presentation
- Morphology: Midline lobular soft tissue mass with osseous destruction

Radiographic Findings
- Radiography
  - Plain films: Lucent lesion with sclerosis
  - Heterogeneous destructive mass of sacrum or vertebral body
    - May extend into disc, involve 2 or more adjacent vertebrae
    - May extend into epidural/perivertebral space, compress cord
    - May extend along nerve roots, enlarge neural foramina
- Myelography: Large extradural mass

CT Findings
- NECT
  - Destructive, lytic lesion
  - Most have associated hypodense soft tissue mass
  - Sclerosis in 40-60%
  - Amorphous intratumoral Ca++
    - Sacrum > 70%
    - Vertebra 30%
- CECT
  - Mild/moderate enhancement
  - +/- Inhomogeneous areas (cystic necrosis)

MR Findings
- T1WI: Heterogeneous hypo- to isointense (compared to marrow)
- T2WI
  - Hyperintense to CSF, intervertebral discs
  - May have low signal septations (fibrous)
- T1 C+: Variable enhancement: Blush ⇒ intense enhancement

Nuclear Medicine Findings
- Bone Scan: Decreased uptake

DDx: Malignant Extradural Masses

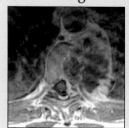

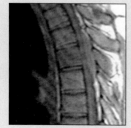

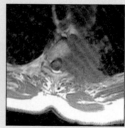

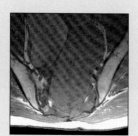

Chondrosarcoma   *Lymphoma*   *Metastasis*   *Giant Cell Tumor*

CHORDOMA

Key Facts

Terminology
- Malignant tumor arising from notochord remnants

Imaging Findings
- Mass is hyperintense to discs on T2WI, with multiple septa
- Histologic identification of physaliphorous cell confirms diagnosis
- Location: Sacrococcygeal > spheno-occipital > > vertebral body
- Size: Several cm at presentation
- Morphology: Midline lobular soft tissue mass with osseous destruction
- May extend into disc, involve 2 or more adjacent vertebrae

- May extend into epidural/perivertebral space, compress cord
- May extend along nerve roots, enlarge neural foramina
- Amorphous intratumoral Ca++

Pathology
- 3 types described
- Typical: Lobules, sheets, and cords of clear cells with intracytoplasmic vacuoles (physaliphorous cells); abundant mucin
- Chondroid: Hyaline cartilage (usually spheno-occipital region)
- Dedifferentiated: Sarcomatous elements (rare, highly malignant)

Imaging Recommendations
- MR for soft tissue (STIR/fat-saturated T2WI, contrast-enhanced T1WI)
- NECT for bone detail

DIFFERENTIAL DIAGNOSIS

Chondrosarcoma
- Neural arch > vertebral body
- Chondroid matrix (rings and arcs)
- Similar MR characteristics

Giant cell tumor
- Heterogeneous MR signal with blood products, low T2 signal

Metastases/multiple myeloma/lymphoma
- Multifocal disease; heterogeneous T2 signal

Sacrococcygeal teratoma
- Heterogeneous MR signal (fat - T1 hyperintense)
- Pediatric patients

Ecchordosis physaliphora (rare)
- Benign, nonneoplastic ectopic notochordal remnant(s)
- Usually at skull base/C2 but can occur anywhere (including intradural)

PATHOLOGY

General Features
- General path comments
  - Location
    - 2-4% of primary malignant bone tumors
    - Sacrococcygeal 50%; spheno-occipital 35%; vertebral body 15%
    - Vertebral body: Cervical (20-50%) > lumbar > thoracic
  - Embryology-anatomy
    - Tumor arises from notochordal remnants
- Genetics

  - Losses on chromosomal arms 3p (50%) and 1p (44%)
  - Gains on 7q (69%), 20 (50%), 5q (38%), and 12q (38%)
- Etiology: Arises from notochord remnants
- Epidemiology
  - 2-4% of primary malignant bone neoplasms
  - Incidence rate of 0.08 per 100,000
  - Rare among patients aged < 40 years

Gross Pathologic & Surgical Features
- Lobulated, soft, grayish gelatinous mass

Microscopic Features
- 3 types described
  - Typical: Lobules, sheets, and cords of clear cells with intracytoplasmic vacuoles (physaliphorous cells); abundant mucin
  - Chondroid: Hyaline cartilage (usually spheno-occipital region)
  - Dedifferentiated: Sarcomatous elements (rare, highly malignant)
- Immunohistochemistry: + Cytokeratin, + epithelial membrane antigen

Staging, Grading or Classification Criteria
- Enneking system for staging musculoskeletal sarcomas
  - Grade of biologic aggressiveness
  - Anatomic setting
  - Presence of metastasis

CLINICAL ISSUES

Presentation
- Most common signs/symptoms
  - Location dependent: Pain, numbness, weakness, incontinence
  - May show autonomic dysfunction
  - Sacral or gluteal mass
- Clinical profile: Middle-aged male presenting with spine pain

CHORDOMA

Demographics
- Age: Peak incidence 5th-6th decades (rare in children)
- Gender: M:F = 2:1 spine (no gender predilection in sacral chordoma)
- Ethnicity: Rare in African-Americans

Natural History & Prognosis
- Slow-growing
- Distant metastases 5-40% (lung, liver, lymph nodes, bone)
- Poor prognostic factors
  - Large size
  - Subtotal resection, local recurrence
  - Microscopic necrosis
  - Ki-67 index > 5%
- 5 year survival up to 67-84%
- 10 year survival 40%

Treatment
- Surgical resection with adjuvant XRT
  - En bloc resection yields best outcome
- Recurrence common
  - Local (90%)
  - Regional lymph nodes (5%)
  - Distant metastases (5%); lung, bone
  - 5 year survival after relapse (5-7%)

DIAGNOSTIC CHECKLIST

Consider
- High signal intensity mass on T2WI with septations, little enhancement is chordoma/chondroid tumor

Image Interpretation Pearls
- Recurrence (seeding) along operative tract is not uncommon, modify field-of-view to include operative approach

SELECTED REFERENCES

1. Smolders D et al: Value of MRI in the diagnosis of non-clival, non-sacral chordoma. Skeletal Radiol. 32(6):343-50, 2003
2. Noel G et al: Radiation therapy for chordoma and chondrosarcoma of the skull base and the cervical spine. Prognostic factors and patterns of failure. Strahlenther Onkol. 179(4):241-8, 2003
3. Baratti D et al: Chordoma: natural history and results in 28 patients treated at a single institution. Ann Surg Oncol. 10(3):291-6, 2003
4. Leone A et al: Chordoma of the low cervical spine presenting with Horner's syndrome. Eur Radiol. 12 Suppl 3:S43-7, 2002
5. Bayar MA et al: Spinal chordoma of the terminal filum. Case report. J Neurosurg. 96(2 Suppl):236-8, 2002
6. Carpentier A et al: Suboccipital and cervical chordomas: the value of aggressive treatment at first presentation of the disease. J Neurosurg. 97(5):1070-7, 2002
7. Steenberghs J et al: Intradural chordoma without bone involvement. Case report and review of the literature. J Neurosurg. 97(1 Suppl):94-7, 2002
8. Delank KS et al: Metastasizing chordoma of the lumbar spine. Eur Spine J. 11(2):167-71, 2002
9. Soo MY: Chordoma: review of clinicoradiological features and factors affecting survival. Australas Radiol. 45(4):427-34, 2001
10. Arnautovic KI et al: Surgical seeding of chordomas. J Neurosurg. 95(5):798-803, 2001
11. Scheil S et al: Genome-wide analysis of sixteen chordomas by comparative genomic hybridization and cytogenetics of the first human chordoma cell line, U-CH1. Genes Chromosomes Cancer. 32(3):203-11, 2001
12. Bosma JJ et al: En bloc removal of the lower lumbar vertebral body for chordoma. Report of two cases. J Neurosurg. 94(2 Suppl):284-91, 2001
13. Crapanzano JP et al: Chordoma: a cytologic study with histologic and radiologic correlation. Cancer. 93(1):40-51, 2001
14. McMaster ML et al: Chordoma: incidence and survival patterns in the United States, 1973-1995. Cancer Causes Control. 12(1):1-11, 2001
15. Bergh P et al: Prognostic factors in chordoma of the sacrum and mobile spine: a study of 39 patients. Cancer. 88:2122-34, 2000
16. Tai PT et al: Management issues in chordoma: a case series. Clin Oncol (R Coll Radiol). 12(2):80-6, 2000
17. Gelabert-Gonzalez M et al: Intradural cervical chordoma. Case report. J Neurosurg Sci. 43(2):159-62, 1999
18. Cheng EY et al: Lumbosacral chordoma. Prognostic factors and treatment. Spine. 24(16):1639-45, 1999
19. Wippold FJ 2nd et al: Clinical and imaging features of cervical chordoma. AJR Am J Roentgenol. 172(5):1423-6, 1999
20. York JE et al: Sacral chordoma: 40-year experience at a major cancer center. Neurosurgery. 44(1):74-9; discussion 79-80, 1999
21. Logroscino CA et al: Chordoma: long-term evaluation of 15 cases treated surgically. Chir Organi Mov. 83(1-2):87-103, 1998
22. Ng SH et al: Cervical ecchordosis physaliphora: CT and MR features. Br J Radiol. 71(843):329-31, 1998
23. Murphy JM et al: CT and MRI appearances of a thoracic chordoma. Eur Radiol. 8(9):1677-9, 1998
24. Boriani S et al: Primary bone tumors of the spine. Terminology and surgical staging. Spine. 22(9):1036-44, 1997
25. Catton C et al: Chordoma: long-term follow-up after radical photon irradiation. Radiother Oncol. 41(1):67-72, 1996
26. Murphey MD et al: From the archives of the AFIP. Primary tumors of the spine: radiologic pathologic correlation. Radiographics. 16(5):1131-58, 1996
27. Boriani S et al: Chordoma of the spine above the sacrum. Treatment and outcome in 21 cases. Spine. 21(13):1569-77, 1996
28. Klekamp J et al: Spinal chordomas--results of treatment over a 17-year period. Acta Neurochir (Wien). 138(5):514-9, 1996
29. Fagundes MA et al: Radiation therapy for chordomas of the base of skull and cervical spine: patterns of failure and outcome after relapse. Int J Radiat Oncol Biol Phys. 33(3):579-84, 1995
30. Hall WA et al: Sacrococcygeal chordoma metastatic to the brain with review of the literature. J Neurooncol. 25(2):155-9, 1995
31. Wojno KJ et al: Chondroid chordomas and low-grade chondrosarcomas of the craniospinal axis. An immunohistochemical analysis of 17 cases. Am J Surg Pathol. 16(12):1144-52, 1992

CHORDOMA

IMAGE GALLERY

Typical

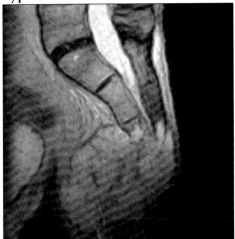
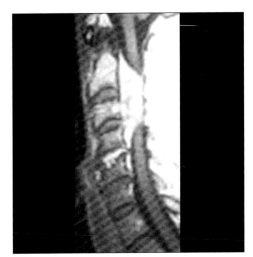

(Left) Sagittal T2WI MR shows large hyperintense mass destroying distal sacrum and extending into pelvis. *(Right)* Sagittal T1 C+ MR shows diffuse enhancement of extradural mass spanning C2 through C4. Enhancement in C4-5 disc relates to disc degeneration.

Typical

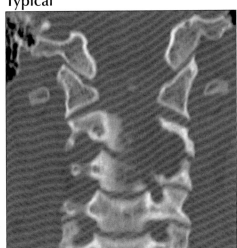
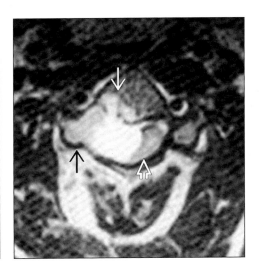

(Left) Coronal NECT shows destruction of left side of C2 and superior aspect of C3, with no internal calcific matrix. *(Right)* Axial T1 C+ MR shows enhancing extradural mass involving posterior vertebral body (white arrow), compressing cord (open arrow) and remodeling bone (black arrow).

Variant

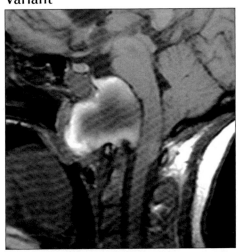
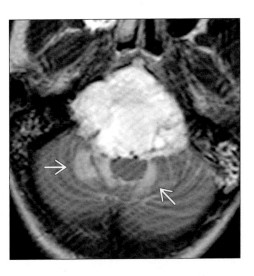

(Left) Sagittal T1WI MR shows large atypically hyperintense mass involving clivus and extending into C1-2 junction. Tumor mass effect compresses medulla and cervical cord. *(Right)* Axial T2WI MR shows typical high signal mass with multiple low signal septations. There are bilateral tonsillar infarcts from mass effect (arrows).

EWING SARCOMA

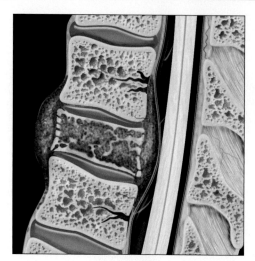

Sagittal graphic shows vertebral body replaced by Ewing sarcoma, resulting in mild collapse. Tumor extends into adjacent soft tissues through small perforations in bone cortex.

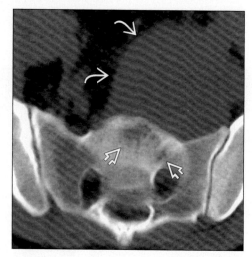

Axial bone CT shows ill-defined sacral Ewing sarcoma (open arrows). Cortex anteriorly is irregular, with tumor extending through cortical perforations into soft tissues (curved arrows).

TERMINOLOGY

Abbreviations and Synonyms
- Ewing's sarcoma, Ewing tumor

Definitions
- Round cell sarcoma of bone

IMAGING FINDINGS

General Features
- Best diagnostic clue: Permeative lytic lesion of vertebral body or sacrum
- Location
  - Spine: 5% of all Ewing tumor
  - Involve vertebral body before neural arch
  - Sacrum more common site than spine
  - May involve adjacent bones: Vertebrae, ribs, or ilium
  - Contiguous spread along peripheral nerves from spine or sacral primary
  - May originate in soft tissues

Radiographic Findings
- Radiography
  - Centered in vertebral body or sacrum
  - Permeative/moth eaten bone destruction
  - Wide zone of transition
  - Tiny perforations of cortex rather than extensive loss or cortical bone radiographically
  - 50% have extraosseous, noncalcified, soft tissue mass
  - 5% sclerotic (represents host reaction, not tumor matrix)
  - May cause vertebra plana
  - May involve 2 or more adjacent bones
  - If adjacent vertebrae involved, do not see disc height loss and peridiscal erosions as in osteomyelitis

CT Findings
- CECT
  - Heterogeneous enhancement
  - Areas of central necrosis common
- Bone CT
  - Permeative intramedullary mass +/- soft tissue mass
  - Tiny perforations through cortex more common than widespread breakthrough
  - Rarely sclerotic; no ossification in soft tissue mass

MR Findings
- T1WI
  - Intermediate to low signal intensity
  - Hypointense compared to surrounding bone marrow
  - Cortex often appears thinned but intact despite extraosseous tumor spread
- T2WI
  - Intermediate to high signal intensity

DDx: Ewing Sarcoma

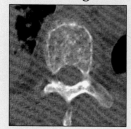

Myeloma

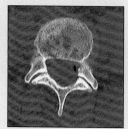

Osteomyelitis

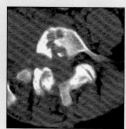

Osteomyelitis

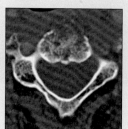

Chondrosarcoma

EWING SARCOMA

Key Facts

Terminology
- Round cell sarcoma of bone

Imaging Findings
- Centered in vertebral body or sacrum
- Permeative/moth eaten bone destruction
- Wide zone of transition
- Tiny perforations of cortex rather than extensive loss or cortical bone radiographically
- 50% have extraosseous, noncalcified, soft tissue mass
- MRI best shows involvement of adjacent bones & soft tissues, which can be underestimated on CT scan

Top Differential Diagnoses
- Primitive neuroectodermal tumor (PNET)
- Langerhans cell histiocytosis
- Other small round cell tumors

- Osteomyelitis
- Osteogenic sarcoma (OGS)
- Other primary sarcomas and metastatic disease

Pathology
- Primitive neuroectodermal tumor (PNET) is closely related tumor
- 6th most common malignant bone tumor

Clinical Issues
- Localized pain
- Fever, leukocytosis, elevated ESR (simulating osteomyelitis)
- Prognosis worse in spinal than peripheral Ewing sarcoma because of difficulty of surgical resection
- Significant risk of second malignancy

- o Cannot reliably distinguish between tumor/peritumor edema
- STIR: Tumor more conspicuous than on T2WI
- T1 C+
  - o Moderate enhancement
  - o Areas of necrosis
  - o Cannot reliably distinguish between tumor/peritumoral edema

Nuclear Medicine Findings
- Bone Scan: Positive 3-phase bone scan
- PET: Increased FDG uptake of tumor, metastases

Imaging Recommendations
- Best imaging tool
  - o MRI best shows involvement of adjacent bones & soft tissues, which can be underestimated on CT scan
  - o May overestimate tumor size due to peritumoral edema
- Protocol advice
  - o MRI to determine extent of tumor
    - ▪ Sagittal T1WI
    - ▪ Axial and Sagittal STIR, post-contrast T1WI
  - o CT useful to confirm absence of tumor matrix, distinguish from OGS

DIFFERENTIAL DIAGNOSIS

Primitive neuroectodermal tumor (PNET)
- Clinically/radiologically identical to Ewing sarcoma
- Greater neuroectodermal differentiation of tumor cells

Langerhans cell histiocytosis
- May have identical radiographic appearance
- May form discrete geographic lytic lesion

Other small round cell tumors
- Lymphoma, leukemia, myeloma, metastatic neuroblastoma
- Have same radiographic appearance as Ewing sarcoma
- Ill-defined lytic lesion showing permeative pattern
- Involve vertebral body more than neural arch

- Often involve multiple vertebrae

Osteomyelitis
- Ill-defined lytic lesion showing permeative pattern
- May be more geographic (intraosseous abscess with peripheral enhancement)
- Involves vertebral body more than neural arch
- Discocentric: Extends from one vertebral body to adjacent vertebra across disc
- Disc height loss, enhancement of disc on MRI, endplate erosions
- Soft tissue mass common

Osteogenic sarcoma (OGS)
- Ill-defined lytic lesion showing permeative pattern
- 80% show bone matrix on radiographs or CT
- Involves vertebral body or neural arch
- May involve adjacent vertebral body

Other primary sarcomas and metastatic disease
- Include: Chondrosarcoma, malignant fibrous histiocytoma, malignant giant cell tumor (GCT)
- Ill defined lytic lesion showing permeative pattern
- Tend to have more focal and complete cortical destruction
- Involve vertebral body, +/- neural arch

PATHOLOGY

General Features
- General path comments
  - o Prototype of non-hematologic small round cell tumor
  - o Primitive neuroectodermal tumor (PNET) is closely related tumor
- Genetics: Reciprocal translocation between EWS gene on chromosome 22 and ETS-like genes on chromosome 11
- Etiology: Undifferentiated mesenchymal cells with slight differentiation toward neuroectodermal cells
- Epidemiology

EWING SARCOMA

○ Annual incidence of Ewing sarcoma all locations: 3/1,000,000 Caucasian children < 15 years old
○ 6th most common malignant bone tumor

Gross Pathologic & Surgical Features

• Grayish white tumor
• Poorly demarcated
• Areas of hemorrhage, cyst formation, necrosis

Microscopic Features

• Small, round cells (2-3 times larger than lymphocytes), meager cytoplasm
• Cell outlines indistinct
• Round nuclei, frequent indentations, high mitotic rate
• Solid sheets of cells divided into irregular masses by fibrous strands
• Features which distinguish PNET from Ewing sarcoma
  ○ PNET forms rosettes of cells
  ○ PNET is positive for 2 or more neuroectodermal markers
  ○ Distinction most reliably made with Fluorescence in Situ Hybridization (FISH)

CLINICAL ISSUES

Presentation

• Most common signs/symptoms
  ○ Localized pain
  ○ Fever, leukocytosis, elevated ESR (simulating osteomyelitis)
  ○ Vertebra plana
  ○ Neurologic symptoms ranging from radiculopathy to paralysis

Demographics

• Age
  ○ 90% of all Ewing sarcoma patients present before 20 years
  ○ Second (smaller) peak at age 50 years
  ○ Spine and sacral lesions often in older patients than peripheral Ewing sarcoma
• Gender: M:F = 2:1

Natural History & Prognosis

• Metastases to lung, regional lymph nodes, and other bones in 30% at presentation
• Prognosis worse in spinal than peripheral Ewing sarcoma because of difficulty of surgical resection
• Significant risk of second malignancy
• Current treatments yield long term survival > 50% of patients with localized disease at presentation
• Complications common > 5 years after treatment
  ○ Local recurrence
  ○ Metastases
  ○ Treatment complications
  ○ Second malignancies

Treatment

• Surgery or radiotherapy; without chemotherapy universally fatal
• Neoadjuvant chemotherapy given prior to surgery
• Surgical resection with wide margins
• Radiation therapy for surgically inaccessible lesions, stage III disease, poor response to chemotherapy

DIAGNOSTIC CHECKLIST

Image Interpretation Pearls

• Always consider osteomyelitis and other small round cell tumors in imaging differential diagnosis

SELECTED REFERENCES

1. Bacci G et al: Long-term outcome for patients with non-metastatic Ewing's sarcoma treated with adjuvant and neoadjuvant chemotherapies. 402 patients treated at Rizzoli between 1972 and 1992. Eur J Cancer. 40(1):73-83, 2004
2. Caksen H et al: A case of metastatic spinal Ewing's sarcoma misdiagnosed as brucellosis and transverse myelitis. Neurol Sci. 24(6):414-6, 2004
3. Fuchs B et al: Complications in long-term survivors of Ewing sarcoma. Cancer. 98(12):2687-92, 2003
4. Burchill SA: Ewing's sarcoma: diagnostic, prognostic, and therapeutic implications of molecular abnormalities. J Clin Pathol. 56(2):96-102, 2003
5. Bacci G et al: Therapy and survival after recurrence of Ewing's tumors: the Rizzoli experience in 195 patients treated with adjuvant and neoadjuvant chemotherapy from 1979 to 1997. Ann Oncol. 14(11):1654-9, 2003
6. Fuchs B et al: Ewing's sarcoma and the development of secondary malignancies. Clin Orthop. (415):82-9, 2003
7. Hawkins DS et al: Evaluation of chemotherapy response in pediatric bone sarcomas by [F-18]-fluorodeoxy-D-glucose positron emission tomography. Cancer. 94:3277-84, 2002
8. Goktepe AS et al: Paraplegia: an unusual presentation of Ewing's sarcoma. Spinal Cord. 40(7):367-9, 2002
9. Hoffer FA: Primary skeletal neoplasms: osteosarcoma and ewing sarcoma. Top Magn Reson Imaging. 13(4):231-9, 2002
10. Paulussen M et al: Ewing tumour: incidence, prognosis and treatment options. Paediatr Drugs. 3(12):899-913, 2001
11. Devoe K et al: Immunohistochemistry of small round-cell tumors. Semin Diagn Pathol. 17:216-24, 2000
12. Llombart-Bosch A et al: Histology, immunohistochemistry, and electron microscopy of small round cell tumors of bone. Semin Diagn Pathol. 13:153-70, 1996
13. Eggli KD et al: Ewing's sarcoma. Radiol Clin North Am. 31:325-37, 1993
14. Downing JR et al: Detection of the (11;22)(q24;q12) translocation of Ewing's sarcoma and peripheral neuroectodermal tumor by reverse transcription polymerase chain reaction. Am J Pathol. 143:1294-300, 1993
15. Boyko OB et al: MR imaging of osteogenic and Ewing's sarcoma. Am J Roentgenol. 148:317-22, 1987

IMAGE GALLERY

Typical

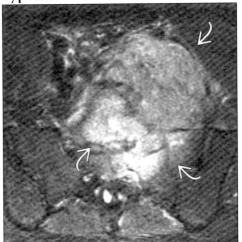 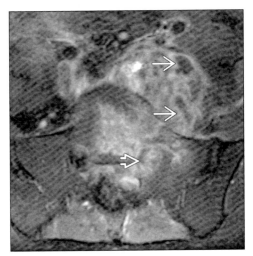

(Left) Axial STIR MR shows sacral Ewing sarcoma with heterogeneous signal intensity mass (arrows) extending through cortical perforations into presacral soft tissues. Patient presented with radiculopathy. *(Right)* Axial T1 C+ MR shows sacral Ewing sarcoma containing areas of necrosis (arrows) within enhancing mass. Note extension of tumor into left S1 neural foramen (open arrow).

Typical

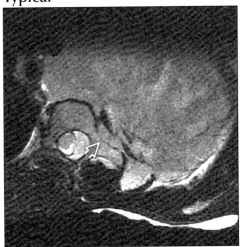 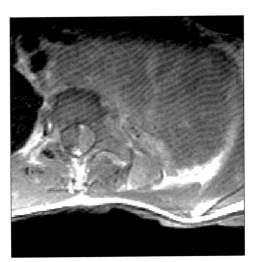

(Left) Axial T2WI MR shows metastatic Ewing sarcoma of thoracic vertebra, spinal canal, adjacent rib, and thoracic cavity. Note cortical thinning and indistinctness in areas of tumor permeation (arrow). *(Right)* Axial T1 C+ MR shows metastatic Ewing sarcoma of thoracic vertebra, spinal canal, adjacent rib, and thoracic cavity. There is moderate, heterogeneous enhancement.

Variant

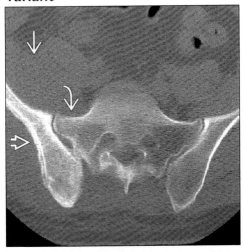 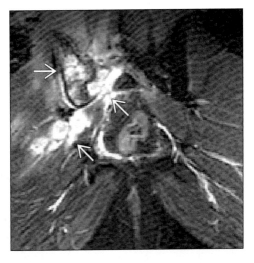

(Left) Axial bone CT shows sclerotic Ewing sarcoma of sacrum (curved arrow) and ilium (open arrow). Sacral involvement was better seen on subsequent MR. Tumor extends into iliacus muscle (arrow). *(Right)* Coronal STIR MR shows Ewing tumor (arrows) in sacrum, paraspinous soft tissues, and along right sciatic nerve. MR appearance is typical, but lesion showed atypical sclerosis on CT scan.

LYMPHOMA

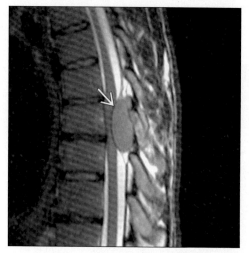

Sagittal T2WI MR demonstrates a focal lymphoma deposit in the spinal epidural space. Note hypointense dura interposed between tumor and cord (arrow).

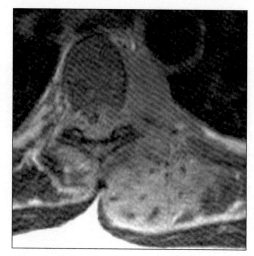

Axial T1 C+ MR shows extensive epidural lymphoma also involving adjacent structures (paraspinal muscles, pleura, rib).

TERMINOLOGY

Definitions
- Lymphoreticular neoplasms with wide variety of specific diseases & cellular differentiation

IMAGING FINDINGS

General Features
- Location
  - Multiple types with variable imaging manifestations
    - Epidural lymphoma (epidural): Thoracic > lumbar > cervical
    - Osseous lymphoma (osseous): Long bones > spine
    - Lymphomatous leptomeningitis (leptomeningitic)
    - Intramedullary lymphoma (intramedullary): Cervical > thoracic > lumbar
  - Secondary > primary involvement
    - 30% of systemic lymphomas have skeletal involvement
    - Primary osseous lymphoma = 3-4% of all malignant bone tumors
  - Extradural > intradural > intramedullary
  - Common: Epidural extension from adjacent vertebral/paraspinous disease
- Best imaging clue(s)
  - Epidural: Enhancing epidural mass +/- vertebral involvement
  - Osseous: Bone destruction ("ivory" vertebra, rare)
  - Leptomeningitic: Smooth/nodular pial enhancement
  - Intramedullary: Poorly-defined enhancing mass

Radiographic Findings
- Radiography
  - Epidural: May see bony erosion
  - Osseous
    - Bone destruction (30-40%)
    - Rare "ivory" vertebral body, vertebra plana

CT Findings
- NECT: Epidural: Homogeneous, slightly dense mass, +/- bone involvement
- CECT: Epidural: Homogeneous enhancement
- Bone CT
  - Osseous
    - Lytic, permeative bone destruction
    - May cross disc spaces
    - +/- Soft tissue mass
    - Often spreads over multiple levels

MR Findings
- T1WI

DDx: Spinal Lymphoma Mimics

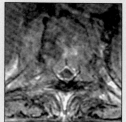

Epidural Mets

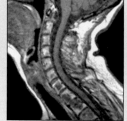

Osseous Mets

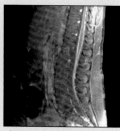

Leptomeningitic Mets

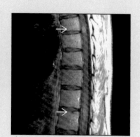

Intramedullary Mets

LYMPHOMA

Key Facts

Terminology
- Lymphoreticular neoplasms with wide variety of specific diseases & cellular differentiation

Imaging Findings
- Epidural: Enhancing epidural mass +/- vertebral involvement
- Osseous: Bone destruction ("ivory" vertebra, rare)
- Leptomeningitic: Smooth/nodular pial enhancement
- Intramedullary: Poorly-defined enhancing mass
- Best imaging tool: MRI + C

Top Differential Diagnoses
- Epidural disease that may mimic epidural lymphoma
- Osseous lymphoma mimics
- Lymphomatous meningitis mimics
- Intramedullary lymphoma mimics

Pathology
- Exact causes are unknown
- NHL > > Hodgkin disease (HD); 80-90% are B cell
- CNS lymphoma > 85% NHL (B cell > > > T cell)
- Hodgkin disease rare

Clinical Issues
- Most common presenting symptom = back pain
- Intramedullary = myelopathy (weakness, numbness)
- Generally poor prognosis for CNS lymphoma
- Best prognosis with primary osseous lymphoma
- XRT +/- chemotherapy

Diagnostic Checklist
- Lymphoma is a great mimicker

- Epidural: Isointense homogeneous epidural mass (often multisegmental +/- extends through foramina)
- Osseous: Hypointense to normal marrow (+/- epidural extension)
- Leptomeningitic: Thick nerve roots +/- focal nodules (isointense with cord)
- Intramedullary: Mass usually isointense to spinal cord
- T2WI
  - Epidural: Iso/hyperintense to cord
  - Osseous: Variable; iso/hyperintense
  - Leptomeningitic: Thick nerve roots +/- focal nodules (isointense with cord)
  - Intramedullary: Hyperintense with surrounding edema
- STIR: Osseous: May show T2 characteristics better
- T1 C+
  - Epidural: Enhances intensely, uniformly
  - Osseous: Diffuse uniform enhancement
  - Leptomeningitic: Roots enhance
  - Intramedullary: Variable: Patchy/confluent, infiltrating/discrete
- Dynamic contrast–enhanced MRI
  - Demonstrates ↑ bone marrow enhancement in patients with lymphoproliferative diseases with diagnostic accuracy of 99%
  - Assess degree of diffuse bone marrow infiltration
  - ↓ After treatment in all patients who respond to treatment; but not in 2/3 patients who did not respond to treatment

Nuclear Medicine Findings
- Bone Scan: Increased uptake
- PET: Fluorine-18 fluorodeoxyglucose (FDG) PET has proven useful for staging, monitoring treatment response, predicting treatment outcomes, & risk stratifying lymphoma patients
- Gallium scan
  - 67Ga scintigraphy has a high sensitivity & specificity for diagnosis of bone lymphoma

- Discriminates between patients who achieve complete response & those who show no or only partial response to induction therapy
- Prognosis can be predicted during treatment, as soon as after 1 cycle of chemotherapy
- Recurrent disease can be diagnosed early during follow-up

Imaging Recommendations
- Best imaging tool: MRI + C
- Protocol advice
  - Fat-saturated T1WI
  - STIR may be helpful

DIFFERENTIAL DIAGNOSIS

Epidural disease that may mimic epidural lymphoma
- Hematoma: Heterogeneous > homogeneous signal
- Abscess: Rim > solid enhancement, central low signal common
- Metastasis: Epidural met without bone involvement rare

Osseous lymphoma mimics
- Metastasis: Destructive, +/- soft tissue mass
- Eosinophilic granuloma: Vertebra plana; younger patients

Lymphomatous meningitis mimics
- Other neoplastic/granulomatous or infectious meningitides

Intramedullary lymphoma mimics
- Ependymoma: Hemorrhage, cysts common
- Astrocytoma: Multisegmental; cysts common
- Metastasis: Usually round, more sharply delineated

PATHOLOGY

General Features
- Etiology

LYMPHOMA

- ○ Exact causes are unknown
- ○ CNS lymphoma may be primary or secondary (hematogenous or direct geographic extension)
- ○ Risk factors
  - ▪ Chemical exposure such as pesticides, fertilizers, or solvents
  - ▪ Epstein-Barr virus plays role in immunocompromised
  - ▪ Infection with HTLV-1
  - ▪ AIDS/transplant immunocompromised patients
  - ▪ Family history of NHL, although no hereditary pattern has been established
- • Epidemiology
  - ○ NHL > > Hodgkin disease (HD); 80-90% are B cell
    - ▪ CNS lymphoma > 85% NHL (B cell > > > T cell)
    - ▪ Hodgkin disease rare
  - ○ Primary epidural = 1-7% of NHL; 10-30% of epidural malignancies
  - ○ Secondary epidural in 5% of patients with systemic lymphoma
  - ○ Primary osseous = 3-4% of malignant bone tumors
  - ○ Bone marrow involvement in 25-50% NHL patients, 5-15% HD
  - ○ Epidural/vertebral involvement related to hematogenous metastatic involvement or local spread from adjacent lymph nodes
  - ○ Intramedullary = 3% of CNS lymphoma
  - ○ Leptomeningitic nearly always occurs as spread from intracranial lymphoma
  - ○ Most common malignancy of the epidural space
  - ○ Lymphoma represents an increasingly important cause of morbidity & mortality in older patients
- • Associated abnormalities: Multisystem/multiorgan involvement

Gross Pathologic & Surgical Features
- • Varies from discrete mass to poorly-marginated infiltrative disease

Microscopic Features
- • Neoplastic lymphocytes in marrow, meninges
- • Pack perivascular spaces

Staging, Grading or Classification Criteria
- • NHL: Ann Arbor staging system
- • Hodgkin: Cotswold system (modified Ann Arbor staging system)

CLINICAL ISSUES

Presentation
- • Most common signs/symptoms
  - ○ Most common presenting symptom = back pain
  - ○ Intramedullary = myelopathy (weakness, numbness)

Demographics
- • Age: Adults; peak = 4th-7th decade
- • Gender: Slight male predominance
- • Ethnicity: All affected

Natural History & Prognosis
- • Cord compression occurs in up to 5-10% of systemic lymphomas
- • Generally poor prognosis for CNS lymphoma

- • Best prognosis with primary osseous lymphoma
  - ○ 5-10 yr survival rates = 91-87%

Treatment
- • XRT +/- chemotherapy
  - ○ Markedly sensitive to chemotherapy/XRT
  - ○ Intrathecal for leptomeningitic
- • +/- Surgery

DIAGNOSTIC CHECKLIST

Consider
- • Lymphoma is a great mimicker

SELECTED REFERENCES

1. Westin EH et al: Lymphoma and myeloma in older patients. Semin Oncol. 31(2):198-205, 2004
2. Rahmouni A et al: Bone marrow with diffuse tumor infiltration in patients with lymphoproliferative diseases: dynamic gadolinium-enhanced MR imaging. Radiology. 229(3):710-7, 2003
3. Israel O et al: Bone lymphoma: 67Ga scintigraphy and CT for prediction of outcome after treatment. J Nucl Med. 43(10):1295-303, 2002
4. Vazquez E et al: Neuroimaging in pediatric leukemia and lymphoma: differential diagnosis. Radiographics. 22(6):1411-28, 2002
5. Guermazi A et al: Extranodal Hodgkin disease: spectrum of disease. Radiographics. 21(1):161-79, 2001
6. Koeller KK et al: Neoplasms of the spinal cord and filum terminale: Radiologic-Pathologic correlation. RadioGraphics. 20:1721-49, 2000
7. Mulligan ME et al: Imaging features of primary lymphoma of bone. AJR. 173:1691-7, 1999
8. White LM et al: MR imaging of primary lymphoma of bone: variability of T2-weighted signal intensity. AJR Am J Roentgenol. 170(5):1243-7, 1998
9. Caruso PA et al: Primary intramedullary lymphoma of the spinal cord mimicking cervical spondylotic myelopathy. AJR Am J Roentgenol. 171(2):526-7, 1998
10. Moulopoulos LA et al: Magnetic resonance imaging of the bone marrow in hematologic malignancies. Blood. 90(6):2127-47, 1997
11. Boukobza M et al: Primary vertebral and spinal epidural non-Hodgkin's lymphoma with spinal cord compression. Neuroradiology. 38:333-7, 1996
12. Yankelevitz DF et al: Effect of radiation therapy on thoracic and lumbar bone marrow: evaluation with MR imaging. AJR Am J Roentgenol. 157(1):87-92, 1991
13. Lim V et al: Spinal cord pial metastases: MR imaging with gadopentetate dimeglumine. AJR Am J Roentgenol. 155(5):1077-84, 1990
14. Lim V et al: Spinal cord pial metastases: MR imaging with gadopentetate dimeglumine. AJNR Am J Neuroradiol. 11(5):975-82, 1990
15. Beres J et al: Spinal epidural lymphomas: CT features in seven patients. AJNR Am J Neuroradiol. 7(2):327-8, 1986

IMAGE GALLERY

Typical

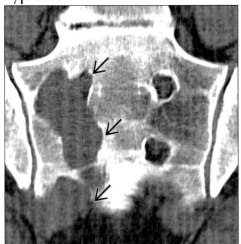 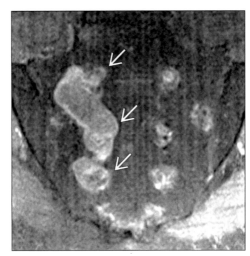

(Left) Coronal bone CT reformat demonstrates osseous lymphoma within the right sacrum, filling involved sacral neural foramina (arrows). *(Right)* Coronal T1 C+ MR with fat-saturation reveals enhancing osseous lymphoma within the right sacrum, filling involved sacral neural foramina (arrows).

Typical

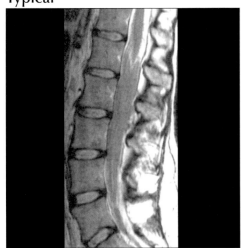 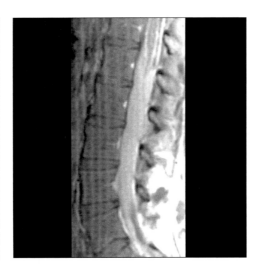

(Left) Sagittal T2WI MR shows diffuse leptomeningitic lymphoma, hypointense to CSF, coating the conus and filling the lumbar canal. *(Right)* Sagittal DWI MR confirms diffuse enhancing leptomeningitic lymphoma coating the conus and filling the lumbar canal.

Typical

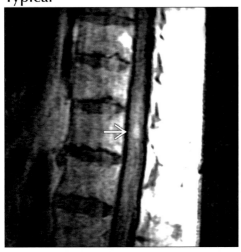 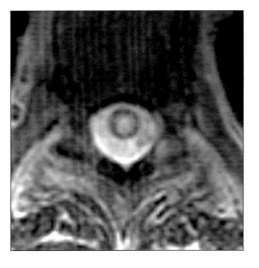

(Left) Sagittal T1 C+ MR demonstrates ill-defined intramedullary enhancing lymphoma (arrow). *(Right)* Axial T2WI MR reveals hyperintensity of intramedullary lymphoma.

LEUKEMIA

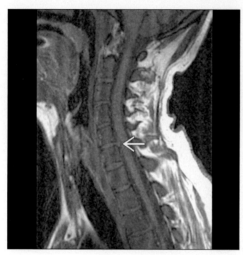

Sagittal T1WI MR in CML patient demonstrates marked diffuse marrow hypointensity relative to adjacent discs. Incidental disc herniation (arrow) was etiology of neck pain prompting imaging.

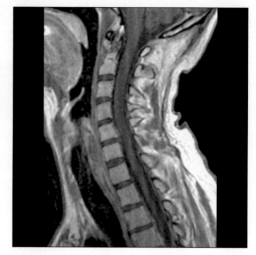

Sagittal T1 C+ MR depicts avid diffuse marrow enhancement reflecting CML marrow infiltration. Normal marrow would be expected to minimally enhance.

TERMINOLOGY

Abbreviations and Synonyms
- Acute lymphocytic leukemia (ALL), chronic lymphocytic leukemia (CLL), acute myelogenous leukemia (AML), chronic myelogenous leukemia (CML), granulocytic sarcoma, chloroma

Definitions
- Acute or chronic myeloid or lymphoid white blood cell neoplasia with spinal involvement as component of systemic disease

IMAGING FINDINGS

General Features
- Best diagnostic clue: Diffuse osteopenia with multiple vertebral fractures +/- lytic spine lesions
- Location
  ○ Children: Multiple long bones and spine (14%)
  ○ Adults: Predominately axial skeleton
- Morphology: Osteopenia +/- moth eaten bone destruction of multiple vertebral bodies, leptomeningeal enhancement, focal mass ("chloroma")

Radiographic Findings
- Radiography
  ○ Diffuse vertebral, long bone osteopenia

- Coarse cancellous trabeculation +/- pathologic vertebral compression fractures
- Radiographs may look normal, even if extensive disease
  ○ +/- "Leukemic lines" (horizontal vertebral bands)
  ○ Granulocytic sarcoma ⇒ focal lytic mass

CT Findings
- NECT
  ○ Isodense soft tissue mass with adjacent bone destruction
  ○ Leptomeningeal disease: ↑ Density of lumbar theca, nerve root enlargement
- CECT: Variable enhancement
- Bone CT
  ○ Permeative bone destruction +/- focal lytic lesions, pathologic vertebral fractures

MR Findings
- T1WI: Leukemic marrow, focal tumor masses relatively hypointense
- T2WI: Increased leukemic marrow signal intensity +/- focal vertebral mass, cord signal abnormality
- STIR: Hyperintense leukemic marrow
- T1 C+: Abnormal enhancement of marrow, focal lesion, or leptomeninges

DDx: Spinal Leukemia

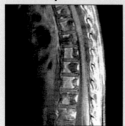

Neuroblastoma

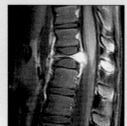

LCH

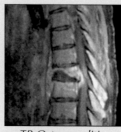

TB Osteomyelitis

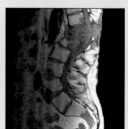

Lymphoma

LEUKEMIA

Key Facts

Terminology
- Acute or chronic myeloid or lymphoid white blood cell neoplasia with spinal involvement as component of systemic disease

Imaging Findings
- Best diagnostic clue: Diffuse osteopenia with multiple vertebral fractures +/- lytic spine lesions
- Radiographs may look normal, even if extensive disease
- Granulocytic sarcoma ⇒ focal lytic mass

Top Differential Diagnoses
- Metastases
- Langerhans cell histiocytosis (LCH)
- Osteomyelitis
- Lymphoma
- Ewing sarcoma

Pathology
- Strong association with chromosomal abnormalities

Clinical Issues
- Chronic leukemia may be asymptomatic
- Symptomatic patients present with fever, ↑ ESR, hepatosplenomegaly, lymphadenopathy, joint effusions, petechial and retinal hemorrhage, anemia, frequent infections

Diagnostic Checklist
- MRI sensitivity for leptomeningeal metastases < < laboratory CSF evaluation
- Consider leukemia in a patient with unexplained compression fractures

Nuclear Medicine Findings
- Bone Scan: +/- ↑ Radiotracer uptake; often underestimates disease extent, especially in absence of significant cortical destruction

Imaging Recommendations
- Best imaging tool: MR imaging
- Protocol advice
  - Multiplanar T1WI, T2WI (+ fat-saturation) or STIR, T1 C+ MRI
  - Whole body STIR MRI (WBMR) proposed for staging, assessing lesion burden
  - Bone CT with multiplanar reformats to clarify osseous lesions, quantitate compression fractures

DIFFERENTIAL DIAGNOSIS

Metastases
- Metastatic neuroblastoma or rhabdomyosarcoma in children, carcinomas in adults
- Multifocal bone involvement similar to leukemia

Langerhans cell histiocytosis (LCH)
- Lytic lesion with periosteal reaction, endosteal scalloping, soft tissue mass
- May have systemic symptoms similar to leukemia

Osteomyelitis
- Granulomatous or pyogenic; TB in particular may (relatively) spare disc spaces
- Periosteal reaction, soft tissue extension
- May have systemic symptoms similar to leukemia

Lymphoma
- Older patient with large soft tissue mass; predilection for paraspinal, epidural locations
- Systemic lymphomatous metastasis or primary vertebral lesion

Ewing sarcoma
- Marked periosteal reaction + associated soft tissue mass
- No metaphyseal lucent lines
- May have systemic symptoms similar to leukemia

PATHOLOGY

General Features
- General path comments
  - Spinal leukemia may involve either single or multiple vertebral bodies
    - Most common spinal presentation is multiple compression fractures
  - Neuropathologic features include manifestations of primary disease, side effects of therapeutic procedures (radiation therapy, chemotherapy, BMT), and complications 2° to immunosuppression
    - Spinal manifestations of primary disease: Fractures, marrow or meningeal infiltration
    - Treatment effects: Secondary neoplasms (usually aggressive CNS tumors), hemorrhage, anterior lumbosacral radiculopathy (intrathecal methotrexate toxicity)
    - Immunosuppression complications: Fungal or other opportunistic infection
  - Granulocytic sarcoma (chloroma): Extramedullary neoplasm of immature granulocytic cells → focal lytic mass
    - Most common in AML (concurrent presentation ≤ 9.1% AML cases); rare aleukemic presentations reported
- Genetics
  - Strong association with chromosomal abnormalities
    - ALL: Trisomy 21, chromosomal translocations
    - CLL: Trisomy 12
    - CML: 90% have Philadelphia chromosome t(9;22)
- Etiology
  - External factors: Alkylating drugs, ionizing radiation, chemicals (benzene)
  - Internal factors: Chromosomal abnormalities
  - Predisposing hematological disorders: Aplastic anemia, chronic myeloproliferative disorders
- Epidemiology
  - Most common malignancy of childhood (ALL: 75%, AML: 15-20%, CML: 5%)
  - 20th most common cause of cancer death (all age groups)

LEUKEMIA

- Associated abnormalities
  - Long bone periostitis (12-25%), "leukemic" metaphyseal lines
  - Focal destruction of flat/tubular bones, pathologic fractures
  - Opportunistic infections, second malignancies
  - Chemotherapy-related complications

Gross Pathologic & Surgical Features
- Hyperemic/hemorrhagic bone marrow with destruction of bony trabeculae, bone infarction

Microscopic Features
- Diffuse bone marrow infiltration by poorly-differentiated hematologic cells
  - ALL: Infiltrates of small blue cells
  - AML: Auer rods (condensed lysosomal cytoplasmic rod shaped structures) diagnostic
  - CLL: Mature lymphocytes, < 55% atypical cells
  - CML: Leukocytosis with increase in basophils, eosinophils, neutrophils; Philadelphia chromosome t(9;22)

CLINICAL ISSUES

Presentation
- Most common signs/symptoms
  - Localized or diffuse bone pain
  - Recurrent para-articular arthralgias (75%)
- Clinical profile
  - Chronic leukemia may be asymptomatic
  - Symptomatic patients present with fever, ↑ ESR, hepatosplenomegaly, lymphadenopathy, joint effusions, petechial and retinal hemorrhage, anemia, frequent infections

Demographics
- Age
  - ALL: Peak 2-10 y
  - AML: Peak > 65 y
  - CML: Rare in childhood (< 5%), peak > 40 y
  - CLL: Peak 50-70 y
- Gender: M:F = 2:1

Natural History & Prognosis
- 5 year survival (all leukemias): 25-30%
  - Children with ALL: 90% complete remission, 80% 5 year disease free survival
  - Adults with ALL: Remission in 60-80%, 20-30% 5 year disease free survival
  - AML: 45% 5 year survival
  - CLL: 6 years median survival
  - CML: 5 years median survival

Treatment
- Chemotherapy
  - Induction phase, consolidation phase, maintenance therapy phase
  - Intrathecal chemotherapy for CNS involvement
- Radiation therapy
- Bone marrow transplant

DIAGNOSTIC CHECKLIST

Consider
- Marrow infiltration in child with osteoporosis raises suspicion for leukemia
- MRI sensitivity for leptomeningeal metastases < < laboratory CSF evaluation

Image Interpretation Pearls
- Consider leukemia in a patient with unexplained compression fractures

SELECTED REFERENCES

1. Kuhn J et al: Caffey's Pediatric Diagnostic Imaging. 10th ed. Philadelphia, Mosby. Pages 710-711, 2004
2. Laffan EE et al: Whole-body magnetic resonance imaging: a useful additional sequence in paediatric imaging. Pediatr Radiol. 34(6):472-80, 2004
3. Chang YW et al: Spinal MRI of vincristine neuropathy mimicking Guillain-Barre syndrome. Pediatr Radiol. 33(11):791-3, 2003
4. Beckers R et al: Acute lymphoblastic leukaemia presenting with low back pain. Eur J Paediatr Neurol. 6(5):285-7, 2002
5. Vazquez E et al: Neuroimaging in pediatric leukemia and lymphoma: differential diagnosis. Radiographics. 22(6):1411-28, 2002
6. Buckland ME et al: Spinal chloroma presenting with triplegia in an aleukaemic patient. Pathology. 33(3):386-9, 2001
7. Carriere B et al: Vertebral fractures as initial signs for acute lymphoblastic leukemia. Pediatr Emerg Care. 17(4):258-61, 2001
8. Shalaby-Rana E et al: (99m)Tc-MDP scintigraphic findings in children with leukemia: value of early and delayed whole-body imaging. J Nucl Med. 42(6):878-83, 2001
9. Yavuz H et al: Transverse myelopathy: an initial presentation of acute leukemia. Pediatr Neurol. 24(5):382-4, 2001
10. Lo LD et al: Are L5 fractures an indicator of metastasis? Skeletal Radiol. 29(8):454-8, 2000
11. Kim HJ et al: Spinal involvement of hematopoietic malignancies and metastasis: differentiation using MR imaging. Clin Imaging. 23(2):125-33, 1999
12. Sandhu GS et al: Granulocytic sarcoma presenting as cauda equina syndrome. Clin Neurol Neurosurg. 100(3):205-8, 1998
13. Aisenberg J et al: Bone mineral density in young adult survivors of childhood cancer. J Pediatr Hematol Oncol. 20(3):241-5, 1998
14. Novick SL et al: Granulocytic sarcoma (chloroma) of the sacrum: initial manifestation of leukemia. Skeletal Radiol. 27(2):112-4, 1998
15. Deme S et al: Granulocytic sarcoma of the spine in nonleukemic patients: report of three cases. Neurosurgery. 40(6):1283-7, 1997
16. Wu CY et al: Detection of dural involvement by magnetic resonance imaging in adult patients with acute leukemias--preliminary experience. Ann Hematol. 70(5):243-9, 1995
17. Heinrich SD et al: The prognostic significance of the skeletal manifestations of acute lymphoblastic leukemia of childhood. J Pediatr Orthop. 14(1):105-11, 1994

LEUKEMIA

IMAGE GALLERY

Typical

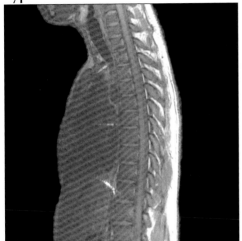
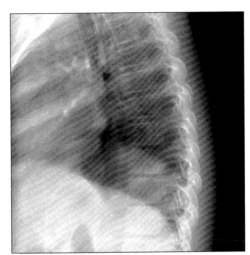

(Left) Sagittal T1WI MR depicts diffuse abnormal marrow replacement characterized by marrow signal hypointense relative to adjacent discs. *(Right)* Lateral radiography shows osteopenia only in a pediatric patient with systemic leukemia.

Typical

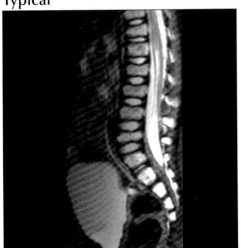
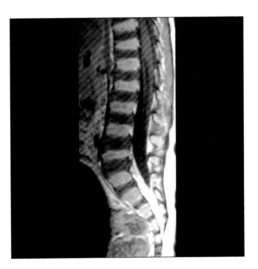

(Left) Sagittal STIR MR depicts marked diffuse abnormal vertebral marrow hyperintensity in a school age child with multiple vertebral compression fractures and confirmed systemic leukemia. *(Right)* Sagittal T1 C+ MR depicts marked abnormal vertebral marrow enhancement in a school age child with multiple vertebral compression fractures and confirmed systemic leukemia.

Variant

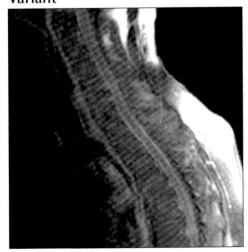
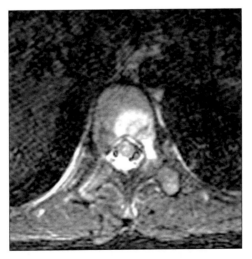

(Left) Sagittal T1 C+ MR with fat-saturation in a symptomatic AML patient shows extensive leptomeningeal neoplastic enhancement replacing normal hypointense CSF signal. *(Right)* Axial T2WI MR with fat-saturation of the T10 vertebra shows a hyperintense focal leukemic metastasis extending into the left pedicle, without epidural extension (Courtesy R. Boyer, MD).

PLASMACYTOMA

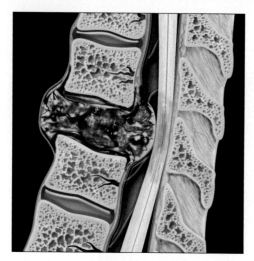

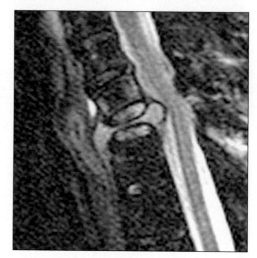

Sagittal graphic shows collapse of thoracic vertebral body due to tumor infiltration with retropulsion of anterior & posterior margins. Dorsal retropulsion & tumor causes cord compression.

Sagittal STIR MR shows C7 severe collapse (vertebra plana) with posterior bony retropulsion and cord compression. There is no associated soft tissue mass.

TERMINOLOGY

Abbreviations and Synonyms

- Solitary bone plasmacytoma (SBP), solitary plasmacytoma, solitary myeloma, solitary plasma cell tumor

Definitions

- Solitary monoclonal plasma cell tumor of bone or soft tissue, with no evidence of multiple myeloma (MM) elsewhere
- Diagnosis requires
  - Solitary lesion, biopsy showing plasma cells
  - Negative skeletal survey, negative MR spine, pelvis, proximal femora/humeri
  - Negative clonal cells in marrow aspirate
  - No anemia, hypercalcemia, or renal involvement suggesting systemic myeloma
- Some variations in definitions such as including 2 bone lesions, or < 10% bone marrow plasmacytosis

IMAGING FINDINGS

General Features

- Best diagnostic clue: T1 hypointense marrow with low-signal, curvilinear areas
- Location: Vertebral body = most common site of SBP

Radiographic Findings

- Radiography
  - Can be normal early
  - Lytic multicystic-appearing lesion +/- vertical dense striations
  - Pathologic compression fracture common
- Myelography: May show extradural defect in contrast column with collapse, contrast block in severe cases

CT Findings

- NECT
  - Common
    - Lytic, destructive vertebral body lesion
    - Compression fracture +/- associated soft tissue mass
  - Uncommon: Osteosclerosis (3%)
  - Rare: Involvement of intervertebral disc, adjacent vertebrae (if present, helpful differentiating feature from metastasis)
- CECT: Usually little/no detectable enhancement

MR Findings

- T1WI
  - Solitary vertebral body lesion
    - Marrow iso/hypointense (compared to muscle)
    - Contains curvilinear low signal areas and/or cortical irregularities ("infoldings" caused by endplate Fxs)

DDx: Vertebral Body Collapse

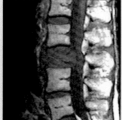

Metastasis

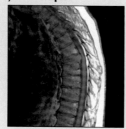

Multiple Myeloma

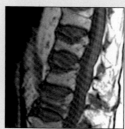

Osteoporosis

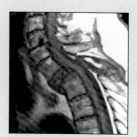

Paget Disease

PLASMACYTOMA

63

Key Facts

Terminology
- Solitary monoclonal plasma cell tumor of bone or soft tissue, with no evidence of multiple myeloma (MM) elsewhere

Imaging Findings
- Best diagnostic clue: T1 hypointense marrow with low-signal, curvilinear areas
- Location: Vertebral body = most common site of SBP
- Bone scintigraphy unreliable for staging and monitoring
- FDG-PET reliably detects active MM
- Standard MR + STIR, scan entire spine

Top Differential Diagnoses
- Multiple myeloma
- Metastasis

- Benign (osteoporotic) compression fracture
- Vertebral hemangioma (VH)

Pathology
- Most patients SBP reflects early (stage I) multiple myeloma (MM), the malignant plasma cell disorder

Clinical Issues
- Age: Mean age = 55 years (younger than age of patients with MM)
- SBPs typically have indolent course (median survival = 10 years)
- Definitive local radiotherapy (4,000 cGy)

Diagnostic Checklist
- Caution: Must exclude second unanticipated lesion (33% of cases)

- Variable degrees of compression
- Posterior elements involved in most cases
- +/- Associated soft tissue mass (paraspinous or epidural with "draped curtain" sign)
- "Mini brain" appearance due to thick cortical struts in expanded vertebral body
  ○ Scanning entire spine reveals second lesion in 1/3 of cases
- T2WI
  ○ Heterogeneous signal
    ▪ Focal hyperintensities (compared to fat)
    ▪ Curvilinear areas of signal void
- STIR: STIR: Hyperintense (corresponds to lytic lesions on NECT)
- T1 C+
  ○ Common: Mild/moderate diffuse enhancement
  ○ Uncommon: Peripheral (rim) enhancement

Nuclear Medicine Findings
- Bone Scan
  ○ Intense uptake, but may be normal early in disease
  ○ Bone scintigraphy unreliable for staging and monitoring
- PET
  ○ FDG-PET reliably detects active MM
  ○ Negative FDG-PET supports diagnosis of monoclonal gammopathy of undetermined significance (MGUS)
- Gallium Scan
  ○ Rare report of Gallium uptake in soft tissue plasmacytoma
- Tc-99m-MIBI
  ○ Increased uptake in MM, with extent and intensity correlated with disease activity

Imaging Recommendations
- Standard MR + STIR, scan entire spine
- CT-guided biopsy/fine needle aspiration

DIFFERENTIAL DIAGNOSIS

Multiple myeloma
- Second lesion found in 33% of cases with presumed spine SBP

Metastasis
- May be indistinguishable from SBP
- Posterior element involvement not useful in differentiating from SBP
- Doesn't involve disc or adjacent vertebrae

Benign (osteoporotic) compression fracture
- Common in older patients, including those with SBP and MM
- 50-60% of compression fractures in MM appear benign on MR
- Signal intensity (subacute/chronic Fxs) like normal marrow

Vertebral hemangioma (VH)
- Aggressive VHs that mimic SBP, metastases are rare
- Marrow signal of aggressive VH may resemble SBP (most benign VHs are hyperintense on both T1 and T2WI)
- Intense enhancement

Paget disease
- Vertebral body expansion with thickened trabeculae

PATHOLOGY

General Features
- General path comments: Marrow infiltrated with neoplastic plasma cells
- Genetics
  ○ Unknown for SBP
  ○ In situ hybridization studies show cytogenetic abnormalities in 80-90% of MM patients
    ▪ Chromosome 13 deletion most common (13q)
    ▪ Other: Chromosome 14q32 deletions/translocations, 11q, miscellaneous translocations

PLASMACYTOMA

- Monosomy 13 correlated with poor prognosis, especially combined with elevated β2 microglobulin, concomitant chromosome 11 aberration
- Etiology
  - Most patients SBP reflects early (stage I) multiple myeloma (MM), the malignant plasma cell disorder
  - Some patients stable for decades, suggesting relationship to MGUS
- Epidemiology
  - Solitary bone plasmacytic lesions represent 3-5% of monoclonal gammopathies
  - Spine is most common site
  - 20% have solitary lesions in rib, sternum, clavicle, scapula

Gross Pathologic & Surgical Features
- Compressed vertebra with gray-purple fatty marrow replacement

Microscopic Features
- Monotonous collection of neoplastic plasma cells
  - Eccentric, round, pleomorphic nuclei with "clock-face" chromatin
  - Rich basophilic cytoplasm

Staging, Grading or Classification Criteria
- SBPs considered clinical stage I Durie/Salmon lesions
- Imaging shows normal bone or only SBP

CLINICAL ISSUES

Presentation
- Most common signs/symptoms
  - Most common symptom = pain
  - Can be asymptomatic
  - Epidural extension, pathologic fracture may cause cord compression
  - Other signs/symptoms
    - Low levels of serum/urine monoclonal proteins (25-75%)
    - Uncommon presentation of demyelinating polyneuropathy
    - In such cases, consider POEMS syndrome: Polyneuropathy, organomegaly, endocrinopathy, M protein, skin changes

Demographics
- Age: Mean age = 55 years (younger than age of patients with MM)
- Gender: M > F

Natural History & Prognosis
- SBPs typically have indolent course (median survival = 10 years)
- Common progression patterns include new bone lesions, increased myeloma protein levels, marrow plasmacytosis
- When MM evolves from SBP, tend to have low tumor mass disease with high chemotherapy response rate

Treatment
- Definitive local radiotherapy (4,000 cGy)
  - Tumors > 5 cm in size at risk for recurrence

- Some asymptomatic patients with stage I MM not treated until more aggressive disease demonstrated at clinical follow-up

DIAGNOSTIC CHECKLIST

Consider
- Caution: Must exclude second unanticipated lesion (33% of cases)

Image Interpretation Pearls
- Classic imaging appearance = hypointense vertebra (T1WI) with cortical "infoldings," curvilinear low signal areas

SELECTED REFERENCES

1. Durr HR et al: Multiple myeloma: surgery of the spine: retrospective analysis of 27 patients. Spine. 27(3):320-4; discussion 325-6, 2002
2. Wilder RB et al: Persistence of myeloma protein for more than one year after radiotherapy is an adverse prognostic factor in solitary plasmacytoma of bone. Cancer. 94(5):1532-7, 2002
3. Gossios K et al: Solitary plasmacytoma of the spine in an adolescent: a case report. Pediatr Radiol. 32(5):366-9, 2002
4. Dimopoulos MA et al: Solitary bone plasmacytoma and extramedullary plasmacytoma. Curr Treat Options Oncol. 3(3):255-9, 2002
5. Tsang RW et al: Solitary plasmacytoma treated with radiotherapy: impact of tumor size on outcome. Int J Radiat Oncol Biol Phys. 50(1):113-20, 2001
6. Soderlund V et al: Diagnosis of skeletal lymphoma and myeloma by radiology and fine needle aspiration cytology. Cytopathology. 12(3):157-67, 2001
7. Alexandrakis MG et al: Value of Tc-99m sestamibi scintigraphy in the detection of bone lesions in multiple myeloma: comparison with Tc-99m methylene diphosphonate. Ann Hematol. 80(6):349-53, 2001
8. Voss SD et al: Solitary osteosclerotic plasmacytoma: association with demyelinating polyneuropathy and amyloid deposition. Skeletal Radiol. 30(9):527-9, 2001
9. Avva R et al: CT-guided biopsy of focal lesions in patients with multiple myeloma may reveal new and more aggressive cytogenetic abnormalities. AJNR. 22: 781-5, 2001
10. Ota K et al: A therapeutic strategy for isolated plasmacytoma of bone. J Int Med Res. 29(4):366-73, 2001
11. Major NM et al: The "mini brain": plasmacytoma in a vertebral body on MR imaging. AJR Am J Roentgenol. 175(1):261-3, 2000
12. Shah BK et al: Magnetic resonance imaging of spinal plasmacytoma. Clin Radiol. 55: 439-45, 2000
13. Dimopoulos MA et al: Solitary plasmacytoma of bone and asymptomatic multiple myeloma. Blood. 96(6):2037-44, 2000
14. Liebross RH et al: Clinical course of solitary extramedullary plasmacytoma. Radiother Oncol. 52(3):245-9, 1999
15. Lecouvet F et al: Vertebral compression fractures in multiple myeloma. Radiol. 204: 195-9, 1997

PLASMACYTOMA

IMAGE GALLERY

Typical

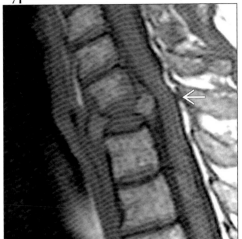
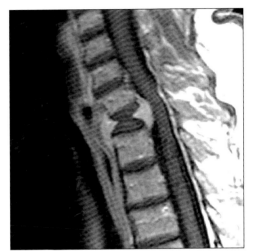

(Left) Sagittal T1WI MR shows severe collapse at C7 level with well-defined margins. There is retropulsion of posterior vertebral body with cord compression (arrow). *(Right)* Sagittal T1 C+ MR shows severe collapse of central portion of C7 body with diffuse enhancement of ventral and dorsal retropulsed segments. There is cord compression due to posterior retropulsion.

Typical

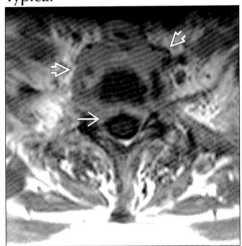
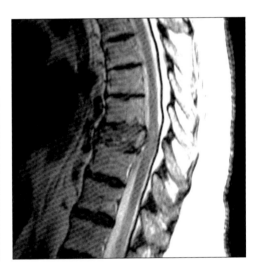

(Left) Axial T1 C+ MR shows plasmacytoma involving C7 body with diffuse axial expansion (open arrows), and retropulsion of posterior vertebral body compressing thecal sac and cord (arrow). *(Right)* Sagittal T2WI MR shows collapse/anterior wedging deformity of lower thoracic vertebral body, showing nonspecific mild signal heterogeneity. Mild posterior retropulsion effaces ventral thecal sac.

Typical

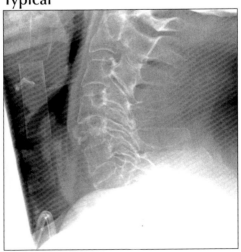
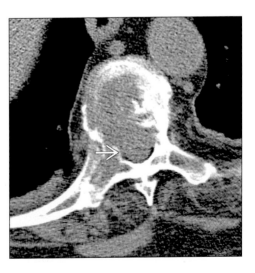

(Left) Lateral radiography shows severe collapse of C5 body with cortical irregularity. *(Right)* Axial NECT shows bone destruction of thoracic body with ventral epidural soft tissue extension, and cord compression (arrow).

MULTIPLE MYELOMA

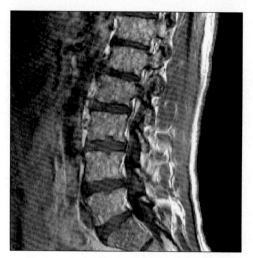

Sagittal T1 C+ MR of lumbar spine shows innumerable small enhancing vertebral myelomatous lesions.

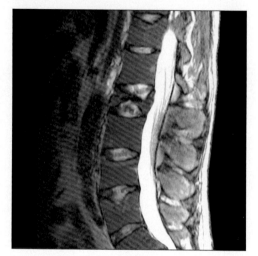

Sagittal T2WI MR shows diffuse marrow hypointensity with severe compression fracture at L2. Fractures also involve superior endplates of T12, L4, and L5.

TERMINOLOGY

Abbreviations and Synonyms
- Multiple myeloma (MM)

Definitions
- Multifocal malignant proliferation of monoclonal plasma cells within bone marrow

IMAGING FINDINGS

General Features
- Best diagnostic clue: Multi-focal, diffuse, or heterogeneous T1 hypointensity
- Location
  - Axial skeleton (red marrow) > long bones
    - Spine, skull (mandible), ribs, pelvis
  - 87% vertebral fractures between T6 and L4
- Size: Variable
- Morphology
  - Well-circumscribed, punched-out lesions on radiography
    - May be expansile

Radiographic Findings
- Radiography
  - Diffuse osteopenia: 85%
  - Multiple lytic lesions: 80%

- Approximately 1% of lesions sclerotic
  - Endosteal scalloping
  - Soft tissue mass adjacent to bone destruction
  - Plasmacytoma
    - Solitary, large, expansile
    - May be septated
  - Vertebral compression fractures
  - POEMS syndrome: Polyneuropathy, organomegaly, endocrine disorders, monoclonal gammopathy, skin changes
    - Enthesopathies of thoracolumbar posterior elements
    - Lytic lesions with surrounding sclerosis
    - Sclerotic lesions

CT Findings
- NECT (bone window)
  - Multi-focal lytic lesions
  - Vertebral destruction and fractures
  - Multidetector CT (MDCT) with sagittal and coronal reformation
    - Cortical disruption, extraosseous soft tissue component, potential instability better evaluated

MR Findings
- Normal
- Focal marrow involvement
  - Low to intermediate signal intensity (SI) compared to marrow on T1WI

DDx: Heterogeneous Marrow Pattern

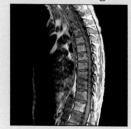

Metastases

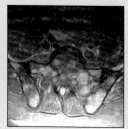

Metastases

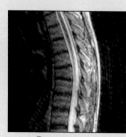

Osteoporosis

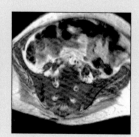

Hyperplastic Marrow

MULTIPLE MYELOMA

Key Facts

Terminology
- Multifocal malignant proliferation of monoclonal plasma cells within bone marrow

Imaging Findings
- Best diagnostic clue: Multi-focal, diffuse, or heterogeneous T1 hypointensity
- Diffuse osteopenia: 85%
- Multiple lytic lesions: 80%
- Focal marrow involvement
- Diffuse marrow involvement
- Variegated pattern
- 67% of vertebral fractures appear benign
- Bone scintigraphy detects 10% of lesions
- MM lesions metabolically active

- MRI or MDCT more sensitive than plain films or bone scintigraphy in MM staging

Top Differential Diagnoses
- Metastases
- Osteoporosis

Pathology
- Most common primary tumor of bone
- Incidence: 3-4 per 100,000 persons per year

Clinical Issues
- Bone pain: 75%
- 20% asymptomatic at presentation
- Median survival rate of 3-5 years with chemotherapy

- ○ Hyperintense on T2WI or STIR
- ○ Post-gadolinium enhancement
- Diffuse marrow involvement
  - ○ Fatty marrow replaced by low SI
    - ■ Iso- or hypointense to intervertebral discs
  - ○ Diffuse marrow enhancement
- Variegated pattern
  - ○ Patchy, heterogeneous, or mottled T1 SI
  - ○ Heterogeneous post-gadolinium enhancement
- Compression fractures with variable central canal narrowing
  - ○ 67% of vertebral fractures appear benign
- Patterns of response
  - ○ Resolved marrow abnormality
  - ○ Persistent abnormality without enhancement or with peripheral enhancement
  - ○ Conversion of diffuse to variegated or focal pattern

Nuclear Medicine Findings
- Bone Scan
  - ○ Typically negative
    - ■ Bone scintigraphy detects 10% of lesions
  - ○ Photopenic areas
- PET
  - ○ MM lesions metabolically active
    - ■ Sensitivity: 84-92%
    - ■ Specificity: 83-100%
  - ○ Useful in monitoring treatment response

Imaging Recommendations
- Best imaging tool
  - ○ MRI or MDCT more sensitive than plain films or bone scintigraphy in MM staging
    - ■ MRI in combination with MDCT as initial staging modalities
- Protocol advice: FSE T2 with fat-saturation, STIR, or post-gadolinium T1WI with fat suppression increases lesion conspicuity

DIFFERENTIAL DIAGNOSIS

Metastases
- Pedicles often involved earlier in metastases
  - ○ Late involvement in MM
- Increased radiotracer uptake on bone scan
- Mandible rarely involved
- No monoclonal gammopathy or Bence Jones proteinuria

Osteoporosis
- No endosteal scalloping on plain film
- No discrete lesions
- Difficult to distinguish from diffuse MM marrow involvement on MRI

Hyperplastic marrow
- Diffuse or patchy T1 hypointensity
- No discrete lesions
- No post-gadolinium enhancement

PATHOLOGY

General Features
- General path comments
  - ○ Accelerated osteoclastic bone resorption
  - ○ Inhibited osteoblastic bone formation
- Genetics: Development of multidrug resistance gene 1 precludes cure with chemotherapy
- Etiology
  - ○ Largely unknown
  - ○ Risk factors
    - ■ Ionizing radiation
    - ■ Exposure to pesticide, herbicide, dioxin
    - ■ Chronic immune stimulation
    - ■ Autoimmune diseases
    - ■ HIV, human herpesvirus 8
  - ○ Cell of origin: Memory B lymphocyte
  - ○ Interleukin-6 promotes growth of MM cells by preventing apoptosis
- Epidemiology
  - ○ Most common primary tumor of bone

MULTIPLE MYELOMA

- 27% of biopsied bone tumors
- Incidence: 3-4 per 100,000 persons per year

Gross Pathologic & Surgical Features
- Confluent or well-circumscribed, red-gray, soft tumor replacing cancellous bone

Microscopic Features
- Aggregates of neoplastic plasma cells
  - Infiltration and replacement of normal marrow
- Myeloma cells
  - Eccentric, round, hyperchromatic nuclei with "cartwheel" distribution of chromatin

Staging, Grading or Classification Criteria
- Durie-Salmon staging system: Based on Hgb and serum calcium levels, monoclonal protein burden, and number of bone lesions
  - Stage I: Low tumor mass
  - Stage II: Intermediate tumor mass
  - Stage III: High tumor mass
  - Each stage divided into A (serum creatinine < 2 mg/dl) or B (serum creatinine > 2 mg/dl)

CLINICAL ISSUES

Presentation
- Most common signs/symptoms
  - Bone pain: 75%
  - Pathologic fractures
  - Marrow failure: Anemia, infection
  - Renal failure
  - Other signs/symptoms
    - Bence Jones proteinuria: Free light chains
    - Electrophoresis: Monoclonal gammopathy
    - Hypercalcemia
    - Amyloidosis (10%)
- Clinical profile
  - 20% asymptomatic at presentation
  - Excessive production of nonfunctional monoclonal immunoglobulins
    - M protein: 60% IgG, 20% IgA, 20% free light chain

Demographics
- Age
  - Peak incidence from 40-80s
    - Peak age mid 60s to early 70s
- Gender: M:F = 3:2
- Ethnicity
  - 2x in African-Americans than Caucasians
  - Less common in Asians

Natural History & Prognosis
- Median survival rate of 3-5 years with chemotherapy
  - 5% complete remission
- Factors portending poor prognosis
  - Low hemoglobin
  - Hypercalcemia
  - Extensive lytic lesions
  - High immunoglobulin production rate
  - Impaired renal function

Treatment
- Supportive care
  - Analgesia
  - Osteoclast inhibiting agents: Bisphosphates
  - Erythropoietin
  - Vertebroplasty
- Local radiation
- Chemotherapy
  - Melphalan and prednisone
  - Thalidomide
- Transplants
  - Autologous hematopoietic stem cell: Patients < 78 years old with newly diagnosed MM
  - Allogeneic bone marrow: Treatment related mortality up to 50%

DIAGNOSTIC CHECKLIST

Consider
- MM when multi-focal, diffuse, or heterogeneous T1 marrow hypointensity present

SELECTED REFERENCES

1. Schirrmeister H et al: Initial results in the assessment of multiple myeloma using 18F-FDG PET. Eur J Nucl Med Mol Imaging. 29(3):361-6, 2002
2. Mahnken AH et al: Multidetector CT of the spine in multiple myeloma: comparison with MR imaging and radiography. AJR Am J Roentgenol. 178(6):1429-36, 2002
3. Jadvar H et al: Diagnostic utility of FDG PET in multiple myeloma. Skeletal Radiol. 31(12):690-4, 2002
4. Zaidi AA et al: Multiple myeloma: an old disease with new hope for the future. CA Cancer J Clin. 51(5):273-85; quiz 286-9, 2001
5. Lecouvet FE et al: Skeletal survey in advanced multiple myeloma: Radiographic versus MR imaging survey. Br J Haematol. 106:35-9, 1999
6. Singer CR: ABC of clinical haematology. Multiple myeloma and related conditions. BMJ. 314(7085):960-3, 1997
7. Lecouvet FE et al: Vertebral compression fractures in multiple myeloma. Part I. Distribution and appearance at MR imaging. Radiology. 204(1):195-9, 1997
8. Moulopoulos LA et al: Multiple myeloma: MR patterns of response to treatment. Radiology. 193(2):441-6, 1994
9. Rahmouni A et al: Detection of multiple myeloma involving the spine: efficacy of fat-suppression and contrast-enhanced MR imaging. AJR Am J Roentgenol. 160(5):1049-52, 1993
10. Libshitz HI et al: Multiple myeloma: Appearance at MR imaging. Radiology. 182:833-7, 1992
11. Moulopoulos LA et al: Multiple myeloma: Spinal MR imaging in patients with untreated newly diagnosed disease. Radiology. 185:833-40, 1992
12. Resnick D et al: Plasma-cell dyscrasia with polyneuropathy, organomegaly, endocrinopathy, M-protein, and skin changes: the POEMS syndrome. Distinctive radiographic abnormalities. Radiology. 140(1):17-22, 1981
13. Woolfenden JM et al: Comparison of bone scintigraphy and radiography in multiple myeloma. Radiology. 134(3):723-8, 1980

MULTIPLE MYELOMA

IMAGE GALLERY

Typical

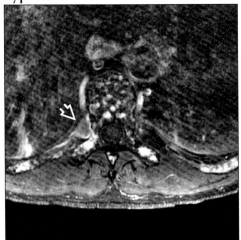 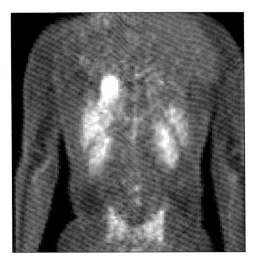

(Left) Axial T1 C+ MR with fat suppression through thoracic spine shows multiple small enhancing vertebral and rib lesions. A larger right rib lesion is partially visible (arrow). *(Right)* Coronal PET with FDG-18 demonstrates the same metabolically active right rib lesion.

Typical

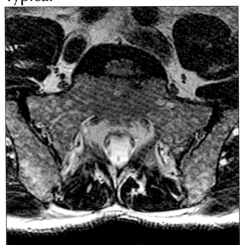 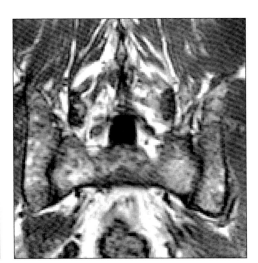

(Left) Axial T2WI MR shows multiple slightly ill-defined hyperintense lesions in the sacrum and iliac wings. *(Right)* Coronal T1WI MR in the same patient shows multi-focal patchy and discrete hypointense myelomatous involvement.

Typical

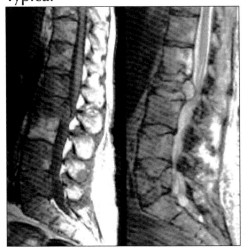 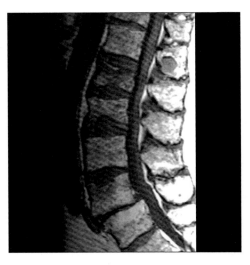

(Left) Sagittal T1WI MR (A) and T2WI MR (B) demonstrate a heterogeneous marrow pattern in thoracolumbar spine and sacrum. Compression fractures involve L2 and L5, narrowing central canal at L2. *(Right)* Sagittal T1WI MR shows typical heterogeneous marrow signal pattern of multiple myeloma throughout lumbar spine. Note focal involvement of T12 spinous process. Compression Fxs present at L4, L2, L1.

NEUROBLASTIC TUMOR

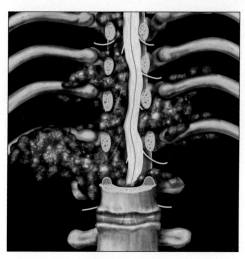

Coronal graphic shows a vascular paraspinal NB originating on the right, with spread through contiguous neural foramina across midline to the left (stage III).

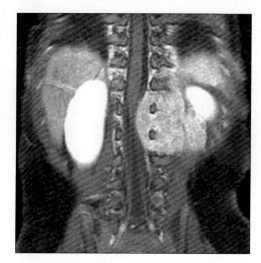

Coronal T1 C+ MR shows an enhancing left paraspinal NB with intraspinal spread through the neural foramina, causing mild cord displacement (Courtesy G. Hedlund, DO).

TERMINOLOGY

Abbreviations and Synonyms
- Neuroblastic tumors (NT) = ganglioneuroma (GN), ganglioneuroblastoma (GNB), and neuroblastoma (NB)

Definitions
- Embryonal tumors derived from neural crest cells

IMAGING FINDINGS

General Features
- Best diagnostic clue: Abdominal or thoracic paraspinal mass +/- intraspinal extension, calcification
- Location: Abdominal (40% adrenal, 25% paraspinal ganglia) > thoracic (15%) >, pelvic (5%) > cervical (3%); miscellaneous (12%)
- Size: Variable: 1-10 cm diameter
- Morphology: Marrow replacement, "dumbbell" paraspinal-intraspinal tumor

Radiographic Findings
- Radiography
  ○ Widened paraspinal soft tissues +/- scoliosis
  ○ +/- Stippled abdominal or mediastinal calcifications

CT Findings
- CECT: Enhancing paraspinal mass +/- epidural extension, finely stippled calcifications
- Bone CT
  ○ Widened neural foramina & intercostal spaces, pedicle erosion, adjacent rib splaying (GN, GNB) or destruction (NB)

MR Findings
- T1WI
  ○ Hypointense → isointense paraspinal mass +/- epidural extension through neural foramina
  ○ +/- Hypointense marrow replacement
- T2WI: Hypointense → hyperintense paraspinal mass +/- epidural extension, spinal cord compression
- T1 C+: Variable enhancement +/- internal hemorrhage, necrosis

Ultrasonographic Findings
- Real Time: Mixed echogenicity paraspinal mass; calcifications → posterior acoustic shadowing

Nuclear Medicine Findings
- Bone Scan: 99mTc MDP uptake in osseous metastatic lesions
- PET: Avid FDG uptake
- MIBG (metaiodobenzylguanidine)
  ○ Uptake by sympathetic catecholaminergic cells

DDx: Neuroblastic Tumors

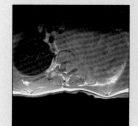

Ewing Sarcoma

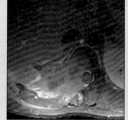

Metastasis

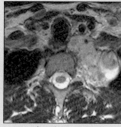

Plexiform NF

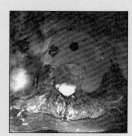

Lymphoma (NHL)

NEUROBLASTIC TUMOR

Key Facts

Terminology
- Neuroblastic tumors (NT) = ganglioneuroma (GN), ganglioneuroblastoma (GNB), and neuroblastoma (NB)

Imaging Findings
- Best diagnostic clue: Abdominal or thoracic paraspinal mass +/- intraspinal extension, calcification
- Location: Abdominal (40% adrenal, 25% paraspinal ganglia) > thoracic (15%) >, pelvic (5%) > cervical (3%); miscellaneous (12%)

Top Differential Diagnoses
- Ewing sarcoma
- Vertebral metastasis
- Nerve sheath tumor

- Lymphoma
- Wilms tumor

Pathology
- Arise from primordial neural crest cell derivatives along sympathetic chain

Clinical Issues
- Abdominal mass/pain, bone pain, fatigue, weight loss, blanching subcutaneous nodules
- Paraparesis/paraplegia (cord compression)

Diagnostic Checklist
- Infants more often present with thoracic, cervical tumors; older children with abdominal tumors
- Critical to recognize epidural extension prior to surgery

- (123)I-MIBG for NB staging, post-therapy surveillance
- (131)I-MIBG shows early therapeutic promise for NB treatment

Imaging Recommendations
- Best imaging tool
  - MR imaging for diagnosis, pre-surgical planning
  - MIBG for staging, post-treatment surveillance
- Protocol advice
  - Multiplanar enhanced MRI for tumor evaluation
  - Bone CT with multiplanar reformats to evaluate bone disease, detect calcifications
  - MIBG +/- bone scan for staging, surveillance

DIFFERENTIAL DIAGNOSIS

Ewing sarcoma
- "Small round blue cell tumor"; relatively T2 hypointense
- Arises from adjacent flat bones (rib, chest wall, pelvis) → 2° vertebral invasion

Vertebral metastasis
- Variable signal intensity; imaging characteristics follow primary tumor
- Multifocal disease common

Nerve sheath tumor
- Contiguous with neural foramen +/- "dumbbell" configuration

Lymphoma
- Systemic metastasis or primary vertebral lesion; predilection for paraspinal, epidural locations

Wilms tumor
- Majority arise from renal parenchyma; distinctive histopathology, slightly older age facilitate distinction from NB

PATHOLOGY

General Features
- General path comments
  - Arise from primordial neural crest cell derivatives along sympathetic chain
    - Ganglioneuroma = best differentiated, most benign, mature ganglion cells
    - Ganglioneuroblastoma = intermediate malignant potential, varying proportions of neuroblastoma and mature ganglion cells
    - Neuroblastoma = poorly differentiated malignant "small round blue cell tumor"
- Genetics: 1p chromosomal deletion in 70-80% of NB patients
- Etiology: No specific environmental exposure or risk factors definitively identified
- Epidemiology: 7-10 new NB cases/1,000,000 children (U.S.); true incidence of GNB, GN unknown because many asymptomatic
- Associated abnormalities: Orbit/skull/mandible osseous/dural metastases, "hair-on-end" periostitis, primary brain neuroblastoma (PNET)

Gross Pathologic & Surgical Features
- GN, GNB: Firm gray-white nodules
- NB: Soft gray-tan nodules +/- hemorrhage, necrosis, calcification

Microscopic Features
- GN: Mature ganglion cells, Schwann cells, neuritic processes
- GNB: Internal spectrum ranging GN → NB
- NB: Undifferentiated neuroblasts, ganglion cells
  - Small uniform round blue cells containing dense hyperchromatic nuclei, scant cytoplasm
  - Homer-Wright pseudorosettes around central neuropil core (15-50%)

Staging, Grading or Classification Criteria
- GN, GNB (intermixed-GNBi or nodular-GNBn), NB
- NB morphologic indicators: Undifferentiated (U), poorly differentiated (PD), differentiating (D)

NEUROBLASTIC TUMOR

- Evans anatomic staging for NB (prognosis - % survival)
  - Locoregional (combines stages 1-3)
    - 1: Confined to organ of interest (90%)
    - 2: Extension beyond organ but not crossing midline (75%)
    - 3: Extension crossing midline (include vertebral column) (30%)
  - Stage 4: Systemic, widespread distal metastases (10%)
  - Stage 4S: < 1 yrs at diagnosis, metastatic disease confined to skin, liver, and bone marrow, may spontaneously regress (nearly 100% survival)

CLINICAL ISSUES

Presentation
- Most common signs/symptoms
  - Abdominal mass/pain, bone pain, fatigue, weight loss, blanching subcutaneous nodules
  - Paraparesis/paraplegia (cord compression)
  - Other signs/symptoms
    - Diarrhea (VIP syndrome)
    - Proptosis, periorbital/conjunctival ecchymoses ("raccoon eyes")
    - Opsoclonus-myoclonus-ataxia (OMA) paraneoplastic syndrome (2-3%)
    - Horner syndrome (cervical NB)
  - Laboratory findings
    - > 90% ↑ urine homovanillic acid (HVA) and/or vanillylmandelic acid (VMA)
    - ↑ Serum neuron-specific enolase (NSE), lactic dehydrogenase (LDH), ferritin
- Clinical profile
  - Kerner-Morrison syndrome → intractable secretory diarrhea 2° VIP secretion (GN, GNB > NB)
  - Pepper syndrome: Infant with overwhelming liver metastatic NB → respiratory compromise
  - "Blueberry muffin baby": Infant with subcutaneous metastatic NB
  - Hutchinson syndrome: Widespread bone metastasis → bone pain, limping, pathologic fractures
  - NAT mimic: Metastatic retrobulbar neuroblastoma → rapidly progressive painless proptosis, periorbital ecchymosis

Demographics
- Age: 40% < 1 yr, 35% 1-2 yr, and 25% > 2 yr at diagnosis; rare after age 10 yr
- Gender: M > F (1.3:1)

Natural History & Prognosis
- GN prognosis excellent after surgical resection
- GNB prognosis dependent on proportion of GN, NB
- NB 5 year survival ≈ 83% for infants, 55% for children 1-5 years, and 40% for children > 5 years
  - Favorable prognostic indicators: Locoregional, stage 4s, ↓ n-myc amplification, hyperdiploid DNA
  - Unfavorable prognostic indicators: Stage 4 disease, ocular involvement, HER2/neu oncogene over-expression, ↑ NSE/LDH/serum ferritin, ↑ urine HVA/VMA, 1p chromosomal deletion

Treatment
- Options include chemotherapy, surgery, radiation, steroids

DIAGNOSTIC CHECKLIST

Consider
- NB presentation depends on patient age, primary site, metastatic burden, metabolically active products
- Infants more often present with thoracic, cervical tumors; older children with abdominal tumors

Image Interpretation Pearls
- Critical to recognize epidural extension prior to surgery

SELECTED REFERENCES

1. Tateishi U et al: Adult neuroblastoma: radiologic and clinicopathologic features. J Comput Assist Tomogr. 27(3):321-6, 2003
2. Rha SE et al: Neurogenic tumors in the abdomen: tumor types and imaging characteristics. Radiographics. 23(1):29-43, 2003
3. Pfluger T et al: Integrated imaging using MRI and 123I metaiodobenzylguanidine scintigraphy to improve sensitivity and specificity in the diagnosis of pediatric neuroblastoma. AJR Am J Roentgenol. 181(4):1115-24, 2003
4. Siegel MJ et al: Staging of neuroblastoma at imaging: report of the radiology diagnostic oncology group. Radiology. 223(1):168-75, 2002
5. Lonergan GJ et al: Neuroblastoma, ganglioneuroblastoma, and ganglioneuroma: radiologic-pathologic correlation. Radiographics. 22(4):911-34, 2002
6. Meyer JS et al: Imaging of neuroblastoma and Wilms' tumor. Magn Reson Imaging Clin N Am. 10(2):275-302, 2002
7. Geoerger B et al: Metabolic activity and clinical features of primary ganglioneuromas. Cancer. 91(10):1905-13, 2001
8. Kushner BH et al: Extending positron emission tomography scan utility to high-risk neuroblastoma: fluorodeoxyglucose positron emission tomography as sole imaging modality in follow-up of patients. J Clin Oncol. 19(14):3397-405, 2001
9. Joshi VJ: Peripheral neuroblastic tumors: Pathological classification based on recommendations of international neuroblastoma committee. Pediatr and Dev Path. 3:184-99, 2000
10. Schwab et al: Neuroblastic tumors of the adrenal gland and sympathetic nervous system, Kleihues and Cavenee (eds): Pathology and Genetics of tumors of the nervous system. IARC press, Lyon. 153-161, 2000
11. Sofka CM et al: Magnetic resonance imaging of neuroblastoma using current techniques. Magn Reson Imaging. 17(2):193-8, 1999
12. Perel Y et al: Clinical impact and prognostic value of metaiodobenzylguanidine imaging in children with metastatic neuroblastoma. J Pediatr Hematol Oncol. 21(1):13-8, 1999
13. Brodeur GM et al: International criteria for diagnosis, staging, and response to treatment in patients with neuroblastoma. J Clin Oncol. 6(12):1874-81, 1988

NEUROBLASTIC TUMOR

IMAGE GALLERY

Typical

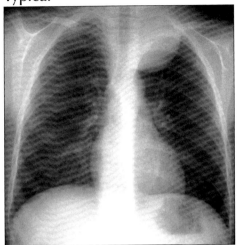
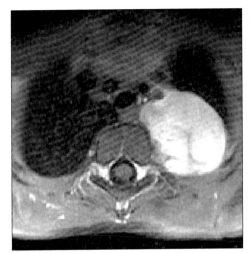

(Left) Anteroposterior radiography shows large posterior mediastinal mass (ganglioneuroma) without rib or vertebral destruction (Courtesy R. Boyer, MD). *(Right)* Axial T1 C+ MR reveals large left (surgically proven) paraspinal ganglioneuroma. No vertebral or neural foraminal invasion was detected (Courtesy G. Hedlund, DO).

Typical

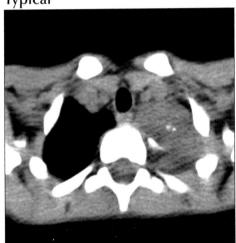
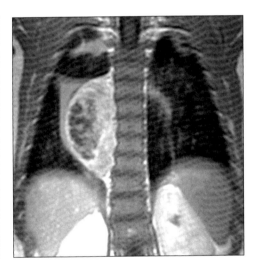

(Left) Axial NECT depicts large left posterior mediastinal mass with stippled internal calcification. Surgical pathology revealed ganglioneuroblastoma (Courtesy R. Boyer, MD). *(Right)* Coronal T1 C+ MR demonstrates heterogeneously enhancing necrotic thoracic neuroblastoma without epidural invasion. The large mass produces atelectasis of adjacent lung (Courtesy G. Hedlund, DO).

Typical

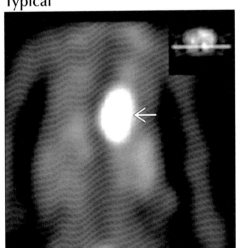
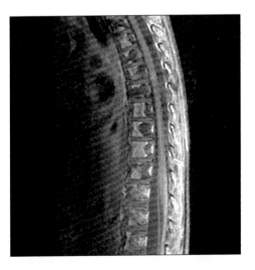

(Left) Coronal I-123 MIBG coronal SPECT scan demonstrates typical avid uptake within large left paraspinal neuroblastoma (arrow) (Courtesy B. Reid, MD). *(Right)* Sagittal T1 C+ MR shows extensive blastic enhancing extradural neuroblastoma metastases to the axial skeleton in child (Courtesy G. Hedlund, DO).

ANGIOLIPOMA

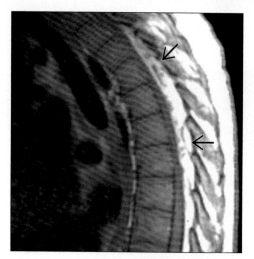

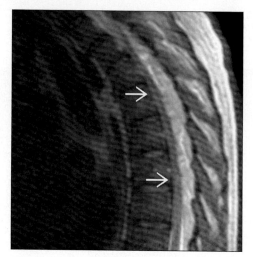

Sagittal T1WI MR shows long segment heterogeneous T1 hyperintense mass within posterior thoracic epidural space causing cord compression. Scattered foci of low signal are present (arrows).

Sagittal T2WI MR shows heterogeneous slight hyperintensity from dorsal epidural mass extending over multiple thoracic segments. Cord compression is well identified (arrows).

TERMINOLOGY

Abbreviations and Synonyms
- Angiolipoma (AL), vascular lipoma, hemangiolipoma, fibromyolipoma

Definitions
- Benign tumor of adipose and vascular elements

IMAGING FINDINGS

General Features
- Best diagnostic clue: Hyperintense mass on unenhanced T1WI, showing enhancement on fat suppressed T1WI
- Location
  ○ Uncommon tumors of extremities, trunk, neck
  ○ Spine involvement uncommon: Extradural >> intramedullary
  ○ C6 ⇒ L4 level
  ○ Rare reports of mediastinal angiolipoma with spinal canal extension
- Size
  ○ Extend over 1-4 vertebral body segments
  ○ Average extent > 2 vertebral body length
- Morphology: Focal or infiltrating mass showing heterogeneous fat signal

Radiographic Findings
- Myelography
  ○ Nonspecific extradural mass
  ○ May show block with aggressive lesion

CT Findings
- NECT
  ○ CT shows extradural mass of fat attenuation (-20 to -60 HU), with scattered soft tissue reticulation
  ○ Slight enhancement
  ○ Rare calcification
  ○ Rare bony remodeling

MR Findings
- T1WI
  ○ Hyperintense on T1WI, with inhomogeneous signal
  ○ Heterogeneity thought related to capillary and venous channels
  ○ Prominence of vascular component may give more isointense T1 signal
- T2WI: Mild increase signal relative to CSF
- PD/Intermediate: Increased signal relative to CSF, but decreased signal relative to fat
- T1 C+: Fat suppressed T1WI most useful for lesion definition, showing heterogeneous enhancement

---

DDx: T1 Hyperintense Masses

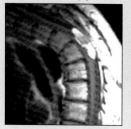

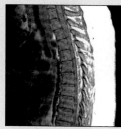

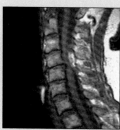

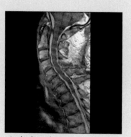

Lipoma   *Epidural Abscess*   *Epidural Hemorrhage*   *Subdural Hemorrhage*

ANGIOLIPOMA

Key Facts

Terminology
- Angiolipoma (AL), vascular lipoma, hemangiolipoma, fibromyolipoma
- Benign tumor of adipose and vascular elements

Imaging Findings
- Best diagnostic clue: Hyperintense mass on unenhanced T1WI, showing enhancement on fat suppressed T1WI
- Spine involvement uncommon: Extradural >> intramedullary
- Extend over 1-4 vertebral body segments
- CT shows extradural mass of fat attenuation (-20 to -60 HU), with scattered soft tissue reticulation
- Hyperintense on T1WI, with inhomogeneous signal

- T1 C+: Fat suppressed T1WI most useful for lesion definition, showing heterogeneous enhancement

Pathology
- May occur as focal or infiltrating forms
- Infiltrating form more common in anterior epidural space, may destroy adjacent bone
- Focal form more common in posterior thoracic epidural space, no bone destruction

Clinical Issues
- Nonspecific back pain
- Progressive paraparesis
- Surgical excision for painful, symptomatic lesions

Diagnostic Checklist
- Angiolipomas do not show vascular flow voids

Imaging Recommendations
- Best imaging tool: Fat suppressed contrast-enhanced T1WI
- Protocol advice
  - Axial, sagittal T1 and T2 weighted images precontrast
  - Axial and sagittal post-contrast fat suppressed T1WI

DIFFERENTIAL DIAGNOSIS

Lipoma
- Little or no enhancement, minimal septations
- May be intradural, extradural or subcutaneous
- Distinguishable microscopically, with AL showing vessels branching pattern and fibrous scarring

Liposarcoma
- May have irregular thickened septa, with areas of T2 hyperintensity
- Liposarcoma show cellular pleomorphism and mitotic activity
- May show considerable T1 isointense tissue

Hematoma
- No suppression with fat-sat
- No enhancement, unless more chronic
- May show low signal on T2* images

Abscess
- May show heterogenous T1 signal within epidural fat, with focal areas of low signal
- Prominent peripheral enhancement
- May show heterogeneous signal and enhancement-like angiolipoma

Epidural lipomatosis
- Homogeneous fat signal, without enhancement
- Typical history of steroid use
- Typical dorsal thoracic epidural location

PATHOLOGY

General Features
- General path comments
  - Benign tumor usually found in extremities, trunk or neck
  - Spine angiolipomas rare
  - May occur as focal or infiltrating forms
    - Infiltrating form more common in anterior epidural space, may destroy adjacent bone
    - Focal form more common in posterior thoracic epidural space, no bone destruction
  - Focal form may occur at multiple sites in subcutaneous tissues
- Genetics
  - Subcutaneous angiolipomas show predominately normal karyotype
    - Contrasted with characteristic chromosomal aberrations in other lipomatous lesions such as lipoma, lipoblastoma, hibernomas
  - Rare familial occurrence of angiolipomas
- Etiology
  - Etiology unknown, with several theories
    - May originate from primitive pluripotential mesenchymal cells
    - Congenital malformation
    - Hamartomatous lesion, enlarging in response to injury/inflammation
- Epidemiology
  - Rare, approximately 0.2-1% of all spinal tumors
  - 2-3% of extradural tumors
  - Focal form more common in spine
  - Typically mid-thoracic level, but can occur any where in spine
  - CNS involvement rare, but 90% occur in spine

Gross Pathologic & Surgical Features
- Gross features of fatty tissue, although may show port wine or dark brown coloration

Microscopic Features
- Presence of fat and vascular tissues
  - Vascular proliferation with microthrombi

ANGIOLIPOMA

- ○ Consistent marker of angiolipomas is presence of fibrin microthrombi in vascular channels associated with disrupted endothelial cells
- Vessels variously described as sinusoids, thin-walled, thick walled with smooth muscle proliferation
- Mitoses and pleomorphism not present
- Features vary
  - ○ Predominately lipomatous with few small angiomatous regions
  - ○ Predominately vascular with small lipomatous component

CLINICAL ISSUES

Presentation
- Most common signs/symptoms
  - ○ Nonspecific back pain
  - ○ Other signs/symptoms: Cord compression
    - Progressive paraparesis
    - Symptoms may progress with pregnancy
    - Acute onset of symptoms may occur due to degeneration, or hemorrhage into lesion
- Clinical profile: Slowly progressive paraparesis with back pain

Demographics
- Age
  - ○ 5th decade, although may occur in children or adults
  - ○ Mean age 42 years
- Gender: M < F

Natural History & Prognosis
- Slowly progressive
- Bone infiltration associated with more aggressive behavior and worse prognosis

Treatment
- Surgical excision for painful, symptomatic lesions
  - ○ Focal form low rate of recurrence following excision
  - ○ Infiltrative form 50% recurrence rate
- Partial resection may give good symptomatic relief in infiltrative form
- Degree of hypointensity on T1WI predictive of degree of vascularity encountered at surgery

DIAGNOSTIC CHECKLIST

Consider
- Not to be confused with angiomyolipoma, which is seen in tuberous sclerosis, and occurs in kidney

Image Interpretation Pearls
- Angiolipomas do not show vascular flow voids

SELECTED REFERENCES

1. Gelabert-Gonzalez M et al: Spinal extradural angiolipoma, with a literature review. Childs Nerv Syst. 18(12): 725-8, 2002
2. Amlashi SF et al: Spinal epidural angiolipoma. J Neuroradiol. 28(4): 253-6, 2001
3. Choi JY et al: Angiolipoma of the posterior mediastinum with extension into the spinal canal: a case report. Korean J Radiol. 1(4): 212-4, 2000
4. Bailey D et al: Dorsal thoracic cord compression from a spinal angiolipoma: case report and brief comment. Conn Med. 64(5): 267-9, 2000
5. Labram EK et al: Revisited: spinal angiolipoma--three additional cases. Br J Neurosurg. 13(1): 25-9, 1999
6. Oge HK et al: Spinal angiolipoma: case report and review of literature. J Spinal Disord. 12(4): 353-6, 1999
7. Klisch J et al: Radiological and histological findings in spinal intramedullary angiolipoma. Neuroradiology. 41(8): 584-7, 1999
8. Sciot R et al: Cytogenetic analysis of subcutaneous angiolipoma: further evidence supporting its difference from ordinary pure lipomas: a report of the CHAMP Study Group. Am J Surg Pathol. 21(4):441-4, 1997
9. Weiss SW: Lipomatous tumors. Monogr Pathol. 38:207-39, 1996
10. Provenzale JM et al: Spinal angiolipomas: MR features. AJNR Am J Neuroradiol. 17(4): 713-9, 1996
11. Fletcher CD et al: Correlation between clinicopathological features and karyotype in lipomatous tumors. A report of 178 cases from the Chromosomes and Morphology (CHAMP) Collaborative Study Group. Am J Pathol. 148(2):623-30, 1996
12. Shibata Y et al: Thoracic epidural angiolipoma--case report. Neurol Med Chir (Tokyo). 33(5): 316-9, 1993
13. Jelinek JS et al: Liposarcoma of the extremities: MR and CT findings in the histologic subtypes. Radiology. 186(2):455-9, 1993
14. Pagni CA et al: Spinal epidural angiolipoma: rare or unreported? Neurosurgery. 31(4): 758-64; discussion 764, 1992
15. Stranjalis G et al: MRI in the diagnosis of spinal extradural angiolipoma. Br J Neurosurg. 6(5): 481-3, 1992
16. Weill A et al: Spinal angiolipomas: CT and MR aspects. J Comput Assist Tomogr. 15(1): 83-5, 1991
17. Quint DJ et al: Epidural lipomatosis. Radiology. 169(2):485-90, 1988
18. Matsushima K et al: Spinal extradural angiolipoma: MR and CT diagnosis. J Comput Assist Tomogr. 11(6):1104-6, 1987
19. Dixon AY et al: Angiolipomas: an ultrastructural and clinicopathological study. Hum Pathol. 12(8):739-47, 1981
20. HOWARD WR et al: Angiolipoma. Arch Dermatol. 82:924-31, 1960

ANGIOLIPOMA

IMAGE GALLERY

Typical

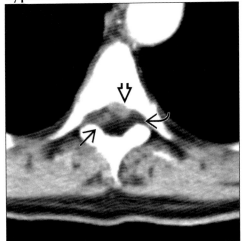
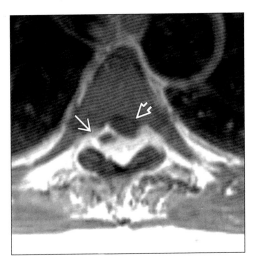

(Left) Axial CECT shows fat attenuation mass within dorsal epidural space (curved arrow), compressing the cord anteriorly (open arrow). Heterogeneous signal present within right side of lesion (arrow). *(Right)* Axial T1 C+ MR shows hyperintense mass within dorsal thoracic epidural space, compressing cord ventrally (open arrow). Focus of low signal present within right side of lesion (arrow).

Typical

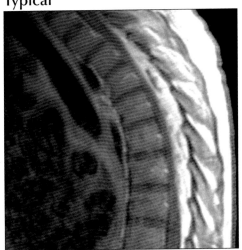
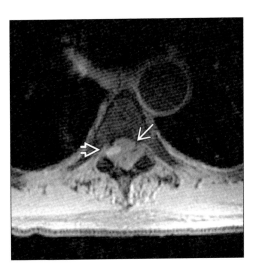

(Left) Sagittal T1 C+ MR shows enhancing heterogeneous signal epidural mass extending over multiple thoracic segments, compressing the cord anteriorly. Adjacent bone intact. *(Right)* Axial T2* GRE MR shows intermediate fat signal mass within the posterior epidural space, displacing cord anteriorly (arrow). Small amount of heterogeneous signal present on right (open arrow).

Typical

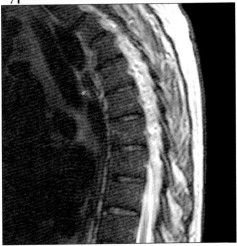
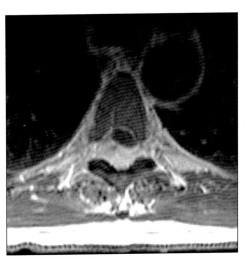

(Left) Sagittal T2WI MR shows slightly heterogeneous signal from fatty mass involving posterior epidural space. Overall, lesion is not significantly hyperintense. *(Right)* Axial T1 C+ MR shows ill-defined high signal mass involving posterior epidural space, compressing cord ventrally, and to left.

MENINGIOMA

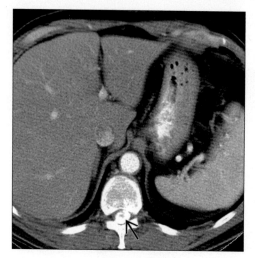

Axial CECT done for abdominal pain, incidentally depicts calcified meningioma within lower thoracic spinal canal (arrow).

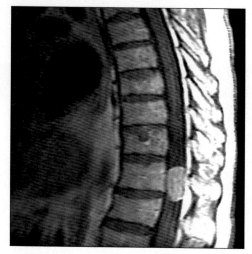

Sagittal T1 C+ MR shows homogeneously enhancing oval lesion in low thoracic canal. Note dural base, well-circumscribed margins.

TERMINOLOGY

Definitions
- Slow growing, benign tumor originating from and based on the dura matter

IMAGING FINDINGS

General Features
- Best diagnostic clue
  - Enhancing intradural/extramedullary mass + dural "tail"
    - 90% intradural (10% extradural and/or "dumbbell")
    - Ca++ < 5%
- Location
  - Typically intradural, extramedullary
    - Can rarely be intraosseous, extradural, even paraspinous
- Size: Variable
- Morphology
  - Typically round
  - Broad base against dura
  - Trailing "tail" into adjacent dura

Radiographic Findings
- Radiography: Focal intraspinal calcification

- Myelography: Intradural, extramedullary mass

CT Findings
- NECT: Iso- to hyperdense mass (compared to muscle)
- CECT: Strong homogeneous enhancement
- Bone CT
  - May see hyperostosis

MR Findings
- T1WI: Isointense (to spinal cord)
- T2WI
  - Majority are isointense to cord
  - Some hyperintense
  - May be hypointense if densely calcified
  - Very vascular meningioma may have prominent "flow voids"
- PD/Intermediate: Typically isointense
- T1 C+
  - Prominent enhancement
  - May see enhancing dural "tail" (less common than intracranial)

Angiographic Findings
- Conventional
  - Early capillary blush
  - Vascular stain well into venous phase

Other Modality Findings
- Myelography, CT myelography

DDx: Meningioma Look-Alikes

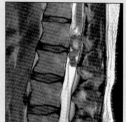

Cauda Ependymoma

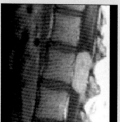

Neurinoma

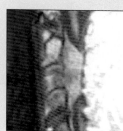

C3 Chordoma

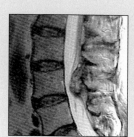

Synovial Cyst

MENINGIOMA

Key Facts

Terminology
- Slow growing, benign tumor originating from and based on the dura mater

Imaging Findings
- Enhancing intradural/extramedullary mass + dural "tail"
- T1WI: Isointense (to spinal cord)
- Majority are isointense to cord
- Prominent enhancement
- Myelography, CT myelography
- Sharp meniscus of contrast caps lesion (classic for intradural, extramedullary mass)
- Ipsilateral subarachnoid space widened (cord, roots displaced away from mass)

Top Differential Diagnoses
- Schwannoma
- Lymphoma
- Extradural masses

Pathology
- Most are solitary, sporadic
- Thoracic (80%) > > cervical (16%) > lumbar (4%)
- NF2
- Multiple meningiomatosis
- Firm, well demarcated, lobulated/rounded mass with dural attachment
- Occasionally cystic

- ○ Sharp meniscus of contrast caps lesion (classic for intradural, extramedullary mass)
- ○ Ipsilateral subarachnoid space widened (cord, roots displaced away from mass)

Imaging Recommendations
- Contrast-enhanced MRI
- CT (if densely calcified)

DIFFERENTIAL DIAGNOSIS

Schwannoma
- Very hyperintense on T2WI
- Cystic change, hemorrhage more common
- No dural attachment
- Very rare posterior to cord

Other intradural extramedullary masses
- Paraganglioma (rare)
- Epidermoid (signal usually = CSF)
- Arachnoid cyst (like CSF, doesn't enhance)
- Intradural metastasis (often multiple)
- Intradural tumors below cord; e.g., cauda equina ependymoma, drop metastases

Lymphoma
- Solitary intradural mass uncommon

Extradural masses
- Can simulate meningioma if big, cannot be compartmentalized
  - ○ Chordoma
  - ○ Cyst

PATHOLOGY

General Features
- General path comments
  - ○ Most are solitary, sporadic
  - ○ Intracranial: Spine meningiomas = 8:1
  - ○ Thoracic (80%) > > cervical (16%) > lumbar (4%)

- ■ Site frequency roughly proportional to surface area of dura in spine
- Genetics
  - ○ Almost all have chromosome 22 abnormalities
  - ○ NF2
    - ■ Multiple meningiomatosis
    - ■ Familial clear cell meningioma syndrome
    - ■ Multiple meningiomas
- Etiology
  - ○ Arise from arachnoid cap cell rests
  - ○ Genetic predisposition in women, NF2
  - ○ Associated with prior radiation
- Epidemiology
  - ○ Second most common intradural extramedullary tumor
    - ■ 25% of primary spinal tumors
  - ○ F:M = 4:1
- Associated abnormalities: Bony sclerosis

Gross Pathologic & Surgical Features
- Firm, well demarcated, lobulated/rounded mass with dural attachment
- Expands centripetally within dural sac
- May rarely have dumbbell morphology simulating neurinoma
- Occasionally cystic

Microscopic Features
- Most are "typical" meningiomas
  - ○ Common histologic subtypes
    - ■ Most common = psammomatous type with Ca++ concretions
    - ■ Meningothelial
    - ■ Fibrous
    - ■ Transitional
  - ○ Less common
    - ■ Angiomatous
    - ■ Microcystic
    - ■ Clear cell
    - ■ Choroid
    - ■ Lipomatous
    - ■ Hemorrhagic
- Rare

MENINGIOMA

- ○ Atypical (increased mitoses, cellularity, etc.)
- ○ Anaplastic (malignant)
  - Angioblastic, difficult to distinguish from hemangiopericytoma
  - Can metastasize or be multicentric

Staging, Grading or Classification Criteria

- \> 95% WHO grade I

CLINICAL ISSUES

Presentation

- Most common signs/symptoms
  - ○ Pain
  - ○ Other signs/symptoms
    - Motor/sensory deficit
    - Gait disturbance
- Clinical profile: Female with onset of myelopathy

Demographics

- Age
  - ○ Peak incidence 5th/6th decade
  - ○ Under 50, more commonly genetic, worse prognosis
- Gender: > 80% female

Natural History & Prognosis

- Slow growing, compresses but doesn't invade adjacent structures
- Excellent prognosis with complete excision
  - ○ Possible in 96%
- Recurrence rate up to 40% at 5 years in patients with incomplete resection, en plaque, and infiltrative meningioma

Treatment

- Complete surgical resection
- +/- XRT (subtotal resection, aggressive tumors)

DIAGNOSTIC CHECKLIST

Consider

- Angiogram for distinguishing meningioma, neurofibroma

Image Interpretation Pearls

- If tumor is dorsal to cord, almost always meningioma, not neurinoma (nerve roots are anterolaterally located)

SELECTED REFERENCES

1. Cohen-Gadol AA et al: Spinal meningiomas in patients younger than 50 years of age: a 21-year experience. J Neurosurg. 98(3 Suppl):258-63, 2003
2. Covert S et al: Magnetic resonance imaging of intramedullary meningioma of the spinal cord: case report and review of the literature. Can Assoc Radiol J. 54(3):177-80, 2003
3. Lucey BP et al: Spinal meningioma causing diffuse leptomeningeal enhancement. Neurology. 60(2):350-1, 2003
4. Doita M et al: Recurrent calcified spinal meningioma detected by plain radiograph. Spine. 26(11):E249-52, 2001
5. Eastwood JD et al: Diffusion-weighted MR imaging in a patient with spinal meningioma. AJR Am J Roentgenol. 177(6):1479-81, 2001
6. Louis DN et al: Meningiomas. In Kleihues P, Cavanee WK (eds), Tumours of the Nervous System, 176-84, IARC Press, 2000
7. Naderi S: Spinal meningiomas. Surg Neurol. 54(1):95, 2000
8. Klekamp J et al: Surgical results for spinal meningiomas. Surg Neurol. 52: 552-62, 1999
9. Yoshiura T et al: Cervical spinal meningioma with unusual MR contrast enhancement. AJNR Am J Neuroradiol. 19(6):1040-2, 1998
10. Sato N et al: Extradural spinal meningioma: MRI. Neuroradiology. 39(6):450-2, 1997
11. Borden NM: Aggressive angioblastic meningioma with multiple sites in the neural axis. AJNR Am J Neuroradiol. 16(4):793-4, 1995
12. Akeson P et al: Radiological investigation of neurofibromatosis type 2. Neuroradiology. 36(2):107-10, 1994
13. Souweidane MM et al: Spinal cord meningiomas. Neurosurg Clin N Am. 5(2):283-91, 1994
14. Kabus D et al: Metastatic meningioma. Hemangiopericytoma or angioblastic meningioma? Am J Surg Pathol. 17(11):1144-50, 1993
15. Kannuki S et al: Coexistence of intracranial and spinal meningiomas--report of two cases. Neurol Med Chir (Tokyo). 31(11):720-4, 1991
16. Solero CL et al: Spinal menigiomas: Review of 174 operated cases. Neurosurg. 125: 153-60, 1989
17. Levy WJ Jr et al: Spinal cord meningioma. J Neurosurg. 57(6):804-12, 1982

MENINGIOMA

IMAGE GALLERY

Typical

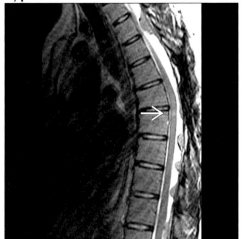
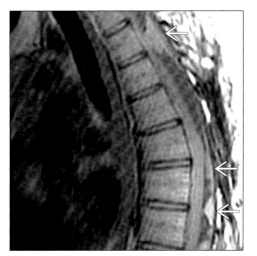

(Left) Sagittal T2WI MR in patient with NF2 shows many dural based tumors - dorsal location, morphology, low signal, and clinical context all typical of meningioma. Note small intramedullary lesion (arrow). *(Right)* Sagittal T1WI MR shows several dural based lesions (arrows), isointense to cord, in patient with NF2, which were hypointense on T2WI, enhanced vividly.

Typical

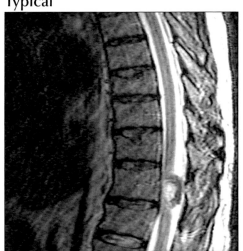
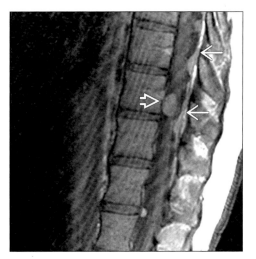

(Left) Sagittal T2WI MR shows intradural (note expanded subarachnoid space) mass with inhomogeneous signal. Calcium content on CT explained low signal of dural base. No significant myelopathy = slow growth. *(Right)* Sagittal T1 C+ MR shows numerous enhancing lesions in NF2 patient. Note dural "tails" (arrows) on several. Ventral lesion (open arrow) impossible to distinguish from neurinoma.

Variant

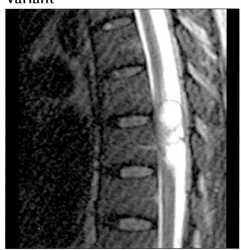
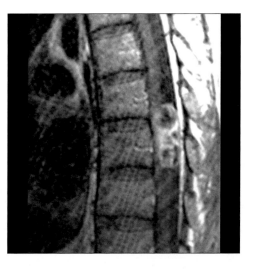

(Left) Sagittal T2WI MR in patient with family history of NF2 shows extramedullary multicystic mass, which enhanced. Despite similarity to neurinoma, dorsal location favors meningioma - proven at surgery. *(Right)* Sagittal T1 C+ MR shows enhancing multicystic mass (family history of NF2): Nonspecific appearance. Dorsal extra-axial location favors meningioma (surgically proven), though cysts unusual.

HEMANGIOPERICYTOMA

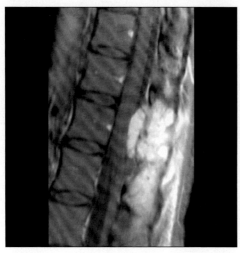

Sagittal T1 C+ MR shows enhancing, dural based intraspinal mass invading the posterior elements.

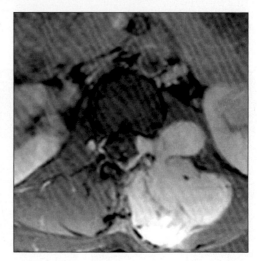

Axial T1 C+ MR shows paraspinous, vividly enhancing mass associated with intraspinal dural component.

TERMINOLOGY

Abbreviations and Synonyms

- Hemangiopericytic meningioma, angioblastic meningioma
  - These are not truly synonymous as the cell of origin is different
  - May be indistinguishable on imaging, and even pathologically
  - Dual differentiation into both cell types (pericyte, meningeal) has been described

Definitions

- Hypervascular neoplasm arising from pericytes

IMAGING FINDINGS

General Features

- Best diagnostic clue: Vividly enhancing lesion expanding/eroding spinal canal, with large soft tissue component
- Location
  - Dural based if primary
  - Epicenter in bone if metastatic
- Size: Variable
- Morphology: Reasonably well-circumscribed, multilobulated

Radiographic Findings

- Radiography: Erosive lesion in spinal column or appendages
- Myelography: Epidural mass effect on contrast column with bone remodeling/erosion

CT Findings

- NECT
  - Replacement/erosion of bone, expansion of canal by isodense mass with reasonably well-circumscribed borders
  - No phleboliths or calcific components
- CECT: Vivid enhancement
- Bone CT
  - Bony expansion/erosion

MR Findings

- T1WI: Hypointense multilobular mass expanding/eroding bone and canal
- T2WI: Mild to moderate hyperintensity
- STIR: Emphasizes high signal compared to normal bone
- T2* GRE: Same as STIR
- T1 C+: Vivid, homogeneous enhancement

Angiographic Findings

- Conventional: Marked hypervascularity in arterial phase with abnormal irregular vessels

DDx: Dural/Extradural Tumors

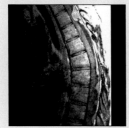

Meningioma

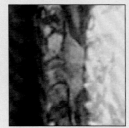

Chordoma

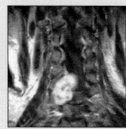

Neurofibroma

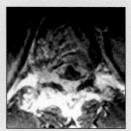

Hemangioma

HEMANGIOPERICYTOMA

Key Facts

Terminology
- Hypervascular neoplasm arising from pericytes

Imaging Findings
- Best diagnostic clue: Vividly enhancing lesion expanding/eroding spinal canal, with large soft tissue component
- Dural based if primary
- Epicenter in bone if metastatic
- T1WI: Hypointense multilobular mass expanding/eroding bone and canal
- T2WI: Mild to moderate hyperintensity
- T1 C+: Vivid, homogeneous enhancement
- Conventional: Marked hypervascularity in arterial phase with abnormal irregular vessels

Top Differential Diagnoses
- Meningioma
- Chordoma and other primary bone malignancies
- Neurinoma
- Aggressive hemangioma
- Vascular metastases

Pathology
- Vascular neoplasm consisting of capillaries outlined by intact basement membrane
- Basement membrane separates capillaries from spindle shaped tumor cells in the extravascular area
- Undifferentiated malignancy, but may see dual differentiation towards hemangiopericytoma and meningioma

Nuclear Medicine Findings
- Bone Scan: "Hot" focal uptake

Imaging Recommendations
- Best imaging tool: T1 C+ with fat-saturation
- Protocol advice: Scan entire neural axis to look for primary, as metastases common, especially in previously treated cases

DIFFERENTIAL DIAGNOSIS

Meningioma
- Usually well-circumscribed, non erosive
- Calcification helpful clue
- Malignant, invasive meningiomas may be very hard to distinguish from hemangiopericytoma

Chordoma and other primary bone malignancies
- Typically epicentered in bone
- Associated with notochord, ventral in canal or in vertebral body with extension beyond

Neurinoma
- Bilobular if through neural foramen
- Expand neural foramen

Aggressive hemangioma
- Spoke wheel pattern of vessels
- Symmetrical extension from vertebral body into epidural space

Vascular metastases
- Renal cell, thyroid carcinoma
- Usually centered in cancellous bone
- If dural based, quite focal

Angiosarcoma
- Very rarely in spine
- More haphazard boundaries

PATHOLOGY

General Features
- General path comments: Discrete, "dumbbell" shaped or multilobular fleshy lesion
- Etiology: Malignant dedifferentiation of pericytes
- Epidemiology: Rare
- Associated abnormalities: Pathologic fracture

Gross Pathologic & Surgical Features
- Discrete dural or epidural red appearing mass

Microscopic Features
- Vascular neoplasm consisting of capillaries outlined by intact basement membrane
- Basement membrane separates capillaries from spindle shaped tumor cells in the extravascular area
- Undifferentiated malignancy, but may see dual differentiation towards hemangiopericytoma and meningioma

CLINICAL ISSUES

Presentation
- Most common signs/symptoms
  - Pain
  - Other signs/symptoms
    - Neuropathy
    - Myelopathy

Demographics
- Age: Any
- Gender: No preference

Natural History & Prognosis
- Progressive growth, prone to late metastases

Treatment
- Options, risks, complications: Resection, radiation

HEMANGIOPERICYTOMA

DIAGNOSTIC CHECKLIST

Consider
• Angiography and embolization for operative planning

Image Interpretation Pearls
• Malignant meningioma more likely to show invasive finger like processes as opposed to lobules of hemangiopericytoma

SELECTED REFERENCES

1. Woitzik J et al: Delayed manifestation of spinal metastasis: a special feature of hemangiopericytoma. Clin Neurol Neurosurg. 105(3):159-66, 2003
2. Musacchio M et al: Posterior cervical haemangiopericytoma with intracranial and skull base extension. Diagnostic and therapeutic challenge of a rare hypervascular neoplasm. J Neuroradiol. 30(3):180-7, 2003
3. Cox DP et al: Myopericytoma of the thoracic spine: a case report. Spine. 28(2):E30-2, 2003
4. Akhaddar A et al: Thoracic epidural hemangiopericytoma. Case report. J Neurosurg Sci. 46(2):89-92; discussion 92, 2002
5. Tayoro K et al: [Imaging of meningeal hemangiopericytomas] J Radiol. 83(4 Pt 1):459-65, 2002
6. Ijiri K et al: Primary epidural hemangiopericytoma in the lumbar spine: a case report. Spine. 27(7):E189-92, 2002
7. Betchen S et al: Intradural hemangiopericytoma of the lumbar spine: case report. Neurosurgery. 50(3):654-7, 2002
8. Nonaka M et al: Metastatic meningeal hemangiopericytoma of thoracic spine. Clin Neurol Neurosurg. 100(3):228-30, 1998
9. Lin YJ et al: Primary hemangiopericytoma in the axis bone: case report and review of literature. Neurosurgery. 39(2):397-9; discussion 399-400, 1996
10. Murphey MD et al: From the archives of the AFIP. Musculoskeletal angiomatous lesions: radiologic-pathologic correlation. Radiographics. 15(4):893-917, 1995
11. Kozlowski K et al: Primary sacral bone tumours in children (report of 16 cases with a short literature review). Australas Radiol. 34(2):142-9, 1990
12. Bridges LR et al: Haemangiopericytic meningioma of the sacral canal: a case report. J Neurol Neurosurg Psychiatry. 51(2):288-90, 1988
13. Cuccurullo L et al: Hemangiopericytoma of the cervical spine. A case report. Acta Neurol (Napoli). 6(6):472-81, 1984
14. Beadle GF et al: Treatment of advanced malignant hemangiopericytoma with combination adriamycin and DTIC: a report of four cases. J Surg Oncol. 22(3):167-70, 1983
15. Muraszko KM et al: Hemangiopericytomas of the spine. Neurosurgery. 10(4):473-9, 1982
16. Cappabianca P et al: Hemangiopericytoma of the spinal canal. Surg Neurol. 15(4):298-302, 1981
17. Stern MB et al: Hemangiopericytoma of the cervical spine: report of an unusual case. Clin Orthop. (151):201-4, 1980
18. Anderson C et al: Skeletal metastases of an intracranial malignant hemangiopericytoma. Report of a case. J Bone Joint Surg Am. 62(1):145-8, 1980
19. Subbarao K et al: Primary malignant neoplasms. Semin Roentgenol. 14(1):44-57, 1979
20. Harris DJ et al: Hemangiopericytoma of the spinal canal. Report of three cases. J Neurosurg. 49(6):914-20, 1978
21. Hart S et al: Haemangiopericytoma of the pre-sacral space. Br J Surg. 60(7):583-4, 1973
22. Baxter PJ et al: Haemangiopericytoma. Light and electron microscopy studies of a cerebral secondary tumour. Acta Neuropathol (Berl). 21(3):253-7, 1972

HEMANGIOPERICYTOMA

IMAGE GALLERY

Typical

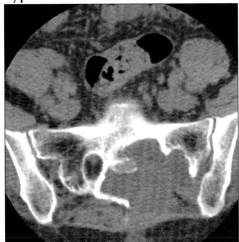 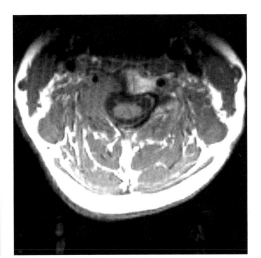

(Left) Axial NECT shows large isodense lesion expanding and eroding the sacral canal and neural foramen in patient with previously treated intracranial hemangiopericytoma. *(Right)* Axial T1WI MR shows replacement of right arch and vb by isointense lesion, encasement of vertebral artery. Lesion showed high signal on T2WI and vivid enhancement. Patient had intracranial primary.

Typical

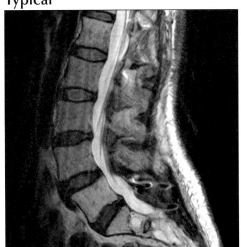 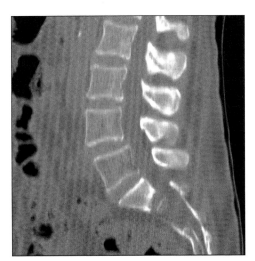

(Left) Sagittal T2WI MR depicts multilobulated high signal lesion in sacrum, extending from bone into spinal canal in patient with intracranial hemangiopericytoma previously treated by surgery and radiation. *(Right)* Sagittal bone CT reformation shows erosive bony lesion of sacrum in patient with previously treated intracranial hemangiopericytoma.

Typical

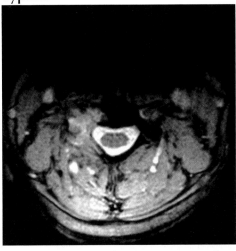 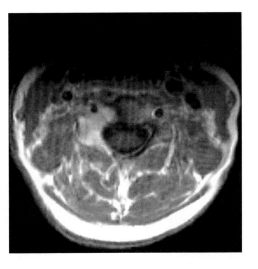

(Left) Axial T2* GRE MR shows high signal lesion expanding right arch of C4 and encasing vertebral artery. Metastatic hemangiopericytoma. *(Right)* Axial T1 C+ MR shows enhancing expansile lesion within arch and vb of C4. Metastatic hemangiopericytoma.

SCHWANNOMA

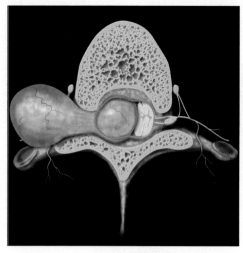

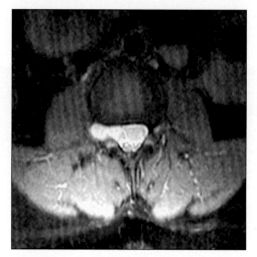

Axial graphic portrays a right-sided "dumbbell" shaped spinal nerve root schwannoma, enlarging neural foramen and compressing spinal cord. Both intra- and extradural components are present.

Axial T2WI MR with fat suppression shows a "dumbbell" shaped schwannoma in right intervertebral foramen.

TERMINOLOGY

Abbreviations and Synonyms

- Neurinoma, neurilemmoma

Definitions

- Neoplasm of nerve sheath in peripheral nervous system

IMAGING FINDINGS

General Features

- Best diagnostic clue: Well-circumscribed, "dumbbell" shaped, enhancing spinal mass
- Location
  - 70-75% intradural extramedullary
    - Most common intradural extramedullary mass
  - 15% completely extradural
  - 15% "dumbbell"
    - Both intra- and extradural
  - Rare intramedullary
  - Thoracic > cervical = lumbar
- Size
  - Most are small: Few mm
  - Giant schwannoma
    - Extend over 2 vertebral segments
    - Paraspinal extension > 2.5 cm

- Posterolateral extension into myofascial planes: Giant invasive schwannoma
- Lumbosacral spine most common
- Morphology
  - Round
  - Lobulated

Radiographic Findings

- Radiography
  - Widened interpediculate distance
  - Posterior vertebral erosion
    - Giant invasive schwannoma
  - Enlarged intervertebral foramen
    - Paraspinal soft tissue mass
  - Thinned pedicle
- Myelography: May block cerebral spinal fluid (CSF) flow

CT Findings

- NECT
  - Well-marginated mass
  - Isodense to cord, nerve roots
    - Cystic change common
    - Gross hemorrhage uncommon
    - Calcifications rare
  - Adjacent bone erosion, remodeling
    - Enlarged neural foramen with "dumbbell" lesion
    - Large lesions may expand canal
    - Posterior vertebral body scalloping

DDx: Spinal Masses

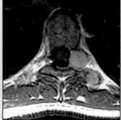

Neurofibroma

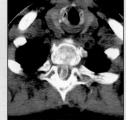

Meningioma

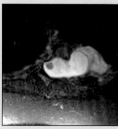

Lateral Meningocele

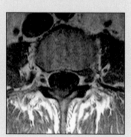

Disc Extrusion

SCHWANNOMA

Key Facts

Terminology
- Neurinoma, neurilemmoma
- Neoplasm of nerve sheath in peripheral nervous system

Imaging Findings
- Best diagnostic clue: Well-circumscribed, "dumbbell" shaped, enhancing spinal mass
- 70-75% intradural extramedullary
- Most common intradural extramedullary mass
- 15% completely extradural
- 15% "dumbbell"
- Enlarged intervertebral foramen
- Thinned pedicle
- Isodense to cord, nerve roots
- Iso/hypointense relative to cord, roots

- 75% hyperintense
- Intense enhancement

Top Differential Diagnoses
- Neurofibroma (NF)
- Meningioma
- Myxopapillary ependymoma

Pathology
- Sporadic: Most common
- Inactivation of NF2 gene
- 30% of primary spine tumors

Clinical Issues
- Clinical profile: Pain associated with movement

- CECT: Moderate solid or peripheral enhancement

MR Findings
- T1WI
  - Iso/hypointense relative to cord, roots
  - Melanotic schwannoma hyperintense
- T2WI
  - 75% hyperintense
  - 40% cystic change
  - 10% hemorrhage
  - Occasional: "Target sign"
    - High signal rim, low intensity center
  - Surrounding cord edema if intramedullary
    - Syringomyelia may be present
- STIR: Hyperintense
- T1 C+
  - Intense enhancement
    - Uniform or heterogeneous
    - Peripheral enhancement

Angiographic Findings
- Conventional: Variable vascularity

Imaging Recommendations
- Best imaging tool: T2WI and T1WI MRI in sagittal and axial planes
- Protocol advice
  - Post-gadolinium imaging with fat suppression
  - Scan entire spine in asymptomatic patients with suspected neurofibromatosis type 2 (NF2)

DIFFERENTIAL DIAGNOSIS

Neurofibroma (NF)
- May be difficult to distinguish by imaging
- NF more often fusiform
- Hemorrhage, cystic degeneration more common with schwannoma

Meningioma
- 90% intradural
- Thoracic spine most common: 80%
- May see enhancing dural "tail"

- T2 hypointensity due to calcification: < 5%

Myxopapillary ependymoma
- Larger, more vascular
- Hemorrhage more common
- May be indistinguishable from giant schwannoma

Meningocele
- CSF signal intensity/density
- Nonenhancing cystic mass
- Expanded intervertebral foramen

Extruded disc fragments
- May extend down root sleeve or into neuroforamen
  - No bony erosion
- Usually hypo- (not hyperintense)
- No enhancement
- Nerve root may be identified as a separate structure

PATHOLOGY

General Features
- General path comments
  - Arising from single nerve fascicle
    - Displacing other fascicles
    - Typically dorsal spinal nerve roots
- Genetics
  - Sporadic: Most common
    - Inactivating mutations of NF2 gene in 60%
  - NF2
    - Autosomal dominant
    - 1:30,000 to 40,000
    - Chromosome 22q mutations
    - Bilateral acoustic schwannomas diagnostic
    - Multiple schwannomas
  - Schwannomatosis
    - Multiple peripheral schwannomas
    - Other NF2 features absent
  - Carney complex
    - Mendelian-dominant: Chromosome 17
    - Melanotic schwannoma, cutaneous myxomas, potentially life-threatening cardiac myxomas, pigmented adrenal tumors

SCHWANNOMA

- Etiology
  - Inactivation of NF2 gene
    - Encoding merlin protein
- Epidemiology
  - 30% of primary spine tumors
  - Typically solitary unless part of inherited tumor syndrome
- Associated abnormalities
  - NF2
    - Spinal meningiomas
    - Intramedullary ependymomas

Gross Pathologic & Surgical Features
- Circumscribed, well-encapsulated
- Light tan/yellow, round/ovoid
- Cysts may occur
  - Gross hemorrhage, frank necrosis uncommon

Microscopic Features
- 3-layered capsule: Fibrous layer, nerve tissue, transitional layer
- Cell of origin: Schwann cells
- Classic "biphasic" pattern
  - Antoni A: Compact, elongated cells with occasional palisading
  - Antoni B: Less cellular, loosely textured, often lipidized
- Hyalinized blood vessels
- Fatty degeneration, cystic change, hemorrhage
- May contain melanin: 50% have Carney complex
- Immunohistochemistry: S100 and anti-leu-7 positive; EMA negative
- Electron microscopy: Basal lamina present

Staging, Grading or Classification Criteria
- WHO grade I

CLINICAL ISSUES

Presentation
- Most common signs/symptoms
  - Radicular pain
    - Mimics sciatica
  - Other signs/symptoms
    - Paresthesia
    - Progressive paraparesis
  - Multiple schwannomas in children with NF2 often asymptomatic
- Clinical profile: Pain associated with movement

Demographics
- Age: 30-60 yr
- Gender: M = F
- Ethnicity: No racial predilection

Natural History & Prognosis
- Slow growing
- Malignant degeneration rare
- No recurrence
  - NF2 and schwannomatosis may develop new lesions
  - Melanotic schwannoma: 15% recurrence, 26% metastasis

Treatment
- Total surgical resection
  - Involved nerve root sacrificed

DIAGNOSTIC CHECKLIST

Consider
- Schwannoma when solitary enhancing "dumbbell" shaped spinal lesion present

Image Interpretation Pearls
- All spinal nerve root tumors are NFs in NF1
- All spinal nerve root tumors are schwannomas or mixed tumors in NF2

SELECTED REFERENCES

1. Conti P et al: Spinal neurinomas: retrospective analysis and long-term outcome of 179 consecutively operated cases and review of the literature. Surg Neurol. 61(1):34-43; discussion 44, 2004
2. Colosimo C et al: Magnetic resonance imaging of intramedullary spinal cord schwannomas. Report of two cases and review of the literature. J Neurosurg. 99(1 Suppl):114-7, 2003
3. Hasegawa M et al: Surgical pathology of spinal schwannomas. Neurosurg. 6: 1388-93, 2001
4. Sridhar K et al: Giant invasive spinal schwannomas: definition and surgical management. J Neurosurg. 94(2 Suppl):210-5, 2001
5. Woodruff JM et al: Schwannoma. In Kleihues P, Cavenee WK (eds). Tumors of the Nervous System, 164-6. IARC Press, 2000
6. Murphey MD et al: Imaging of musculoskeletal neurogenic tumors: Radiologic-pathologic correlation. Radiographics. 19: 1253-80, 1999
7. Vallat-Decouvelaere AV et al: Spinal melanotic schwannoma: a tumour with poor prognosis. Histopathology. 35(6):558-66, 1999
8. Mautner VF et al: Spinal tumors in patients with neurofibromatosis type 2: MR imaging study of frequency, multiplicity, and variety. AJR Am J Roentgenol. 165(4):951-5, 1995
9. Akeson P et al: Radiological investigation of neurofibromatosis type 2. Neuroradiology. 36(2):107-10, 1994
10. Grossman RI et al: Neuroradiology The Requisites. 489-90. Mosby-Year Book, Inc., 1994
11. Matsumoto S et al: MRI of intradural-extramedullary spinal neurinomas and meningiomas. Clin Imaging. 17(1):46-52, 1993
12. Friedman DP et al: Intradural schwannomas of the spine: MR findings with emphasis on contrast-enhancement characteristics. AJR Am J Roentgenol. 158(6):1347-50, 1992
13. Shen WC et al: Cystic spinal neurilemmoma on magnetic resonance imaging. Neuroradiology. 34(5):447-8, 1992
14. Demachi H et al: MR imaging of spinal neurinomas with pathological correlation. J Comput Assist Tomogr. 14(2):250-4, 1990

SCHWANNOMA

IMAGE GALLERY

Typical

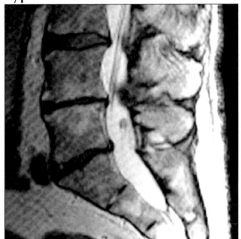
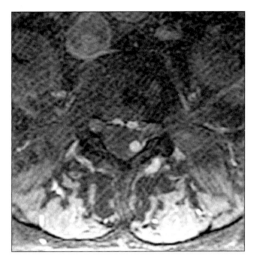

(Left) Sagittal T2WI MR shows an isointense nodule within cauda equina at L5, proven to be a schwannoma. *(Right)* Axial T1WI MR with fat suppression shows the same lesion with homogeneous enhancement.

Typical

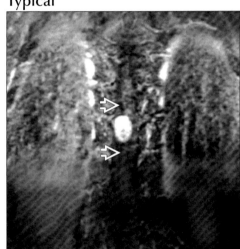
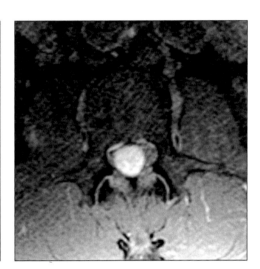

(Left) Coronal T1 C+ MR with fat suppression shows an enhancing intradural schwannoma deviating thoracic cord to the left *(arrows)*. *(Right)* Axial T1 C+ MR with fat suppression shows an intradural extramedullary homogeneously enhancing schwannoma compressing spinal cord.

Typical

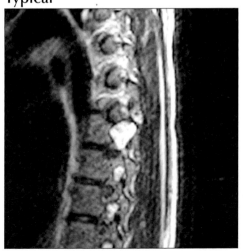
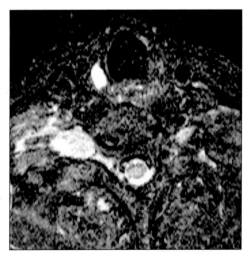

(Left) Sagittal T2WI MR of thoracic spine shows a schwannoma enlarging intervertebral foramen. *(Right)* Axial T2WI MR with fat suppression through cervical spine demonstrates a right paraspinal hyperintense fusiform mass contiguous with spinal nerve root, proven to be a schwannoma.

NEUROFIBROMA

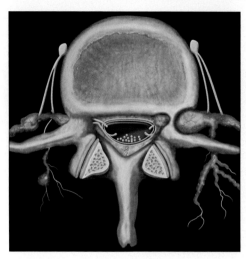

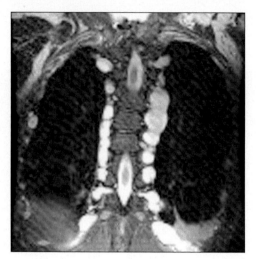

Axial graphic portrays bilateral lobulated plexiform neurofibromas in NF1. There is erosion of the left pedicle.

Coronal T2WI MR shows bilateral multi-level thoracic spinal neurofibromas in a patient with NF1.

TERMINOLOGY

Abbreviations and Synonyms
- Neurofibroma (NF)
- Nerve sheath tumor

Definitions
- Localized, diffuse, or plexiform neoplasm of nerve sheath

IMAGING FINDINGS

General Features
- Best diagnostic clue: Bulky multilevel spinal nerve root tumors in patient with stigmata of neurofibromatosis type 1 (NF1)
- Location
  - Intradural extramedullary
  - Paraspinal
  - Variable involvement of spinal root, neural plexus, peripheral nerve, or end organs
  - NF1
    - Cervical > thoracic and lumbar
    - Uni- or bilateral
- Size
  - Variable
    - Largest in lumbar spine in NF1

- Morphology
  - Three NF morphologic features
    - Localized
    - Diffuse
    - Plexiform

Radiographic Findings
- Radiography
  - Bone erosion
    - Neuroforaminal widening
    - Thinned pedicles
    - Vertebral scalloping in NF1

CT Findings
- NECT
  - Isodense to spinal cord
  - +/- Enlarged neural foramina
  - Calcifications rare
- CECT: Mild/moderate enhancement

MR Findings
- T1WI: Similar signal intensity (SI) to cord and nerve roots
- T2WI
  - Iso/hyperintense
  - "Target sign"
    - Periphery high SI
    - Central low/intermediate SI
    - Suggestive but not pathognomonic for NF

DDx: Spinal Masses

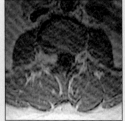

Schwannoma

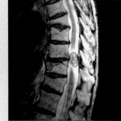

Meningioma

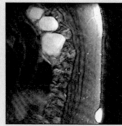

Meningoceles

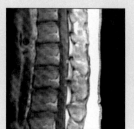

Leptomeningeal Mets

NEUROFIBROMA

Key Facts

Terminology
- Localized, diffuse, or plexiform neoplasm of nerve sheath

Imaging Findings
- Best diagnostic clue: Bulky multilevel spinal nerve root tumors in patient with stigmata of neurofibromatosis type 1 (NF1)
- Localized
- Diffuse
- Plexiform
- Isodense to spinal cord
- T1WI: Similar signal intensity (SI) to cord and nerve roots
- "Target sign"
- Hypointense septations throughout plexiform NF

- Malignant peripheral nerve sheath tumor (MPNST) metabolically active

Top Differential Diagnoses
- Schwannoma
- Spinal meningioma
- Meningocele

Pathology
- 5% of all benign soft tissue tumors
- 90% of NFs occur as sporadic, solitary tumors
- 13-65% of NF1 patients have spinal NFs

Clinical Issues
- Clinical profile: Rapid growth of NF suggestive of malignant transformation

---

- ○ Hypointense septations throughout plexiform NF
- STIR: Hyperintense
- T1 C+
  - ○ Variable
    - ▪ Mild, moderate
    - ▪ Relatively homogeneous
- Hemorrhage uncommon
- Variable cord compression

Nuclear Medicine Findings
- PET
  - ○ Malignant peripheral nerve sheath tumor (MPNST) metabolically active
  - ○ Useful in distinguishing benign from malignant nerve sheath tumor
    - ▪ Cutoff value of 1.8 SUV 1hr post-FDG injection
    - ▪ Sensitivity: 100%
    - ▪ Specificity: 83%

Imaging Recommendations
- Best imaging tool: T2WI and T1WI MRI in sagittal and coronal planes with gadolinium
- Protocol advice: T2WI with fat suppression or STIR improves lesion detection

DIFFERENTIAL DIAGNOSIS

Schwannoma
- Indistinguishable from solitary NF by imaging
- "Target sign" more common with NF than schwannoma
- Hemorrhage, fatty degeneration more common

Spinal meningioma
- 90% intradural
- May see enhancing dural "tail"
- T2 hypointensity due to calcification: < 5%

Meningocele
- Cystic nonenhancing mass
  - ○ CSF density/signal intensity
- Opacified by intrathecal contrast

Chronic interstitial demyelinating polyneuropathy (CIDP)
- Caused by repeated episodes of demyelination, remyelination
- "Onion" skin layered enlargement of spinal, peripheral nerves
- Mimics plexiform NF on imaging studies
- Features of NF1 absent

Other causes of multiple, enlarged, enhancing spinal nerves
- Inflammatory neuritis
  - ○ CMV radiculopathy in HIV+
  - ○ Mechanical/chemical nerve root irritation
    - ▪ Disc herniation
    - ▪ Post surgery
- Neoplastic neuritis
  - ○ Lymphoma
  - ○ Leptomeningeal metastases

PATHOLOGY

General Features
- General path comments: Variable appearance from circumscribed nodular masses to diffusely infiltrating tumors
- Genetics
  - ○ NF1
    - ▪ Autosomal dominant
    - ▪ von Recklinghausen disease
    - ▪ 50% cases from spontaneous mutation
    - ▪ Incidence: 1:3,000
  - ○ Mutation or loss of NF1 gene
    - ▪ Long arm of chromosomal 17
    - ▪ Only one gene needs to be affected
    - ▪ Gene product: Neurofibromin
    - ▪ Tumor suppressor function
  - ○ Sporadic NFs
    - ▪ Probably due to NF1 gene alteration
- Epidemiology
  - ○ 5% of all benign soft tissue tumors

NEUROFIBROMA

- ○ 90% of NFs occur as sporadic, solitary tumors
- ○ 13-65% of NF1 patients have spinal NFs
  - ▪ 57% single lesions
- ○ 3-5% of NF1 patients develop MPNST
- ○ 50-60% of MPNSTs are associated with NF1
- • Associated abnormalities
  - ○ NF1
    - ▪ Short segment thoracic scoliosis ± kyphosis: 40-60%
    - ▪ Vertebral anomalies
    - ▪ Meningocele
    - ▪ Dural ectasia
    - ▪ Intramedullary astrocytomas

Microscopic Features

- • No true capsule
- • Neoplastic Schwann cells + fibroblasts
- • Tumor, nerve fascicles intermixed
  - ○ Presence of axons characteristic of NFs
- • Collagen common
  - ○ Rare in schwannoma
- • Mucoid/myxoid matrix
  - ○ Rare hemorrhage, fatty degeneration, or vascular change
- • Mitotic figures rare in NFs
  - ○ High mitotic rate in MPNSTs
- • Immunohistochemistry
  - ○ S-100 and anti-leu 7 positive

Staging, Grading or Classification Criteria

- • NFs: WHO grade I
- • MPNSTs: WHO grade III/IV

CLINICAL ISSUES

Presentation

- • Most common signs/symptoms
  - ○ Pain
  - ○ Weakness
  - ○ Sensory deficit
    - ▪ Associated with plexiform NFs
  - ○ Other signs/symptoms
    - ▪ Myelopathy
    - ▪ NF1 patients: Café-au-lait spots, skin fold freckling, cutaneous NFs, Lisch nodules
- • Clinical profile: Rapid growth of NF suggestive of malignant transformation

Demographics

- • Age: Peak presentation: 20-30 y
- • Gender: No gender predilection
- • Ethnicity: No racial predilection

Natural History & Prognosis

- • Slow-growing
- • Malignant transformation to MPNSTs
  - ○ Rapid growth of NFs
  - ○ Rare with sporadic NFs
  - ○ 3-5% of plexiform NFs

Treatment

- • Resection of sporadic/solitary NF
  - ○ > 80% cure rate
- • Plexiform NFs difficult to resect

- ○ high recurrence rate
- • MR surveillance of asymptomatic spinal NFs in NF1 of doubtful benefit

DIAGNOSTIC CHECKLIST

Image Interpretation Pearls

- • All spinal nerve root tumors are NFs in NF1
- • They are schwannomas or mixed tumors in NF2
- • Solitary spinal lesion most likely schwannoma

SELECTED REFERENCES

1. Khong PL et al: MR imaging of spinal tumors in children with neurofibromatosis 1. AJR Am J Roentgenol. 180(2):413-7, 2003
2. Cardona S et al: Evaluation of F18-deoxyglucose positron emission tomography (FDG-PET) to assess the nature of neurogenic tumours. Eur J Surg Oncol. 29(6):536-41, 2003
3. Simoens WA et al: MR features of peripheral nerve sheath tumors: can a calculated index compete with radiologist's experience? Eur Radiol. 11: 250-7, 2001
4. Woodruff JM et al: Neurofibroma. In: Kleihues P, Cavenee WK (eds), Tumors of the Nervous System, 167-8, IARC Press, 2000
5. Ferner RE et al: Evaluation of (18)fluorodeoxyglucose positron emission tomography ((18)FDG PET) in the detection of malignant peripheral nerve sheath tumours arising from within plexiform neurofibromas in neurofibromatosis 1. J Neurol Neurosurg Psychiatry. 68(3):353-7, 2000
6. Thakkar SD et al: Spinal tumours in neurofibromatosis type 1: an MRI study of frequency, multiplicity and variety. Neuroradiology. 41(9):625-9, 1999
7. Murphey MD et al: Imaging of musculoskeletal neurogenic tumors: Radiologic-pathologic correlation. RadioGraphics. 19: 1253-80, 1999
8. Klekamp J et al: Surgery of spinal nerve sheath tumors with special reference to neurofibromatosis. Neurosurgery. 42(2):279-89; discussion 289-90, 1998
9. Yagi T et al: Intramedullary spinal cord tumour associated with neurofibromatosis type 1. Acta Neurochir (Wien). 139(11):1055-60, 1997
10. Shariff SY et al: Intraspinal tumours in children--clinical presentation. Ir Med J. 90(7):264-5, 1997
11. Grossman RI et al: Neuroradiology The Requisites. 489-90. Mosby-Year Book, Inc., 1994
12. Tatagiba M et al: Involvement of spinal nerves in neurofibromatosis. Neurosurg Rev. 17(1):43-9, 1994
13. Shu HH et al: Neurofibromatosis: MR imaging findings involving the head and spine. AJR Am J Roentgenol. 160(1):159-64, 1993
14. Clinchot DM et al: The spectrum of neurofibromatosis: neurologic manifestations with malignant transformation. J Am Paraplegia Soc. 16(2):81-3, 1993
15. Egelhoff JC et al: Spinal MR findings in neurofibromatosis types 1 and 2. AJNR Am J Neuroradiol. 13(4):1071-7, 1992
16. Ros PR et al: Plexiform neurofibroma of the pelvis: CT and MRI findings. Magn Reson Imaging. 9(3):463-5, 1991
17. Li MH et al: MR imaging of spinal neurofibromatosis. Acta Radiol. 32(4):279-85, 1991

NEUROFIBROMA

IMAGE GALLERY

Typical

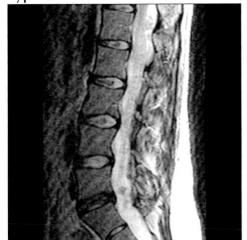 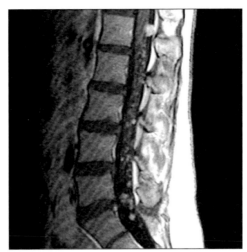

(Left) Sagittal T2WI MR of lumbar spine shows multiple ill-defined isointense nodules within cauda equina, obscuring lumbar nerve roots. *(Right)* Sagittal T1 C+ MR of the same patient shows innumerable enhancing neurofibromas within cauda equina.

Typical

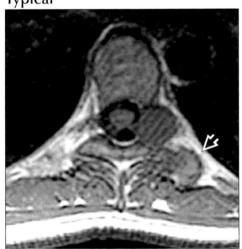 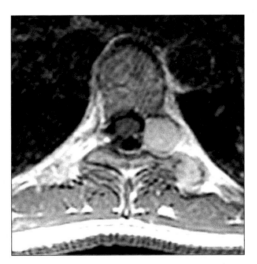

(Left) Axial T1WI MR through thoracic spine shows an isointense mass within left neuroforamen. A second mass is present more laterally and dorsally (arrow). *(Right)* Axial T1 C+ MR shows two neurofibromas with diffuse enhancement.

Typical

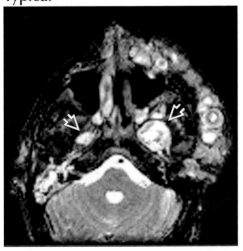 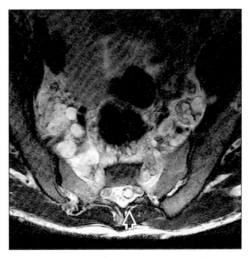

(Left) Axial T2WI MR with fat suppression shows an infiltrating neurofibroma in left malar soft tissue. Bilateral parapharyngeal neurofibromas are evident (arrows). *(Right)* Axial T2WI MR shows plexiform neurofibromas involving sacral plexus bilaterally with intraspinal extension (arrow).

MALIGNANT NERVE SHEATH TUMORS

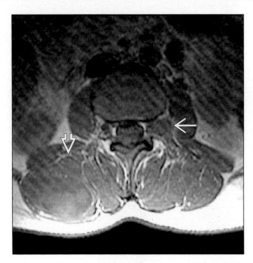

Axial T1WI MR in a patient with NF1 shows a large isointense mass within right paraspinous muscle (open arrow). A second smaller mass resides in left neuroforamen (arrow).

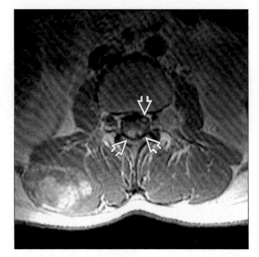

Axial T1 C+ MR shows right paraspinous MPNST with heterogenous enhancement. The left neurofibroma also enhances. In addition, multiple intrathecal neurofibromas are present (arrows).

TERMINOLOGY

Abbreviations and Synonyms
- Malignant peripheral nerve sheath tumors (MPNST) divided into
  - Malignant schwannoma
  - Neurofibrosarcoma

Definitions
- Malignant lesion of neural origin involving spinal root, neural plexus, peripheral nerve, or end organs

IMAGING FINDINGS

General Features
- Best diagnostic clue: Large infiltrative, often hemorrhagic, soft tissue mass related to neurovascular bundle
- Location
  - Paravertebral, rare intraspinal
    - Posterior mediastinum
    - Retroperitoneum
  - Proximal portion of extremities
- Size: > 5 cm
- Morphology: Circumscribed or infiltrative soft tissue mass

Radiographic Findings
- Radiography
  - Deep or superficial soft tissue mass
  - Intervertebral foraminal widening

CT Findings
- NECT
  - Soft tissue mass iso- or hypodense to muscle
  - Heterogeneous areas correspond to hemorrhage and necrosis
  - Calcifications
- CECT: Marked enhancement

MR Findings
- T1WI: Soft tissue mass isointense to muscle
- T2WI: Hyperintense compared to surrounding fat
- STIR: Hyperintense
- T1 C+: Marked enhancement
- Heterogeneous soft tissue mass with indistinct margins
- Infiltration of surrounding soft tissues
- Areas of hemorrhage
- Nerve entering and exiting mass
- Muscle atrophy may be present
- Spinal involvement
  - Intradural extramedullary mass
    - Dumbbell configuration
  - Widening of intervertebral foramina
    - Erosion of pedicles

DDx: Masses Resembling MPNST

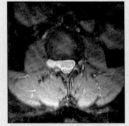

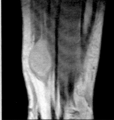

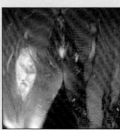

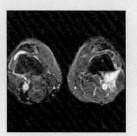

Spinal Schwannoma   *Ulnar Schwannoma*   *Liposarcoma*   *Hematoma*

MALIGNANT NERVE SHEATH TUMORS

Key Facts

Terminology
- Malignant lesion of neural origin involving spinal root, neural plexus, peripheral nerve, or end organs

Imaging Findings
- Best diagnostic clue: Large infiltrative, often hemorrhagic, soft tissue mass related to neurovascular bundle
- Intervertebral foraminal widening
- Heterogeneous areas correspond to hemorrhage and necrosis
- T1WI: Soft tissue mass isointense to muscle
- T2WI: Hyperintense compared to surrounding fat
- T1 C+: Marked enhancement
- Difficult to distinguish from benign spinal schwannomas

Top Differential Diagnoses
- Benign peripheral nerve sheath tumor
- Soft tissue sarcoma

Pathology
- Incidence in general population: 0.001%
- 50-60% of MPNST patients have NF1

Clinical Issues
- Involves major nerve trunks
- Sudden enlargement of preexisting neurofibroma in NF1
- Local recurrence: 26-65%
- Metastases: 20-65%
- Surgical resection
- Improved resectability with distal lesions

- Scalloping of vertebral bodies
  - Difficult to distinguish from benign spinal schwannomas

Angiographic Findings
- Hypervascular soft tissue mass

Nuclear Medicine Findings
- Bone Scan: Increased radiotracer uptake on blood pool and delayed images
- PET
  - Increased FDG uptake
  - To detect malignant transformation in plexiform neurofibroma

Imaging Recommendations
- Best imaging tool: MRI: Best soft tissue delineation
- Protocol advice: T1WI, T2WI , and T1 C+ MR in multiple planes

DIFFERENTIAL DIAGNOSIS

Benign peripheral nerve sheath tumor
- No invasion of surrounding structures
- Well-circumscribed
- Variable enhancement
- Sudden enlargement of pre-existing neurofibroma in neurofibromatosis type 1 (NF1) suspicious for MPNST

Soft tissue sarcoma
- Not related to neurovascular bundle
- No spinal involvement
- Hemorrhagic and necrotic components
- Intense enhancement

Hematoma
- No enhancing solid components
- T2 hypointensity invariably present
- Surrounding edema

PATHOLOGY

General Features
- General path comments
  - Spindle cell sarcoma of nerve sheath
    - Composed of Schwann cells and perineurial cells
- Genetics
  - NF1: von Recklinghausen disease
    - Autosomal dominant
    - High rate of penetrance
    - 50% of cases from new mutations
    - Genetic abnormality on chromosome 17
    - Increased Ras activity due to loss of NF1 gene product, neurofibromin
  - Increased expression of CD44 family transaminase glycoproteins
    - Might be responsible for tumor invasion and metastatic potential
- Etiology
  - Tissue of neuroectodermal or neural crest origin: Schwann cell
  - Vast majority arises from neurofibroma
    - 50-60% associated with NF1
    - MPNST in patients without NF1 also associated with neurofibroma
  - 11% radiation-induced
    - Latency: 10-20 years
- Epidemiology
  - Incidence in general population: 0.001%
    - 3-5% of NF1 patients develop MPNST
  - 50-60% of MPNST patients have NF1
  - 5-10% of all malignant soft tissue tumors
  - 2-3% of spinal schwannomas malignant
- Associated abnormalities
  - NF1
    - Kyphoscoliosis
    - Rib deformities
    - Meningoceles
    - Optic nerve glioma, astrocytoma

Gross Pathologic & Surgical Features
- Large globoid or fusiform mass associated with major nerve

MALIGNANT NERVE SHEATH TUMORS

- No true capsule
- Tan-gray, fleshy
- Areas of hemorrhage and necrosis
- Infiltrates surrounding soft tissue
- Spreads along perineurium and epineurium

Microscopic Features

- Fasciculated hyperchromatic mitotically active spindle cells
- Epithelioid and mesenchymal differentiation: 12-27%
  - Due to pluripotent nature of neural crest
  - Epithelial glands, foci of mature bone and cartilage
  - Features of chondrosarcoma, rhabdomyosarcoma (malignant Triton tumor), osteosarcoma, angiosarcoma
- Immunohistochemistry stains for S-100 protein, Leu-7, Vimentin, and neuron specific enolase

Staging, Grading or Classification Criteria

- Surgical staging
  - Stage I: Low grade
  - Stage II: High grade
  - Stage III: Low or high grade, metastases
    - Within each Stage: A = intracompartmental; B = extracompartmental
- Low grade: Perineurial cell differentiation
- High grade: High mitotic rate, ± necrosis, sarcomatous divergent differentiation

CLINICAL ISSUES

Presentation

- Most common signs/symptoms
  - Local or radicular pain
  - Enlarging soft tissue mass
  - Paraparesis
  - Paresthesia
- Clinical profile
  - Involves major nerve trunks
    - Sciatic nerve, brachial or lumbosacral plexus
  - Sudden enlargement of preexisting neurofibroma in NF1
  - Usually presents as stage IIb lesion: 85%

Demographics

- Age
  - 40-50 years
  - If associated with NF1: 26-42 years
- Gender
  - M = F
  - In NF1: M > F

Natural History & Prognosis

- Local recurrence: 26-65%
  - 71% in primary spinal malignant schwannoma
- Metastases: 20-65%
  - Lung, bone, pleura, liver
- 5 year survival: 10-50%
- NF1 patients have worse prognosis
  - Higher recurrence rate
  - Shorter survival
- Better prognosis associated with
  - Diameter < 5 cm
  - Gross total resection

  - Younger age

Treatment

- Surgical resection
  - Improved resectability with distal lesions
    - 20% in paraspinal MPNST vs. 95% in extremity lesions
  - Amputation often necessary
  - Resection with wide margins
    - Margin of at least 3 cm recommended
- Pre- or post-operative radiation therapy
- Chemotherapy for metastatic disease
  - Effectiveness unproven

DIAGNOSTIC CHECKLIST

Consider

- Malignant transformation when preexisting neurofibroma enlarges

SELECTED REFERENCES

1. Baehring JM et al: Malignant peripheral nerve sheath tumor: the clinical spectrum and outcome of treatment. Neurology. 61(5):696-8, 2003
2. Su W et al: Malignant peripheral nerve sheath tumor cell invasion is facilitated by Src and aberrant CD44 expression. Glia. 42:350-8, 2003
3. Asavamongkolkul A et al: Malignant peripheral nerve sheath tumor with neurofibromatosis type 1: a 2-case report and review of the literature. J Med Assoc Thai. 84(2):285-93, 2001
4. Weiss SW et al: Enzinger and Weiss's soft tissue tumors. 4th ed. St.Louis MO, CV Mosby, 1209-63, 2001
5. Ferner RE et al: Evaluation of (18) fluorodeoxyglucose positron emission tomography ((18) FDG PET) in the detection of malignant peripheral nerve sheath tumors arising from within plexiform neurofibromas in neurofibromatosis 1. J Neurol Neurosurg Psychiatry. 68:353-7, 2000
6. Woodruff JM: Pathology of tumors of the peripheral nerve sheath in type 1 neurofibromatosis. Am J Med Genet. 89(1):23-30, 1999
7. Beggs I: Pictorial review: Imaging of peripheral nerve tumors. Clin Radiol. 52:8-17, 1997
8. Kransdorf MJ et al: Imaging of soft tissue tumors, 1st ed. Philadelphia PA, W.B. Saunders. 240-54, 1997
9. Celli P et al: Primary spinal malignant schwannomas: clinical and prognostic remarks. Acta Neurochir (Wien). 135(1-2):52-5, 1995
10. Bass JC et al: Retroperitoneal plexiform neurofibromas: CT findings. Am J Roentgenol. 163:617-20, 1994
11. Suh JS et al: Peripheral (extracranial) nerve tumors: Correlation of MR imaging and histologic findings. Radiology. 183:341-6, 1992
12. Stull M et al: Magnetic resonance appearance of peripheral nerve sheath tumors. Skeletal Radiol. 20:9-14,1991
13. Riccardi VM et al: Neurofibrosarcoma as a complication of von Recklinghausen neurofibromatosis. Neurofibromatosis. 2:152-65, 1989

MALIGNANT NERVE SHEATH TUMORS

IMAGE GALLERY

Typical

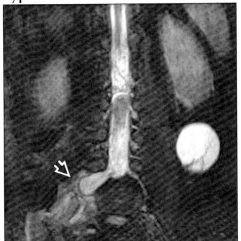
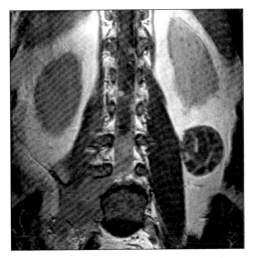

(Left) Coronal STIR MR shows an intraspinal mass extending through neuroforamen with a large extra-spinal component (arrow). A round left-sided retroperitoneal mass is also present. *(Right)* Coronal T1 C+ MR shows the same enhancing MPNST with intra- and extra-spinal components. The left retroperitoneal neurofibroma is predominantly cystic with linear enhancement.

Typical

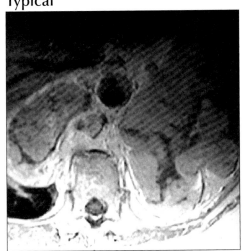
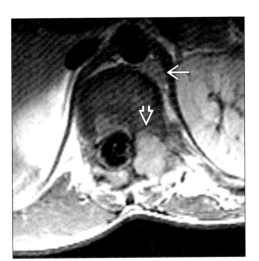

(Left) Axial T1 C+ MR shows a large lobulated heterogeneously enhancing retroperitoneal MPNST, displacing abdominal aorta and liver. *(Right)* Axial T1 C+ MR shows an enhancing neurofibrosarcoma (open arrow) eroding left vertebral body and posterior element. A left retrocrural neurofibroma (arrow) also enhances.

Typical

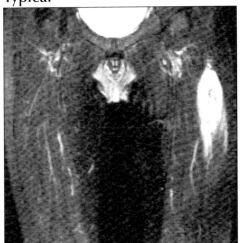
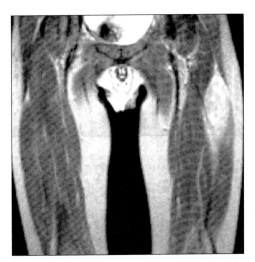

(Left) Coronal STIR MR shows a fusiform heterogenous hyperintense lesion in proximal left thigh with indistinct margins distally. *(Right)* Coronal T1 C+ MR shows the same MPNST with diffuse post-gadolinium enhancement.

CSF DISSEMINATED METASTASES

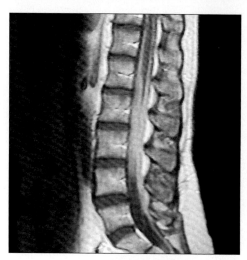

Sagittal T1 C+ MR shows diffuse, sheet-like enhancement of leptomeninges along conus and cauda equina in patient with severe polyradiculopathy due to metastic melanoma.

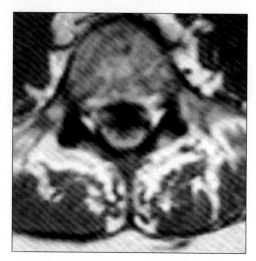

Axial T1 C+ MR shows enhancing, thickened, coalescent nerve roots in patient with polyradiculopathy, metastatic melanoma.

TERMINOLOGY

Abbreviations and Synonyms
- Leptomeningeal carcinomatosis
- Leptomeningeal tumor spread
- Drop metastases

Definitions
- Spread of malignant tumors through the subarachnoid space

IMAGING FINDINGS

General Features
- Best diagnostic clue: Smooth/nodular enhancement along cord, roots
- Location: Any point along CSF pathway (including central canal)
- Size: Variable
- Morphology
  - Four basic patterns
    - Solitary focal mass at bottom of thecal sac or along cord surface
    - Diffuse, thin, sheet-like coating of cord/roots ("carcinomatous meningitis")
    - "Rope-like" thickening of cauda equina
    - Multifocal discrete nodules along cord/roots

  - Intramedullary nodule(s)
    - Rarely due to CSF spread, impossible to distinguish from hematogenous met(s) to cord

Radiographic Findings
- Myelography
  - Myelography, CT myelography
    - "Filling defects"

CT Findings
- NECT: Often normal; +/- bony/extradural tumor present
- CECT
  - May be normal
  - Enhancement of cauda equina

MR Findings
- T1WI
  - Metastases usually isointense with cord, roots
  - Extensive disease may fill thecal sac, elevating normally low CSF signal
    - CSF in sac has "ground glass" appearance
    - Nerve roots appear blurred, "smudged"
- T2WI
  - Focal metastases usually isointense with cord, roots (hypointense to CSF)
  - Thickened nerve roots
- T1 C+
  - Obvious enhancement

DDx: Leptomeningeal Enhancement

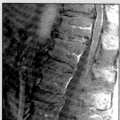
Post-Operative

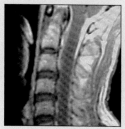
TB Meningitis

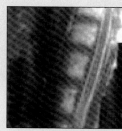
Subdural Empyema

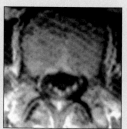
Guillain-Barre

CSF DISSEMINATED METASTASES

Key Facts

Terminology
- Leptomeningeal carcinomatosis
- Drop metastases

Imaging Findings
- Obvious enhancement
- Pattern varies
- "Sugar coating" of cord, roots
- Single/multiple enhancing nodular masses
- Round/ovoid intramedullary mass, often with ring-like pattern
- Image entire neuraxis!
- Contrast-enhanced, fat suppressed T1WI

Top Differential Diagnoses
- Multifocal primary tumor
- Pyogenic meningitis (clinical/laboratory findings helpful)
- Granulomatous meningitis
- Chemical meningitis
- Congenital hypertrophic polyradiculoneuropathies

Clinical Issues
- Most common signs/symptoms: Severe pain, polyradiculopathy
- Typically seen in advanced cancer cases

Diagnostic Checklist
- MRI more sensitive than CSF cytology; especially fat-saturated T1 C+
- Post-operative enhancement of meninges can mimic leptomeningeal tumor spread

---

- Pattern varies
  - "Sugar coating" of cord, roots
  - Single/multiple enhancing nodular masses
  - Round/ovoid intramedullary mass, often with ring-like pattern

Imaging Recommendations
- Image entire neuraxis!
  - High-resolution T2WI
  - Contrast-enhanced, fat suppressed T1WI
  - STIR (look for bony metastases)
- Do it prior to craniotomy!

DIFFERENTIAL DIAGNOSIS

Multifocal primary tumor
- Hemangioblastoma
- Astrocytoma (uncommon)
- Myxopapillary ependymoma

Pyogenic meningitis (clinical/laboratory findings helpful)
- Typically chronic bacterial or fungal meningitis
- Subdural empyema

Granulomatous meningitis
- Tubercular meningitis
- Sarcoidosis

Chemical meningitis
- Post-operative change
  - Subarachnoid blood, adhesions can mimic leptomeningeal mets

Congenital hypertrophic polyradiculoneuropathies
- Charcot-Marie-Tooth
- Dejerine-Sottas

Thick nerve roots/cauda equina
- Guillain-Barré syndrome
  - Post-viral or vaccinial ascending paralysis
  - Predominantly motor signs
- AIDS-associated polyneuropathy (e.g., CMV)
- Chemotherapy-associated polyneuropathy
- Chronic interstitial demyelinating polyneuropathy (CIDP)

PATHOLOGY

General Features
- General path comments: Broad spectrum of primary neoplasms
- Etiology
  - Hematogenous dissemination from extracranial neoplasm
    - Most are adenocarcinomas (lung, breast)
    - Other: Melanoma, non-Hodgkin lymphoma, leukemia
  - "Drop" metastases from CNS primary tumor
    - Adults: Anaplastic astrocytoma, GBM (0.5-1% of cases), ependymoma
    - Children: Most common - PNETs (medulloblastoma)
    - Other in children: Germinoma, ependymoma, choroid plexus papilloma/carcinoma
- Epidemiology
  - 5% of all spinal metastases
  - Prevalence increasing as cancer patients living longer
- Associated abnormalities
  - Elevated CSF protein
  - Increased signal from CSF on T1WI (pre-contrast)

Gross Pathologic & Surgical Features
- Varies with pattern, type of metastasis

Microscopic Features
- Varies with histology of primary neoplasm
- CSF usually positive in leptomeningeal metastatic disease; negative in intramedullary tumors
  - Multiple CSF samplings may be necessary to get + cytology

CSF DISSEMINATED METASTASES

CLINICAL ISSUES

Presentation
- Most common signs/symptoms: Severe pain, polyradiculopathy
- Clinical profile
  - Typically seen in advanced cancer cases
  - May be asymptomatic early
  - Radiculopathy > myelopathy
  - Other signs/symptoms
    - Nuchal rigidity
    - Myelopathy

Natural History & Prognosis
- Relentless progression typical
- Survival usually < 1 year

Treatment
- Radiation, chemotherapy

DIAGNOSTIC CHECKLIST

Consider
- MRI more sensitive than CSF cytology; especially fat-saturated T1 C+

Image Interpretation Pearls
- Post-operative enhancement of meninges can mimic leptomeningeal tumor spread

SELECTED REFERENCES

1. Lindsay A et al: Spinal leptomeningeal metastases following glioblastoma multiforme treated with radiotherapy. J Clin Neurosci. 9(6): 725-8, 2002
2. Singh SK et al: MR imaging of leptomeningeal metastases: comparison of three sequences. AJNR Am J Neuroradiol. 23(5): 817-21, 2002
3. Straathof CS et al: The diagnostic accuracy of magnetic resonance imaging and cerebrospinal fluid cytology in leptomeningeal metastasis. J Neurol. 246(9): 810-4, 1999
4. Collie DA et al: Imaging features of leptomeningeal metastases. Clin Radiol. 54(11): 765-71, 1999
5. van der Ree TC et al: Leptomeningeal metastasis after surgical resection of brain metastases. J Neurol Neurosurg Psychiatry. 66(2): 225-7, 1999
6. Gomori JM et al: Leptomeningeal metastases: evaluation by gadolinium enhanced spinal magnetic resonance imaging. J Neurooncol. 36(1): 55-60, 1998
7. Kallmes DF et al: High-dose gadolinium-enhanced MRI for diagnosis of meningeal metastases. Neuroradiology. 40(1): 23-6, 1998
8. Formaglio F et al: Meningeal metastases: clinical aspects and diagnosis. Ital J Neurol Sci. 19(3): 133-49, 1998
9. Chamberlain MC et al: Carcinomatous meningitis secondary to breast cancer: predictors of response to combined modality therapy. J Neurooncol. 35(1): 55-64, 1997
10. Chamberlain MC: Comparative spine imaging in leptomeningeal metastases. J Neurooncol. 23(3): 233-8, 1995
11. Heinz R et al: Detection of CSF metastasis: CT myelography or MR? AJNR. 16: 1147-51, 1995
12. Freilich RJ et al: Neuroimaging and cerebrospinal fluid cytology in the diagnosis of leptomeningeal metastasis. Ann Neurol. 38(1): 51-7, 1995
13. Watanabe M et al: Correlation of MRI and clinical features in meningeal carcinomatosis. Neuroradiology. 35(7): 512-5, 1993
14. Chua SL et al: Magnetic resonance imaging of leptomeningeal metastases to the spine. Singapore Med J. 34(3): 253-6, 1993
15. Schuknecht B et al: Spinal leptomeningeal neoplastic disease. Eur Neurol. 32: 11-6, 1992
16. Lossos A et al: Spinal subarachnoid hemorrhage associated with leptomeningeal metastases. J Neurooncol. 12(2): 167-71, 1992
17. Yousem DM et al: Leptomeningeal metastases: MR evaluation. J Comput Assist Tomogr. 14(2): 255-61, 1990
18. Davis PC et al: Leptomeningeal metastasis: MR imaging. Radiology. 163(2): 449-54, 1987
19. Weissman DE et al: Simultaneous leptomeningeal and intramedullary spinal metastases in small cell lung carcinoma. Med Pediatr Oncol. 14(1): 54-6, 1986
20. Freeman CR et al: Primary malignant lymphoma of the central nervous system. Cancer. 58(5): 1106-11, 1986

IMAGE GALLERY

Typical

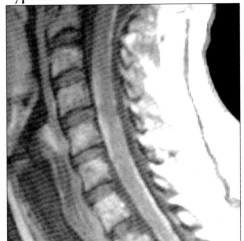
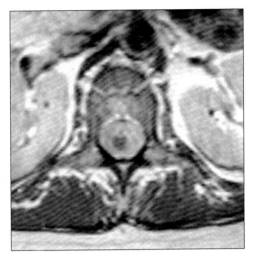

(Left) Sagittal T1 C+ MR shows thickened, enhancing surface of the cord in patient with metastatic breast cancer, severe pain and cervical polyradiculopathy. *(Right)* Axial T1 C+ MR at the level of the conus shows diffuse enhancing rind of tumor in patient with metastatic melanoma. Sagittal images depicted extensive spread along entire canal.

Typical

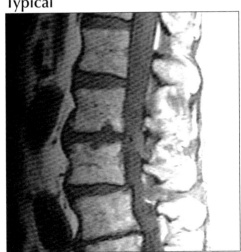
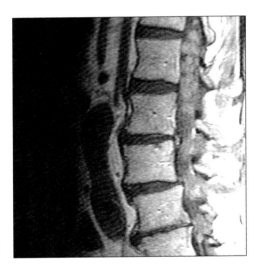

(Left) Sagittal T1WI MR shows "muddy" spinal fluid, higher signal intensity than expected for nonenhanced T1WI, in patient with metastatic adenocarcinoma. Post-contrast images showed leptomeningeal spread. *(Right)* Sagittal T1 C+ MR depicts numerous, coalescent enhancing nodules in cauda equina region. Patient had severe pain, polyradiculopathy, and end-stage metastatic adenocarcinoma of lung.

Variant

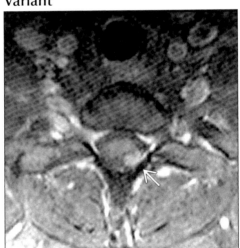
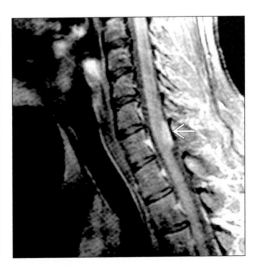

(Left) Axial T1 C+ MR demonstrates enhancing nodule on posterolateral cord surface (arrow) in patient recently treated for pineal germinoma, indicating single "drop" metastasis: Resolved with radiation. *(Right)* Sagittal T1WI MR with fat-saturation depicts a plaque-like mass on cord surface (arrow) in patient with recently treated pineal germinoma, new cervical radiculopathy due to "drop" met.

ASTROCYTOMA, SPINAL CORD

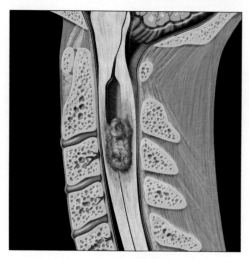

Sagittal graphic of cervical spine shows solid mass with cystic component within cervical cord.

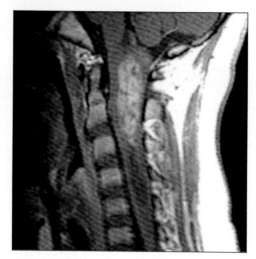

Sagittal T1 C+ MR shows enhancing, exophytic cord mass. Note cystic, low signal component inferiorly.

TERMINOLOGY

Abbreviations and Synonyms
- Intramedullary glioma

Definitions
- Primary neoplasm of astrocytic origin within spinal cord

IMAGING FINDINGS

General Features
- Best diagnostic clue: Enhancing infiltrating mass expanding cord
- Location: Cervical > thoracic
- Size
  - Usually 4 segments or less
  - May be extensive, especially with pilocytic histology
- Morphology
  - Fusiform expansion of cord, with enhancing component of variable morphology
  - Occasionally asymmetric, even exophytic

Radiographic Findings
- Radiography
  - May see scoliosis
  - May see expansion of canal

- Myelography: Enlarged cord shadow, effacing contrast in surrounding thecal sac

CT Findings
- NECT
  - Big cord
  - +/- Expansion, remodeling of bony canal
- CECT: Mild/moderate enhancement, rarely done

MR Findings
- T1WI
  - Cord expansion
    - Usually < 4 segments
    - Occasionally multisegmental, even holocord (more common with pilocytic astrocytoma)
  - +/- Cyst/syrinx (fluid slightly hyperintense to CSF)
  - Solid portion hypo/isointense
  - In minority of cases, hyperintensity due to methemoglobin
- T2WI: Hyperintense on PD, T2WI
- T2* GRE
  - Hyperintense
  - Low signal if hemorrhagic by-products in minority of cases
- T1 C+
  - Almost always enhances
    - Mild/moderate > intense enhancement
    - Partial > total enhancement

DDx: Enlarged Cord

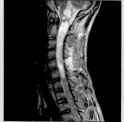
Ependymoma

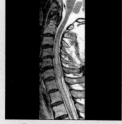
Breast Metastasis

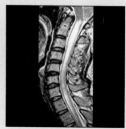
TB Meningitis

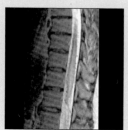
Dural AVM

ASTROCYTOMA, SPINAL CORD

Key Facts

Terminology
- Intramedullary glioma

Imaging Findings
- Best diagnostic clue: Enhancing infiltrating mass expanding cord
- Location: Cervical > thoracic
- Occasionally asymmetric, even exophytic
- Cord expansion
- Usually < 4 segments
- Occasionally multisegmental, even holocord (more common with pilocytic astrocytoma)
- +/- Cyst/syrinx (fluid slightly hyperintense to CSF)
- T2WI: Hyperintense on PD, T2WI
- Almost always enhances
- Focus of enhancement is target for biopsy

Top Differential Diagnoses
- Ependymoma
- Other neoplasms
- Metastasis (older patients)
- Hemangioblastoma
- Syringohydromyelia
- Autoimmune or inflammatory myelitis
- Cord ischemia/infarction
- Dural vascular malformation

Pathology
- Second most common cord neoplasm
- 80-90% low grade

Clinical Issues
- Slow onset of myelopathy

- Inhomogeneous/infiltrating > homogeneous/sharply-delineated
- Focus of enhancement is target for biopsy

Imaging Recommendations
- Contrast-enhanced MR is single best test for any form of myelopathy

DIFFERENTIAL DIAGNOSIS

Ependymoma
- Patients often older
- Intense, sharply delineated enhancement
- Central > eccentric growth pattern
- Hemorrhage more common
- More often seen in low thoracic cord
- Cystic or necrotic component often seen

Other neoplasms
- Ganglioglioma, mixed glioma (may be indistinguishable)
- Lymphoma
- Metastasis (older patients)
  - Nidus of enhancement much more focal, if intramedullary
  - Pial met can simulate hemangioblastoma
- Hemangioblastoma
  - Focal, enhancing pial/sub-pial nodule
  - Associated syrinx in cord simulates astrocytoma

Syringohydromyelia
- Cyst fluid like CSF; no enhancement

Autoimmune or inflammatory myelitis
- Demyelinating disease (+/- patchy, ill-defined enhancement if acute)
  - Multiple sclerosis
    - Typically multifocal
    - Cord may show focal swelling, flame shaped
  - Transverse myelitis
    - Long cord segment
    - Patchy enhancement
  - Infectious myelitis

- TB or other granulomatous disease
- Bacterial meningitis
- Infectious vasculitis causes cord swelling and edema
- Rapid onset
- Constitutional signs
- Cord ischemia/infarction
  - Abrupt onset
  - Risk factors of atherosclerosis, hypertension, diabetes
  - Aortic dissection predisposes
  - Abdominal aortic aneurysm or surgery for it poses particular risk
- Dural vascular malformation
  - Mild edema and enlargement
  - Typically in distal cord
  - Slow onset of upper leg weakness
  - Prominent pial vessels

PATHOLOGY

General Features
- General path comments
  - Eccentric > central growth pattern
  - Bony canal often enlarged, remodeled in pediatric cases
  - Cervical > thoracic
- Etiology: No specific cause known
- Epidemiology
  - Second most common cord neoplasm
  - Intramedullary spinal cord tumors (IMSCTs) = 5-10% of all CNS tumors
    - 20% of intraspinal neoplasms in adults
    - 30-35% of intraspinal neoplasms in children
  - 90-95% of IMSCTs are gliomas
    - Overall, ependymomas outnumber astrocytomas 2:1
    - Diffuse fibrillary > pilocytic astrocytoma
  - M:F = 1.3:1
  - Association with NF2

ASTROCYTOMA, SPINAL CORD

Gross Pathologic & Surgical Features
- Expanded cord

Microscopic Features
- Fibrillary astrocytoma
  - Increased cellularity, variable atypia/mitoses
  - Parenchymal infiltration
- Pilocytic astrocytoma
  - Rosenthal fibers, glomeruloid/hyalinized vessels
  - Low prevalence of nuclear atypia/mitoses

Staging, Grading or Classification Criteria
- 80-90% low grade
  - Fibrillary astrocytoma = WHO II
  - Pilocytic astrocytoma = WHO I
  - Ganglioglioma, mixed gliomas also occur
- 10-15% high grade
  - Most are anaplastic astrocytomas (WHO III)
  - Glioblastoma (WHO IV) uncommon

CLINICAL ISSUES

Presentation
- Most common signs/symptoms
  - Slow onset of myelopathy
  - Other signs/symptoms
    - May cause painful scoliosis
- Clinical profile: Insidious onset of myelopathy in adolescent or young adult

Demographics
- Age
  - Most common intramedullary tumor in children/young adults
  - 60% of IMSCTs in children are astrocytomas, 30% ependymomas
- Gender: M > F = 1.3:1

Natural History & Prognosis
- Most are slow-growing
- Malignant tumors may cause rapid neurologic deterioration
- Survival varies with tumor histology/grade, & gross total resection
  - 80% 5 year for low grade; 30% for high grade
- Post-operative neurologic function determined largely by degree of pre-operative deficit

Treatment
- Obtain tissue diagnosis
- Microsurgical resection (low grade tumors)
  - Intraoperative US, evoked potentials helpful
- Adjuvant therapy
  - No evidence that XRT, chemotherapy improve long term outcome

DIAGNOSTIC CHECKLIST

Consider
- MR at first suggestion of myelopathy

Image Interpretation Pearls
- Axial, sagittal fat-saturated T1WI after contrast to exclude dural or pial lesion inciting syringomyelia

SELECTED REFERENCES

1. Sun B et al: MRI features of intramedullary spinal cord ependymomas. J Neuroimaging. 13(4):346-51, 2003
2. Saito R et al: Symptomatic spinal dissemination of malignant astrocytoma. J Neurooncol. 61(3):227-35, 2003
3. Santi M et al: Spinal cord malignant astrocytomas. Clinicopathologic features in 36 cases. Cancer. 98(3):554-61, 2003
4. Arslanoglu A et al: MR imaging characteristics of pilomyxoid astrocytomas. AJNR Am J Neuroradiol. 24(9):1906-8, 2003
5. Brotchi J: Intrinsic spinal cord tumor resection. Neurosurgery. 50(5):1059-63, 2002
6. Kim MS et al: Intramedullary spinal cord astrocytoma in adults: postoperative outcome. J Neurooncol. 52(1):85-94, 2001
7. Constantini S et al: Radical excision of intramedullary spinal cord tumors: surgical morbidity and long-term follow-up evaluation in 164 children and young adults. J Neurosurg (Spine 2). 93: 183-93, 2000
8. Houten JK et al: Spinal cord astrocytomas: presentation, management and outcome. J Neurooncol. 47: 219-4, 2000
9. Lowe GM: Magnetic resonance imaging of intramedullary spinal cord tumors. J Neurooncol. 47(3):195-210, 2000
10. Miller DC: Surgical pathology of intramedullary spinal cord neoplasms. J Neurooncol. 47(3):189-94, 2000
11. Strik HM et al: A case of spinal glioblastoma multiforme: immunohistochemical study and review of the literature. J Neurooncol. 50(3):239-43, 2000
12. Nishio S et al: Spinal cord gliomas: management and outcome with reference to adjuvant therapy. J Clin Neurosci. 7(1):20-3, 2000
13. Houten JK et al: Spinal cord astrocytomas: presentation, management and outcome. J Neurooncol. 47(3):219-24, 2000
14. Houten JK et al: Pediatric intramedullary spinal cord tumors: special considerations. J Neurooncol. 47(3):225-30, 2000
15. Baleriaux DL: Spinal cord tumors. Eur Radiol. 9(7):1252-8, 1999
16. Bourgouin PM et al: A pattern approach to the differential diagnosis of intramedullary spinal cord lesions on MR imaging. AJR Am J Roentgenol. 170(6):1645-9, 1998
17. Squires LA et al: Diffuse infiltrating astrocytoma of the cervicomedullary region: clinicopathologic entity. Pediatr Neurosurg. 27(3):153-9, 1997
18. Minehan KJ et al: Spinal cord astrocytoma: pathological and treatment considerations. J Neurosurg. 83: 590-5, 1996
19. Nemoto Y et al: Intramedullary spinal cord tumors: significance of associated hemorrhage at MR imaging. Radiology. 182(3):793-6, 1992
20. Li MH et al: MR imaging of spinal intramedullary tumors. Acta Radiol. 32(6):505-13, 1991
21. Scotti G et al: Magnetic resonance diagnosis of intramedullary tumors of the spinal cord. Neuroradiology. 29(2):130-5, 1987

IMAGE GALLERY

Typical

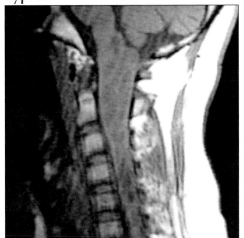 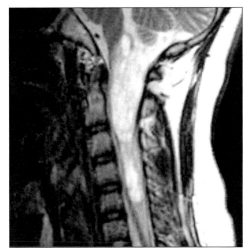

(Left) Sagittal T1WI MR shows exophytic mass expanding high cervical cord, with cystic component inferiorly. *(Right)* Sagittal T2WI MR shows high signal intensity of exophytic high cervical mass, cystic component inferiorly, and diffuse abnormal signal increase in lowest component.

Typical

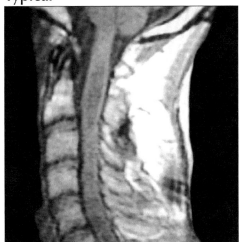 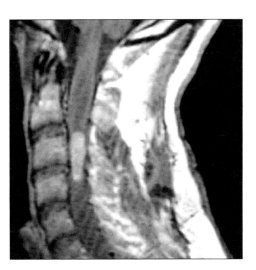

(Left) Sagittal T1WI MR shows fusiform expansion of cord at C1-C2, and isointense enlargement of cord below. *(Right)* Sagittal T1 C+ MR shows cystic expansion of cord at C1-C2, enhancing lesion below, and iso/hypointense cord below. Biopsy was targeted to enhancing lesion, proving astrocytoma.

Typical

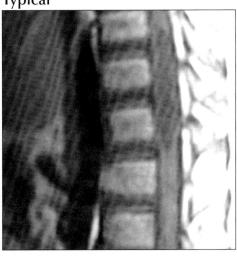 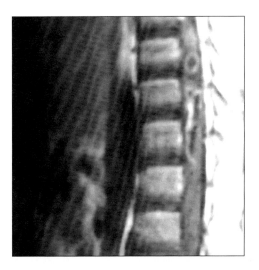

(Left) Sagittal T1WI MR shows multisegmental cystic expansion within diffusely enlarged distal thoracic cord in patient with pilocytic astrocytoma. *(Right)* Sagittal T1 C+ MR shows haphazard enhancement of multilocular cystic lesion within diffusely enlarged distal thoracic cord. Biopsy showed pilocytic astrocytoma.

EPENDYMOMA, CELLULAR, SPINAL CORD

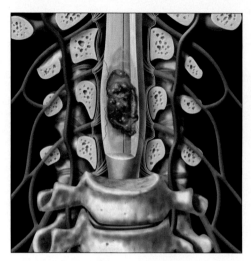

Coronal graphic depicts an ependymoma centered in cervical cord with mild cord expansion. Cranial and rostral cyst as well as hemorrhagic products are associated with this mass.

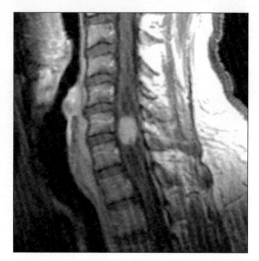

Sagittal T1 C+ MR shows solid enhancing component of ependymoma at C6 level. Note the rostral + caudal nonenhancing tumor associated cysts.

TERMINOLOGY

Abbreviations and Synonyms
- Cord ependymoma

Definitions
- Neoplasm of ependyma lining spinal cord central canal

IMAGING FINDINGS

General Features
- Best diagnostic clue: Circumscribed, enhancing cord mass with hemorrhage
- Location: Cervical > thoracic > conus
- Size
  - Multisegmental
    - Typically 3-4 segments
- Morphology
  - Well-circumscribed
  - Symmetric cord expansion
  - May have exophytic component

Radiographic Findings
- Radiography
  - Central canal widening: 20%
  - Posterior vertebral scalloping
  - Scoliosis

- Myelography
  - Fusiform cord enlargement
  - Partial or complete block of intrathecal contrast

CT Findings
- NECT
  - Spinal canal widening
    - Thinned pedicles
    - Widened interpediculate distance
    - Posterior vertebral scalloping
- CECT: Symmetrically enlarged spinal cord with well-circumscribed enhancement

MR Findings
- T1WI
  - Isointense or slightly hypointense to spinal cord
  - Hemorrhage hyperintense
  - Cord atrophy may be present
    - Correlates with surgical morbidity
- T2WI
  - Hyperintense
  - Polar (rostral or caudal) or intratumoral cysts: 50-90%
    - Similar to CSF intensity
  - Syrinx
  - Focal hypointensity: Hemosiderin
    - "Cap sign": Hemosiderin at cranial or caudal margin
    - 20-64% of cord ependymomas

DDx: Intramedullary Lesions

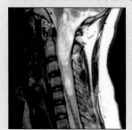

Astrocytoma

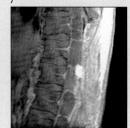

Hemangioblastoma

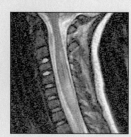

Cord Ischemia

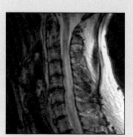

Idio. Trans. Myelitis

EPENDYMOMA, CELLULAR, SPINAL CORD

Key Facts

Terminology
- Neoplasm of ependyma lining spinal cord central canal

Imaging Findings
- Best diagnostic clue: Circumscribed, enhancing cord mass with hemorrhage
- Central canal widening: 20%
- Fusiform cord enlargement
- Hyperintense
- Polar (rostral or caudal) or intratumoral cysts: 50-90%
- Focal hypointensity: Hemosiderin
- Intense, well-delineated homogeneous enhancement: 50%

Top Differential Diagnoses
- Astrocytoma

- Hemangioblastoma
- Demyelinating disease (MS, ADEM)

Pathology
- Most common primary spinal cord tumor in adults
- Second most common primary spinal cord tumor in children

Clinical Issues
- Neck or back pain
- Delay in diagnosis due to slow growth
- 5 year survival: 85%
- Surgical resection

Diagnostic Checklist
- Associated peripheral hemorrhage suggestive of cord ependymoma

---

- ○ Surrounding cord edema
- STIR: Hyperintense
- T1 C+
  - ○ Intense, well-delineated homogeneous enhancement: 50%
  - ○ Nodular, peripheral, heterogeneous enhancement
  - ○ Minimal or no enhancement rare

Imaging Recommendations
- Best imaging tool: T2WI and T1WI MR in sagittal and axial planes with gadolinium
- Protocol advice: Fat suppression with T2WI and T1WI plus gadolinium

DIFFERENTIAL DIAGNOSIS

Astrocytoma
- May be indistinguishable
- Often longer
  - ○ Can be holocord
- More often eccentric, infiltrative
  - ○ Indistinct margins
- Hemorrhage uncommon
- Tumor cysts and syrinx less common
- Most common primary cord neoplasm in children

Hemangioblastoma
- Cyst with enhancing highly vascular nodule
  - ○ Flow voids may be present
- More extensive surrounding edema
- Thoracic > cervical
- Older patients
- 1/3 with von Hippel-Lindau disease

Demyelinating disease (MS, ADEM)
- Often multifocal
  - ○ 90% have brain lesions
- Lesions more often peripheral, posterolateral
- Typically < 2 vertebral segments in length
- Ill-defined
- Faint nodular or patchy enhancement

Spinal cord ischemia and infarct
- Sudden onset of symptoms
- Posterior columns typically spared in anterior spinal infarct

Idiopathic transverse myelitis
- Cord expansion less pronounced
- Centrally located
- 3-4 vertebral segments in length
- Thoracic > cervical
- Variable enhancement
- Diagnosis of exclusion

PATHOLOGY

General Features
- General path comments
  - ○ Four subtypes: Cellular, papillary, clear-cell, tanycytic
    - Cellular most common intramedullary tumor subtype
    - Tanycytes: Precursors of astrocytes and ependymal cells
- Genetics
  - ○ Myriad tumoral genetic abnormalities
  - ○ Cord ependymomas genetically different from intracranial lesions
    - Chromosome copy number aberrations using comparative genomic hybridization: Gain on chromosomes 2, 7, 12, etc.
    - Structural abnormalities on chromosomes 1, 6, 17, etc.
  - ○ Ependymoma associated with NF2
    - Deletions, translocations of chromosome 22
- Etiology: Arises from ependymal cells of central canal
- Epidemiology
  - ○ Ependymomas: 4% of all primary central nervous system neoplasms in adults
    - 30% of ependymomas are spinal
  - ○ Most common primary spinal cord tumor in adults
    - 60% of primary spinal cord neoplasms

EPENDYMOMA, CELLULAR, SPINAL CORD

○ Second most common primary spinal cord tumor in children
• Associated abnormalities
  ○ Subarachnoid hemorrhage
  ○ Superficial siderosis
  ○ NF2
    ▪ Schwannomas
    ▪ Meningiomas

Gross Pathologic & Surgical Features
• Soft red or grayish-purple mass
  ○ Small blood vessels on tumor surface
• Well-circumscribed
  ○ May be encapsulated
• Cystic change common
• Hemorrhage at tumor periphery

Microscopic Features
• Perivascular pseudorosettes
• True ependymal rosettes less common
• Moderate cellularity with low mitotic activity
• Occasional nuclear atypia
• Rare to no mitoses
• Immunohistochemistry: Positive for GFAP, S-100, vimentin

Staging, Grading or Classification Criteria
• Most are WHO grade II
• Rare: WHO grade III
  ○ Anaplastic ependymoma

CLINICAL ISSUES

Presentation
• Most common signs/symptoms
  ○ Neck or back pain
  ○ Other signs/symptoms
    ▪ Progressive paraparesis
    ▪ Paresthesia
• Clinical profile
  ○ Delay in diagnosis due to slow growth
    ▪ Average duration of symptoms before diagnosis: 2.5 yrs

Demographics
• Age
  ○ 35-45 yo
    ▪ Mean age at presentation: 39 yo
• Gender: Slight female predilection
• Ethnicity: No racial predilection

Natural History & Prognosis
• Less pre-operative neurologic deficit at presentation, better post-operative outcome
• Thoracic tumors have worse surgical outcome
• Rarely metastasis
  ○ Lung, skin, kidney, lymph nodes
• 5 year survival: 85%

Treatment
• Surgical resection
  ○ Gross total resection in > 85% of cases
• Radiotherapy for subtotal resection or recurrent disease
• Chemotherapy for failed surgery and radiotherapy
  ○ Unproven benefit

DIAGNOSTIC CHECKLIST

Image Interpretation Pearls
• Associated peripheral hemorrhage suggestive of cord ependymoma

SELECTED REFERENCES

1. Chamberlain MC: Ependymomas. Curr Neurol Neurosci Rep. 3(3):193-9, 2003
2. Sun B et al: MRI features of intramedullary spinal cord ependymomas. J Neuroimaging. 13(4):346-51, 2003
3. Carter M et al: Genetic abnormalities detected in ependymomas by comparative genomic hybridisation. Br J Cancer. 86(6):929-39, 2002
4. Jeuken JW et al: Correlation between localization, age, and chromosomal imbalances in ependymal tumours as detected by CGH. J Pathol. 197(2):238-44, 2002
5. Chang UK et al: Surgical outcome and prognostic factors of spinal intramedullary ependymomas in adults. J Neurooncol. 57(2):133-9, 2002
6. Hanbali F et al: Spinal cord ependymoma: radical surgical resection and outcome. Neurosurgery. 51(5):1162-72; discussion 1172-4, 2002
7. Choi JY et al: Intracranial and spinal ependymomas: review of MR images in 61 patients. Korean J Radiol. 3(4):219-28, 2002
8. Hirose Y et al: Chromosomal abnormalities subdivide ependymal tumors into clinically relevant groups. Am J Pathol. 158(3):1137-43, 2001
9. Wiestler OD et al: Ependymoma. In Kleihues P, Cavanee WK (eds), Pathology & Genetics of Tumors of the Central Nervous System, 72-7. IARC Press, 2000
10. Lagares A et al: Spinal cord ependymoma presenting with acute paraplegia due to tumoral bleeding. J Neurosurg Sci. 44(2):95-7; discussion 97-8, 2000
11. Koeller KK et al: Neoplasms of the spinal cord and filum terminale: Radiologic-pathologic correlation. Radiographics 20: 1721-49, 2000
12. Miyazawa N et al: MRI at 1.5 T of intramedullary ependymoma and classification of pattern of contrast enhancement. Neuroradiology. 42(11):828-32, 2000
13. Mazewski C et al: Karyotype studies in 18 ependymomas with literature review of 107 cases. Cancer Genet Cytogenet. 113(1):1-8, 1999
14. Graf M et al: Extraneural metastasizing ependymoma of the spinal cord. Pathol Oncol Res. 5(1):56-60, 1999
15. Bourgouin PM et al: A pattern approach to the differential diagnosis of intramedullary spinal cord lesions on MR imaging. AJR Am J Roentgenol. 170(6):1645-9, 1998
16. Kahan H et al: MR characteristics of histopathologic subtypes of spinal ependymoma. AJNR 17: 143-50, 1996
17. Fine MJ et al: Spinal cord ependymomas: MR imaging features. Radiology. 197(3):655-8, 1995
18. Waldron JN et al: Spinal cord ependymomas: a retrospective analysis of 59 cases. Int J Radiat Oncol Biol Phys. 27(2):223-9, 1993
19. Nemoto Y et al: Intramedullary spinal cord tumors: significance of associated hemorrhage at MR imaging. Radiology. 182(3):793-6, 1992

IMAGE GALLERY

Typical

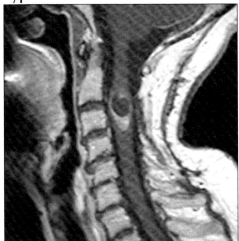 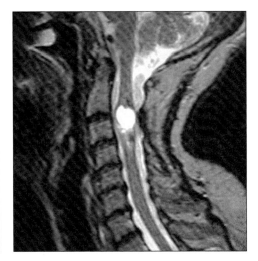

(Left) Sagittal T1 C+ MR of cervical spine shows well-defined cystic & solid mass at C2-C3 level w/focal cord expansion. Note the tumor cyst w/peripheral enhancement + more solid inferior nodular component. *(Right)* Sagittal T2WI MR of cervical spine shows focal cord enlargement w/predominating cyst at C2-C3 level. Note evidence of hemorrhage + hemosiderin deposition both cranial plus caudal to cystic component.

Typical

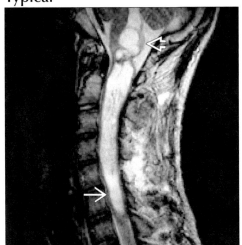 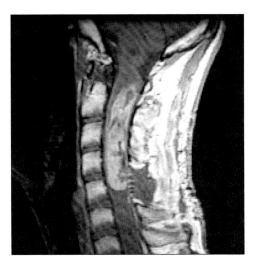

(Left) Sagittal T2WI MR of cervical spine shows a hyperintense expansile intramedullary mass with caudal edema (arrow). A cystic component is present in the medulla (open arrow). *(Right)* Sagittal T1 C+ MR in the same patient shows a heterogenously enhancing mass from C2-5. Biopsy reveals an ependymoma.

Typical

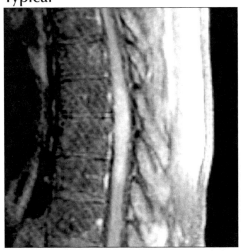 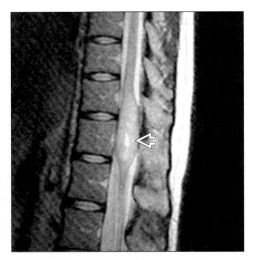

(Left) Sagittal T1 C+ MR with fat suppression shows a thoracic homogeneously enhancing intramedullary mass, with slight cord expansion. An ependymoma was found at surgery. *(Right)* Sagittal T2WI MR shows enlargement of the conus with a hyperintense mass with intra-tumoral cystic change (arrow).

EPENDYMOMA, MYXOPAPILLARY, SPINAL CORD

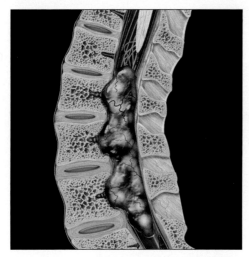

Sagittal graphic shows cauda equina myxopapillary ependymoma, enlarging spinal canal & remodeling vertebral cortex. Mass is vascular, w/old intratumoral hemorrhage & acute SAH.

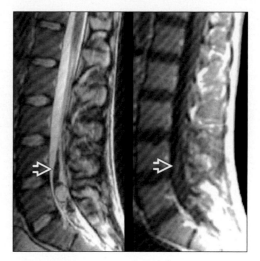

Sagittal T2WI MR (left) and T1 C+ MR (right) show a predominantly cystic cauda equina mass with associated subacute hemorrhage (arrows). A ME was found at surgery (Courtesy A. Osborn, MD).

TERMINOLOGY

Abbreviations and Synonyms
- Ependymoma, myxopapillary (ME)

Definitions
- Slow growing glioma arising from ependymal cells of filum terminale

IMAGING FINDINGS

General Features
- Best diagnostic clue: Enhancing cauda equina mass with hemorrhage
- Location
  - Almost exclusively in conus, filum terminale, cauda equina
  - Ependymomas outside of CNS rare
    - Metastases or direct extension of primary CNS lesion after surgery
    - Direct extension to sacrococcygeal area from cord ependymoma or ME
    - Primary presacral, pelvic, or abdominal lesion
    - Primary ME of skin or subcutaneous tissue in sacrococcygeal region
- Size
  - Usually spans 2-4 vertebral segments
    - May fill entire lumbosacral thecal sac
- Morphology
  - Well-circumscribed
  - Ovoid, lobular, sausage shaped

Radiographic Findings
- Radiography
  - Vertebral changes
    - Widened interpediculate distance
    - Eroded pedicles
    - Posterior vertebral scalloping
    - Intervertebral foraminal widening
- Myelography
  - Well-demarcated lobular mass extending from conus
    - Nerve roots draped around the mass
  - "Meniscus" of contrast delineates intradural extramedullary mass

CT Findings
- NECT
  - Isodense intradural mass
  - +/- Bony canal expansion
    - Thinned pedicles
    - Widened interpediculate distance
    - Scalloped vertebral bodies
    - May enlarge and extend through neural foramina
- CECT: Homogeneous, avid enhancement

DDx: Intradural Extramedullary Mass

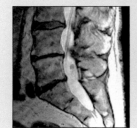

Schwannoma

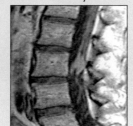

Metastasis

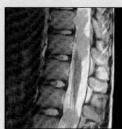

Metastases

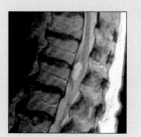

Acquired Epidermoid

EPENDYMOMA, MYXOPAPILLARY, SPINAL CORD

Key Facts

Terminology
- Slow growing glioma arising from ependymal cells of filum terminale

Imaging Findings
- Best diagnostic clue: Enhancing cauda equina mass with hemorrhage
- Almost exclusively in conus, filum terminale, cauda equina
- Well circumscribed
- Isodense intradural mass
- +/- Bony canal expansion
- Hyperintensity due to accumulation of mucin
- Hypointensity at tumor margin: Hemosiderin
- T1 C+: Intense enhancement

Top Differential Diagnoses
- Nerve sheath tumor (NST)
- Intradural metastases
- Acquired epidermoid

Pathology
- ME most common subtype to hemorrhage
- 90% of filum terminale tumors
- Acute non-aneurysmal subarachnoid hemorrhage
- Superficial siderosis

Clinical Issues
- Back pain
- Average duration of symptoms prior to diagnosis: 2 yr

MR Findings
- T1WI
  - Usually isointense with cord
  - Hyperintensity due to accumulation of mucin
- T2WI
  - Almost always hyperintense to cord
  - Hypointensity at tumor margin: Hemosiderin
    - 70% of intradural spine tumors with hemorrhage are ependymomas
  - May see flow voids
- STIR: Hyperintense
- T1 C+: Intense enhancement
- Rare: Destructive extradural sacrococcygeal lesion

Imaging Recommendations
- Best imaging tool: Sagittal and axial T2WI and T1WI MRI with gadolinium
- Protocol advice: Always include the conus in patients with back pain

DIFFERENTIAL DIAGNOSIS

Nerve sheath tumor (NST)
- Large, multilevel NST may be indistinguishable
- Small tumor associated with nerve root rather than filum terminale
- Usually extends through neural foramina
- Hemorrhage less common

Intradural metastases
- Smooth or nodular enhancement along conus and nerve roots
- Enhancing masses
  - Usually multiple

Acquired epidermoid
- Hypointense on T1WI
- Hyperintense on T2WI: Similar to CSF
- No enhancement
- Typically small

Meningioma
- Usually isointense with cord on T1 and T2WI
- More common in thoracic, cervical spine
  - Conus/filum location unusual
- Hemorrhage uncommon
- Bony changes rare

Paraganglioma
- Rare tumor of cauda equina
- May be highly vascular
  - Indistinguishable from myxopapillary ependymoma
- Usually smaller

PATHOLOGY

General Features
- General path comments
  - Four epemdymoma subtypes: Cellular, myxopapillary, clear-cell, tanycytic
    - Cellular most common intramedullary tumor subtype
    - ME most common subtype to hemorrhage
    - 10-40% of MEs are multiple
- Genetics
  - Spinal ependymomas genetically different from intracranial ependymomas
  - No consistent alterations
    - Tumor genetics: Extra copies of chromosomes 9 and 18 have been reported
- Etiology
  - ME originates from ependymal cells of filum terminale
  - Subcutaneous sacrococcygeal ME arises from coccygeal medullary vestige
    - Ependyma lined cavity of caudal neural tube at the postanal pit
- Epidemiology
  - Ependymoma: 4% of all primary central nervous system neoplasms in adults
    - 30% of ependymomas are spinal

EPENDYMOMA, MYXOPAPILLARY, SPINAL CORD

○ Cord ependymoma: Most common primary spinal cord tumor in adults
  ▪ 60% of primary spinal cord neoplasms
○ ME: 27-30% of all ependymomas
  ▪ Most common tumor of conus, filum terminale, cauda equina
  ▪ 90% of filum terminale tumors
• Associated abnormalities
  ○ Acute non-aneurysmal subarachnoid hemorrhage
  ○ Superficial siderosis

Gross Pathologic & Surgical Features
• Soft, lobulated, ovoid
• Grayish white surface
• Noninfiltrating, often encapsulated
• May be highly vascular

Microscopic Features
• Spindle, columnar, cuboidal tumor cells with radial perivascular arrangement
• Fibrous, mucoid matrix
• Cysts, hemorrhage, calcifications common
• Absent, low mitotic activity
  ○ MIB 0.4-1.6%
• Immunohistochemistry: GFAP, S-100, vimentin positive
  ○ Cytokeratin negative

Staging, Grading or Classification Criteria
• WHO grade I/IV
• May have local seeding
  ○ Subarachnoid dissemination
• No malignant degeneration

CLINICAL ISSUES

Presentation
• Most common signs/symptoms
  ○ Back pain
  ○ Other signs/symptoms
    ▪ Paraparesis
    ▪ Radiculopathy
    ▪ Bladder and bowel dysfunction: 20-25%
• Clinical profile
  ○ Symptoms mimic disc herniation
  ○ Delay in diagnosis due to slow tumor growth
    ▪ Average duration of symptoms prior to diagnosis: 2 yr

Demographics
• Age
  ○ Broad age range: Reported at all ages
    ▪ Peak: 30-40 yo
• Gender: M:F = 2:1
• Ethnicity: No racial predilection

Natural History & Prognosis
• Late recurrence, distant metastases uncommon after complete resection
• Risk of local recurrence if incomplete resection
• Excellent prognosis with complete resection

Treatment
• Resection

○ Gross total resection in > 85% of cases
• Radiotherapy in recurrence or subtotal resection
• Adjuvant therapy for multifocal lesions

DIAGNOSTIC CHECKLIST

Consider
• Scanning up to at least mid-thoracic spine if conus lesion found

Image Interpretation Pearls
• T1 hyperintense, enhancing, hemorrhagic mass associated with filum terminale highly suggestive of ME

SELECTED REFERENCES

1. Mahler-Araujo MB et al: Structural genomic abnormalities of chromosomes 9 and 18 in myxopapillary ependymomas. J Neuropathol Exp Neurol. 62(9):927-35, 2003
2. Sun B et al: MRI features of intramedullary spinal cord ependymomas. J Neuroimaging. 13(4):346-51, 2003
3. Akpolat N et al: Sacrococcygeal extraspinal ependymoma: a case report. Turk J Pediatr. 45(3):276-9, 2003
4. Hanbali F et al: Spinal cord ependymoma: radical surgical resection and outcome. Neurosurgery. 51(5):1162-72; discussion 1172-4, 2002
5. Choi JY et al: Intracranial and spinal ependymomas: review of MR images in 61 patients. Korean J Radiol. 3(4):219-28, 2002
6. Bavbek M et al: Lumbar myxopapillary ependymoma mimicking neurofibroma. Spinal Cord. 39(8):449-52, 2001
7. Wiestler OD et al: Myxopapillary ependymoma. In Kleihues P, Cavenee WK (eds): Tumors of the Central Nervous System, 78-9. IARC Press, 2000
8. Wager M et al: Cauda equina tumors: a French multicenter retrospective review of 231 adult cases and review of the literature. Neurosurg Rev. 23(3):119-29; discussion 130-1, 2000
9. Chung JY et al: Subcutaneous sacrococcygeal myxopapillary ependymoma. AJNR Am J Neuroradiol. 20(2):344-6, 1999
10. Asazuma T et al: Ependymomas of the spinal cord and cauda equina: An analysis of 26 cases and a review of the literature. Spinal Cord. 37(11):753-9, 1999
11. Rickert CH et al: Ependymoma of the cauda equina. Acta Neurochir (Wien). 141(7):781-2, 1999
12. Friedman DP et al: Neuroradiology case of the day. Radiographics. 18: 794-8, 1998
13. Yamada CY et al: Myxopapillary ependymoma of the filum terminale. AJR Am J Roentgenol. 168(2):366, 1997
14. Kahan H et al: MR characteristics of histopathologic subtypes of spinal ependymoma. AJNR Am J Neuroradiol. 17(1):143-50, 1996
15. Kline MJ et al: Extradural myxopapillary ependymoma: report of two cases and review of the literature. Pediatr Pathol Lab Med. 16(5):813-22, 1996
16. Wippold FJ II et al: MR imaging of myxopapillary ependymoma. AJR. 165: 1263-7, 1995
17. Shen WC et al: Ependymoma of the cauda equina presenting with subarachnoid hemorrhage. AJNR Am J Neuroradiol. 14(2):399-400, 1993
18. Parenti G et al: Primary cauda equina tumors. J Neurosurg Sci. 37(3):149-56, 1993

IMAGE GALLERY

Typical

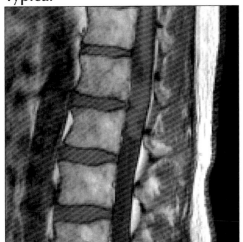 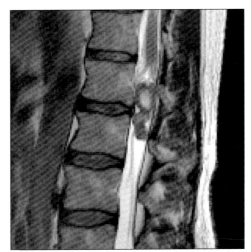

(Left) Sagittal T1WI MR shows a lobulated intradural mass caudal to conus medullaris. *(Right)* Sagittal T2WI MR in same patient shows the mass to be predominantly hyperintense, with hypointense foci compatible with hemorrhage. Nerve roots drape around the mass.

Typical

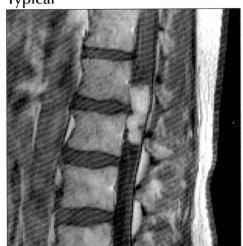 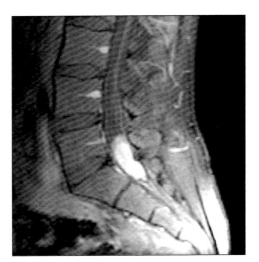

(Left) Sagittal T1 C+ MR in same patient demonstrates homogeneous enhancement in the cauda equina mass, proven to be a myxopapillary ependymoma. *(Right)* Sagittal T1WI MR with fat suppression in another patient shows an intensely enhancing myxopapillary ependymoma in lumbosacral thecal sac.

Typical

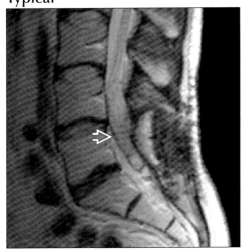 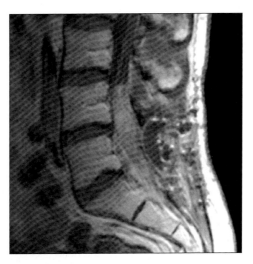

(Left) Sagittal PD/Intermediate MR shows a subtle mass filling thecal sac from L4 to L5, with a linear hypointense signal (arrow). Post-surgical changes are evident posteriorly. *(Right)* Sagittal T1 C+ MR in same patient demonstrates the mass with diffuse enhancement. Biopsy showed a myxopapillary ependymoma.

HEMANGIOBLASTOMA, SPINAL CORD

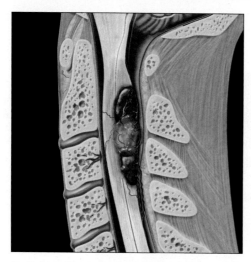

Sagittal graphic shows focal intramedullary mass in cervical cord with prominent feeding vessels, associated cyst, and cord expansion/edema.

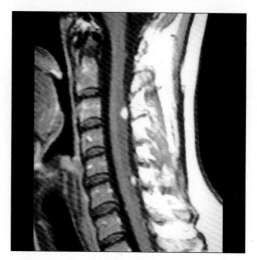

Sagittal T1 C+ MR shows two small enhancing intradural nodules on dorsal pial surface of cervical cord.

TERMINOLOGY

Abbreviations and Synonyms

- Capillary hemangioblastoma (HB); von Hippel-Lindau syndrome (VHL)

Definitions

- Low grade, capillary rich neoplasms of cerebellum and spinal cord that occur sporadically or in setting of von Hippel-Lindau syndrome

IMAGING FINDINGS

General Features

- Best diagnostic clue: Intramedullary mass with serpentine "flow voids"
- Location
  - Subpial
  - Posterior aspect of the spinal cord, often associated with intraspinal cyst
  - Rarely anterior aspect of cord
- Size
  - Few mm to several cm
  - Multiple tumors (often small) in VHL
- Morphology: Round, well-defined margins

CT Findings

- NECT: Intramedullary mass +/- expanded/remodeled spinal canal
- CECT: May demonstrate enhancing nodule
- CTA: May show enlarged feeding vessels, enhancing mass

MR Findings

- T1WI
  - Depends on lesion size, presence of syrinx
  - Small
    - Isointense with cord (may be invisible unless hemorrhage has occurred)
    - Well-delineated syrinx (hypointense) present in > 50%
  - Large
    - Mixed hypo/isointense
    - Lesions = > 2.5 cm almost always show "flow voids" (enlarged feeding arteries and/or draining veins)
- T2WI
  - Small lesions usually uniformly hyperintense
  - +/- Peritumoral edema
  - Syrinx fluid often slightly hyperintense to CSF
  - Mixed hyperintense (flow voids, hemorrhage common)
  - May show extensive, long segment cord edema without syrinx

DDx: Enhancing Intradural Lesions

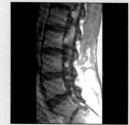

NF2

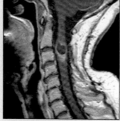

Ependymoma

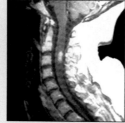

Metastasis

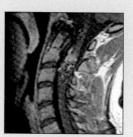

AVM

Key Facts

Terminology
- Low grade, capillary rich neoplasms of cerebellum and spinal cord that occur sporadically or in setting of von Hippel-Lindau syndrome

Imaging Findings
- Best diagnostic clue: Intramedullary mass with serpentine "flow voids"
- Subpial
- Posterior aspect of the spinal cord, often associated with intraspinal cyst
- May show extensive, long segment cord edema without syrinx

Top Differential Diagnoses
- Arteriovenous malformation (AVM)
- Cavernous malformation

- Hypervascular cord neoplasms
- Intradural/extramedullary tumors

Pathology
- 1-5% of all spinal cord neoplasms
- 75% of spinal HBs are sporadic (25% VHL-associated)
- Often multiple (VHL usually has one large +/- many small HBs)
- Cerebellar HBs, retinal angiomas, pheochromocytoma, renal cell carcinoma, angiomatous or cystic lesions of the kidneys, pancreas, and epididymis
- HBs are WHO grade I

Clinical Issues
- Does not undergo malignant degeneration

- T1 C+
  - Small
    - Subpial nodule (often on surface of dorsal cord)
    - Well-demarcated, intense, homogeneous enhancement
  - Large
    - Heterogeneous enhancement
    - If syrinx present, wall doesn't enhance

Angiographic Findings
- Conventional
  - Intense, prolonged vascular stain
  - +/- A-V shunting
  - Enlarged spinal arteries (anterior > posterior) supply mass

Other Modality Findings
- Intraoperative sonography may be useful in locating nodule

Imaging Recommendations
- Contrast-enhanced MR
  - Scan brain, entire spine in patients with known/suspected VHL
- DSA for large lesions/pre-operative embolization

DIFFERENTIAL DIAGNOSIS

Arteriovenous malformation (AVM)
- Cord often normal/small, gliotic
- Syrinx, focal nodule absent

Cavernous malformation
- Mottled or speckled pattern of prior hemorrhage, hemosiderin rim
- Minimal enhancement

Hypervascular cord neoplasms
- Ependymoma (mass centrally located; no syrinx)
- Astrocytoma (usually not hypervascular; peritumoral edema common)
- Vascular metastasis (known primary, e.g., renal cell carcinoma)

Intradural/extramedullary tumors
- Meningioma/schwannoma rare associated syrinx, uncommon flow voids
- Paraganglioma (filum > > cord but may be indistinguishable)

PATHOLOGY

General Features
- General path comments
  - VHL phenotypes
    - Type 1 = without pheochromocytoma
    - Type 2A = with pheochromocytoma, renal cell carcinoma (RCC)
    - Type 2B = with pheochromocytoma, no RCC
- Genetics
  - Familial HB (VHL)
    - Autosomal dominant
    - Chromosome 3p, other gene mutations common
    - VEGF highly expressed
    - Erythropoietin often upregulated
    - Tumors arise after the loss or inactivation of wild type allele in a cell
    - 20% of VHL families no deletion or mutation can be detected
  - Sporadic HB (unknown origin)
- Etiology: Suppressor gene product (VHL protein) causes neoplastic transformation
- Epidemiology
  - 1-5% of all spinal cord neoplasms
  - 75% of spinal HBs are sporadic (25% VHL-associated)
  - Often multiple (VHL usually has one large +/- many small HBs)
- Associated abnormalities
  - VHL
    - Cerebellar HBs, retinal angiomas, pheochromocytoma, renal cell carcinoma, angiomatous or cystic lesions of the kidneys, pancreas, and epididymis

HEMANGIOBLASTOMA, SPINAL CORD

Gross Pathologic & Surgical Features
- Well-circumscribed vascular nodule
  - Dorsal surface of cord
  - Extramedullary spinal HBs occur but are rare
- Prominent arteries, veins
- +/- Syrinx
- Rare extensive involvement of leptomeninges "leptomeningeal hemangioblastomatosis"

Microscopic Features
- Large vacuolated stromal cells + rich capillary network
- If present, cyst wall usually compressed cord (not tumor)

Staging, Grading or Classification Criteria
- HBs are WHO grade I

CLINICAL ISSUES

Presentation
- Most common signs/symptoms
  - Nonspecific clinical symptoms
  - Sensory/motor > pain
  - VHL patients usually have one dominant symptomatic lesion; may have other smaller, asymptomatic lesions
    - 95% symptom-producing spinal HBs associated with syringomyelia
  - Other signs/symptoms
    - May cause secondary polycythemia (erythropoietin upregulated)
- Clinical profile: Young adult with family history of VHL

Demographics
- Age: Mean age at presentation = 30 years
- Gender: M = F

Natural History & Prognosis
- Grows slowly
- Does not undergo malignant degeneration
- Life expectancy of VHL patients = 50 years
- CNS hemangioblastomas most common cause of death
- Renal cell carcinoma second most common cause of death

Treatment
- Microsurgical resection

DIAGNOSTIC CHECKLIST

Consider
- VHL: Annual physical and ophthalmologic examinations should begin in infancy
  - Imaging of abdominal organs, CNS (brain and spine) added in teenagers and adults

Image Interpretation Pearls
- Typical patten of intensely enhancing small mass on dorsal pial surface of cord
- Large lesions have vessel flow voids

SELECTED REFERENCES

1. Lee DK et al: Spinal cord hemangioblastoma: surgical strategy and clinical outcome. J Neurooncol. 61(1):27-34, 2003
2. Pluta RM et al: Comparison of anterior and posterior surgical approaches in the treatment of ventral spinal hemangioblastomas in patients with von Hippel-Lindau disease. J Neurosurg. 98(1):117-24, 2003
3. Wanebo JE et al: The natural history of hemangioblastomas of the central nervous system in patients with von Hippel-Lindau disease. J Neurosurg. 98(1):82-94, 2003
4. Hamazaki S et al: Metastasis of renal cell carcinoma to central nervous system hemangioblastoma in two patients with von Hippel-Lindau disease. Pathol Int. 51(12):948-53, 2001
5. Chu BC et al: MR findings in spinal hemangioblastoma: correlation with symptoms and with angiographic and surgical findings. AJNR Am J Neuroradiol. 22(1):206-17, 2001
6. Conway JE et al: Hemangioblastomas of the central nervous system in von Hippel-Lindau syndrome and sporadic disease. Neurosurgery. 48(1):55-62; discussion 62-3, 2001
7. Miller DJ et al: Hemangioblastomas and other uncommon intramedullary tumors. J Neurooncol. 47(3):253-70, 2000
8. Couch V et al: von Hippel-Lindau disease. Mayo Clin Proc. 75(3):265-72, 2000
9. Baker KB et al: MR imaging of spinal hemangioblastoma. AJR Am J Roentgenol. 174(2):377-82, 2000
10. Friedrich CA: Von Hippel-Lindau syndrome. A pleomorphic condition. Cancer. 86(11 Suppl):2478-82, 1999
11. Roessler K et al: Multiple spinal "miliary" hemangioblastomas in von Hippel-Lindau (vHL) disease without cerebellar involvement. A case report and review of the literature. Neurosurg Rev. 22(2-3):130-4, 1999
12. Irie K et al: Spinal cord hemangioblastoma presenting with subarachnoid hemorrhage. Neurol Med Chir (Tokyo). 38(6):355-8, 1998
13. Bakshi R et al: Spinal leptomeningeal hemangioblastomatosis in von Hippel-Lindau disease: magnetic resonance and pathological findings. J Neuroimaging. 7(4):242-4, 1997
14. Spetzger U et al: Hemangioblastomas of the spinal cord and the brainstem: diagnostic and therapeutic features. Neurosurg Rev. 19(3):147-51, 1996
15. Wizigmann-Voos S et al: Pathology, genetics and cell biology of hemangioblastomas. Histol Histopathol. 11(4):1049-61, 1996
16. Richards FM et al: Expression of the von Hippel-Lindau disease tumour suppressor gene during human embryogenesis. Hum Mol Genet. 5(5):639-44, 1996
17. Eskridge JM et al: Preoperative endovascular embolization of craniospinal hemangioblastomas. AJNR Am J Neuroradiol. 17(3):525-31, 1996
18. Crossey PA et al: Identification of intragenic mutations in the von Hippel-Lindau disease tumour suppressor gene and correlation with disease phenotype. Hum Mol Genet. 3(8):1303-8, 1994
19. Resche F et al: Haemangioblastoma, haemangioblastomatosis, and von Hippel-Lindau disease. Adv Tech Stand Neurosurg. 20:197-304, 1993
20. Lunardi P et al: Isolated haemangioblastoma of spinal cord: report of 18 cases and a review of the literature. Acta Neurochir (Wien). 122(3-4):236-9, 1993
21. Neumann HP et al: Central nervous system lesions in von Hippel-Lindau syndrome. J Neurol Neurosurg Psychiatry. 55(10):898-901, 1992

IMAGE GALLERY

Typical

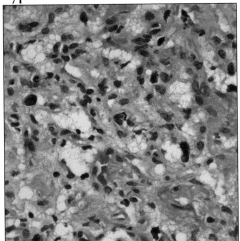
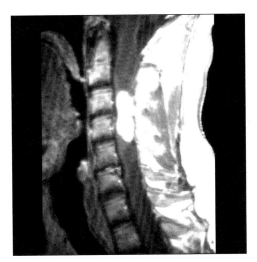

(Left) Micropathology, low power, H&E shows typical "stromal cells" (neoplastic component of the tumor) with pale vacuolated cytoplasm (clear cells) containing lipid droplets. *(Right)* Sagittal T1 C+ MR shows focal, well-defined enhancing intramedullary tumor. There is diffuse expansion of cord above and below tumor. Low signal edema in cervical cord could be mistaken for syrinx.

Typical

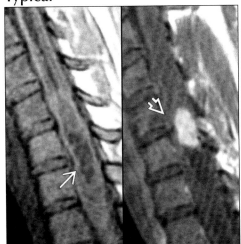
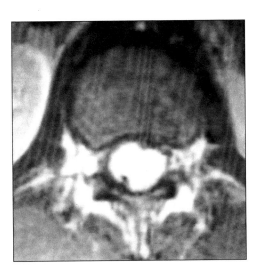

(Left) Sagittal T1WI MR (left side) show diffuse cord enlargement, heterogeneous signal with cord cysts (arrow). T1WI with contrast (right side) shows focal enhancing cord mass (open arrow). *(Right)* Axial T1 C+ MR shows an intensely enhancing intradural mass involving the conus, with peripheral flow voids seen as punctate low signal.

Typical

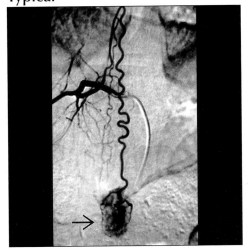
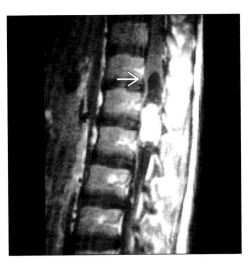

(Left) Anteroposterior angiography shows enlarged anterior spinal artery feeding hypervascular mass at the the thoracic lumbar junction (arrow). *(Right)* Sagittal T1 C+ MR shows focal enhancing intradural mass with superior cyst (arrow) within conus.

SPINAL CORD METASTASES

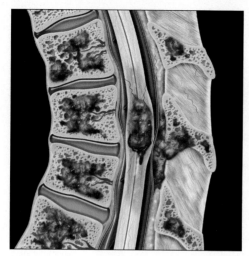

Metastatic involvement of skeleton dorsal, epidural space and cord: Note the hemorrhagic intramedullary metastasis expanding the cord.

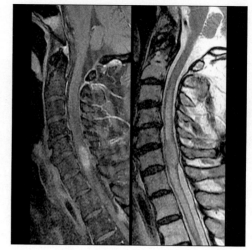

Sagittal T1 C+ MR (L) and sagittal T2WI MR (R) show focal enhancing oval lesion in cord with edema above and below. Patient had breast metastases and developed paresis.

TERMINOLOGY

Abbreviations and Synonyms
- Intramedullary spinal cord metastatic disease
- ISCM, ISM

Definitions
- Metastatic lesion from primary carcinoma in another organ (including brain)

IMAGING FINDINGS

General Features
- Best diagnostic clue: Focal, enhancing cord lesion(s) with extensive edema
- Location
  - Any cord segment
  - Conus least common
- Size: Typically small (< 1.5 cm)
- Morphology
  - Well-circumscribed
  - Spherical or oval

Radiographic Findings
- Myelography
  - May miss the lesion in substantial minority of cases
  - When positive, depicts focal cord swelling

CT Findings
- CECT: May rarely depict hypervascular mets as enhancing intraspinal foci (e.g., from hypernephroma)

MR Findings
- T1WI
  - Enlarged cord
  - Rarely, syrinx cavity
- T2WI
  - Focal high signal
  - Diffuse edema
  - Rarely syrinx
  - Rarely, low signal due to hemorrhagic metastasis (e.g., from thyroid, melanoma)
- PD/Intermediate: As T2WI
- T2* GRE: Highlights hemorrhagic focus
- T1 C+: Focal enhancement

Ultrasonographic Findings
- Real Time
  - Helps in surgical removal
  - Focal hyperechoic lesion

Angiographic Findings
- Conventional: Helps differentiate AVM or hemangioblastoma from metastasis

DDx: Met-Like Cord Lesions

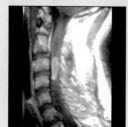

Astrocytoma

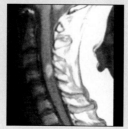

Multiple Sclerosis

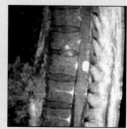

Hemangioblastoma

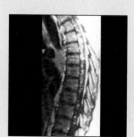

Sarcoidosis

SPINAL CORD METASTASES

Key Facts

Imaging Findings
- Best diagnostic clue: Focal, enhancing cord lesion(s) with extensive edema
- Spherical or oval

Top Differential Diagnoses
- Demyelinating disease
- Primary cord tumor
- Cord arteriovenous malformation
- Inflammatory granuloma
- Inflammatory myelitis

Pathology
- Seen in less than 1% of general autopsies
- Only 5% diagnosed antemortem
- Lung most common primary
- Breast second most common

Epidemiology
- Epidemiology: IMSM represents only 4-8.5% of all CNS mets

Clinical Issues
- Rapidly progressive flaccid paraparesis
- Other signs/symptoms
- Sphincter disturbance
- Pain
- Hypesthesia
- Brown-Sequard syndrome
- In 20% of ISCM, this is first presentation of cancer

Diagnostic Checklist
- Full craniospinal imaging when focal cord lesion found
- Edema out of proportion to focal small cord lesion suggests metastasis, even if solitary

Nuclear Medicine Findings
- PET: Has been anecdotally reported to detect metastases

Other Modality Findings
- CT with intrathecal contrast (post-myelography)
  - As myelography, can miss lesion
  - Focal cord swelling

Imaging Recommendations
- Best imaging tool
  - MRI
    - T2WI and T1 C+
    - Fat-saturation helps conspicuity
- Protocol advice: Double-contrast or delayed contrast T1WI in clinically suspected cases

DIFFERENTIAL DIAGNOSIS

Demyelinating disease
- Multiple sclerosis (MS)
  - Usually in dorsal cord, flame shaped on T2WI
  - Less cord swelling and edema compared to metastasis
  - Multiple lesions
  - Lesion(s) may not enhance
  - Most have brain involvement
- Acute disseminated encephalomyelitis (ADEM)
  - Multiple lesions
  - Simulates MS

Primary cord tumor
- Astrocytoma
- Ependymoma
- Hemangioblastoma
- Neurofibroma

Cord arteriovenous malformation
- Vascular flow voids leading to and from high-flow lesions
- Angiographically occult AVMs have hemosiderin stain, no edema

Inflammatory granuloma
- Tuberculosis (TB)
- Sarcoidosis
  - Look for pretracheal nodes

Inflammatory myelitis
- Transverse myelitis
  - Usually very long cord segment involved
  - Haphazard, if any, enhancement
- Viral myelitis
  - Pre-existing illness
  - CSF viral titres may prove diagnosis

PATHOLOGY

General Features
- General path comments
  - Seen in less than 1% of general autopsies
  - Only 5% diagnosed antemortem
- Etiology
  - Lung most common primary
    - Small cell > non-small cell
  - Breast second most common
  - Virtually any primary, including brain, can be source
- Epidemiology: IMSM represents only 4-8.5% of all CNS mets
- Associated abnormalities
  - Hemorrhage
  - Syrinx
    - Fluid in cavity typically higher in signal compared to developmental syringohydromyelia
  - Brain mets in approximately 20%

Gross Pathologic & Surgical Features
- Well-circumscribed fleshy lesion

Microscopic Features
- Typically reflect primary source

SPINAL CORD METASTASES

CLINICAL ISSUES

Presentation
- Most common signs/symptoms
  - Rapidly progressive flaccid paraparesis
  - Other signs/symptoms
    - Sphincter disturbance
    - Pain
    - Hypesthesia
    - Brown-Sequard syndrome
- Clinical profile
  - Most cases have known primary CA and develop sudden myelopathy
  - In 20% of ISCM, this is first presentation of cancer

Demographics
- Age: Any, typically over 50
- Gender: No gender preference

Natural History & Prognosis
- ISCM heralds poor prognosis
- Minority survive more than one year

Treatment
- Options, risks, complications
  - Steroids, chemotherapy, radiation therapy
  - Surgery an option in solitary cases
- Goal of therapy is stabilization or reversal of myelopathy, and preservation of ambulation

DIAGNOSTIC CHECKLIST

Consider
- Full craniospinal imaging when focal cord lesion found

Image Interpretation Pearls
- Edema out of proportion to focal small cord lesion suggests metastasis, even if solitary

SELECTED REFERENCES

1. Aryan HE et al: Intramedullary spinal cord metastasis of lung adenocarcinoma presenting as Brown-Sequard syndrome. Surg Neurol. 61(1):72-6, 2004
2. Reddy P et al: Intramedullary spinal cord metastases: case report and review of literature. J La State Med Soc. 155(1):44-5, 2003
3. Ogino M et al: Successful removal of solitary intramedullary spinal cord metastasis from colon cancer. Clin Neurol Neurosurg. 104(2):152-6, 2002
4. Potti A et al: Intramedullary spinal cord metastases (ISCM) and non-small cell lung carcinoma (NSCLC): clinical patterns, diagnosis and therapeutic considerations. Lung Cancer. 31(2-3):319-23, 2001
5. Fakih M et al: Intramedullary spinal cord metastasis (ISCM) in renal cell carcinoma: a series of six cases. Ann Oncol. 12(8):1173-7, 2001
6. Mortimer N et al: Intramedullary spinal cord metastasis. Lancet Oncol. 2(10):607, 2001
7. Mathur S et al: Late intramedullary spinal cord metastasis in a patient with lymphoblastic lymphoma: case report. J Clin Neurosci. 7(3):264-8, 2000
8. Schijns OE et al: Intramedullary spinal cord metastasis as a first manifestation of a renal cell carcinoma: report of a case and review of the literature. Clin Neurol Neurosurg. 102(4):249-254, 2000
9. Ateaque A et al: Intramedullary spinal cord metastases from a hypernephroma 11 years following the diagnosis and treatment of the primary lesion. Br J Neurosurg. 14(5):474-6, 2000
10. Keung YK et al: Secondary syringomyelia due to intramedullary spinal cord metastasis. Case report and review of literature. Am J Clin Oncol. 20(6):577-9, 1997
11. Phuphanich S et al: Magnetic resonance imaging of syrinx associated with intramedullary metastases and leptomeningeal disease. J Neuroimaging. 6(2):115-7, 1996
12. Honma Y et al: Intramedullary spinal cord and brain metastases from thyroid carcinoma detected 11 years after initial diagnosis--case report. Neurol Med Chir (Tokyo). 36(8):593-7, 1996
13. Schiff D et al: Intramedullary spinal cord metastases: clinical features and treatment outcome. Neurology. 47(4):906-12, 1996
14. Connolly ES Jr et al: Intramedullary spinal cord metastasis: report of three cases and review of the literature. Surg Neurol. 46(4):329-37; discussion 337-8, 1996
15. Shibamoto Y et al: Spinal metastasis from occult intracranial germinoma mimicking primary intramedullary tumour. Neuroradiology. 36(2):137-8, 1994
16. Raco A et al: Intramedullary metastasis of unknown origin: a case report. Neurosurg Rev. 15(2):135-8, 1992
17. Tognetti F et al: Metastases of the spinal cord from remote neoplasms. Study of five cases. Surg Neurol. 30(3):220-7, 1988
18. Van Velthoven V et al: Intramedullary spread of a cerebral oligodendroglioma. Surg Neurol. 30(6):476-81, 1988
19. Winkelman MD et al: Intramedullary spinal cord metastasis. Diagnostic and therapeutic considerations. Arch Neurol. 44(5):526-31, 1987
20. Foster O et al: Syrinx associated with intramedullary metastasis. J Neurol Neurosurg Psychiatry. 50(8):1067-70, 1987

IMAGE GALLERY

Typical

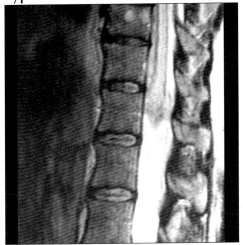 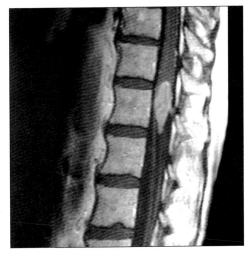

(Left) Sagittal T2WI MR shows diffuse distal cord edema and bulbous lesion (which enhanced) at tip of conus. Patient had sphincter disruption, weak legs, and metastatic non-small cell lung cancer. *(Right)* Sagittal T1 C+ MR shows vivid enhancement of conus metastasis in patient with non-small cell metastatic lung cancer. Note slight enhancement of cauda roots.

Typical

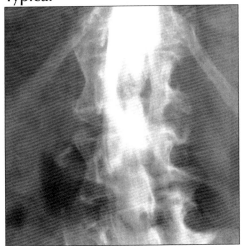 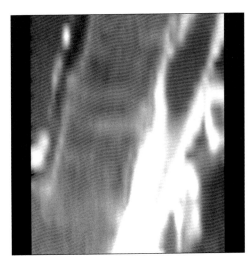

(Left) Anteroposterior myelography demonstrates focal swelling of the conus in paretic patient with subsequently found breast metastases from primary tumor treated 10 years ago. *(Right)* Sagittal CT reformation post myelography shows focally swollen conus in paretic patient with history of breast cancer treated 10 years ago. Metastases elsewhere were found after conus biopsy.

Variant

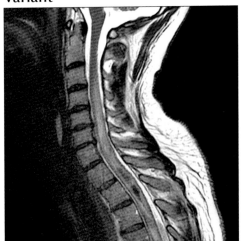 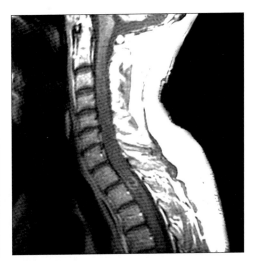

(Left) Sagittal T2WI MR shows diffuse swelling of cervico-thoracic cord with high signal and focal low signal zones indicating hemorrhage. Patient had metastatic lung adenocarcinoma. *(Right)* Sagittal T1 C+ MR shows diffuse cervico-thoracic cord swelling and focal enhancing lesion at T2 in patient with metastatic adenocarcinoma of the lung.

PARAGANGLIOMA

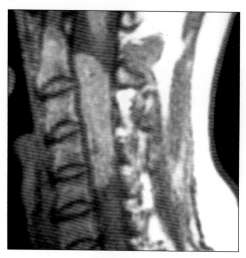

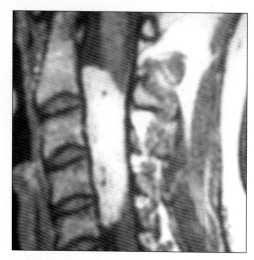

Sagittal T1WI MR shows well-defined intradural extramedullary mass spanning multiple cervical segments, with cord compression.

Sagittal T1 C+ MR shows intradural extramedullary mass markedly enhancing.

TERMINOLOGY

Abbreviations and Synonyms
- Paraganglioma (PG), chemodectoma, glomus tumor (terminology based on anatomic site)

Definitions
- Extra adrenal, spinal paraganglioma composed of chromaffin cells (groups of cells associated to the autonomous system)

IMAGING FINDINGS

General Features
- Best diagnostic clue: Vascular cauda equina mass
- Location
  - Spine is rare extra-adrenal site of paraganglioma
  - Most common in cauda equina
  - Rarely occur cervical, thoracic spine
- Size: 10 ⇒ > 50 mm
- Morphology: Well-defined intradural extramedullary mass

Radiographic Findings
- Myelography
  - Smooth/lobulated intradural extramedullary mass
  - +/- Serpentine filling defects (large arteries, draining veins)

CT Findings
- NECT
  - Large tumors may show bony remodeling, even erosion
  - Rare presentation = destructive intraosseous mass (usually in sacrum)
- CECT: May demonstrate enhancing mass below conus/along filum

MR Findings
- T1WI
  - Imaging features nonspecific (vascular intradural extramedullary mass)
  - Well-delineated round/ovoid/lobulated mass
  - Isointense, mixed isointense/hypointense compared to cord
  - Prominent "flow voids" common
- T2WI
  - Hyperintense +/- blood products, hemosiderin rim or "cap"
  - Prominent flow voids
- T1 C+
  - Intense homogeneous enhancement
    - Rare: Demonstrates multiple "uphill" intradural metastases

Angiographic Findings
- Conventional: Hypervascular mass

DDx: Intradural Tumor

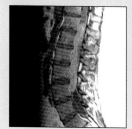

Ependymoma

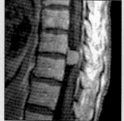

Meningioma

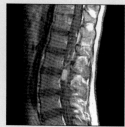

Schwannoma

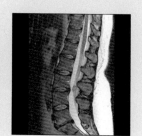

Leptomeningeal Mets

PARAGANGLIOMA

Key Facts

Terminology
- Paraganglioma (PG), chemodectoma, glomus tumor (terminology based on anatomic site)
- Extra adrenal, spinal paraganglioma composed of chromaffin cells (groups of cells associated to the autonomous system)

Imaging Findings
- Best diagnostic clue: Vascular cauda equina mass
- Morphology: Well-defined intradural extramedullary mass

Top Differential Diagnoses
- Myxopapillary ependymoma
- Schwannoma
- Meningioma
- Metastasis

Pathology
- General path comments: Can be difficult to distinguish PG from ependymoma using only light microscopy, standard H&E stains
- PGs originate from neural crest cells associated with segmental or collateral autonomic ganglia ("paraganglia") throughout body
- "APUD" cell tumors (Amine Precursor Uptake and Decarboxylation)
- Most neural crest tumors occur in adrenal medulla (pheochromocytoma)
- 80-90% of extra-adrenal paragangliomas occur in/near carotid body, jugular bulb
- Spine is uncommon site

Nuclear Medicine Findings
- I-123 or I-131 MIBG uptake with in metastatic paraganglioma
- Octreotide may also show uptake due to somatostatin receptors

Imaging Recommendations
- Contrast-enhanced MRI (do entire spine)

DIFFERENTIAL DIAGNOSIS

Myxopapillary ependymoma
- May be indistinguishable on imaging studies, standard light microscopy
- Immunohistochemistry distinguishes PG from ependymoma, other tumors

Schwannoma
- Usually less vascular, hemorrhage less common than PG
- Vascular schwannoma may be indistinguishable

Meningioma
- Thoracic > lumbar (even less common in cauda equina)
- Dural-based mass +/- reactive thickening ("tail" sign)

Metastasis
- Vascular intradural extramedullary metastasis may be indistinguishable
- Malignant paraganglioma may metastasize to spine

PATHOLOGY

General Features
- General path comments: Can be difficult to distinguish PG from ependymoma using only light microscopy, standard H&E stains
- Genetics
  - Sporadic: Cytogenetics, molecular genetics unknown
  - Familial

  - No reports of familial cauda equina PGs
  - Other extra-adrenal PGs can occur with MEN types 2A/2B, von Hipple Lindau
- Etiology
  - PGs originate from neural crest cells associated with segmental or collateral autonomic ganglia ("paraganglia") throughout body
  - "APUD" cell tumors (Amine Precursor Uptake and Decarboxylation)
  - Histogenesis of spinal PGs debatable
    - Paraganglionic tissue not normally found in cauda equina
    - Peripheral neuroblasts in filum may undergo paraganglionic differentiation
- Epidemiology
  - Most neural crest tumors occur in adrenal medulla (pheochromocytoma)
  - 80-90% of extra-adrenal paragangliomas occur in/near carotid body, jugular bulb
  - Spine is uncommon site

Gross Pathologic & Surgical Features
- Encapsulated, soft, dark red-brown tumor
- Richly vascular

Microscopic Features
- Well-differentiated tumor (resembles normal paraganglia)
  - Chief (type I) cells arranged in compact nests ("zellballen")
  - Surrounded by inconspicuous single layer of sustentacular (type II) cells
- Round/oval nuclei with finely stippled chromatin, indistinct nucleoli
- Sinusoidal blood vessels (occasionally thick-walled, hyalinized)
- Immunohistochemistry
  - Neuron-specific enolase 23/23 (100%)
  - S100 protein (95%)
  - Synaptophysin (90%)
  - Somatostatin (30%)
  - Glial fibrillary acidic protein (30%)

PARAGANGLIOMA

- Electron microscopy shows dense core neurosecretory granules

Staging, Grading or Classification Criteria
- WHO grade I
- Rare aggressive, malignant spinal paragangliomas have been reported

CLINICAL ISSUES

Presentation
- Most common signs/symptoms
  - Spinal paragangliomas have little/no secretory activity
  - Most common symptom = back/lower extremity pain
  - Symptom duration varies from days to years
  - Other signs/symptoms
    - Sensory/motor loss, bowel/bladder dysfunction
- Clinical profile: Middle-aged patient with myelopathy, intradural extramedullary enhancing mass

Demographics
- Age
  - Range from 13 ⇒ 70 years
  - Average = 45-50 years
- Gender: M = F

Natural History & Prognosis
- Slow-growing, generally benign behavior
- Varies with tumor location (generally excellent for spinal PGs)
- Recurrence < 5% after gross total removal

Treatment
- May require pre-operative embolization
- Surgical excision usually curative

DIAGNOSTIC CHECKLIST

Consider
- MR features nonspecific

Image Interpretation Pearls
- Prominent flow voids with intradural extramedullary enhancing lesion most often ependymoma

SELECTED REFERENCES

1. Lazaro B et al: Malignant paraganglioma with vertebral metastasis: case report. Arq Neuropsiquiatr. 61(2B):463-7, 2003
2. Jeffs GJ et al: Functioning paraganglioma of the thoracic spine: case report. Neurosurgery. 53(4):992-4; discussion 954-5, 2003
3. U-King-Im JM et al: Vertebral metastatic chemodectoma: imaging and therapeutic octreotide. Case report. J Neurosurg. 97(1 Suppl):106-9, 2002
4. Houten JK et al: Thoracic paraganglioma presenting with spinal cord compression and metastases. J Spinal Disord Tech. 15(4):319-23, 2002
5. Kim SH et al: Oncocytoma of the spinal cord. Case report. J Neurosurg. 94(2 Suppl):310-2, 2001
6. Shin JY et al: MR findings of the spinal paraganglioma :
report of three cases. J Korean Med Sci. 16(4):522-6, 2001
7. Masuoka J et al: Germline SDHD mutation in paraganglioma of the spinal cord. Oncogene. 20(36):5084-6, 2001
8. Lalloo ST et al: Clinics in diagnostic imaging (68). Intradural extramedullary spinal paraganglioma. Singapore Med J. 42(12):592-5, 2001
9. Hamilton MA et al: Metastatic paraganglioma causing spinal cord compression. Br J Radiol. 73(872):901-4, 2000
10. Sundgren P et al: Paragangliomas of the spinal canal. Neuroradiology. 41(10):788-94, 1999
11. Herman M et al: Paraganglioma of the cauda equina: case report and review of the MRI features. Acta Univ Palacki Olomuc Fac Med. 141:27-30, 1998
12. Ashkenazi E et al: Paraganglioma of the filum terminale: case report and literature review. J Spinal Disord. 11(6):540-2, 1998
13. Herman M et al: Paraganglioma of the cauda equina: case report and review of the MRI features. Acta Univ Palacki Olomuc Fac Med. 141:27-30, 1998
14. Hopster DJ et al: Widespread neuroendocrine malignancy within the central nervous system: a diagnostic conundrum. J Clin Pathol. 50(5):440-2, 1997
15. Moran CA et al: Primary spinal paragangliomas: a clinicopathological and immunohistochemical study of 30 cases. Histopathology. 31(2):167-73, 1997
16. Faro SH et al: Paraganglioma of the cauda equina with associated intramedullary cyst: MR findings. AJNR Am J Neuroradiol. 18(8):1588-90, 1997
17. Roche PH et al: Cauda equina paraganglioma with subsequent intracranial and intraspinal metastases. Acta Neurochir (Wien). 138(4):475-9, 1996
18. Rees JH et al: Paragangliomas of the cauda equina. IJNR 2: 242-50, 1996
19. Fitzgerald LF et al: Paraganglioma of the thoracic spinal cord. Clin Neurol Neurosurg. 98(2):183-5, 1996
20. Campbell L et al: Improved detection of disseminated pheochromocytoma using post therapy I-131 MIBG scanning. Clin Nucl Med. 21(12):960-3, 1996
21. Brodkey JA et al: Metastatic paraganglioma causing spinal cord compression. Spine. 20(3):367-72, 1995
22. Patel SR et al: A 15-year experience with chemotherapy of patients with paraganglioma. Cancer. 76(8):1476-80, 1995
23. Steel TR et al: Paraganglioma of the cauda equina with associated syringomyelia: case report. Surg Neurol. 42(6):489-93, 1994
24. Boukobza M et al: Paraganglioma of the cauda equina: magnetic resonance imaging. Neuroradiology. 35(6):459-60, 1993
25. Singh RV et al: Paraganglioma of the cauda equina: a case report and review of the literature. Clin Neurol Neurosurg. 95(2):109-13, 1993
26. Massey V et al: Treatment of metastatic chemodectoma. Cancer. 69(3):790-2, 1992
27. Pande AK: Malignant pheochromocytoma. Int J Cardiol. 34(3):346-8, 1992
28. Cybulski GR et al: Spinal cord compression from a thoracic paraganglioma: case report. Neurosurgery. 28(2):306-9, 1991
29. Yoshida A et al: Paraganglioma of the cauda equina. A case report and review of the literature. Acta Pathol Jpn. 41(4):305-10, 1991
30. North CA et al: Multiple spinal metastases from paraganglioma. Cancer. 66(10):2224-8, 1990
31. Parnell AP et al: Extradural metastases from paraganglionomas, report of two cases. Clin Radiol. 39(1):65-8, 1988
32. Sato Y et al: Hippel-Lindau disease: MR imaging. Radiology. 166(1 Pt 1):241-6, 1988

IMAGE GALLERY

Typical

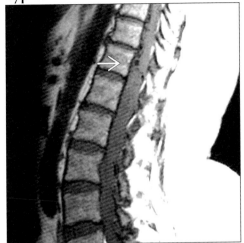
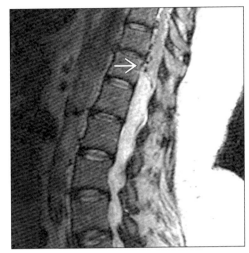

(Left) Sagittal T1WI MR shows isointense mass filling thecal sac and obliterating normal CSF signal. Large flow voids present along superior margin (arrow). *(Right)* Sagittal T2WI MR shows mass of increased T2 signal, filling the lumbar thecal sac. Flow voids again prominent along superior margin (arrow).

Typical

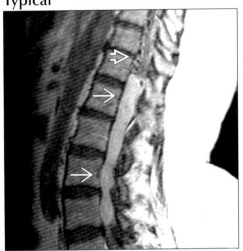
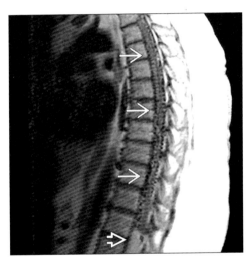

(Left) Sagittal T1 C+ MR shows enhancement of intradural mass extending throughout lumbar spine to thoracic junction (arrows). Multiple feeding vessel flow voids present at superior margin (open arrow). *(Right)* Sagittal T1 C+ MR shows extensive feeding vessels with prominent flow voids throughout the thoracic spine (arrows). Superior aspect of enhancing intradural tumor also seen (open arrow).

Typical

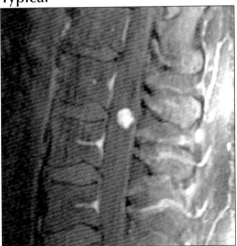
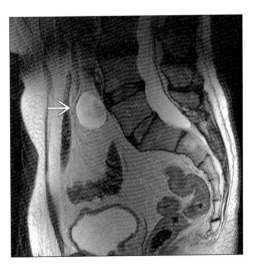

(Left) Sagittal T1 C+ MR with fat suppression shows focal enhancing intradural mass at L1-2 level. *(Right)* Sagittal T2WI MR shows focal hyperintense mass in retroperitoneum (arrow) at level of aortic bifurcation (organ of Zuckerkandel).

MELANOCYTOMA

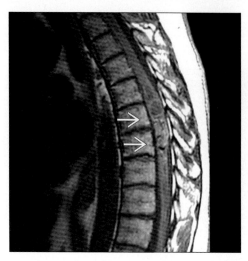

Sagittal T1WI MR shows intramedullary thoracic mass with heterogeneous T1 hyperintensity (arrows).

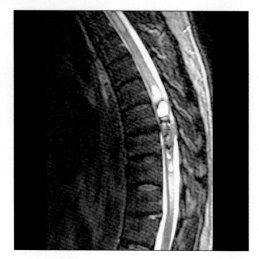

Sagittal T2WI MR shows heterogeneous solid and cystic mass intramedullary mass involving thoracic spine. Multple foci of low signal present within lesion.

TERMINOLOGY

Abbreviations and Synonyms
- Primary melanocytoma of cord, meningeal melanocytoma

Definitions
- Pigmented primary neoplasm of the CNS, involving cord or meninges
- Distinct from other melanotic lesions such as meningioma, schwannoma, melanoma

IMAGING FINDINGS

General Features
- Best diagnostic clue: Intradural enhancing mass showing T1 hyperintensity, not fat suppressing
- Location: Intradural mass, either intradural/extramedullary or rarely intramedullary
- Size: May extend over several vertebral body segments
- Morphology: Heterogeneous signal mass lesion

Radiographic Findings
- Myelography: Nonspecific intradural mass, may show block with larger lesion

CT Findings
- NECT: Nonspecific intradural mass, poorly visualized by CT

MR Findings
- T1WI: Isointense to hyperintense intradural lesion
- T2WI: Isointense to hypointense to normal cord
- T2* GRE: May show blooming of low signal related to melanin susceptibility effect
- T1 C+: Heterogeneous enhancement

Imaging Recommendations
- Best imaging tool: MR C+ of entire spine, brain to exclude additional lesions and possiblity of metastatic melanoma
- Protocol advice: T1, T2WI and post-contrast T1WI

DIFFERENTIAL DIAGNOSIS

Hemorrhagic cord neoplasm
- Ependymoma may show hemorrhage, hemosiderin
- Astrocytoma (usually not hypervascular; peritumoral edema common)
- Vascular metastasis such as renal cell carcinoma

Cavernous malformation
- Mottled or speckled pattern of prior hemorrhage, hemosiderin rim

DDx: Hemorrhagic Cord Masses

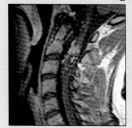

AVM

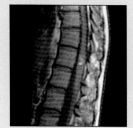

Cav. Malformation

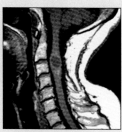

Ependymoma

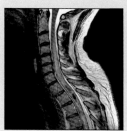

Metastasis

MELANOCYTOMA

Key Facts

Terminology
- Pigmented primary neoplasm of the CNS, involving cord or meninges
- Distinct from other melanotic lesions such as meningioma, schwannoma, melanoma

Top Differential Diagnoses
- Hemorrhagic cord neoplasm
- Cavernous malformation

- Arteriovenous malformation
- Pigmented intradural/extramedullary tumors

Pathology
- General path comments: Melanotic lesions probably constitute spectrum from well-differentiated melanocytoma ⇒ overtly malignant melanoma
- Immunoreactive for antimelanoma antibody HMB-45 and S-100 protein, vimentin antibodies and negative for epithelial membrane antigen

Arteriovenous malformation
- Cord may be small, gliotic
- Multiple flow voids

Pigmented intradural/extramedullary tumors
- Meningiomas and schwanommas rarely may show increased T1 signal due to melanin

PATHOLOGY

General Features
- General path comments: Melanotic lesions probably constitute spectrum from well-differentiated melanocytoma ⇒ overtly malignant melanoma
- Genetics: Heterogeneous with diploid, tetraploid, aneuploid lesions
- Etiology: Unknown, may arise from neoplastic transformation of meningeal melanocytes, or cord lesions from melanocytes in Virchow-Robin spaces
- Epidemiology: Cervico-thoracic region most common

Gross Pathologic & Surgical Features
- Most lesions appear black, but other colorations seen such as red, brown and tan

Microscopic Features
- Spindle cells arranged in fascicles and sheets
- Minimal nuclear pleomorphism, and minimal to absent mitotic activity
- Variable amounts of melanin pigment
- Immunoreactive for antimelanoma antibody HMB-45 and S-100 protein, vimentin antibodies and negative for epithelial membrane antigen

Staging, Grading or Classification Criteria
- Melanocytoma MIB-1 staining low (< 1-2%)
- Melanoma MIB-1 labeling indices (mean, 8.1%) higher than melanocytomas
- Intermediate grade lesions occasional mitoses, MIB-1 staining 1-4%

CLINICAL ISSUES

Presentation
- Most common signs/symptoms
  - Progressive back pain, extremety numbness, weakness
  - Other signs/symptoms

- Rare cases of subarachoid hemorrhage as presenting finding

Demographics
- Age: Wide age range (25-75 years)
- Gender: M = F

Natural History & Prognosis
- Progressive, low grade lesions curable by resection
- Generally lack metastaic potential

Treatment
- Treated by resection

DIAGNOSTIC CHECKLIST

Consider
- Signal relates to paramagnetic free radicals in melanin, with shortening of T1, T2 by proton-proton dipole-dipole interaction

SELECTED REFERENCES

1. Brat DJ et al: Primary melanocytic neoplasms of the central nervous systems. Am J Surg Pathol. 23(7):745-54, 1999
2. Alameda F et al: Meningeal melanocytoma: a case report and literature review. Ultrastruct Pathol. 22(4):349-56, 1998
3. Czarnecki EJ et al: MR of spinal meningeal melanocytoma. AJNR Am J Neuroradiol. 18(1):180-2, 1997
4. Chen CJ et al: Intracranial meningeal melanocytoma: CT and MRI. Neuroradiology. 39(11):811-4, 1997

IMAGE GALLERY

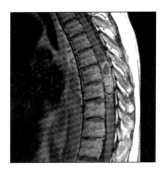 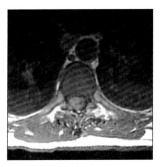

(Left) Sagittal T1 C+ MR shows heterogeneous enhancement of intramedullary thoracic lesion. (Right) Axial T1WI MR shows slightly hyperintense intramedullary mass within thoracic cord.

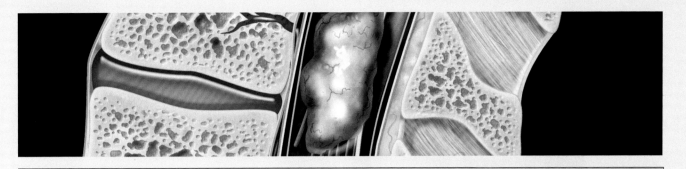

SECTION 2: Non-Neoplastic Cysts and Tumor Mimics

Cysts

Non-Neoplastic Masses and Tumor Mimics

ARACHNOID CYST

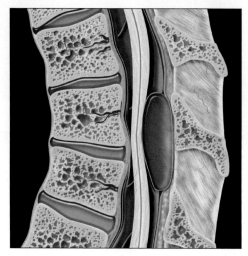

Sagittal graphic demonstrates a type III intradural arachnoid cyst in mild dorsal thoracic canal, with moderate mass effect on spinal cord.

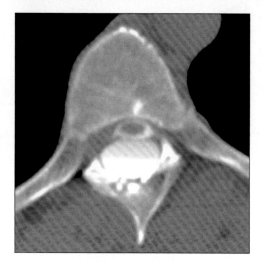

Axial bone CT following myelography shows dorsal epidural contrast containing cystic mass displacing thecal sac, characteristic of an extradural AC. Spinal canal is mildly expanded.

TERMINOLOGY

Abbreviations and Synonyms
- Arachnoid cyst (AC)
- Spinal meningeal cyst (MC)

Definitions
- Intraspinal extramedullary loculated cerebral spinal fluid (CSF) collection

IMAGING FINDINGS

General Features
- Best diagnostic clue: Nonenhancing extramedullary loculated CSF intensity collection displacing cord or nerve roots
- Location
  - Extradural or intradural extramedullary
  - Primary AC
    - Extradural: Posterior or posterolateral lower thoracic spine
    - Intradural: Dorsal midthoracic spine
    - Anterior location uncommon
  - Secondary AC without specific location
- Size
  - Variable
    - Average between 2-4 vertebral segments

- Morphology
  - Well-circumscribed
  - Oval, elongated
  - "Dumbbell" lesion: Extension through neural foramen

Radiographic Findings
- Radiography
  - +/- Bony canal expansion
    - Posterior vertebral scalloping
    - Thinned pedicles
    - Widened interpedicular distance
    - May enlarge and extend through intervertebral foramina
- Myelography
  - Intradural AC: Intrathecal filling defect
  - Extradural AC: Effaced subarachnoid space
  - Spinal cord compression
  - Variable myelographic block
  - Filling of AC
    - Often on delayed imaging

CT Findings
- NECT
  - Axial post-myelography CT may delineate communication between extradural AC and subarachnoid space
  - Contrast filled intradural AC difficult to visualize
    - Suggested by mass effect on cord and nerve roots

DDx: Intraspinal Fluid Collections

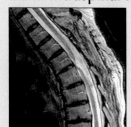

Cord Herniation

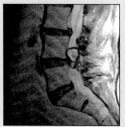

Facet Synovial Cyst

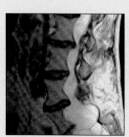

Dural Ectasia

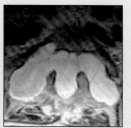

Dural Ectasia

ARACHNOID CYST

Key Facts

Terminology
- Spinal meningeal cyst (MC)
- Intraspinal extramedullary loculated cerebral spinal fluid (CSF) collection

Imaging Findings
- Best diagnostic clue: Nonenhancing extramedullary loculated CSF intensity collection displacing cord or nerve roots
- Extradural or intradural extramedullary
- +/- Bony canal expansion
- Axial post-myelography CT may delineate communication between extradural AC and subarachnoid space
- Contrast filled intradural AC difficult to visualize
- Suggested by mass effect on cord and nerve roots

- Typically CSF intensity
- T1 C+: No enhancement
- Variable mass effect on spinal cord

Top Differential Diagnoses
- Idiopathic spinal cord herniation
- Facet synovial cyst
- Dural ectasia

Pathology
- Primary AC: Diverticulum of dura, arachnoid, or nerve root sheath
- Nabors classification of spinal MC

Clinical Issues
- Pain may worsen with Valsalva maneuver
- Laminectomy with complete cyst wall resection

- Bone CT
  - Vertebral changes better characterized

MR Findings
- T1WI: CSF intensity
- T2WI
  - Typically CSF intensity
  - May be more hyperintense than CSF
    - Lack of CSF flow
  - Hypointensity related to flow related signal loss
- PD/Intermediate: CSF intensity
- T1 C+: No enhancement
- Cyst wall may be imperceptible
  - Presence of intradural AC suggested by mass effect on spinal cord
  - 2D cine phase contrast CSF flow study may show abrupt change in flow at cyst magin
- Solitary, multiple, or multiloculated
- Extradural AC may extend through enlarged neural foramina
- "Cap sign": Extradural AC outlined by rostral and caudal epidural fat
- Variable mass effect on spinal cord
  - Myelomalacia
- Syringohydromyelia at or away from site of AC

Imaging Recommendations
- Best imaging tool: Sagittal and axial T2WI and T1WI MR with gadolinium
- Protocol advice: Delayed imaging on post-myelography CT to allow filling of AC

DIFFERENTIAL DIAGNOSIS

Idiopathic spinal cord herniation
- Upper to midthoracic level most common
- Focal cord atrophy and ventral deviation
  - No dorsal intradural AC on myelography
  - Herniation through ventral dural defect
- May be associated with intra- or extradural AC

Facet synovial cyst
- Typically lumbosacral spine

  - L4-5 most common
- Posterolateral aspect of spinal canal
  - Adjacent to facet joint
- Associated facet arthropathy

Dural ectasia
- Associated with Marfan syndrome, neurofibromatosis, etc.
- Diffuse dilatation of thecal sac
- Spinal cord not distorted
- No block on myelography

Spinal nerve root avulsion
- Contiguous with subarachnoid space
- No discrete intraspinal lesion
- History of trauma

PATHOLOGY

General Features
- General path comments
  - Primary or congenital vs. secondary or acquired
  - Primary AC: Diverticulum of dura, arachnoid, or nerve root sheath
- Genetics: Multiple ACs may be associated with adult polycystic kidney disease
- Etiology
  - Primary intradural AC thought to arise from diverticulum of arachnoid
    - Arachnoid membrane splits to form cyst wall
  - Possible etiologies of primary extradural AC
    - Congenital diverticulum of dura
    - Arachnoid protrusion through a dural defect
  - Both ± communication with arachnoid space through a neck
    - Enlargement possibly due to "ball valve" mechanism
  - Secondary AC result from prior trauma, surgery, infection, or hemorrhage
    - Post-traumatic dural tear with arachnoid herniation

ARACHNOID CYST

- Post-inflammatory or surgical adhesions compartmentalize subarachnoid space
- Epidemiology: Primary extradural AC relatively rare
- Associated abnormalities
  - Kyphoscoliosis
  - Syrinx
  - Spinal dysraphism

Gross Pathologic & Surgical Features
- Smooth-walled cystic mass
- Clear, colorless fluid

Microscopic Features
- Primary AC ± arachnoid lining inner cyst wall
  - Sometimes duplicated
  - Variable connective tissue also present
  - Typically avascular
  - No significant inflammatory changes
- Secondary AC formed by fibrous connective tissue

Staging, Grading or Classification Criteria
- Nabors classification of spinal MC
  - Type I: Extradural MC without spinal nerve root fibers
    - A: Extradural MC/AC
    - B: Sacral meningocele
  - Type II: Extradural MC with spinal nerve root fibers
    - Tarlov perineural cyst
    - Spinal nerve root diverticulum
  - Type III: Intradural MC
    - Intradural AC
    - Acquired intradural AC also known as subarachnoid cyst

CLINICAL ISSUES

Presentation
- Most common signs/symptoms
  - Most patients asymptomatic
    - Especially type II MC
  - Other signs/symptoms
    - Pain
    - Paraparesis
    - Paresthesia
    - Hyperreflexia
    - Bladder and bowel incontinence
- Clinical profile
  - Pain may worsen with Valsalva maneuver
    - Increased intracystic pressure

Demographics
- Age
  - May present at any age
    - Type I thoracic AC more common in adolescents
    - Others more common in adults
- Gender: No gender predilection
- Ethnicity: No racial predilection

Natural History & Prognosis
- Worsening neurologic deficits with enlarging cyst
- Excellent prognosis
  - Complete relief of symptoms > 80%
- Degree of cord atrophy predictive of neurological outcome

Treatment
- Laminectomy with complete cyst wall resection
- If complete resection not possible
  - Wide marsupialization of cyst
  - Shunting

DIAGNOSTIC CHECKLIST

Consider
- Thin-section axial post-myelography CT to define communication between extradural AC and subarachnoid space

Image Interpretation Pearls
- Nonenhancing thoracic extramedullary CSF intensity collection highly suggestive of spinal AC

SELECTED REFERENCES

1. Wang MY et al: Intradural spinal arachnoid cysts in adults. Surg Neurol. 60(1):49-55; discussion 55-6, 2003
2. Takeuchi A et al: Spinal arachnoid cysts associated with syringomyelia: report of two cases and a review of the literature. J Spinal Disord Tech. 16(2):207-11, 2003
3. Abou-Fakhr FS et al: Thoracic spinal intradural arachnoid cyst: report of two cases and review of literature. Eur Radiol. 12(4):877-82, 2002
4. Krings T et al: Diagnostic and therapeutic management of spinal arachnoid cysts. Acta Neurochir (Wien). 143(3):227-34; discussion 234-5, 2001
5. Lee HJ et al: Symptomatic spinal intradural arachnoid cysts in the pediatric age group: description of three new cases and review of the literature. Pediatr Neurosurg. 35(4):181-7, 2001
6. Watters MR et al: Transdural spinal cord herniation: imaging and clinical spectra. AJNR Am J Neuroradiol. 19(7):1337-44, 1998
7. Silbergleit R et al: Imaging of spinal intradural arachnoid cysts: MRI, myelography and CT. Neuroradiology. 40(10):664-8, 1998
8. Congia S et al: Myelographic and MRI appearances of a thoracic spinal extradural arachnoid cyst of the spine with extra- and intraspinal extension. Neuroradiology. 34(5):444-6, 1992
9. Rabb CH et al: Spinal arachnoid cysts in the pediatric age group: an association with neural tube defects. J Neurosurg. 77(3):369-72, 1992
10. Gindre-Barrucand T et al: Magnetic resonance imaging contribution to the diagnosis of spinal cord compression by a subdural arachnoid cyst. Neuroradiology. 33(1):87-9, 1991
11. Dietemann JL et al: Thoracic intradural arachnoid cyst: possible pitfalls with myelo-CT and MR. Neuroradiology. 33(1):90-1, 1991
12. Boisserie-Lacroix M et al: The value of MRI in the study of spinal extradural arachnoid cysts. Comput Med Imaging Graph. 14(3):221-3, 1990
13. Sklar E et al: Acquired spinal subarachnoid cysts: Evaluation with MR, CT myelography, and intraoperative sonography. AJNR. 10:1097-104, 1989
14. Gray L et al: MR imaging of thoracic extradural arachnoid cysts. JACT. 4:664-8, 1988
15. Nabors MW et al: Updated assessment and current classification of spinal meningeal cysts. J Neurosurg. 68(3):366-77, 1988

ARACHNOID CYST

IMAGE GALLERY

Typical

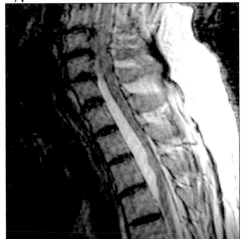

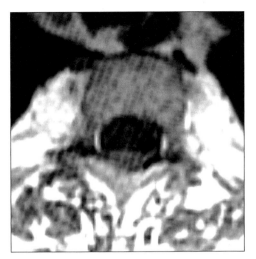

(Left) Sagittal T2WI MR shows a ventral multi-segmental intraspinal CSF intensity collection. It displaces spinal cord and produces a scalloped appearance on ventral cord surface. *(Right)* Axial T1WI MR in same patient confirms its intradural location. Note the cord is flattened. An intradural AC was found at surgery.

Typical

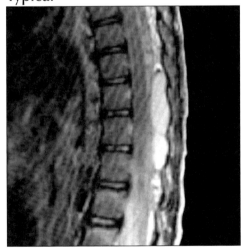

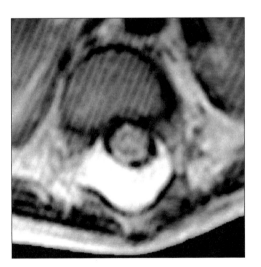

(Left) Sagittal PD/Intermediate MR through thoracic spine demonstrates a dorsal epidural fluid intensity mass with mild mass effect. *(Right)* Axial T2WI MR in same patient shows expanded spinal canal. Dorsal cystic mass proved to be an extradural AC at surgery.

Typical

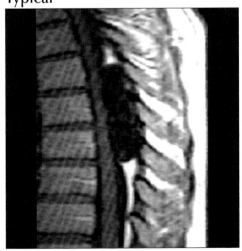

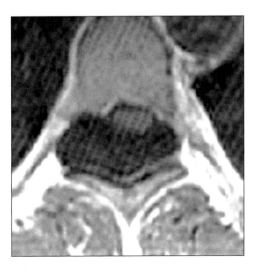

(Left) Sagittal T1 C+ MR through thoracic spine shows a nonenhancing dorsal epidural fluid intensity mass outlined by surrounding fat. There is mass effect on spinal cord (Courtesy M. Modic, MD). *(Right)* Axial T1WI MR in same patient shows dorsal extradural AC enlarging and extending through neural foramina, and compressing spinal cord (Courtesy M. Modic, MD).

POSTERIOR SACRAL MENINGOCELE

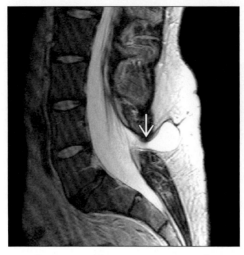

Sagittal T2WI MR demonstrates a meningocele at L5, extending into posterior subcutaneous tissue. Filum terminale appears thickened (arrow), tethered at the neck of herniation sac.

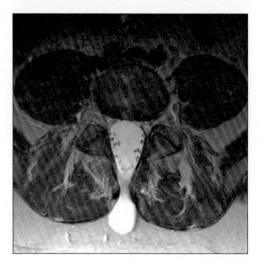

Axial T2WI MR shows a midline defect in vertebral arch of L5. There is direct communication between thecal sac, which contains sacral nerve roots, and the meningocele.

TERMINOLOGY

Abbreviations and Synonyms
- Posterior sacral meningocele (PSM)

Definitions
- PSM: Posterior herniation of dural sac through vertebral arch defect in lumbosacral spine
- Spina bifida: Spinal dysraphism involving bony elements of spine
  - Non-union of neural arch > unfused vertebral body

IMAGING FINDINGS

General Features
- Best diagnostic clue: Focal outpouching of thecal sac through defect in posterior arch of a vertebra
- Location: Lumbosacral > cervical or thoracic
- Size: Variable
- Morphology
  - Well-circumscribed
  - Round or elongated
  - Thin-walled
  - Cystic mass

Radiographic Findings
- Radiography
  - Spectrum of bony abnormalities
    - Absent single spinous process
    - Single level spina bifida
    - Multisegmental spina bifida
  - Spinal canal may be widened

CT Findings
- NECT
  - Cerebral spinal fluid (CSF) density
  - Variable extension into posterior subcutaneous soft tissue
    - Covered by skin
- CECT: No enhancement
- Bone CT
  - Deficient posterior elements in one or two spinal segments

MR Findings
- T1WI: Isointense to CSF
- T2WI: Isointense to CSF
- PD/Intermediate: Isointense to CSF
- STIR: CSF intensity
- T1 C+: No enhancement
- Communicates with subarachnoid space
- Typically without neural elements
  - Nerve root may enter and exit meningocele before leaving neural foramen
  - Filum terminale may extend into sac
- Midline defect in vertebral posterior elements

DDx: Cystic Sacral Masses

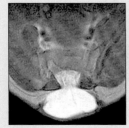

Myelomeningocele

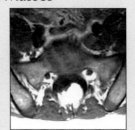

Lipomyelomeningocele

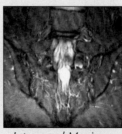

Intrasacral Mening.

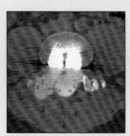

Pseudomeningocele

POSTERIOR SACRAL MENINGOCELE

Key Facts

Terminology
- PSM: Posterior herniation of dural sac through vertebral arch defect in lumbosacral spine

Imaging Findings
- Best diagnostic clue: Focal outpouching of thecal sac through defect in posterior arch of a vertebra
- Lumbosacral > cervical or thoracic
- Cystic mass
- Cerebral spinal fluid (CSF) density
- Variable extension into posterior subcutaneous soft tissue
- T2WI: Isointense to CSF
- T1 C+: No enhancement
- Communicates with subarachnoid space
- Typically without neural elements

- Midline defect in vertebral posterior elements

Top Differential Diagnoses
- Myelomeningocele
- Lipomyelomeningocele
- Distal sacral or intrasacral meningocele

Pathology
- PSM: Least common form of spina bifida

Clinical Issues
- Subcutaneous mass may be palpable
- Usually asymptomatic

Diagnostic Checklist
- Careful evaluation of spinal cord to exclude associated anomalies

Ultrasonographic Findings
- Real Time
  - Posterior midline bony defect
  - Anechoic herniation sac contiguous with thecal sac
    - Changing size with Valsalva maneuver

Imaging Recommendations
- Best imaging tool: Sagittal and axial T2WI and T1WI MRI
- Protocol advice: Image entire spine to exclude other congenital spinal lesions

DIFFERENTIAL DIAGNOSIS

Myelomeningocele
- Neural elements within meningocele
- Protruding beyond sacral soft tissue
- Not covered by skin
- Wide spinal dysraphism
- Low lying cord
- Chiari II anomalies
- Presents at birth or in utero

Lipomyelomeningocele
- Lipoma-neural placode complex within meningocele
- Contiguous with subcutaneous fat
- Covered by skin
- Osseous spinal dysraphism
- Cord always tethered

Distal sacral or intrasacral meningocele
- Type IB meningeal cyst
- CSF intensity mass filling sacral canal
- Connected to distal thecal sac by a pedicle
- No bony defects

Tarlov perineural cyst
- No osseous dysraphism
- Enlarged neural foramen
- Usually more than one
- Contains nerve fibers

Post-surgical pseudomeningocele
- History and findings of prior lumbar surgery
- Outpouching of meninges

PATHOLOGY

General Features
- General path comments: Mildest form of spina bifida cystica
- Genetics: Multifactorial genetic inheritance in spinal bifida
- Etiology
  - Failure of neural tube closure due to a combination of complex genetic and environmental influences
  - Environmental factors
    - Folic acid deficiency
    - Antiepileptic medications during pregnancy
- Epidemiology
  - Spina bifida: 1 per 1,000 live births
  - PSM: Least common form of spina bifida
    - Most common of all simple meningoceles
- Associated abnormalities
  - Split cord malformation
  - Hydromyelia
  - Low lying conus
  - Tight filum terminale
  - Epidermoid
  - Dorsal lipoma
  - Intracranial hypotension associated with rupture
- Embryology
  - Neural tube closure occurs during 3rd and 4th week of gestational age

Gross Pathologic & Surgical Features
- Does not contain neural elements

Microscopic Features
- Lined by arachnoid and dura

Staging, Grading or Classification Criteria
- Spina bifida: Spina bifida cystica and occulta
  - Spina bifida cystica: 83%

POSTERIOR SACRAL MENINGOCELE

- Myelomeningocele
- PSM
  - Spina bifida occulta: 17%
    - Non-union of vertebral arch
    - Asymptomatic
    - Cutaneous findings overlying bony defect: Skin dimpling, patch of hair
    - L5, S1, C1 most common
- Spinal dysraphism: Open or closed
  - Open spinal dysraphism
    - Myelomeningocele
    - Myeloschisis
    - Hemimyelo(meningo)cele
  - Closed spinal dysraphism: ± Back mass
    - With mass: PSM, lipomyelo(meningo)cele
    - Without mass: Simple or complex
    - Simple: Tight filum terminale, intradural lipoma, etc.
    - Complex: Split cord malformation, caudal regression, neurenteric cyst, etc.

CLINICAL ISSUES

Presentation
- Most common signs/symptoms
  - If large, may see posterior lumbosacral contour bulge
  - Subcutaneous mass may be palpable
  - Other signs/symptoms
    - Neurologic symptoms if cord tethered
    - Back pain
    - Scoliosis
    - Lower extremity weakness
    - Sensory loss
    - Gait disturbance
    - Bladder and bowel dysfunction
    - Decreased deep tendons reflexes
- Clinical profile
  - Usually asymptomatic
  - Symptoms, if present, develop after first few years of life

Demographics
- Age
  - Usually presents in first two decades of life
  - May present as late as fourth decade
- Gender: M = F
- Ethnicity: Spina bifida: Hispanics, Caucasians > Asians, African-Americans

Natural History & Prognosis
- Good prognosis
- Surgical complications
  - Meningitis
  - Cord tethering
    - May present later in life

Treatment
- Surgical resection of PSM
- Closure of dura
- Myocutaneous flap

DIAGNOSTIC CHECKLIST

Consider
- Careful evaluation of spinal cord to exclude associated anomalies

Image Interpretation Pearls
- Skin covered posterior outpouching of thecal sac through lumbosacral bony defect characteristic of PSM

SELECTED REFERENCES

1. Barazi SA et al: High and low pressure states associated with posterior sacral meningocele. Br J Neurosurg. 17(2):184-7, 2003
2. Khanna AJ et al: Magnetic resonance imaging of the pediatric spine. J Am Acad Orthop Surg. 11(4):248-59, 2003
3. Dick EA et al: Spinal ultrasound in infants. Br J Radiol. 75(892):384-92, 2002
4. Evans A et al: Magnetic resonance imaging of intraspinal cystic lesions: a pictorial review. Curr Probl Diagn Radiol. 31(3):79-94, 2002
5. Diel J et al: The sacrum: pathologic spectrum, multimodality imaging, and subspecialty approach. Radiographics. 21(1):83-104, 2001
6. Ersahin Y et al: Is meningocele really an isolated lesion? Childs Nerv Syst. 17:487-90, 2001
7. Tortori-Donati P et al: Magnetic resonance imaging of spinal dysraphism. Top Magn Reson Imaging. 12(6):375-409, 2001
8. Tortori-Donati P et al: Spinal dysraphism: a review of neuroradiological features with embryological correlations and proposal for a new classification. Neuroradiology. 42(7):471-91, 2000
9. Northrup H et al: Spina bifida and other neural tube defects. Curr Probl Pediatr. 30(10):313-32, 2000
10. Egelhoff JC: MR imaging of congenital anomalies of the pediatric spine. Magn Reson Imaging Clin N Am. 7(3):459-79, 1999
11. Cornette L et al: Closed spinal dysraphism: a review on diagnosis and treatment in infancy. Eur J Paediatr Neurol. 2(4):179-85, 1998
12. Babcook CJ: Ultrasound evaluation of prenatal and neonatal spina bifida. Neurosurg Clin N Am. 6(2):203-18, 1995
13. Barkovich AJ: Pediatric Neuroimaging. 2nd ed. 491-496, 1995
14. Byrd SE et al: Developmental disorders of the pediatric spine. Radiol Clin North Am. 29:711-52, 1991
15. Brunberg JA et al: Magnetic resonance imaging of spinal dysraphism. Radiol Clin North Am. 26(2):181-205, 1988
16. Fitz CR: Diagnostic imaging in children with spinal disorders. Pediatr Clin North Am. 32(6):1537-58, 1985
17. Raghavendra BN et al: Sonography of the spine and spinal cord. Radiol Clin North Am. 23(1):91-105, 1985
18. Bale PM: Sacrococcygeal developmental abnormalities and tumors in children. Perspect Pediatr Pathol. 8(1):9-56, 1984
19. Levine E et al: Computed tomography of sacral and perisacral lesions. Crit Rev Diagn Imaging. 21(4):307-74, 1984
20. Campbell S et al: Ultrasound in the diagnosis of spina bifida. Lancet. 1(7915):1065-8, 1975

IMAGE GALLERY

Typical

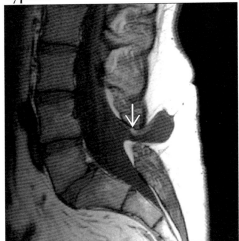
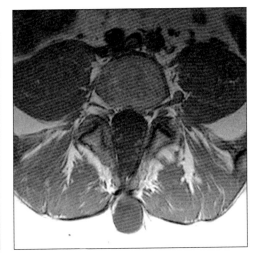

(Left) Sagittal T1WI MR shows a posterior meningocele at L5. Focal fat *(arrow)* is present in the filum terminale, tethered at the neck of herniation sac. Distal spinal canal is widened. *(Right)* Axial T1WI MR shows meningocele and midline defect in neural arch of L5.

Typical

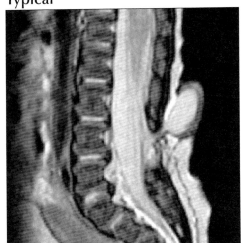
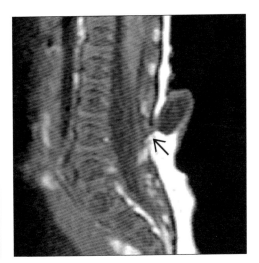

(Left) Sagittal PD/Intermediate MR demonstrates simple meningocele in lower lumbar spine. It is well-circumscribed and of CSF intensity. *(Right)* Sagittal T1WI MR shows meningocele connected to distal thecal sac through a thin pedicle *(arrow)*.

Typical

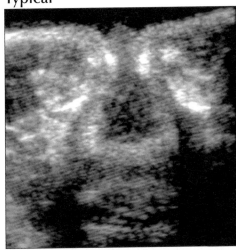
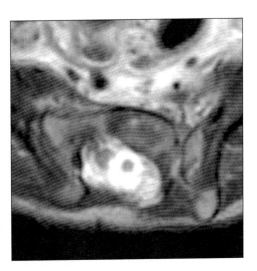

(Left) Transverse ultrasound real time reveals parallel sacral laminae with associated midline osseous defect. *(Right)* Axial T2WI MR in another patient demonstrates deficient posterior elements in upper sacrum, with meningocele covered by skin and subcutaneous tissue.

PERINEURAL ROOT SLEEVE CYST

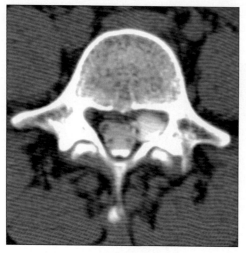

Axial NECT post-myelography through L5 shows contrast filling a left perineural cyst.

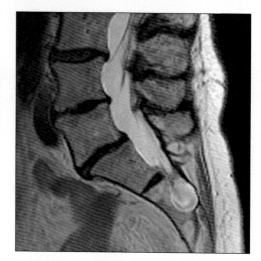

Sagittal T2WI MR through lumbar spine demonstrates a well-circumscribed hyperintense Tarlov cyst remodeling posterior aspect of S2. Intrinsic low intensity represents CSF flow.

TERMINOLOGY

Abbreviations and Synonyms
- Spinal nerve root diverticulum
- Tarlov perineural cyst
- Type II extradural meningeal cyst (MC)

Definitions
- Dilatation of arachnoid and dura of spinal posterior nerve root sheath, containing nerve fibers

IMAGING FINDINGS

General Features
- Best diagnostic clue: Cerebral spinal fluid (CSF) density/intensity masses enlarging sacral neural foramina
- Location
  - Anywhere along spine
    - More common in lower lumbar spine and sacrum
    - S2 and S3 nerve roots most commonly involved
- Size: Variable
- Morphology
  - Well-circumscribed
  - Thin-walled
  - Round, lobular, multiloculated
  - Cystic mass

- Often multiple and bilateral

Radiographic Findings
- Radiography
  - Widened canal
  - Enlarged foramen
  - Thinned pedicles
  - Posterior vertebral scalloping
- Myelography: Rounded sacral intraspinal filling defect

CT Findings
- NECT
  - Discrete CSF density mass
  - Enlarged sacral canal
  - Expanded neural foramen
  - Post-myelography CT
    - Opacification of cyst by intrathecal contrast
    - Sometimes on delayed imaging
- CECT: No enhancement

MR Findings
- T1WI: Hypointense
- T2WI: Hyperintense
- PD/Intermediate: Hyperintense
- STIR: Hyperintense
- T1 C+: No enhancement
- Flow sensitive sequence may demonstrate signal loss within cyst
  - Inflow of CSF from subarachnoid space

DDx: Cystic Spinal Masses

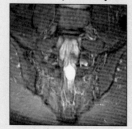
Sacral Meningocele

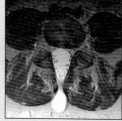
Post. Sac. Meningocele

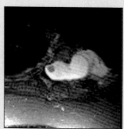
Lat. Th. Meningocele

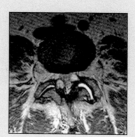
Facet Synovial Cysts

PERINEURAL ROOT SLEEVE CYST

Key Facts

Terminology
- Spinal nerve root diverticulum
- Type II extradural meningeal cyst (MC)
- Dilatation of arachnoid and dura of spinal posterior nerve root sheath, containing nerve fibers

Imaging Findings
- Best diagnostic clue: Cerebral spinal fluid (CSF) density/intensity masses enlarging sacral neural foramina
- S2 and S3 nerve roots most commonly involved
- Widened canal
- Enlarged foramen
- Posterior vertebral scalloping
- Opacification of cyst by intrathecal contrast
- T1 C+: No enhancement

- Flow sensitive sequence may demonstrate signal loss within cyst

Top Differential Diagnoses
- Meningocele
- Facet synovial cyst

Pathology
- Common, incidental, and usually asymptomatic
- No reliable imaging method to differentiate symptomatic from asymptomatic lesions
- Rupture may cause spontaneous intracranial hypotension
- Nabors classification of spinal MC

- Bone erosion
- Neural foraminal widening

Imaging Recommendations
- Best imaging tool: Sagittal and axial T2WI and T1WI MRI
- Protocol advice: Gadolinium to exclude solid mass if signal intensity not entirely cystic

DIFFERENTIAL DIAGNOSIS

Meningocele
- Anterior sacral meningocele
  - Solitary, CSF intensity lesion in pelvis
    - Protrusion of meninges through anterior sacral defect
  - ± Sacral anomaly (scimitar) and anorectal malformation
    - Currarino triad
- Distal, or occult intrasacral meningocele
  - Type IB MC
    - No neural elements
  - CSF intensity mass filling sacral canal
  - Connected to caudal tip of thecal sac by a pedicle
- Posterior sacral meningocele
  - Posterior herniation of dural sac through spina bifida
  - No neural elements
- Lateral thoracic meningocele
  - Neurofibromatosis type I in 75-85% of cases
  - Sharp angle thoracic scoliosis

Facet synovial cyst
- Posterolateral lumbosacral spine
  - L4-5 most common
  - Abutting facet joint
- Associated facet arthropathy

Spinal nerve root avulsion
- Pseudomeningocele
- Usually unilateral and at contiguous levels
- More common in lower cervical and upper thoracic spine

- No bony erosion
- Immediate filling of intrathecal contrast on myelography
- History of trauma

Nerve sheath tumor (NST), metastases, other neoplasms
- Soft tissue intensity
- Intradural extramedullary
  - NST may expand and extend through neural foramen
- Intense post-gadolinium enhancement

PATHOLOGY

General Features
- General path comments
  - Common, incidental, and usually asymptomatic
  - No reliable imaging method to differentiate symptomatic from asymptomatic lesions
  - Spinal nerve root diverticulum shown to communicate with subarachnoid space
    - Likely the same lesion as Tarlov perineural cyst
- Genetics: No genetic predisposition
- Etiology
  - Controversial
  - Congenital arachnoid proliferation within root sleeve, versus
  - Post-traumatic rupture of perineurium and epineurium
  - Typical finding of stenotic cyst ostium
    - Valve-like mechanism allowing pulsatile CSF inflow, limiting egress
    - Other possible mechanisms of cyst formation include osmotic pressure and secretory activity of cyst wall
- Epidemiology: 4.6-9% of adults
- Associated abnormalities
  - Rupture may cause spontaneous intracranial hypotension
  - Sacral insufficiency fracture

PERINEURAL ROOT SLEEVE CYST

Gross Pathologic & Surgical Features
- Origin at junction of dorsal nerve root and its ganglion
- Spinal nerve root traverses through cyst or within cyst wall
- ± Communication with subarachnoid space

Microscopic Features
- Outer wall with epineurium lined by arachnoid
- Inner wall lined with pia mater
- Fibrocollagenous tissue also present
- Old hemorrhage
- Nerve fibers (75%) or ganglionic cells (25%) within cyst or cyst wall

Staging, Grading or Classification Criteria
- Nabors classification of spinal MC
- Type I: Extradural MC without spinal nerve root fibers
  - IA: Extradural MC
    - Also known as extradural arachnoid cyst
    - Relatively rare
    - Dorsal or dorsal-lateral lower thoracic spine
    - May extend into neural foramina
  - IB: Occult sacral meningocele
- Type II: Extradural MC with spinal nerve root fibers
  - Tarlov perineural cyst
  - Spinal nerve root diverticulum
- Type III: Intradural MC
  - Also known as intradural arachnoid cyst
  - Posterior aspect of midthoracic spine

CLINICAL ISSUES

Presentation
- Most common signs/symptoms
  - Majority asymptomatic: > 80%
  - Other signs/symptoms
    - Low back or sacral pain
    - Radicular or perineal pain
    - Paresthesia
    - Weakness
    - Bladder or bowel dysfunction
- Clinical profile
  - Symptoms simulate disc herniation and spinal stenosis
  - Symptoms may worsen with postural changes and Valsalva maneuvers

Demographics
- Age: 30-40 yo
- Gender: M = F
- Ethnicity: No racial predilection

Natural History & Prognosis
- Progressive cyst enlargement
- Cyst recurs following aspiration or partial resection
- Symptomatic relief after complete resection: > 70%
  - Better outcome associated with
    - Cysts < 1.5 cm
    - Radicular pain
    - Bladder/bowel dysfunction
    - Worsening symptoms with Valsalva maneuver

Treatment
- Medical treatment
  - Anti-inflammatory medication
  - Physical therapy
- Temporary relief with cyst aspiration
  - Usually several months
- Sacral laminectomies with microsurgical cyst fenestration and imbrication
- Complete cyst/nerve root resection

DIAGNOSTIC CHECKLIST

Consider
- Delayed CT (30-60 minutes) after intrathecal contrast injection to visualize filling of perineural cyst

Image Interpretation Pearls
- Sacral CSF intensity mass enlarging neural foramen characteristic of perineural root sleeve cyst

SELECTED REFERENCES

1. Kumar K et al: Symptomatic spinal arachnoid cysts: report of two cases with review of the literature. Spine. 28(2):E25-9, 2003
2. Caspar W et al: Microsurgical excision of symptomatic sacral perineurial cysts: a study of 15 cases. Surg Neurol. 59(2):101-5; discussion 105-6, 2003
3. Acosta FL et al: Diagnosis and management of sacral Tarlov cysts. Case report and review of the literature. Neurosurg Focus. 15 (2):Article 15, 2003
4. Voyadzis JM et al: Tarlov cysts: a study of 10 cases with review of the literature. J Neurosurg. 95(1 Suppl):25-32, 2001
5. Mummaneni PV et al: Microsurgical treatment of symptomatic sacral Tarlov cysts. Neurosurgery. 47(1):74-8; discussion 78-9, 2000
6. ArunKumar MJ et al: Sacral nerve root cysts: A review on pathophysiology. Neurol India. 47(1):61-4, 1999
7. Paulsen RD et al: Prevalence and percutaneous drainage of cysts of the sacral nerve root sheath (Tarlov cysts). AJNR. 15:293-7, 1994
8. Davis SW et al: Sacral meningeal cysts: Evaluation with MR imaging. Radiology. 187:445-8, 1993
9. Araki Y et al: MRI of symptomatic sacral perineural cyst. Radiat Med. 10(6):250-2, 1992
10. Nabors MW et al: Updated assessment and current classification of spinal meningeal cysts. J Neurosurg. 68:366-77, 1988
11. Goyal RN et al: Intraspinal cysts: a classification and literature review. Spine. 12(3):209-13, 1987
12. Willinsky RA et al: Computed tomography of a sacral perineural cyst. J Comput Assist Tomogr. 9(3):599-601, 1985
13. Dastur HM: The radiological appearances of spinal extradural arachnoid cysts. J Neurol Neurosurg Psychiatry. 26:231-235, 1963
14. Abbott KH et al: The role of perineurial sacral cysts in the sciatic and sacrococcygeal syndromes. A review of the literature and report of 9 cases. J Neurosurg. 14:5-21, 1957
15. Tarlov IM: Perineural cysts of the spinal nerve roots. Arch Neurol Psychiatry. 40:1067-1074, 1938

PERINEURAL ROOT SLEEVE CYST

IMAGE GALLERY

Typical

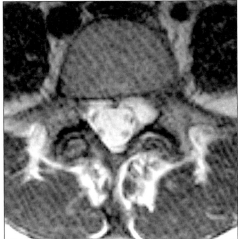
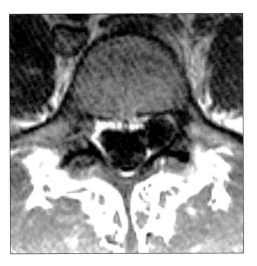

(Left) Axial T2WI MR through L5 shows a CSF intensity mass in left lateral recess. *(Right)* Axial T1 C+ MR demonstrates left lateral recess lesion without enhancement, compatible with a Tarlov perineural cyst.

Typical

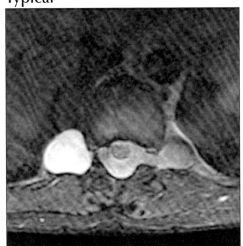
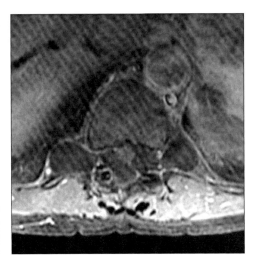

(Left) Axial T2WI MR with fat suppression shows bilateral thoracic paraspinal hyperintense masses. Left-sided mass communicates with and is of same intensity as CSF. Right-sided mass is more hyperintense. *(Right)* Axial T1 C+ MR with fat suppression demonstrates nonenhancing nature of cysts, consistent with bilateral nerve sheath diverticula.

Typical

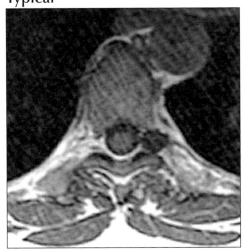
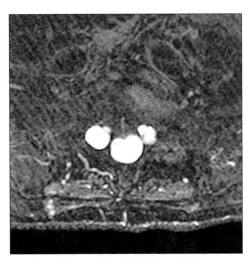

(Left) Axial T1WI MR through thoracic spine shows a left foraminal CSF intensity perineural cyst. *(Right)* Axial T2WI MR with fat suppression shows bilateral sacral Tarlov perineural cysts, remodeling neural foramina.

SYRINGOMYELIA

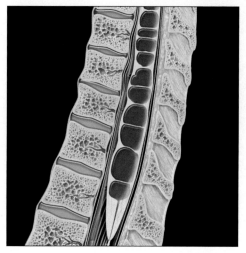

Sagittal graphic demonstrates a large, sacculated, "beaded" syrinx extending to the conus.

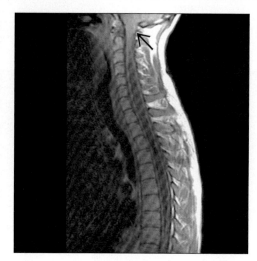

Sagittal T1WI MR depicts a large longstanding sacculated syrinx associated with severe tonsillar ectopia (Chiari 1, arrow) and mild posterior cervical vertebral scalloping.

TERMINOLOGY

Abbreviations and Synonyms
- Synonyms: Hydromyelia, syringohydromyelia, syrinx

Definitions
- Hydromyelia = cystic central canal dilatation
- Syringomyelia = cystic spinal cord cavity not contiguous with central cord canal
  - Syringobulbia = brainstem syrinx extension
  - Syringocephaly = brain/cerebral peduncle syrinx extension
- Syringohydromyelia = features of both syringomyelia and hydromyelia

IMAGING FINDINGS

General Features
- Best diagnostic clue: Expanded spinal cord with dilated, beaded, or sacculated cystic cavity
- Location: Intramedullary spinal cord
- Size: Small → markedly dilated
- Morphology: Cystic intramedullary lesion; small syrinxes are tubular, large are "beaded" or "loculated with septations"

Radiographic Findings
- Radiography

  - Normal or wide osseous canal
  - +/- Atrophic neuroarthropathy (cervical syrinx)
- Myelography
  - Expanded spinal cord +/- spinal canal widening
  - Delayed syrinx contrast uptake

CT Findings
- CECT: Cord expansion, nonenhancing CSF density spinal cord cavitation
- Bone CT
  - Normal or canal enlargement, vertebral scalloping (severe, longstanding syrinx)

MR Findings
- T1WI
  - Hypointense spinal cord cleft
    - Sagittal images demonstrate longitudinal extent
    - Axial images confirm syrinx topology, clarify relationship to adjacent structures
- T2WI
  - Hyperintense intramedullary cavity +/- adjacent gliosis, myelomalacia
    - +/- Arachnoidal adhesions, cord tethering or edema
- T1 C+: Nonenhancing cavity; enhancement suggests inflammatory or neoplastic lesion

DDx: Spinal Cord Cysts

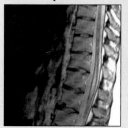

Ventriculus Terminalis

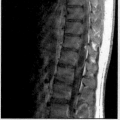

Hemangioblastoma

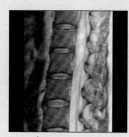

Astrocytoma

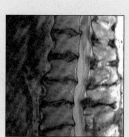

Myelomalacia

SYRINGOMYELIA

Key Facts

Terminology
- Synonyms: Hydromyelia, syringohydromyelia, syrinx
- Hydromyelia = cystic central canal dilatation
- Syringomyelia = cystic spinal cord cavity not contiguous with central cord canal

Imaging Findings
- Best diagnostic clue: Expanded spinal cord with dilated, beaded, or sacculated cystic cavity
- Sagittal images demonstrate longitudinal extent
- Axial images confirm syrinx topology, clarify relationship to adjacent structures

Top Differential Diagnoses
- Ventriculus terminalis
- Cystic spinal cord tumor
- Myelomalacia

Pathology
- Longitudinally oriented CSF-filled cavity +/- surrounding gliosis, myelomalacia

Clinical Issues
- "Cloak-like" pain and temperature sensory loss with preservation of position sense, proprioception, light touch
- Distal upper extremity weakness, gait instability
- Mechanical spinal pain, radicular pain, spastic paraparesis, scoliosis

Diagnostic Checklist
- Despite septated appearance, large syrinx cavities usually contiguous
- Contrast administration essential to exclude tumor in complicated cavitary lesions

Ultrasonographic Findings
- Real Time: Hypoechoic intramedullary cavitation or central canal dilatation

Other Modality Findings
- 2D MR cine phase contrast (PC) CSF flow study
  - +/- Abnormal CSF dynamics across tonsils (Chiari I)
  - Normal conus motion argues against tethered cord
  - Larger syrinx commonly shows internal CSF flow

Imaging Recommendations
- Best imaging tool: MR imaging
- Protocol advice
  - Sagittal and axial T1WI, T2WI, T1 C+ MR
  - Cine PC CSF flow MRI

DIFFERENTIAL DIAGNOSIS

Ventriculus terminalis
- Asymptomatic (normal) dilatation of terminal cord central canal only

Cystic spinal cord tumor
- Cord expansion, cystic cavity surrounded by abnormal T2 signal, nodular enhancement

Myelomalacia
- Cord volume loss, gliosis
- No CSF signal cavitation on T1WI

PATHOLOGY

General Features
- General path comments
  - Longitudinally oriented CSF-filled cavity +/- surrounding gliosis, myelomalacia
  - Associated with scoliosis (↑ with left curve, high or low apex/end vertebra, male sex, Chiari I or II malformation)
  - Hydromyelia: Dilated ependymal-lined central canal
    - "Spinal cord hydrocephalus"
    - Central canal patency determines syrinx location, extent
    - Slit-like central canal remnant detected in small percentage of asymptomatic adults
  - Syringomyelia: Paracentral spinal cord cavitation lined by gliotic parenchyma independent of central canal
    - +/- Eccentric extension into anterior commissure, posterior horn
    - ↑ Intramedullary pressure → neurological dysfunction 2° to compression of long tracts, neurons, and microcirculation
- Etiology
  - Etiology actively debated; two most popular theories not mutually exclusive
    - Abnormal subarachnoid space (arachnoid adhesions, mass, Chiari malformation, spinal dysraphism, diastematomyelia) drives CSF into cord through perivascular spaces → formation, enlargement of syrinx
    - Cord destruction 2° to primary disease process (trauma, infectious or inflammatory myelitis, spondylosis) → cord cavitation
- Epidemiology
  - Primary syrinx usually in young patients
    - ↑ Prevalence with basilar invagination, Chiari 1 or 2 malformation
  - Secondary syrinx at any age; timing of appearance determined by primary disease behavior
    - 25% spinal cord injury (SCI) patients → syrinx
- Associated abnormalities: Hydrocephalus, Chiari 1 or 2 malformation, myelomeningocele or other spinal dysraphism, tethered cord, congenital scoliosis

Gross Pathologic & Surgical Features
- Dilated cavity +/- contiguous with central canal
- +/- Arachnoid adhesions, mass lesion, tethered cord, Chiari malformation, blood products/trauma detritus

Microscopic Features
- Central canal dilatation communicates directly with IVth ventricle

SYRINGOMYELIA

- Cavity lined by ependyma; length influenced by age-related central canal stenosis
- Noncommunicating (isolated) central canal dilation below syrinx-free cord segment
  - Variable distance below IVth ventricle; cavity margins defined by adjacent central canal stenosis
  - +/- Paracentral dissection into parenchyma, gliosis
- Extracanalicular (parenchymal) syrinx non-contiguous with central canal
  - Watershed spinal cord area +/- myelomalacia, paracentral dissection lined by glial or fibroglial tissue, rupture into spinal subarachnoid space, central chromatolysis, neuronophagia, Wallerian degeneration

CLINICAL ISSUES

Presentation
- Most common signs/symptoms
  - "Cloak-like" pain and temperature sensory loss with preservation of position sense, proprioception, light touch
  - Distal upper extremity weakness, gait instability
  - Other signs/symptoms
    - Mechanical spinal pain, radicular pain, spastic paraparesis, scoliosis
    - Cranial neuropathy (2° to syringobulbia)
- Clinical profile
  - Symmetrically enlarged central cavity asymptomatic or presents with nonspecific neurological signs (spasticity, weakness, segmental pain)
  - Paracentral cavitation associated with combination of long tract and segmental signs referable to level, side, and quadrant of spinal cord cavitation

Demographics
- Age: Usual presentation in late adolescence or early adulthood; uncommon in childhood
- Gender: M = F

Natural History & Prognosis
- Variable; dependent on underlying etiology
  - Chronic, slow progression usual; occasional acute course
  - Spontaneous resolution rare
- +/- Reversibility after Chiari decompression, mass removal, adhesion lysis, or cord untethering
  - Long term improvement < 50%
  - Sensory disturbances, dysesthesias, pain more likely to improve than motor weakness or gait disturbance
- CSF diastolic flow determines cyst size, biological behavior
  - Diastolic flow velocity ↓ after successful surgery; persistent ↑ implies poor outcome

Treatment
- Primarily address underlying causative etiology
  - Correct osseous deformities, decompress/untether spinal cord, lyse adhesions
  - Consider syrinx drainage with indwelling catheter only if not possible to restore normal cord CSF dynamics

DIAGNOSTIC CHECKLIST

Consider
- Syrinx etiology influences treatment approach
- Despite septated appearance, large syrinx cavities usually contiguous

Image Interpretation Pearls
- Simple syringomyelia rarely enhances or produces diagnostic dilemma
- Contrast administration essential to exclude tumor in complicated cavitary lesions

SELECTED REFERENCES

1. Aryan HE et al: Syringocephaly. J Clin Neurosci. 11(4):421-3, 2004
2. Piatt JH Jr: Syringomyelia complicating myelomeningocele: review of the evidence. J Neurosurg. 100(2 Suppl):101-9, 2004
3. Kyoshima K et al: Spontaneous resolution of syringomyelia: report of two cases and review of the literature. Neurosurgery. 53(3):762-8; discussion 768-9, 2003
4. Brodbelt AR et al: Post-traumatic syringomyelia: a review. J Clin Neurosci. 10(4):401-8, 2003
5. Ozerdemoglu RA et al: Scoliosis associated with syringomyelia: clinical and radiologic correlation. Spine. 28(13):1410-7, 2003
6. Klekamp J et al: Syringomyelia associated with foramen magnum arachnoiditis. J Neurosurg. 97(3 Suppl):317-22, 2002
7. Holly LT et al: Slitlike syrinx cavities: a persistent central canal. J Neurosurg. 97(2 Suppl):161-5, 2002
8. Klekamp J: The pathophysiology of syringomyelia - historical overview and current concept. Acta Neurochir (Wien). 144(7):649-64, 2002
9. Vinas FC et al: Spontaneous resolution of a syrinx. J Clin Neurosci. 8(2):170-2, 2001
10. Klekamp J et al: Spontaneous resolution of Chiari I malformation and syringomyelia: case report and review of the literature. Neurosurgery. 48(3):664-7, 2001
11. Unsinn KM et al: US of the spinal cord in newborns: spectrum of normal findings, variants, congenital anomalies, and acquired diseases. Radiographics. 20(4):923-38, 2000
12. Brugieres P et al: CSF flow measurement in syringomyelia. AJNR. 21(10): 1785-92, 2000
13. Levy LM: MR imaging of cerebrospinal fluid flow and spinal cord motion in neurologic disorders of the spine. Magn Reson Imaging Clin N Am. 7(3):573-87, 1999
14. Fischbein NJ et al: The "presyrinx" state: a reversible myelopathic condition that may precede syringomyelia. AJNR Am J Neuroradiol. 20(1):7-20, 1999
15. Milhorat TH et al: Intramedullary pressure in syringomyelia: clinical and pathophysiological correlates of syrinx distension. Neurosurgery. 41(5):1102-10, 1997
16. Tanghe HL: Magnetic resonance imaging (MRI) in syringomyelia. Acta Neurochir (Wien). 134(1-2):93-9, 1995
17. Milhorat TH et al: Pathological basis of spinal cord cavitation in syringomyelia: analysis of 105 autopsy cases. J Neurosurg. 82(5):802-12, 1995

SYRINGOMYELIA

IMAGE GALLERY

Typical

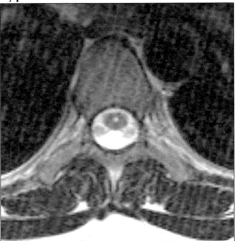 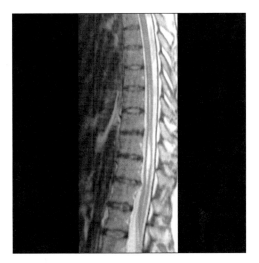

(Left) Axial T2WI MR demonstrates mild central canal dilatation (hydromyelia) in conjunction with Chiari 1 malformation (not shown). (Right) Sagittal T2WI MR shows thoracic cord syringohydromyelia extending into conus medullaris. Extensive cord involvement distinguishes from ventriculus terminalis.

Variant

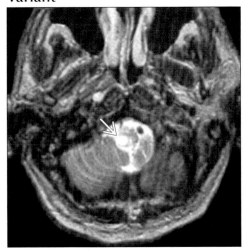 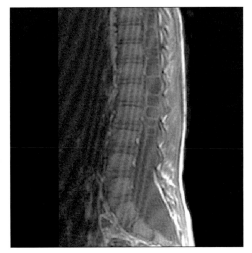

(Left) Axial T2WI MR demonstrates asymmetric syrinx extension into right medulla (syringobulbia) with surrounding gliosis (arrow). (Right) Sagittal T1WI MR depicts a large sacculated syrinx extending entire length of cord into conus. The syrinx cavity is contiguous despite septated appearance (Courtesy R. Boyer, MD).

Variant

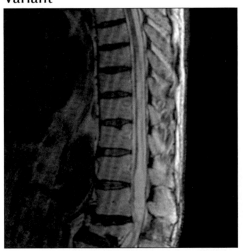 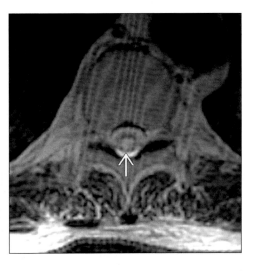

(Left) Sagittal T2WI MR shows an extensive post-traumatic syrinx in conjunction with healed thoracolumbar burst fracture. (Right) Axial T2WI MR of post-traumatic syrinx shows extensive irregular cord T2 hyperintensity with asymmetric extension into dorsal cord (arrow).

EPIDURAL LIPOMATOSIS

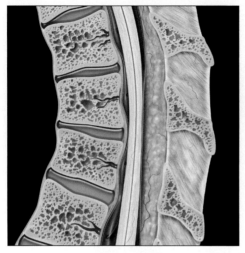
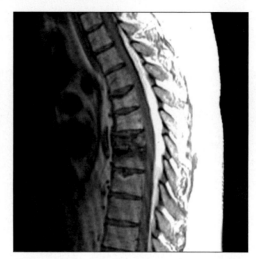

Sagittal graphic illustrates confluent abundant epidural fat in dorsal thoracic canal, with mild mass effect on spinal cord.

Sagittal T1WI MR shows prominent dorsal epidural fat from T1 to T9, narrowing central canal. Compression fractures involve T4 through T8 vertebrae. Patient has Cushing disease.

TERMINOLOGY

Abbreviations and Synonyms
- Spinal epidural lipomatosis (SEL)

Definitions
- Excessive accumulation of intraspinal fat causing cord compression and neurologic deficits

IMAGING FINDINGS

General Features
- Best diagnostic clue: Abundant epidural fat in mid-thoracic and distal lumbar spinal canal compressing thecal sac
- Location
  - Thoracic spine: 58-61%
    - T6-8
    - Dorsal to spinal cord
  - Lumbar spine: 39-42%
    - L4-5
    - Circumferential surrounding thecal sac
- Size
  - Epidural fat ≥ 7 mm thick in thoracic spine
  - Over multiple vertebral segments
- Morphology
  - "Y" sign

- "Y" shaped configuration to lumbar thecal sac on axial imaging

Radiographic Findings
- Radiography
  - Osteopenia from exogenous or endogenous steroids
  - Vertebral compression fractures
- Myelography
  - Often normal
  - Effacement of cerebral spinal fluid (CSF)

CT Findings
- NECT
  - Increased fat density in spinal canal
  - Cord compression
  - Tapered caudal thecal sac
- CECT: No enhancement
- Bone CT
  - No bony erosion

MR Findings
- T1WI
  - Hyperintense
  - Hypointense with fat suppression
- T2WI: Intermediate signal intensity
- STIR: Hypointense
- T1 C+: No enhancement
- Homogeneous
- Mass effect on thecal sac and nerve roots

DDx: Epidural Masses

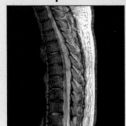 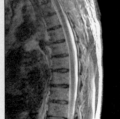 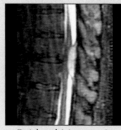 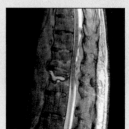

Epidural Hematoma   *Epidural Hematoma*   *Epidural Metastasis*   *Epidural Abscess*

EPIDURAL LIPOMATOSIS

Key Facts

Terminology
- Excessive accumulation of intraspinal fat causing cord compression and neurologic deficits

Imaging Findings
- Best diagnostic clue: Abundant epidural fat in mid-thoracic and distal lumbar spinal canal compressing thecal sac
- Thoracic spine: 58-61%
- Lumbar spine: 39-42%
- Epidural fat ≥ 7 mm thick in thoracic spine
- "Y" shaped configuration to lumbar thecal sac on axial imaging
- Increased fat density in spinal canal
- Homogeneous
- Mass effect on thecal sac and nerve roots

Top Differential Diagnoses
- Subacute epidural hematoma
- Spinal angiolipoma
- Epidural metastasis, lymphoma

Pathology
- Long term exogenous steroid administration
- Excessive endogenous steroid production

Clinical Issues
- Weakness: > 85%
- Back pain: 64%
- > 80% with post-surgical symptomatic relief

Diagnostic Checklist
- Excessive extradural fat in dorsal midthoracic spine and caudal lumbar spine diagnostic of SEL

- ○ Obliterated CSF
- ○ Cord compression
- ○ Crowded cauda equina

Imaging Recommendations
- Best imaging tool: Sagittal and axial T1WI and T2WI MRI
- Protocol advice: Fat suppression to confirm adipose tissue

DIFFERENTIAL DIAGNOSIS

Subacute epidural hematoma
- Hyperintense on T1WI
  - ○ Hyperintense even with fat suppression
- Heterogeneous with hypointense foci on T2WI
- Acute onset of symptoms

Spinal angiolipoma
- Benign neoplasm with varying proportion of adipose and vascular elements
- Mid-thoracic region most common
- Infiltrative type invades surrounding bone
- Hyperintense on T1WI
  - ○ Slightly or moderately hypointense to epidural fat
  - ○ Heterogeneous due to vascular elements
- Iso- to slightly hypointense to epidural fat on T2WI
- Diffuse post-contrast-enhancement
  - ○ Better visualized with fat suppression

Epidural metastasis, lymphoma
- Hypointense to epidural fat on T1WI and T2WI
  - ○ Soft tissue signal intensity
- Vertebral and paraspinal involvement
  - ○ Not limited to spinal canal
- Avid post-gadolinium enhancement

Epidural abscess
- Most common in ventral epidural space
  - ○ Associated with discitis/osteomyelitis
- Posterolateral spinal canal from septic facet joint
- Hypointense on T1WI
- Hyperintense on T2WI

- Diffuse or peripheral enhancement

PATHOLOGY

General Features
- General path comments
  - ○ Increased fat tissue in spinal canal
  - ○ Typically in thoracic and lumbar regions
- Genetics: No genetic predisposition
- Etiology
  - ○ Long term exogenous steroid administration
    - ▪ 75% of reported cases
    - ▪ Treatment of obstructive airways disease, systemic lupus erythematosus, etc.
    - ▪ No definite correlation between dosage and duration of steroid use and development of SEL
    - ▪ Mean dosage between 30 mg/d and 100 mg/d for 5-11 years in reported cases
  - ○ Association with epidural steroid injection also reported
  - ○ Excessive endogenous steroid production
    - ▪ Cushing disease
    - ▪ Hypothyroidism
    - ▪ Other endocrinopathies
  - ○ General obesity
  - ○ Idiopathic
- Epidemiology: Uncommon entity
- Associated abnormalities
  - ○ Vertebral compression fractures
    - ▪ Steroid related osteoporosis
  - ○ Syrinx
- Anatomy
  - ○ Meningovertebral ligaments in lumbar spine
    - ▪ Median, paramedian, lateral aspects of ventral and dorsal epidural space
    - ▪ Anchor dura to spinal canal
    - ▪ May form septum, partitioning epidural space
    - ▪ May explain triangular or "Y" shaped configuration of lumbar thecal sac on axial imaging

EPIDURAL LIPOMATOSIS

Gross Pathologic & Surgical Features
- Abundant adipose tissue external to thecal sac
- No capsule

Microscopic Features
- Hypertrophied fat cells

CLINICAL ISSUES

Presentation
- Most common signs/symptoms
  - Weakness: > 85%
  - Other signs/symptoms
    - Back pain: 64%
    - Sensory loss
    - Polyradiculopathy
    - Altered reflexes
    - Incontinence
    - Ataxia
- Clinical profile: Gradual progression of symptoms

Demographics
- Age
  - Mean age at presentation: 43 yo
    - Slightly younger for thoracic SEL
    - Older (50s) for lumbar SEL
- Gender: M > F
- Ethnicity: No racial predilection

Natural History & Prognosis
- Excellent
  - > 80% with post-surgical symptomatic relief
  - Pre-surgical low steroid dose and idiopathic SEL have better prognosis
- Post-surgical mortality: 22%
  - Immunocompromised state from chronic steroid use

Treatment
- Correction of underlying endocrinopathies
- Discontinuing exogenous steroids
- Weight reduction in case of general obesity
- Surgical intervention
  - Indicated when cord compression and radiculopathy present
  - Multilevel laminectomy
  - Fat debulking
  - Posterolateral fusion to maintain stability

DIAGNOSTIC CHECKLIST

Consider
- Fat suppression to distinguish SEL from epidural hematoma

Image Interpretation Pearls
- Excessive extradural fat in dorsal midthoracic spine and caudal lumbar spine diagnostic of SEL

SELECTED REFERENCES

1. Fassett DR et al: Spinal epidural lipomatosis: a review of its causes and recommendations for treatment. Neurosurg Focus. 16(4):Article 11, 2004
2. Payer M et al: Idiopathic symptomatic epidural lipomatosis of the lumbar spine. Acta Neurochir (Wien). 145(4):315-20; discussion 321, 2003
3. Geers C et al: Polygonal deformation of the dural sac in lumbar epidural lipomatosis: anatomic explanation by the presence of meningovertebral ligaments. AJNR Am J Neuroradiol. 24(7):1276-82, 2003
4. Dumont-Fischer D et al: Spinal epidural lipomatosis revealing endogenous Cushing's syndrome. Joint Bone Spine. 69(2):222-5, 2002
5. Lisai P et al: Cauda Equina Syndrome Secondary to Idiopathic Spinal Epidural Lipomatosis. Spine. Vol 26:307-9, 2001
6. Citow JS et al: Thoracic epidural lipomatosis with associated syrinx: case report. Surg Neurol. 53(6):589-91, 2000
7. McCullen GM et al: Epidural lipomatosis complicating lumbar steroid injections. J Spinal Disord. 12(6):526-9, 1999
8. Robertson SC et al: Idiopathic spinal epidural lipomatosis. Neurosurgery. 41(1):68-74; discussion 74-5, 1997
9. Fiirgaard B et al: Spinal epidural lipomatosis. Case report and review of the literature. Scand J Med Sci Sports. 7(6):354-7, 1997
10. Benamou PH et al: Epidural lipomatosis not induced by corticosteroid therapy. Three cases including one in a patient with primary Cushing's disease (review of the literature). Rev Rhum Engl Ed. 63(3):207-12, 1996
11. Hierholzer J et al: Epidural lipomatosis: case report and literature review. Neuroradiology. 38(4):343-8, 1996
12. Kumar K et al: Symptomatic Epidural lipomatosis Secondary to Obesity. J Neurosurg. Vol 85: 348-50, 1996
13. Provenzale JM et al: Spinal angiolipomas: MR features. AJNR Am J Neuroradiol. 17(4):713-9, 1996
14. Zentner J et al: Spinal epidural lipomatosis as a complication of prolonged corticosteroid therapy. J Neurosurg Sci. 39(1):81-5, 1995
15. Beges C et al: Epidural lipomatosis. Interest of magnetic resonance imaging in a weight-reduction treated case. Spine. 19(2):251-4, 1994
16. Kuhn MJ et al: Lumbar epidural lipomatosis: the "Y" sign of thecal sac compression. Comput Med Imaging Graph. 18(5):367-72, 1994
17. Preul MC et al: Spinal angiolipomas. Report of three cases. J Neurosurg. 78(2):280-6, 1993
18. Roy-Camille R et al: Symptomatic spinal epidural lipomatosis induced by a long-term steroid treatment. Review of the literature and report of two additional cases. Spine. 16(12):1365-71, 1991
19. Healy ME et al: Demonstration by magnetic resonance of symptomatic spinal epidural lipomatosis. Neurosurgery. 21(3):414-5, 1987
20. Randall BC et al: Epidural lipomatosis with lumbar radiculopathy: CT appearance. J Comput Assist Tomogr. 10(6):1039-41, 1986

EPIDURAL LIPOMATOSIS

IMAGE GALLERY

Typical

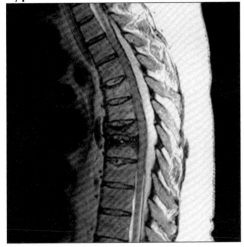
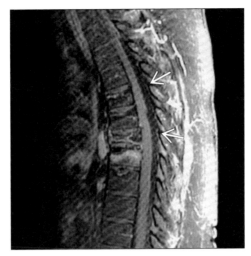

(Left) Sagittal T2WI MR of thoracic spine shows smooth and homogeneous dorsal epidural tissue, isointense to subcutaneous fat. Vertebral compression fractures are due to steroid induced osteoporosis. *(Right)* Sagittal T1 C+ MR with fat suppression demonstrates hypointense epidural tissue, identical to subcutaneous fat, compatible with epidural lipomatosis (arrows).

Typical

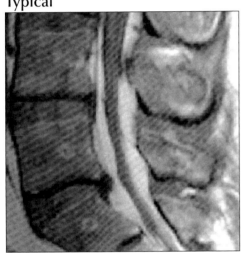
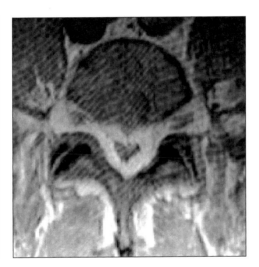

(Left) Sagittal T1WI MR shows increased extradural fat in lumbar canal, narrowing thecal sac. *(Right)* Axial T1WI MR shows excessive epidural fat surrounding thecal sac, with a triangular configuration.

Typical

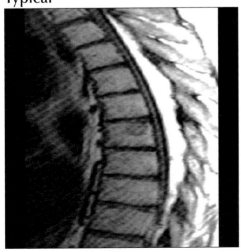
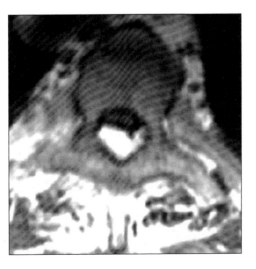

(Left) Sagittal T1WI MR of thoracic spine demonstrates abundant dorsal extradural fat, narrowing central canal. *(Right)* Axial T1WI MR shows increased epidural fat compressing thecal sac and flattening thoracic cord (Courtesy M. Modic, MD).

HETEROGENEOUS FATTY MARROW

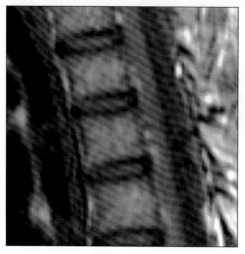

Sagittal T1WI MR shows stippled appearance of normal hematopoietic and fatty marrow in 10 year old child.

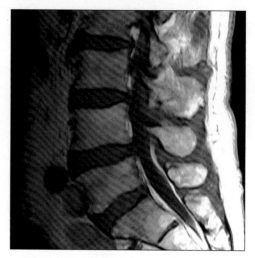

Sagittal T1WI MR shows marbled appearance of fatty and erythropoietic marrow in middle-aged adult.

TERMINOLOGY

Abbreviations and Synonyms
- Red marrow reconversion

Definitions
- Irregularly distributed fatty, hematopoietic and fibrous elements in bone marrow
- Red marrow: Hematopoietic marrow
- Yellow marrow: Fatty marrow

IMAGING FINDINGS

General Features
- Best diagnostic clue: Red marrow signal intensity equal or higher than intervertebral disc on T1WI
- Location
  - Vertebral bodies
  - Yellow marrow often distributed around central perforating vein
  - Yellow marrow adjacent to endplates in degenerative disc disease
  - After bone marrow transplantation: Fat centrally in vertebral body, red marrow at periphery
  - Loss of red marrow in regions of radiation therapy
- Morphology: Stippled or marbled appearance of vertebral body

CT Findings
- Bone CT
  - Normal trabecular pattern preserved

MR Findings
- T1WI
  - High signal intensity fat intermingled with low to intermediate signal intensity red marrow
  - Red marrow equal or higher signal than disc
- T2WI: Heterogeneity less apparent than on T1WI, STIR
- STIR: Low signal intensity fat intermingled with intermediate signal intensity marrow
- DWI: Not shown to be of use in distinguishing red marrow from tumor
- T1 C+: Erythropoietic marrow enhances slightly
- In phase and out of phase gradient echo imaging
  - Contribution of fat and water to signal cycle in and out of phase with increasing TE
  - Erythropoietic marrow contains fat and water: Low signal on out of phase images
  - Neoplasm usually doesn't contain fat: High signal on out of phase images
  - No large series to validate this concept
    - Early myeloma has same appearance as red marrow

Nuclear Medicine Findings
- Bone Scan: Normal

DDx: Heterogeneous Fatty Marrow on T1 WI

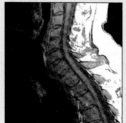

Early Myeloma

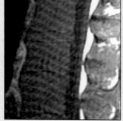

Leukemia

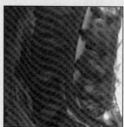

Metastasis

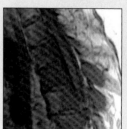

Metastasis

HETEROGENEOUS FATTY MARROW

Terminology
- Irregularly distributed fatty, hematopoietic and fibrous elements in bone marrow

Imaging Findings
- Best diagnostic clue: Red marrow signal intensity equal or higher than intervertebral disc on T1WI
- Yellow marrow often distributed around central perforating vein

Key Facts
- Yellow marrow adjacent to endplates in degenerative disc disease
- After bone marrow transplantation: Fat centrally in vertebral body, red marrow at periphery
- Loss of red marrow in regions of radiation therapy

Top Differential Diagnoses
- Multiple myeloma, leukemia
- Metastasis
- Myelofibrosis

Imaging Recommendations
- Best imaging tool: CT in questionable cases to exclude lytic lesions
- Protocol advice: 1-3 mm helical scans with sagittal, coronal reformations

DIFFERENTIAL DIAGNOSIS

Multiple myeloma, leukemia
- Early: May appear identical on MRI
- Late: Lower signal on T1WI than intervertebral disc
- CT scan shows focal trabecular destruction

Metastasis
- Lower signal on T1WI than intervertebral disc
- In phase/out of phase MRI: High signal
- Often enhance avidly with gadolinium
- Usually high signal on STIR, but intermediate in sclerotic metastasis

Myelofibrosis
- Low signal intensity on all MRI sequences

PATHOLOGY

General Features
- Etiology
  - Increased red marrow
    - Anemia, obesity, high athletic activity, bone marrow transplantation
  - Increased yellow marrow
    - Radiation therapy, degenerative disc disease
- Epidemiology: Very common

Gross Pathologic & Surgical Features
- Admixture of red and yellow marrow

Microscopic Features
- Admixture of hematopoietic elements and fat

CLINICAL ISSUES

Presentation
- Most common signs/symptoms: Asymptomatic

Demographics
- Age
  - Fat content of marrow increases with patient age

- Process begins in hands, feet, progresses centrally
- Gender: No gender predominance

DIAGNOSTIC CHECKLIST

Consider
- Mimic of metastasis and myeloma

SELECTED REFERENCES

1. Montazel JL et al: Normal spinal bone marrow in adults: dynamic gadolinium-enhanced MR imaging. Radiology. 229(3):703-9, 2003
2. Castillo M: Diffusion-weighted imaging of the spine: is it reliable? AJNR Am J Neuroradiol. 24(6):1251-3, 2003
3. Otake S et al: Radiation-induced changes in MR signal intensity and contrast enhancement of lumbosacral vertebrae: do changes occur only inside the radiation therapy field? Radiology. 222(1):179-83, 2002
4. Baur A et al: Diffusion-weighted magnetic resonance imaging of spinal bone marrow. Semin Musculoskelet Radiol. 5(1):35-42, 2001
5. Kim HJ et al: Spinal involvement of hematopoietic malignancies and metastasis: differentiation using MR imaging. Clin Imaging. 23(2):125-33, 1999

IMAGE GALLERY

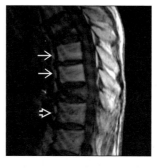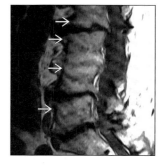

(Left) Sagittal T1WI MR shows completely fatty marrow (arrows) due to radiation therapy. There are pathologic fractures at adjacent levels. Open arrow points to normal vertebral body for comparison. *(Right)* Sagittal T1WI MR shows fatty marrow (arrows) beneath vertebral endplates in severe degenerative disc disease.

LANGERHANS CELL HISTIOCYTOSIS

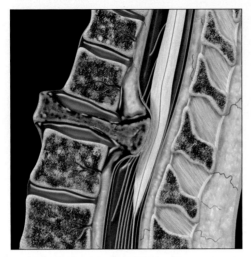

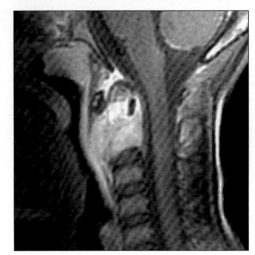

Sagittal graphic shows diffuse vertebral marrow infiltration with pathologic fracture producing vertebra plana sparing the disc spaces. Epidural extension produces ventral cord compression.

Sagittal T1 C+ MR in a child shows an avidly enhancing destructive C2 mass with posterior epidural spread. The adjacent disc space is spared, typical of LCH (Courtesy G. Hedlund, DO).

TERMINOLOGY

Abbreviations and Synonyms
- Synonyms: Langerhans cell histiocytosis (LCH), Langerhans cell granulomatosis, eosinophilic granuloma (EG), histiocytosis X

Definitions
- Abnormal histiocyte proliferation producing granulomatous skeletal lesions

IMAGING FINDINGS

General Features
- Best diagnostic clue: Child presenting with vertebra plana sparing disc space
- Location
  - Calvarium > mandible > long bones > ribs > pelvis > vertebrae
  - Spinal involvement
    - Thoracic (54%) > lumbar (35%) > cervical (11%)
    - Children > adults
- Morphology: Destructive lytic lesion +/- pathologic fracture, soft tissue mass, spinal canal extension

Radiographic Findings
- Radiography
  - Lytic non-sclerotic destructive vertebral lesion

- +/- Vertebra plana (adjacent discs, posterior elements rarely involved)
- +/- Scoliosis; kyphosis uncommon

CT Findings
- CECT: Lytic (non-sclerotic) destructive vertebral lesion with enhancing soft tissue mass +/- paraspinal, epidural extension
- Bone CT
  - Lytic vertebral lesion +/- collapsed vertebral body (vertebra plana)

MR Findings
- T1WI: Hypointense vertebral soft tissue mass +/- pathologic fracture
- T2WI
  - Heterogeneously hyperintense soft tissue mass +/- pathologic fracture
  - Disc spaces generally spared
- T1 C+: Homogeneous enhancement

Nuclear Medicine Findings
- Bone Scan
  - Variable uptake; bone lesions may be hot, cold, or mixed ("ring") activity
  - False negatives common (35%)

Imaging Recommendations
- Best imaging tool: MR imaging

DDx: Langerhans Cell Histiocytosis

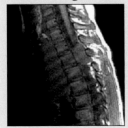

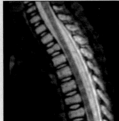

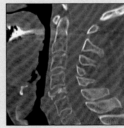

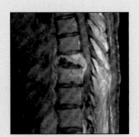

Ewing Sarcoma   *Leukemia*   *Multiple Myeloma*   *TB Osteomyelitis*

LANGERHANS CELL HISTIOCYTOSIS

Key Facts

Terminology
- Synonyms: Langerhans cell histiocytosis (LCH), Langerhans cell granulomatosis, eosinophilic granuloma (EG), histiocytosis X
- Abnormal histiocyte proliferation producing granulomatous skeletal lesions

Imaging Findings
- Best diagnostic clue: Child presenting with vertebra plana sparing disc space
- Calvarium > mandible > long bones > ribs > pelvis > vertebrae
- Thoracic (54%) > lumbar (35%) > cervical (11%)
- Children > adults
- Morphology: Destructive lytic lesion +/- pathologic fracture, soft tissue mass, spinal canal extension

Top Differential Diagnoses
- Ewing sarcoma
- Metastases, neuroblastoma, hemopoietic malignancies
- Osteomyelitis
- Giant cell tumor

Pathology
- Expanding erosive histiocyte accumulation within medullary cavity

Diagnostic Checklist
- Vertebra plana much more common in children than adults
- Unexplained vertebral compression fractures in children or adolescents merit evaluation to exclude LCH or leukemia

- Protocol advice
  - Multiplanar enhanced MRI to evaluate soft tissues, determine epidural extension
  - Bone algorithm CT with multiplanar reformats to define osseous destruction, vertebral height loss

DIFFERENTIAL DIAGNOSIS

Ewing sarcoma
- Permeative bone destruction +/- pathological fracture
- More likely than LCH to have large soft tissue mass, adjacent bone destruction

Metastases, neuroblastoma, hemopoietic malignancies
- Multifocal disease; may be indistinguishable from LCH
- Widespread abnormal marrow signal, enhancement with extensive disease

Osteomyelitis
- Abnormal marrow signal +/- vertebral collapse
- Hyperintense narrowed disc +/- fluid signal

Giant cell tumor
- Expansile, lytic vertebral lesion + soft tissue mass
- Usually older patient (> 30 y)

PATHOLOGY

General Features
- General path comments
  - Expanding erosive histiocyte accumulation within medullary cavity
  - < 1% of biopsy-proven primary bone lesions; vertebral involvement (6%)
    - Most common cause of vertebra plana in children
    - Variable vertebral body restoration occurs over months to years
    - Pedicles often involved; posterior elements, adjacent disc spaces usually spared

  - PCR-based assay demonstrates all LCH forms are clonal ⇒ LCH probably clonal neoplastic rather than reactive disorder as previously believed
  - Solitary > multiple lesions; new osseous lesions appear ≤ 1-2 years
- Etiology: Cause not known; infectious agents (especially viruses), immune system dysfunction, neoplastic mechanisms, genetic factors, cellular adhesion molecules proposed but not confirmed
- Epidemiology: Incidence 0.05-0.5/100,000 children/year
- Associated abnormalities
  - Pituitary-hypothalamic axis → diabetes insipidus
  - Purulent otitis media → deafness
  - Orbital involvement → proptosis
  - Cutaneous LCH (≤ 50%)
  - Pulmonary involvement (20-40%); male predominance, older age (20-40 y), smoking association
  - Gastrointestinal (GI) bleeding, liver/spleen abnormalities
  - Lymph node enlargement +/- suppuration, chronic drainage (30%)

Gross Pathologic & Surgical Features
- Yellow, gray, or brown mass, +/- hemorrhage, cystic components

Microscopic Features
- Light microscopy ⇒ abnormal granulomatous histiocytes (Langerhans cells) with folded nuclei, cytoplasmic S-100 reactivity, areas of bone necrosis
- EM: Birbeck granule cytoplasmic inclusions

Staging, Grading or Classification Criteria
- Classically LCH divided into 3 named disease categories based on age, severity, extent of involvement
  - Eosinophilic granuloma (EG)
  - Hand-Schüller-Christian disease
  - Letterer-Siwe disease
- Revised criteria classify LCH according to disease extent
  - Restricted LCH

LANGERHANS CELL HISTIOCYTOSIS

- Skin lesions without other site of involvement
- Monostotic lesion +/- diabetes insipidus (DI), adjacent lymph node involvement, or rash
- Polyostotic lesions involving several bones or ≥ 2 lesions in one bone +/- DI, adjacent lymph node involvement, or rash
  - ○ Extensive LCH
    - Visceral organ involvement +/- bone lesions, DI, adjacent lymph node involvement, and/or rash without lung, liver, or hemopoietic organ system dysfunction
    - Visceral organ involvement +/- bone lesions, DI, adjacent lymph node involvement, and/or rash with lung, liver, or hemopoietic organ system dysfunction

CLINICAL ISSUES

Presentation

- Most common signs/symptoms
  - ○ Asymptomatic
  - ○ Localized pain 2° medullary expansion or pathologic fracture, reduced mobility, swelling, fever, leukocytosis
  - ○ Other signs/symptoms
    - Myelopathy or radiculopathy
- Clinical profile
  - ○ EG (70%)
    - Localized form (bone lesions only), older children (5-15 y), good prognosis
    - Back pain, stiffness, scoliosis, neurologic complications, fever, leukocytosis
  - ○ Hand-Schüller-Christian disease (20%)
    - Chronic disseminated osseous and visceral lesions, younger children (1-5 y), intermediate prognosis (fatal 10-30%)
    - Triad of diabetes insipidus, exophthalmos, bone destruction
  - ○ Letterer-Siwe disease (10%)
    - Acute form, rapid visceral organ dissemination, infants (< 3 y), poor prognosis
    - Fever, cachexia, anemia, hepatosplenomegaly, lymphadenopathy, rash, gum hyperplasia
    - Most patients die ≤ 1-2 years

Demographics

- Age
  - ○ Predominantly affects children, adolescents, or young adults, but may occur at any age
    - Most severe manifestations peak at younger ages
- Gender: M:F = 2:1

Natural History & Prognosis

- Variable depending on presentation age, extent of systemic disease
  - ○ Spontaneous remission of lesions common, but relapse or reactivation possible
  - ○ Lesions usually begin to regress after ≈ 3 months, may take up to 2 years to resolve
  - ○ Vertebra plana prognosis favorable for symptomatic improvement, vertebral height restoration with conservative orthopedic treatment

- Vertebral height restoration varies 18.2% → 63.8% before, 72.2% → 97% after skeletal maturity

Treatment

- Conservative management initially with observation +/- bracing
- +/- Surgical intervention (partial intralesional curettage, fusion), external beam radiotherapy, chemotherapy, steroids in patients with neurological deficits, conservative treatment failure

DIAGNOSTIC CHECKLIST

Consider

- Vertebra plana much more common in children than adults
- Unexplained vertebral compression fractures in children or adolescents merit evaluation to exclude LCH or leukemia

Image Interpretation Pearls

- Vertebra plana with relative absence of epidural mass, disc abnormalities classic for LCH

SELECTED REFERENCES

1. Kuhn J et al: Caffey's Pediatric Diagnostic Imaging. 10th ed. Philadelphia, Mosby. Page 704, 2004
2. Simanski C et al: The Langerhans' cell histiocytosis (eosinophilic granuloma) of the cervical spine: a rare diagnosis of cervical pain. Magn Reson Imaging. 22(4):589-94, 2004
3. Bavbek M et al: Spontaneous resolution of lumbar vertebral eosinophilic granuloma. Acta Neurochir (Wien). 146(2):165-7, 2004
4. Puertas EB et al: Surgical treatment of eosinophilic granuloma in the thoracic spine in patients with neurological lesions. J Pediatr Orthop B. 12(5):303-6, 2003
5. Fernando Ugarriza L et al: Solitary eosinophilic granuloma of the cervicothoracic junction causing neurological deficit. Br J Neurosurg. 17(2):178-81, 2003
6. Graham D et al: Greenfield's Neuropathology. 7th ed. London, Arnold. 1017-1018, 2002
7. Bertram C et al: Eosinophilic granuloma of the cervical spine. Spine. 27(13):1408-13, 2002
8. Plasschaert F et al: Eosinophilic granuloma. A different behaviour in children than in adults. J Bone Joint Surg Br. 84(6):870-2, 2002
9. Kamimura M et al: Eosinophilic granuloma of the spine: early spontaneous disappearance of tumor detected on magnetic resonance imaging. Case report. J Neurosurg. 93(2 Suppl):312-6, 2000
10. Reddy PK et al: Eosinophilic granuloma of spine in adults: a case report and review of literature. Spinal Cord. 38(12):766-8, 2000
11. Yeom JS et al: Langerhans' cell histiocytosis of the spine. Analysis of twenty-three cases. Spine. 24(16):1740-9, 1999
12. Kandoi M et al: Rapidly progressive polyostotic eosinophilic granuloma involving spine: a case report. Indian J Med Sci. 52(1):22-4, 1998
13. Raab P et al: Vertebral remodeling in eosinophilic granuloma of the spine. A long-term follow-up. Spine. 23(12):1351-4, 1998

LANGERHANS CELL HISTIOCYTOSIS

IMAGE GALLERY

Typical

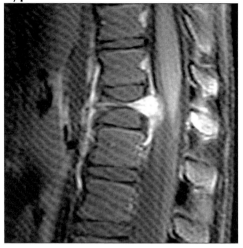

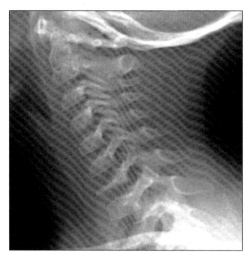

(Left) Sagittal T1 C+ MR shows pathological vertebral collapse with enhancing epidural mass. Vertebral endplates and adjacent discs are intact (Courtesy S. Blaser MD, and A. Illner, MD). (Right) Lateral radiography demonstrates marked C7 vertebral compression ("vertebra plana") without endplate destruction or kyphosis.

Typical

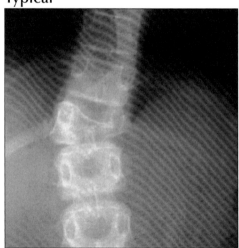

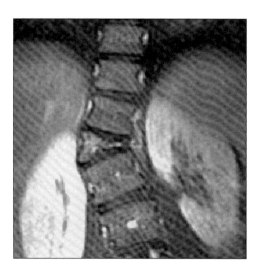

(Left) Anteroposterior radiography shows left lateral collapse of the T12 vertebra producing acute angle scoliosis. Vertebral endplates and pedicles are preserved (Courtesy R. Boyer, MD). (Right) Coronal T1 C+ MR depicts lateral T12 vertebral collapse with focal scoliosis and small paraspinal enhancing mass. Vertebral endplates and adjacent disc spaces are preserved (Courtesy R. Boyer, MD).

Typical

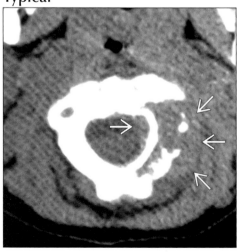

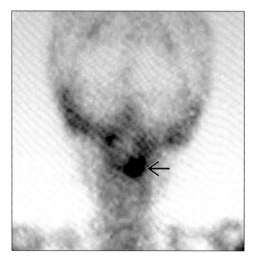

(Left) Axial NECT shows a destructive lytic process of the left C2 vertebra, with paraspinal and epidural soft tissue mass (arrows). Cord is mildly displaced to the right (Courtesy R. Boyer, MD). (Right) Coronal bone scan shows marked 99-Tc MDP uptake (arrow) in C2 vertebral EG lesion (Courtesy R. Boyer, MD).

ACQUIRED EPIDERMOID TUMOR

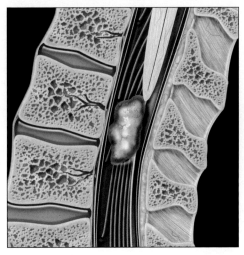

Sagittal graphic depicts a small well-circumscribed pearly white tumor within cauda equina, compatible with an epidermoid.

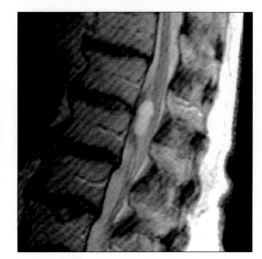

Sagittal T2WI MR through lumbar spine shows a well-circumscribed lesion, hyperintense to CSF, adherent to cauda equina.

TERMINOLOGY

Abbreviations and Synonyms
- Epidermoid cyst

Definitions
- Acquired intraspinal mass arising from iatrogenically implanted epithelial elements

IMAGING FINDINGS

General Features
- Best diagnostic clue: Nonenhancing intradural mass similar to cerebral spinal fluid (CSF) intensity within cauda equina
- Location: Lumbar spine most common
- Size: Variable
- Morphology: Well-circumscribed

Radiographic Findings
- Myelography: Intradural extramedullary mass

CT Findings
- NECT: Low density: Similar to CSF
- CECT: No or faint peripheral enhancement

MR Findings
- T1WI: Isointense to CSF or cord

- T2WI: Iso- to hyperintense to CSF
- DWI: More hyperintense than CSF
- T1 C+: No or faint peripheral enhancement
- Adherent to spinal cord, cauda equina, or thecal sac
- Can be very subtle: Suggested by nerve root or cord displacement

Imaging Recommendations
- Best imaging tool: Sagittal and axial T2WI and T1WI MR with gadolinium
- Protocol advice
  ○ Heavily T1 weighted sequence may distinguish subtle extramedullary mass from CSF
    ▪ Inversion recovery or SPGR
  ○ CT myelography can supplement MRI in delineating extramedullary CSF-isointense mass
  ○ Navigated diffusion imaging may be helpful in diagnosing epidermoid tumor

DIFFERENTIAL DIAGNOSIS

Congenital epidermoid
- Focal incorporation of cutaneous ectoderm into neural ectoderm during disjunction
- Evenly distributed throughout spine
- Similar to CSF intensity
- 20% associated with dermal sinus
  ○ May present with meningitis or abscess

DDx: Intradural Masses

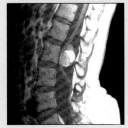

Congenital Epidermoid

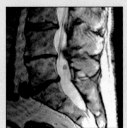

Schwannoma

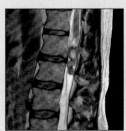

Myxo. Ependymoma

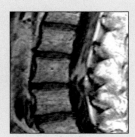

Intradural Met

ACQUIRED EPIDERMOID TUMOR

Key Facts

Terminology
- Acquired intraspinal mass arising from iatrogenically implanted epithelial elements

Imaging Findings
- Best diagnostic clue: Nonenhancing intradural mass similar to cerebral spinal fluid (CSF) intensity within cauda equina
- NECT: Low density: Similar to CSF
- T1WI: Isointense to CSF or cord
- T2WI: Iso- to hyperintense to CSF
- T1 C+: No or faint peripheral enhancement

Top Differential Diagnoses
- Intradural extramedullary neoplasms

Pathology
- Epithelial cells iatrogenically introduced into thecal sac during lumbar puncture

Intradural extramedullary neoplasms
- Nerve sheath tumor, meningioma, ependymoma, metastasis, paraganglioma
- Isointense to cord on T1WI
- Hyperintense on T2WI
- Intense post-gadolinium enhancement
- Carcinomatous meningitis may show smooth or nodular enhancement

Intradural lipoma
- Fat intensity on all pulse sequences
- Typically midline
- Cervical and thoracic spine most common

PATHOLOGY

General Features
- General path comments: Slow growing tumor
- Etiology
  ○ Epithelial cells iatrogenically introduced into thecal sac during lumbar puncture
    ▪ Without or with ill-fitting stylets
    ▪ Reported time between apparent implantation and development of epidermoid: 2-23 years
  ○ Sequela of dysraphism repair in some reports
- Epidemiology
  ○ Epidermoid: 0.5-1% of spinal tumors
    ▪ 40% acquired

Gross Pathologic & Surgical Features
- Discrete pearly white tumor

Microscopic Features
- Desquamated epithelium

CLINICAL ISSUES

Presentation
- Most common signs/symptoms
  ○ Low back pain
  ○ Other signs/symptoms
    ▪ Radicular pain
    ▪ Paraparesis
    ▪ Paresthesia
    ▪ Sphincter dysfunction

Demographics
- Age: All ages reported

Natural History & Prognosis
- Surgery curative in most cases

Treatment
- Laminectomy with complete resection

DIAGNOSTIC CHECKLIST

Image Interpretation Pearls
- Nonenhancing CSF intensity mass in cauda equina of patients with history of lumbar puncture suggestive of acquired epidermoid

SELECTED REFERENCES

1. Kikuchi K et al: The utility of diffusion-weighted imaging with navigator-echo technique for the diagnosis of spinal epidermoid cysts. AJNR Am J Neuroradiol. 21(6):1164-6, 2000
2. Potgieter S et al: Epidermoid tumours associated with lumbar punctures performed in early neonatal life. Dev Med Child Neurol. 40(4):266-9, 1998
3. Toro VE et al: MRI of iatrogenic spinal epidermoid tumor. JACT. 17:970-2, 1993
4. Visciani A et al: Iatrogenic intraspinal epidermoid tumor: myelo-CT and MRI diagnosis. Neuroradiology. 31(3):273-5, 1989

IMAGE GALLERY

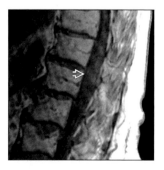 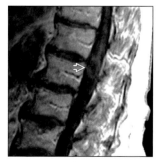

(Left) Sagittal T1WI MR through lumbar spine demonstrates a subtle intradural lesion (arrow) distal to conus medullaris, slightly hyperintense to CSF. *(Right)* Sagittal T1 C+ MR shows the same lesion without enhancement (arrow). An epidermoid was found at surgery.

FIBROUS DYSPLASIA

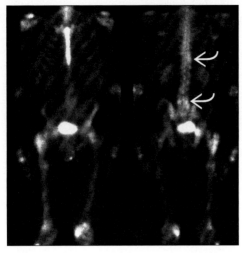

Anteroposterior and posteroanterior bone scans show polyostotic fibrous dysplasia. Note scoliosis and multifocal involvement of spine (arrows).

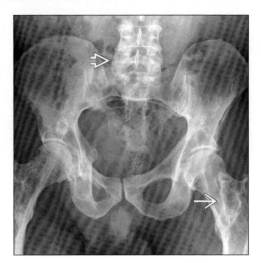

Anteroposterior radiography shows polyostotic FD. Arrow shows femoral lesion. Right L5 pedicle is involved (open arrow), but this might be missed without positive BS in this region.

TERMINOLOGY

Abbreviations and Synonyms
- Fibrous dysplasia (FD)

Definitions
- Monostotic: Single lesion
- Polyostotic: Multiple lesions, often associated with growth disturbances
- McCune Albright Syndrome: Polyostotic FD, precocious puberty, café-au-lait skin lesions

IMAGING FINDINGS

General Features
- Best diagnostic clue: Mildly expansile lesion with "ground glass" bone matrix
- Location
  - Rarely involves spine
    - Neural arch > vertebral body
    - Spine involvement almost always with polyostotic disease
  - Commonly involves pelvis
    - Innominate bone much more frequently involved than sacrum
- Morphology
  - Round or ovoid destructive lesion

- May have associated aneurysmal bone cyst (ABC)
  - Balloon-like expansion of bone
  - Fluid-fluid levels on CT, MR

Radiographic Findings
- Radiography
  - Fusiform expansion of bone
  - Enlarged or sclerotic pedicle
  - Solitary lesions usually have sclerotic rim
  - Although bilateral, multiple lesions tend to predominate on one side of body
  - Commonly "ground glass" matrix
  - Scoliosis

CT Findings
- Bone CT
  - Mildly expansile
  - "Ground glass" matrix characteristic
  - However, may range from purely lytic to purely sclerotic lesion
  - May contain islands of cartilage

MR Findings
- T1WI: Low to intermediate signal intensity
- T2WI: Heterogeneous intermediate to high signal intensity
- STIR: Heterogeneous intermediate to high signal intensity
- T1 C+: Heterogeneous enhancement

DDx: Fibrous Dysplasia

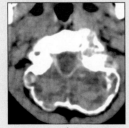

Aneurysmal Bone Cyst

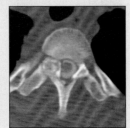

Osteoid Osteoma

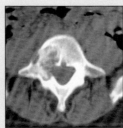

Osteoblastoma

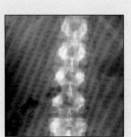

Tuberous Sclerosis

FIBROUS DYSPLASIA

Key Facts

Terminology
- McCune Albright Syndrome: Polyostotic FD, precocious puberty, café-au-lait skin lesions

Imaging Findings
- Best diagnostic clue: Mildly expansile lesion with "ground glass" bone matrix
- Spine involvement almost always with polyostotic disease

- Best imaging tool: CT scan, 1-3 mm sections

Top Differential Diagnoses
- Aneurysmal bone cyst (ABC)
- Osteoid osteoma
- Osteoblastoma

Pathology
- Endocrine abnormalities

Nuclear Medicine Findings
- Bone Scan
  - Mild to marked increase in radionuclide uptake
  - Asymptomatic spine foci commonly found on bone scan in polyostotic FD

Imaging Recommendations
- Best imaging tool: CT scan, 1-3 mm sections

DIFFERENTIAL DIAGNOSIS

Aneurysmal bone cyst (ABC)
- Balloon-like expansion of neural arch
- Fluid/fluid levels on CT or MRI
- Can be associated with fibrous dysplasia

Osteoid osteoma
- Central lucent or sclerotic nidus
- Surrounded by sclerotic reactive bone

Osteoblastoma
- Usually shows more discrete bone matrix
- May mimic "ground glass" matrix

Tuberous sclerosis
- Sclerotic bone lesions
- Characteristic brain abnormalities

Neurofibromatosis
- Scoliosis, café-au-lait spots
- Peripheral nerve sheath tumors

PATHOLOGY

General Features
- Genetics: Sporadic mutation in GNAS1 gene
- Epidemiology
  - Solitary lesions common
  - Polyostotic form less common
- Associated abnormalities
  - Endocrine abnormalities
    - Hyperparathyroidism
    - Acromegaly
    - Premature puberty
    - Phosphaturia

Gross Pathologic & Surgical Features
- White or tan lesion with gritty consistency

Microscopic Features
- Stroma of bland fibrous tissue
- Small spicules of woven bone ("alphabet soup")
- Occasionally has foci of cartilage

CLINICAL ISSUES

Demographics
- Age
  - Polyostotic disease presents in first or second decade
  - Monostotic disease usually an incidental finding
- Gender: M = F

Natural History & Prognosis
- Growth disturbance, pathologic fracture common in polyostotic form
- Rarely undergoes sarcomatous transformation

SELECTED REFERENCES

1. Leet AI et al: Fibrous dysplasia in the spine: prevalence of lesions and association with scoliosis. J Bone Joint Surg Am. 86-A(3):531-7, 2004
2. Arazi M et al: Monostotic fibrous dysplasia of the thoracic spine: clinopathological description and follow up. Case report. J Neurosurg. 100(4 Suppl):378-81, 2004

IMAGE GALLERY

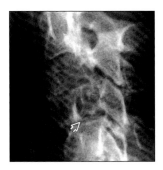 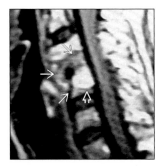

(Left) Lateral radiography shows lytic lesions at C3 and C4 due to FD and associated ABC. Balloon-like expansion of C4 reflects ABC component (arrow) (Courtesy L. Lomasney, MD). *(Right)* Sagittal T1WI MR shows FD (arrows) and associated ABC (open arrow) involving C3 and C4. Blood products in ABC component result in high signal intensity on T1WI.

KUMMELL DISEASE

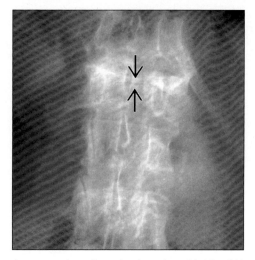

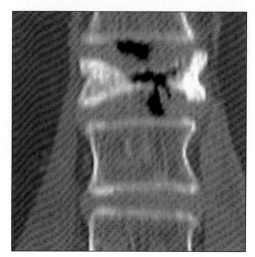

Anteroposterior radiography shows loss of height of L1 vertebral body, and sclerosis beneath endplate. A thin band of gas is visible (arrows).

Coronal bone CT shows gas within collapsed, sclerotic vertebral body. Gas is also present in adjacent disc spaces.

TERMINOLOGY

Abbreviations and Synonyms
- Post-traumatic avascular necrosis

Definitions
- Delayed, post-traumatic collapse of vertebral body

IMAGING FINDINGS

General Features
- Best diagnostic clue: Gas-filled cleft in vertebral body
- Location: Thoracic or lumbar vertebral body

Radiographic Findings
- Radiography
  - Loss of height, sclerosis of vertebral body
  - Narrow, horizontally oriented band of gas in vertebral body

CT Findings
- Bone CT
  - Horizontal band of gas filling cleft in vertebral body
  - Gas often in adjacent disc space

MR Findings
- T1WI
  - Signal void in area of gas
  - Low signal intensity in vertebral body
  - Fracture line may be visible
- T2WI
  - Signal void in area of gas
  - Intermediate to high signal intensity in vertebral body
- STIR
  - Signal void in area of gas
  - Intermediate to high signal intensity in vertebral body
  - Fracture line may be visible
- T1 C+: Heterogeneous enhancement
- Gas collection may be mimicked by calcium

Nuclear Medicine Findings
- Bone Scan: Positive 3 phase bone scan

Imaging Recommendations
- Best imaging tool: CT scan
- Protocol advice: 1-3 mm thick helical images with sagittal and coronal reformations

DIFFERENTIAL DIAGNOSIS

Infection
- Small bubbles of gas sometimes present, but not a cleft
- Endplate destruction

DDx: Kummell Disease

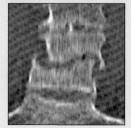

Infection

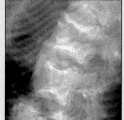

Sickle Cell

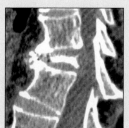

Metastasis

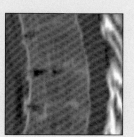

Degenerated Discs

KUMMELL DISEASE

Key Facts

Terminology
- Delayed, post-traumatic collapse of vertebral body

Imaging Findings
- Location: Thoracic or lumbar vertebral body
- Loss of height, sclerosis of vertebral body
- Narrow, horizontally oriented band of gas in vertebral body
- Best imaging tool: CT scan

Top Differential Diagnoses
- Infection
- Nontraumatic bone infarction
- Gas within degenerated discs
- Gas in metastasis

- Heterogeneous enhancement of disc and vertebral body
- Fluid collections

Nontraumatic bone infarction
- Heterogeneous low signal on T1WI, high signal T2WI, STIR
- Serpentine contour of infarct with peripheral enhancement
- Associated with steroids, sickle cell disease, pancreatitis, vasculitis, emboli, caisson disease

Gas within degenerated discs
- Gas forms in degenerated discs, may enter Schmorl nodes

Gas in metastasis
- Small bubbles of gas rarely seen in metastasis with vertebral body collapse

PATHOLOGY

General Features
- General path comments: Kyphoplasty data suggests radiographically occult vertebral body clefts are common in patients with fracture
- Etiology
  ○ Nonunited vertebral body fracture undergoes secondary necrosis and collapse
  ○ Nitrogen accumulates in fracture cleft
- Epidemiology: Uncommon

CLINICAL ISSUES

Presentation
- Most common signs/symptoms: Pain, kyphosis

Demographics
- Age: Usually elderly, osteoporotic patients
- Gender: More common in females

Natural History & Prognosis
- Progressive vertebral body collapse if untreated

Treatment
- Options, risks, complications: Vertebroplasty or kyphoplasty relieves pain

DIAGNOSTIC CHECKLIST

Image Interpretation Pearls
- Air better seen on AP than on lateral radiographs

SELECTED REFERENCES

1. Jang JS et al: Efficacy of percutaneous vertebroplasty in the treatment of intravertebral pseudarthrosis associated with noninfected avascular necrosis of the vertebral body. Spine. 28(14):1588-92, 2003
2. Lane JI et al: Intravertebral clefts opacified during vertebroplasty: pathogenesis, technical implications, and prognostic significance. AJNR Am J Neuroradiol. 23(10):1642-6, 2002
3. Young WF et al: Delayed post-traumatic osteonecrosis of a vertebral body (Kummell's disease). Acta Orthop Belg. 68(1):13-9, 2002
4. Chou LH et al: Idiopathic avascular necrosis of a vertebral body. Case report and literature review. Spine. 22(16):1928-32, 1997
5. The intravertebral vacuum phenomenon ("vertebral osteonecrosis"): intradiscal gas in a fractured vertebral body? Spine. 22(16):1885-91, 1997
6. Dupuy DE et al: Vertebral fluid collection associated with vertebral collapse. AJR Am J Roentgenol. 167(6):1535-8, 1996
7. Malghem J et al: Intravertebral vacuum cleft: changes in content after supine positioning. Radiology. 187(2):483-7, 1993
8. Naul LG et al: Avascular necrosis of the vertebral body: MR imaging. Radiology. 172(1):219-22, 1989

IMAGE GALLERY

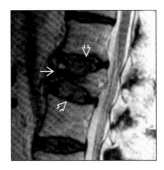 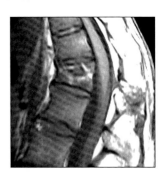

(Left) Sagittal T2WI MR shows band-like gas in vertebral body (arrow), and gas in intervertebral discs (open arrows). Findings less conspicuous and less specific than on CT. *(Right)* Sagittal T1WI MR shows fluid filled vertebral cleft 5 months following fracture, precursor to gas-filled cleft of Kümmell disease.

PART V

Vascular and Systemic Disorders

Vascular Lesions **1**

Spinal Manifestations of Systemic Diseases **2**

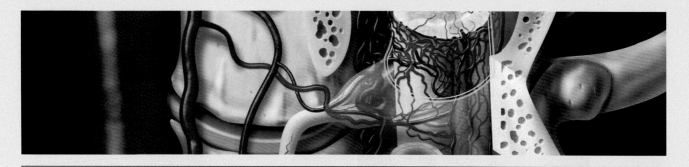

SECTION 1: Vascular Lesions

SECTION 1
Vascular Lesions

Introduction and Overview

Vascular Lesions

VASCULAR ANATOMY

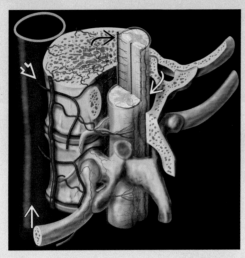

Coronal oblique graphic shows source of thoracic vascular supply from aorta (arrow) derived from segmental feeders (open arrow). ASA (curved black arrow), PSA shown (curved white arrow).

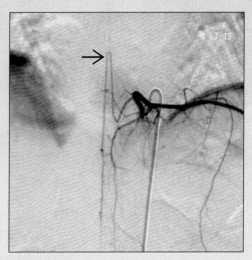

Anteroposterior angiography of left T9 intercostal artery shows classic hairpin turn of anterior spinal artery (Adamkiewicz) (arrow).

TERMINOLOGY

Abbreviations and Synonyms
- Abbreviations: Anterior spinal artery (ASA); posterior spinal artery (PSA); artery of Adamkiewicz (AA)
- Synonyms: Great anterior radicular artery, arteria radicularis magna = artery of Adamkiewicz

Definitions
- Anatomic definition of blood supply to spinal structures

IMAGING ANATOMY

Internal Structures-Critical Contents
- Spinal cord circulation derived from
  - Branches of vertebral arteries
  - Multiple radicular arteries arising from segmental vessels at multiple levels
    - Ascending cervical
    - Deep cervical
    - Intercostal
    - Lumbar
    - Sacral
- Anterior spinal artery (ASA)
  - Arises at junction of intradural segment of vertebral arteries, below basilar artery
  - Descends in midline without interruption form foramen magnum to filum terminale
  - Reinforced by segmental feeders
  - Gives rise to sulcal (central) branches supplying anterior 2/3 of cord
    - Supply includes anterior horns, spinothalamic tracts, corticospinal tracts
  - Lies in midline on ventral aspect of cord in groove of anterior median fissure of cord
- Posterior spinal arteries (PSAs)
  - Arise from posterior rami of vertebral artery, or from posterior inferior cerebellar artery

- Paired longitudinal system on dorsal cord medial to dorsal roots
- Plexiform and variable venous network between two dorsal arteries
- Supply posterior 1/3 of cord
  - Supply includes posterior columns, and variable supply of corticospinal tracts
- Segmental supply
  - ASA, PSA supply derived from segmental anastomoses
  - Segmental vessels arise as dorsal rami from vertebral, subclavian, thoracic intercostal, lumbar intercostal
    - Dorsal rami enter canal through foramen, penetrates dura and divides ⇒
    - 1. Dural artery supplying nerve root sleeve and dura
    - 2. Radiculomedullary branch ⇒
    - a. Radicular artery penetrating subarachnoid space to supply anterior and posterior roots
    - b. Variable medullary artery which joins ASA, PSA
- Radicular arteries
  - Division of radiculomedullary arteries along anterior & posterior nerve roots
  - Anterior radicular artery ⇒ anterior surface of cord
  - Posterior radicular artery ⇒ posterior surface of cord
  - Fetal segmental vessels regress with variable number in adult
    - 2-14 (average 6) anterior radicular arteries persist in adult
    - 11-16 posterior radicular arteries persist in adult
- Cervical
  - Major radicular feeders between C5-C7 level
  - 2-3 anterior cervical cord feeders (400-600 μ)
    - No right-left lateralization preference
  - 3-4 posterior cervical cord feeders (150-400 μ)
- Thoracic
  - Anterior thoracic cord feeders ⇒ 2-3
  - Usually left sided (550-1,200 μ)
    - Small ventral feeders may also be present (200 μ)
  - Inverse relationship between number and caliber of ventral radicular vessels

VASCULAR ANATOMY

DIFFERENTIAL DIAGNOSIS

Anterior spinal artery
- Descends in midline without interruption form foramen magnum to filum terminale
- Reinforced by segmental feeders
- Gives rise to sulcal (central) branches supplying anterior 2/3 of cord
- Dominant thoracic anterior radicular = artery of Adamkiewicz (left side, T9-T12 origin most common)

Posterior spinal arteries
- Paired longitudinal system on dorsal cord medial to dorsal roots
- Plexiform and variable venous network between two dorsal arteries
- Supply posterior 1/3 of cord

Prominent intradural vessels and mimics
- Normal variant (particularly dorsal veins, & near conus)
- CSF flow dephasing mimics vessel flow voids (particularly dorsal thoracic)
- Collateral flow (IVC occlusion)
- Enlarged nerve roots with chronic inflammatory demyelinating polyneuropathy (CIDP)
- Central canal stenosis with nerve root redundancy
- Tumor: Hemangioblastoma, schwannoma, meningioma, ependymoma, paraganglioma
- Spinal dural fistulas (type I)
- Spinal cord arteriovenous malformations (types II, III)
- Spinal intradural-perimedullary fistula (type IV)

- "Pauci-segmental" fewer vessels (< 5) with larger caliber
- "Pluri-segmental" more vessels with smaller caliber
- Dominant thoracic anterior radicular = artery of Adamkiewicz
  - Left side origin (73%)
  - T9-T12 origin (62%)
  - Lumbar origin (26%)
  - T6-T8 (12%)
- Posterior thoracic cord feeders ⇒ 9-12 (average 8)
  - No right-left lateralization preference
  - Vessel caliber 150-400 μ
  - Variable reporting of "great posterior radicular artery"
- Lumbosacral & pelvic
  - 0-1 major cord feeders
  - Anterior spinal artery ends at conus with communicating branches "rami cruciantes" to posterior spinal artery
  - Posterior division of iliac artery ⇒ inferior & superior lateral sacral branches ⇒ spinal arteries via anterior sacral foramina
  - Anterior division iliac artery ⇒ inferior gluteal artery ⇒ supplies sciatic nerve
  - Posterior division internal iliac artery ⇒ iliolumbar artery artery supplies femoral nerve at iliac wing level
- Cord nutrient vessels
  - Central & peripheral systems
  - Central ⇒ ASA & flow centrifugal
  - Peripheral ⇒ PSA, pial plexus & flow centripetal
  - Dense capillary network in gray matter of cord
- Veins
  - Parallels spinal arteries
    - Very symmetrical pattern of venous drainage (compared with highly asymmetric arterial supply) with minimal anterior-posterior, right-left, segmental variation
  - Two sets of intrinsic radial draining veins drain into anastomoses on cord surface

- Central group provides return for anterior horns & surrounding white matter ⇒ drain into central veins in anterior median fissure ⇒ form anterior median vein
- Peripheral dorsal & lateral cord drainage via small valveless radial vein plexus ⇒ coronal venous plexus on cord surface ⇒ epidural venous plexus of Batson
- Epidural plexus connects with superior, inferior vena cavae, azygos & hemiazygos systems, intracranial dural sinuses
- 30-70 medullary radicular veins
  - No anterior or posterior dominance of veins
- Anterior median vein continues caudally along filum terminale to end of dural sac
- Coronal & median veins drain ⇒ medullary veins which leave intradural space at root sleeve into epidural plexus
  - Medullary veins have functional valve-like mechanism at dural margin preventing epidural reflux into intradural space
  - No intradural valves

EMBRYOLOGY

Embryologic Events
- Spinal cord vessels originate from capillary network on ventrolateral surface of cord connected with segmental aortic branches
- Two primitive longitudinal systems formed
- End of 2nd month ventrolateral systems transformed into longitudinal solitary anteromedian anterior spinal artery
- Plexus-like pattern remains more prominent on dorsal side
- ASA formation followed by variable regression of segmental feeders (initially 31), completed by 4th month
  - Reduction most pronounced in thoracic & lumbar areas
- Segmental arteries persist as intercostal and lumbar arteries

VASCULAR ANATOMY

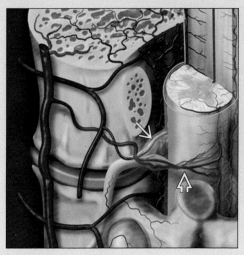

Oblique coronal graphic of thoracic cord supply shows anterior (arrow) & posterior (open arrow) radicular arteries which anastomose to ASA, PSA.

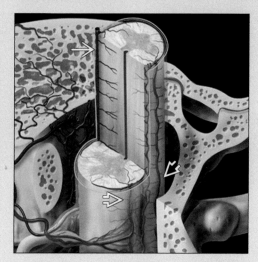

Coronal oblique graphic shows detail of dominant anterior spinal artery in anterior sulcus (arrow), & two posterior spinal arteries (open arrows).

- Cervical
  - Dorsal intersegmental anastomoses persist as components of vertebral arteries
  - Ventral anastomoses persist as thyrocervical trunk

CUSTOM DIFFERENTIAL DIAGNOSIS

Normal CSF pulsations
- Typically dorsal to cord on T2WI, ill-defined margins

Tortuous roots from spinal stenosis
- Distinguished by presence of severe central stenosis

Spinal cord tumor
- Distinguishable by imaging with intramedullary mass showing focal enhancement

Collateral venous flow
- IVC occlusion may give epidural/intradural prominent veins

Spinal cord arteriovenous malformation (SCAVM)
- Usually acute presentation (compared to insidious presentation of DAVF), subarachnoid hemorrhage
- Spinal arteriography is gold standard for confirming diagnosis
  - Provides precise localization of anterior spinal artery
  - Provides access for interventional therapy/embolization
  - Permits identification of exact level of arteriovenous shunting

SELECTED REFERENCES

1. Caglar S et al: Extraforaminal lumbar arterial anatomy. Surg Neurol. 61(1):29-33; discussion 33, 2004
2. Williams GM et al: Preoperative selective intercostal angiography in patients undergoing thoracoabdominal aneurysm repair. J Vasc Surg. 39(2):314-21, 2004
3. Marinkovic S et al: Microsurgical anatomy of the perforating branches of the vertebral artery. Surg Neurol. 61(2):190-7; discussion 197, 2004
4. Biglioli P et al: Upper and lower spinal cord blood supply: the continuity of the anterior spinal artery and the relevance of the lumbar arteries. J Thorac Cardiovasc Surg. 127(4):1188-92, 2004
5. Anatomical study of blood supply to the spinal cord: Ann Thorac Surg. 76(6):1967-71, 2003
6. Kudo K et al: Anterior spinal artery and artery of Adamkiewicz detected by using multi-detector row CT. AJNR Am J Neuroradiol. 24(1):13-7, 2003
7. Kulkarni SS et al: Arterial complications following anterior lumbar interbody fusion: report of eight cases. Eur Spine J. 12(1):48-54; discussion 55-6, 2003
8. Suzuki T et al: Vertebral body ischemia in the posterior spinal artery syndrome: case report and review of the literature. Spine. 28(13):E260-4, 2003
9. Shamji MF et al: Circulation of the spinal cord: an important consideration for thoracic surgeons. Ann Thorac Surg. 76(1):315-21, 2003
10. Prestigiacomo CJ et al: Three-dimensional rotational spinal angiography in the evaluation and treatment of vascular malformations. AJNR Am J Neuroradiol. 24(7):1429-35, 2003
11. Yoshioka K et al: MR angiography and CT angiography of the artery of Adamkiewicz: noninvasive preoperative assessment of thoracoabdominal aortic aneurysm. Radiographics. 23(5):1215-25, 2003
12. Jellema K et al: Spinal dural arteriovenous fistulas: clinical features in 80 patients. J Neurol Neurosurg Psychiatry. 74(10):1438-40, 2003
13. Bowen BC et al: MR angiography of the spine: update. Magn Reson Imaging Clin N Am. 11(4):559-84, 2003

IMAGE GALLERY

Typical

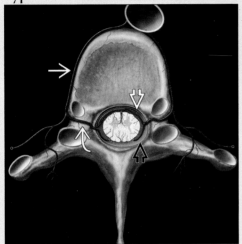
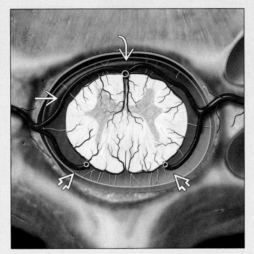

(Left) Axial graphic shows intercostal (arrow) arising from aorta, giving spinal branch (curved arrow), dividing into ventral (open white arrow), & dorsal (open black arrow) radiculomedullary arteries. (Right) Axial graphic shows ventral radiculomedullary artery (RM) (arrow) supplying anterior spinal artery (curved arrow), & posterior RM artery supplying paired posterior spinal arteries (open arrows).

Typical

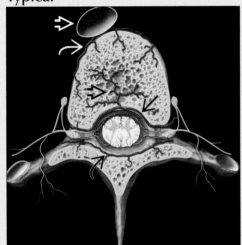
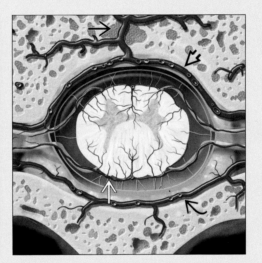

(Left) Axial graphic shows ventral (black arrow) & dorsal (curved black arrow) epidural plexus, basivertebral vein (open black arrow), ventral external plexus (curved white arrow), IVC (open white arrow). (Right) Axial graphic shows normal coronal plexus on cord surface (white arrow), ventral (open arrow) & dorsal (curved arrow) epidural plexus, basivertebral vein (black arrow).

Typical

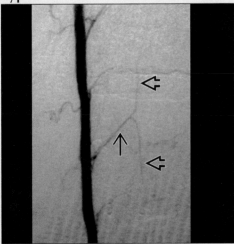
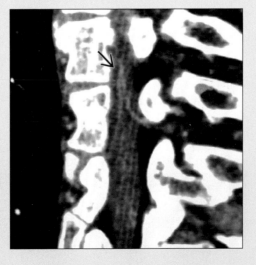

(Left) Anteroposterior angiography of R vertebral shows prominent segmental feeder (arrow), so-called "artery of cervical enlargement" supplying anterior spinal artery (open arrows)(Courtesy M. Ahmed, MD). (Right) Coronal oblique CTA shows normal hairpin turn of artery of Adamkiewicz (arrow) in thoracic spine.

TYPE I DAVF

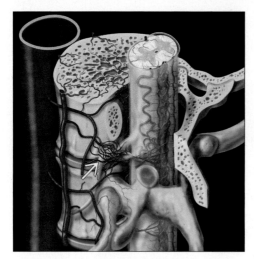

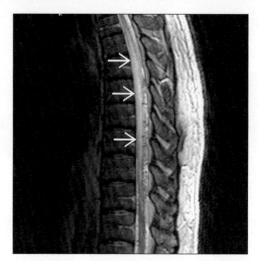

Sagittal Oblique graphic of thoracic cord shows site of type I dural fistula at dural root sleeve level (arrow), with secondary dilatation of intradural venous plexus.

Sagittal T2WI MR shows multiple flow voids on dorsal surface of cord due to enlarged veins. Extensive increased signal in cord reflecting edema from venous hypertension (arrows).

TERMINOLOGY

Abbreviations and Synonyms
- Synonyms: Dural fistula; type I spinal vascular malformation; radiculomeningeal fistula
- Abbreviations: DAVF, dural AVF, type I AVM

Definitions
- Spinal arteriovenous (AV) fistula, present within dura, with intradural distended draining veins

IMAGING FINDINGS

General Features
- Best diagnostic clue: Abnormally enlarged, hyperintense distal cord covered with dilated pial veins
- Location
  - Intradural, extramedullary flow voids from distended draining veins
  - Most commonly occur at level of conus
- Size: Variable
- Morphology: Serpentine vessels on cord surface

Radiographic Findings
- Myelography: Multiple curvilinear filling defects due to dilated veins

CT Findings
- CECT
  - Enlarged distal spinal cord
  - Enhancing pial veins on cord surface
  - Much more difficult to diagnose on routine CT than MR imaging
- CTA
  - Nidus in neural foramen shows focal enhancement, with prominent intradural draining dilated veins
  - Postprocessing with multiplanar reformats mandatory

MR Findings
- T1WI
  - Cord enlarged, hypointense
    - Abnormal small enhancing vessels on cord pial surface
- T2WI
  - Cord enlarged, hypointense
    - Multiple small abnormal vessel flow voids (dilated pial veins) on cord pial surface
    - Edema spares cord periphery
    - Edema has "flame shaped" margins superiorly and inferiorly
    - Low signal cord periphery on T2WI consistent with venous hypertensive myelopathy
- STIR: Cord enlarged, hypointense
- T1 C+

DDx: Prominent "Flow Voids" and Mimics

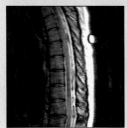

Normal CSF Flow

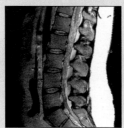

IVC Occlusion

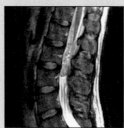

Schwannoma

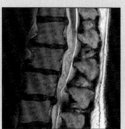

Tortuous Roots

TYPE I DAVF

Key Facts

Terminology
- Spinal arteriovenous (AV) fistula, present within dura, with intradural distended draining veins

Imaging Findings
- Best diagnostic clue: Abnormally enlarged, hyperintense distal cord covered with dilated pial veins
- Cord enlarged, hypointense
- Multiple small abnormal vessel flow voids (dilated pial veins) on cord pial surface
- Edema spares cord periphery
- Edema has "flame shaped" margins superiorly and inferiorly

- MRA: Dynamic contrast-enhanced MRA capable of defining dilated intradural veins; may guide catheter angiography
- Fistula may arise anywhere from vertebral artery to internal iliac superiorly
- CTA technically less demanding than MRA; is capable of superior resolution of nidus location, draining veins
- Use selective spinal arteriography to confirm diagnosis and direct treatment planning

Clinical Issues
- Middle-aged male with progressive lower extremity weakness exacerbated by exercise

---

- ○ Multiple enhancing serpentine veins on cord surface
- ○ May show patchy, ill-defined enhancement within cord
- MRA: Dynamic contrast-enhanced MRA capable of defining dilated intradural veins; may guide catheter angiography
- Occasionally MR imaging normal or demonstrates only abnormal cord signal

Angiographic Findings
- Conventional
  - ○ Spinal arteriography is gold standard for confirming diagnosis
    - ▪ Permits identification of exact level of arteriovenous shunt
    - ▪ Provides precise localization of anterior spinal artery
    - ▪ Provides access for interventional therapy/embolization
    - ▪ Fistula may arise anywhere from vertebral artery to internal iliac superiorly

Imaging Recommendations
- First perform focused MR imaging with small field of view, thin-slices in both sagittal (3 mm/0 mm gap) and axial planes (4 mm/0 mm gap)
  - ○ T1WI, T2WI, T1 C+ sequences in both planes
- CTA technically less demanding than MRA; is capable of superior resolution of nidus location, draining veins
- Use selective spinal arteriography to confirm diagnosis and direct treatment planning
- Myelography no longer primary or secondary diagnostic tool with availability of MRA, CTA

DIFFERENTIAL DIAGNOSIS

Normal CSF pulsations
- Typically dorsal to cord on T2WI, ill-defined margins

Spinal cord tumor
- Distinguishable by imaging with intramedullary mass showing focal enhancement

- May be associated with prominent feeding intradural vessels

Collateral venous flow
- IVC occlusion may cause prominent epidural/intradural veins
- Check for small or ill-defined IVC, or metal artifact in IVC region due to filter

Spinal cord arteriovenous malformation (SCAVM)
- Usually acute presentation (compared to insidious presentation of DAVF)
- Intramedullary or subarachnoid hemorrhage relatively common

Tortuous roots from spinal stenosis
- Distinguished by presence of severe central stenosis

PATHOLOGY

General Features
- General path comments
  - ○ Lesions are extramedullary AVFs, not true AVMs
    - ▪ No intervening small vessel network
    - ▪ Fistula drains directly into venous outflow tract
    - ▪ Usually intradural
  - ○ Supplied by small tortuous arteries originating from dura mater
- Genetics: No association with other CNS vascular malformations
- Etiology
  - ○ Postulated to be acquired lesions, possibly from thrombosis of extradural venous system
  - ○ Venous drainage from the DAVF results in increased pial vein pressure that is transmitted to intrinsic cord veins
  - ○ Venous hypertension from engorgement reduces intramedullary AV pressure gradient, causing reduced tissue perfusion & cord ischemia
- Epidemiology
  - ○ 80% of all spinal vascular malformations

TYPE I DAVF

- 80% of patients are male
- Usually presents in 5th or 6th decade (range 20-80)

Gross Pathologic & Surgical Features

- Most commonly occurs at thoracolumbar level (T5-L3)
- Usually located either adjacent to intervertebral foramen or within dural root sleeve
- Arterial supply arises from dural branch of radicular artery
- Intradural vein drains directly into cord pial veins
- Frequently poor correlation between location of AV shunt and clinical level of spinal dysfunction
- Rarely, clinically manifests as "subacute necrotizing myelopathy" ("Foix-Alajounine syndrome")

Microscopic Features

- True arteriovenous fistula, no intervening small vessel network

Staging, Grading or Classification Criteria

- Previously categorized as type IV spinal arteriovenous malformation
- Anson-Spetzler classification into type IA (single feeder) and IIB (multiple feeders)

CLINICAL ISSUES

Presentation

- Most common signs/symptoms
  - Most common presentation is progressive lower extremity weakness with both upper + lower motor neuron involvement
  - Other signs/symptoms
    - Additional symptoms include back pain, bowel/bladder dysfunction, impotence
    - Thoracolumbar fistula location spares upper extremities
    - Very rarely presents with subarachnoid hemorrhage
- Clinical profile
  - Middle-aged male with progressive lower extremity weakness exacerbated by exercise
  - Time from symptom onset to diagnosis often delayed

Demographics

- Age: Usually presents in 5th or 6th decade
- Gender: M > F

Natural History & Prognosis

- Slowly progressive clinical course over several years leading to paraplegia
- Cord ischemia/venous congestive myelopathy is reversible if treated early, but may become irreversible when untreated
- Bowel/bladder dysfunction & impotence rarely improve, even after successful obliteration of fistula

Treatment

- Endovascular fistula occlusion with permanent embolic agents
- Surgical fistula obliteration
  - 40-60% improve following obliteration of fistula, 40-50% stabilize myelopathic symptoms

- T2WI cord edema decreases over 1-4 months following successful embolization
- Improved cord appearance on MR following treatment does not necessarily correlate with improved symptoms

DIAGNOSTIC CHECKLIST

Consider

- Other type of spinal vascular malformation if evidence of intramedullary flow voids
- CTA effective for defining nidus, draining veins with high spatial resolution
- Cervical type I AVM may drain intracranially with high flow, varix formation and SAH

Image Interpretation Pearls

- Imaging & clinical findings are frequently subtle or nonspecific; early diagnosis requires high level of suspicion

SELECTED REFERENCES

1. Spetzler RF et al: Modified classification of spinal cord vascular lesions. J Neurosurg (Spine 2). 96: 145-156, 2002
2. Van Dijk JM et al: Multidisciplinary management of spinal dural arteriovenous fistulas: clinical presentation and long-term follow-up in 49 patients. Stroke. 33(6): 1578-83, 2002
3. Farb RI et al: Spinal dural arteriovenous fistula localization with a technique of first-pass gadolinium-enhanced MR angiography: initial experience. Radiology. 222(3): 843-50, 2002
4. Mascalchi M et al: Spinal vascular malformations: MR angiography after treatment. Radiology. 219(2): 346-53, 2001
5. Song JK et al: Surgical and endovascular treatment of spinal dural arteriovenous fistulas: long-term disability assessment and prognostic factors. J Neurosurg. 94(2 Suppl): 199-204, 2001
6. Hurst RW et al: Peripheral spinal cord hypointensity on T2-weighted MR images: a reliable imaging sign of venous hypertensive myelopathy. AJNR Am J Neuroradiol. 21(4): 781-6, 2000
7. Bowen BC et al: MR angiography of the spine. Magn Reson Imaging Clin N Am. 6(1): 165-78, 1998
8. Anson J et al: Classification of spinal arteriovenous malformations and implications for treatment. BNI Quarterly. 8: 2-8, 1992

IMAGE GALLERY

Typical

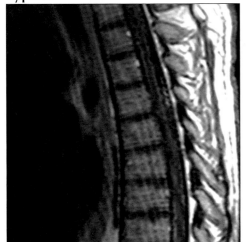 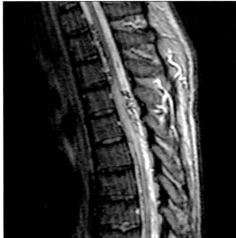

(Left) Sagittal T1 C+ MR shows multiple enhancing serpentine vessels on thoracic cord surface, both ventral and dorsal, due to enlarged draining veins. *(Right)* Sagittal T2WI MR shows enlarged draining veins as multiple flow voids surrounding cord. High T2 signal in cord tapers at both ends, and tends to spare periphery typical of venous hypertensive edema.

Typical

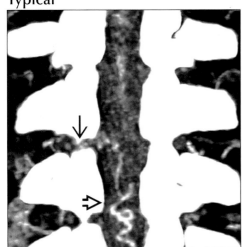 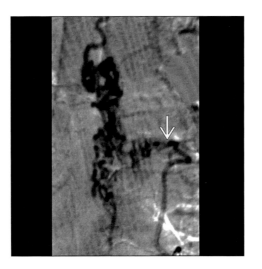

(Left) Coronal CTA shows type I fistula in right thoracic neural foramen (arrow), with enlarged inferior draining veins (open arrow). *(Right)* Anteroposterior angiography of intercostal artery shows peripheral fistula on the left (arrow) draining centrally into dilated venous plexus surrounding cord.

Typical

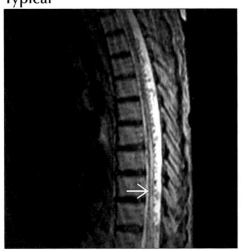 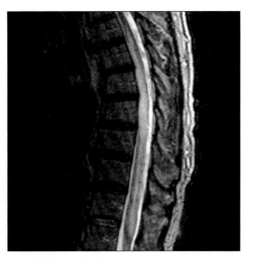

(Left) Sagittal T2WI MR shows typical intradural flow voids from distended & enlarged draining veins, with cord edema (arrow). *(Right)* Sagittal T2WI MR shows diffuse thoracic cord edema & enlargement, but no prominent flow voids within thecal sac. Angiography revealed left T12 fistula.

TYPE II AVM

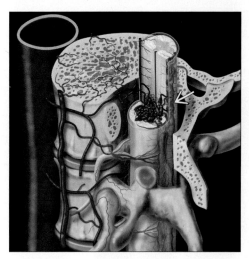

Sagittal oblique graphic of thoracic cord shows focal, compact intramedullary nidus of type II arteriovenous malformation (arrow).

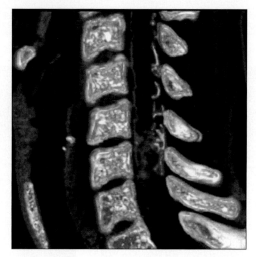

Sagittal CTA shows focal enhancing nidus within cord at C6 level, with anterior and posterior draining veins.

TERMINOLOGY

Abbreviations and Synonyms
- Synonyms: Glomus AVM

Definitions
- Direct arterial/venous communications forming compact nidus within cord
- Spine vascular malformation classification
  - Type I: Dural arteriovenous fistula (DAVF)
    - Most common = type I (up to 80%)
  - Type II: Intramedullary glomus type AVM (similar to brain AVM)
  - Type III: Juvenile-type AVM (intramedullary, extramedullary)
  - Type IV: Intradural extra/perimedullary AVF

IMAGING FINDINGS

General Features
- Best diagnostic clue
  - Type I: Flow voids with cord T2 hyperintensity
  - Type II: Intramedullary nidus (may extend to dorsal subpial surface)
  - Type III: Nidus may have extramedullary and extraspinal extension

  - Type IV: Ventral fistula (venous varices displace, distort cord)
- Location: Type II: Intramedullary nidus within cervical or thoracic cord
- Size: Variable
- Morphology: Multiple well-defined serpentine flow voids within substance of cord

Radiographic Findings
- Myelography
  - Serpentine filling defects in the contrast column from draining veins, enlarged feeding vessels
  - May see slight cord expansion at nidus level

CT Findings
- NECT: Usually normal
- CECT: May show enlarged cord with enhancing nidus
- CTA: Shows enhancing nidus, position with respect to cord, & multiple feeding vessels, draining veins

MR Findings
- T1WI: Large cord, heterogeneous signal (blood products), flow voids
- T2WI: Cord hyperintense (edema, gliosis, ischemia) or mixed (blood)
- STIR: Shows flow voids, edema within cord
- T2* GRE: More sensitive to blood byproducts of AVM hemorrhage
- T1 C+: Variable enhancement of nidus, cord, vessels

DDx: Intramedullary Disease

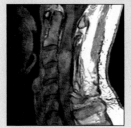

Astrocytoma

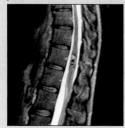

Cavernous Angioma

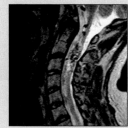

Type III AVM

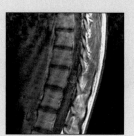

Type IV AVF

TYPE II AVM

Key Facts

Terminology
- Synonyms: Glomus AVM
- Type I: Dural arteriovenous fistula (DAVF)
- Type II: Intramedullary glomus type AVM (similar to brain AVM)
- Type III: Juvenile-type AVM (intramedullary, extramedullary)
- Type IV: Intradural extra/perimedullary AVF

Imaging Findings
- Type I: Flow voids with cord T2 hyperintensity
- Type II: Intramedullary nidus (may extend to dorsal subpial surface)
- Type III: Nidus may have extramedullary and extraspinal extension

- Type IV: Ventral fistula (venous varices displace, distort cord)
- Type II: Supplied by anterior spinal artery (ASA) or posterior spinal artery (PSA); nidus drains to coronal venous plexus (on cord surface) which in turn drains anterograde to extradural space

Pathology
- Associated abnormalities: Aneurysms of feeding vessels in type II AVMs (40%)

Clinical Issues
- Good outcome in type II (glomus) and IV (perimedullary)
- Type II: Surgical resection, + pre-op embolization (aneurysms, nidus)

- MRA: Dynamic enhanced MRA capable of defining feeding enlarged arteries, nidus, & enlarged draining veins
- Compare: Types I, IV fistulas
  - T1WI: Ventral type IV fistula, large flow voids distort/displace cord
  - T2WI: Type I fistula with T2 hyperintense cord + flow voids
  - Contrast: Enhancing pial vessels, epidural plexus, +/- patchy enhancement distal cord

Angiographic Findings
- Conventional
  - Type I: Peripheral dural fistula may arise anywhere from vertebral artery superiorly to internal iliac inferiorly
  - Type II: Supplied by anterior spinal artery (ASA) or posterior spinal artery (PSA); nidus drains to coronal venous plexus (on cord surface) which in turn drains anterograde to extradural space
  - Type III: Large complex nidus, multiple feeding vessels; may be intramedullary and extramedullary and even extraspinal
  - Type IV: Feeding vessel from ASA or PSA connects directly with spinal vein (no nidus)

Imaging Recommendations
- Contrast-enhanced MRI; consider spinal angiography +/- embolization

DIFFERENTIAL DIAGNOSIS

Intramedullary neoplasm
- Ependymoma: Heterogeneous (cysts, blood products)
- Astrocytoma: Multisegmental enhancing mass, no enlarged vessels

Intradural extramedullary tumor with prominent vascular supply
- Paraganglioma: Markedly enhancing intradural/extramedullary mass

Cavernous angioma
- Well-defined lesion showing speckled pattern on T1WI and T2WI like brain
- No prominent vessels

Type IV perimedullary fistula
- Prominent high flow feeders with varices may compress cord & simulate intramedullary lesion

Type III (juvenile) AVM
- Also shows intramedullary flow voids
- Larger and more extensive cord involvement than in type II AVM

PATHOLOGY

General Features
- General path comments
  - Causes of neurologic deterioration include SAH, ischemia from vascular steal, cord compression and venous hypertension
  - Location
    - Type I: Lower thoracic/conus common
    - Type II (glomus): Cervical/upper thoracic (may occur anywhere)
    - Type III (juvenile): Cervical/upper thoracic (may occur anywhere)
    - Type IV: Conus medullaris (type A, B), thoracic (type C)
  - Embryology
    - Persistence of primitive direct communications between arterial and venous channels, without intervening capillary bed
- Genetics
  - Sporadic or syndromic
    - Type I: None
    - Type II: Associated with cutaneous angiomas, Klippel-Trenaunay-Weber, Rendu-Osler-Weber syndromes
    - Type III: Associated with Cobb syndrome (metameric vascular malformation involving triad of spinal cord, skin, bone involvement)

- ▪ Type IV: Associated with Rendu-Osler-Weber syndrome
- Etiology
  - ○ Type II: Compact nidus, high flow, aneurysms common (20-44%)
  - ○ Type III: Large diffuse nidus, cord ischemia, venous hypertension
  - ○ Type IV: Congenital; may be acquired after trauma; (A) venous hypertension, (B, C) arterial steal, (C) cord compression
- Epidemiology
  - ○ Intramedullary (type II, III):15-20% of spinal AVMs
  - ○ AVMs account for 10% of spinal masses
- Associated abnormalities: Aneurysms of feeding vessels in type II AVMs (40%)

Gross Pathologic & Surgical Features

- Type I: Peripheral direct fistula in dura
- Type II: Compact intramedullary nidus lacks normal capillary bed
  - ○ No parenchyma within nidus; (nidus may have pial extension)
- Type III: Large, complex intramedullary lesion, normal neural parenchyma inside nidus (may involve extramedullary, extradural)
- Type IV: Direct fistula between ASA/PSA & draining vein, no nidus

Microscopic Features

- Type II: Abnormal vessels with variable wall thickness, internal elastic lamina
- Reactive change in surrounding tissue: Gliosis, cytoid bodies, Rosenthal fibers; hemosiderin deposition common; +/- Ca++

Staging, Grading or Classification Criteria

- Newest classification of AVMs into extra-intradural; intradural (intramedullary, compact, diffuse, conus; subtyped by flow, size)

CLINICAL ISSUES

Presentation

- Most common signs/symptoms
  - ○ Type I: Progressive myelopathy
  - ○ Type II: SAH most common symptom; pain, myelopathy
  - ○ Type III: Progressive neurologic decline (weakness), SAH
  - ○ Type IV: Progressive conus/cauda equina syndrome, SAH
- Clinical profile: Type II: Adult with acute subarachnoid hemorrhage, myelopathy
- Pregnancy associated with worsening symptoms

Demographics

- Age: Adult
- Gender: M = F

Natural History & Prognosis

- Good outcome in type II (glomus) and IV (perimedullary)
- Poor prognosis for juvenile (type III) AVM

Treatment

- Type I: Embolization or surgical resection
- Type II: Surgical resection, + pre-op embolization (aneurysms, nidus)
- Type III: Complete resection generally not possible, palliative therapy
- Type IV: Embolization or surgical resection depending upon staging and feeding vessels

DIAGNOSTIC CHECKLIST

Consider

- CTA as localization tool prior to catheter angiography
  - ○ Can define malformation type, location of ASA

Image Interpretation Pearls

- Definition of intramedullary involvement critical for classification, prognosis, treatment options

SELECTED REFERENCES

1. Spetzler RF et al: Modified classification of spinal cord vascular lesions. J Neurosurg (Spine 2) 96: 145-156, 2002
2. Mascalchi M et al: Spinal vascular malformations: MR angiography after treatment. Radiology. 219(2): 346-53, 2001
3. Bemporad JA et al: Magnetic resonance imaging of spinal cord vascular malformations with an emphasis on the cervical spine. In Neuropathic basis for imaging. Neuroimaging Clinics of North America 11:111-29, 2001
4. Mascalchi M et al: Contrast-enhanced time-resolved MR angiography of spinal vascular malformations. J Comput Assist Tomogr. 23(3): 341-5, 1999
5. Hasegawa M et al: The efficacy of CT arteriography for spinal arteriovenous fistula surgery: technical note. Neuroradiology. 41(12): 915-9, 1999
6. Morgan MK: Outcome from treatment for spinal arteriovenous malformation. Neurosurg Clin N Am. 10(1):113-9, 1999
7. Bao YH et al: Classification and therapeutic modalities of spinal vascular malformations in 80 patients. Neurosurgery. 40(1):75-81, 1997
8. Hasuo K et al: Contrast-enhanced MRI in spinal arteriovenous malformations and fistulae before and after embolisation therapy. Neuroradiology. 38(7):609-14, 1996
9. Mourier KL et al: Intradural perimedullary arteriovenous fistulae: results of surgical and endovascular treatment in a series of 35 cases. Neurosurgery. 32(6):885-91; discussion 891, 1993
10. Theron J et al: Spinal arteriovenous malformations: advances in therapeutic embolization. Radiology. 158(1):163-9, 1986
11. Horton JA et al: Embolization of intramedullary arteriovenous malformations of the spinal cord. AJNR Am J Neuroradiol. 7(1):113-8, 1986
12. Scialfa G et al: Embolization of vascular malformations of the spinal cord. J Neurosurg Sci. 29(1):1-9, 1985
13. Riche MC et al: Embolization of spinal cord vascular malformations via the anterior spinal artery. AJNR Am J Neuroradiol. 4(3):378-81, 1983

TYPE II AVM

IMAGE GALLERY

Typical

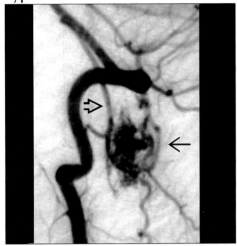

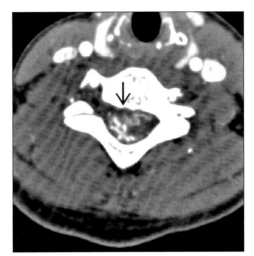

(Left) Lateral angiography of vertebral injection shows dense blush of compact AVM nidus (arrow), being fed from anterior spinal artery (open arrow). (Right) Axial CTA shows multiple serpentine enhancing vessels within substance of cervical cord, eccentric to right representing AVM nidus (arrow).

Typical

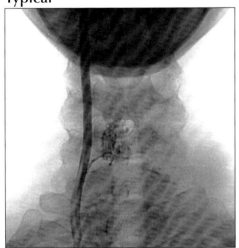

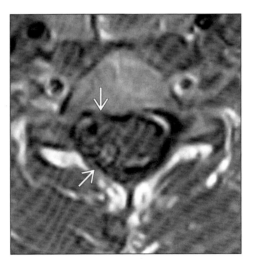

(Left) Anteroposterior angiography of right vertebral injection shows feeding vessels supplying compact AVM nidus involving cervical cord. (Right) Axial T1 C+ MR shows enhancing vessels within right side of the cervical cord, and extending to pial surface (arrows).

Typical

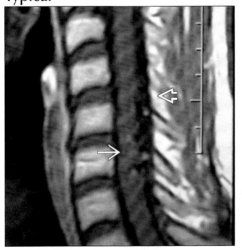

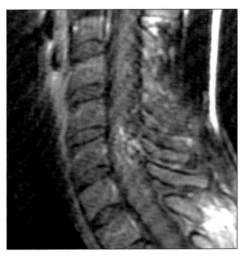

(Left) Sagittal T1WI MR shows multiple flow voids within cord at C6 level (arrow), extending to dorsal pial surface where they merge with draining veins (open arrow) (Right) Sagittal T1 C+ MR with fat suppression shows multiple punctate & linear areas of enhancement within cord from AVM nidus, flow voids dorsal to cord surface from draining veins.

TYPE III AVM

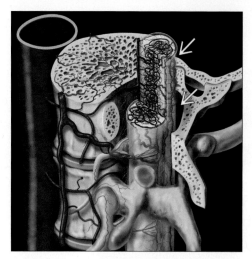

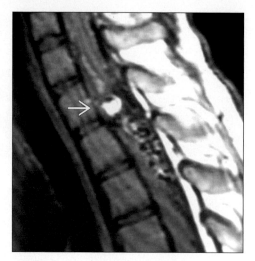

Sagittal oblique graphic of thoracic cord shows large complex intramedullary nidus of type III arteriovenous malformation (arrows), with multiple feeding vessels.

Sagittal T1 C+ MR shows multiple flow voids in cervical cord, and along leptomeninges in this type III AVM. Focal enhancement is within nidal aneurysm (arrow) (Courtesy J. Egelhoff, DO).

TERMINOLOGY

Abbreviations and Synonyms

- Synonyms: Juvenile AVM; intramedullary - extramedullary AVM

Definitions

- Direct arterial/venous communications without capillary bed involving cord
- Spine AVM classification
  - Type I: Dural arteriovenous fistula (DAVF)
    - Most common = type I (up to 80%)
  - Type II: Intramedullary glomus type AVM (similar to brain AVM)
  - Type III: Juvenile-type AVM (large complex intramedullary, extramedullary AVMs)
    - Rarest of spinal AVMs (7%)
  - Type IV: Intradural extra/perimedullary AVF

IMAGING FINDINGS

General Features

- Best diagnostic clue
  - Type I: Flow voids with cord hyperintensity
  - Type II: Intramedullary nidus (may extend to dorsal subpial surface)
  - Type III: Nidus may have extramedullary and extraspinal extension
  - Type IV: Pial fistula (venous varices displace, distort cord)
- Location: Type III: Intramedullary - extramedullary
- Size: Type III tend to be large, complex
- Morphology: Multiple well defined serpentine flow voids within substance of cord

Radiographic Findings

- Myelography
  - Serpentine filling defects from draining veins, enlarged feeding vessels
  - Cord expansion due to edema

CT Findings

- NECT: Usually normal (rare = widened interpedicular distance, posterior vertebral scalloping)
- CECT: May show enlarged cord with enhancing nidus, pial vessels (rare)
- CTA: Shows enhancing nidus, position with respect to cord, and multiple feeding vessels

MR Findings

- T1WI: Large cord, heterogeneous signal (blood products), flow voids
- T2WI: Cord hyperintense (edema, gliosis, ischemia) or mixed (blood)
- STIR: Shows flow voids, edema within cord

DDx: Cervical Intramedullary Disease

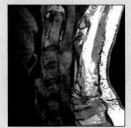

Astrocytoma

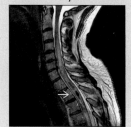

Hemorrhagic Met

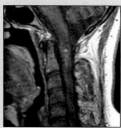

Cavernous Angioma

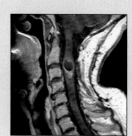

Ependymoma

TYPE III AVM

Key Facts

Terminology
- Synonyms: Juvenile AVM; intramedullary - extramedullary AVM
- Type I: Dural arteriovenous fistula (DAVF)
- Type II: Intramedullary glomus type AVM (similar to brain AVM)
- Type III: Juvenile-type AVM (large complex intramedullary, extramedullary AVMs)
- Type IV: Intradural extra/perimedullary AVF

Imaging Findings
- Type I: Flow voids with cord hyperintensity
- Type II: Intramedullary nidus (may extend to dorsal subpial surface)
- Type III: Nidus may have extramedullary and extraspinal extension

- Type IV: Pial fistula (venous varices displace, distort cord)
- MRA: Dynamic enhanced MRA capable of defining feeding enlarged arteries, nidus, and enlarged draining veins

Pathology
- Associated abnormalities: Type III associated with Cobb syndrome (metameric vascular malformation with triad of spinal cord, skin, bone)

Clinical Issues
- Poor prognosis for juvenile (type III) AVM
- Type III: Complete resection generally not possible, palliative therapy

---

- T2* GRE: More sensitive to blood byproducts of AVM hemorrhage
- T1 C+: Variable enhancement of nidus, cord, vessels
- MRA: Dynamic enhanced MRA capable of defining feeding enlarged arteries, nidus, and enlarged draining veins
- Compare: Types I, IV fistulas
  - T1WI: Ventral or dorsal fistula type IV fistula, large flow voids distort/displace cord
  - T2WI: Type I fistula with T2 hyperintense cord + flow voids
  - Contrast: Enhancing pial vessels, epidural plexus, +/- patchy enhancement distal cord

Angiographic Findings
- Conventional
  - Type I: Peripheral dural fistula may arise anywhere from vertebral artery inferiorly to internal iliac supply
  - Type II: Supplied by anterior spinal artery (ASA) or posterior spinal artery (PSA); nidus drains to coronal venous plexus (on cord surface) which in turn drains anterograde to extradural space
  - Type III: Large complex nidus, multiple feeding vessels; may be intramedullary and extramedullary and even extraspinal
  - Type IV: Feeding vessel from ASA or PSA connects directly with spinal vein (no nidus)

Imaging Recommendations
- Contrast-enhanced MRI; CTA; consider spinal angiography +/- embolization

DIFFERENTIAL DIAGNOSIS

Intramedullary neoplasm
- Ependymoma: Heterogeneous (cysts, blood products)
- Astrocytoma: Multisegmental enhancing mass, no enlarged vessels
- Uncommon: Metastasis with hemorrhage (renal cell)

Intradural extramedullary tumor with prominent vascular supply
- Paraganglioma: Markedly enhancing intradural/extramedullary mass

Cavernous angioma
- Well defined lesion showing speckled pattern on T1WI and T2WI like brain
- No prominent vessels

Type IV perimedullary fistula
- Prominent high flow feeders with varices may compress cord, simulate intramedullary lesion

PATHOLOGY

General Features
- General path comments
  - Location
    - Type I: Lower thoracic/conus common
    - Type II (glomus): Cervical/upper thoracic (may occur anywhere)
    - Type III (juvenile): Cervical/upper thoracic (may occur anywhere)
    - Type IV: Conus medullaris (type A, B), thoracic (type C)
  - Embryology
    - Persistence of primitive direct communications between arterial/venous channels, without intervening capillary bed
- Genetics
  - Sporadic or syndromic
    - Type I: None
    - Type II: Associated with cutaneous angiomas, Klippel-Trenaunay-Weber, Rendu-Osler-Weber syndromes
    - Type III: Associated with Cobb syndrome (metameric vascular malformation with triad of spinal cord, skin, bone)
    - Type IV: Associated with Rendu-Osler-Weber syndrome

TYPE III AVM

- Etiology
  - Type II: Compact nidus, high flow, aneurysms common (20-44%), congenital
  - Type III: Large diffuse nidus, cord ischemia, venous hypertension, congenital
  - Type IV: Congenital; may be acquired after trauma; (A) venous hypertension, (B, C) arterial steal, (C) cord compression
- Epidemiology
  - Intramedullary (type II, III):15-20% of spinal AVM; type IV:10-20%
  - AVMs account for < 10% of spinal masses
- Associated abnormalities: Type III associated with Cobb syndrome (metameric vascular malformation with triad of spinal cord, skin, bone)

Gross Pathologic & Surgical Features
- Type I: Peripheral direct fistula in dura
- Type II: Compact intramedullary nidus lacks normal capillary bed; no parenchyma within nidus; (nidus may have pial extension)
- Type III: Large, complex intramedullary lesion, normal neural parenchyma inside nidus (may involve extramedullary, extradural)
- Type IV: Direct fistula between ASA/PSA & draining vein, no nidus
  - IV-A: Small AVF with slow flow, mild venous enlargement
  - IV-B: Intermediate AVF, dilated arteries; high flow rate
  - IV-C: Large AVF, dilated arteries, veins

Microscopic Features
- Abnormal vessels with variable wall thickness, internal elastic lamina
- Reactive change in surrounding tissue: Gliosis, cytoid bodies, Rosenthal fibers; hemosiderin deposition common; +/- Ca++

CLINICAL ISSUES

Presentation
- Most common signs/symptoms
  - Type I: Progressive myelopathy
  - Type II: SAH most common symptom; pain, myelopathy
  - Type III: Progressive neurologic decline (weakness), SAH
  - Type IV: Progressive conus/cauda equina syndrome, SAH
- Clinical profile: Type III: Young adult with acute SAH, myelopathy

Demographics
- Age: 1st-3rd decades
- Gender: M = F

Natural History & Prognosis
- Poor prognosis for juvenile (type III) AVM
- Good outcome in type II (glomus) and IV (perimedullary)

Treatment
- Type I: Embolization or surgical resection

- Type II: Surgical resection, + pre-op embolization (aneurysms, nidus)
- Type III: Complete resection generally not possible, palliative therapy
- Type IV: Embolization or surgical resection depending upon staging and feeding vessels

DIAGNOSTIC CHECKLIST

Consider
- CTA as localization tool prior to catheter angiography
  - Can define malformation type, location of ASA

Image Interpretation Pearls
- Definition of intramedullary involvement critical for classification, prognosis, treatment options

SELECTED REFERENCES

1. Saraf-Lavi E et al: Detection of spinal dural arteriovenous fistulae with MR imaging and contrast-enhanced MR angiography: sensitivity, specificity, and prediction of vertebral level. AJNR Am J Neuroradiol. 23(5): 858-67, 2002
2. Van Dijk JM et al: Multidisciplinary management of spinal dural arteriovenous fistulas: clinical presentation and long-term follow-up in 49 patients. Stroke. 33(6): 1578-83, 2002
3. Rodesch G et al: Classification of spinal cord arteriovenous shunts: proposal for a reappraisal--the Bicetre experience with 155 consecutive patients treated between 1981 and 1999. Neurosurgery. 51(2): 374-9; discussion 379-80, 2002
4. Spetzler RF et al: Modified classification of spinal cord vascular lesions. J Neurosurg. 96(2 Suppl): 145-56, 2002
5. Mascalchi M et al: Spinal vascular malformations: MR angiography after treatment. Radiology. 219(2): 346-53, 2001
6. Bemporad JA et al: Magnetic resonance imaging of spinal cord vascular malformations with an emphasis on the cervical spine. In Neuropathic basis for imaging. Neuroimaging Clinics of North America 11:111-29, 2001
7. Bemporad JA et al: Magnetic resonance imaging of spinal cord vascular malformations with an emphasis on the cervical spine. Neuroimaging Clin N Am. 11(1): viii, 111-29, 2001
8. Ferch RD et al: Spinal arteriovenous malformations: a review with case illustrations. J Clin Neurosci. 8(4): 299-304, 2001
9. Rosenow J et al: Type IV spinal arteriovenous malformation in association with familial pulmonary vascular malformations: case report. Neurosurgery. 46(5): 1240-4; discussion 1244-5, 2000
10. Mandzia JL et al: Spinal cord arteriovenous malformations in two patients with hereditary hemorrhagic telangiectasia. Childs Nerv Syst. 15(2-3): 80-3, 1999
11. Hasegawa M et al: The efficacy of CT arteriography for spinal arteriovenous fistula surgery: technical note. Neuroradiology. 41(12): 915-9, 1999
12. Bao YH et al: Classification and therapeutic modalities of spinal vascular malformations in 80 patients. Neurosurgery 40:75-81, 1997

IMAGE GALLERY

Typical

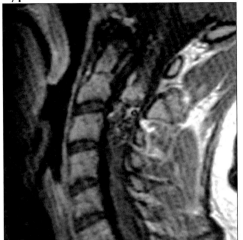 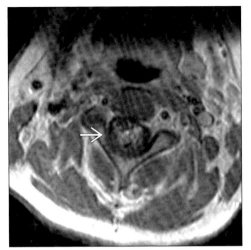

(Left) Sagittal T1 C+ MR shows multiple vascular flow voids within the substance of the cord reflecting intramedullary AVM. There is patchy enhancement of the cord, and cord expansion. *(Right)* Axial T1 C+ MR shows multiple intramedullary flow voids, and enhancing vessels within substance of cord (arrow).

Typical

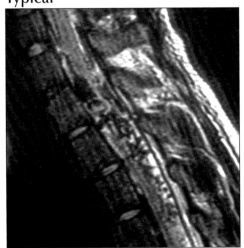 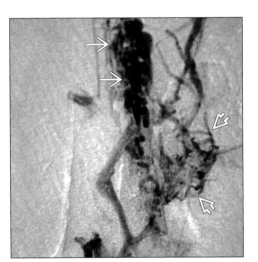

(Left) Sagittal T2WI MR of cervical spine shows long segment of multiple intramedullary flow voids extending onto cord surface (Courtesy J. Egelhoff, DO). *(Right)* Anteroposterior angiography of type III AVM with extradural involvement (Cobb syndrome) shows large draining veins both intradural (arrows) and extradural (open arrows)(Courtesy J. Egelhoff, DO).

Typical

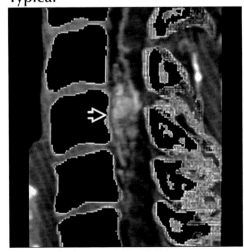 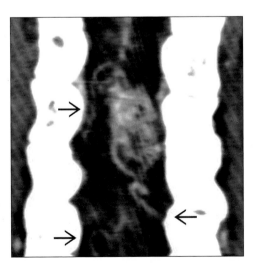

(Left) Sagittal CTA with bone subtraction shows intramedullary nidus (arrow) nearly encompassing entire bony canal. *(Right)* Coronal CTA shows nidus within left side of cord, with multiple feeding vessels (arrows).

TYPE IV AVF

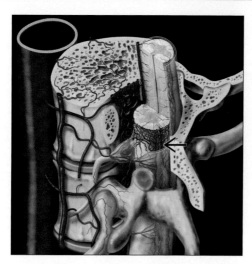

Coronal oblique graphic of thoracic cord shows intradural site of arteriovenous fistula (type IV) on dorsal cord surface with diffuse venous engorgment (arrow).

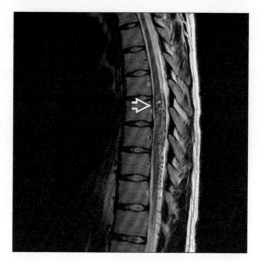

Sagittal T2WI MR shows multiple serpentine intradural/extramedullary flow voids dorsal to thoracic cord, plus focal cord abnormality (arrow) due to high flow aneurysm.

TERMINOLOGY

Abbreviations and Synonyms

- Synonyms: Perimedullary fistula; type IV spinal vascular malformation

Definitions

- Type IV: Direct intradural, extramedullary arterial/venous communication from ASA, or PSA to draining vein without capillary bed
- Spine vascular malformation classification
  - Type I: Dural arteriovenous fistula (DAVF)
    - Most common = type I (up to 80%)
  - Type II: Intramedullary glomus type AVM (similar to brain AVM)
  - Type III: Juvenile-type AVM (intramedullary, extramedullary)
    - Second most common = intramedullary, type II, III (15-20%)
  - Type IV: Intradural extra/perimedullary AVF (types A, B, C)

IMAGING FINDINGS

General Features

- Best diagnostic clue
  - Type I: Flow voids with cord hyperintensity

- Type II: Intramedullary nidus (may extend to dorsal subpial surface)
- Type III: Nidus may have extramedullary and extraspinal extension
- Type IV: Ventral fistula (venous varices displace, distort cord)
- Location
  - Type IV: Intradural location for fistula, adjacent to the cord
  - Draining veins may be pronounced on dorsal or ventral surface of cord
- Size: Variable depending on number of feeding vessels, size of draining veins, presence of aneurysms
- Morphology: Multiple well-defined serpentine flow voids

Radiographic Findings

- Myelography: Serpentine filling defects along cord

CT Findings

- NECT: Usually normal (rare = widened interpediculate distance, posterior vertebral scalloping)
- CECT: May show enlarged cord with enhancing nidus, pial vessels (rare)
- CTA
  - Intradural draining veins identifiable; precise fistula site more difficult
  - Postprocessing mandatory for best anatomic display

DDx: Prominent Intradural "Flow Voids" and Mimics

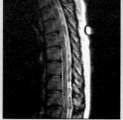

Normal CSF Motion

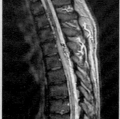

Type I Dural Fistula

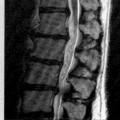

Tortuous Roots

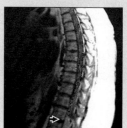

Intradural Tumor

TYPE IV AVF

Key Facts

Terminology

- Synonyms: Perimedullary fistula; type IV spinal vascular malformation
- Type I: Dural arteriovenous fistula (DAVF)
- Type II: Intramedullary glomus type AVM (similar to brain AVM)
- Type III: Juvenile-type AVM (intramedullary, extramedullary)
- Type IV: Intradural extra/perimedullary AVF (types A, B, C)

Imaging Findings

- Type I: Flow voids with cord hyperintensity
- Type II: Intramedullary nidus (may extend to dorsal subpial surface)

- Type III: Nidus may have extramedullary and extraspinal extension
- Type IV: Ventral fistula (venous varices displace, distort cord)
- Type IV: Feeding vessel from ASA or PSA connects directly with spinal vein (no nidus)

Clinical Issues

- Type IV-A tends to surgical resection since normal caliber ASA is inaccessible to embolization
- Type IV-B have dilated feeding vessels allowing embolization, or surgery
- Type IV-C have high flow state, and most emendable to embolization

MR Findings

- T1WI
  - Type IV (perimedullary)
  - Ventral fistula, large flow voids distort/displace cord
- T2WI: Hyperintense cord + flow voids
- T1 C+: Enhancing pial vessels, epidural plexus, +/- patchy enhancement distal cord
- MRA
  - Dynamic enhanced MRA capable of defining distending draining veins.
  - Spatial resolution generally inadequate for arterial feeders
- Compare: Types II, III (intramedullary AVMs)
  - T1WI: Large cord, heterogeneous signal (blood products), flow voids
  - T2WI: Cord hyperintense (edema, gliosis, ischemia) or mixed (blood)
  - Contrast enhanced T1WI: Variable enhancement of nidus, cord, vessels

Angiographic Findings

- Conventional
  - Type I: Peripheral dural fistula may arise anywhere from vertebral artery inferiorly to internal iliac supply
  - Type II: Supplied by anterior spinal artery (ASA) or posterior spinal artery (PSA); nidus drains to coronal venous plexus (on cord surface) which in turn drains anterograde to extradural space
  - Type III: Large complex nidus, multiple feeding vessels; may be intramedullary and extramedullary and even extraspinal
  - Type IV: Feeding vessel from ASA or PSA connects directly with spinal vein (no nidus)

Imaging Recommendations

- Contrast-enhanced MRI; CTA; consider spinal angiography +/- embolization

DIFFERENTIAL DIAGNOSIS

Normal CSF flow artifact

- Most prominent dorsal to thoracic cord
- Ill-defined margins, appearance varies with different sequences

Lumbar canal stenosis with tortuous intradural roots

- Distinguished by presence of severe central stenosis
- Redundant serpentine roots stop at conus

Intramedullary neoplasm

- Ependymoma: Heterogeneous (cysts, blood products)
- Astrocytoma: Multisegmental enhancing mass, no enlarged vessels

Intradural/extramedullary tumor with prominent vascular supply

- Paraganglioma: Markedly enhancing intradural/extramedullary mass

Type I dural fistula

- May be indistinguishable from type IV by MR, CTA

PATHOLOGY

General Features

- General path comments
  - Location
    - Type I: Lower thoracic/conus common
    - Type II (glomus): Cervical/upper thoracic (may occur anywhere)
    - Type III (juvenile): Cervical/upper thoracic (may occur anywhere)
    - Type IV: Conus medullaris (type A, B), thoracic (type C)
  - Embryology
    - Persistence of primitive direct communications between arterial & venous channels, without intervening capillary bed
- Genetics

TYPE IV AVF

- ○ Sporadic or syndromic
  - Type I: None
  - Type II: Associated with cutaneous angiomas, Klippel-Trenaunay-Weber, Rendu-Osler-Weber syndromes
  - Type III: Associated with Cobb syndrome (metameric vascular malformation involving triad of spinal cord, skin, bone)
  - Type IV: Associated with Rendu-Osler-Weber syndrome
- • Etiology
  - ○ Type IV: Congenital
  - ○ May be acquired after trauma
- • Epidemiology
  - ○ Intramedullary (type II, III): 15-20% of spinal AVM
  - ○ Type IV: 10-20% of spinal AVMs
  - ○ AVMs account for < 10% of spinal masses
- • Associated abnormalities: Type IV: Associated with Rendu-Osler-Weber syndrome

Gross Pathologic & Surgical Features
- • Type I: Peripheral direct fistula in dura
- • Type II: Compact intramedullary nidus lacks normal capillary bed; no parenchyma within nidus; (nidus may have pial extension)
- • Type III: Large, complex intramedullary lesion, normal neural parenchyma inside nidus (may involve extramedullary, extradural)
- • Type IV: Direct fistula between ASA/PSA & draining vein, no nidus

Microscopic Features
- • Abnormal vessels with variable wall thickness, internal elastic lamina
- • Reactive change in surrounding tissue: Gliosis, cytoid bodies, Rosenthal fibers; hemosiderin deposition common; +/- Ca++

Staging, Grading or Classification Criteria
- • IV-A: Small AVF with slow flow, mild venous enlargement
- • IV-B: Intermediate AVF, dilated feeding arteries; high flow rate
- • IV-C: Large AVF, dilated feeding arteries; dilated, tortuous veins

CLINICAL ISSUES

Presentation
- • Most common signs/symptoms
  - ○ Type I: Progressive myelopathy
  - ○ Type II: SAH most common symptom; pain, myelopathy
  - ○ Type III: Progressive neurologic decline (weakness), SAH
  - ○ Type IV: Progressive conus/cauda equina syndrome, SAH
    - Type IV-A with slow flow, venous hypertension primary cause of symptoms, no SAH
    - Types IV-B, C show arterial steal and cord compression from venous varices, SAH

Demographics
- • Age: Child and adult

- • Gender: M = F

Natural History & Prognosis
- • Type I: 40-60% improve following obliteration of fistula, 40-50% stabilize myelopathic symptoms
- • Type II, IV: Generally good outcome
- • Type III: Poor prognosis

Treatment
- • Type IV: Embolization or surgical resection based upon anatomy and size: (A) surgical resection, (B) surgical resection or embolization, (C) embolization
  - ○ Type IV-A tends to surgical resection since normal caliber ASA is inaccessible to embolization
  - ○ Type IV-B have dilated feeding vessels allowing embolization, or surgery
  - ○ Type IV-C have high flow state, and most emendable to embolization

DIAGNOSTIC CHECKLIST

Consider
- • CTA as localization tool prior to catheter angiography
  - ○ Can define malformation type, location of ASA

SELECTED REFERENCES
1. Hida K et al: Corpectomy: a direct approach to perimedullary arteriovenous fistulas of the anterior cervical spinal cord. J Neurosurg. 96(2 Suppl): 157-61, 2002
2. Rodesch G et al: Classification of spinal cord arteriovenous shunts: proposal for a reappraisal--the Bicetre experience with 155 consecutive patients treated between 1981 and 1999. Neurosurgery. 51(2): 374-9; discussion 379-80, 2002
3. Spetzler RF et al: Modified classification of spinal cord vascular lesions. J Neurosurg. 96(2 Suppl): 145-56, 2002
4. Mascalchi M et al: Spinal vascular malformations: MR angiography after treatment. Radiology. 219(2): 346-53, 2001
5. Vates GE et al: Conus perimedullary arteriovenous fistula with intracranial drainage: case report. Neurosurgery. 49(2): 457-61; discussion 461-2, 2001
6. Sugiu K et al: Successful embolization of a spinal perimedullary arteriovenous fistula with cellulose acetate polymer solution: technical case report. Neurosurgery. 49(5): 1257-60; discussion 1260-1, 2001
7. Sure U et al: Spinal type IV arteriovenous malformations (perimedullary fistulas) in children. Childs Nerv Syst. 16(8): 508-15, 2000
8. Grote EH et al: Clinical syndromes, natural history, and pathophysiology of vascular lesions of the spinal cord. Neurosurg Clin N Am. 10(1): 17-45, 1999
9. Hida K et al: Results of the surgical treatment of perimedullary arteriovenous fistulas with special reference to embolization. J Neurosurg. 90(4 Suppl): 198-205, 1999
10. Mascalchi M et al: Contrast-enhanced time-resolved MR angiography of spinal vascular malformations. J Comput Assist Tomogr. 23(3): 341-5, 1999
11. Bao YH et al: Classification and therapeutic modalities of spinal vascular malformations in 80 patients. Neurosurgery. 40:75-81, 1997
12. Ricolfi F et al: Giant perimedullary arteriovenous fistulas of the spine: clinical and radiologic features and endovascular treatment. AJNR Am J Neuroradiol. 18(4): 677-87, 1997

IMAGE GALLERY

Typical

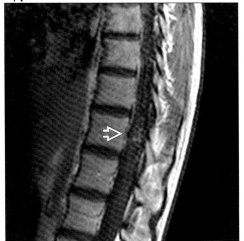 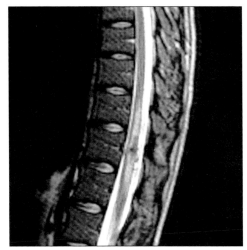

(Left) Sagittal T1 C+ MR shows multiple enhancing intradural vessels surrounding distal cord. *(Right)* Sagittal T2WI MR shows high signal within distal cord due to edema, & more focal low signal reflecting compressing perimedullary vessels.

Typical

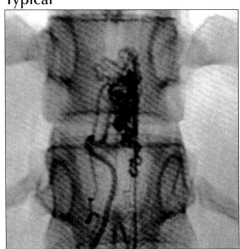 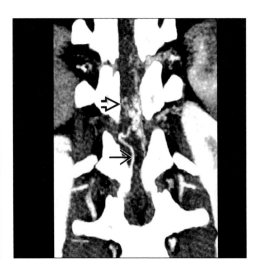

(Left) Anteroposterior angiography shows vascular malformation supplied by radicular artery on pial surface of cord. Shunting is at cord level (type IV), not at dural level (type I). *(Right)* Coronal CTA shows similar pattern to vascular malformation, fed by right radicular artery (arrow) with dilated veins on the dorsal cord (open arrow).

Typical

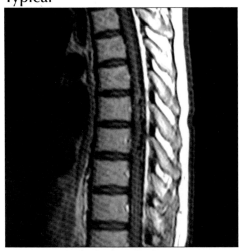 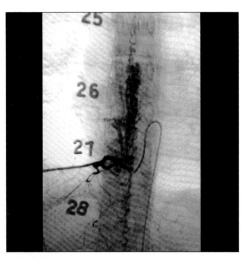

(Left) Sagittal T1WI MR shows multiple serpentine flow voids dorsal to the thoracic cord from the intradural type IV fistula. *(Right)* Anteroposterior angiography shows the fistular fed by right radicular artery, with multiple dilated perimedullary veins.

CAVERNOUS MALFORMATION, SPINAL CORD

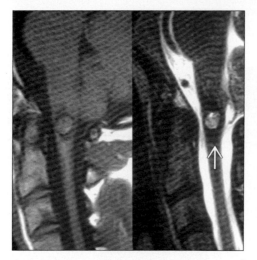

Sagittal T1WI MR (left) and T2WI (right) show well defined lesion with typical heterogeneous signal of cavernous malformation. Note prominent hemosiderin rim on T2WI (arrow).

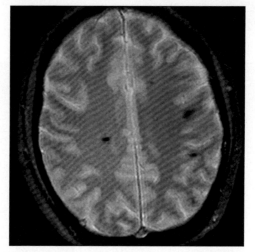

Axial T2* GRE MR shows associated multiple low signal intracranial cavernous malformations in patient with spinal cord cavernous malformation.

TERMINOLOGY

Abbreviations and Synonyms
- Cavernous malformation (CM)
- Synonyms include cavernous angioma, cavernous hemangioma, "cryptic" vascular malformation

Definitions
- Vascular lesion with lobulated, thin sinusoidal vascular channels, no interspersed neural tissue

IMAGING FINDINGS

General Features
- Best diagnostic clue: Locules of blood with fluid-fluid levels surrounded by very T2 hypointense rim
- Location: Spinal cord uncommon site, 3-5% of all cavernous malformations
- Size: Few mm, punctate to > 1 cm
- Morphology: Round heterogeneous signal abnormality, well-defined margins

CT Findings
- NECT: Often normal; cord may appear widened
- CECT: +/- Faint enhancement (rare)

MR Findings
- T1WI
  - Heterogeneous (blood products, varying ages)
  - Typical speckled "popcorn" heterogeneous signal
  - Small lesion may not show obvious heterogeneous signal
- T2WI
  - Heterogeneous, hypointense rim (hemosiderin)
  - Small lesion may not show obvious heterogeneous signal, may only show focal low signal
  - No edema, unless recent hemorrhage
- T2* GRE: Prominent "blooming" due to susceptibility effects
- T1 C+: Enhancement absent/minimal

Angiographic Findings
- Conventional: Negative (one of "angiographically occult" vascular malformations)

Imaging Recommendations
- MRI spine (use gradient echo, contrast sequences to exclude other etiologies)
- Scan the brain (may show other lesions)

DIFFERENTIAL DIAGNOSIS

Intramedullary neoplasm
- Ependymoma: Enhancing mass with cysts, blood products; flow foids rare

---

DDx: Hemorrhagic Cord Lesions

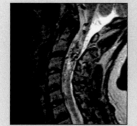

AVM

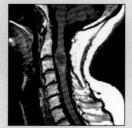

Ependymoma

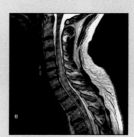

Hemorrhagic Met

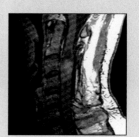

Astrocytoma

Key Facts

Terminology

- Cavernous malformation (CM)
- Synonyms include cavernous angioma, cavernous hemangioma, "cryptic" vascular malformation
- Vascular lesion with lobulated, thin sinusoidal vascular channels, no interspersed neural tissue

Imaging Findings

- Best diagnostic clue: Locules of blood with fluid-fluid levels surrounded by very T2 hypointense rim
- Location: Spinal cord uncommon site, 3-5% of all cavernous malformations

Top Differential Diagnoses

- Intramedullary neoplasm
- AVM
- Multiple sclerosis

Pathology

- Thoracic (50%)
- Cervical (40%)
- Conus (10%)
- Multiple (familial) CM syndrome (20%)
- Autosomal dominant, variable penetrance
- Familial CMs at high risk for hemorrhage, forming new lesions

Clinical Issues

- Sensorimotor deficits, progressive paraparesis
- Gender: M:F = 1:2

Diagnostic Checklist

- Scan brain for additional lesions!

- Astrocytoma: Multisegmental enhancing mass (hemorrhage uncommon)
- Hemangioblastoma: Vascular nodule; "flow voids" common
- Metastatis: Enhancing mass with edema, hemorrhage

AVM

- Enlarged flow voids with vascular nidus
- DSA reveals enlarged feeding arteries, nidus, early draining veins

Multiple sclerosis

- Clinical course of spinal cavernous malformations resembles multiple sclerosis with chronicity, exacerbations
- No blood byproducts/hemosiderin in MS

PATHOLOGY

General Features

- General path comments
  - Identical to intracranial cavernous malformations
  - Location
    - Thoracic (50%)
    - Cervical (40%)
    - Conus (10%)
- Genetics
  - Multiple (familial) CM syndrome (20%)
    - Autosomal dominant, variable penetrance
    - Mutation in chromosomes 3, 7q (Hispanic-Americans)
  - Familial CMs at high risk for hemorrhage, forming new lesions
    - Familial characterized by higher frequency multiple CMs, infratentorial location, lower age at clinical presentation
- Etiology: Angiogenically immature lesions with endothelial proliferation, increased neoangiogenesis; VEGF, βFGF, TGFα expressed
- Epidemiology
  - 10-30% multiple, familial
  - 70% of spinal CMs in females
  - Cranial irradiation suspected risk factor for cerebral CMs

Gross Pathologic & Surgical Features

- Discrete, lobulated blue-reddish brown ("mulberry-like") nodule
- Pseudocapsule (gliotic, hemosiderin-stained cord)

Microscopic Features

- Vascular spaces with single layer of endothelial cells
- Vascular spaces separated by collagenous walls without smooth muscle or elastin
- Histologic features of arteries, capillaries and vein generally lacking
- No intervening neural tissue between vascular spaces
  - Ca++ rare (common in brain cavernous malformations)
  - Blood products in different stages of evolution
  - Areas of partial & complete thrombosis
- No true surrounding capsule
  - Surrounding neural tissue shows gliosis, atrophy, hemosiderin, calcium & iron deposits

CLINICAL ISSUES

Presentation

- Most common signs/symptoms
  - Sensorimotor deficits, progressive paraparesis
  - Four clinical patterns
    - Multiple episodes of neurological deterioration, intermittent recovery
    - Slowly progressive neurological decline
    - Sudden symptom onset with rapid decline (hours-days)
    - Mild symptoms with acute onset, gradual decline (weeks-months)
  - Extremely rare: Subarachnoid hemorrhage
- Clinical profile: Young adult with sudden paraplegia

Demographics

- Age
  - Between 3rd and 6th decade
    - Range = 12-88 years

- ▪ Peak = 4th decade
- Gender: M:F = 1:2

Natural History & Prognosis
- Broad range of dynamic behavior (may progress, enlarge, regress)
- De novo lesions may develop (especially in familial CM syndrome)
- Clinical course varies from slow progression to acute quadriplegia
- Bleeding rate ~ 1-5% per lesion per year

Treatment
- Conservative management if asymptomatic
  ○ Follow with serial MRI
- Surgical resection for symptomatic lesions
  ○ Long pre-treatment duration (~ 3 years)
  ○ Post-operative outcome related to pre-operative neurologic status
  ○ 66% improve, 28% stable, 6% deterioration post-operatively

DIAGNOSTIC CHECKLIST

Consider
- Other hemorrhagic lesions if no classic speckled pattern, or hemosiderin margins

Image Interpretation Pearls
- Heterogeneous mass ("locules" of blood with "popcorn" appearance) surrounded by dark rim (hemosiderin)
- Scan brain for additional lesions!
- Screen with GRE

SELECTED REFERENCES

1. Sandalcioglu IE et al: Intramedullary spinal cord cavernous malformations: clinical features and risk of hemorrhage. Neurosurg Rev. 26(4):253-6, 2003
2. Musunuru K et al: Widespread central nervous system cavernous malformations associated with cafe-au-lait skin lesions. Case report. J Neurosurg. 99(2):412-5, 2003
3. Nagib MG et al: Intramedullary cavernous angiomas of the spinal cord in the pediatric age group: a pediatric series. Pediatr Neurosurg. 36(2):57-63, 2002
4. Chen DH et al: Cerebral cavernous malformation: novel mutation in a Chinese family and evidence for heterogeneity. J Neurol Sci. 196(1-2):91-6, 2002
5. Mottolese C et al: Central nervous system cavernomas in the pediatric age group. Neurosurg Rev. 24(2-3):55-71; discussion 72-3, 2001
6. Balaban H et al: Multiple spinal intramedullary cavernous angioma: case report. Clin Neurol Neurosurg. 103(2):120-2, 2001
7. Sure U et al: Endothelial proliferation, neoangiogenesis, and potential de novo generation of cerebrovascular malformations. J Neurosurg 94:972-7, 2001
8. Clatterbuck RE et al: The nature and fate of punctate (Type IV) cavernous malformations. Neurosurg 49:26-32, 2001
9. Deutsch H et al: Pediatric intramedullary spinal cavernous malformations. Spine. 26(18):E427-31, 2001
10. Zacharia TT et al: Co-existing spinal cord and brain cavernous angiomas. J Assoc Physicians India. 49:835-7, 2001
11. Deutsch H et al: Spinal intramedullary cavernoma: clinical presentation and surgical outcome. J Neurosurg. 93(1

Suppl):65-70, 2000
12. Vishteh AG et al: Patients with spinal cord cavernous malformations are at an increased risk for multiple neuraxis cavernous malformations. Neurosurgery. 45(1):30-2; discussion 33, 1999
13. Moriarity JL et al: The natural history of cavernous malformations. Neurosurg Clin N Am. 10(3):411-7, 1999
14. Chabert E et al: Intramedullary cavernous malformations. J Neuroradiol. 26(4):262-8, 1999
15. Zevgaridis D et al: Cavernous haemangiomas of the spinal cord. A review of 117 cases. Acta Neurochir (Wien). 141(3):237-45, 1999
16. Duke BJ et al: Cavernous angiomas of the cauda equina: case report and review of the literature. Surg Neurol. 50(5):442-5, 1998
17. Naim-Ur-Rahman et al: Intramedullary ossified cavernous angioma of the spinal cord: case report. Br J Neurosurg. 12(3):267-70, 1998
18. Huffmann BC et al: Treatment strategies and results in spinal vascular malformations. Neurol Med Chir (Tokyo). 38 Suppl:231-7, 1998
19. Padovani R et al: Cavernous angiomas of the spinal district: surgical treatment of 11 patients. Eur Spine J. 6(5):298-303, 1997
20. Turjman F et al: MRI of intramedullary cavernous haemangiomas. Neuroradiology. 37(4):297-302, 1995
21. Harrison MJ et al: Symptomatic cavernous malformations affecting the spine and spinal cord. Neurosurgery. 37(2):195-204; discussion 204-5, 1995
22. Spetzger U et al: Cavernous angiomas of the spinal cord clinical presentation, surgical strategy, and postoperative results. Acta Neurochir (Wien). 134(3-4):200-6, 1995
23. Canavero S et al: Spinal intramedullary cavernous angiomas: a literature meta-analysis. Surg Neurol. 41(5):381-8, 1994
24. Acciarri N et al: Surgical treatment of spinal cavernous angiomas. J Neurosurg Sci. 37(4):209-15, 1993
25. Acciarri N et al: Spinal cavernous angioma: a rare cause of subarachnoid hemorrhage. Surg Neurol. 37(6):453-6, 1992
26. Bourgouin PM et al: Multiple occult vascular malformations of the brain and spinal cord: MRI diagnosis. Neuroradiology. 34(2):110-1, 1992

IMAGE GALLERY

Typical

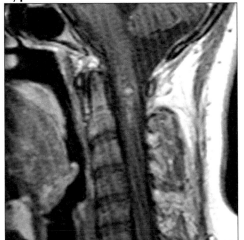 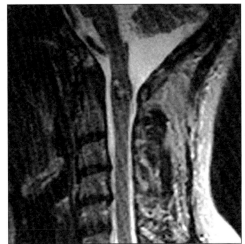

(Left) Sagittal T1WI MR shows focal high signal within cord at C2 due to hemorrhage, which extends inferiorly to C2-3. Superior portion has well-defined margins. *(Right)* Sagittal T2WI MR shows heterogeneous signal from lesion in cord at C2, with peripheral low signal (hemosiderin).

Typical

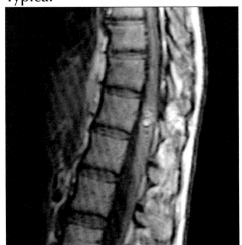 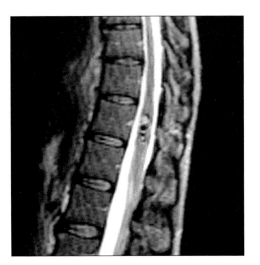

(Left) Sagittal T1WI MR shows focal hemorrhage within distal thoracic cord, with heterogeneous signal. *(Right)* Sagittal T2WI MR shows well-defined region of heterogeneous signal within cord due to various ages of blood byproducts. There is no adjacent cord hyperintensity.

Typical

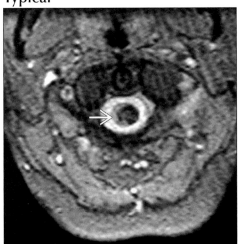 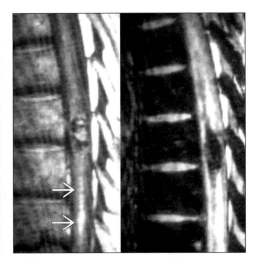

(Left) Axial T2* GRE MR shows cavernous malformation as patchy low signal within cervical cord (arrow). *(Right)* Sagittal T1WI MR (left side) shows mixed signal within thoracic cord with well-defined margins. Hemorrhage extends inferiorly into distal cord (arrows). T2* GE study (right side) shows blooming.

SPINAL CORD INFARCTION

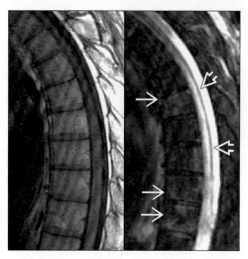

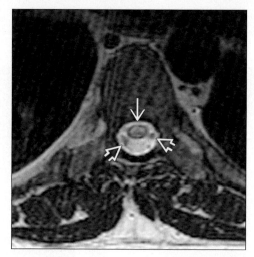

Sagittal T1WI MR (left side) is unremarkable. STIR MR (right side) shows hyperintense foci in thoracic bodies (arrows) & cord (open arrows) due to bone + parenchymal infarcts.

Axial T2WI MR shows central hyperintensity involving gray matter of cord (arrow), typical for infarction. Low signal foci surrounding cord is CSF pulsation artifact (open arrows).

TERMINOLOGY

Abbreviations and Synonyms
- Spinal cord infarction (SCI); cord ischemia

Definitions
- Permanent tissue loss in spinal cord due to vessel occlusion, typically radicular branch of vertebral artery (cervical cord) or aorta (thoracic & lumbar cord)

IMAGING FINDINGS

General Features
- Best diagnostic clue: Focal hyperintensity on T2WI in slightly expanded cord
- Location: Most frequent in thoracic cord because of arterial border zone
- Size: Variable, but usually > 1 vertebral body segment
- Morphology: Central hyperintensity on T2WI

CT Findings
- NECT: Noncontributory
- CTA
  - Generally noncontributory
  - Wide variability in presence of intercostals arteries with aortic aneurysm with thrombosis
  - Definition of anterior spinal artery (ASA) possible, but technically challenging

MR Findings
- T1WI
  - Sight cord expansion, & decreased signal
  - Early may have no significant T1 signal abnormality
  - Atrophy in late stage
  - Focal hemorrhage conversion may occur with hyperintensity on T1WI & hypointensity on T2WI
  - May see large vessel abnormalities such as aortic aneurysm or dissection
- T2WI
  - T2 hyperintensity in gray matter, gray matter with adjacent white matter, or entire cross sectional area of cord
  - Marrow T2 hyperintensity in anterior vertebral body or in deep medullary portion near endplate may be present due to vertebral body infarct
- STIR
  - Nonspecific increased signal in cord
  - Marrow hyperintensity may be present due to vertebral body infarct
- DWI: Shows abnormal restricted diffusion (as in brain with infarct)
- T1 C+: May show patchy ill-defined enhancement in subacute phase
- MRA: Noncontributory since resolution of dynamic enhanced MRA not sufficient to define ASA

DDx: Cord T2WI Hyperintensity

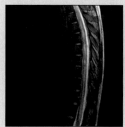

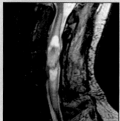

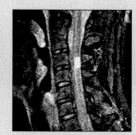

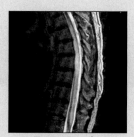

| *ADEM* | *Astrocytoma* | *MS* | *Type I Fistula* |

SPINAL CORD INFARCTION

Key Facts

Terminology
- Spinal cord infarction (SCI); cord ischemia
- Permanent tissue loss in spinal cord due to vessel occlusion, typically radicular branch of vertebral artery (cervical cord) or aorta (thoracic & lumbar cord)

Imaging Findings
- Best diagnostic clue: Focal hyperintensity on T2WI in slightly expanded cord
- Location: Most frequent in thoracic cord because of arterial border zone
- Focal hemorrhage conversion may occur with hyperintensity on T1WI & hypointensity on T2WI
- May see large vessel abnormalities such as aortic aneurysm or dissection

- T2 hyperintensity in gray matter, gray matter with adjacent white matter, or entire cross sectional area of cord
- Marrow T2 hyperintensity in anterior vertebral body or in deep medullary portion near endplate may be present due to vertebral body infarct
- DWI: Shows abnormal restricted diffusion (as in brain with infarct)
- T2WI sagittal and axial, 3 mm slice thickness; DWI of cord

Top Differential Diagnoses
- Multiple sclerosis (MS)
- Spinal cord neoplasm
- Idiopathic transverse myelitis
- Type I dural fistula

Angiographic Findings
- Conventional: Spinal artery occlusion

Imaging Recommendations
- T2WI sagittal and axial, 3 mm slice thickness; DWI of cord

DIFFERENTIAL DIAGNOSIS

Multiple sclerosis (MS)
- Peripheral in location
- Less than two vertebral segments in length
- Less than half cross-sectional area of cord
- 90% incidence of associated intracranial lesions
- Relapsing & remitting clinical course

Spinal cord neoplasm
- Cord expansion invariably present
- Diffuse or nodular contrast enhancement
- Extensive peri-tumoral edema
- Associated cystic changes
- Slower clinical onset

Idiopathic transverse myelitis
- Lesion centrally located
- 3 to 4 segments in length
- Occupying more than two-thirds of cord's cross-sectional area
- No associated intracranial lesions
- Onset not quite as sudden

Type I dural fistula
- May rarely show only cord expansion and edema on T2WI, without prominent vessels
- Typical findings include prominent enlarged serpentine pial veins on cord surface

PATHOLOGY

General Features
- General path comments

- Embryology-anatomy
  - Seven to eight of 62 (31 pairs) radicular arteries supply spinal cord in three territories
  - Cervicothoracic territory includes the cervical cord & first two or three thoracic segments, supplied by anterior spinal artery from vertebral artery + branches of the costocervical trunk
  - Midthoracic territory includes fourth to eighth thoracic segments, supplied by radicular branch from aorta at T7 level
  - Thoracolumbar territory includes remainder of thoracic segments + lumbar cord, supplied by artery of Adamkiewicz
  - Artery of Adamkiewicz usually originates from 9th, 10th, 11th, or 12th intercostal artery (75%), less commonly from higher intercostal artery or lumbar artery
  - Radicular arteries form one anterior & two posterior spinal arteries
  - Anterior spinal arteries + branches supply gray matter + an adjacent mantle of white matter
  - Posterior spinal arteries + branches supply one-third to one-half of periphery of cord
- Genetics
  - Rare: CADASIL (cerebral autosomal dominant arteriopathy with subcortical infarcts and leukoencephalopathy)
    - Mapped to chromosome 19q12
    - Subarachnoid vessel abnormalities including concentric thickening of media and adventitia
- Etiology
  - Idiopathic
  - Atherosclerosis
  - Thoracoabdominal aneurysm
  - Aortic surgery
  - Systemic hypotension
  - Infection
  - Embolic disease
  - Spinal arteriovenous malformation
  - Vasculitis
  - Dissection (vertebral or aortic)
  - Decompression sickness
  - Coagulopathy

SPINAL CORD INFARCTION

○ Post anesthesia complication (epidural injection, celiac plexus block)
- Epidemiology: Rare, usually patients > 50
- Associated abnormalities: Atherosclerotic risk factors such as hypertension, diabetes, cigarette smoking

Gross Pathologic & Surgical Features
- Change with time
- Soft pale, swollen tissue with increasingly distinct margin with more normal tissue over time

Microscopic Features
- Acute: Ischemic neurons with cytotoxic + vasogenic edema, swelling of endothelial cells + astrocytes
- Subacute: Increasing numbers of phagocytic cells, activated microglia
- Chronic: Macrophages contain myelin breakdown products, progression of astrocytic reaction with protoplasmic extensions

CLINICAL ISSUES

Presentation
- Most common signs/symptoms
  ○ Anterior spinal syndrome presents with paralysis, loss of pain and temperature sensation, bladder & bowel dysfunction
  ○ Posterior spinal cord infarction characterized by loss of proprioception + vibration sense, paresis, sphincter dysfunction
  ○ Sudden onset of neurologic deficits helps to make diagnosis
  ○ Other signs/symptoms
    ▪ Anterior sulcus artery occlusion presents with Brown-Sequard syndrome
- Clinical profile
  ○ Abrupt onset of weakness, loss of sensation
  ○ Rapid progression of neurologic deficits, reaching maximum impairment within hours

Demographics
- Age: > 50
- Gender: M = F

Natural History & Prognosis
- Acute spinal cord ischemia syndrome has severe prognosis with permanent disabling sequelae
- > 20% in-hospital mortality rate

Treatment
- Anticoagulation
- Intravenous corticosteroids
- Maintain systemic perfusion
- Physical rehabilitation

DIAGNOSTIC CHECKLIST

Consider
- Associated vertebral infarction seen as T2 hyperintensity allowing specific diagnosis of nonspecific cord signal change

Image Interpretation Pearls
- Classic imaging appearance: T2 hyperintensity involving the anterior horn cells
- Check for aortic aneurysm or dissection

SELECTED REFERENCES

1. Weidauer S et al: Spinal cord infarction: MR imaging and clinical features in 16 cases. Neuroradiology. 44(10): 851-7, 2002
2. Bornke C et al: Vertebral body infarction indicating midthoracic spinal stroke. Spinal Cord. 40(5): 244-7, 2002
3. White ML et al: Neurovascular injuries of the spinal cord. Eur J Radiol. 42(2): 117-26, 2002
4. Chan LL et al: Post-epidural analgesia spinal cord infarction: MRI correlation. Acta Neurol Scand. 105(4): 344-8, 2002
5. Salvador de la Barrera S et al: Spinal cord infarction: prognosis and recovery in a series of 36 patients. Spinal Cord. 39(10): 520-5, 2001
6. de Seze J et al: Acute myelopathies: Clinical, laboratory and outcome profiles in 79 cases. Brain. 124(Pt 8): 1509-21, 2001
7. Pathak M et al: Spinal cord infarction following vertebral angiography: clinical and pathological findings. J Spinal Cord Med. 23(2): 92-5, 2000
8. Bowen BC et al: Vascular anatomy and disorders of the lumbar spine and spinal cord. Magn Reson Imaging Clin N Am. 7(3): 555-71, 1999
9. Amano Y et al: Spinal cord infarcts with contrast enhancement of the cauda equina: two cases. Neuroradiology. 40(10): 669-72, 1998
10. Suzuki K et al: Anterior spinal artery syndrome associated with severe stenosis of the vertebral artery. AJNR Am J Neuroradiol. 19(7): 1353-5, 1998
11. Mascalchi M et al: Posterior spinal artery infarct. AJNR Am J Neuroradiol. 19(2): 361-3, 1998
12. Faig J et al: Vertebral body infarction as a confirmatory sign of spinal cord ischemic stroke: report of three cases and review of the literature. Stroke. 29(1): 239-43, 1998
13. Cheshire WP et al: Spinal cord infarction: etiology and outcome. Neurology. 47(2): 321-30, 1996
14. Suh DC et al: MRI in presumed cervical anterior spinal artery territory infarcts. Neuroradiology. 38(1): 56-8, 1996
15. Gaeta TJ et al: Anterior spinal artery infarction. Ann Emerg Med. 26(1): 90-3, 1995
16. Fortuna A et al: Spinal cord ischemia diagnosed by MRI. Case report and review of the literature. J Neuroradiol. 22(2): 115-22, 1995
17. Yuh WT et al: MR imaging of spinal cord and vertebral body infarction. AJNR 13:145-154, 1992
18. Berlit P et al: Spinal cord infarction: MRI and MEP findings in three cases. Journal of Spinal Disorders 5:212-216, 1992
19. Mawad ME et al: Spinal cord ischemia after resection of thoracoabdominal aortic aneurysms: MR findings in 24 patients. AJNR 11:987-991, 1990

IMAGE GALLERY

Typical

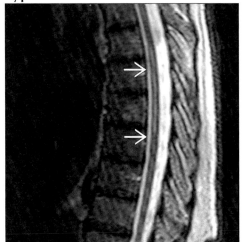
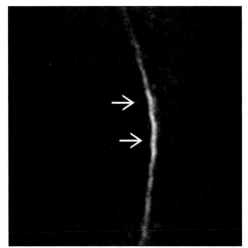

(Left) Sagittal T2WI MR shows linear hyperintensity within central thoracic cord due to infarction *(arrows)*. *(Right)* Sagittal DWI MR shows abnormal increased signal (restricted diffusion) from thoracic cord infarct *(arrows)*. Adjacent soft tissue not visible due to high b value utilized.

Typical

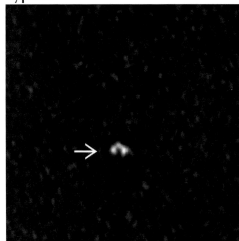
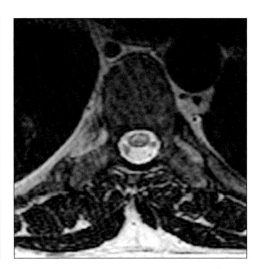

(Left) Axial DWI MR shows restricted diffusion (high signal) from central gray matter of cord *(arrow)*. Remainder of extramedullary tissues low in signal due to high b value utilized. *(Right)* Axial T2WI MR shows increased signal from central gray matter, sparing cord periphery. Patient also had positive diffusion study for acute infarct.

Typical

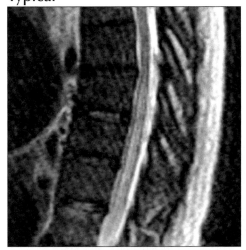
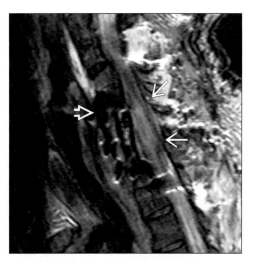

(Left) Sagittal T2WI MR in a patient following aortic aneurysm surgery shows increased signal within distal cord/conus due to infarct. *(Right)* Sagittal T2WI MR following multilevel corpectomy *(open arrow)* for spondylosis shows diffuse hyperintensity + enlargement of cervical cord due to infarct *(arrows)*.

SUBARACHNOID HEMORRHAGE

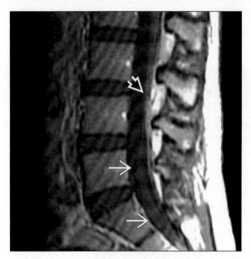

Sagittal T1 C+ MR shows variable appearance of spinal subarachnoid hemorrhage with nonenhancing clot in caudal thecal sac (arrows) & mild inflammatory nerve root enhancement (open arrow).

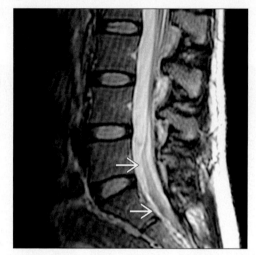

Sagittal T2WI MR shows spinal subarachnoid hemorrhage with intermediate signal linear clot in distal thecal sac (arrows).

TERMINOLOGY

Abbreviations and Synonyms
- Subarachnoid hemorrhage (SAH)

Definitions
- Hemorrhage into spinal subarachnoid space from variety of etiologies
  - Trauma (> 50%)
    - MVA, occupational, etc.
    - Post-operative
    - Lumbar puncture, epidural or intradural catheter placement
  - Related to brain pathology
    - Aneurysmal SAH with spinal extension
  - Spinal arteriovenous malformations
  - Spinal dural fistula (rare)
  - Tumor
    - Spinal ependymoma
    - Spinal neurinoma
    - Hemangioblastoma
    - Astrocytoma (rare)
    - Endometriosis (rare)
  - Bleeding diatheses
  - Anticoagulant therapy
  - Infection (pneumococcal meningitis, herpes)
  - Spinal artery aneurysm (rare)

- Usually associated with AVM, or coarctation of aorta
  - Systemic disease
    - Lupus erythematosus, polyarteritis nodosa
  - Spontaneous idiopathic (rare)

IMAGING FINDINGS

General Features
- Best diagnostic clue: Fluid-fluid level within thecal sac
- Location: Intrathecal: Lumbar > thoracic > cervical
- Size: Variable
- Morphology: Variable depending upon degree of clot formation; mass-like to fluid-fluid level

CT Findings
- NECT: High attenuation in subarachnoid space
- CECT: May show enhancement of underlying etiology (AVM, tumor)
- CTA: Useful in defining underlying spinal vascular malformation (nidus, enlarged draining veins)

MR Findings
- T1WI
  - Variable depending upon stage of blood breakdown and byproducts
    - Slight to pronounced increased signal within thecal sac

DDx: Other Hemorrhage Locations

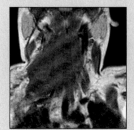

Paraverterbral

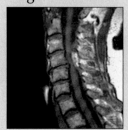

Cervical Epidural

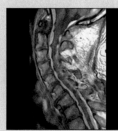

Cervical Subdural

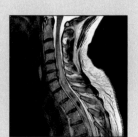

Intramedullary

Key Facts

Terminology
- Hemorrhage into spinal subarachnoid space from variety of etiologies
- Trauma (> 50%)
- Lumbar puncture, epidural or intradural catheter placement
- Aneurysmal SAH with spinal extension
- Spinal arteriovenous malformations
- Spinal ependymoma
- Spinal neurinoma
- Bleeding diatheses
- Anticoagulant therapy
- Infection (pneumococcal meningitis, herpes)

Imaging Findings
- Best diagnostic clue: Fluid-fluid level within thecal sac
- Scan whole spinal axis, + brain if unknown etiology

Pathology
- Incidence of SAH 6/100,000 people annually
- 85% relate to aneurysm rupture
- Non-aneurysmal perimesencephalic hemorrhage 10%
- Primary spinal SAH 1%

Clinical Issues
- Spinal SAH characterized by sudden headache, acute sciatic pain, xanthochromic CSF, meningeal irritation, sensory deficit or paralysis

---

- Fluid-fluid level, or more focal globular clot within cauda equina
- May show indistinct CSF/cord/root distinction within thecal sac due to diffuse SAH
- T2WI: Variable depending upon stage of blood breakdown and byproducts
- T2* GRE: Low signal from blood breakdown products
- T1 C+
  - May show mild enhancement of cauda equina due to 2° inflammatory reaction
  - Look for enhancement of underlying pathology
- MRA: Dynamic enhanced MRA useful as screen for spinal vascular malformation (enlarged draining veins)

Angiographic Findings
- Conventional: Spinal angiography for elucidation of underlying pathology (spinal vascular malformation)

Imaging Recommendations
- Best imaging tool: MRI for evaluation of underlying etiology (AVM, tumor)
- Protocol advice
  - Sagittal, axial T1WI, T2WI, Gradient echo + post-contrast T1WI
  - Scan whole spinal axis, + brain if unknown etiology

DIFFERENTIAL DIAGNOSIS

Epidural hemorrhage
- Linear mass displacing low signal dural margin, cord
- Variable signal depending upon age, may be isointense in acute phase

Subdural hemorrhage
- Lobulated extramedullary signal abnormality, with well preserved outer dural margin
- Axial may show lobulation as "Mercedes-Benz" sign

Intramedullary hemorrhage
- Focal increase signal within cord on T1WI
- Focal low signal on T2WI within cord
- Increase in size with gradient echo imaging

PATHOLOGY

General Features
- General path comments
  - Incidence of SAH 6/100,000 people annually
  - 85% relate to aneurysm rupture
    - Non-aneurysmal perimesencephalic hemorrhage 10%
    - Primary spinal SAH 1%
- Etiology
  - Anticoagulant induced hemorrhage
    - Any part of spine: Epidural, subdural or subarachnoid spaces
    - May occur without antecedent trauma
    - May occur with PT, PTT, clotting times are within therapeutic range
    - Spinal presentation most commonly epidural
  - Traumatic lumbar puncture (LP) vs. true SAH
    - Estimated 20% LPs are traumatic
    - No consensus as to what constitutes traumatic tap
    - General guideline of < 1,000 cells/mm3
    - Opening pressure normal with traumatic tap, elevated opening pressure in 60% true SAH cases
    - Traumatic tap initially bloody with clearing over 3 tubes, true SAH persistently bloody
    - Xanthochromia (RBC catabolism of hemoglobin ⇒ methemoglobin & bilirubin) with true SAH
    - Spectrophotometry + in true SAH for hemoglobin breakdown products
    - Persistence of ↑ RBC count over multiple tubes with true SAH
    - WBC count proportional to peripheral blood with traumatic tap
    - CSF from true SAH should not clot (defibrination)
    - D-dimer + with true SAH (problem with false ±)
- Epidemiology
  - Trauma major cause of spinal hemorrhage
    - 10,000 new cases of spinal cord injury in US per year
- Associated abnormalities: Rare reports of thoracic arachnoiditis developing following spinal SAH

SUBARACHNOID HEMORRHAGE

Staging, Grading or Classification Criteria

- Hunt and Hess scale for SAH
  - I: Asymptomatic
  - II: Severe headache or nuchal rigidity, no neurologic deficit
  - III: Drowsy, minimal neurologic deficit
  - IV: Stuporous, hemiparesis
  - V: Coma, decerebrate posturing

CLINICAL ISSUES

Presentation

- Most common signs/symptoms
  - Acute back or radicular pain ± signs of cord compression (numbness, weakness)
    - Spinal SAH characterized by sudden headache, acute sciatic pain, xanthochromic CSF, meningeal irritation, sensory deficit or paralysis
    - Massive spinal SAH may give acute cord compression, paraplegia, fecal & urinary incontinence

Demographics

- Age: Adult > children
- Gender: Predilection related to underlying etiology
- Ethnicity: Predilection related to underlying etiology

DIAGNOSTIC CHECKLIST

Consider

- CT brain > 95% sensitive to SAH during first 24 hours
  - Sensitivity at 1 week 50%

SELECTED REFERENCES

1. Pancu D et al: EPs do not accept the strategy of "lumbar puncture first" in subarachnoid hemorrhage. Am J Emerg Med. 22(2):115-7, 2004
2. Yahiro T et al: Pseudoaneurysm of the thoracic radiculomedullary artery with subarachnoid hemorrhage. Case report. J Neurosurg. 100(3 Suppl):312-5, 2004
3. Koch C et al: Dural arteriovenous fistula of the lumbar spine presenting with subarachnoid hemorrhage. Case report and review of the literature. J Neurosurg. 100(4 Suppl):385-91, 2004
4. Shah KH et al: Incidence of traumatic lumbar puncture. Acad Emerg Med. 10(2):151-4, 2003
5. Kastenbauer S et al: Pneumococcal meningitis in adults: spectrum of complications and prognostic factors in a series of 87 cases. Brain. 126(Pt 5):1015-25, 2003
6. Chatterjee T et al: Pneumococcal meningitis masquerading as subarachnoid haemorrhage. Med J Aust. 178(10):505-7, 2003
7. Yamaguchi S et al: Spinal subdural hematoma: a sequela of a ruptured intracranial aneurysm? Surg Neurol. 59(5):408-12; discussion 412, 2003
8. Bertalanffy H et al: Isolated paramedullary hemangioblastoma originating from the first cervical nerve root: case report. Spine. 28(10):E191-3, 2003
9. Rabinov JD et al: Endovascular management of vertebrobasilar dissecting aneurysms. AJNR Am J Neuroradiol. 24(7):1421-8, 2003
10. Nozaki K et al: Spinal intradural extramedullary cavernous angioma. Case report. J Neurosurg. 99(3 Suppl):316-9, 2003
11. Berlis A et al: Subarachnoid haemorrhage due to cervical spinal cord haemangioblastomas in a patient with von Hippel-Lindau disease. Acta Neurochir (Wien). 145(11):1009-13; discussion 1013, 2003
12. Wells JB et al: Subarachnoid hemorrhage presenting as post-dural puncture headache: a case report. Mt Sinai J Med. 69(1-2):109-10, 2002
13. Wityk RJ et al: Neurovascular complications of marfan syndrome: a retrospective, hospital-based study. Stroke. 33(3):680-4, 2002
14. Fahy BG et al: Current concepts in neurocritical care. Anesthesiol Clin North America. 20(2):441-62, viii, 2002
15. Pai SB et al: Post lumbar puncture spinal subarachnoid hematoma causing paraplegia: a short report. Neurol India. 50(3):367-9, 2002
16. Ruelle A et al: Spinal subarachnoid bleeding of unknown etiology. Case reports. J Neurosurg Sci. 45(1):53-7, 2001
17. Hausmann et al: Coagulopathy induced spinal intradural extramedullary hematoma: report of three cases and review of the literature. Acta Neurochir (Wien). 143(2):135-40, 2001
18. Hosoda H et al: Mediastinal neurilemmoma complicated with spinal subarachnoid hemorrhage. Jpn J Thorac Cardiovasc Surg. 49(6):384-7, 2001
19. Cihangiroglu M et al: Spinal subarachnoid hemorrhage complicating oral anticoagulant therapy. Eur J Radiol. 39(3):176-9, 2001
20. Cruickshank AM: ACP Best Practice No 166: CSF spectrophotometry in the diagnosis of subarachnoid haemorrhage. J Clin Pathol. 54(11):827-30, 2001

SUBARACHNOID HEMORRHAGE

IMAGE GALLERY

Typical

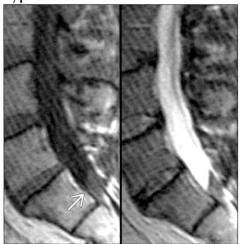 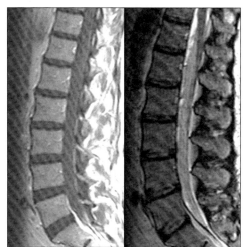

(Left) Sagittal T1WI MR (left) and T2WI MR (right) shows CSF fluid level (arrow) related to subarachnoid hemorrhage (intracranial aneurysm rupture). *(Right)* Sagittal T1 C+ MR (left) shows poor discrimination of conus/cauda equina but no intradural enhancement. T2WI MR (right) shows subarachnoid hemorrhage as low signal (post lumbar catheter placement).

Typical

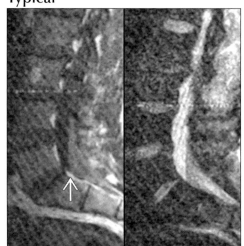 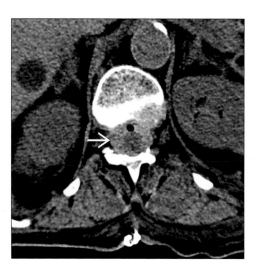

(Left) Sagittal T1WI MR (left) show high signal subarachnoid hemorrhage layering dependently within caudal thecal sac (arrow). T2WI (right) shows blood as decreased signal relative to CSF. *(Right)* Axial NECT following posterior fossae tumor surgery shows extensive subarachnoid blood as intradural high attenuation (arrow). Note intrathecal post-operative gas.

Typical

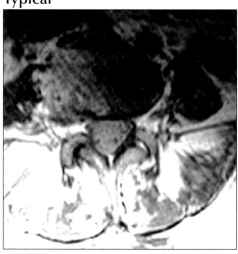 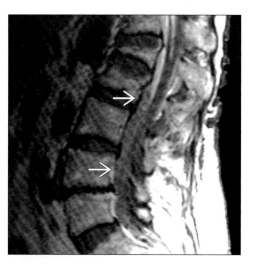

(Left) Axial T1WI MR shows subarachnoid blood as diffuse increased signal within thecal sac, with preserved dural margin & no extra dural mass. Normal nerve roots are defined by high signal blood. *(Right)* Sagittal T1WI MR shows extensive subarachnoid hemorrhage as increased signal throughout lumbar thecal sac (arrows), outlining conus & cauda equina.

SPONTANEOUS EPIDURAL HEMATOMA

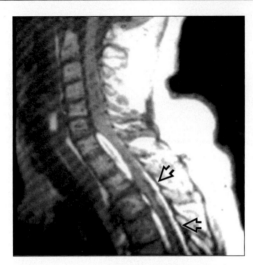

Sagittal T1WI MR through cervicothoracic spine shows two lentiform shaped hyperintense ventral epidural hematomas with central stenosis. Thoracic dorsal epidural fat is noted (arrows).

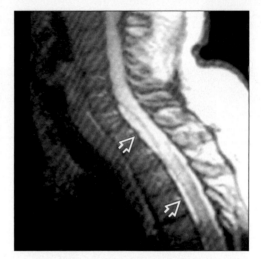

Sagittal T2WI MR in same case demonstrates subacute hyperintense epidural hematomas (arrows). Patient had no history of trauma, & underwent emergent laminectomy & evacuation of hematomas.

TERMINOLOGY

Abbreviations and Synonyms
- Spontaneous spinal epidural hematoma: SSEDH

Definitions
- Accumulation of hemorrhage between dura & spine not caused by significant trauma or iatrogenic procedures

IMAGING FINDINGS

General Features
- Best diagnostic clue: Extradural multisegmental T1 hyperintense fluid collection
- Location
  - Thoracic, lumbar > cervical
    - Cervicothoracic region more common in children
  - Dorsal > ventral > circumferential
- Size: Multi-level > single level
- Morphology
  - Broad-based
  - Lentiform or biconvex
  - Outlined by dorsal epidural fat cranially and rostrally

Radiographic Findings
- Radiography: Noncontributory

- Myelography
  - Block of cerebral spinal fluid
    - Post-myelography CT confirms epidural location

CT Findings
- NECT
  - Hyperdense epidural mass
  - Variable cord compression
  - Sagittal reformation better evaluates craniocaudal extent

MR Findings
- T1WI
  - Variable signal intensity with age of SSEDH
  - Acute: < 48 hrs
    - Isointense > hypo- or hyperintense
  - Subacute and chronic
    - Hyperintense > isointense
  - Fat suppressed T1WI to distinguish blood vs. fat
- T2WI
  - Heterogeneously hyperintense
  - Hypointense foci due to deoxyhemoglobin or fibrous septae in epidural fat
- PD/Intermediate: Diffusely hyperintense
- T2* GRE: Hyperintense with prominent hypointense deoxyhemoglobin
- T1 C+
  - Focal enhancement in acute SSEH represents active extravasation of contrast-enhanced blood

DDx: Epidural Masses

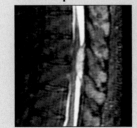

Metastasis

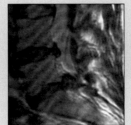

Disc Extrusion

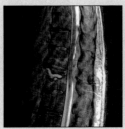

Abscess

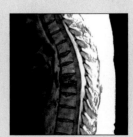

Lipomatosis

SPONTANEOUS EPIDURAL HEMATOMA

Key Facts

Terminology
- Accumulation of hemorrhage between dura & spine not caused by significant trauma or iatrogenic procedures

Imaging Findings
- Best diagnostic clue: Extradural multisegmental T1 hyperintense fluid collection
- Thoracic, lumbar > cervical
- Dorsal > ventral > circumferential
- Hyperdense epidural mass
- Variable signal intensity with age of SSEDH
- T2* GRE: Hyperintense with prominent hypointense deoxyhemoglobin
- Focal enhancement in acute SSEH represents active extravasation of contrast-enhanced blood

Top Differential Diagnoses
- Epidural metastasis, lymphoma
- Disc extrusion, migration

Pathology
- General path comments: Epidural venous hemorrhage ± minimal trauma

Clinical Issues
- Acute onset of neck, back pain
- Rapid progression of neurologic impairment
- Favorable clinical and imaging outcome with conservative management
- Severity and duration of neurologic deficit predictive of post-operative neurologic recovery

---

- ○ Peripheral enhancement due to adjacent dural hyperemia
- ○ Linear enhancement may represent epidural septa or vessels
- Cord compression
  - ○ ± Cord edema

Imaging Recommendations
- Best imaging tool
  - ○ Sagittal and axial T1WI and T2WI MR
    - ▪ NECT may be helpful in confirming acute T1 isointense SSEDH with focal enhancement
    - ▪ Post-myelography CT in patients with instrumentation
  - ○ Spinal angiography not indicated unless findings of arteriovenous malformation present

DIFFERENTIAL DIAGNOSIS

Epidural metastasis, lymphoma
- Well circumscribed extra-osseous soft tissue mass
  - ○ Hypointense on T1WI
  - ○ Hyperintense on T2WI
  - ○ Diffuse enhancement unless necrotic
  - ○ Often contiguous with vertebral lesion
    - ▪ Destruction of posterior vertebral body, pedicle
- Pathologic compression fractures
- Spinal column may be spared in some cases
  - ○ Spinal epidural lymphoma

Disc extrusion, migration
- Associated parent disc height loss, dessication, protrusion; anular tear
- More focal appearance
  - ○ < Half vertebral height in craniocaudal dimension
- Similar signal intensity as parent disc
  - ○ Isointense on T1WI
  - ○ Iso- to hypointense on T2WI
  - ○ ± Mild peripheral enhancement
- SSEDH may be associated with disc extrusion
  - ○ Difficult to distinguish by imaging

Epidural abscess
- More common in ventral epidural space
- Typically associated with infectious spondylodiscitis
- Iso- to hypointense on T1WI
- Hyperintense on T2WI
- Diffuse or peripheral enhancement

Subdural hematoma
- Other than trauma, lumbar puncture in patients with coagulopathy is the most common cause
- More common in lumbar or thoracolumbar region
- Conforms to thecal sac
- Predominantly hypointense on T2WI or gradient echo
  - ○ Isointense on T1WI
- No post-contrast-enhancement

Epidural fat lipomatosis
- Prominent epidural fat in thoracic spine normal
- Excessive epidural fat in spinal canal = lipomatosis
  - ○ Thoracic spine most common
- Homogeneous and hyperintense on T1WI and T2WI
- Signal loss with fat suppression
- No post-contrast-enhancement

PATHOLOGY

General Features
- General path comments: Epidural venous hemorrhage ± minimal trauma
- Genetics: No genetic predilection
- Etiology
  - ○ Minor trauma
    - ▪ Rupture of valveless epidural venous plexus
  - ○ Anticoagulation
  - ○ Coagulopathy
  - ○ Transient venous hypertension
    - ▪ Coughing, sneezing, or other sudden Valsalva maneuvers
  - ○ Disk herniation
    - ▪ 78% of lumbar SSEH in one series
    - ▪ Rupture of adjacent epidural veins
  - ○ Vascular anomaly

SPONTANEOUS EPIDURAL HEMATOMA

○ Pregnancy
○ Paget disease
○ Idiopathic: 40-50%
• Epidemiology
○ Incidence of approximately 0.1 per 100,000 per year
○ Less than 1% of spinal space-occupying lesions
  ▪ Leading cause of spinal epidural hematoma
• Associated abnormalities
○ Disc herniation
○ Anular tear
○ Arteriovenous malformation

Gross Pathologic & Surgical Features

• Isolated hematoma in epidural space

CLINICAL ISSUES

Presentation

• Most common signs/symptoms
○ Acute onset of neck, back pain
○ Radicular pain
○ Other signs/symptoms
  ▪ Progressive paraparesis
  ▪ Sensory deficit
  ▪ Altered deep tendon reflexes
  ▪ Bladder or bowel dysfunction
• Clinical profile
○ Mimics acute disc herniation
○ Rapid progression of neurologic impairment

Demographics

• Age
○ Bimodal distribution
  ▪ Childhood
  ▪ 50s and 60s
• Gender
○ M:F = 4:1
○ M = F in children
• Ethnicity: No racial predilection

Natural History & Prognosis

• May resolve spontaneously
• Favorable clinical and imaging outcome with conservative management
• Severity and duration of neurologic deficit predictive of post-operative neurologic recovery
○ Return to neurologic baseline after surgery
  ▪ 89-95% of patients with incomplete neurologic deficit vs 38-45% of patients with complete impairment
○ Improved outcome when surgery performed ≤ 36 hrs in patients with complete sensorimotor loss
  ▪ ≤ 48 hrs in patients with incomplete deficit
○ Localization in lumbosacral spine or single level involvement also has favorable surgical prognosis
• Mortality rate: 6%

Treatment

• Decompressive laminectomy with hematoma evacuation
• Management
○ Correction of underlying coagulopathy with vitamin K, protamine sulfate, platelet transfusions, etc.

○ Intravenous dexamethasone to decrease inflammatory reaction and cord edema
○ In cases of mild symptoms at presentation
  ▪ Regardless of the degree of cord compression on MRI
○ In cases of rapid and progressive neurologic recovery

DIAGNOSTIC CHECKLIST

Image Interpretation Pearls

• Biconvex epidural mass hyperintense on T1WI and T2WI with hypointense foci highly suggestive of spinal epidural hematoma

SELECTED REFERENCES

1. Liao CC et al: Experience in the surgical management of spontaneous spinal epidural hematoma. J Neurosurg. 100(1 Suppl):38-45, 2004
2. Dorsay TA et al: MR imaging of epidural hematoma in the lumbar spine. Skeletal Radiol. 31(12):677-85, 2002
3. Nawashiro H et al: Contrast enhancement of a hyperacute spontaneous spinal epidural hematoma. AJNR Am J Neuroradiol. 22(7):1445, 2001
4. Duffill J et al: Can spontaneous spinal epidural haematoma be managed safely without operation? A report of four cases. 69(6):816-9, 2000
5. Kuker W et al: Spinal subdural and epidural haematomas: diagnostic and therapeutic aspects in acute and subacute cases. Acta Neurochir (Wien). 142(7):777-85, 2000
6. Sklar EM et al: MRI of acute spinal epidural hematomas. J Comput Assist Tomogr. 23(2):238-43, 1999
7. Fukui MB et al: Acute spontaneous spinal epidural hematomas. AJNR Am J Neuroradiol. 20(7):1365-72, 1999
8. Alexiadou-Rudolf C et al: Acute nontraumatic spinal epidural hematomas: An important differential diagnosis in spinal emergencies. Spine. 23:1810-1813, 1998
9. Patel H et al: Spontaneous spinal epidural hematoma in children. Pediatr Neurol. 19(4):302-7, 1998
10. Chen CJ et al: Imaging findings of spontaneous spinal epidural hematoma. J Formos Med Assoc. 96(4):283-7, 1997
11. Holtas S et al: Spontaneous spinal epidural hematoma: findings at MR imaging and clinical correlation. Radiology. 199(2):409-13, 1996
12. Groen RJ et al: Operative treatment of spontaneous spinal epidural hematomas: a study of the factors determining postoperative outcome. Neurosurgery. 39(3):494-508; discussion 508-9, 1996
13. Lawton MT et al: Surgical management of spinal epidural hematoma: relationship between surgical timing and neurological outcome. J Neurosurg. 83(1):1-7, 1995
14. Gundry CR et al: Epidural hematoma of the lumbar spine: 18 surgically confirmed cases. Radiology. 187(2):427-31, 1993
15. Groen RJ et al: The spontaneous spinal epidural hematoma. A study of the etiology. J Neurol Sci. 98(2-3):121-38, 1990
16. Rothfus WE et al: MR imaging in the diagnosis of spontaneous spinal epidural hematomas. J Comput Assist Tomogr. 11(5):851-4, 1987
17. Levitan LH et al: Chronic lumbar extradural hematoma: CT findings. Radiology. 148(3):707-8, 1983
18. Foo D et al: Preoperative neurological status in predicting surgical outcome of spinal epidural hematomas. Surg Neurol. 15(5):389-401, 1981

SPONTANEOUS EPIDURAL HEMATOMA

IMAGE GALLERY

Typical

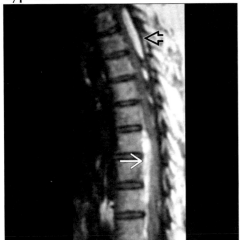

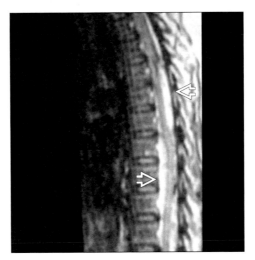

(Left) Sagittal T1WI MR through thoracic spine shows two subacute hyperintense SSEDHs, one ventral *(arrow)* and one dorsal *(open arrow)*. Isointense foci are present at rostral aspect of dorsal SSEDH. *(Right)* Sagittal T2WI MR shows multisegmental epidural hematomas *(arrows)*, which are hyperintense. Spinal stenosis and cord compression are evident.

Typical

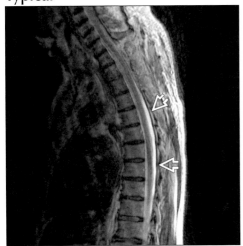

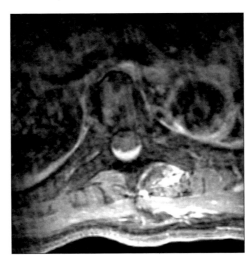

(Left) Sagittal T1WI MR through thoracic spine demonstrates an extensive homogenous hyperintense dorsal epidural collection *(arrows)*. *(Right)* Axial T1WI MR with fat-saturation in same patient demonstrates persistent hyperintensity, compatible with a subacute epidural hematoma.

Typical

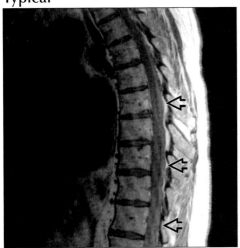

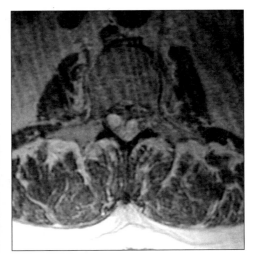

(Left) Sagittal T1WI MR through thoracolumbar spine in patient with acute onset of myelopathy shows subtle diffuse isointense epidural collection *(arrows)*. *(Right)* Axial T2WI MR through lumbar vertebra in same patient confirms predominantly hyperintense epidural collection, with severe central stenosis. An epidural hematoma was found at surgery.

SUBDURAL HEMATOMA

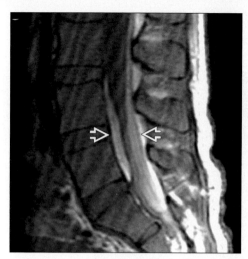

Sagittal T1WI MR through lumbosacral spine shows distal ventral and dorsal intraspinal hyperintense collections (arrows). The dorsal collection is outlined by cauda equina and epidural fat.

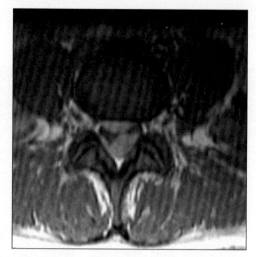

Axial T1WI MR confirms the subdural location of both ventral and dorsal subacute hematomas, causing severe central stenosis.

TERMINOLOGY

Abbreviations and Synonyms
- Spinal subdural hematoma (SSDH)

Definitions
- Accumulation of blood between dura, arachnoid

IMAGING FINDINGS

General Features
- Best diagnostic clue: Intradural collection hyperintense on T1WI, predominantly hypointense on T2WI or gradient-echo imaging
- Location
  - Thoracolumbar > lumbar or lumbosacral > cervical
  - Ventral, dorsal, lateral, or circumferential
- Size
  - Variable cranial-caudal extension
    - Typically over multiple levels
- Morphology
  - Clumped, loculated masses of hemorrhagic density/intensity
  - Conforms to dura
  - Distinct from epidural fat & adjacent osseous structures

Radiographic Findings
- Radiography: Noncontributory except in setting of trauma
- Myelography
  - Effaced subarachnoid space over multiple levels
  - Cord compression

CT Findings
- NECT
  - Hyperdense intradural collection
    - Outlined by epidural fat & relatively low density cord
  - Sagittal reformation best depicts craniocaudal extent
  - Cord compression
- CECT: No significant enhancement
- Bone CT
  - Vertebral fractures in trauma patients

MR Findings
- T1WI
  - Heterogeneous, variable signal intensity depending on duration of SSDH
    - Acute: Iso- to slightly hyperintense
    - Subacute to chronic: Hyperintense
- T2WI
  - Heterogeneously hyperintense
    - Significant hypointense portion
- PD/Intermediate: Hyperintense

DDx: Intraspinal Collections

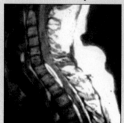

Epidural Hematomas

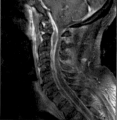

Subdural Abscess

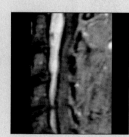

CSF Leakage Syndrome

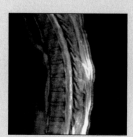

Spinal Meningitis

SUBDURAL HEMATOMA

Key Facts

Terminology
- Accumulation of blood between dura, arachnoid

Imaging Findings
- Best diagnostic clue: Intradural collection hyperintense on T1WI, predominantly hypointense on T2WI or gradient-echo imaging
- Thoracolumbar > lumbar or lumbosacral > cervical
- Clumped, loculated masses of hemorrhagic density/intensity
- Outlined by epidural fat & relatively low density cord
- Heterogeneous, variable signal intensity depending on duration of SSDH
- T2* GRE: Significant hypointense portion due to deoxyhemoglobin
- T1 C+: ± Slight enhancement

Top Differential Diagnoses
- Epidural hematoma
- Subdural abscess
- CSF leakage syndrome

Pathology
- Iatrogenic cause factor in 2/3 of those with abnormal coagulation parameters

Clinical Issues
- Acute onset of neck or back pain
- Radicular pain
- May resolve spontaneously
- Decompressive laminectomy with clot evacuation

- STIR: Hyperintense
- T2* GRE: Significant hypointense portion due to deoxyhemoglobin
- T1 C+: ± Slight enhancement
- Variable mass effect on spinal cord and cauda equina
  - Hyperintense cord edema on T2WI

Imaging Recommendations
- Best imaging tool
  - Sagittal and axial T2WI and T1WI MR
  - Spinal angiography not indicated unless findings of arteriovenous malformation present

DIFFERENTIAL DIAGNOSIS

Epidural hematoma
- Thoracolumbar spine most common
- "Capping" of hematoma by dorsal epidural fat on sagittal imaging
- Directly adjacent to osseous structures with effacement of epidural fat
  - Not limited by dura
- Iso- to hyperintense on T1WI acute, hyperintense subacute to chronic
- Hyperintense on T2WI with hypointense deoxyhemoglobin
- ± Central or peripheral enhancement

Subdural abscess
- Thoracolumbar spine most common
- Multi-segmental dural/subdural thickening
- Obliterated CSF
- Isointense on T1WI, hyperintense on T2WI
- Diffuse vs. rim-enhancement

CSF leakage syndrome
- Spontaneous or from prior spinal trauma, diagnostic or interventional procedure, or spontaneous
- Low opening pressure on lumbar puncture
- Dural venous engorgement and enhancement
- Diffuse smooth meningeal thickening, enhancement
- May see cerebellar tonsillar descent, effaced pre-pontine space in posterior fossa

Spinal meningitis
- Normal or increased CSF intensity on T1WI
- Indistinct cord-CSF interface
- Diffusely enhancing CSF
- Smooth or nodular meningeal/nerve root enhancement
- ± Cord edema/swelling

Idiopathic hypertrophic spinal pachymeningitis
- Diagnosis of exclusion
- Unknown etiology
- Fibrous inflammatory thickening of dura mater
- Thickened dura iso- to hypointense on T1WI and T2WI
  - Marked post-contrast-enhancement

PATHOLOGY

General Features
- General path comments
  - Embryology-anatomy
    - Inner dura (dural border cell layer) structurally weaker than outer layer
    - May tear during trauma
    - Creating potential space within dural border cell layer
    - SSDH forms between strong external dura and arachnoid
    - True spinal subdural space demonstrated in human autopsy studies
  - Other proposed mechanisms of SSDH formation
    - Rupture of valveless radiculomedullary veins that cross subdural and subarachnoid spaces
    - Rupture of extra-arachnoidal vessels on inner dural surface
- Genetics: No genetic predilection
- Etiology
  - Trauma
  - Bleeding diathesis: 54% of reported cases
    - Anticoagulation

SUBDURAL HEMATOMA

- Coagulopathy: Hemophilia, leukemia, thrombocytopenia, polycythemia, etc.
  o Iatrogenic cause factor in 2/3 of those with abnormal coagulation parameters
    - Lumbar puncture
    - Spinal anesthesia
  o Neoplasm
  o Arteriovenous malformation
  o Post-operative complication
  o Spontaneous: 15%
- Epidemiology: Much less common than spinal epidural hematoma
- Associated abnormalities
  o In the setting of trauma
    - Vertebral fracture-dislocation
    - Posttraumatic disc herniation
    - Hemorrhagic cord contusion: Hyperintense on T2WI with focal hypointensity
  o Subarachnoid and epidural hemorrhage

Gross Pathologic & Surgical Features
- Subdural (partially) organized blood clot under pressure
  o Bluish tense dura
- ± Subarachnoid/epidural hemorrhage

Microscopic Features
- Hemosiderin
- Fibrin and histiocytes
- Little or no fibroadipose tissue

CLINICAL ISSUES

Presentation
- Most common signs/symptoms
  o Acute onset of neck or back pain
  o Radicular pain
  o Other signs/symptoms
    - Headache
    - Meningismus
    - Paraplegia
    - Paresthesia
    - Bladder/bowel dysfunction
    - Diminished deep tendon reflexes
- Clinical profile
  o Neurologic impairment may be delayed
    - Onset of neurologic deficits varies from hours to > 1 week
  o Chronic SSDH may not have significant pain
  o Mimics subarachnoid hemorrhage clinically

Demographics
- Age
  o All ages affected
  o Slightly increased incidence in those ≥ 60
- Gender: M = F
- Ethnicity: No racial predilection

Natural History & Prognosis
- May resolve spontaneously
- Favorable clinical and imaging outcome in those suitable for conservative management
- > 40% of patients undergoing surgery have near complete neurologic recovery

- Concurrent subarachnoid hemorrhage portends poor outcome

Treatment
- Decompressive laminectomy with clot evacuation
  o Indicated with severe & progressive deterioration of neurologic symptoms
- Non-operative management
  o In cases of mild symptoms at presentation
  o In patients with rapid neurologic recovery
  o Analgesics
  o ± Intravenous dexamethasone to decrease inflammatory reaction and cord edema

DIAGNOSTIC CHECKLIST

Consider
- NECT to confirm intradural location + hyperdense acute hematoma if MR findings equivocal

Image Interpretation Pearls
- Intradural extramedullary collection hyperintense on T1WI and predominantly hypointense on T2WI or gradient-echo imaging without significant enhancement characteristic of SSDH

SELECTED REFERENCES

1. Hung KS et al: Traumatic spinal subdural hematoma with spontaneous resolution. Spine. 27(24):E534-8, 2002
2. Boukobza M et al: Spinal subdural haematoma: a study of three cases. Clin Radiol. 56(6):475-80, 2001
3. Adler MD et al: Acute hemorrhagic complication of diagnostic lumbar puncture. Pediatr Emerg Care. 17(3):184-8, 2001
4. Hausmann et al: Coagulopathy induced spinal intradural extramedullary haematoma: report of three cases and review of the literature. Acta Neurochir (Wien). 143(2):135-40, 2001
5. Maeda M et al: Nonsurgical treatment of an upper thoracic spinal subdural hemorrhage. Spinal Cord. 39(12):657-61, 2001
6. Abla AA et al: Spinal chronic subdural hematoma. Neurosurg Clin N Am. 11(3):465-71, 2000
7. Egede LE et al: Spinal subdural hematoma: a rare complication of lumbar puncture. Case report and review of the literature. Md Med J. 48(1):15-7, 1999
8. Domenicucci M et al: Nontraumatic acute spinal subdural hematoma: report of five cases and review of the literature. J Neurosurg. 91(1 Suppl):65-73, 1999
9. Longatti PL et al: Spontaneous spinal subdural hematoma. Journal of Neurosurgical Sciences. 38:197-9, 1994
10. Donovan MJ et al: Acute spinal subdural hematoma: MR and CT findings with pathologic correlates. AJNR. 15:1895-905, 1994
11. Haines DE et al: The "subdural" space: a new look at an outdated concept. Neurosurgery. 32(1):111-20, 1993
12. Calhoun JM et al: Spontaneous spinal subdural hematoma: case report and review of the literature. Neurosurgery. 29(1):133-4, 1991
13. Spanu G et al: Spinal subdural haematoma: a rare complication of lumbar puncture. Case report and review of the literature. Neurochirurgia (Stuttg). 31(5):157-9, 1988

SUBDURAL HEMATOMA

IMAGE GALLERY

Typical

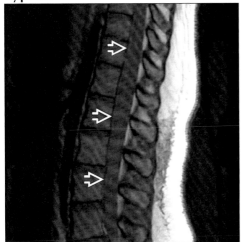
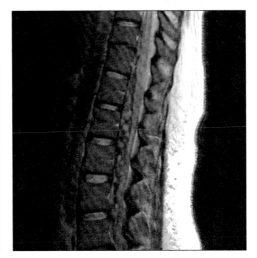

(Left) Sagittal T1WI MR through thoracolumbar spine in patient with leukemia + recent lumbar puncture demonstrates diffuse subtle ventral intraspinal collection (arrows), iso- to slightly hyperintense. *(Right)* Sagittal T2WI MR shows same ventral collection, with loculation and prominent hypointense areas.

Typical

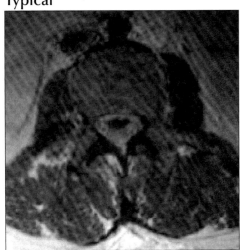
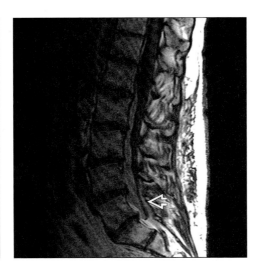

(Left) Axial T2WI MR through lumbar vertebra shows subdural location of this acute hematoma, with mass effect in thecal sac. *(Right)* Sagittal T1WI MR through lumbosacral spine in another patient shows extensive ventral and minimal dorsal (arrow) hyperintense subdural hematomas.

Typical

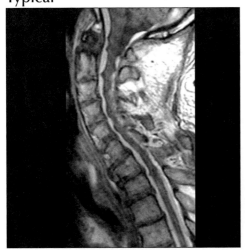
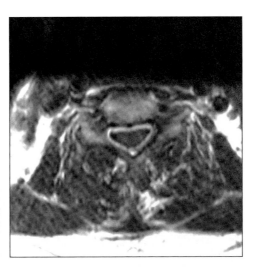

(Left) Sagittal T1WI MR in patient with chronic neck pain demonstrates diffuse ventral and dorsal intraspinal hyperintense collections, with intracranial extension. *(Right)* Axial T1WI MR through cervical vertebra shows thin circumferential hyperintense chronic subdural hematoma.

SUPERFICIAL SIDEROSIS

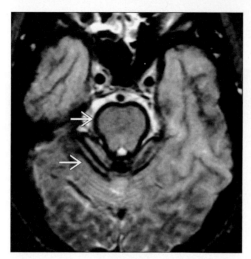

Axial T2WI MR shows multiple areas of curvilinear low signal coating surface of brainstem & cerebellar folia (arrows) due to hemosiderin deposition.

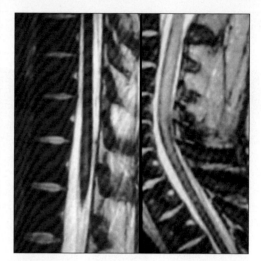

Sagittal T2WI MR of conus (left) & cervical cord (right) shows diffuse low signal involving surface of cord, with relative hyperintensity of normal central cord.

TERMINOLOGY

Abbreviations and Synonyms
- Synonyms: Central nervous system siderosis, hemosiderosis
- Abbreviation: Superficial siderosis (SS), sensorineural hearing loss (SNHL)

Definitions
- Recurrent subarachnoid hemorrhage (multiple etiologies) causing hemosiderin deposition on cord, nerve surface

IMAGING FINDINGS

General Features
- Best diagnostic clue: Diffuse hypointensity of cord/brain surface on T2WI, gradient echo images
- Location: Cerebellum, brainstem, cerebrum, cord, cranial nerves
- Size: Linear low signal < few mm in thickness
- Morphology: Curvilinear, following surface contour of involved CNS structure

CT Findings
- NECT: Cord, brain volume loss
- CECT: No enhancement

MR Findings
- T1WI: Usually normal, occasional low signal on cord surface
- T2WI
  - Linear low signal involving cord surface, nerve roots
  - Look for typical surface involvement of cerebellum, brainstem
- T2* GRE
  - Linear low signal involving cord surface, nerve roots
  - Findings more pronounced than with T2WI, T1WI
- T1 C+: No enhancement of leptomeninges

Imaging Recommendations
- Best imaging tool
  - MR brain/spine
  - Diagnosis of siderosis necessitates search for underlying cause of repetitive subarachnoid hemorrhage
- Protocol advice
  - Brian MR: T1WI, T2WI, FLAIR, post-contrast T1WI, T2* GRE
  - Spine: Scan total spine with sagittal T2WI, T2* GRE, post-contrast T1WI

DDx: Peripheral Cord Low T2 Signal & Mimics

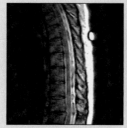

CSF Dephasing

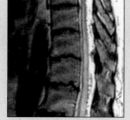

Dural Fistula

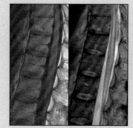

Infarct

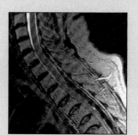

Subdural Hemorrhage

SUPERFICIAL SIDEROSIS

Key Facts

Terminology
- Synonyms: Central nervous system siderosis, hemosiderosis
- Recurrent subarachnoid hemorrhage (multiple etiologies) causing hemosiderin deposition on cord, nerve surface

Imaging Findings
- Best diagnostic clue: Diffuse hypointensity of cord/brain surface on T2WI, gradient echo images

Top Differential Diagnoses
- MR artifact
- Subdural hemorrhage
- Cord central T2 hyperintensity
- Cord peripheral T2 hypointensity in dural fistula

Pathology
- Hemosiderin coating surface of cerebellum, brainstem, spinal cord
- Extends to & involves pial, subpial, subependymal surfaces
- Variable neuronal loss, reactive gliosis, demyelination
- Rare, insidious, progressive abnormality

Clinical Issues
- Bilateral sensorineural hearing loss (95%)
- Ataxia (88%)
- Pyramidal signs (76%)
- Dementia (20%)
- Nystagmus (19%)
- Idiopathic (25-46%)

DIFFERENTIAL DIAGNOSIS

MR artifact
- Low signal adjacent to cord, related to CSF flow dephasing
- Appearance varies with different sequences, plane of acquisition

Subdural hemorrhage
- Lobulated low T2 signal adjacent to cord, not on cord surface

Cord central T2 hyperintensity
- Variety of pathologies may give cord central T2 hyperintensity, causing periphery of cord to look abnormally low signal
- Look for cord expansion, enhancement with demyelinating disease or tumor which does not occur with SS
- Cord infarction - acute symptoms onset

Cord peripheral T2 hypointensity in dural fistula
- True cord decreased T2 signal with type I dural fistula, thought related to venous hypertensive myelopathy

Underlying etiology of subarachnoid hemorrhage
- Intramedullary neoplasm (ependymoma, astrocytoma)
- Cavernous malformation(s)
- Arteriovenous malformations
- Cranial pathology (post-operative)

PATHOLOGY

General Features
- General path comments
  - Hemosiderin coating surface of cerebellum, brainstem, spinal cord
  - Extends to & involves pial, subpial, subependymal surfaces
  - Variable neuronal loss, reactive gliosis, demyelination
    - Cerebellum typically shows loss of Purkinje cells and Bergmann gliosis
- Etiology
  - Repeated subarachnoid hemorrhage ⇒ hemosiderin encrustation of surface of CNS
    - Hemosiderin is cytotoxic
  - Involvement of brain, cord surface is active process requiring glial tissues (microglia, Bergmann glia, subpial astrocytes)
    - Peripheral myelinated structures much less involved
    - Long length of "central" myelination of CN8 explains preferential involvement, along with CN1, 2 involvement
  - Hemosiderin deposition may extend into cord gray matter to affect neurons
    - Ferritin biosynthesis overwhelmed by large iron load ⇒ excess free iron ⇒ stimulation of lipid peroxidation ⇒ local tissue necrosis
- Epidemiology
  - Rare, insidious, progressive abnormality
  - 0.15% patients undergoing MR imaging
    - 85% showed no symptoms
- Associated abnormalities: Hydrocephalus

Gross Pathologic & Surgical Features
- Dark brown/black staining of pial/subpial surface of cord, nerve roots

Microscopic Features
- Staining of cord surface by hemosiderin, thickened leptomeninges

CLINICAL ISSUES

Presentation
- Most common signs/symptoms
  - Bilateral sensorineural hearing loss (95%)
    - Ataxia (88%)
    - Pyramidal signs (76%)

SUPERFICIAL SIDEROSIS

- Dementia (20%)
- Nystagmus (19%)
- Anosmia (17%)
  - Poor correlation of MR findings with clinical symptoms
  - Cause of recurrent subarachnoid hemorrhage found in 50%
    - Post-operative change with friable surgical cavity (hemispherectomy)
    - Traumatic nerve root avulsion
    - Neoplastic hemorrhage (35%); ependymoma most common tumoral cause
    - Arteriovenous malformation
    - Aneurysm
    - Cavernous malformation (0.5-0.9% of population affected)
  - Idiopathic (25-46%)
- Clinical profile
  - Classic description: Sensorineural hearing loss, cerebellar ataxia, dementia, myelopathy (uncommon to see all manifestations)
  - CSF analysis
    - Xanthochromia
    - Elevated RBC count
    - Elevated iron & ferritin levels
    - May be normal

Demographics
- Age: Adult and children (average age 50 years)
- Gender: M:F = 3:1
- Ethnicity: No predilection

Natural History & Prognosis
- Preclinical phase often prolonged (> 10 years)
  - Reports of SS developing > 30 years following initial surgical procedure

Treatment
- Treat underlying abnormality by surgical or endovascular means
  - AVM, aneurysm, tumor
- Cochlear implant for SNHL
- Iron/copper chelates unsuccessful for treatment

DIAGNOSTIC CHECKLIST

Consider
- Superficial siderosis is secondary to repetitive subarachnoid hemorrhage
  - Look for underlying etiology in brain/spine

SELECTED REFERENCES
1. Messori A et al: The importance of suspecting superficial siderosis of the central nervous system in clinical practice. J Neurol Neurosurg Psychiatry. 75(2):188-90, 2004
2. Anderson NE: Late complications in childhood central nervous system tumour survivors. Curr Opin Neurol. 16(6):677-83, 2003
3. Yoshida S et al: Superficial siderosis from spinal teratoma. Lancet. 360(9345):1539, 2002
4. Polidori MC et al: Superficial siderosis of the central nervous system: a 70-year-old man with ataxia, depression and visual deficits. Gerontology. 47(2):93-5, 2001
5. Padberg M et al: Cerebral siderosis: deafness by a spinal tumor. J Neurol. 247(6):473, 2000
6. Bostantjopoulou S et al: Superficial CNS siderosis and spinal pilocytic astrocytoma. Neurology. 55(3):450, 2000
7. Pelak VS et al: Evidence for preganglionic pupillary involvement in superficial siderosis. Neurology. 53(5):1130-2, 1999
8. Manfredi M et al: Superficial siderosis of the central nervous system and anticoagulant therapy: a case report. Ital J Neurol Sci. 20(4):247-9, 1999
9. Lemmerling M et al: Secondary superficial siderosis of the central nervous system in a patient presenting with sensorineural hearing loss. Neuroradiology. 40(5):312-4, 1998
10. Schievink WI et al: Surgical treatment of superficial siderosis associated with a spinal arteriovenous malformation. Case report. J Neurosurg. 89(6):1029-31, 1998
11. Pyhtinen J et al: Superficial siderosis in the central nervous system. Neuroradiology. 37(2):127-8, 1995
12. Lai MT et al: Superficial siderosis of the central nervous system: a case with an unruptured intracranial aneurysm. J Laryngol Otol. 109(6):549-52, 1995
13. Bonito V et al: Superficial siderosis of the central nervous system after brachial plexus injury. Case report. J Neurosurg. 80(5):931-4, 1994
14. Pribitkin EA et al: Superficial siderosis of the central nervous system: an underdiagnosed cause of sensorineural hearing loss and ataxia. Am J Otol. 15(3):415-8, 1994
15. River Y et al: Superficial hemosiderosis of the central nervous system. Mov Disord. 9(5):559-62, 1994
16. Bracchi M et al: Superficial siderosis of the CNS: MR diagnosis and clinical findings. AJNR Am J Neuroradiol. 14(1):227-36, 1993
17. Kumar A et al: Posterior fossa surgery: an unusual cause of superficial siderosis. Neurosurgery. 32(3):455-7; discussion 457, 1993
18. Grunshaw ND et al: Superficial siderosis of the central nervous system--diagnosis by magnetic resonance imaging. Clin Radiol. 48(3):186-8, 1993
19. Parnes SM et al: Superficial siderosis of the central nervous system: a neglected cause of sensorineural hearing loss. Otolaryngol Head Neck Surg. 107(1):69-77, 1992

IMAGE GALLERY

Typical

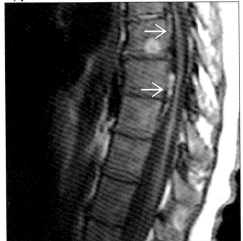
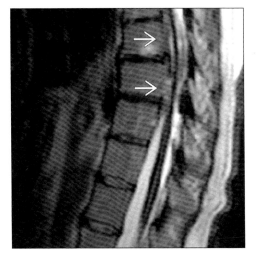

(Left) Sagittal T1WI MR of thoracolumbar junction in superficial siderosis shows ossification of posterior longitudinal ligament compressing cord (arrow), but no significant cord surface signal abnormality. *(Right)* Sagittal T2WI MR of thoracolumbar junction shows OPLL (arrows) causing repetitive cord trauma, with abnormal linear low signal on surface of distal cord reflecting superficial siderosis.

Typical

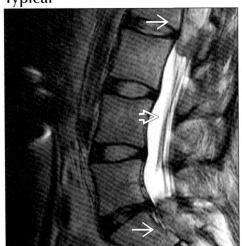
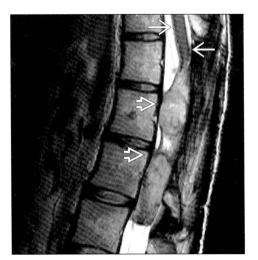

(Left) Sagittal T2WI MR shows large filum terminale ependymoma with drop metastases (arrows), superficial siderosis of cauda equina with linear low signal (open arrow). *(Right)* Sagittal T2WI MR of recurrent ependymoma (open arrows) shows superficial siderosis extending cephalad along cord (arrows).

Typical

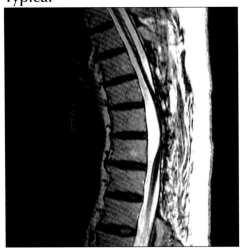
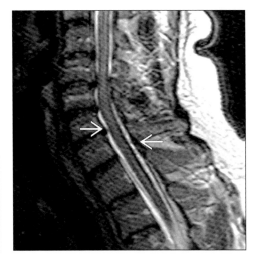

(Left) Sagittal T2WI MR in patient following thoracic ependymoma resection shows diffuse hemosiderin staining of thoracic cord with diffuse low signal, volume loss, and local tethering to laminectomy site. *(Right)* Sagittal T2WI MR shows linear low signal on cervical cord surface from repeated subarachnoid hemorrhage (arrows).

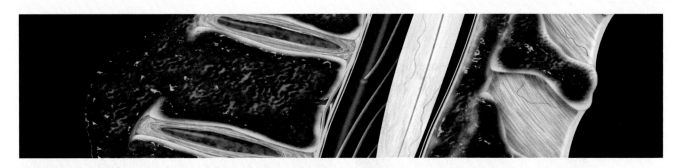

SECTION 2: Spinal Manifestations of Systemic Diseases

PAGET DISEASE

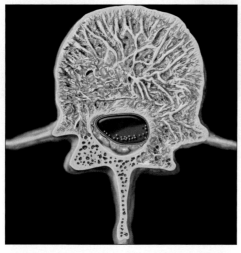

Axial graphic of Pagetic vertebra demonstrates enlarged vertebral body, pedicles, and left facet with trabellular thickening and increased fatty marrow.

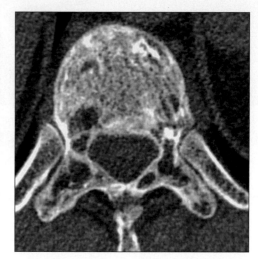

Axial NECT shows thoracic body with coarse & thickened trabeculae, focal areas or fat attenuation.

TERMINOLOGY

Abbreviations and Synonyms
- Osteitis deformans

Definitions
- Chronic metabolic disorder of abnormal bone remodeling in adult skeleton

IMAGING FINDINGS

General Features
- Best diagnostic clue: Enlarged vertebra with trabecular coarsening and cortical thickening
- Location: Lumbar spine most common: L3, L4
- Size: Single or multiple levels
- Morphology
  ○ Vertebra expanded, "squared"
    ▪ Loss of anterior concave margin
    ▪ Thickened cortex
  ○ Coarse trabeculae in vertical orientation
  ○ Both vertebral body, neural arch involved

Radiographic Findings
- Radiography
  ○ "Picture frame" vertebra
    ▪ Coarse and sclerotic peripheral trabecular pattern
    ▪ Central osteopenia

  ○ Diffusely dense "ivory" vertebra
  ○ Rare solitary discrete lytic lesion

CT Findings
- CECT: Significant marrow enhancement in active phase
- Bone CT
  ○ Better characterization of sclerotic cortex & disorganized trabeculae

MR Findings
- T1WI: Hypointense cortex + thickened trabeculae
- T2WI: Cortex hypointense
- STIR: Hypointense bone
- Variable degree of spinal stenosis + foraminal narrowing
- Marrow pattern
  ○ Fibrovascular marrow in active phase
    ▪ Heterogeneous but predominantly hypointense on T1WI, hyperintense on T2WI
    ▪ Foci of fatty marrow
    ▪ Post-gadolinium enhancement
  ○ Fatty marrow in mixed phase
    ▪ Hyperintense on T1WI and T2WI
    ▪ Most often imaged
    ▪ May be increased compared to normal vertebrae

Nuclear Medicine Findings
- Bone Scan

DDx: Abnormal Marrow/Bone Simulating Paget Disease

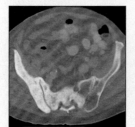

Metastasis

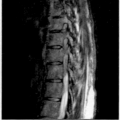

Metastasis

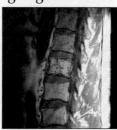

Vertebral Hemangioma

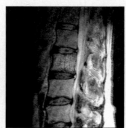

Vertebral Hemangioma

PAGET DISEASE

Key Facts

Terminology
- Osteitis deformans
- Chronic metabolic disorder of abnormal bone remodeling in adult skeleton

Imaging Findings
- Best diagnostic clue: Enlarged vertebra with trabecular coarsening and cortical thickening
- Location: Lumbar spine most common: L3, L4
- "Picture frame" vertebra
- Diffusely dense "ivory" vertebra
- T1WI: Hypointense cortex + thickened trabeculae
- Variable degree of spinal stenosis + foraminal narrowing
- Diffusely increased uptake in enlarged vertebra

Top Differential Diagnoses
- Osteoblastic metastases
- Vertebral hemangioma

Pathology
- Possible viral etiology
- 3-4% of adults over 40
- Sarcomatous transformation: < 1%
- Uncommon in skull & spine relative to high prevalence of disease in axial skeleton

Clinical Issues
- Deep, dull bone pain
- Disease process may be halted with return of normal osseous architecture after medical treatment

---

- ○ Diffusely increased uptake in enlarged vertebra
- ○ May be normal in inactive phase
  - ▪ Radiographic abnormality persists
- PET
  - ○ Most cases not hypermetabolic
    - ▪ Low to high grade uptake without sarcomatous transformation has been reported

Imaging Recommendations
- Best imaging tool
  - ○ Radiography cost effective
  - ○ CT if question of metastasis/bone destruction
  - ○ MR best in evaluating neurologic symptoms
  - ○ Bone scan best in determining extent of disease, assessing disease activity, monitoring response to treatment

DIFFERENTIAL DIAGNOSIS

Osteoblastic metastases
- Multi-focal, patchy, or diffuse
- Hyperintense on T2WI with fat suppression or STIR
  - ○ Hypointense on T1WI
- Post-gadolinium enhancement
- "Picture frame" appearance uncommon
- May be indistinguishable if "ivory" vertebra present
  - ○ Lymphoma, metastases
- Epidural, paravertebral soft tissue mass common
- Pathologic compression fractures

Vertebral hemangioma
- Typically hyperintense on T1WI & T2WI
  - ○ Post-gadolinium enhancement
- Stippled appearance on axial CT
- Striated appearance on plain film
  - ○ Trabecular condensation more delicate than that in Paget disease
- No vertebral enlargement or cortical thickening

PATHOLOGY

General Features
- General path comments: Overactive osteoclasts, osteoblasts resulting in abnormal and disordered bone remodeling
- Genetics
  - ○ Familial incidence reported
    - ▪ 40% with family history of disease
  - ○ No single gene implicated
- Etiology
  - ○ Possible viral etiology
    - ▪ Measles virus of paramyxovirus family found in osteoclasts
    - ▪ Upregulation of interleukin-6 and its receptor gene reported
- Epidemiology
  - ○ 3-4% of adults over 40
  - ○ 10-11% of adults over 80
  - ○ Vertebral involvement
    - ▪ 30-75% of patients with Paget disease
- Associated abnormalities
  - ○ Other sites of osseous involvement
    - ▪ Pelvis = spine > femur > skull > tibia > clavicle > humerus > ribs
    - ▪ Polyostotic, asymmetric > monostotic
  - ○ Pathologic compression fracture
  - ○ Kyphoscoliosis
  - ○ Spondylosis
  - ○ Basilar invagination
    - ▪ Narrowing at foramen magnum due to cervical spine prolapsing into Pagetic calvarium
  - ○ Cord ischemia
    - ▪ Hyperemic bone shunts blood away from spinal cord
    - ▪ Vascular compression
  - ○ Extramedullary hematopoiesis
  - ○ Sarcomatous transformation: < 1%
    - ▪ Increased risk with polyostotic disease
    - ▪ Hip, pelvis, shoulder most common
    - ▪ Uncommon in skull & spine relative to high prevalence of disease in axial skeleton

- Osteosarcoma: 50-60%
- Fibrosarcoma/MFH: 20-25%
- Chondrosarcoma: 10%
- Histologic distinction of secondary sarcoma not critical due to high degree of anaplasia
- Osseous destruction, enhancing soft tissue mass with necrosis, metastases

Gross Pathologic & Surgical Features

- Newly formed bone abnormally enlarged, deformed, weak

Microscopic Features

- Active phase: Osteolytic phase
  - Aggressive bone resorption
  - Giant osteoclasts with multiple nuclei and inclusion bodies
  - Osteoclastic > osteoblastic activity
  - Replacement of hematopoietic bone marrow by fibrous connective tissue
  - Increased vascular channels
- Mixed blastic-lytic phase
  - Increasing osteoblastic activity eventually surpasses bone resorption
  - Disorganized trabecular pattern
    - "Mosaic" or "jigsaw": Multiple remodeling lines
  - "Pumice" bone
    - Weak bone lacking normal interconnections
- Inactive quiescent phase
  - Decreased bone turnover
    - Diminishing osteoblasts, osteoclasts
  - Loss of excessive vascularity
  - Fatty marrow

CLINICAL ISSUES

Presentation

- Most common signs/symptoms
  - Deep, dull bone pain
  - Other signs/symptoms
    - Asymptomatic: 20%
    - Myelopathy, cauda equina syndrome from canal narrowing
    - Radiculopathy from foraminal stenosis
    - Elevated serum alkaline phosphatase, urine hydroxyproline
- Clinical profile
  - Sarcomatous transformation
    - Severe pain at site of previous asymptomatic disease with large lytic lesion + soft tissue mass

Demographics

- Age
  - 55-85 yo
    - Rare < 40 yo
- Gender: M:F = 3-4:2
- Ethnicity
  - Caucasians of Northern Europeans descent
  - Rare in Asians and African-Americans

Natural History & Prognosis

- Disease process may be halted with return of normal osseous architecture after medical treatment
  - Long term remission expected

- Poor prognosis when sarcomatous degeneration present
  - 3 year mortality rate: > 90%

Treatment

- Analgesic medications
- Medications to inhibit osteoclastic bone resorption & relieve pain
  - Bisphosphates: Alendronate (Fosamax), Pamidronate (Aredia), etc.
  - Calcitonin
  - Mithramycin
- Surgical decompression of spinal stenosis

DIAGNOSTIC CHECKLIST

Image Interpretation Pearls

- Expanded and square vertebra with cortical thickening and central lucency ("picture frame") highly suggestive of Paget disease

SELECTED REFERENCES

1. Spieth ME et al: Positron emission tomography and Paget disease: hot is not necessarily malignant. Clin Nucl Med. 28(9):773-4, 2003
2. Saifuddin A et al: Paget's disease of the spine: unusual features and complications. Clin Radiol. 58(2):102-11, 2003
3. Whitehouse RW: Paget's disease of bone. Semin Musculoskelet Radiol. 6(4):313-22, 2002
4. Smith SE et al: From the archives of the AFIP. Radiologic spectrum of Paget disease of bone and its complications with pathologic correlation. Radiographics. 22(5):1191-216, 2002
5. Vande Berg BC et al: Magnetic resonance appearance of uncomplicated Paget's disease of bone. Semin Musculoskelet Radiol. 5(1):69-77, 2001
6. Hadjipavlou AG et al: Paget's disease of the spine and its management. Eur Spine J. 10(5):370-84, 2001
7. Poncelet A: The neurologic complications of Paget's disease. J Bone Miner Res. 14 Suppl 2:88-91, 1999
8. Boutin RD et al: Complications in Paget disease at MR imaging. Radiology. 209:641-51, 1998
9. Cook GJ et al: Fluorine-18-FDG PET in Paget's disease of bone. J Nucl Med. 38(9):1495-7, 1997
10. Klein RM et al: Diagnostic procedures for Paget's disease. Radiologic, pathologic, and laboratory testing. Endocrinol Metab Clin North Am. 24(2):437-50, 1995
11. Mirra JM et al: Paget's disease of bone: review with emphasis on radiologic features, Part I. Skeletal Radiol. 24(3):163-71, 1995
12. Mirra JM et al: Paget's disease of bone: review with emphasis on radiologic features, Part II. Skeletal Radiol. 24(3):173-84, 1995
13. Hadjipavlou A et al: Malignant transformation in Paget disease of bone. Cancer. 70(12):2802-8, 1992
14. Ryan MD et al: Spinal manifestations of Paget's disease. Aust N Z J Surg. 62(1):33-8, 1992
15. Roberts MC et al: Paget disease: MR imaging findings. Radiology. 173:341-5, 1989
16. Vellenga CJ et al: Bone scintigraphy and radiology in Paget's disease of bone: a review. Am J Physiol Imaging. 3(3):154-68, 1988
17. Frame B et al: Paget disease: A review of current knowledge. Radiology. 141:21-4, 1981

PAGET DISEASE

IMAGE GALLERY

Typical

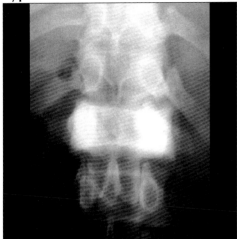 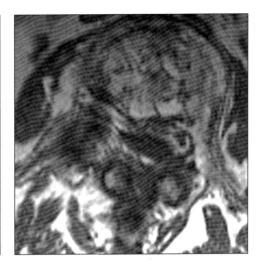

(Left) Anteroposterior radiography of thoracolumbar shows a diffusely dense "ivory" L1 vertebra. Differential diagnoses also include lymphoma and sclerotic metastasis. *(Right)* Axial T1WI MR in another patient through a lumbar vertebra shows coarse and irregular trabeculae with mild vertebral expansion (Courtesy M. Modic, MD).

Typical

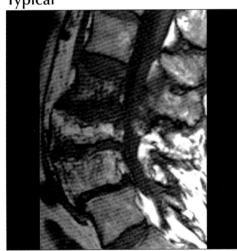 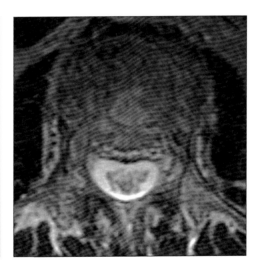

(Left) Sagittal T1WI MR through lumbar spine demonstrates abnormal L2-4 vertebrae. There is mild vertebral enlargement with coarse trabeculae. Increased fatty marrow is present in L3 and L4. *(Right)* Axial T2WI MR in same patient demonstrates a diffusely coarse and haphazard trabecular pattern, in vertebral body and posterior elements.

Typical

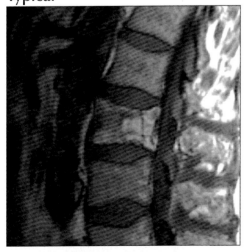 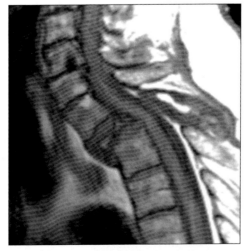

(Left) Sagittal T1WI MR of lumbar spine shows a slightly enlarged L2 vertebra in anterior-posterior dimension. Increased fatty marrow and mild compression are present. *(Right)* Sagittal T1WI MR shows low signal with thickened cortex from T1 body and spinous process. Fatty marrow signal and expansion most obvious for spinous process.

HYPERPARATHYROIDISM

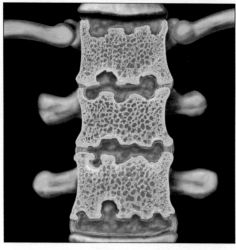

Coronal graphic shows severe hyperparathyroidism with extensive endplate erosions and thinned trabeculae.

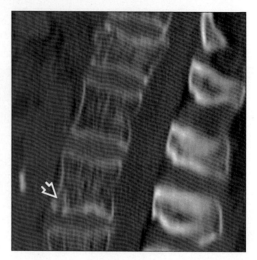

Sagittal bone CT shows diffuse osteopenia and endplate erosion (arrow).

TERMINOLOGY

Abbreviations and Synonyms
- Hyperparathyroidism (HPT)

Definitions
- Increased levels of hyperparathyroid hormone
- Osteitis fibrosa cystica: Florid bony changes due to longstanding HPT
- Brown tumor: Reactive giant cell lesion due to HPT
- HPT may be primary, secondary or tertiary

IMAGING FINDINGS

General Features
- Best diagnostic clue: Osteopenia
- Location: Peripheral skeleton > spine

Radiographic Findings
- Radiography
  - Osteopenia
    - 30-50% bone loss necessary to detect osteopenia
  - Resorption of secondary trabeculae (interlinking, non-weight-bearing trabeculae)
  - Accentuation of primary trabeculae (weight-bearing trabeculae)
  - Cortical thinning

- Sharp distinction between cortex, medullary cavity
  - Subperiosteal bone resorption
  - Sacroiliac joint erosions
  - Schmorl nodes
  - Rare: Vertebral endplate erosions
  - Rare: Brown tumor (osteoclastoma)
    - Lytic, expansile lesion without matrix production
    - Histologically identical to giant cell tumor
  - Soft tissue calcifications
    - Usually involve extremities

CT Findings
- Bone CT
  - More sensitive than radiographs to detect osteopenia, bone resorption

Nuclear Medicine Findings
- Bone Scan: Increased bone turnover

Other Modality Findings
- Bone densitometry most sensitive in detection of osteopenia

Imaging Recommendations
- Best imaging tool
  - Radiography of hands
    - Subperiosteal bone resorption, cortical thinning, acro-osteolysis

DDx: Hyperparathyroidism

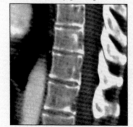

Myeloma

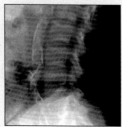

Renal Osteodystrophy

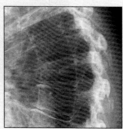

Senile Osteoporosis

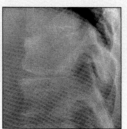

Spondyloarthropathy

HYPERPARATHYROIDISM

Key Facts

Terminology
- Increased levels of hyperparathyroid hormone

Imaging Findings
- Osteopenia
- Cortical thinning
- Subperiosteal bone resorption
- Sacroiliac joint erosions
- Rare: Brown tumor (osteoclastoma)
- Soft tissue calcifications

Top Differential Diagnoses
- Multiple myeloma
- Renal osteodystrophy
- Senile osteoporosis
- Seronegative spondyloarthropathy

DIFFERENTIAL DIAGNOSIS

Multiple myeloma
- Most frequently presents as diffuse osteopenia of spine
- Focal lytic lesions often visible on CT but not radiographs

Renal osteodystrophy
- Secondary HPT plus osteomalacia, bone sclerosis
- "Rugger jersey" spine, blurred trabeculae
- Erosions sacroiliac joints

Senile osteoporosis
- Cortical thinning, resorption primary bone trabeculae
- Compression fractures common

Seronegative spondyloarthropathy
- Erosions sacroiliac joints, vertebral corners
- Syndesmophytes

PATHOLOGY

General Features
- Etiology
  - Primary
    - Parathyroid adenoma, hyperplasia or carcinoma
  - Secondary
    - Due to renal failure, or rarely intestinal malabsorption
    - Hyperplasia of parathyroid glands
  - Tertiary
    - Longstanding secondary HPT leads to autonomous function of parathyroid glands
- Associated abnormalities: Hypophosphatemia, renal calculi, peptic ulcer disease, pancreatitis

Microscopic Features
- Increased osteoclastic activity
- Vascularized fibrous tissue

CLINICAL ISSUES

Presentation
- Most common signs/symptoms: Bone pain, renal colic

Natural History & Prognosis
- Many cases remain mild, stable

Treatment
- Options, risks, complications: Major risk parathyroidectomy: = Recurrent laryngeal n. injury
- Mild cases can be followed conservatively

DIAGNOSTIC CHECKLIST

Image Interpretation Pearls
- Hand radiographs useful to corroborate diagnosis

SELECTED REFERENCES

1. Paderni S et al: Vertebral localization of a brown tumor: description of a case and review of the literature. Chir Organi Mov. 88(1):83-91, 2003
2. Cormier C et al: Hyperparathyroidism: the limits of surgery in cases of bone or cardiovascular involvement. Curr Opin Rheumatol. 12(4):349-53, 2000
3. Adami S et al: Bone measurements in asymptomatic primary hyperparathyroidism. Bone. 22(5):565-70, 1998
4. Barzilay J et al: Erosive spondyloarthropathy in primary hyperparathyroidism without renal failure. Am J Kidney Dis. 20(1):90-3, 1992
5. Lafferty FW et al: Primary hyperparathyroidism. A review of the long-term surgical and nonsurgical morbidities as a basis for a rational approach to treatment. Arch Intern Med. 149(4):789-96, 1989

IMAGE GALLERY

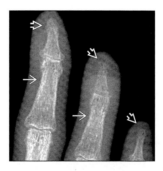 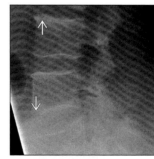

(Left) Anteroposterior radiography shows subperiosteal bone resorption at middle phalanges (arrows), and resorption of terminal tufts (open arrows). *(Right)* Lateral radiography shows diffuse, nonspecific osteopenia. Endplate erosions (arrows) are clue to diagnosis.

RENAL OSTEODYSTROPHY

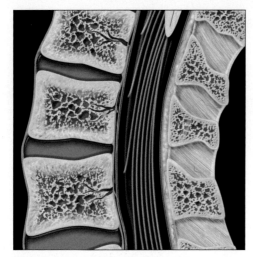

Sagittal graphic shows thickened, sclerotic vertebral endplates. Trabeculae are scanty and irregular in morphology.

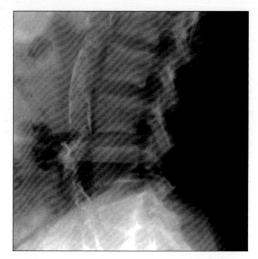

Lateral radiography shows blurring of trabeculae and ill-defined sclerosis adjacent to vertebral endplates in young patient on hemodialysis. Note premature aortoiliac atherosclerosis.

TERMINOLOGY

Abbreviations and Synonyms
- Renal osteodystrophy (OD)

Definitions
- Bony changes due to chronic, end-stage renal disease
  - Secondary hyperparathyroidism (HPT), osteomalacia, bone sclerosis, aluminum toxity contribute to findings

IMAGING FINDINGS

General Features
- Best diagnostic clue: "Rugger jersey" spine
- Location: Involves axial and appendicular skeleton

Radiographic Findings
- Radiography
  - Osteosclerosis and/or osteopenia
  - Rugger jersey spine
    - Bands of hazy sclerosis paralleling endplates
  - Changes of hyperparathyroidism
    - Resorption secondary trabeculae
    - Cortical thinning
    - Erosions at entheses, endplates, signal intensity (SI) joints
    - Subperiosteal bone resorption

  - Brown tumors: Lytic lesion, no matrix, sharp zone transition
  - Changes of osteomalacia/rickets
    - Blurred, coarse bone trabeculae
    - Children: Fraying, cupping metaphyses
  - Retarded skeletal age
  - Pathologic fracture

MR Findings
- Bone marrow has heterogeneous, nonspecific appearance
- Brown tumor
  - T1WI: Low signal intensity focal mass
  - T2WI: High signal intensity focal mass

Nuclear Medicine Findings
- Bone scan may show diffusely increased uptake ("super scan")

Imaging Recommendations
- Best imaging tool: Radiography

DIFFERENTIAL DIAGNOSIS

Primary hyperparathyroidism
- Osteopenia, resorption secondary trabeculae
- Erosions vertebral endplates, sacroiliac joints

DDx: Endplate Sclerosis

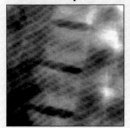
Osteopetrosis

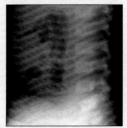
Rickets

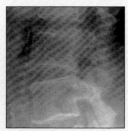
Paget Disease

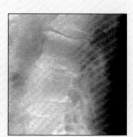
Discogenic Sclerosis

RENAL OSTEODYSTROPHY

Key Facts

Terminology
- Bony changes due to chronic, end-stage renal disease
- Secondary hyperparathyroidism (HPT), osteomalacia, bone sclerosis, aluminum toxity contribute to findings

Imaging Findings
- Osteosclerosis and/or osteopenia
- Rugger jersey spine

- Changes of hyperparathyroidism
- Changes of osteomalacia/rickets

Top Differential Diagnoses
- Primary hyperparathyroidism
- Osteomalacia and rickets
- Dialysis arthropathy
- Osteopetrosis
- Paget disease
- Discogenic sclerosis

Osteomalacia and rickets
- Blurring of trabeculae
- Loss of distinction between cortex, medullary bone
- "Bone within bone" appearance of vertebrae

Dialysis arthropathy
- Arthritis due to deposition of crystals or amyloid
- Only in patients on dialysis, usually hemodialysis
- Endplate erosions, destruction
- Soft tissue masses due to amyloid or crystal deposits
- Co-existing renal osteodystrophy in most of these patients

Osteopetrosis
- Sharply demarcated sclerotic bands adjacent to endplates

Paget disease
- Thickening of cortex around vertebra
- Thickened, disorganized trabeculae

Discogenic sclerosis
- May involve multiple levels
- Not as diffuse as renal OD
- Osteophytes, disc space narrowing also present

PATHOLOGY

General Features
- General path comments: A complex of abnormalities with variable appearance
- Etiology
  - Secondary hyperparathyroidism
    - Hyperplasia of parathyroid glands in chronic renal failure
    - Due to phosphate retention, low serum calcium
  - Osteomalacia
    - Abnormal vitamin D metabolism
    - Aluminum intoxication
- Epidemiology: Common in chronic renal failure

Gross Pathologic & Surgical Features
- Trabeculae thickened, disorganized; or thinned

Microscopic Features
- Osteoblastic, osteoclastic activity may be increased or decreased

CLINICAL ISSUES

Presentation
- Most common signs/symptoms: Pathologic fracture

Natural History & Prognosis
- Increased fracture risk
- Hemodialysis may result in hemodialysis arthropathy

Treatment
- Options, risks, complications
  - Vitamin D analogs
  - Phosphate binders

SELECTED REFERENCES

1. Paderni S et al: Vertebral localization of a brown tumor: description of a case and review of the literature. Chir Organi Mov. 88(1):83-91, 2003
2. Spasovski GB et al: Spectrum of renal bone disease in end-stage renal failure patients not yet on dialysis. Nephrol Dial Transplant. 18(6):1159-66, 2003
3. Jevtic V: Imaging of renal osteodystrophy. Eur J Radiol. 46(2):85-95, 2003
4. Bardin T: Musculoskeletal manifestations of chronic renal failure. Curr Opin Rheumatol. 15(1):48-54, 2003

IMAGE GALLERY

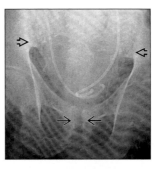 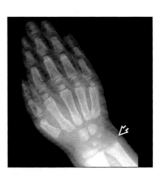

(Left) Anteroposterior radiography of pelvis shows sacroiliac joint erosions (open arrows) + pubic symphysis erosions (arrows). Note blurred trabeculae throughout pelvis. *(Right)* Anteroposterior radiography of hand shows renal OD manifest primarily as rickets. Note fraying, cupping of ulnar metaphysis (arrow) + coarsened trabecular pattern.

HYPERPLASTIC VERTEBRAL MARROW

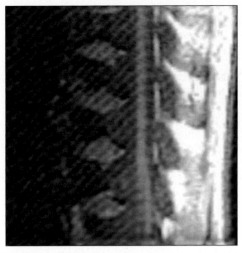

Sagittal T1WI MR in a patient with sickle cell anemia demonstrates biconcave vertebrae with diffuse marrow hypointensity. Intervertebral discs appear hyperintense compared to marrow.

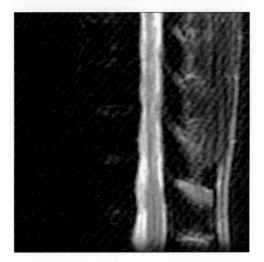

Sagittal T2WI MR in same patient shows homogeneous marrow hypointensity, compatible with hyperplastic cellular marrow.

TERMINOLOGY

Abbreviations and Synonyms
- Marrow reconversion
- Hypercellular marrow expansion

Definitions
- Physiologic process where fatty marrow is converted to red marrow in response to systemic stress

IMAGING FINDINGS

General Features
- Best diagnostic clue: Intervertebral discs hyperintense compared to vertebral marrow on T1WI
- Location
  - Calvarium, spine, ribs, pelvis initially involved
    - Followed by extremities
- Size: Entire spinal column typically affected
- Morphology
  - Diffuse, homogeneous
  - Patchy, geographic

Radiographic Findings
- Radiography
  - Hemolytic anemias
    - Medullary expansion in ribs, calvarium, long bones

- Cortical thinning
- "Hair-on-end" striations in calvarium
- Biconcave vertebrae in sickle cell anemia

CT Findings
- Bone CT
  - H-shaped vertebrae due to endplate infarction in sickle cell anemia

MR Findings
- T1WI
  - Intermediate to low signal intensity (SI)
    - Where fatty marrow is expected
    - Similar to, hypointense, or slightly hyperintense to muscle
    - Normal vertebral marrow SI significantly higher than muscle
- T2WI
  - Intermediate to low SI
    - Similar to, but not higher than, muscle on fat-suppressed T2WI
- STIR: Similar, but not hyperintense, compared to muscle
- T1 C+: Mild post-gadolinium enhancement

Nuclear Medicine Findings
- Tc-99m diphosphonate or Tc-99m sulfur colloid scan
  - Sites of increased uptake due to marrow expansion
    - Distal appendicular skeleton

DDx: Hypointense Vertebral Marrow

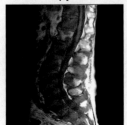

Metastases

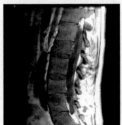

Multiple Myeloma

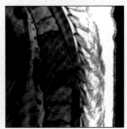

Osteomyelitis

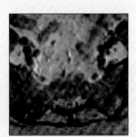

Myelofibrosis

HYPERPLASTIC VERTEBRAL MARROW

Key Facts

Terminology
- Marrow reconversion
- Physiologic process where fatty marrow is converted to red marrow in response to systemic stress

Imaging Findings
- Best diagnostic clue: Intervertebral discs hyperintense compared to vertebral marrow on T1WI
- Intermediate to low signal intensity (SI)
- STIR: Similar, but not hyperintense, compared to muscle
- T1 C+: Mild post-gadolinium enhancement
- MRI modality of choice in marrow imaging

Top Differential Diagnoses
- Marrow infiltration/replacement
- Myeloproliferative disorder

- Marrow edema

Pathology
- Process of reconversion starts in axial skeleton
- Beginning with calvarium, then vertebrae, ribs, sternum, and pelvis
- Followed by extremities, from proximal to distal

Diagnostic Checklist
- Fat-suppressed T2WI (or STIR) & T1WI with gadolinium when hypointense marrow present on T1WI
- Diffuse marrow T1 hypointensity without marked post-gadolinium enhancement or cortical disruption suggests hyperplastic marrow

---

    ▪ Calvarium

Other Modality Findings
- Iron-oxide-enhanced MR marrow imaging
  ○ Normal and hypercellular reconverted marrow accumulate supermagnetic iron oxides
    ▪ Significant signal loss on STIR 45-60 minutes after iron oxide infusion
  ○ May be useful in distinguishing tumor infiltration from marrow reconversion

Imaging Recommendations
- Best imaging tool
  ○ MRI modality of choice in marrow imaging
    ▪ High sensitivity in detecting increased marrow cellularity on T1WI
- Protocol advice
  ○ STIR or T2WI MRI with fat-saturation
    ▪ To distinguish hematopoietic elements from marrow edema or neoplastic infiltration
  ○ Pre-, post-gadolinium T1WI with fat suppression also helpful

DIFFERENTIAL DIAGNOSIS

Normal hematopoetic marrow
- Children up to ~ 10 years

Marrow infiltration/replacement
- Leukemia, lymphoma, multiple myeloma, or metastases
- Diffuse or focal T1 hypointensity
  ○ Multifocal disease more easily distinguished from hyperplastic normal marrow
  ○ Diffuse marrow infiltration may appear very similar
- SI usually great than muscle on STIR or fat suppressed T2WI
- Post-gadolinium enhancement
- Increased metabolic activity on PET scan
- Pathologic compression fractures
- Epidural/paravertebral tumor extension

Myeloproliferative disorder
- Polycythemia vera, chronic myelogenous leukemia, primary thrombocythemia, myelofibrosis with myeloid metaplasia
- Uncontrolled proliferation of hematopoietic stem cells
- May overlap, evolve into one another, or transform into acute leukemia
- MR appearance overlaps with hyperplastic normal marrow

Marrow edema
- Trauma, osteomyelitis, marrow surrounding tumors
- Hypointensity on T1WI
  ○ Typically less than muscle SI
- Focal or multisegmental hyperintensity on STIR
- Associated cortical disruption
- Soft tissue and intraspinal hematoma in trauma
- Discitis intraspinal ± phlegmon/abscess in osteomyelitis

PATHOLOGY

General Features
- General path comments
  ○ Circulatory demands exceed available cellular marrow
    ▪ Recruitment of yellow marrow to produce red marrow
  ○ Embryology-anatomy
    ▪ At birth, marrow space in entire skeleton occupied with red marrow
    ▪ Conversion of red to yellow marrow occurs in first two decades of life
    ▪ From peripheral and distal to central and proximal
    ▪ Adult marrow pattern by 25 years of age
    ▪ Red marrow (40% fat, 40% water, 20% protein) predominantly in axial skeleton, proximal humeri and femora

- With age, red marrow decreases from 58% of total marrow volume in 1st decade to 29% by 8th decade
- Amount of fatty marrow (80% fat, 15% water, 5% protein) increases
- Also to replace bone loss
  - ○ Process of reconversion starts in axial skeleton
    - Beginning with calvarium, then vertebrae, ribs, sternum, and pelvis
    - Followed by extremities, from proximal to distal
    - Epiphyses usually spared unless extreme needs present
    - Extensive reconversion in appendicular skeleton suggests severe anemia or neoplastic involvement of axial skeleton
  - ○ Adults < 40 yo have better marrow reconversion capacity than older adults
- Etiology
  - ○ Iron deficiency anemia
    - Most common cause of anemia
    - Chronic blood loss
    - Increased requirements (pregnancy, adolescence etc.)
    - Inadequate diet
  - ○ Anemia of chronic disease
    - Second most common cause of anemia
    - Infections (e.g., AIDS), inflammatory disease (e.g., rheumatoid arthritis), cancer most common
    - Interferons, interleukins from monocytes inhibit erythropoietin production, erythroid proliferation
    - Inadequate release of iron from reticulum cells to plasma
    - Increased destruction of red blood cells by reticuloendothelial system
  - ○ Hemolytic anemia
    - Accelerated destruction of red blood cells
    - Sickle cell disease, thalassemia, etc.
  - ○ Chronic hypoxemia
    - Cyanotic heart disorder, heart failure
    - Heavy smoking: > 1 pack per day
    - High altitude
    - Obesity
    - Marathon athletes
  - ○ Hematopoietic growth factors
    - E.g., granulocyte colony-stimulating factor
    - Adjunct in chemotherapy
    - May simulate marrow tumor progression
- Associated abnormalities
  - ○ Increased marrow cellularity in diaphyses of long bones
  - ○ Osteonecrosis in sickle cell anemia

Microscopic Features

- Capillary proliferation
- Increased sinusoids
- Expanded cellular marrow
- Anemia of chronic disease
  - ○ Normal or increased reticuloendothelial iron storage
- Iron deficiency anemia
  - ○ Decreased reticuloendothelial iron storage

CLINICAL ISSUES

Presentation

- Most common signs/symptoms
  - ○ May not have symptoms referable to spine
  - ○ Other signs/symptoms related to anemia, hypoxemia
    - Skin and mucous membrane pallor
    - Weakness and fatigue
    - Dyspnea
    - Congestive heart failure

Demographics

- Age
  - ○ All ages reported
  - ○ More evident in adults > 25 yo
- Ethnicity
  - ○ No racial predilection except certain anemias
    - Sickle cell disease: African-Americans
    - Thalassemia: Races along Eastern Mediterranean Sea; Greek, Italian, Persian, etc.

Natural History & Prognosis

- Dependent on underlying etiology causing marrow reconversion

Treatment

- Treatment of underlying disease
- Transfusions
- Recombinant erythropoietin

DIAGNOSTIC CHECKLIST

Consider

- Fat-suppressed T2WI (or STIR) & T1WI with gadolinium when hypointense marrow present on T1WI

Image Interpretation Pearls

- Diffuse marrow T1 hypointensity without marked post-gadolinium enhancement or cortical disruption suggests hyperplastic marrow

SELECTED REFERENCES

1. Daldrup-Link HE et al: Iron-oxide-enhanced MR imaging of bone marrow in patients with non-Hodgkin's lymphoma: differentiation between tumor infiltration and hypercellular bone marrow. Eur Radiol. 12(6):1557-66, 2002
2. Plecha DM: Imaging of bone marrow disease in the spine. Semin Musculoskelet Radiol. 4(3):321-7, 2000
3. Baur A et al: MRI gadolinium enhancement of bone marrow: age-related changes in normals and in diffuse neoplastic infiltration. Skeletal Radiol. 26(7):414-8, 1997
4. Carroll KW et al: Useful internal standards for distinguishing infiltrative marrow pathology from hematopoietic marrow at MRI. J Magn Reson Imaging. 7(2):394-8, 1997
5. Poulton TB et al: Bone marrow reconversion in adults who are smokers: MR Imaging findings. AJR Am J Roentgenol. 161(6):1217-21, 1993

HYPERPLASTIC VERTEBRAL MARROW

IMAGE GALLERY

Typical

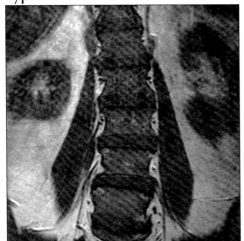
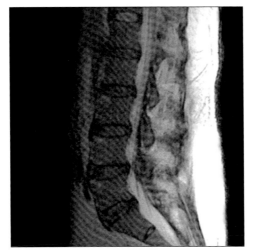

(Left) Coronal T1WI MR through lumbar spine in a patient with anemia of chronic disease shows homogeneously hypointense marrow, similar to muscle. (Right) Sagittal T2WI MR in the same patient shows intermediate to low marrow signal intensity. Degenerative changes are present at anterior and superior endplates of L3-5.

Typical

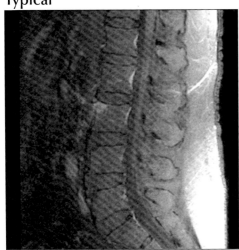
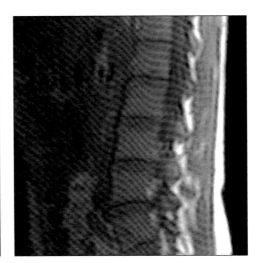

(Left) Sagittal T1 C+ MR with fat suppression in the patient demonstrates lack of enhancement in lumbar vertebral marrow, except for degenerative change at anterior and superior endplate of L3. (Right) Sagittal T1WI MR through lumbar spine in patient with chronic anemia shows a homogeneous hypointense marrow pattern, consistent with marrow reconversion.

Typical

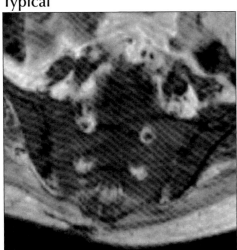
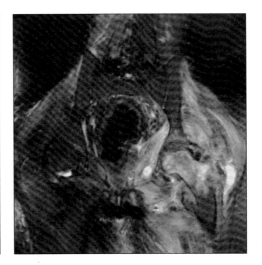

(Left) Axial T1WI MR through sacrum in a patient with chronic anemia & osteomyelitis demonstrates diffuse hypointense marrow signal intensity, lower than surrounding muscle. (Right) Coronal T2WI MR with fat suppression shows left hip osteomyelitis and surrounding myositis and abscesses. Remainder of the marrow is hypointense.

MYELOFIBROSIS

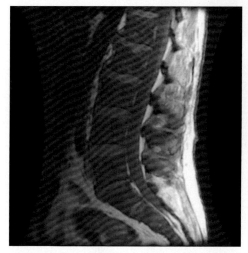

Sagittal T1WI MR shows uniform low signal intensity marrow replacement in patient with primary myelofibrosis (Courtesy L. Steinbach, MD).

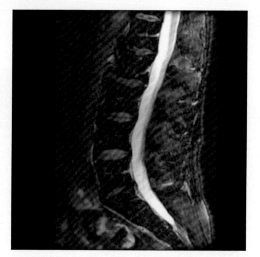

Sagittal STIR MR shows marrow signal intensity almost equal to cortical bone in patient with primary myelofibrosis (Courtesy L. Steinbach, MD).

TERMINOLOGY

Abbreviations and Synonyms
• Myelosclerosis

Definitions
• Histomorphologic pattern of fibrosis in bone marrow which may be associated with various disorders
• Myelodysplastic syndromes: Myeloproliferative disorders which may show myelofibrosis at some point in their evolution

IMAGING FINDINGS

General Features
• Best diagnostic clue: Very low signal intensity in bone marrow on all sequences of MRI

Radiographic Findings
• Radiography: Usually normal; bone sometimes diffusely sclerotic

CT Findings
• Bone CT
  ○ May see diffuse bone sclerosis

MR Findings
• T1WI: Very low signal intensity marrow

• T2WI: Very low signal intensity marrow
• STIR: Very low signal intensity marrow

Imaging Recommendations
• Best imaging tool: MRI
• Protocol advice: Sagittal T1WI, T2WI, STIR

DIFFERENTIAL DIAGNOSIS

Leukemia and lymphoma
• Low signal intensity on T1WI and T2WI
• Usually higher signal than myelofibrosis

Erythropoietic marrow
• Low signal intensity on T1WI and T2WI
• Usually higher signal than myelofibrosis

Sclerotic metastases
• Very low signal intensity on T1WI and T2WI

Osteopetrosis
• Very low signal intensity on T1WI and T2WI
• "Bone-in-bone" appearance

PATHOLOGY

General Features
• General path comments

DDx: Myelofibrosis

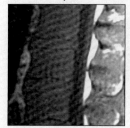

Hairy Cell Leukemia

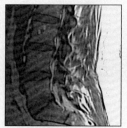

Nl Red Marrow

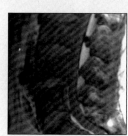

Metastasis

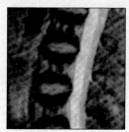

Osteopetrosis

MYELOFIBROSIS

Key Facts

Terminology
- Histomorphologic pattern of fibrosis in bone marrow which may be associated with various disorders

Imaging Findings
- Best diagnostic clue: Very low signal intensity in bone marrow on all sequences of MRI

Top Differential Diagnoses
- Leukemia and lymphoma
- Erythropoietic marrow
- Sclerotic metastases

Diagnostic Checklist
- Cannot exclude concomitant tumor by MRI; biopsy needed for diagnosis

- Most commonly a secondary phenomenon due to leukemia, lymphoma or metastatic tumor
- "Primary" form may be a precursor to polycythemia vera and chronic myeloid leukemia
- Etiology: May be single or multiple lineage dysplasias of hematopoiesis

Gross Pathologic & Surgical Features
- Bone marrow biopsy difficult due to fibrosis

Microscopic Features
- Increased reticulin fibers in bone marrow; other findings variable

Staging, Grading or Classification Criteria
- Primary: Indolent process
- Secondary: Associated with leukemia, lymphoma or metastatic disease
- Acute myelofibrosis: Abrupt onset, anemia, panmyeloid proliferation, rapidly fatal
- 5q-syndrome myelofibrosis associated with increased atypical megakaryocytes
- Some cases are autoimmune-mediated

CLINICAL ISSUES

Presentation
- Most common signs/symptoms
  - Anemia
  - Other signs/symptoms
    - Splenomegaly due to extramedullary hematopoiesis

Demographics
- Age: Primary: 50-70

Natural History & Prognosis
- Variable, depending on causative disease entity

Treatment
- Options, risks, complications: Androgens, prednisone, thalidomide, bone marrow transplants have some effectiveness

DIAGNOSTIC CHECKLIST

Image Interpretation Pearls
- Cannot exclude concomitant tumor by MRI; biopsy needed for diagnosis

SELECTED REFERENCES

1. Rosai, J Rosai &Ackerman's Surgical Pathology, vol. 2, 9th ed., Edinburgh, Mosby. 2048-2068, 2004
2. Barosi G: Myelofibrosis with myeloid metaplasia. Hematol Oncol Clin North Am. 17(5):1211-26, 2003
3. Barosi G: Myelofibrosis with myeloid metaplasia. Hematol Oncol Clin North Am. 17(5):1211-26, 2003
4. Mesa RA: The therapy of myelofibrosis: targeting pathogenesis. Int J Hematol. 76 Suppl 2:296-304, 2002
5. Diamond T et al: Syndrome of myelofibrosis and osteosclerosis: a series of case reports and review of the literature. Bone. 30(3):498-501, 2002
6. Bass RD et al: Pathology of autoimmune myelofibrosis. A report of three cases and a review of the literature. Am J Clin Pathol. 116(2):211-6, 2001
7. Smith BD et al: Biology and management of idiopathic myelofibrosis. Curr Opin Oncol. 13(2):91-4, 2001

IMAGE GALLERY

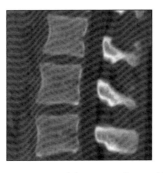 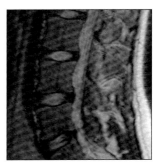

(Left) Sagittal bone CT shows diffusely increased bone density in myelofibrosis associated with Hodgkin lymphoma. Individual trabeculae are not discernible in dense bone meshwork. (Right) Sagittal T2WI MR shows decreased bone marrow signal intensity in myelofibrosis associated with Hodgkin lymphoma.

EXTRAMEDULLARY HEMATOPOIESIS

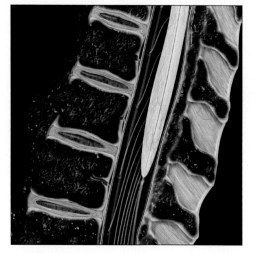

Sagittal graphic of extramedullary hematopoiesis depicts abundant hematopoietic marrow in lumbar vertebrae, extending into prevertebral and dorsal epidural space.

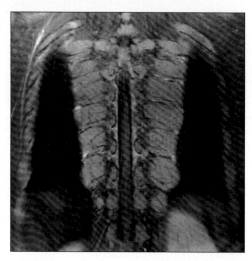

Coronal T1 C+ MR with fat suppression in patient with beta-thalassemia shows mildly enhancing bilateral paraspinal masses, proven extramedullary hematopoiesis at biopsy.

TERMINOLOGY

Abbreviations and Synonyms
- Extramedullary hematopoiesis (EMH)

Definitions
- Epidural ± paravertebral proliferation of hematopoietic tissue in response to profound chronic anemia

IMAGING FINDINGS

General Features
- Best diagnostic clue: Minimally enhancing isointense thoracic intra- or paraspinal masses with associated diffuse marrow hypointensity
- Location
  ○ Mid thoracic > cervical, lumbar
    ▪ Epidural
    ▪ Paravertebral
- Size: Multi-segmental
- Morphology
  ○ Well-circumscribed
  ○ Homogeneous
  ○ Lobular soft tissue mass

Radiographic Findings
- Radiography: Bilateral (a)symmetrically widened paraspinal stripe on frontal radiograph

- Myelography: Nonspecific epidural mass effacing central canal

CT Findings
- NECT
  ○ Soft tissue density
  ○ Central canal narrowing
  ○ Cord displacement and compression
- CECT: Mild enhancement
- Bone CT
  ○ No bony erosion
  ○ No calcifications

MR Findings
- T1WI: Isointense to cord
- T2WI
  ○ Iso- to mildly hyperintense to cord
    ▪ Hypointensity may represent increased iron content in hematopoietic tissue
- STIR: Iso- to hyperintense
- T1 C+: Minimal, mild, or moderate
- Variable mass effect on spinal cord
  ○ Cord compression most commonly reported with β-thalassemia
  ○ Intramedullary T2 hyperintensity may be present
    ▪ Edema or myelomalacia
- Nerve root compression
- Diffuse vertebral marrow hypointensity on all sequences

DDx: Epidural Masses

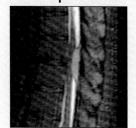
Metastasis

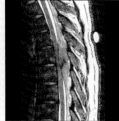
Lymphoma

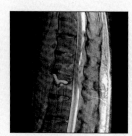
Phlegmon

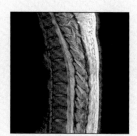
Hematoma

EXTRAMEDULLARY HEMATOPOIESIS

Key Facts

Terminology
- Epidural ± paravertebral proliferation of hematopoietic tissue in response to profound chronic anemia

Imaging Findings
- Best diagnostic clue: Minimally enhancing isointense thoracic intra- or paraspinal masses with associated diffuse marrow hypointensity
- Mid thoracic > cervical, lumbar
- Soft tissue density
- T1WI: Isointense to cord
- T1 C+: Minimal, mild, or moderate
- Variable mass effect on spinal cord
- Nerve root compression

- Diffuse vertebral marrow hypointensity on all sequences

Top Differential Diagnoses
- Epidural/paraspinal metastasis
- Spinal epidural lymphoma

Pathology
- Ectopic hematopoietic rests stimulated in response to chronic anemic states
- Spinal involvement most common after hepatosplenic EMH

Clinical Issues
- Cord compression from epidural EMH should be suspected in patients with chronic anemia who present with neurologic complaints

Nuclear Medicine Findings
- Technetium sulfur colloid scan
  - Foci of epidural/paraspinal uptake correspond to EMH

Imaging Recommendations
- Best imaging tool: Sagittal, axial T2WI + T1 C+ MR

DIFFERENTIAL DIAGNOSIS

Epidural/paraspinal metastasis
- Extension from adjacent vertebral lesions
  - Posterior cortex typically involved
    - High intensity on STIR
  - Compression fractures
- Isolated epidural/paraspinal disease sparing spinal column rare
- Moderate enhancement invariably present

Spinal epidural lymphoma
- Isointense to cord on T1WI
  - Iso- to hyperintense on T2WI
- Intense homogeneous post-gadolinium enhancement
- ± Adjacent vertebral involvement
- Diffuse marrow hypointensity may be present

Epidural/paravertebral phlegmon/abscess
- Associated with infectious spondylitis
  - Destructive changes in adjacent vertebrae
- Hyperintense on STIR
  - Especially liquified components
- Diffuse or peripheral enhancement

Neurogenic tumor
- Often at a single level
- Multiple neurofibromas in neurofibromatosis type 1
- Isointense to cord on T1WI
  - Hyperintense on T2WI
- Avid post-contrast-enhancement
- Widened intervertebral foramina

Epidural hematoma
- Often hyperintense on T1WI

- Iso- to hypointense on T2WI
- No post-gadolinium enhancement
- Sudden onset of symptoms

PATHOLOGY

General Features
- General path comments
  - Compensatory mechanism when normal marrow insufficient to meet circulatory demands in chronic anemia
  - Typical sites of EMH
    - Liver, spleen, kidneys
    - Sites of fetal hematopoiesis
  - Lymph node, retroperitoneum, cardiac, thymic involvement also reported
- Etiology
  - Ectopic hematopoietic rests stimulated in response to chronic anemic states
    - Intermediate β-thalassemia: Most common
    - Sickle cell anemia
    - Polycythemia vera
    - Myelofibrosis with myeloid metaplasia
  - Source of extra-vertebral hematopoiesis controversial
    - Embryonic hematopoietic rests in epidural space
    - Direct extension of hematopoietic marrow from vertebrae into epidural space
    - Fetal hematopoietic capacity of dura
  - Other possible theory: Stem cells differentiate into hematopoietic cells
    - Stimulated by unknown factors
- Epidemiology
  - Spinal involvement most common after hepatosplenic EMH
    - Spinal EMH: 27% of non-hepatosplenic involvement
- Associated abnormalities
  - Marrow expansion in ribs
  - Small infarcted spleen in patients with sickle cell disease
  - Splenomegaly in other causes
  - Hemothorax with paraspinal EMH

EXTRAMEDULLARY HEMATOPOIESIS

Gross Pathologic & Surgical Features
- Discrete flesh colored mass

Microscopic Features
- Resembles bone marrow on biopsy
  - Trilineage hematopoiesis
    - Erythroid and granulocytic precursors
    - Megakaryocytes

CLINICAL ISSUES

Presentation
- Most common signs/symptoms
  - Back ± radicular pain
  - Other signs/symptoms
    - Paraparesis
    - Sensory deficit
    - Gait disturbance
    - Bladder, bowel dysfunction
    - Diminished deep tendon reflexes
    - Anemia, pancytopenia
- Clinical profile: Cord compression from epidural EMH should be suspected in patients with chronic anemia who present with neurologic complaints

Demographics
- Age: More common in adults
- Gender: No gender predilection
- Ethnicity
  - Some hemoglobinopathies more common in certain ethnic groups
    - Sickle cell disease: African-Americans
    - Thalassemia: Races along Eastern Mediterranean Sea; Greek, Italian, Persian, etc.
  - Myeloproliferative disorders: No ethnic predilection

Natural History & Prognosis
- Excellent prognosis: Resolution of symptoms 3-7 days after radiotherapy
  - Overall prognosis limited by underlying hemoglobinopathy or myeloproliferative disorder

Treatment
- Intravenous steroids
  - Decrease cord edema
- Radiation therapy
  - Treatment of choice
    - Ectopic hematopoietic tissue extremely radio-sensitive
  - Alone or in conjunction with surgery
  - Risk of marrow suppression
- Decompressive laminectomy with surgical resection
  - Indicated when significant myelopathy present
- Transfusions
  - When radiation or surgery contraindicated
  - Hematopoietic tissues regress as stress of anemia relieved
  - Frequent recurrences
- Hydroxyurea
  - Increases production of hemoglobin-F

DIAGNOSTIC CHECKLIST

Image Interpretation Pearls
- Spinal EMH should be considered when thoracic epidural/paraspinal isointense masses are present in patients with hemoglobinopathies or myeloproliferative disorders

SELECTED REFERENCES

1. Salehi SA et al: Spinal cord compression in beta-thalassemia: case report and review of the literature. Spinal Cord. 42(2):117-23, 2004
2. Koch CA et al: Nonhepatosplenic extramedullary hematopoiesis: associated diseases, pathology, clinical course, and treatment. Mayo Clin Proc. 78(10):1223-33, 2003
3. Chehal A et al: Hypertransfusion: a successful method of treatment in thalassemia intermedia patients with spinal cord compression secondary to extramedullary hematopoiesis. Spine. 28(13):E245-9, 2003
4. Cario H et al: Treatment with hydroxyurea in thalassemia intermedia with paravertebral pseudotumors of extramedullary hematopoiesis. Ann Hematol. 81(8):478-82, 2002
5. Chourmouzi D et al: MRI findings of extramedullary haemopoiesis. Eur Radiol. 11(9):1803-6, 2001
6. Alorainy IA et al: MRI features of epidural extramedullary hematopoiesis. Eur J Radiol. 35(1):8-11, 2000
7. Aydingoz U et al: Spinal cord compression due to epidural extramedullary haematopoiesis in thalassaemia: MRI. Neuroradiology. 39(12):870-2, 1997
8. Guermazi A et al: Imaging of spinal cord compression due to thoracic extramedullary haematopoiesis in myelofibrosis. Neuroradiology. 39(10):733-6, 1997
9. Dibbern DA Jr et al: MR of thoracic cord compression caused by epidural extramedullary hematopoiesis in myelodysplastic syndrome. AJNR Am J Neuroradiol. 18(2):363-6, 1997
10. Kalina P et al: Cord compression by extramedullary hematopoiesis in polycythemia vera. AJR Am J Roentgenol. 164(4):1027-8, 1995
11. Papavasiliou C: Clinical expressions of the expansion of the bone marrow in the chronic anemias: the role of radiotherapy. Int J Radiat Oncol Biol Phys. 28(3):605-12, 1994
12. Kalina P et al: MR of extramedullary hematopoiesis causing cord compression in beta-thalassemia. AJNR Am J Neuroradiol. 13(5):1407-9, 1992
13. Konstantopoulos K et al: A case of spinal cord compression by extramedullary haemopoiesis in a thalassaemic patient: a putative role for hydroxyurea? Haematologica. 77(4):352-4, 1992
14. Kaufmann T et al: The role of radiation therapy in the management of hematopoietic neurologic complications in thalassemia. Acta Haematol. 85(3):156-9, 1991
15. Gouliamos A et al: Low back pain due to extramedullary hemopoiesis. Neuroradiology. 33(3):284-5, 1991
16. Papavasiliou C et al: Masses of myeloadipose tissue: radiological and clinical considerations. Int J Radiat Oncol Biol Phys. 19(4):985-93, 1990

EXTRAMEDULLARY HEMATOPOIESIS

IMAGE GALLERY

Typical

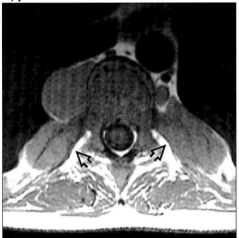
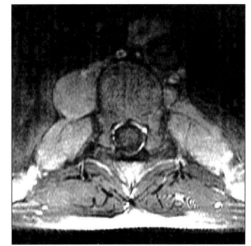

(Left) Axial T1WI MR in a patient with beta-thalassemia shows bilateral paraspinal masses, isointense to cord. Bilateral rib marrow expansion is evident (arrows). *(Right)* Axial T1 C+ MR demonstrates moderate enhancement of bilateral paraspinal masses in patient with beta-thalassemia.

Typical

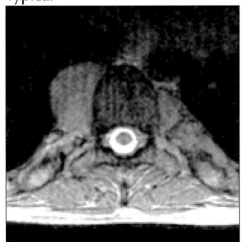
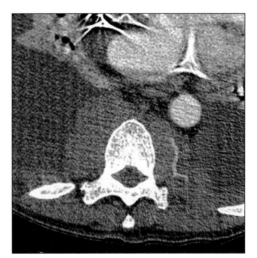

(Left) Axial T2* GRE MR shows paravertebral masses, isointense to spinal cord. Biopsy reveals EMH. *(Right)* Axial CECT in patient with EMH shows bilateral mildly enhancing paravertebral masses. A vessel traverses through left paraspinal mass. Bilateral pleural effusions are present.

Typical

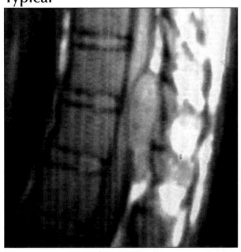
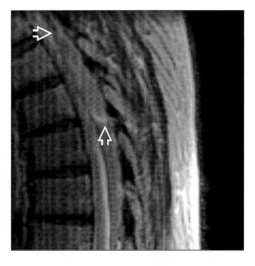

(Left) Sagittal T1WI MR in a patient with thoracic EMH shows elliptical well-circumscribed dorsal epidural mass, isointense to cord, narrowing spinal canal and compressing thoracic cord. *(Right)* Sagittal T2WI MR with fat suppression in another patient with spinal EMH shows mildly hyperintense dorsal extradural mass (arrows) in upper thoracic spine with cord compression.

TUMORAL CALCINOSIS

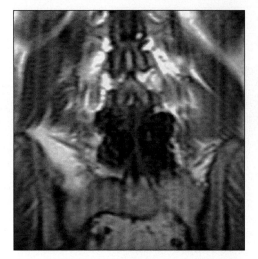

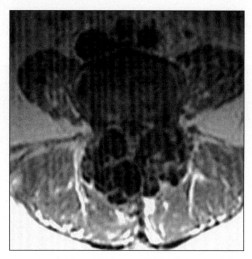

Coronal T1WI MR shows large lobulated masses of low signal involving posterior elements at L4, L5, with no associated intermediate or soft tissue component.

Sagittal T1WI MR shows multiple, well-defined low signal lesions encompassing posterior elements at L4-5. There is moderate canal stenosis due to tumoral calcinosis mass effect.

TERMINOLOGY

Abbreviations and Synonyms
- Lipocalcinogranulomatosis
- Calcifying collagenolysis
- Tumoral lipocalcinosis

Definitions
- Benign periarticular soft tissue hyperplasia, calcification

IMAGING FINDINGS

General Features
- Best diagnostic clue
  - Nonaggressive appearing calcific mass centered about large synovial joints
    - Rare
    - Commonly misdiagnosed
- Location
  - Predilection for large joints
    - Hip
    - Shoulder
    - Elbow
    - Spinal involvement uncommon
- Size: Variable
- Morphology: Well-defined calcific mass

Radiographic Findings
- Radiography
  - Calcific mass with clustered calcific aggregates surrounding joint
  - May show bone remodeling
  - No bone destruction

CT Findings
- NECT
  - Calcific mass with clustered calcific aggregates surrounding joint
  - Occasional bone remodeling
  - No evidence of bone destruction
  - No significant soft tissue mass which is not calcified

MR Findings
- T1WI
  - Lobulated low signal masses centered on facet joint
  - May extend into adjacent paraspinal soft tissue
  - May extend beyond midline to involve dorsal elements, ligamentum flavum
  - Diagnosis very difficult on MR, need CT confirmation
- T2WI
  - Low signal masses, lobulated
  - Mass effect on high signal adjacent thecal sac
- STIR: Low signal, lobulated

DDx: Masses Centered on Posterior Elements

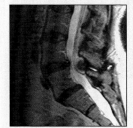

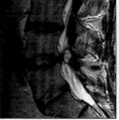

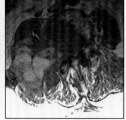

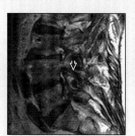

Baastrup *Synovial Cyst* *Osteosarcoma* *Septic Facet*

TUMORAL CALCINOSIS

Key Facts

Terminology
- Benign periarticular soft tissue hyperplasia, calcification

Imaging Findings
- Predilection for large joints
- Hip
- Shoulder
- Elbow
- Spinal involvement uncommon
- Calcific mass with clustered calcific aggregates surrounding joint
- Occasional bone remodeling
- No evidence of bone destruction
- No significant soft tissue mass which is not calcified

Top Differential Diagnoses
- Calcium pyrophosphate deposition disease
- Primary bone tumor
- Synovial chondromatosis
- Neuropathic joint
- Baastrup disease
- Synovial cyst
- Infection/septic facet

Pathology
- Most cases spontaneous and sporadic
- Autosomal recessive and dominant patterns occasionally found
- Unknown - several theories

Diagnostic Checklist
- Tumoral calcinosis is diagnosis of exclusion

- T2* GRE: Low signal from expansile dorsal element lobulated masses
- T1 C+
  - Minimal enhancement
  - No associated enhancing soft tissue component

Nuclear Medicine Findings
- Bone Scan: Markedly increased uptake

Imaging Recommendations
- Best imaging tool: CT shows calcific lesions, extent, presence or absence of bone destruction
- Protocol advice: Axial thin section CT, multiplanar reformats

DIFFERENTIAL DIAGNOSIS

Calcium pyrophosphate deposition disease
- Calcification involving ligamentum flavum
- May compress dorsal thecal sac
- Confined to ligamentum flavum
- No facet joint involvement

Primary bone tumor
- Ill-defined margins, infiltrative
- Large soft tissue component separate from calcific mass
- Enhancement of soft tissue component
- Bone destruction

Synovial chondromatosis
- Usually affects larger joints as does tumoral calcinosis
- Monoarticular involvement, unknown cause
- Middle aged patients, M < F
- Progressive periarticular swelling and pain
- Multiple intra-articular densities on CT, plain film

Neuropathic joint
- Bone destruction, as well as bone proliferation

Baastrup disease
- Degeneration of interspinous ligament, ligamentum flavum
- Thickening, buckling of dorsal spinal ligaments

- "Kissing" spinous processes
- Cystic degeneration of interspinous ligament with high signal on T2WI

Synovial cyst
- Well-defined mass arising from ventral margin of facet joint/ligamentum flavum
- Central high signal on T2WI
- Peripheral low signal on T2WI, peripheral enhancement
- Commonly associated with joint effusion

Infection/septic facet
- Abnormal low signal from facet, with irregular adjacent soft tissue extension
- Joint effusion
- Bone destruction
- Peripheral enhancement of epidural abscess

PATHOLOGY

General Features
- General path comments
  - Calcific masses about large joints, with spine involvement uncommon
  - Need to exclude other causes of soft tissue calcification
    - Collagen vascular disease, hypervitaminosis D, chronic renal disease
- Genetics
  - Most cases spontaneous and sporadic
  - Autosomal recessive and dominant patterns occasionally found
  - Cases of familial hyperphosphatemia with tumoral calcinosis
  - Some overlap of clinical features with pseudoxanthoma elasticum (PXE)
    - PXE shows degenerated dermal elastic fibers
    - PXE shows vasculopathy, and there are rare cases of peripheral aneurysm formation in tumoral calcinosis
- Etiology

TUMORAL CALCINOSIS

- Unknown - several theories
  - Inborn error of phosphorus metabolism
  - "Traumatic theory": Microtrauma of connective tissues around the joints, bleeding + formation of rudimentary bursae initial event
  - Variation of calcium pyrophosphate deposition disease
- Laboratory values generally normal
  - Elevated renal phosphate absorption
  - Elevated serum 1, 25-dihydroxy-vitamin D levels
- Epidemiology: 2nd to 3rd decades of life
- Associated abnormalities
  - Chronic renal failure
  - Hyperphosphatemia occasionally
  - CPPD

Gross Pathologic & Surgical Features
- Calcific mass, with solid & "milk of calcium" components

Microscopic Features
- Hydroxyapatite + calcium pyrophosphate dihydrate crystals identified
- Chronic inflammatory cells, multinucleated giant cells, granulation tissue

CLINICAL ISSUES

Presentation
- Most common signs/symptoms
  - Painless enlargement of joint
  - Other signs/symptoms
    - Usually lesions at other large synovial joints when spinal involvement present
- Clinical profile: Painless growth about large joint in adult

Demographics
- Age: Adult
- Gender: M = F
- Ethnicity: African-American > Caucasian

Natural History & Prognosis
- Progressive
- Multiple locations may be involved

Treatment
- Options, risks, complications
  - Symptomatic treatment
  - Wide surgical excision
  - Recurrence common
  - Evaluate for underlying metabolic abnormality
  - Drug treatment with phosphorus deprivation by oral aluminum hydroxide, or acetazolamide

DIAGNOSTIC CHECKLIST

Consider
- Tumoral calcinosis is diagnosis of exclusion
- Look for lesions in other large joints by CT

Image Interpretation Pearls
- Recognition of this entity important

- Benign nature
- Potential for confusion with malignant lesions such as sarcoma
- No enhancement

SELECTED REFERENCES

1. Martinez S: Tumoral calcinosis: 12 years later. Semin Musculoskelet Radiol. 6(4): 331-39, 2002
2. Blay P et al: Vertebral involvement in hyperphosphatemic tumoral calcinosis. Bone. 28(3): 316-8, 2001
3. Durant DM et al: Tumoral calcinosis of the spine: a study of 21 cases. Spine. 26(15): 1673-9, 2001
4. Matsukado K et al: Tumoral calcinosis in the upper cervical spine causing progressive radiculomyelopathy--case report. Neurol Med Chir (Tokyo). 41(8): 411-4, 2001
5. Watanabe A et al: Tumoral calcinosis of the lumbar meninges: case report. Neurosurgery. 47(1): 230-2, 2000
6. Reginato AJ et al: Familial and clinical aspects of calcium pyrophosphate deposition disease. Curr Rheumatol Rep. 1(2): 112-20, 1999
7. Adams WM et al: Familial tumoral calcinosis: association with cerebral and peripheral aneurysm formation. Neuroradiology. 41(5):351-5, 1999
8. Kokubun S et al: Tumoral calcinosis in the upper cervical spine: a case report. Spine. 21(2): 249-52, 1996
9. Ohashi K et al: Idiopathic tumoral calcinosis involving the cervical spine. Skeletal Radiol. 25(4): 388-90, 1996
10. Geirnaerdt MJ et al: Tumoral calcinosis. Skeletal Radiol. 24(2):148-51, 1995
11. Yamaguchi T et al: Successful treatment of hyperphosphatemic tumoral calcinosis with long-term acetazolamide. Bone. 16(4 Suppl):247S-250S, 1995
12. McGuinness FE: Hyperphosphataemic tumoral calcinosis in Bedouin Arabs--clinical and radiological features. Clin Radiol. 50(4):259-64, 1995
13. McGregor DH et al: Nonfamilial tumoral calcinosis associated with chronic renal failure and secondary hyperparathyroidism: report of two cases with clinicopathological, immunohistochemical, and electron microscopic findings. Hum Pathol. 26(6):607-13, 1995
14. Steinbach LS et al: Tumoral calcinosis: radiologic-pathologic correlation. Skeletal Radiol. 24(8):573-8, 1995
15. Shaffrey CI et al: Tumoral calcium pyrophosphate dihydrate deposition disease mimicking a cervical spine neoplasm: case report. Neurosurgery. 37(2): 335-9, 1995
16. Noyez JF et al: Tumoral calcinosis, a clinical report of eleven cases. Acta Orthop Belg. 59(3):249-54, 1993
17. Calloway DM et al: Combined modality treatment for tumoral calcinosis. Orthop Rev. 22(3):365-9, 1993
18. Tezelman S et al: Tumoral calcinosis. Controversies in the etiology and alternatives in the treatment. Arch Surg. 128(7):737-44; discussion 744-5, 1993
19. Peller PJ et al: Extraosseous Tc-99m MDP uptake: a pathophysiologic approach. Radiographics. 13(4):715-34, 1993
20. Slavin RE et al: Familial tumoral calcinosis. A clinical, histopathologic, and ultrastructural study with an analysis of its calcifying process and pathogenesis. Am J Surg Pathol. 17(8):788-802, 1993
21. Fam AG: Calcium pyrophosphate crystal deposition disease and other crystal deposition diseases. Curr Opin Rheumatol. 4(4):574-82, 1992

TUMORAL CALCINOSIS

IMAGE GALLERY

Typical

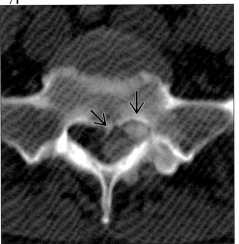
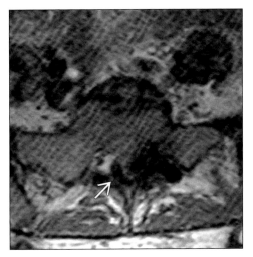

(Left) Axial NECT shows lobulated masses of high attenuation centered around left L5-S1 facet joint, extending into dorsal epidural space (arrows). *(Right)* Axial T1WI MR in the same patient shows extensive lobulated low signal surrounding the left L5-S1 facet joint. There is mass effect upon left side of the thecal sac (arrow).

Typical

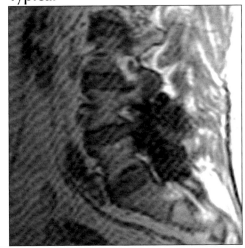
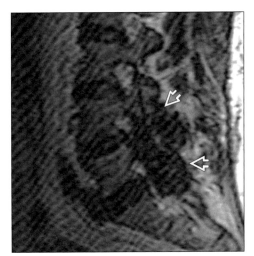

(Left) Sagittal T1WI MR shows lobulated low signal mass involving posterior elements from L4-5 to L5-S1 level, with well-defined margin. Lesion expansion produces foraminal stenosis at L5-S1. *(Right)* Sagittal T2WI MR shows large area of low signal from tumoral mass of posterior elements at L4-5, and L5-S1.

Variant

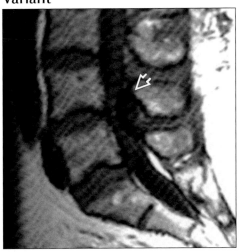
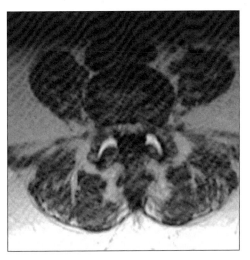

(Left) Sagittal T1WI MR shows well-defined low signal mass involving ligamentum flavum, with severe compression of dorsal thecal sac at L4-5 (arrow). *(Right)* Axial T2WI MR in the same patient shows the low signal mass in the midline of the dorsal elements, effacing the dorsal thecal sac. There are bilateral facet effusions.

PART VI

Peripheral Nerve and Plexus

Plexus & Peripheral Nerve Lesions 1

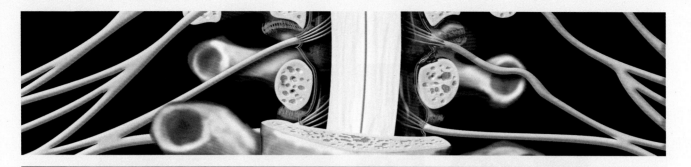

SECTION 1: Plexus & Peripheral Nerve Lesions

NORMAL PLEXUS AND NERVE ANATOMY

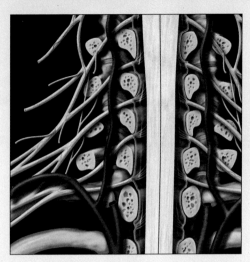

Coronal graphic demonstrates right brachial plexus in relation to vertebra, vertebral and subclavian arteries. C5, C6, & C7 rami exit above same-numbered vertebra, C8 & T1 below.

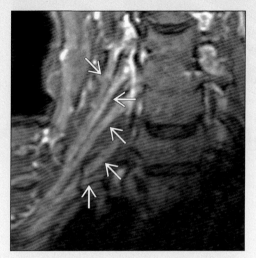

Coronal STIR MR depicts normal mildly hyperintense brachial plexus roots/rami (arrows). C5 & C6 form the superior (upper) trunk, C7 the middle trunk, and C8 & T1 the inferior (lower) trunk.

TERMINOLOGY

Definitions
- Nerve rootlets
  - Individual neural filaments of dorsal & ventral roots exiting from spinal cord
  - Rootlets coalesce → nerve roots
- Nerve root
  - Dorsal sensory root: Exits dorsolateral cord, cell bodies reside within DRG
  - Ventral motor root: Arises from anterior gray matter
- Dorsal root ganglion (DRG): Sensory ganglion of dorsal nerve root
- Spinal nerve (proper): Union of dorsal & ventral roots
  - 31 pairs; 8 cervical, 12 thoracic, 5 lumbar, 5 sacral, 1 coccygeal
- Ramus: First branches of spinal nerve
  - Ventral primary ramus (VPR) larger branch → ventral musculature, facet
  - Dorsal primary ramus (DPR) smaller branch → paraspinal muscles, facet
- Plexus: Neural network of anastomosing nerves
- Peripheral nerve: Combination of ≥ 1 rami into single neural conduit +/- Schwann cell myelin sheath

IMAGING ANATOMY

- Cervical plexus (ventral rami of C1-C4 +/- minor branch of C5)
  - Ascending superficial, descending superficial, and deep branches
  - Supplies nuchal muscles, diaphragm, cutaneous H&N tissues
- Brachial plexus (ventral rami of C5 - T1 +/- minor branches from C4, T2)
  - Minor peripheral branches originating above plexus proper: Dorsal scapular nerve, long thoracic nerve, nerves to scalene and longus colli muscles, phrenic nerve

- Remaining minor and all major peripheral branches arise from brachial plexus proper
- Classically divided anatomically into 5 segments (roots/rami, trunks, divisions, cords, terminal branches)
  - Anterior divisions innervate anterior (flexor) muscles, while posterior divisions innervate posterior (extensor) muscles
  - Lateral, medial cords innervate anterior (flexor) muscles, while posterior cord innervates posterior (extensor) muscles
- Clinically, BP divided into supraclavicular (roots, trunks), retroclavicular (divisions), and infraclavicular (cords, terminal branches) plexus
- Roots/rami (supraclavicular)
  - Originate from spinal cord C5 → T1
- Trunks (supraclavicular)
  - Superior (C5-C6), middle (C7), inferior (T1) trunks
  - Minor nerves arising directly from trunks: Suprascapular nerve, nerve to subclavius
- Divisions (retroclavicular)
  - Anterior and posterior divisions
- Cords (infraclavicular)
  - Lateral cord (anterior divisions of superior, middle trunks)
  - Medial cord (anterior division of inferior trunk)
  - Posterior cord (posterior divisions of all 3 trunks)
- Terminal branches (infraclavicular)
  - Musculocutaneous nerve (C5-C6), lateral root of median nerve (lateral cord)
  - Ulnar nerve (C8-T1), medial root of median nerve (medial cord)
  - Axillary nerve (C5-C6), radial nerve (C5-T1), thoracodorsal nerve (C6-C8), upper (C6-C7) and lower (C5-C6) subscapular nerves (posterior cord)
- Lumbar plexus (LP): Ventral rami of L1-L4 + minor branch of T12
  - Minor branches: Iliohypogastric, ilioinguinal, genitofemoral, lateral femoral cutaneous (L2-L3), superior (L4-S1) and inferior (L5-S2) gluteal nerves

DIFFERENTIAL DIAGNOSIS

Normal nerve/plexus
- Normal nerve size, course, contour, internal architecture

Nerve/plexus mass
- Metastasis (systemic or local extension)
- Nerve sheath tumor
- Neurolymphomatosis

Trauma
- Stretch/avulsion injury (traction)
- Laceration (fracture fragment, projectile)
- Direct compression (hematoma, fracture)

Entrapment syndrome
- Retinacular or muscular compression at specific locations

HMSN
- Charcot-Marie-Tooth, Dejerine-Sottas

Inflammatory disease
- Infectious neuritis (usually viral)
- Tabes dorsalis (Syphilis)
- Leprosy
- Sarcoidosis
- Guillain-Barré syndrome
- CIDP
- Idiopathic (Parsonage-Turner syndrome)

Vascular insult
- Ischemic neuropathy (peripheral vascular disease, vascular trauma)
- Vasculitis (diabetic, Churg-Strauss, polyarteritis nodosa, Wegener granulomatosis)

  - ○ Major branches: Femoral (posterior division L2-L4), obturator (anterior division L2-L4) nerves
- Lumbosacral trunk (LST): Ventral rami of L4 (minor branch), L5
- Sacral plexus (SP): LST + ventral rami of S1-S3, minor branch of S4
  - ○ May be directly visualized using MR imaging
  - ○ Sacral rami, LST converge to form upper and lower sacral neural bands
    - ▪ Upper band: LST + S1-S3 → sciatic nerve
    - ▪ Lower band: S3-S4 → pudendal nerve
- Coccygeal plexus: S5-Cx1
  - ○ Ventral rami of S5, Cx1 + minor branch of S4 → anococcygeal nerve
- Radial nerve (RN)
  - ○ Terminal branch of posterior BP cord
    - ▪ Most important branch: Posterior interosseous nerve (PIN)
  - ○ Innervates extensor muscles of arm, forearm (triceps, brachioradialis, extensor forearm muscles)
- Median nerve (MN)
  - ○ Terminal branch of lateral and medial cords
    - ▪ Most important branch: Anterior interosseous nerve (AIN)
  - ○ Innervates flexor muscles of forearm, thumb, 1st/2nd lumbricals
- Ulnar nerve (UN)
  - ○ Terminal branch of medial cord
  - ○ Innervates flexor carpi ulnaris, 3rd/4th lumbricals, majority of intrinsic hand muscles
- Musculocutaneous nerve (MuscN)
  - ○ Terminal branch of lateral cord
  - ○ Innervates arm flexor muscles (coracobrachialis, biceps, brachialis muscles)
- Axillary nerve (AxN)
  - ○ Terminal branch of posterior cord
  - ○ Innervates deltoid, teres minor muscles
- Obturator nerve (ObN)
  - ○ Terminal branch of lumbar plexus
  - ○ Innervates thigh adductor muscles
- Femoral nerve (FN)
  - ○ Terminal branch of lumbar plexus
  - ○ Innervates iliacus, psoas, quadriceps muscles

- Sciatic nerve (SN)
  - ○ Major branch of sacral plexus
  - ○ Innervates posterior thigh (biceps femoris, semitendinosus, semimembranosus, adductor magnus) & all leg muscles (via CPN, TN)
- Common peroneal nerve (CPN)
  - ○ Major anterior terminal branch of SN; innervates anterior leg muscles
    - ▪ Superficial peroneal nerve (SPN): Peroneus muscles, extensor digitorum brevis
    - ▪ Deep peroneal nerve (DPN): Tibialis anterior, extensor digitorum longus, extensor hallucis longus
- Tibial nerve (TN)
  - ○ Major posterior terminal branch of SN
  - ○ Innervates posterior leg muscles (gastrocnemius, soleus, tibialis posterior, flexor digitorum longus, flexor hallucis longus)

ANATOMY-BASED IMAGING ISSUES

Key Concepts or Questions
- Normal nerve findings
  - ○ Round/ovoid shape with well-defined internal fascicular architecture
  - ○ No abrupt change in nerve caliber or course
  - ○ Uniform mildly hyperintense fascicles with interspersed hypointense fibrofatty connective tissue (STIR, fat-saturated T2WI MR)
- Abnormal nerve findings
  - ○ Enlargement +/- loss of normal internal fascicular architecture
  - ○ Abrupt change in caliber or course
  - ○ Hyperintense fascicles approach signal intensity of regional vessels (STIR, fat-saturated T2WI MR)

Imaging Pitfalls
- Nerves & vessels occasionally difficult to differentiate
  - ○ Nerves: Round/ovoid linear structure, no flow voids, branch at relatively acute angles, enhance minimally, distinctive fascicular architecture on transverse imaging

NORMAL PLEXUS AND NERVE ANATOMY

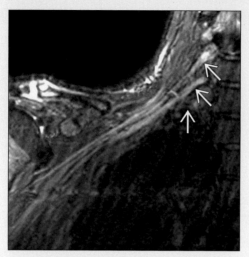

Coronal STIR MR demonstrates normal lower (C7, C8, T1) brachial plexus roots/rami (arrows) sequentially forming trunks, divisions, and cords. Normal brachial plexus courses retroclavicular into the axilla.

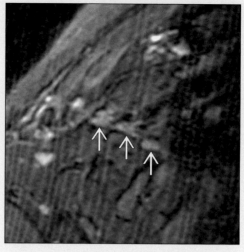

Sagittal oblique STIR MR shows normal anatomy & internal fasicular architecture of superior, middle, and inferior trunks (arrows). Normal fascicles are regular and slightly hyperintense (STIR, fat-saturated T2WI).

○ Vessels: Round/ovoid linear structure, + internal flow void, branch at large angles, intense contrast-enhancement

CLINICAL IMPLICATIONS

Clinical Importance
• Working knowledge of nerve & plexus anatomy critical to image clinical neuropathy syndromes
  ○ Larger major nerves readily visualized using high resolution MR technique to evaluate internal architecture
  ○ Many smaller major and essentially all minor peripheral nerves too small to image directly; knowing expected location & course predicts lesion location

CUSTOM DIFFERENTIAL DIAGNOSIS

Normal nerve/plexus
• Normal nerve course, contour, internal architecture
• Consider myopathy or other non-neural etiology

Nerve/plexus mass
• Metastasis (systemic or local extension)
• Nerve sheath tumor (solitary or plexiform neurofibroma, schwannoma, MPNST)
• Neurolymphomatosis

Trauma
• Stretch/avulsion injury (traction)
• Laceration (fracture fragment, projectile)
• Direct compression (hematoma, fracture)

Entrapment syndrome
• Compression at characteristic locations
• Often related to poor ergonomics, overuse injury

Hereditary motor & sensory neuropathy (HMSN)
• Charcot-Marie-Tooth, Dejerine-Sottas syndromes
• Nerve enlargement, histological "onion bulb" formations

Infection/inflammation
• Infectious neuritis (usually viral)
• Tabes dorsalis (Syphilis)
• Leprosy
• Sarcoidosis
• Guillain-Barré syndrome (GBS)
• Chronic immune demyelinating polyneuropathy (CIDP)
• Idiopathic (Parsonage-Turner syndrome)

Drug/toxic injury
• Vinca alkaloids, therapeutic gold, amiodarone, dapsone, thalidomide, lead or mercury intoxication

Vascular insult
• Nerve ischemia (peripheral vascular disease, vascular trauma)
• Vasculitis (diabetic, Churg-Strauss, polyarteritis nodosa, Wegener granulomatosis most common)

SELECTED REFERENCES

1. Bowen B et al: The brachial plexus: normal anatomy, pathology, and MR imaging. Neuroimag Clin N Am. 14:59-85, 2004
2. Cros et al: Peripheral neuropathy: a practical approach to diagnosis and management. Philadelphia. Lippincott Williams & Wilkins, 2001
3. Jinkins JR: Atlas of neuroradiologic embryology, anatomy, and variants. Philadelphia. Lippincott Williams & Wilkins. 586-590, 2000
4. Blake L et al: Sacral plexus: optimal imaging planes for MR assessment. Radiology. 199:767-772, 1996
5. Gray H: Gray's Anatomy, 1901 classic edition. Philadelphia, Running press. 764-798, 1974

IMAGE GALLERY

Typical

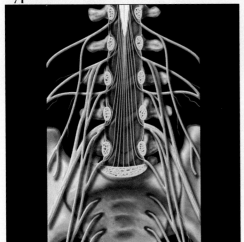

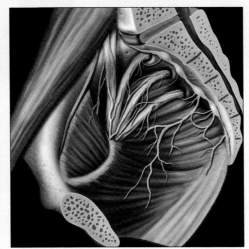

(Left) Coronal graphic reveals normal anatomy of the bilateral lumbar and sacral plexi. The lumbosacral trunk (LST) crosses the sacral ala and joins the S1-S3 ventral rami to form the sacral plexus. *(Right)* Sagittal graphic shows the lumbosacral trunk and sacral rami coalescing into the sacral plexus along the ventral piriformis muscle surface.

Typical

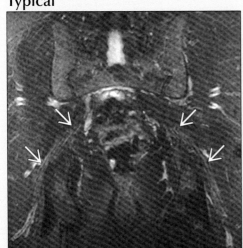

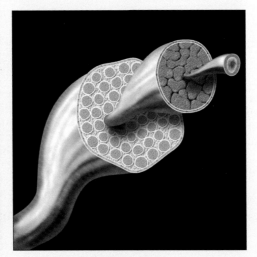

(Left) Coronal fat-saturated T2WI MR reveals normal longitudinal sacral plexus & sciatic nerve anatomy (arrows) as they course through the greater sciatic foramen (GSF) into the thigh. *(Right)* 3D graphic depicts normal peripheral nerve anatomy. The nerve is surrounded by epineurium. The perineurium surrounds the fascicles, each of which contains many endoneurium wrapped axons.

Typical

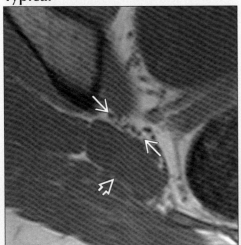

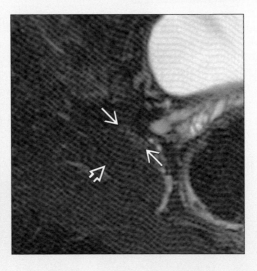

(Left) Sagittal T1WI MR oblique shows normal sciatic nerve internal architecture (arrows) at piriformis muscle (open arrow). Note isointense fascicles within hyperintense fibrofatty connective tissue. *(Right)* Sagittal oblique fat-saturated T2WI MR shows normal sciatic nerve (arrows) at piriformis muscle (open arrow). Mildly hyperintense fascicles interspersed with hypointense fibrofatty connective tissue.

SUPERIOR SULCUS TUMOR

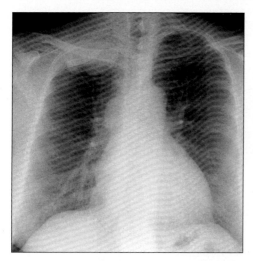

Anteroposterior radiography of chest shows right apical lung mass, with rib destruction from bronchogenic carcinoma.

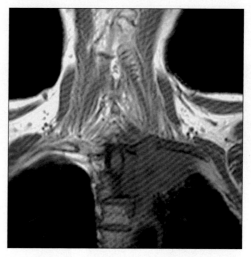

Coronal T1WI MR shows large left apical soft tissue mass involving left first rib, left side of upper thoracic vertebral bodies with epidural extension.

TERMINOLOGY

Abbreviations and Synonyms
- Synonym: Pancoast tumor

Definitions
- Benign or malignant tumor extending to superior thoracic inlet with severe shoulder/arm pain along C8, T1, T2 nerve trunks, Horner syndrome, weakness + atrophy of intrinsic hand muscles (Pancoast syndrome)
  - Non-small cell lung carcinoma (NSCLC) most frequent cause

IMAGING FINDINGS

General Features
- Best diagnostic clue: Soft tissue mass involving lung apex with rib destruction
- Location: Lung apex and adjacent chest wall, brachial plexus, cervicothoracic junction vertebral bodies
- Size: Variable ⇒ several centimeters in size
- Morphology: Soft tissue mass with ill-defined margins, bone destruction

Radiographic Findings
- Radiography: Soft tissue density at lung apex, +/- 1st or 2nd rib destruction

- Myelography: In advanced cases with epidural tumor extension, may show typical extradural defect in contrast column at cervicothoracic junction

CT Findings
- CECT
  - Soft tissue attenuation mass involving lung apex, with variable extension into chest wall and adjacent bone destruction
    - 1st, 2nd rib bone destruction
    - May show vertebral body invasion with epidural/foraminal extension
- CTA: May show encasement or narrowing of subclavian artery and branches

MR Findings
- T1WI
  - Intermediate signal mass involving lung apex, with chest wall/paravertebral extension
    - Will show encasement of subclavian vessels, and relationship of mass to brachial plexus
- T2WI: +/- T2 hyperintense mass
- T1 C+
  - Variable enhancing mass
    - Fat suppressed C+ may improved definition of epidural/foraminal extension
- MRA: 2D and 3D TOF techniques may show aortic arch/proximal great vessel involvement

DDx: Upper Thoracic Masses

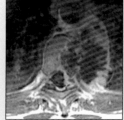

Primary Bone Tumor

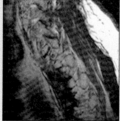

Radiation Fibrosis

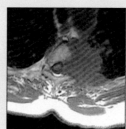

Metastasis

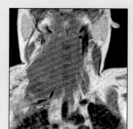

Trauma

Key Facts

Terminology
- Synonym: Pancoast tumor
- Benign or malignant tumor extending to superior thoracic inlet with severe shoulder/arm pain along C8, T1, T2 nerve trunks, Horner syndrome, weakness + atrophy of intrinsic hand muscles (Pancoast syndrome)
- Non-small cell lung carcinoma (NSCLC) most frequent cause

Imaging Findings
- Mediastinoscopy performed regardless of PET positive nodes since N2, 3 node involvement is negative prognostic factor
- MR demonstrates apical soft tissue involvement & relationship to brachial plexus/subclavian vessels
- CT shows mediastinal nodes, pulmonary, hepatic or adrenal metastases

Top Differential Diagnoses
- Metastatic disease
- Other thoracic tumors besides NSCLC
- Hematologic neoplasms
- Infections
- Radiation fibrosis

Clinical Issues
- Median survival with pre-operative radiation and resection 22 months, with 5 year survival 27%
- Classic approach is preoperative radiotherapy followed by surgical resection
- Pain palliation with radiation alone successful in 75%

Angiographic Findings
- Conventional: Generally superceded by MRA/CTA in evaluation of great vessel encasement by tumor

Nuclear Medicine Findings
- Bone Scan: Positive with rib/vertebral body involvement, or diffuse bone metastases
- PET
  - Positive with primary cancer, & nodal involvement
    - Mediastinoscopy performed regardless of PET positive nodes since N2, 3 node involvement is negative prognostic factor

Imaging Recommendations
- Best imaging tool
  - MR and CT complementary
    - MR demonstrates apical soft tissue involvement & relationship to brachial plexus/subclavian vessels
    - CT shows mediastinal nodes, pulmonary, hepatic or adrenal metastases
- Protocol advice: 3 plane T1W, T2W images, post-contrast axial to define bone, epidural extension, relationship to vessels/scalene musculature

DIFFERENTIAL DIAGNOSIS

Metastatic disease
- Usually from breast or lung cancer

Other thoracic tumors besides NSCLC
- Mesothelioma
- Hemangiopericytoma, sarcomas

Brachial plexus tumor
- Schwannoma shows enhancing mass tracking between anterior + middle scalene muscles
- Lymphangioma/hemangioma show T2 hyperintensity, lobulated margins

Hematologic neoplasms
- Lymphoma, plasmacytoma

Infections
- Staphylococcal pneumonia, aspergillosis, cryptococcosis
- Rare: Tuberculosis, hydatid cyst

Radiation fibrosis
- Low signal on T2 weighted images in field of treatment
- Show low levels of contrast-enhancement
- May insinuate into brachial plexus

Myositis ossificans
- Typical post-traumatic history
- May show large irregular mass with variable blood byproducts
- Benign calcification develops over time

PATHOLOGY

General Features
- General path comments
  - Carcinoma invades parietal pleura, endothoracic fascia, subclavian vessels, brachial plexus, vertebral bodies, and upper ribs
  - Clinical features related to location of thoracic inlet involvement relative to scalene muscles
    - Tumors in front of anterior scalene may involve sternocleidomastoid, jugular veins, subclavian veins & first intercostal nerve giving pain in upper chest wall
    - Tumors between anterior and middle scalene may involve subclavian artery, trunks of brachial plexus giving pain/paresthesias to shoulder and upper limb
    - Tumors posterior to middle scalene invade T1 roots, paravertebral sympathetic chain, stellate ganglion and prevertebral muscles
- Genetics
  - EGFR overexpressed in 40-80% NSCLC

- Response to tyrosine kinase inhibitor chemotherapy (which targets epidermal growth factor receptor) dependent upon specific mutation in EGFR gene
  - Mutations lead to increased growth factor signaling conferring susceptibility to the inhibitor molecule
- Variety of other genetic abnormalities in lung cancer
  - p53 tumor suppressor gene mutation most common, clustered around codon 157
  - K-ras mutations associated with smoking (ras oncogenes encode for GDP/GTP binding proteins)
  - COX-2, HER-2, VEGF overexpressions
- Etiology
  - Bronchogenic carcinomas arising from either upper lobe
  - Cigarette smoking major cause of lung cancer
    - 80% of lung cancer attributed to tobacco exposure
    - 20 fold increase risk with smokers vs. nonsmokers
- Epidemiology
  - Superior sulcus lesions are less than 5% of all bronchogenic carcinomas
  - Lung carcinoma leading cause of cancer deaths in U.S. in both men and women
  - Overall 5 year survival rate with lung cancer is < 15%

Gross Pathologic & Surgical Features
- Firm, gray-white polypoid mass infiltrating lung & chest wall

Microscopic Features
- Variety of bronchogenic carcinoma cell types: Squamous > adenocarcinoma > large cell
  - Vary from well differentiated with keratin production/intercellular bridges to undifferentiated pattern

Staging, Grading or Classification Criteria
- Staging/diagnosis by chest x-ray, CT chest, bronchoscopy, needle biopsy
- Tumor extent in brachial plexus by examination/EMG
- Vascular involvement by CTA, MRA, or catheter angiography (arterial and venous)

CLINICAL ISSUES

Presentation
- Most common signs/symptoms
  - Unrelenting pain in shoulder/arm in C8-T2 distribution
    - Pain in upper chest wall with first intercostal nerve involvement
  - Other signs/symptoms
    - Horner syndrome (ptosis, anhidrosis, miosis)
    - Atrophy of hand muscles
  - Tumors are peripheral in lung location
    - Pulmonary symptoms such as cough, hemoptysis, dyspnea are uncommon early in disease course

Demographics
- Age: Adult
- Gender
  - M > F

- Estimated 91,000 men + 68,000 women died of lung cancer in 1999 in U.S.
- Lung cancer 2nd in incidence in men to prostate
- Lung cancer 2nd in incidence in women to breast
- Ethnicity
  - Marked variation in lung cancer incidence + mortality by ethnicity
    - Lung cancer mortality 66.8/100,000 population for Caucasian, 94/100,000 for African-American men
    - 5 year survival rates: 12.7% Caucasian men, 10% African-American men, 16% Caucasian women, 14% African-American women

Natural History & Prognosis
- Median survival with pre-operative radiation and resection 22 months, with 5 year survival 27%
- N2, 3 lymph node involvement major negative prognostic factor
- Horner syndrome associated with poor survival
- Involvement of vertebral bodies or subclavian vessels associated with poor survival after resection

Treatment
- Classic approach is pre-operative radiotherapy followed by surgical resection
- Other treatments include radiation alone, pre-operative chemotherapy with resection, or chemotherapy without resection
- Pain palliation with radiation alone successful in 75%
  - Radiation alone long term survival 5%
- Absolute surgical contraindications include extrathoracic metastatic disease, or mediastinal node involvement
  - Involvement of brachial plexus above T1 also contraindication

DIAGNOSTIC CHECKLIST

Consider
- Apical mass with bone destruction always bronchogenic carcinoma, until proven otherwise; rare cases of benign tumors or infection giving similar imaging pattern

SELECTED REFERENCES
1. Detterbeck FC et al: Lung cancer. Special treatment issues. Chest. 123(1 Suppl):244S-258S, 2003
2. Kichari JR et al: MR imaging of the brachial plexus: current imaging sequences, normal findings, and findings in a spectrum of focal lesions with MR-pathologic correlation. Curr Probl Diagn Radiol. 32(2):88-101, 2003
3. Detterbeck FC: Changes in the treatment of Pancoast tumors. Ann Thorac Surg. 75(6):1990-7, 2003
4. Dartevelle P et al: Surgical management of superior sulcus tumors. Oncologist. 4(5):398-407, 1999
5. Ducic Y et al: A logical approach to the thoracic inlet: the Dartevelle approach revisited. Head Neck. 21(8):767-71, 1999
6. Jones DR et al: Pancoast tumors of the lung. Curr Opin Pulm Med. 4(4):191-7, 1998
7. Kuhlman JE et al: CT and MR imaging evaluation of chest wall disorders. Radiographics. 14(3):571-95, 1994

IMAGE GALLERY

Typical

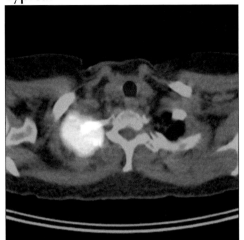 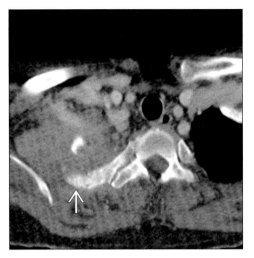

(Left) Axial PET (FDG) CT fusion shows marked increased uptake involving the right upper lobe bronchogenic carcinoma involving right 1st and 2nd ribs. *(Right)* Axial CECT shows soft tissue mass involving right upper lobe with extension beyond the chest wall, involvement + destruction of right T1, T2 ribs (arrow).

Typical

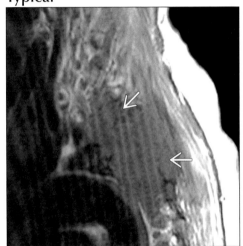 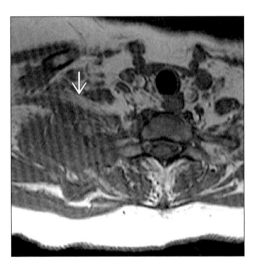

(Left) Sagittal T1WI MR shows large soft tissue mass arising from right upper lobe with extension through chest wall and involvement of paravertebral space and ribs (arrows). *(Right)* Axial T1WI MR shows soft tissue mass involving right lung apex with extension to thoracic inlet adjacent to subclavian vessels (arrow).

Typical

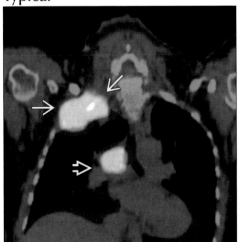 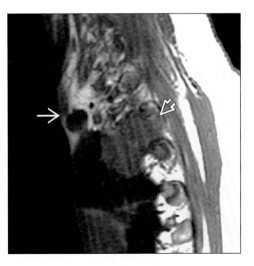

(Left) Coronal PET (FDG) CT fusion shows intense glucose uptake involving the right upper lobe mass, extending beyond the chest wall (arrows), as well as metastatic right hilar lymphadenopathy (open arrow). *(Right)* Sagittal T1WI MR shows extension of the upper lobe bronchogenic carcinoma through chest wall involving upper ribs (open arrow) posterior to subclavian vessels (arrow).

MUSCLE DENERVATION, SPINE

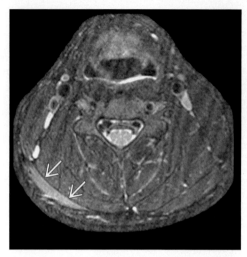

Axial STIR MR shows asymmetric T2 hyperintensity of right trapezius muscle (arrows) indicating acute denervation following spinal accessory nerve injury.

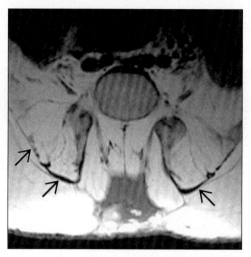

Axial T1WI MR in myelomeningocele patient demonstrates marked fatty replacement and atrophy of paraspinal muscles (arrows) secondary to chronic denervation + disuse.

TERMINOLOGY

Definitions
- Muscle signal/density alteration and volume change following denervation

IMAGING FINDINGS

General Features
- Best diagnostic clue: Asymmetric muscle volume loss with fatty replacement ⇒ chronic denervation
- Location: Paraspinal +/- iliopsoas muscles
- Size: Enlarged 2° muscle edema (acute) or atrophied (chronic)

CT Findings
- CECT
  ○ +/- Mild muscle enlargement +/- enhancement (acute)
  ○ Volume loss, hypodense fatty replacement (chronic)

MR Findings
- T1WI
  ○ Acute denervation ⇒ isointense T1 signal +/- ↑ muscle volume
  ○ Chronic denervation ⇒ ↓ muscle volume, interspersed ↑ T1 signal (fatty replacement)
- T2WI
  ○ Acute denervation ⇒ T2 hyperintense, +/- ↑ muscle volume
    ■ Not reliably identified < 4 days post nerve injury
  ○ Chronic denervation ⇒ ↓ muscle volume, interspersed ↑ T2 signal (fatty replacement)
- STIR: Similar to T2WI
- T1 C+: +/- Muscle enhancement in acute denervation

Other Modality Findings
- Needle electromyography (EMG)
  ○ Up to 3 weeks before abnormal
  ○ Correlates closely with ↑ STIR/T2 signal intensity

Imaging Recommendations
- Best imaging tool: MR imaging
- Protocol advice: Axial T1WI, fat-saturated T2WI or STIR MR best to assess for muscle denervation

DIFFERENTIAL DIAGNOSIS

Muscle trauma or disuse atrophy
- Disuse atrophy appears similar to chronic denervation, but usually more symmetric, widespread
- History, physical exam help make diagnosis

Muscle inflammation or infection
- Ex: Polymyositis/dermatomyositis, infectious myositis, diabetic myonecrosis, rhabdomyolysis, sickle cell crisis

DDx: Spinal Muscle Denervation

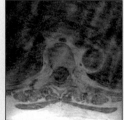

Disuse Atrophy (MS)

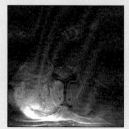

Myonecrosis

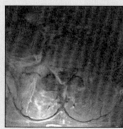

Pyogenic Myositis

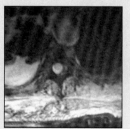

Radiation Myopathy

MUSCLE DENERVATION, SPINE

Key Facts

Terminology
- Muscle signal/density alteration and volume change following denervation

Imaging Findings
- Best diagnostic clue: Asymmetric muscle volume loss with fatty replacement ⇒ chronic denervation
- Size: Enlarged 2° muscle edema (acute) or atrophied (chronic)

Top Differential Diagnoses
- Muscle trauma or disuse atrophy
- Muscle inflammation or infection
- Radiation myopathy

Diagnostic Checklist
- Acute and chronic denervation changes commonly co-exist on MR imaging, and may persist for considerable time periods

---

- History, physical exam help make diagnosis

Radiation myopathy
- Vasculitis, tissue injury → uniform muscle edema
- Straight, sharp edema margins

PATHOLOGY

General Features
- General path comments
  - Acute
    - Muscle injury 2° denervation ⇒ ↑ proteolysis, ↓ glucose uptake, ↑ glycolysis
    - Fluid changes from intra- to extracellular space postulated responsible for ↑ T2 signal
  - Chronic
    - Rapid ↓ muscle diameter after acute phase
    - Fatty infiltration ⇒ abnormal diffuse fat deposition within muscle
- Etiology: Nerve root, plexus, or peripheral nerve injury/lesion

Microscopic Features
- Marked acute capillary enlargement
- Denervation +/- re-innervation ⇒ atrophic fibers

CLINICAL ISSUES

Presentation
- Most common signs/symptoms
  - Weakness, muscle volume loss in distribution of injured nerve
  - +/- Pain
- Clinical profile
  - Patient may present first with either nerve injury or muscle symptoms
  - Pattern of muscle involvement helps identify abnormal nerve

Demographics
- Age: Entire spectrum

Natural History & Prognosis
- Acute denervation may partially or totally recover depending on nerve injury severity
- Chronic denervation changes permanent

Treatment
- Address cause of nerve injury if applicable
- Physical therapy to strengthen residual muscle mass

DIAGNOSTIC CHECKLIST

Consider
- Muscle volume, signal intensity on MRI may detect acute or chronic denervation that confirms suspected nerve injury

Image Interpretation Pearls
- Acute and chronic denervation changes commonly co-exist on MR imaging, and may persist for considerable time periods

SELECTED REFERENCES

1. Haig AJ: Paraspinal denervation and the spinal degenerative cascade. Spine J. 2(5):372-80, 2002
2. Airaksinen O et al: Density of lumbar muscles 4 years after decompressive spinal surgery. Eur Spine J. 5(3):193-7, 1996
3. Kotilainen E et al: Cross-sectional areas of lumbar muscles after surgical treatment of lumbar disc herniation. A study with magnetic resonance imaging after microdiscectomy or percutaneous nucleotomy. Acta Neurochir (Wien). 133(1-2):7-12, 1995

IMAGE GALLERY

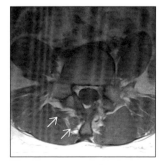 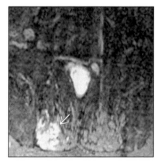

(Left) Axial T1WI MR reveals mild fatty atrophy (chronic denervation) of right paraspinal muscles (arrows) following laminectomy at another level. (Right) Axial STIR MR shows marked T2 hyperintensity indicating acute/ongoing denervation of the right paraspinal muscles (arrow) in patient with lymphomatous infiltration of the right lumbar plexus.

BRACHIAL PLEXUS TRACTION INJURY

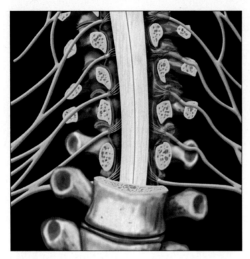

Coronal graphic demonstrates avulsion of left C5 - C8 nerve roots with avulsion pseudomeningoceles.

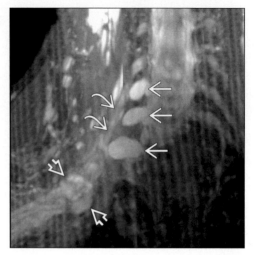

Coronal STIR MR reformat shows multiple pseudomeningoceles (arrows) and "nerve retraction ball" (open arrows). Attenuated, partially avulsed nerve rami are indicated by curved arrows.

TERMINOLOGY

Abbreviations and Synonyms
- Synonyms: Brachial plexus stretch injury, brachial plexus avulsion, avulsion pseudomeningocele

Definitions
- Stretch injury or avulsion of ≥ 1 cervical roots, brachial plexus

IMAGING FINDINGS

General Features
- Best diagnostic clue: Lateral CSF-containing dural sac outpouching(s) devoid of neural elements
- Location: Brachial plexus, pre- or post-ganglionic nerve roots
- Morphology
  - Stretch injury: Enlargement or attenuation of stretched (but contiguous) plexus elements
  - Avulsion injury: Attenuated or disrupted proximal roots/rami within or immediately distal to diverticulum +/- retracted distal nerve roots, nerve "retraction ball"

Radiographic Findings
- Myelography: +/- Dilated empty root sleeves, CSF/contrast leak, spinal cord "divot" at avulsion site

CT Findings
- NECT
  - Difficult CT diagnosis
  - +/- Pseudomeningocele(s), paraspinal hematoma
  - Most useful following myelography
- Bone CT
  - +/- Vertebral fracture(s)

MR Findings
- T1WI
  - Enlargement, hypo- to isointense signal of neural elements (stretch injury)
  - Dilated hypointense CSF signal intensity within empty thecal diverticulum (avulsion)
- T2WI
  - Enlargement, hyperintense signal of neural elements (stretch injury)
  - Hyperintense CSF signal intensity within empty thecal diverticulum (avulsion)
  - +/- Spinal cord edema, myelomalacia, syringomyelia
    - Central spinal cord edema in acute stage 2° root avulsion
  - Denervation changes in posterior cervical paraspinal muscles (especially multifidus) ⇒ pre-ganglionic injury
- STIR: Similar to fat-saturated T2WI
- T1 C+

DDx: Plexus Traction Injuries

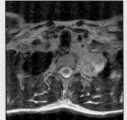
Neurofibroma

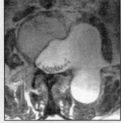
Lateral Meningocele

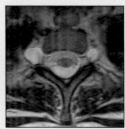
Nerve Root Cysts

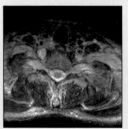
CIDP

BRACHIAL PLEXUS TRACTION INJURY

Key Facts

Terminology
- Synonyms: Brachial plexus stretch injury, brachial plexus avulsion, avulsion pseudomeningocele
- Stretch injury or avulsion of ≥ 1 cervical roots, brachial plexus

Imaging Findings
- Best diagnostic clue: Lateral CSF-containing dural sac outpouching(s) devoid of neural elements

Top Differential Diagnoses
- Nerve sheath tumor
- Lateral meningocele
- Nerve root sleeve cyst
- CIDP

Pathology
- Majority of adult brachial plexus palsies are posttraumatic injuries 2° high-energy force

Clinical Issues
- Pain, paralysis of ipsilateral limb +/- phrenic nerve palsy
- Clinical examination cannot reliably distinguish between pre- and post-ganglionic injuries

Diagnostic Checklist
- MRI may distinguish pre- from post-ganglionic injury for surgical planning, prognostication
- Search for soft tissue trauma (edema, hemorrhage) or fracture to support diagnosis
- Muscle denervation pattern predicts abnormal nerves

  - Enhancement absent in acute injury; chronic may show enhancing scar tissue
  - Enhancing muscle implies denervation

Imaging Recommendations
- Best imaging tool: High-resolution MR imaging (MR neurography)
- Protocol advice
  - Coronal, sagittal oblique T1WI and STIR MR
  - CT myelography if MR inconclusive

DIFFERENTIAL DIAGNOSIS

Nerve sheath tumor
- Plexiform neurofibroma (NF1), solitary nerve sheath tumor mimics root avulsion(s)
- + Tumoral enhancement
- Look for clinical, genetic, or imaging stigmata of NF1

Lateral meningocele
- Marfan syndrome, Ehlers-Danlos syndrome, NF1
- Lateral meningocele mimics pseudomeningocele, but contains neural elements
- Clinical history/stigmata +/- dural dysplasia distinguish from trauma

Nerve root sleeve cyst
- Usually incidental finding; may be large
- Intact nerve root peripherally displaced by cyst
- Spontaneous rupture ⇒ intracranial hypotension
- Clinical history helps distinguish from avulsion

CIDP
- Characteristic clinical, laboratory findings; often bilateral

PATHOLOGY

General Features
- General path comments
  - Brachial plexus traction avulses one or more nerve roots from spinal cord

  - Injury level critical to treatment planning, prognosis
    - Pre-ganglionic injury: Lesion central to dorsal root ganglion, worse prognosis
    - Post-ganglionic injury: Injury peripheral to ganglion, better prognosis
- Etiology
  - Majority of adult brachial plexus palsies are posttraumatic injuries 2° high-energy force
    - Forced abduction or downward displacement of arm, gunshot wound
    - Lacerations (knives, glass, automobile metal, chain saw, or animal bite)
  - In infants, brachial plexus palsy 2° excessive traction on plexus during difficult (breech or forceps) delivery
- Epidemiology
  - Strong association with off-road vehicle, motorcycle accidents
    - Incidence follows trauma epidemiological patterns
- Associated abnormalities
  - +/- Co-existing soft tissue or vascular injury, vertebral fractures
  - +/- Muscle denervation; pattern predicts abnormal nerve roots
  - Transdural spinal cord herniation (rare)

Gross Pathologic & Surgical Features
- Evidence for root avulsion includes spinal cord displacement or edema, hemorrhage or scarring within spinal canal, absence of roots in intervertebral foramina, and pseudomeningocele

Microscopic Features
- Nerve discontinuity, axonal loss, demyelination, hemorrhage, scar

Staging, Grading or Classification Criteria
- Bonney classification (1998)
  - Type A: Roots torn central to transition zone (true avulsion)
  - Type B: Roots torn distal to transition zone
    - Type 1: Dura torn within spinal canal, DRG displaced into neck

BRACHIAL PLEXUS TRACTION INJURY

- ▪ Type 2: Dura torn at mouth of foramen, DRG more or less displaced
- ▪ Type 3: Dura not torn, DRG not displaced
- ▪ Type 4: Dura not torn, DRG not displaced, either ventral or dorsal roots intact

CLINICAL ISSUES

Presentation
- Most common signs/symptoms
  - ○ Pain, paralysis of ipsilateral limb +/- phrenic nerve palsy
    - ▪ Complete brachial plexus avulsion produces useless "flail arm"
    - ▪ Incomplete paralysis common with complete root avulsion(s) because of redundant muscle innervation from multiple roots
  - ○ Clinical examination cannot reliably distinguish between pre- and post-ganglionic injuries
- Clinical profile
  - ○ Erb-Duchenne palsy
    - ▪ Upper plexus injury (C5, C6 roots, upper trunk) → proximal muscle weakness
    - ▪ Direct blow to shoulder, birth traction injury
  - ○ Middle radicular syndrome
    - ▪ C7 root, middle trunk → radial nerve abnormalities
  - ○ Klumpke palsy
    - ▪ Lower plexus injury (C8, T1 roots, lower trunk) → distal muscle weakness
    - ▪ Fall with overhead grasp slowing descent

Demographics
- Age: Young to middle-age adult > infants, children
- Gender: M > F; follows trauma epidemiology

Natural History & Prognosis
- Variable; generally poor in avulsion, better with stretch injury + nerve contiguity
- Post-ganglionic better prognosis than pre-ganglionic injury
- Obstetrical injury better prognosis than adult stretch injuries
- Integrity of nerve roots critical for surgical decision making, prognostication
  - ○ Stretched (but contiguous) nerves may recover some function, while avulsed nerve roots produce irreversible sensory and motor deficits
  - ○ Pre-ganglionic avulsions usually not amenable to surgical repair; function of some denervated muscles restored with nerve transfers from accessory nerves, cervical plexus, or intercostal nerves
  - ○ Post-ganglionic avulsions repaired with excision of damaged segment and nerve autograft between nerve ends

Treatment
- Conservative management
  - ○ Physical therapy, rehabilitation
- Surgical management
  - ○ Re-anastomosis of avulsed roots to spinal cord not generally advocated, but new microsurgical techniques prompting re-review
  - ○ Nerve bypass or graft, reconstruction with neurolysis, nerve graft, nerve transfer, functioning muscle/tendon transfer
  - ○ Amputation of non-functional or painful "flail arm"
  - ○ Dorsal root entry zone (DREZ) lesion palliation for intractable pain

DIAGNOSTIC CHECKLIST

Consider
- Familiarity with normal brachial plexus anatomy essential for MR interpretation
- MRI may distinguish pre- from post-ganglionic injury for surgical planning, prognostication

Image Interpretation Pearls
- Search for soft tissue trauma (edema, hemorrhage) or fracture to support diagnosis
- Muscle denervation pattern predicts abnormal nerves

SELECTED REFERENCES

1. Carlstedt T et al: Restoration of hand function and so called "breathing arm" after intraspinal repair of C5-T1 brachial plexus avulsion injury. Case report. Neurosurg Focus. 16(5):E7, 2004
2. Haerle M et al: Management of complete obstetric brachial plexus lesions. J Pediatr Orthop. 24(2):194-200, 2004
3. Ferraresi S et al: Reinnervation of the biceps in C5-7 brachial plexus avulsion injuries: results after distal bypass surgery. Neurosurg Focus. 16(5):E6, 2004
4. Kim DH et al: Mechanisms of injury in operative brachial plexus lesions. Neurosurg Focus. 16(5):E2, 2004
5. Filler AG et al: MR neurography and muscle MR imaging for image diagnosis of disorders affecting the peripheral nerves and musculature. Neurol Clin. 22(3):643-82, 2004
6. Chen HJ et al: Combined dorsal root entry zone lesions and neural reconstruction for early rehabilitation of brachial plexus avulsion injury. Acta Neurochir Suppl. 87:95-7, 2003
7. Bertelli JA et al: Brachial plexus avulsion injury repairs with nerve transfers and nerve grafts directly implanted into the spinal cord yield partial recovery of shoulder and elbow movements. Neurosurgery. 52(6):1385-9; discussion 1389-90, 2003
8. DaSilva VR et al: Upper thoracic spinal cord herniation after traumatic nerve root avulsion. Case report and review of the literature. J Neurosurg. 99(3 Suppl):306-9, 2003
9. Gei AF et al: Brachial plexus paresis associated with fetal neck compression from forceps. Am J Perinatol. 20(6):289-91, 2003
10. Doi K et al: Cervical nerve root avulsion in brachial plexus injuries: magnetic resonance imaging classification and comparison with myelography and computerized tomography myelography. J Neurosurg. 96(3 Suppl):277-84, 2002
11. Dubuisson AS et al: Brachial plexus injury: a survey of 100 consecutive cases from a single service. Neurosurgery. 51(3):673-82; discussion 682-3, 2002
12. Hems TE et al: The role of magnetic resonance imaging in the management of traction injuries to the adult brachial plexus. J Hand Surg [Br]. 24(5):550-5, 1999

IMAGE GALLERY

Typical

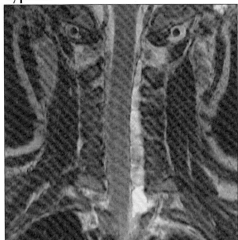
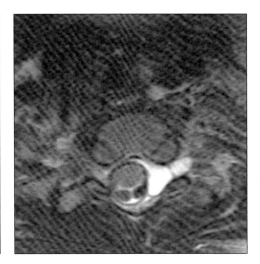

(Left) Coronal T2WI MR demonstrates multiple left sided nerve root avulsions with extradural fluid displacing cord to right (Courtesy P. Chapman, MD). *(Right)* Axial T2WI MR shows left sided C8 nerve root avulsion pseudomeningocele with extradural fluid displacing cord and thecal sac to the right (Courtesy P. Chapman, MD).

Typical

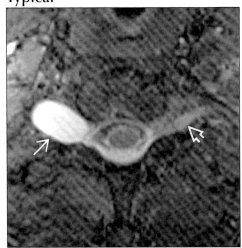
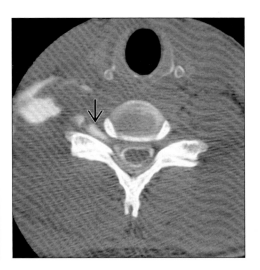

(Left) Axial STIR MR shows a large right C8 avulsion pseudomeningocele (arrow). No internal neural elements identified. Normal left ventral primary ramus indicated with open arrow for comparison. *(Right)* Axial bone CT following myelography depicts contrast surrounding dural sac and leaking through right neural foramen (arrow) into scalene muscles along brachial plexus.

Variant

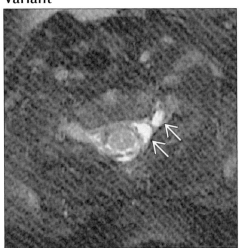
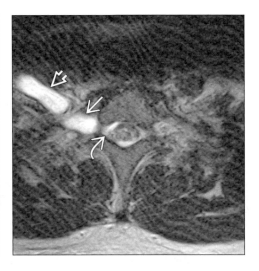

(Left) Axial T2WI MR with fat-saturation shows left brachial plexus obstetrical traction injury (arrows) in a infant following shoulder dystocia & difficult vaginal birth (Courtesy G. Hedlund, DO). *(Right)* Axial T2WI MR shows avulsion pseudomeningocele of T1 (curved arrow) with marked enlargement of the C8 (open arrow) and T1 (arrow) ventral primary rami secondary to stretch injury.

TRAUMATIC NEUROMA

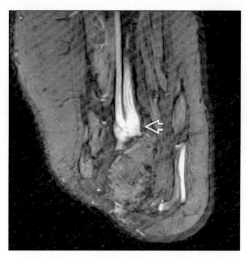

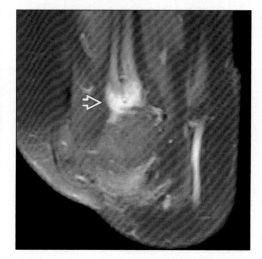

Coronal STIR MR shows enlargement of sciatic nerve, with a bulbous mass (arrow) at tip of severed nerve, representing traumatic neuroma. Note spiculated margins of mass due to scarring.

Coronal T1 C+ MR shows avid contrast-enhancement by traumatic neuroma (arrow) of sciatic nerve. Nerve proximal to focal neuroma shows slight enhancement also.

TERMINOLOGY

Abbreviations and Synonyms
- Amputation neuroma: Subtype of traumatic neuroma following traumatic or surgical amputation
- Morton neuroma: Traumatic neuroma between metatarsal heads

Definitions
- Non-neoplastic nerve growth 2° major or minor trauma

IMAGING FINDINGS

General Features
- Best diagnostic clue: Mass arising in nerve at stump or site of nerve injury
- Location
  - Post amputation
  - Head and neck 2° to tooth extraction
  - Brachial plexus
  - Morton neuroma: Interdigital plantar n., usually between 3rd and 4th toes
  - Biliary system: Post-surgical or blunt trauma
- Morphology
  - Amputated nerve: Bulbous, irregular mass at nerve end
  - Injured but continuous nerve: Fusiform nerve swelling

CT Findings
- NECT: Nerve enlargement

MR Findings
- T1WI: Isointense to nerve
- T2WI
  - Heterogeneous intermediate to high signal intensity
    - May discern nerve fascicles
  - Blends with fat unless fat suppression used
- PD/Intermediate: Isointense to nerve
- STIR: High signal intensity, greater than nerve
- T1 C+
  - Avid enhancement
  - May be uniform or heterogeneous
    - May outline nerve fascicles

Imaging Recommendations
- Best imaging tool: MR imaging
- Protocol advice
  - T1 and T2WI along long and short axes of nerve
  - T1 C+ in two planes to confirm enhancement, origin in nerve

DDx: Traumatic Neuroma

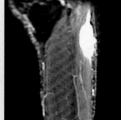

Neurofibroma

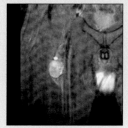

MPNST

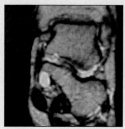

Ganglion Cyst

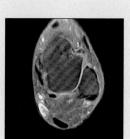

Tumor Recurrence

TRAUMATIC NEUROMA

Key Facts

Terminology
- Amputation neuroma: Subtype of traumatic neuroma following traumatic or surgical amputation
- Morton neuroma: Traumatic neuroma between metatarsal heads
- Non-neoplastic nerve growth 2° major or minor trauma

Imaging Findings
- Best diagnostic clue: Mass arising in nerve at stump or site of nerve injury

Top Differential Diagnoses
- Benign peripheral nerve tumor
- Malignant peripheral nerve sheath tumor (MPNST)
- Perineural cyst, ganglion cyst
- Soft tissue metastasis or recurrent malignancy

DIFFERENTIAL DIAGNOSIS

Benign peripheral nerve tumor
- History, location useful
- Signal characteristics may be identical

Malignant peripheral nerve sheath tumor (MPNST)
- Usually present at larger size
- Heterogeneous signal intensity on T2WI, STIR, T1 C+

Perineural cyst, ganglion cyst
- Mass centered on nerve or adjacent to it
- Will not enhance with gadolinium
- May compress nerve and cause neurologic symptoms

Soft tissue metastasis or recurrent malignancy
- Usually envelopes or displaces nerve
- Mass arising in nerve stump probably traumatic neuroma even in patient with tumor

PATHOLOGY

General Features
- Etiology
  - Secondary to nerve injury
    - Severed nerve
    - Crush injury
    - Deep burns
    - Tooth extraction
    - May occur with minor trauma
    - Morton neuroma associated with tight shoes
- Epidemiology: Arise 1-12 months after nerve injury

Gross Pathologic & Surgical Features
- Glistening gray-white enlargement of tumor

Microscopic Features
- All elements of nerve present, as well as scar tissue

CLINICAL ISSUES

Presentation
- Most common signs/symptoms: Severe pain or paresthesias

Treatment
- Steroid injection, physical therapy, resection

DIAGNOSTIC CHECKLIST

Consider
- Important entity to consider in MRI surveillance following tumor resection

Image Interpretation Pearls
- Morton neuroma may be inapparent on MRI without gadolinium administration

SELECTED REFERENCES
1. Rosai J: Surgical Pathology, vol 2. 9th ed. Edinburgh, Mosby. 2263, 2004
2. Huang LF et al: Traumatic neuroma after neck dissection: CT characteristics in four cases. AJNR Am J Neuroradiol. 21(9):1676-80, 2000
3. Henrot P et al: Imaging of the painful lower limb stump. Radiographics. 20 Spec No:S219-35, 2000
4. Murphey MD et al: From the archives of the AFIP. Imaging of musculoskeletal neurogenic tumors: radiologic-pathologic correlation. Radiographics. 19(5):1253-80, 1999
5. Hoskins CL et al: Magnetic resonance imaging of foot neuromas. J Foot Surg. 31(1):10-6, 1992
6. Ono T et al: Traumatic neuroma: multiple lesions in the fingers occurring after deep burns. J Dermatol. 17(12):760-3, 1990

IMAGE GALLERY

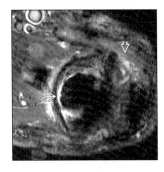 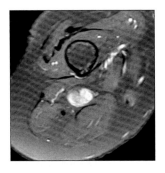

(Left) Axial STIR MR shows traumatic ulnar nerve neuroma (open arrow) in patient following total elbow arthroplasty (curved arrow). Images are diagnostic despite metal artifact. (Right) Axial T1 C+ MR shows heterogeneous enhancement of traumatic neuroma of sciatic n. in patient status post amputation for osteogenic sarcoma. Enhancement outlines nerve fascicles.

THORACIC OUTLET SYNDROME

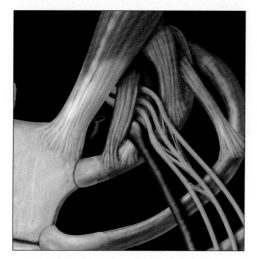

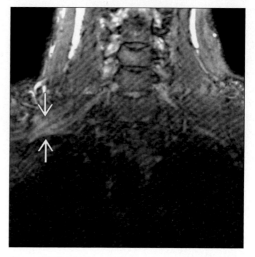

Coronal graphic of thoracic outlet demonstrates brachial plexus compression + subclavian artery aneurysm arising secondary to cervical rib and anterior scalene muscle compression.

Coronal STIR MR in a professional musician (drummer) with symptomatic TOS shows abnormal brachial plexus T2 hyperintensity at the thoracic outlet.

TERMINOLOGY

Abbreviations and Synonyms
- Thoracic outlet syndrome (TOS)

Definitions
- Neural, venous, and/or arterial compressive syndrome at thoracic outlet (TO)

IMAGING FINDINGS

General Features
- Best diagnostic clue
  - Radiography: Cervical rib in symptomatic patient
  - MRI: Neural or vascular compression within interscalene or costocervical tunnels
- Location: Interscalene, costoclavicular space, retropectoralis minor space (subcoracoid tunnel)

Radiographic Findings
- Radiography
  - Cervical radiographs usually normal
    - +/- Cervical rib, elongated C7 transverse process

CT Findings
- CECT: Usually normal; +/- abnormal soft tissue process, vascular anomaly within TO

- CTA: +/- Vascular compression, subclavian artery (SCA) aneurysm or subclavian vein (SCV) thrombosis
- Bone CT
  - +/- Cervical rib, elongated C7 transverse process

MR Findings
- T1WI: Often normal; abnormal cases ⇒ brachial plexus (BP) compression or distortion, abnormal vascular flow void at TO
- T2WI
  - +/- Focal abnormal brachial plexus T2 hyperintensity in TO
  - +/- Brachial plexus compression or distortion, scalene muscle inflammation or fibrosis, abnormal vascular flow voids within TO
- STIR: Similar to fat-saturated T2WI
- T1 C+: +/- Focal enhancement at TO
- MRA
  - +/- SCA compression, aneurysm on MRA
  - Positional occlusion or narrowing of SCA with arm hyperabduction, external rotation
- MRV: +/- Subclavian vein compression or thrombosis, positional occlusion or narrowing of SCV

Ultrasonographic Findings
- Real Time: Muscular or osseous compression of brachial plexus, SCA, or SCV
- Color Doppler: +/- SCA aneurysm, SCV thrombosis

DDx: Thoracic Outlet Syndrome

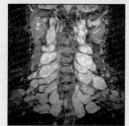

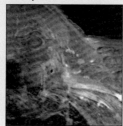

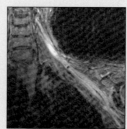

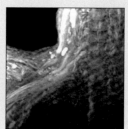

| *Plexiform NF* | *Pancoast Tumor* | *XRT Plexopathy* | *BP Stretch Injury* |

THORACIC OUTLET SYNDROME

Key Facts

Terminology

- Thoracic outlet syndrome (TOS)
- Neural, venous, and/or arterial compressive syndrome at thoracic outlet (TO)

Imaging Findings

- +/- Cervical rib, elongated C7 transverse process
- +/- brachial plexus compression or distortion, scalene muscle inflammation or fibrosis, abnormal vascular flow voids within TO
- Positional occlusion or narrowing of SCA with arm hyperabduction, external rotation

Top Differential Diagnoses

- Primary and secondary plexus tumors
- Radiation plexopathy
- Trauma

Pathology

- Cervical ribs, abnormal transverse processes, fibrous bands, scalene compression of TO contents
- Neural injury with fibrosis, axonal loss

Clinical Issues

- "True" neurological TOS: Intermittent arm pain, numbness, and weakness with hyperabduction, external rotation
- Vascular TOS: Paresthesias 2° to ischemia

Diagnostic Checklist

- TOS probably end result of diverse symptomatic etiologies rather than a single disease process
- SCA aneurysm, SCV thrombosis, brachial plexus compression with abnormal T2 hyperintensity at TO strongly suggest TOS

Angiographic Findings

- Conventional: Positional occlusion/narrowing of SCV or SCA with arm hyperabduction +/- mural thrombi, emboli, aneurysm

Imaging Recommendations

- Best imaging tool: MR imaging
- Protocol advice
  - Multiplanar T1WI and STIR MR through TO
  - Plain radiography or CT ⇒ cervical rib, aberrant transverse process
  - MRA/MRV in neutral, abducted arm position

DIFFERENTIAL DIAGNOSIS

Primary and secondary plexus tumors

- E.g., superior sulcus tumor, metastatic breast carcinoma, nerve sheath tumor
- History helpful

Radiation plexopathy

- Diffuse plexus T2 hyperintensity +/- enhancement
- Most common following radiation therapy for breast carcinoma, Hodgkin disease
- Clinical history makes diagnosis

Trauma

- Stretch injury or avulsion
- Trauma history, clinical findings make diagnosis

PATHOLOGY

General Features

- General path comments
  - TO consists of interscalene triangle, costoclavicular space, and retropectoralis minor space (subcoracoid tunnel)
    - Compression of neural, arterial, or venous structures crossing these tunnels → TOS

- Narrowing of costoclavicular distance may be most important abnormality in symptomatic patients
  - Neuropathic TOS: Symptomatology 2° to brachial plexus compression (most symptomatic patients)
    - Up to 98% symptomatic patients have plexus compression; minority 2° to arterial or venous impingement
  - Vascular TOS: Compression of subclavian vessels
    - Repetitive arterial trauma → focal stenosis, aneurysm formation, micro-embolization, tissue loss
    - Venous compression → SCV thrombosis
  - Interscalene triangle bordered by anterior scalene muscle anteriorly, middle and posterior scalene muscles posteriorly, and 1st rib inferiorly
    - SCA passes through lower portion of interscalene triangle, superior (C5–C6) and middle (C7) trunks of brachial plexus pass through upper portion, and lower (C8–T1) trunk crosses inferior portion behind SCA
    - SCV courses between clavicle anteriorly and anterior scalene muscle posteriorly
  - Congenital bony/fibromuscular anomalies, trauma, phenotype and posture contribute to compression or elongation of neurovascular bundle as it passes through these compartments
    - Raising arms above head further compresses already narrowed thoracic outlet
- Etiology: Neural > > vascular compression
- Epidemiology
  - TOS incidence, prevalence disputed; may be ≤ 1/1,000,000
  - Cervical ribs: 6% of general population → 13% of TOS patients, up to 90% of patients receiving surgery for SCA aneurysm
- Associated abnormalities
  - Cervical ribs
  - Unusually large or elongated C7 transverse process
  - Klippel-Feil syndrome

THORACIC OUTLET SYNDROME

Gross Pathologic & Surgical Features

- Vascular compression, SCA aneurysm, SCV thrombosis may be noted at surgery
- Nerves may be swollen and edematous, or atrophic and fibrotic
- Cervical ribs, abnormal transverse processes, fibrous bands, scalene compression of TO contents

Microscopic Features

- Neural injury with fibrosis, axonal loss

CLINICAL ISSUES

Presentation

- Most common signs/symptoms
  ○ Paresthesias, numbness in forearm/ hand
  ○ Pain in shoulder, proximal upper extremity ⇒ neck
  ○ Obliteration of brachial, radial pulses with arm hyperabduction and elevation
- Clinical profile
  ○ "True" neurological TOS: Intermittent arm pain, numbness, and weakness with hyperabduction, external rotation
    ▪ Lower trunk (C8, T1) ≥ upper, middle trunks
    ▪ Nearly always 2° to fibrous band extending from cervical rib compressing lower trunk
    ▪ Hand wasting, concordant EMG findings
  ○ "Disputed" neurological TOS: No consistent clinical or laboratory findings
  ○ Vascular TOS: Paresthesias 2° to ischemia
    ▪ More diffuse than neurological TOS
    ▪ +/- Obliteration of brachial, radial pulses

Demographics

- Age: Adult > > children; average age at diagnosis 26 yrs
- Gender: M < F

Natural History & Prognosis

- Symptomatic patients rarely recover spontaneously without treatment
- Post-operative prognosis of vascular TOS better than neurological TOS

Treatment

- Initial conservative treatment with physical therapy
- Consider TOS decompression/1st rib resection for conservative treatment failures

DIAGNOSTIC CHECKLIST

Consider

- TOS probably end result of diverse symptomatic etiologies rather than a single disease process

Image Interpretation Pearls

- SCA aneurysm, SCV thrombosis, brachial plexus compression with abnormal T2 hyperintensity at TO strongly suggest TOS

SELECTED REFERENCES

1. Charon JP et al: Evaluation of MR angiographic technique in the assessment of thoracic outlet syndrome. Clin Radiol. 59(7):588-95, 2004
2. Samarasam I et al: Surgical management of thoracic outlet syndrome: a 10-year experience. ANZ J Surg. 74(6):450-4, 2004
3. Konstantinou DT et al: Klippel-Feil syndrome presenting with bilateral thoracic outlet syndrome. Spine. 29(9):E189-92, 2004
4. Ambrad-Chalela E et al: Recurrent neurogenic thoracic outlet syndrome. Am J Surg. 187(4):505-10, 2004
5. Yanaka K et al: Diagnosis of vascular compression at the thoracic outlet using magnetic resonance angiography. Eur Neurol. 51(2):122-3, 2004
6. Demondion X et al: Thoracic outlet: assessment with MR imaging in asymptomatic and symptomatic populations. Radiology. 227(2):461-8, 2003
7. Reid JR et al: Thoracic outlet syndrome with subclavian aneurysm in a very young child: the complementary value of MRA and 3D-CT in diagnosis. Pediatr Radiol. 32(1):22-4, 2002
8. Athanassiadi K et al: Treatment of thoracic outlet syndrome: long-term results. World J Surg. 25(5):553-7, 2001
9. Demondion X et al: Thoracic outlet: anatomic correlation with MR imaging. AJR Am J Roentgenol. 175(2):417-22, 2000
10. Hagspiel KD et al: Diagnosis of vascular compression at the thoracic outlet using gadolinium-enhanced high-resolution ultrafast MR angiography in abduction and adduction. Cardiovasc Intervent Radiol. 23(2):152-4, 2000
11. Dymarkowski S et al: Three-dimensional MR angiography in the evaluation of thoracic outlet syndrome. AJR Am J Roentgenol. 173(4):1005-8, 1999
12. Esposito MD et al: Thoracic outlet syndrome in a throwing athlete diagnosed with MRI and MRA. J Magn Reson Imaging. 7(3):598-9, 1997
13. Remy-Jardin M et al: Functional anatomy of the thoracic outlet: evaluation with spiral CT. Radiology. 205: 843–851, 1997
14. Matsumura JS et al: Helical computed tomography of the normal thoracic outlet. J Vasc Surg. 26: 776–783, 1997
15. Longley DG et al: Thoracic outlet syndrome: evaluation of the subclavian vessels by color duplex sonography. AJR Am J Roentgenol. 158:623–630, 1992

IMAGE GALLERY

Typical

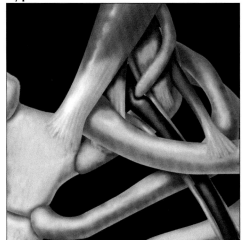
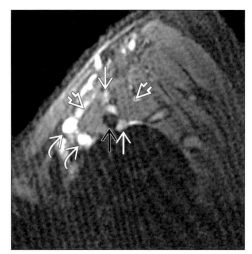

(Left) Graphic demonstrates TOS variant with predominately SCA compression from cervical rib. *(Right)* Sagittal oblique STIR MR shows normal anatomy of interscalene triangle. BP trunks (white arrows), anterior and middle scalene muscles (open arrows), SCA (black arrow), SCV (curved arrows).

Typical

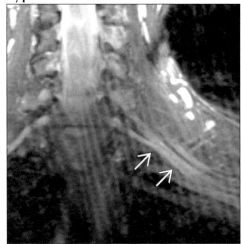
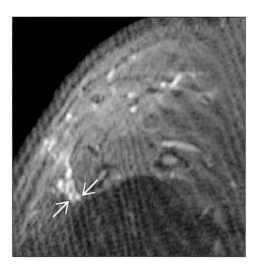

(Left) Coronal STIR MR depicts mild T2 hyperintensity involving BP elements at TOS (arrows). *(Right)* Sagittal oblique STIR MR reveals mild T2 hyperintensity of several fascicles within lower trunk (arrows) in a symptomatic TOS patient.

Typical

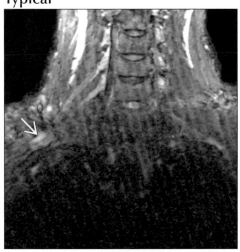
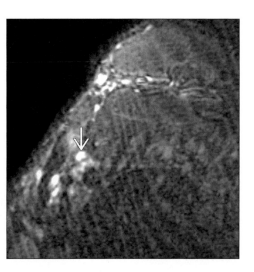

(Left) Coronal STIR MR demonstrates focal T2 hyperintensity of upper trunk (arrow) within thoracic outlet. *(Right)* STIR MR Sagittal oblique depicts focal T2 hyperintensity in BP upper trunk (arrow) corresponding to clinical TOS symptoms.

IDIOPATHIC BRACHIAL PLEXUS NEURITIS

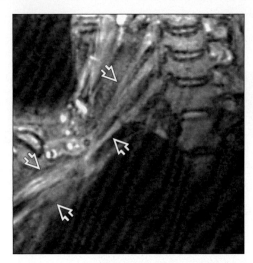

Coronal STIR MR shows diffusely increased signal intensity in brachial plexus (arrows) due to idiopathic brachial neuritis.

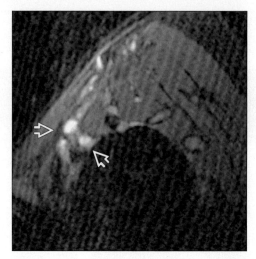

Sagittal oblique STIR MR shows abnormal signal intensity in brachial plexus (arrows) due to idiopathic brachial neuritis.

TERMINOLOGY

Abbreviations and Synonyms
- Parsonage-Turner syndrome
- Acute brachial neuritis
- Neuralgic amyotrophy

Definitions
- Immune-mediated neuropathy of brachial plexus

IMAGING FINDINGS

General Features
- Best diagnostic clue: Homogeneously increased signal on T2WI in one or more muscles of shoulder
- Location
  - Any muscle innervated by brachial plexus
    - Most common: Rotator cuff, deltoid, biceps, triceps
    - Uncommon: Brachialis, forearm muscles, diaphragm, serratus anterior (long thoracic nerve)
  - Sometimes bilateral
  - May cause pure sensory nerve deficit
- Size
  - Mild, uniform enlargement of affected muscles
  - Muscle atrophy seen in chronic cases

- Morphology: Diffuse involvement of muscle without focal mass

CT Findings
- NECT
  - Muscle atrophy, fatty infiltration evident in chronic cases
  - Used to exclude mass involving brachial plexus or peripheral nerves

MR Findings
- T1WI
  - Images through brachial plexus
    - Smooth enlargement of brachial plexus components
    - No evidence of mass and surrounding structures normal
  - Images through affected muscles
    - Acute or subacute: Muscles normal in appearance
    - Chronic: Muscle may be atrophic and show high signal fatty streaks interspersed between muscle fibers
- T2WI
  - Images through brachial plexus
    - Smooth, uniform plexus enlargement
    - Diffuse high T2 signal in affected nerves
    - No evidence of mass, surrounding soft tissue structures normal
  - Images through affected muscles

DDx: Idiopathic Brachial Neuritis

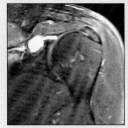

Nerve Entrapment

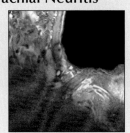

Metastasis

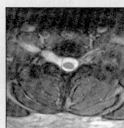

Nerve Trauma

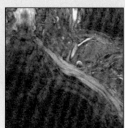

Radiation

Key Facts

Terminology
- Immune-mediated neuropathy of brachial plexus

Imaging Findings
- Any muscle innervated by brachial plexus
- Most common: Rotator cuff, deltoid, biceps, triceps
- Uncommon: Brachialis, forearm muscles, diaphragm, serratus anterior (long thoracic nerve)
- Sometimes bilateral

Top Differential Diagnoses
- Cervical radiculopathy
- Suprascapular nerve entrapment
- Brachial plexus neoplasm
- Brachial plexus or cervical nerve root avulsion
- Radiation neuritis/myositis
- Quadrilateral space syndrome
- Diabetic neuropathy
- Pancoast tumor
- Myositis

Pathology
- Often associated with viral or bacterial infection
- Can occur post-vaccination
- Can also be post-traumatic or post-surgical

Clinical Issues
- Sudden onset of pain, followed by weakness, paresthesias
- May have sensory abnormalities only

Diagnostic Checklist
- Abnormal muscle signal often involves more than one peripheral nerve distribution

---

- Diffuse, homogeneous high signal within muscle bellies
- Tendons normal in appearance
- No evidence of mass
- Often affects muscles from two or more different peripheral nerves
- E.g., infraspinatus (suprascapular nerve) + teres minor (axillary nerve)
- PD/Intermediate: Similar findings to T2WI, but high signal in nerves and muscles less pronounced
- STIR: Similar findings to T2WI, but high signal in nerves and muscles more prominent
- T1 C+: Mild, diffuse enhancement of nerves and affected muscles

Other Modality Findings
- Nerve conduction studies show nerve abnormalities

Imaging Recommendations
- Best imaging tool: MR imaging
- Protocol advice
  - T1WI, T2WI or STIR along long and short axes of symptomatic muscles
  - MRI of shoulder should have 16-18 cm FOV on coronal images
    - Include spinoglenoid notch, quadrilateral space to exclude mass in these regions
  - Imaging of brachial plexus excludes brachial plexus mass
    - Not needed if patient gives characteristic history, unless symptoms do not resolve

DIFFERENTIAL DIAGNOSIS

Cervical radiculopathy
- Evaluate with cervical spine MRI
- Most commonly see involvement of single nerve root
- Brachial neuritis involves multiple nerve roots
- Severe cases may have denervation changes in affected muscles

Suprascapular nerve entrapment
- Affects infraspinatus +/- supraspinatus muscles
- Mass seen in spinoglenoid or suprascapular notch

Brachial plexus neoplasm
- Presents with pain, muscle weakness
- Mass seen on MRI of brachial plexus
- Usually metastasis; primary tumor uncommon

Brachial plexus or cervical nerve root avulsion
- Severe, high velocity injury
- Loss of nerve continuity, fluid around nerve course seen on MRI

Radiation neuritis/myositis
- Diffusely enlarged nerves showing increased T2 signal
- Diffusely enlarged muscles showing increased T2 signal
- Geographic distribution
- History of radiation therapy

Quadrilateral space syndrome
- Mass between teres minor and teres major muscles
- Compresses axillary nerve, affects deltoid, teres minor muscles

Diabetic neuropathy
- Usually distal, symmetric
- Sometimes involves one or more proximal muscles

Pancoast tumor
- Bronchogenic carcinoma at lung apex ("superior sulcus")
- May directly extend to involve brachial plexus

Myositis
- Diffuse T2 signal abnormalities in muscle
- Edema in surrounding fat

Muscle injury
- Heterogeneous signal abnormalities in muscle belly
- Blood products often evident
- Surrounding soft tissues usually show edema/hematoma

IDIOPATHIC BRACHIAL PLEXUS NEURITIS

Rotator cuff tear
- Fluid in tendon defect on MRI
- Chronic, large tears show muscle atrophy

Burner/stinger syndrome
- Common athletic injury in contact sports
- Pain, paresthesias, muscle weakness
- Direct blow to brachial plexus in supraclavicular region
- Alternatively caused by traction to brachial plexus or cervical nerve root
- Usually transient but may persist for weeks
- MRI may be performed to exclude nerve avulsion

PATHOLOGY

General Features
- Etiology
  - Often associated with viral or bacterial infection
    - EBV, CMV, HIV among viral infections
  - Can occur post-vaccination
  - Can also be post-traumatic or post-surgical
    - Surgery may not be in same region (e.g., hip arthroplasty has been reported as cause)
- Epidemiology: M > F

Gross Pathologic & Surgical Features
- Perineural edema, edema in affected muscles

Microscopic Features
- Perineural inflammatory infiltrate
- Thinning of myelin sheath
- Axonal degeneration

CLINICAL ISSUES

Presentation
- Most common signs/symptoms
  - Sudden onset of pain, followed by weakness, paresthesias
  - May have sensory abnormalities only
  - Long thoracic nerve involvement: Winging of scapula
  - Phrenic nerve involvement: Shortness of breath

Demographics
- Age: May occur at any age
- Gender: M > F

Natural History & Prognosis
- Most cases resolve in 3 months to 2 years

Treatment
- Options, risks, complications: Physical therapy to preserve range of motion

DIAGNOSTIC CHECKLIST

Consider
- Shoulder MRI in patient with shoulder weakness and sensory loss, normal cervical spine MRI

- Brachial plexus MRI to exclude other causes in atypical cases
  - Muscles outside of shoulder girdle
  - Respiratory compromise
  - Pure sensory loss

Image Interpretation Pearls
- Abnormal muscle signal often involves more than one peripheral nerve distribution
- Distribution of signal abnormalities helps to distinguish from nerve entrapment syndromes

SELECTED REFERENCES

1. Safran MR: Nerve injury about the shoulder in athletes, part 2: long thoracic nerve, spinal accessory nerve, burners/stingers, thoracic outlet syndrome. Am J Sports Med. 32(4):1063-76, 2004
2. Safran MR: Nerve injury about the shoulder in athletes, part 1: suprascapular nerve and axillary nerve. Am J Sports Med. 32(3):803-19, 2004
3. Gourie-Devi M et al: Long-term follow-up of 44 patients with brachial monomelic amyotrophy. Acta Neurol Scand. 107(3):215-20, 2003
4. Janes SE et al: Brachial neuritis following infection with Epstein-Barr virus. Eur J Paediatr Neurol. 7(6):413-5, 2003
5. Cruz-Martinez A et al: Neuralgic amyotrophy: variable expression in 40 patients. J Peripher Nerv Syst. 7(3):198-204, 2002
6. Gonzalez-Alegre P et al: Idiopathic brachial neuritis. Iowa Orthop J. 22:81-5, 2002
7. Carroll KW et al: Magnetic resonance imaging of the shoulder: a review of potential sources of diagnostic errors. Skeletal Radiol. 31(7):373-83, 2002
8. Watson BV et al: Isolated brachialis wasting: an unusual presentation of neuralgic amyotrophy. Muscle Nerve. 24(12):1699-702, 2001
9. Simon JP et al: Parsonage-Turner syndrome after total-hip arthroplasty. J Arthroplasty. 16(4):518-20, 2001
10. Antoniou J et al: Suprascapular neuropathy. Variability in the diagnosis, treatment, and outcome. Clin Orthop. (386):131-8, 2001
11. Miller JD et al: Acute brachial plexus neuritis: an uncommon cause of shoulder pain. Am Fam Physician. 62(9):2067-72, 2000
12. Bredella MA et al: Denervation syndromes of the shoulder girdle: MR imaging with electrophysiologic correlation. Skeletal Radiol. 28(10):567-72, 1999
13. Helms CA et al: Acute brachial neuritis (Parsonage-Turner syndrome): MR imaging appearance--report of three cases. Radiology. 207(1):255-9, 1998

IMAGE GALLERY

Typical

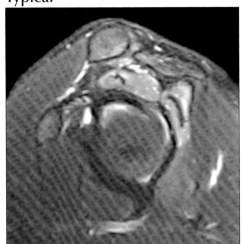 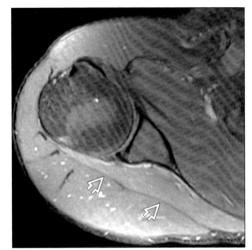

(Left) Sagittal T2WI MR shows diffusely abnormal signal intensity in the infraspinatus and supraspinatus muscles due to idiopathic brachial neuritis. *(Right)* Axial PD/Intermediate MR shows mild increase in signal intensity throughout infraspinatus (arrows). Deltoid is slightly higher signal than subscapularis due to signal drop-off from surface coil.

Typical

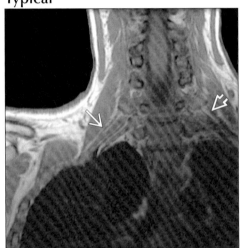 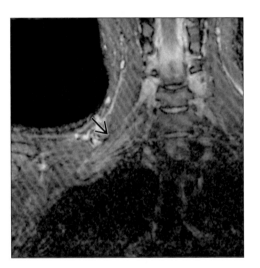

(Left) Coronal T1WI MR shows uniform, smooth enlargement of visualized portions of right brachial plexus (arrow) in patient with brachial neuritis, compared to normal left side (open arrow). *(Right)* Coronal STIR MR shows uniform, tubular nerve enlargement (arrow) and increased signal intensity which is primarily at the periphery of the nerves.

Typical

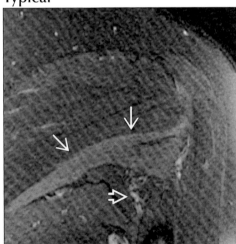 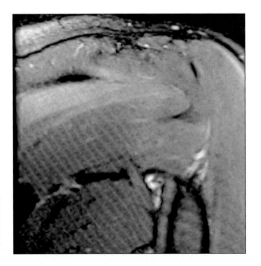

(Left) Coronal oblique T2WI MR shows signal abnormality throughout teres minor (arrows) due to brachial neuritis. Quadrilateral space (open arrow) shows no evidence of mass involving axillary nerve. *(Right)* Coronal oblique T2WI MR shows diffuse increase in signal intensity throughout superior fibers of infraspinatus muscle due to brachial neuritis.

RADIATION PLEXOPATHY

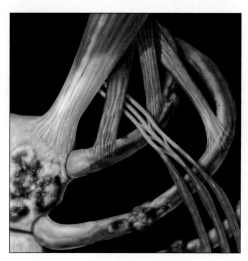

Coronal graphic shows diffuse edema of brachial plexus elements in breast cancer patient with skeletal metastases following radiation therapy.

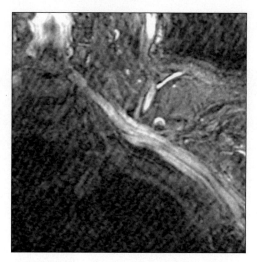

Coronal STIR MR (breast cancer post-XRT with vague symptoms) shows mild diffuse brachial plexus T2 hyperintensity without focal nodular involvement.

TERMINOLOGY

Abbreviations and Synonyms
- Synonyms: Radiation plexitis, XRT plexitis, radiation-induced fibrosis (RIF)

Definitions
- Post-radiation brachial plexus (BP) or lumbosacral plexus inflammation

IMAGING FINDINGS

General Features
- Best diagnostic clue: Smooth, diffuse T2 hyperintensity +/- enhancement of multiple plexus elements
- Location
  - Upper BP (C5-7) > lower BP (C8, T1)
  - Lumbosacral plexus following XRT for prostate, cervical carcinoma
- Size: Mild diffuse enlargement of abnormal nerves
- Morphology: Smooth, diffuse T2 hyperintensity of multiple trunks/divisions

CT Findings
- CECT
  - Difficult CT diagnosis
  - +/- Diffuse plexus enlargement, enhancement (acute)
  - +/- Distortion of tissue planes, ↑ density of axillary fat

MR Findings
- T1WI
  - Acute: Diffuse nerve enlargement, mild T1 hypointensity +/- diffuse enhancement without focal nodularity, muscle denervation changes
  - Chronic: Nerves normal or architectural distortion +/- surrounding tissue scarring, fibrosis, muscle denervation changes
- T2WI
  - Acute: Diffuse plexus enlargement, relatively homogeneous T2 hyperintensity, preservation of plexus internal architecture +/- muscle denervation changes
  - Chronic: Nerves normal or architectural distortion +/- surrounding tissue scarring, fibrosis, muscle denervation changes
- STIR: Similar to fat-saturated T2WI
- T1 C+: +/- Mild homogeneous enhancement

Nuclear Medicine Findings
- PET: +/- Mild diffuse FDG uptake; avid focal uptake implies neoplasm

Other Modality Findings
- Electromyography: Subacute to chronic plexopathy with myokymic discharges in affected muscles

---

DDx: Radiation Plexopathy

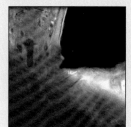
Breast CA Met.

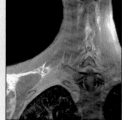
Pancreatic CA Met.

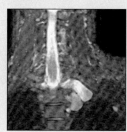
Plexiform NF

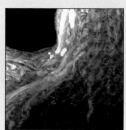
BP Traction Injury

RADIATION PLEXOPATHY

Key Facts

Terminology

- Synonyms: Radiation plexitis, XRT plexitis, radiation-induced fibrosis (RIF)
- Post-radiation brachial plexus (BP) or lumbosacral plexus inflammation

Imaging Findings

- Best diagnostic clue: Smooth, diffuse T2 hyperintensity +/- enhancement of multiple plexus elements

Top Differential Diagnoses

- Malignant brachial plexus infiltration
- Plexiform neurofibroma
- Plexus traction injury

Pathology

- Connective tissue response spectrum from edema, acute inflammation → chronic inflammation, progressive fibrosis, & neovascularization, disruption of vascular supply to nerve

Clinical Issues

- Pain, paresthesia, motor deficits of ipsilateral extremity

Diagnostic Checklist

- Important to correctly diagnosis to avoid inappropriate additional radiation therapy
- May be difficult to distinguish XRT plexitis from recurrent tumor on imaging studies
- Smooth T2 hyperintensity, linear enhancement of upper BP favors XRT plexitis > malignancy

---

Imaging Recommendations

- Best imaging tool: High-resolution MRI (MR neurography)
- Protocol advice: Coronal, sagittal oblique T1WI, STIR, fat-saturated T1 C+ MR

DIFFERENTIAL DIAGNOSIS

Malignant brachial plexus infiltration

- Most commonly involves inferior BP (C8, T1), pain usually more severe than XRT plexopathy
- Direct extension from axillary adenopathy (breast cancer) or lung apex (Pancoast tumor) > systemic metastasis
- More focal, nodular than radiation plexopathy

Plexiform neurofibroma

- More nodular, focal than radiation plexopathy
- Clinical phenotype, genetic testing usually distinguish

Plexus traction injury

- Usually more focal, involves fewer plexus elements
- +/- Avulsion pseudomeningocele
- Search for trauma history, diagnostic clinical and imaging findings

PATHOLOGY

General Features

- General path comments
  - Pathogenesis poorly understood
    - Connective tissue response spectrum from edema, acute inflammation → chronic inflammation, progressive fibrosis, & neovascularization, disruption of vascular supply to nerve
    - Acute edema may resolve if injury minor & becomes subclinical, but frequently some level of nerve injury persists pathologically
    - Damaged neural tissue replaced by fibrosis in chronic plexopathies

- Incidence of complications ↑ with time following radiation
- Etiology
  - Combination of direct cell damage 2° ionizing radiation → free radicals + progressive radiation - induced ischemia (vascular damage to vaso nervosum)
  - Uncommon < 60 Gray dose; dose-dependent, more common with large daily fractions or brachytherapy
  - Potentiated by chemotherapy
- Epidemiology
  - Rare (< 1% incidence)
  - Delayed onset 6 months to > 20 years post-XRT
    - Peak onset at 10–20 months post-XRT, median 1.5 years
- Associated abnormalities
  - +/- Residual malignant tissue, fibrotic scar tissue
  - Unilateral left vocal cord paralysis (5%)
  - Radiation arteritis, accelerated atherosclerotic plaque formation

Gross Pathologic & Surgical Features

- Edema, demyelination, neural tissue atrophy, fibrous nerve sheath thickening, fibrous replacement of nerve fibers, connective tissue fibrosis

Microscopic Features

- Acute: Excessive extracellular matrix deposition, inflammatory infiltrate
- Chronic: Dense, noninflammatory fibrous matrix with fewer cells

Staging, Grading or Classification Criteria

- Modified LENT-SOMA scale (brachial plexopathy)
  - Grade 1: Mild sensory deficits, no pain
  - Grade 2: Moderate sensory deficits, tolerable pain, mild arm weakness
  - Grade 3: Continuous paresthesia with incomplete paresis
  - Grade 4: Complete paresis, excruciating pain, muscle atrophy

RADIATION PLEXOPATHY

CLINICAL ISSUES

Presentation

- Most common signs/symptoms
  - Pain, paresthesia, motor deficits of ipsilateral extremity
    - BP plexopathy usually referable to upper (C5-7) > lower BP (C8-T1)
    - Lumbosacral plexopathy most commonly affects sciatic nerve distribution
    - Pain often relatively mild compared to malignant plexopathy
  - Other signs/symptoms
    - Horner syndrome (rare; more common with malignant plexopathy)
- Clinical profile
  - Unilateral BP plexopathy following radiotherapy for breast cancer, Pancoast tumor, systemic metastasis
  - Bilateral brachial plexopathy after mantle radiotherapy for Hodgkin disease
  - Lumbosacral plexopathy following radiotherapy for prostate, cervical cancer

Demographics

- Age: Age at onset parallels demographics of initial cancer diagnosis + development time for radiation plexopathy
- Gender: M < F (reflects pertinent cancer demographics)

Natural History & Prognosis

- Variable; related to dose delivered to plexus, severity of nerve injury
  - Some patients resolve spontaneously
  - Others slowly progress despite treatment
- Risk of brachial plexopathy remains for considerable portion of patient's life
- All patients have potential to develop delayed symptoms, worsening of grade

Treatment

- Avoid inappropriate additional radiation therapy
- Corticosteroids +/- combined pentoxifylline and tocopherol (Vit E) therapy
- No traditional role for surgery
  - Transferred myocutaneous flap + BP neurolysis may improve blood supply to fibrotic brachial plexus
- Palliative long-term narcotics, sympathectomy for pain relief

DIAGNOSTIC CHECKLIST

Consider

- Important to correctly diagnosis to avoid inappropriate additional radiation therapy

Image Interpretation Pearls

- May be difficult to distinguish XRT plexitis from recurrent tumor on imaging studies
- Smooth T2 hyperintensity, linear enhancement of upper BP favors XRT plexitis > malignancy

SELECTED REFERENCES

1. Bajrovic A et al: Is there a life-long risk of brachial plexopathy after radiotherapy of supraclavicular lymph nodes in breast cancer patients? Radiother Oncol. 71(3):297-301, 2004
2. Schierle C et al: Radiation-induced brachial plexopathy: review. Complication without a cure. J Reconstr Microsurg. 20(2):149-52, 2004
3. Lu L et al: Diagnosis and operative treatment of radiation-induced brachial plexopathy. Chin J Traumatol. 5(6):329-32, 2002
4. Ferrante MA et al: Electrodiagnostic approach to the patient with suspected brachial plexopathy. Neurol Clin. 20(2):423-50, 2002
5. Johansson S et al: Dose response and latency for radiation-induced fibrosis, edema, and neuropathy in breast cancer patients. Int J Radiat Oncol Biol Phys. 52(5):1207-19, 2002
6. Fathers E et al: Radiation-induced brachial plexopathy in women treated for carcinoma of the breast. Clin Rehabil. 16(2):160-5, 2002
7. Rubin DI et al: Arteritis and brachial plexus neuropathy as delayed complications of radiation therapy. Mayo Clin Proc. 76(8):849-52, 2001
8. Cros D: Peripheral Neuropathy. First ed, Philadelphia: Lippincott Williams & Wilkins. 185-7, 2001
9. Johansson S et al: Timescale of evolution of late radiation injury after postoperative radiotherapy of breast cancer patients. Int J Radiat Oncol Biol Phys. 48(3):745-50, 2000
10. Wittenberg KH et al: MR imaging of nontraumatic brachial plexopathies: frequency and spectrum of findings. Radiographics. 20(4):1023-32, 2000
11. Johansson S et al: Brachial plexopathy after postoperative radiotherapy of breast cancer patients--a long-term follow-up. Acta Oncol. 39(3):373-82, 2000
12. Churn M et al: Early onset of bilateral brachial plexopathy during mantle radiotherapy for Hodgkin's disease. Clin Oncol (R Coll Radiol). 12(5):289-91, 2000
13. Qayyum A et al: Symptomatic brachial plexopathy following treatment for breast cancer: utility of MR imaging with surface-coil techniques. Radiology. 214(3):837-42, 2000
14. Wadd NJ et al: Brachial plexus neuropathy following mantle radiotherapy. Clin Oncol (R Coll Radiol). 10(6):399-400, 1998
15. Wouter van Es H et al: Radiation-induced brachial plexopathy: MR imaging. Skeletal Radiol. 26(5):284-8, 1997
16. Bowen BC et al: Radiation-induced brachial plexopathy: MR and clinical findings. AJNR Am J Neuroradiol. 17(10):1932-6, 1996
17. Iyer RB et al: MR imaging of the treated brachial plexus. AJR Am J Roentgenol. 167(1):225-9, 1996

IMAGE GALLERY

Typical

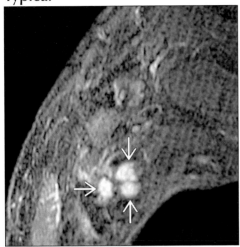 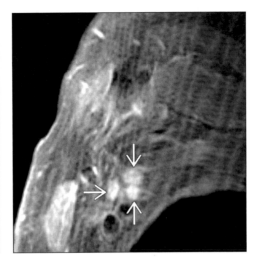

(Left) STIR MR Sagittal oblique (radiation therapy for breast cancer, acute symptoms) depicts diffuse enlargement, fascicular swelling, abnormal T2 hyperintensity of three BP cords (arrows). *(Right)* T1 C+ MR Sagittal oblique (radiation therapy for breast cancer, acute symptoms) demonstrates diffuse enlargement, mild enhancement of abnormal BP cords (arrows).

Typical

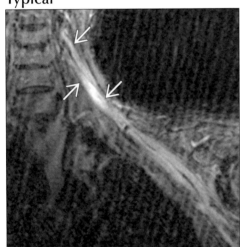 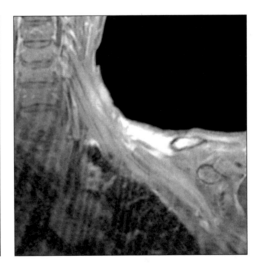

(Left) Coronal STIR MR (radiation therapy for breast cancer, acute symptoms) shows diffuse linear T2 hyperintensity of upper brachial plexus (arrows). *(Right)* Coronal T1 C+ MR (radiation therapy for breast cancer, acute symptoms) reveals patchy mild enhancement of upper brachial plexus elements.

Typical

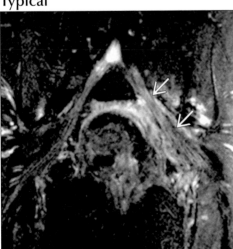 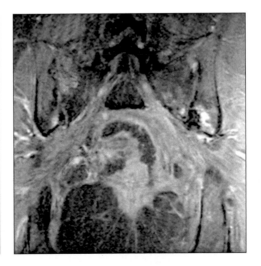

(Left) Coronal STIR MR (radiation therapy for cervical cancer, chronic symptoms) shows mild left lumbosacral plexus T2 hyperintensity (arrows) surrounded by hyperintense fibrovascular scar tissue. *(Right)* Coronal T1 C+ MR (radiation therapy for cervical cancer, chronic symptoms) shows mild surrounding fibrovascular scar tissue enhancement of lumbosacral plexus .

HYPERTROPHIC NEUROPATHY

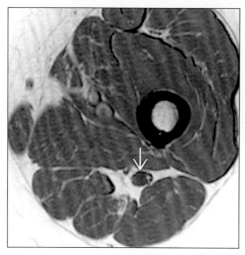

Axial T1WI MR (focal hypertrophic neuropathy, path proven) demonstrates focal enlargement of tibial division (arrow) of sciatic nerve. Histology revealed typical "onion-bulb" formations.

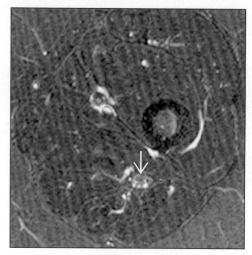

Axial STIR MR (focal HN) confirms mild T2 hyperintensity, partial loss of normal fascicular architecture (arrow). Fascicles adjacent to mass are abnormally enlarged and T2 hyperintense.

TERMINOLOGY

Abbreviations and Synonyms
- Synonyms: Hereditary motor-sensory neuropathy (HMSN), hypertrophic neuropathy (HN), Charcot-Marie-Tooth (CMT) syndrome

Definitions
- Hereditary disorder characterized by focal or diffuse peripheral nerve enlargement
  - HMSN I (Charcot-Marie-Tooth syndrome type I, CMT 1)
  - HMSN II (neuronal type peroneal muscular atrophy, CMT 2)
  - HMSN III (Dejerine-Sottas disease (DSD), hypertrophic neuropathy of infancy, congenital hypomyelinated neuropathy)

IMAGING FINDINGS

General Features
- Best diagnostic clue: Focal or diffuse peripheral nerve enlargement + distal extremity atrophy
- Location: Peripheral nerves +/- spinal nerve roots

Radiographic Findings
- Myelography: +/- Nerve root thickening, myelographic block 2° spinal stenosis

CT Findings
- CECT: Enlarged nerves +/- enhancement

MR Findings
- T1WI
  - Fusiform T1 hypointense mass(es) of peripheral nerves +/- cauda equina nerve roots
  - +/- Abnormal muscle T1 hyperintensity, volume loss (chronic denervation → fatty atrophy)
- T2WI
  - Fusiform T1 hyperintense mass(es) of peripheral nerves +/- cauda equina nerve roots
  - Internal fascicular architecture disrupted over abnormal segment
  - +/- Abnormal muscle hyperintensity, swelling on fat-saturated T2WI (acute denervation)
- STIR: Similar to fat saturated T2WI
- T1 C+: +/- Abnormal enhancement of enlarged nerves (most commonly HMSN I, III)

Other Modality Findings
- Nerve conduction velocities (NCVs)
  - HMSN I: Severe diffuse motor NCV slowing
  - HMSN II: Relatively normal motor NCV, reduced/absent sensory nerve action potentials
  - HMSN III: Markedly reduced motor NCV

DDx: Hypertrophic Neuropathy

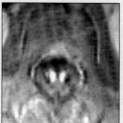
Guillain-Barré

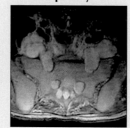
CIDP

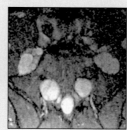
Plexiform

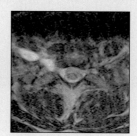
BP Traction Injury

HYPERTROPHIC NEUROPATHY

Key Facts

Terminology
- Synonyms: Hereditary motor-sensory neuropathy (HMSN), hypertrophic neuropathy (HN), Charcot-Marie-Tooth (CMT) syndrome
- Hereditary disorder characterized by focal or diffuse peripheral nerve enlargement

Imaging Findings
- Best diagnostic clue: Focal or diffuse peripheral nerve enlargement + distal extremity atrophy
- Internal fascicular architecture disrupted over abnormal segment

Top Differential Diagnoses
- Guillain-Barré syndrome
- Chronic inflammatory demyelinating polyneuropathy (CIDP)

- Nerve sheath tumor
- Traumatic nerve stretch injury

Pathology
- Enlargement of peripheral nerves +/- spinal nerve roots, "onion-bulb" formations common in HMSN I, III but uncommon in HMSN II
- Histologic features of demyelination, remyelination

Clinical Issues
- Similarly affected relatives common
- Normal life expectancy

Diagnostic Checklist
- Consider HMSN when abnormally enlarged peripheral nerves or nerve roots identified on MR imaging

Imaging Recommendations
- Best imaging tool: High-resolution MR imaging (MR neurography)
- Protocol advice: Axial T1WI, fat-saturated T2WI or STIR, fat-saturated T1 C+ MR

DIFFERENTIAL DIAGNOSIS

Guillain-Barré syndrome
- Acute onset of ascending paralysis with relative sensory preservation
- Symptom onset, progression characteristic
- Pial, nerve root enhancement similar to CIDP

Chronic inflammatory demyelinating polyneuropathy (CIDP)
- Repeated episodes of demyelination, remyelination ⇒ "onion skin" spinal, peripheral nerve enlargement
- Mimics HMSN, plexiform neurofibroma on MRI
- Inflammatory infiltrate (histology) helps distinguishes from HMSN

Nerve sheath tumor
- Schwannoma, solitary neurofibroma, plexiform neurofibroma
- Diffuse nerve root enlargement, enhancement
- +/- Cutaneous stigmata of NF1 on physical exam
- Genetic testing, distinctive clinical stigmata distinguish from CIDP, HMSN

Traumatic nerve stretch injury
- Nerve enlargement, architectural distortion
- History, trauma imaging findings make diagnosis

PATHOLOGY

General Features
- General path comments
  - CMT is most common inherited neurologic disorder

  - Enlargement of peripheral nerves +/- spinal nerve roots, "onion-bulb" formations common in HMSN I, III but uncommon in HMSN II
- Genetics
  - HMSN IA (CMT 1A): Autosomal dominant, short arm of chromosome 17
  - HMSN IB (CMT 1B): Long arm of chromosome 1
  - HMSN II: Chromosome 1
  - HMSN III: Autosomal recessive (controversial), chromosome 17
- Etiology
  - HMSN I (CMT 1): Disorder of peripheral myelination
    - Mutation in peripheral myelin protein-22 (PMP-22) gene → unstable myelin that spontaneously demyelinates
    - Schwann cells proliferate and remyelinate axons
    - Repeated cycles of demyelination, remyelination produce concentric myelin layers around axons ("onion bulb" formations)
  - HMSN II (CMT 2): Primary axonal loss, Wallerian degeneration without remyelination/demyelination cycles
  - HMSN III (Dejerine-Sottas disease): Severe segmental demyelination, myelin thinning around nerve
- Epidemiology
  - HMSN I: Incidence 15/100,000
    - CMT IA incidence 10.5/100,000 (70% of HMSN I cases)
  - HMSN II: Incidence 7/100,000
  - HMSN III: Rare

Gross Pathologic & Surgical Features
- Hypertrophic thickened nerve roots, peripheral nerves
- Roots may fill thecal sac at surgery

Microscopic Features
- Histologic features of demyelination, remyelination
  - HMSN I: Primary hypertrophic myelin pathology → demyelination/remyelination, S-100-positive concentric "onion-bulb" formations, secondary axonal changes

HYPERTROPHIC NEUROPATHY

○ HMSN II: Primary axonal pathology, axon loss + Wallerian degeneration
○ HMSN III: Severe hypomyelination/demyelination, axonal loss, myelin sheath thinning

Staging, Grading or Classification Criteria
• HMSN types IA, IB (CMT 1A, 1B)
• HMSN type II (neuronal type peroneal muscular atrophy)
• HMSN type III (hypertrophic neuropathy of infancy, Dejerine-Sottas disease)
• HMSN type 4 (hypertrophic neuropathy associated with phytanic acid excess)
• HMSN type 5 (associated with spastic paraplegia)
• HMSN type 6 (associated with optic atrophy)
• HMSN type 7

CLINICAL ISSUES

Presentation
• Most common signs/symptoms
  ○ HMSN I
    ■ Similarly affected relatives common
    ■ Distal extremity muscle weakness/atrophy (motor > sensory), foot deformities (pes cavus, hammer toes), ↓ tendon reflexes, +/- palpable extremity nerve masses
    ■ Relative lack of pain (in contrast to acquired neuropathies)
  ○ HMSN II: Often minimally symptomatic
  ○ HMSN III: Clinical symptoms similar but more severe than HMSN I, earlier presentation
    ■ Delayed motor development, progressive muscular weakness of legs and arms
  ○ Other signs/symptoms
    ■ Back/lower extremity radicular pain +/- myelopathy
    ■ Sensory loss, focal tenderness, dysesthesias
    ■ +/- Palpable nerve mass
    ■ Cold feet, hair loss, leg edema
• Clinical profile
  ○ HMSN type I: Distal extremity weakness, muscle atrophy (legs > arms)
    ■ Sensation often normal until adulthood
    ■ Hyporeflexia or areflexia, orthopedic foot deformities, scoliosis (37-50%), tremor (≤ 25%)
  ○ HMSN type II: Peripheral nerves not clinically enlarged, lower extremity > hand weakness, sensory loss in distal extremities, foot deformities (< HMSN I)
  ○ HMSN type III: Infant with hyporeflexia, palpable enlarged peripheral nerves, sensory loss +/- ataxia

Demographics
• Age
  ○ HMSN I: Onset in 1st decade typical, delayed in some patients until young or mid adulthood
  ○ HMSN II: Often diagnosed later in life; symptoms commonly begin during 2nd decade
  ○ HMSN III: Onset typically during infancy or early childhood
• Gender: M = F

Natural History & Prognosis
• Normal life expectancy
• Slowly progressive condition; disability severity highly variable

Treatment
• Conservative: Injury prevention (lifestyle adjustment, avoidance of occupational injury), treatment of acquired neuropathies, physical therapy, ankle-foot orthoses, anti-inflammatory medications
• Surgical: Correction of orthopedic deformities

DIAGNOSTIC CHECKLIST

Consider
• MR imaging currently plays a limited role in the work-up of HMSN
• Genetic consultation for patients with fusiform nerve enlargement identified on MR imaging

Image Interpretation Pearls
• Consider HMSN when abnormally enlarged peripheral nerves or nerve roots identified on MR imaging

SELECTED REFERENCES

1. Kretzer RM et al: Hypertrophic neuropathy of the cauda equina: case report. Neurosurgery. 54(2):515-8; discussion 518-9, 2004
2. Graham D et al: Greenfield's Neuropathology. 7th ed. London, 628-632, 2002
3. Moore KR et al: The value of MR neurography for evaluating extraspinal neuropathic leg pain: a pictorial essay. AJNR Am J Neuroradiol. 22(4):786-94, 2001
4. Cellerini M et al: MR imaging of the cauda equina in hereditary motor sensory neuropathies: correlations with sural nerve biopsy. AJNR Am J Neuroradiol. 21(10):1793-8, 2000
5. Keller MP et al: Inherited peripheral neuropathy. Semin Neurol. 19(4):353-62, 1999
6. Hahn M et al: Hypertrophied cauda equina presenting as intradural mass: case report and review of literature. Surg Neurol. 49(5):514-8; discussion 518-9, 1998
7. Calore EE et al: Hypertrophic motor and sensory neuropathy type I (Charcot-Marie-Tooth disease): ultrastructural study of sural nerve biopsy in members of a family. Pathologica. 86(3):279-83, 1994
8. Vasilescu C: Hereditary motor and sensory neuropathy. Clinical, genetic and electrodiagnostic studies. Rom J Neurol Psychiatry. 31(3-4):207-19, 1993
9. Gemignani F et al: Peroneal muscular atrophy with hereditary spastic paraparesis (HMSN V) is pathologically heterogeneous. Report of nerve biopsy in four cases and review of the literature. Acta Neuropathol (Berl). 83(2):196-201, 1992
10. Chou SM: Immunohistochemical and ultrastructural classification of peripheral neuropathies with onion-bulbs. Clin Neuropathol. 11(3):109-14, 1992
11. Choi SK et al: MR imaging in hypertrophic neuropathy: a case of hereditary motor and sensory neuropathy, type I (Charcot-Marie-Tooth). Clin Imaging. 14(3):204-7, 1990
12. Bird TD: Hereditary motor-sensory neuropathies. Charcot-Marie-Tooth syndrome. Neurol Clin. 7(1):9-23, 1989

IMAGE GALLERY

Typical

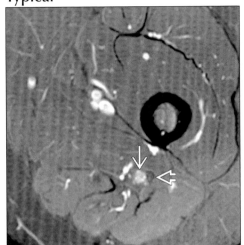 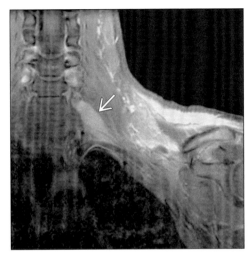

(Left) Axial T1 C+ MR with fat-saturation (focal hypertrophic neuropathy) shows focal enhancement in tibial division of sciatic nerve (arrow). Adjacent peroneal division (open arrow) is uninvolved. *(Right)* Coronal T1 C+ MR with fat-saturation demonstrates fusiform enlargement and enhancement of left C7 root (arrow).

Variant

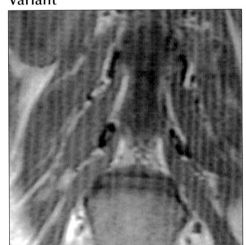 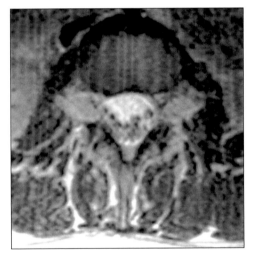

(Left) Coronal T1WI MR (Charcot-Marie-Tooth) demonstrates diffuse bilateral enlargement of spinal nerve roots and lumbar plexus in a patient imaged for symptomatic scoliosis. *(Right)* Axial T2WI MR (Charcot-Marie-Tooth) depicts cauda equina and bilateral spinal nerve root hypertrophy.

Variant

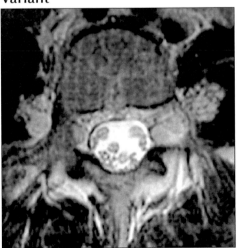 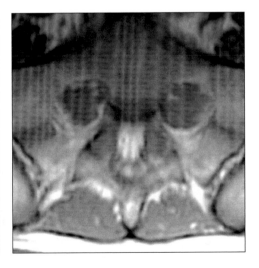

(Left) Axial T2WI MR (Charcot-Marie-Tooth) demonstrates prominent enlargement of cauda equina and bilateral spinal nerves. *(Right)* Axial T1 C+ MR (Charcot-Marie-Tooth) shows prominent enlargement without abnormal enhancement of sacral spinal nerve roots.

PERIPHERAL NERVE TUMOR

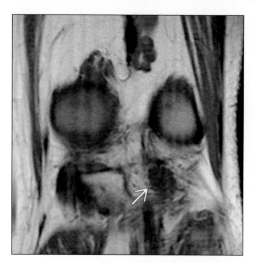

Coronal T1WI MR shows perineuroma of peroneal n. (arrow) found during evaluation for peroneal n. palsy. Mass was contiguous with n. in all imaging planes.

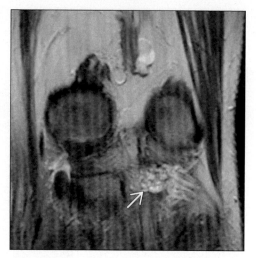

Coronal T2WI MR shows perineuroma of peroneal n. Mass is multilobulated and heterogeneous in signal intensity (arrow). T1 C+ (not shown) revealed avid enhancement.

TERMINOLOGY

Abbreviations and Synonyms
- Peripheral nerve sheath tumor previously used term but less accurate description
- Malignant peripheral nerve sheath tumor (MPNST) replaces earlier terms: Malignant schwannoma, neurofibrosarcoma, neurogenic sarcoma

Definitions
- A grouping of benign and malignant primary tumors of peripheral nerves (nn.)

IMAGING FINDINGS

General Features
- Best diagnostic clue: Mass along course of peripheral nerve
- Morphology
  - Eccentric to nerve: Schwannoma
  - Enlarged nerve in lobulated or cord-like configuration: Neurofibroma
  - Ovoid enlargement of nerve: N. sheath myxoma, perineuroma, MPNST

CT Findings
- NECT: Fusiform, lobulated or ovoid mass along course of nerve

MR Findings
- T1WI
  - Low signal intensity mass
  - May see high signal fatty atrophy in innervated muscles (mm.)
- T2WI
  - Heterogeneous, intermediate to high signal intensity
  - May see denervation edema, diffuse high signal in innervated mm.
- STIR: Same as T2WI but more pronounced
- T1 C+: Avidly enhance with contrast
- Schwannoma often contains areas of cystic degeneration
- MPNST usually shows extensive central necrosis

Imaging Recommendations
- Best imaging tool: MRI
- Protocol advice: T2WI or STIR, T1 C+ long and short axis of tumor

DIFFERENTIAL DIAGNOSIS

Traumatic neuroma
- History of trauma or amputation
- Enlargement, enhancement of nerve

DDx: Peripheral Nerve Tumor

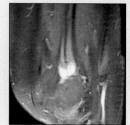

Traumatic Neuroma

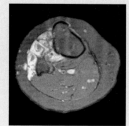

Hemangioma

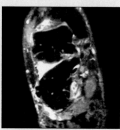

Neuritis

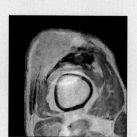

Sarcoma (MFH)

PERIPHERAL NERVE TUMOR

Key Facts

Terminology
- A grouping of benign and malignant primary tumors of peripheral nerves (nn.)

Imaging Findings
- Eccentric to nerve: Schwannoma
- Enlarged nerve in lobulated or cord-like configuration: Neurofibroma
- Ovoid enlargement of nerve: N. sheath myxoma, perineuroma, MPNST
- NECT: Fusiform, lobulated or ovoid mass along course of nerve
- Low signal intensity mass
- Heterogeneous, intermediate to high signal intensity
- May see denervation edema, diffuse high signal in innervated mm.

- T1 C+: Avidly enhance with contrast
- Best imaging tool: MRI
- Protocol advice: T2WI or STIR, T1 C+ long and short axis of tumor

Top Differential Diagnoses
- Traumatic neuroma
- Hemangioma
- Neuritis
- Other soft tissue sarcomas

Pathology
- General path comments: Malignant degeneration seen in neurofibroma, but rare in schwannoma
- Associated abnormalities: 5-13% of patients with neurofibromatosis develop MPNST

Hemangioma
- Enlarged vessels may mimic multilobulated neurofibroma
- Draining veins visible

Neuritis
- Increased T2 signal in affected n., muscles, without mass

Other soft tissue sarcomas
- Not centered along n.

PATHOLOGY

General Features
- General path comments: Malignant degeneration seen in neurofibroma, but rare in schwannoma
- Associated abnormalities: 5-13% of patients with neurofibromatosis develop MPNST

Gross Pathologic & Surgical Features
- Schwannoma: Encapsulated; solid areas, edematous areas, cysts
- Neurofibroma: Not encapsulated, glistening, tan-white
- Nerve sheath myxoma: Gelatinous
- Perineuroma: Circumscribed white mass
- MPNST: Usually large, white-tan, hemorrhage and necrosis

Microscopic Features
- Schwannoma: 2 types of cells, Antoni A (spindle cells) and Antoni B (tumor cells surrounded by fluid)
- Neurofibroma: All elements of peripheral n. proliferate
- Nerve sheath myxoma: Myxoid material, cells arranged in bundles
- Perineuroma: Elongated cells in parallel bundles; storiform growth
- MPNST: Serpentine shape of tumor cells, arranged in whorls or palisades

Staging, Grading or Classification Criteria
- Benign tumors
  - Schwannoma (neurilemoma)
  - Neurofibroma
    - Plexiform neurofibroma: Arborizing tumor of peripheral nerves occurring in neurofibromatosis
  - Nerve sheath myxoma (neurothekeoma)
  - Perineuroma
- Malignant tumors
  - Malignant peripheral nerve sheath tumor (MPNST)
  - Lymphoma

CLINICAL ISSUES

Presentation
- Most common signs/symptoms
  - Palpable, painless mass
  - Other signs/symptoms
    - May cause neurologic symptoms

Demographics
- Age
  - Localized neurofibroma usually ages 20-30
  - Nerve sheath myxoma, perineuroma: Childhood to early adulthood
  - Schwannoma and MPNST ages 20-50

Treatment
- Options, risks, complications
  - Some amenable to surgical excision
  - Radiation, chemotherapy for MPNST

DIAGNOSTIC CHECKLIST

Image Interpretation Pearls
- Often can see tapered transition to normal contiguous n. at margin of mass

SELECTED REFERENCES
1. Rosai J: Surgical Pathology, vol 2. 9th ed. Edinburgh, Mosby. 2629-2662, 2004
2. Skubitz KM, Skubitz AP. Characterization of sarcomas by means of gene expression. J Lab Clin Med. 144(2):78-91, 2004

3. Lin V, Daniel S, Forte V. Is a plexiform neurofibroma pathognomonic of neurofibromatosis type I? Laryngoscope. 114(8):1410-4, 2004

4. He Y, Zhang Z, Tian Z, Zhang C, Zhu H. The application of magnetic resonance imaging-guided fine-needle aspiration cytology in the diagnosis of deep lesions in the head and neck. J Oral Maxillofac Surg. 62(8):953-8, 2004

5. Forthman CL, Blazar PE. Nerve tumors of the hand and upper extremity. Hand Clin. 20(3):233-42, 2004

6. Beekman R, Slooff WB, Van Oosterhout MF, Lammens M, Van Den Berg LH. Bilateral intraneural perineurioma presenting as ulnar neuropathy at the elbow. Muscle Nerve. 30(2):239-43, 2004

7. Robertson TC, Buck DA, Schmidt-Ullrich R, Powers CN, Reiter ER. Isolated plexiform neurofibroma: treatment with three-dimensional conformal radiotherapy. Laryngoscope. 114(7):1139-42, 2004

8. Shapiro SL. Endoscopic decompression of the intermetatarsal nerve for Morton's neuroma. Foot Ankle Clin. 9(2):297-304, 2004

9. Stamatis ED, Karabalis C. Interdigital neuromas: current state of the art--surgical. Foot Ankle Clin. 9(2):287-96, 2004

10. Kim DH, Murovic JA, Tiel RL, Kline DG. Management and outcomes in 318 operative common peroneal nerve lesions at the Louisiana State University Health Sciences Center. Neurosurgery. 54(6):1421-8; discussion 1428-9, 2004

11. Stemmer-Rachamimov AO, Louis DN, Nielsen GP, Antonescu CR, Borowsky AD, Bronson RT, Burns DK, Cervera P, McLaughlin ME, Reifenberger G, Schmale MC, MacCollin M, Chao RC, Cichowski K, Kalamarides M, Messerli SM, McClatchey AI, Niwa-Kawakita M, Ratner N, Reilly KM, Zhu Y, Giovannini M. Comparative pathology of nerve sheath tumors in mouse models and humans. Cancer Res. 15;64(10):3718-24, 2004

12. Dellon AL, Kim J, Ducic I. Painful neuroma of the posterior cutaneous nerve of the forearm after surgery for lateral humeral epicondylitis. J Hand Surg [Am]. 29(3):387-90, 2004

13. Velagaleti GV, Miettinen M, Gatalica Z. Malignant peripheral nerve sheath tumor with rhabdomyoblastic differentiation (malignant triton tumor) with balanced t(7;9)(q11.2;p24) and unbalanced translocation der(16)t(1;16)(q23;q13). Cancer Genet Cytogenet. 149(1):23-7, 2004

14. Hochman MG, Zilberfarb JL. Nerves in a pinch: imaging of nerve compression syndromes. Radiol Clin North Am. 42(1):221-45, 2004

15. Beaulieu S, Rubin B, Djang D, Conrad E, Turcotte E, Eary JF. Positron emission tomography of schwannomas: emphasizing its potential in preoperative planning. AJR Am J Roentgenol. 182(4):971-4, 2004

16. Huang JH, Zaghloul K, Zager EL. Surgical management of brachial plexus region tumors. Surg Neurol. 61(4):372-8, 2004

17. Arun D, Gutmann DH. Recent advances in neurofibromatosis type 1. Curr Opin Neurol. 17(2):101-5, 2004

18. Mohan H, Nada R, Tahlan A, Punia RS, Mukherjee KK. Peripheral nerve sheath tumours--a short series with some uncommon variants. Indian J Pathol Microbiol. 46(2):204-6, 2003

19. Weiss SW, Goldblum JR: Soft Tissue Tumors. 4th ed. St Louis, Mosby. 1111-1263, 2001

IMAGE GALLERY

Typical

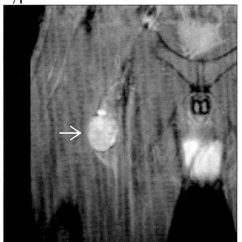
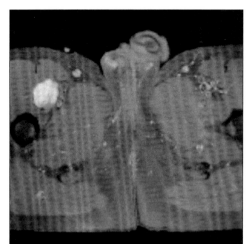

(Left) Coronal STIR MR shows MPNST (arrow) of thigh. Mass is heterogeneous in signal intensity. Appearance is nonspecific, and location adjacent to vessels is best clue to diagnosis. *(Right)* Axial T1 C+ MR shows avid enhancement of MPNST arising in superficial femoral n.

Typical

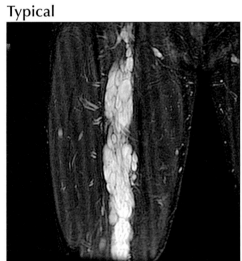
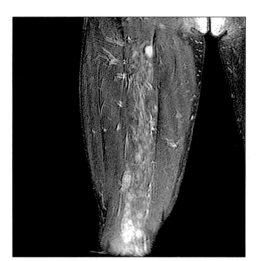

(Left) Coronal STIR MR shows neurofibromatosis of sciatic nerve, forming a multilobulated cascade of oval, heterogeneous signal intensity masses. *(Right)* Coronal T1 C+ MR shows neurofibromatosis diffusely affecting sciatic n. Tumors show variable enhancement pattern.

Variant

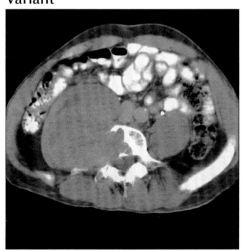
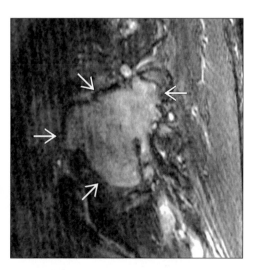

(Left) Axial CECT shows neurofibroma centered in right L4 neural foramen, extending into abdomen, and eroding bone. Patient had vague pain for 14 years before undergoing radiography, which showed mass. *(Right)* Sagittal T2WI MR through lumbar vertebral body and pedicle shows heterogeneous signal intensity in neurofibroma (arrows) causing unusually extensive bone erosion of 2 adjacent spinal levels.

PERIPHERAL NEUROLYMPHOMATOSIS

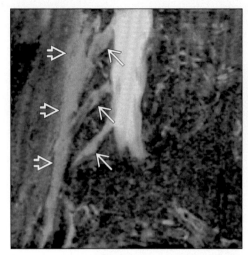

Coronal STIR MR shows L2-L4 dorsal root ganglia enlargement (arrows) & abnormal thickening & hyperintensity of the right lumbar plexus (open arrows).

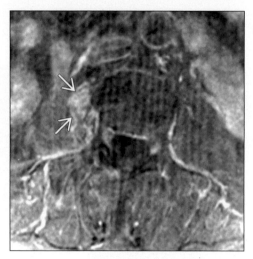

Axial T1 C+ MR in neurolymphomatosis reveals thickening & abnormal enhancement of infiltrated right lumbar plexus (arrows).

TERMINOLOGY

Abbreviations and Synonyms
- Synonyms: Peripheral neurolymphomatosis (NL), Perineural lymphomatosis

Definitions
- Perineural plexus or peripheral nerve lymphomatous infiltration

IMAGING FINDINGS

General Features
- Best diagnostic clue: Diffusely infiltrating plexus or peripheral nerve lesion in patient with lymphoma
- Location: Plexus or peripheral nerve
- Morphology
  - Abnormal plexus/nerve thickening
  - Disruption/distortion of normal fascicular morphology

Radiographic Findings
- Radiography: Usually normal unless bone metastases

CT Findings
- CECT: Often normal; abnormal cases show fusiform or nodular thickening + variable enhancement

MR Findings
- T1WI: Hypo- to isointense nerve/plexus thickening
- T2WI: Abnormal nerve T2 hyperintensity, disruption/distortion of normal fascicular morphology
- STIR: Abnormal nerve T2 hyperintensity, disruption/distortion of normal fascicular morphology
- T1 C+: Variable enhancement

Imaging Recommendations
- Best imaging tool: MR imaging
- Protocol advice: Multiplanar high-resolution MRI (T1WI, fat-saturated T2WI or STIR, fat-saturated T1 C+)

DIFFERENTIAL DIAGNOSIS

Peripheral nerve metastasis
- Usually more focal; signal intensity mimics primary nerve tumor
- Clinical history of known malignancy makes diagnosis

CIDP
- Fusiform nerve/plexus thickening
- Often bilateral, symmetric
- Clinical, history, and laboratory findings distinguish

Hypertrophic neuropathy
- Fusiform nerve/plexus thickening

DDx: Neurolymphomatosis

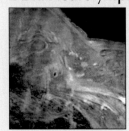

Lung Cancer Metastasis

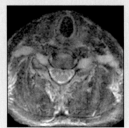

CIDP

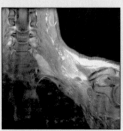

Hyp. Neuropathy

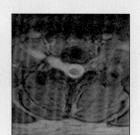

BP Stretch Injury

Key Facts

Terminology
- Synonyms: Peripheral neurolymphomatosis (NL), Perineural lymphomatosis

Imaging Findings
- Abnormal plexus/nerve thickening

Top Differential Diagnoses
- Peripheral nerve metastasis

- CIDP
- Hypertrophic neuropathy
- Nerve/plexus stretch injury

Clinical Issues
- Progressive sensorimotor neuropathy +/- plexopathy

Diagnostic Checklist
- Often subtle; carefully scrutinize clinically abnormal nerves and plexi for thickening, abnormal T2 signal

---

- Often bilateral, symmetric
- Clinical, history, and laboratory findings distinguish

Nerve/plexus stretch injury
- Most commonly brachial plexus; often asymmetric
- Clinical findings, history, soft tissue injury imaging features assure diagnosis

PATHOLOGY

General Features
- General path comments
  - Careful evaluation of NL patients usually reveals subclinical systemic lymphoma
  - Confirmed by histopathogical examination ⇒ lymphomatous infiltration
- Etiology: Isolated disease entity or in association with systemic or primary CNS lymphoma
- Epidemiology
  - More common than generally appreciated
  - Autopsy study showed NL ≈ 40% lymphoma patients

Gross Pathologic & Surgical Features
- Perineural lymphomatous nerve infiltration ⇒ thickened neural elements

Microscopic Features
- Perineural lymphomatosis infiltration ("small blue cell tumor")

CLINICAL ISSUES

Presentation
- Most common signs/symptoms: Pain +/- motor weakness, sensory deficit
- Clinical profile
  - Progressive sensorimotor neuropathy +/- plexopathy
  - Laboratory abnormalities
    - Electrodiagnostic studies: Plexopathy/neuropathy +/- superimposed axonal peripheral neuropathy
    - CSF studies: +/- Elevated protein, malignant cells

Demographics
- Age: Adults
- Gender: M = F

Natural History & Prognosis
- Relentlessly progressive; +/- response to chemotherapy, radiotherapy

Treatment
- Biopsy to establish diagnosis (if findings of systemic lymphoma lacking)
- Chemotherapy, external beam radiation

DIAGNOSTIC CHECKLIST

Consider
- Careful evaluation of NL patients often reveals evidence for subclinical systemic lymphoma

Image Interpretation Pearls
- Often subtle; carefully scrutinize clinically abnormal nerves and plexi for thickening, abnormal T2 signal

SELECTED REFERENCES

1. Moore K et al: The value of MR neurography for evaluating extraspinal neuropathic leg pain: a pictorial essay. AJNR Am J Neuroradiol. 22:786-794, 2001
2. Diaz-Arrastia R et al: Neurolymphomatosis: a clinicopathologic syndrome re-emerges. Neurology. 42:1136-1141, 1992
3. Krendel D et al: Lymphomatous polyneuropathy. Biopsy of clinical involved nerves and successful treatment. Arch Neurol. 48:330-332, 1991
4. Jellinger K et al: Involvement of the central nervous system in malignant lymphomas. VIrchows Arch. 370:345-362, 1976

IMAGE GALLERY

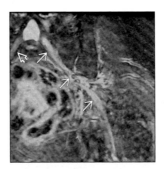 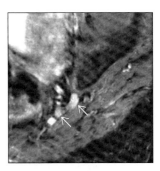

(Left) Coronal STIR MR demonstrates left S1 nerve thickening and abnormal hyperintensity extending into proximal sciatic nerve (arrows). Right S1 root (open arrow) is normal. (Right) Sagittal Oblique T1 C+ MR with fat-saturation shows abnormal sciatic nerve enlargement & enhancement (arrows).

RADIAL NEUROPATHY

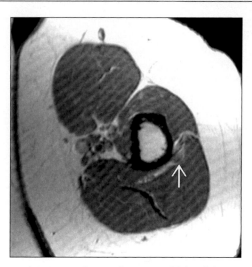

Axial T1WI MR shows enlargement of left radial nerve (arrow) as it crosses humeral spiral groove in Parkinson patient who awoke with radial nerve deficit.

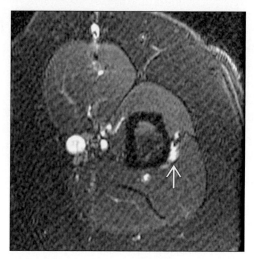

Axial STIR MR shows enlargement, marked T2 hyperintensity of left radial nerve (arrow) as it crosses humeral spiral groove. Abnormal signal intensity equals that of regional vessels.

TERMINOLOGY

Abbreviations and Synonyms
• Radial neuropathy (RN), radial nerve entrapment, posterior interosseous nerve (PIN) syndrome

Definitions
• Radial nerve injury at one of several characteristic locations along nerve course

IMAGING FINDINGS

General Features
• Best diagnostic clue: Focal radial nerve enlargement, abnormal T2 hyperintensity
• Location
  ○ Radial nerve may be injured proximally (brachial plexus) → distally (posterior interosseous, radial sensory nerves)
  ○ Most commonly entrapped at mid humeral shaft or fibrous arch of Frohse above elbow
• Size: Affected nerve, muscles range from acutely enlarged → chronically atrophic

MR Findings
• T1WI: +/- Isointense (to muscle) nerve enlargement, fatty muscle atrophy

• T2WI: +/- Hyperintense nerve enlargement, acute or chronic muscle denervation changes
• STIR: Similar to fat-saturated T2WI
• T1 C+: +/- Enhancement

Other Modality Findings
• Electromyography (EMG): Helps localizes likely level of nerve injury

Imaging Recommendations
• Best imaging tool: MR imaging
• Protocol advice: Axial T1WI, fat-saturated T2WI or STIR, T1 C+ MR

DIFFERENTIAL DIAGNOSIS

Median neuropathy
• Anterior interosseous nerve (AIN) syndrome (clinically distinctive from PIN syndrome)

Ulnar neuropathy
• Symptoms referable to medial elbow (cubital tunnel) +/- anconeus epitrochlearis

Lateral epicondylitis
• Tenderness over lateral epicondyle; clinically distinctive from neuropathy

DDx: Radial Nerve Palsy

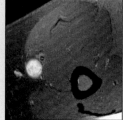 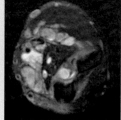 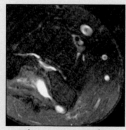 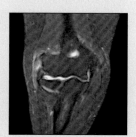

Schwannoma   *Plexiform NF*   *Ulnar Neuropathy*   *Lat. Epicondylitis*

RADIAL NEUROPATHY

Key Facts

Terminology
- Radial neuropathy (RN), radial nerve entrapment, posterior interosseous nerve (PIN) syndrome

Imaging Findings
- Best diagnostic clue: Focal radial nerve enlargement, abnormal T2 hyperintensity
- Most commonly entrapped at mid humeral shaft or fibrous arch of Frohse above elbow

Top Differential Diagnoses
- Median neuropathy
- Ulnar neuropathy
- Lateral epicondylitis

Diagnostic Checklist
- Radial nerve palsy is common complication of humeral fracture

---

PATHOLOGY

General Features
- General path comments
  - Most common compression locations at spiral groove, arcade of Frohse (PIN syndrome)
  - Severity ranges neuropraxia → axonotmesis → neurotmesis (least → most severe)
- Etiology: Compression, entrapment, inflammatory or neoplastic infiltration
- Epidemiology: Rare
- Associated abnormalities
  - Fracture-dislocation of humeral shaft (Holstein-Lewis fracture)
  - Forearm fracture (especially Monteggia fracture)

Gross Pathologic & Surgical Features
- Swollen nerve +/- fibrous scarring, muscle denervation

Microscopic Features
- Histologic examination of resected nerve shows concentration of inflammatory cells around vessels in perineurium
- Nerve edema (acute), axonal loss (chronic)

CLINICAL ISSUES

Presentation
- Most common signs/symptoms: Supracondylar humeral fracture, extensor muscle weakness, pain
- Clinical profile
  - Axillary compression (crutch misuse, poor arm position during drunken sleep) → weakness of triceps, distal muscles innervated by radial nerve
  - Mid-arm compression ("Saturday night palsy") ⇒ compression in humeral spiral groove, humeral fracture, poor positioning during drunken sleep, general anesthesia mishap
  - PIN syndrome: Rheumatoid arthritis, entrapment, total elbow arthroplasty
  - Supinator entrapment: Radial nerve entrapment following forced supination, "tennis elbow"

Demographics
- Age: Children → adults
- Gender: M > F

Natural History & Prognosis
- Occasionally resolves spontaneously with conservative management
- Usually progressive, requires surgical decompression
  - Prognosis after surgery inversely proportional to symptom duration
  - Best prognosis when recovery starts < 6 months

Treatment
- Decompression, division of fibrous bands +/- neurolysis, nerve graft

---

DIAGNOSTIC CHECKLIST

Consider
- Radial nerve palsy is common complication of humeral fracture
- Late, chronic presentations often require surgery

Image Interpretation Pearls
- Recognition of muscle denervation in radial nerve distribution may enable diagnosis without identifying nerve imaging abnormality

---

SELECTED REFERENCES

1. Gosens T et al: Neurovascular complications and functional outcome in displaced supracondylar fractures of the humerus in children. Injury. 34(4):267-73, 2003
2. Spinner RJ et al: The origin of "Saturday night palsy"? Neurosurgery. 51(3):737-41; discussion 741, 2002
3. Lowe JB 3rd et al: Current approach to radial nerve paralysis. Plast Reconstr Surg. 110(4):1099-113, 2002

IMAGE GALLERY

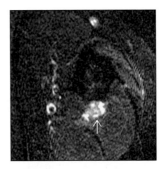 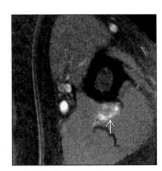

(Left) Axial STIR MR in a peripheral neurolymphomatosis patient shows radial nerve enlargement, abnormal T2 hyperintensity at spiral groove (arrow). *(Right)* Axial T1 C+ MR shows radial nerve enlargement & heterogeneous enhancement (arrow) secondary to lymphomatous infiltration.

FEMORAL NEUROPATHY

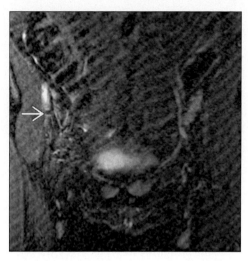

Coronal STIR MR shows a hyperintense enlarged femoral nerve at right femoral canal. Symptoms arose following inguinal herniorrhaphy, and exploration revealed suture (arrow) around nerve.

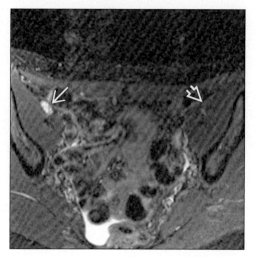

Axial STIR MR shows marked right femoral nerve enlargement, fascicular hyperintensity within iliopsoas groove (arrow). Normal left femoral nerve indicated by open arrow.

TERMINOLOGY

Abbreviations and Synonyms
- Synonyms: Femoral neuropathy, femoral mononeuropathy, femoral nerve (FN) palsy

Definitions
- Femoral nerve (FN) entrapment or injury 2° to direct trauma, compression, stretch injury, or ischemia

IMAGING FINDINGS

General Features
- Best diagnostic clue: Femoral nerve enlargement, abnormal T2 hyperintensity
- Location: Injury most common in psoas muscle body, iliopsoas groove, or femoral canal
- Morphology: Nerve enlargement +/- loss of internal fascicular architecture, abnormal T2 hyperintensity

CT Findings
- CECT: +/- Retroperitoneal/psoas mass, hematoma, lymphadenopathy

MR Findings
- T1WI
  - Iso → hypointense nerve enlargement +/- retroperitoneal/psoas mass

  - +/- Hyperintense quadriceps muscle fatty atrophy (chronic denervation)
- T2WI
  - Hyperintense nerve (+/- fascicular) enlargement
  - +/- Abnormal quadriceps muscle T2 hyperintensity (acute/ongoing denervation)
- STIR: Similar to fat-saturated T2WI
- T1 C+: +/- Enhancement (if neoplastic/inflammatory component)

Other Modality Findings
- Electromyography (EMG): Denervation of anterior thigh muscles

Imaging Recommendations
- Best imaging tool: High-resolution MR imaging
- Protocol advice: Axial T1WI, fat-saturated T2WI or STIR MR, fat-saturated T1 C+ MR

DIFFERENTIAL DIAGNOSIS

Neoplastic femoral nerve infiltration
- Neurolymphomatosis, systemic metastasis, local regional tumor extension

Nerve sheath tumor
- Solitary/plexiform neurofibroma (NF1), schwannoma
- Neural mass + variable tumoral enhancement

DDx: Femoral Neuropathy

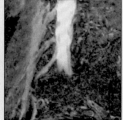

Neurolymphomatosis

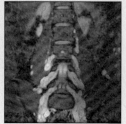

Plexiform NF

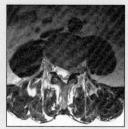

Far Lateral HNP

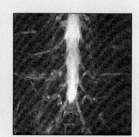

Rt. L4 Radiculopathy

Key Facts

Terminology
- Synonyms: Femoral neuropathy, femoral mononeuropathy, femoral nerve (FN) palsy
- Femoral nerve (FN) entrapment or injury 2° to direct trauma, compression, stretch injury, or ischemia

Imaging Findings
- Best diagnostic clue: Femoral nerve enlargement, abnormal T2 hyperintensity

Top Differential Diagnoses
- Neoplastic femoral nerve infiltration
- Nerve sheath tumor
- Lumbosacral disk syndromes
- Lumbar plexopathy

Diagnostic Checklist
- Look carefully for lesion or hematoma in iliopsoas groove or femoral canal

---

Lumbosacral disk syndromes
- Disc herniation compresses L2, L3, or L4 root
- EMG → radiculopathy, not mononeuropathy

Lumbar plexopathy
- Diabetic, ischemic, traumatic, neoplastic etiologies
- EMG → plexopathy

PATHOLOGY

General Features
- General path comments
  - FN arises from L2–L4 ventral rami, descends in iliopsoas groove, exits pelvis below inguinal ligament
  - Innervates iliacus, sartorius & quadriceps muscles
- Etiology: Reported causes include self-retaining retractor, thigh tourniquet, heparin anticoagulation (retroperitoneal hematoma), obstetrical complication, diabetic neuropathy
- Epidemiology: Uncommon

CLINICAL ISSUES

Presentation
- Most common signs/symptoms
  - Acute symptom onset, pain/weakness in FN distribution, diminished/absent knee jerk reflex, thigh muscle atrophy
  - Severe back/groin pain (retroperitoneal hematoma)

Demographics
- Age: All ages
- Gender: M = F

Natural History & Prognosis
- Recovery is rule over few days → months in most cases

Treatment
- Physical therapy, avoidance of excessive hip abduction/external rotation, knee bracing, treatment of causative mass lesions

DIAGNOSTIC CHECKLIST

Consider
- Femoral neuropathy is uncommon

Image Interpretation Pearls
- Look carefully for lesion or hematoma in iliopsoas groove or femoral canal

SELECTED REFERENCES

1. Kornbluth ID et al: Femoral, saphenous nerve palsy after tourniquet use: a case report. Arch Phys Med Rehabil. 84(6):909-11, 2003
2. Seijo-Martinez M et al: Acute femoral neuropathy secondary to an iliacus muscle hematoma. J Neurol Sci. 209(1-2):119-22, 2003
3. Nogues MA et al: Unilateral femoral neuropathy. Muscle Nerve. 21(1):126-7, 1998
4. Kuntzer et al: Clinical and prognostic features in unilateral femoral neuropathies. Muscle Nerve. 20, 205–211, 1997
5. Brasch RC et al: Femoral neuropathy secondary to the use of a self-retaining retractor. Report of three cases and review of the literature. Dis Colon Rectum. 38(10):1115-8, 1995
6. Kent KC et al: Retroperitoneal hematoma after cardiac catheterization: prevalence, risk factors, and optimal management. J Vasc Surg. 20(6):905-10; discussion 910-3, 1994

IMAGE GALLERY

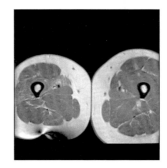 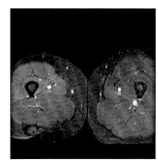

(Left) Axial T1WI MR of both legs in femoral neuropathy patient shows marked volume loss and fatty replacement of right quadriceps muscles (chronic denervation). (Right) Axial STIR MR in femoral neuropathy patient shows marked right quadriceps muscle volume loss, T2 hyperintensity indicating component of acute (ongoing) denervation on top of chronic denervation.

ULNAR NEUROPATHY

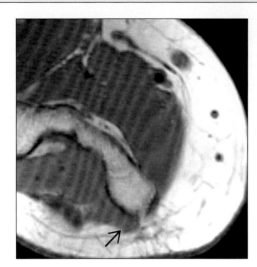

Axial T1WI MR in patient with clinically symptomatic ulnar neuropathy shows focal enlargement of ulnar nerve (arrow) within cubital tunnel.

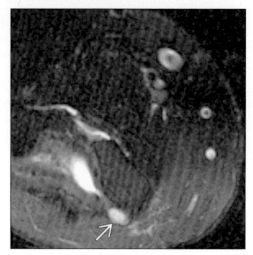

Axial T2WI MR with fat-saturation of ulnar nerve at medial epicondyle (arrow) shows focal enlargement, T2 hyperintensity, loss of internal architecture (axonotmesis).

TERMINOLOGY

Abbreviations and Synonyms
- Synonyms: Ulnar nerve entrapment, cubital tunnel syndrome

Definitions
- Partial fixation, compression, or distortion of ulnar nerve (UN)
  - Most commonly occurs within cubital tunnel at elbow; uncommon within Guyon tunnel at wrist, or 2° to brachial plexus inflammation

IMAGING FINDINGS

General Features
- Best diagnostic clue: UN enlargement +/- T2 hyperintensity at cubital or Guyon tunnel in symptomatic patient
- Location: Most common at elbow near medial epicondyle (cubital tunnel), less common at ulnar wrist (Guyon tunnel)
- Size: Usually enlarged 1.5-2x, with change from mildly flattened → rounded

- Morphology: Nerve swelling +/- enlarged hyperintense fascicles (neuropraxic injury), axonal injury with loss of internal architecture (axonotmesis), or complete anatomic/functional transection (neurotmesis)

CT Findings
- NECT
  - Acute: +/- Soft tissue nerve mass, anconeus epitrochlearis
  - Chronic: Fatty atrophy of affected muscles (volume loss, hypodense fat infiltration)
- CECT: +/- UN enhancement

MR Findings
- T1WI
  - UN thickening +/- architectural distortion
  - Thickened cubital tunnel retinaculum
- T2WI
  - UN enlargement, abnormal T2 hyperintensity
  - Loss of internal UN architecture in more severe cases
- STIR: Similar to fat-saturated T2WI
- T1 C+: +/- UN enhancement (focal fascicles or diffusely)

Ultrasonographic Findings
- Real Time: Enlarged UN +/- loss of reticular fascicular pattern (round hypoechoic areas surrounded by hyperechoic lines)

DDx: Ulnar Neuropathy

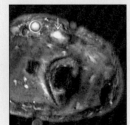
UN Transection

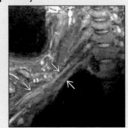
Brachial Plexitis

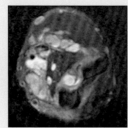
Plexiform NF

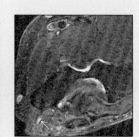
Perineural Vein

Key Facts

Terminology
- Synonyms: Ulnar nerve entrapment, cubital tunnel syndrome
- Partial fixation, compression, or distortion of ulnar nerve (UN)

Imaging Findings
- Best diagnostic clue: UN enlargement +/- T2 hyperintensity at cubital or Guyon tunnel in symptomatic patient

Top Differential Diagnoses
- Acute direct nerve trauma
- Idiopathic brachial plexitis (Parsonage-Turner syndrome)
- Nerve sheath tumor
- Enlarged perineural vein
- Medial epicondylitis

Pathology
- Edematous/indurated UN +/- thickened retinaculum, fibrous stranding
- +/- Anconeus epitrochlearis, enlarged medial triceps head

Clinical Issues
- Pain, paresthesias in ulnar nerve distribution

Diagnostic Checklist
- MR imaging is more sensitive for acute than chronic neuropraxia
- Focal ulnar nerve enlargement, abnormal T2 hyperintensity at retinaculum just distal to medial epicondyle diagnostic for UN neuropathy

Other Modality Findings
- Electromyography (EMG): Helps localizes most likely level of nerve injury

Imaging Recommendations
- Best imaging tool: High-resolution MR peripheral nerve imaging (MR neurography)
- Protocol advice: Axial T1WI, fat-saturated T2WI, and STIR imaging using surface coil

DIFFERENTIAL DIAGNOSIS

Acute direct nerve trauma
- Appropriate history, traumatic soft tissue findings

Idiopathic brachial plexitis (Parsonage-Turner syndrome)
- BP inflammation, multiple nerve/muscle denervation patterns
- +/- Viral prodrome: Pain → weakness

Nerve sheath tumor
- Focal nerve enlargement, displacement/obliteration of internal fascicle architecture
- Tumoral enhancement, T2/STIR hyperintensity

Enlarged perineural vein
- Mimics enlarged UN
- Flow void, contrast-enhancement similar to other veins

Medial epicondylitis
- "Thrower's, golfer's elbow"
- Chronic valgus stress → +/- MCL tear, hyperintensity within flexor pronatus muscle belly

PATHOLOGY

General Features
- General path comments
  - Important normal anatomy
    - UN lies in anterior proximal arm compartment along intermuscular septum
    - Enters posterior compartment at mid-humerus, piercing arcade of Struthers
    - Passes distally through posterior/medial intermuscular septum → cubital tunnel
    - Distal to cubital tunnel, UN passes between two heads of flexor carpi ulnaris (FCU) muscle (most frequent compression site)
  - Cause of abnormal high signal on T2WI/ STIR sequences not definitively known
    - Speculated that axoplasmic flow alterations or edema from increased endoneurial fluid 2° to disordered endoneurial fluid flow, local venous obstruction → T2 hyperintensity
- Etiology
  - Intermuscular septum (arcade of Struthers) → compression 2° to musculofascial band 5-8 cm proximal to medial epicondyle
  - Thickened cubital tunnel retinaculum → entrapment with dynamic elbow flexion
  - Congenitally shallow groove, absent/dysfunctional retinaculum
  - Repeated valgus stress → medial epicondylitis (throwing athletes)
  - Malunion, callus around condylar fracture
  - Fascial compression at FCU heads
- Epidemiology
  - Second most common upper extremity entrapment syndrome (after carpal tunnel syndrome)
    - Up to 22% of U.S. population may have chronic compression during flexion 2° thickened retinaculum
    - 10% static compression in association with anconeus epitrochlearis muscle
- Associated abnormalities
  - Anconeus epitrochlearis muscle
  - Enlarged medial triceps head
  - +/- Medial elbow osteophyte, condylar osseous abnormality

ULNAR NEUROPATHY

Gross Pathologic & Surgical Features
- Edematous/indurated UN +/- thickened retinaculum, fibrous stranding
- +/- Anconeus epitrochlearis, enlarged medial triceps head

Microscopic Features
- Nerve edema +/- inflammatory cells, fibrous infiltration, fascicular atrophy/loss

Staging, Grading or Classification Criteria
- Three severities of nerve injury
  - Neuropraxic injury (mildest)
    - Focal myelin sheath damage without axonal disruption
    - Contiguous swollen/T2 hyperintense nerve fascicles
  - Axonotmetic injury (intermediate)
    - Axon/myelin sheath disruption; subsequent Wallerian degeneration leaves Schwann cells and endoneurium intact
    - Homogeneously increased T2 signal intensity, loss of fascicular architecture at injury site
  - Neurotmetic injury (most severe)
    - Functional +/- anatomical transection
    - Axon, myelin sheath disruption with discontinuity of some/all of surrounding connective tissues → Wallerian degeneration, regeneration failure
    - Cannot always distinguish from axonotmesis

CLINICAL ISSUES

Presentation
- Most common signs/symptoms
  - Range of symptoms; mild transient paresthesias of 4th and fifth digits → claw hand/digits, intrinsic muscle atrophy
  - +/- Severe elbow/wrist pain radiating proximally or distally
- Clinical profile
  - Pain, paresthesias in ulnar nerve distribution
  - Throwing athletes with elbow pain of medial epicondylitis + paresthesias

Demographics
- Age: Adults > children
- Gender: M ≤ F

Natural History & Prognosis
- Rest, avoidance of provocative activities may produce remission in mild cases
- More severe cases show variable response to surgical decompression
  - Chronic pain, muscle weakness, atrophy portend worse prognosis

Treatment
- Conservative: Physical therapy, avoidance of provocative maneuvers
- Surgical: Osteophyte or anconeus resection, decompression +/- nerve transposition
  - In situ decompression brings rapid relief, but transposition may bring longer symptom remission

DIAGNOSTIC CHECKLIST

Consider
- MR imaging is more sensitive for acute than chronic neuropraxia
- Search for anatomic abnormalities (enlarged medial head of triceps, anconeus muscle, osteophyte, thickened retinaculum)

Image Interpretation Pearls
- Focal ulnar nerve enlargement, abnormal T2 hyperintensity at retinaculum just distal to medial epicondyle diagnostic for UN neuropathy

SELECTED REFERENCES
1. Matsuzaki H et al: Long-term clinical and neurologic recovery in the hand after surgery for severe cubital tunnel syndrome. J Hand Surg [Am]. 29(3):373-8, 2004
2. Hochman MG et al: Nerves in a pinch: imaging of nerve compression syndromes. Radiol Clin North Am. 42(1):221-45, 2004
3. Park GY et al: The ultrasonographic and electrodiagnostic findings of ulnar neuropathy at the elbow. Arch Phys Med Rehabil. 85(6):1000-5, 2004
4. Thornton R et al: Magnetic resonance imaging of sports injuries of the elbow. Top Magn Reson Imaging. 14(1):69-86, 2003
5. Kim DH et al: Surgical outcomes of 654 ulnar nerve lesions. J Neurosurg. 98(5):993-1004, 2003
6. Murata K et al: Causes of ulnar tunnel syndrome: a retrospective study of 31 subjects. J Hand Surg [Am]. 28(4):647-51, 2003
7. Dellon AL et al: Results of the musculofascial lengthening technique for submuscular transposition of the ulnar nerve at the elbow. J Bone Joint Surg Am. 85-A(7):1314-20, 2003
8. Matev B: Cubital tunnel syndrome. Hand Surg. 8(1):127-31, 2003
9. Kato H et al: Cubital tunnel syndrome associated with medial elbow Ganglia and osteoarthritis of the elbow. J Bone Joint Surg Am. 84-A(8):1413-9, 2002
10. Chung CB et al: Magnetic resonance imaging of the upper extremity: advances in technique and application. Clin Orthop. (383):162-74, 2001
11. Arle JE et al: Surgical treatment of common entrapment neuropathies in the upper limbs. Muscle Nerve. 23(8):1160-74, 2000
12. Martinoli C et al: US of nerve entrapments in osteofibrous tunnels of the upper and lower limbs. Radiographics. 20 Spec No:S199-213; discussion S213-7, 2000
13. Ruocco MJ et al: MR imaging of ulnar nerve entrapment secondary to an anomalous wrist muscle. Skeletal Radiol. 27(4):218-21, 1998
14. Chiou HJ et al: Cubital tunnel syndrome: diagnosis by high-resolution ultrasonography. J Ultrasound Med. 17(10):643-8, 1998
15. Britz GW et al: Ulnar nerve entrapment at the elbow: correlation of magnetic resonance imaging, clinical, electrodiagnostic, and intraoperative findings. Neurosurgery. 38(3):458-65; discussion 465, 1996
16. Zeiss J et al: The ulnar tunnel at the wrist (Guyon's canal): normal MR anatomy and variants. AJR Am J Roentgenol. 158(5):1081-5, 1992

ULNAR NEUROPATHY

IMAGE GALLERY

Typical

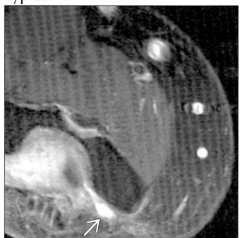
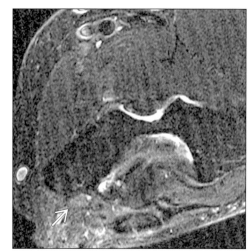

(Left) Axial T1 C+ MR with fat-saturation depicts uniform enhancement of left ulnar nerve (arrow) at elbow with loss of internal architecture (axonotmesis). *(Right)* Axial STIR MR shows normal appearance of ulnar nerve (arrow) despite chronic clinical symptoms.

Variant

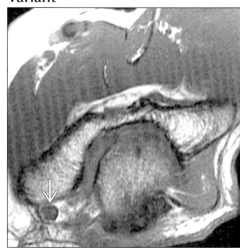
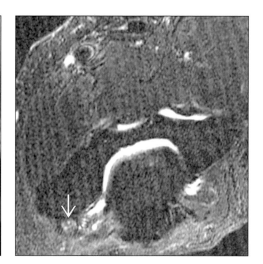

(Left) Axial T1WI MR shows mild abnormal UN rounding (arrow) with associated perineural inflammatory changes of subcutaneous fat (mild neuropraxic injury). *(Right)* Axial STIR MR shows rounding of UN at elbow (arrow) with mild hyperintensity of several fascicles (mild neuropraxic injury).

Variant

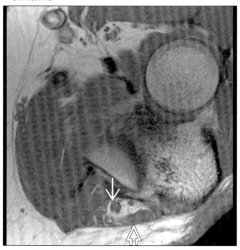
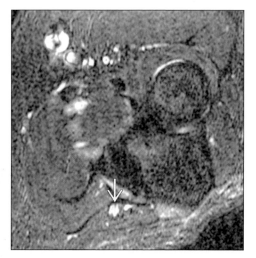

(Left) Axial T1WI MR distal to medial epicondyle shows focal UN rounding (arrow) and anconeus epitrochlearis muscle (open arrow) covering cubital tunnel. *(Right)* Axial STIR MR distal to medial epicondyle shows focal ulnar nerve rounding (arrow) & mild fascicular hyperintensity (neuropraxic injury).

SUPRASCAPULAR NERVE ENTRAPMENT

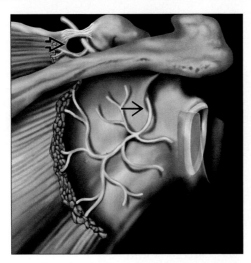

Coronal graphic shows suprascapular nerve coursing through suprascapular notch (open arrow) & spinoglenoid notch (arrow).

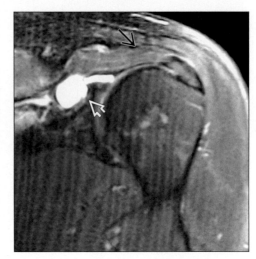

Coronal T2WI MR shows cyst extending from torn labrum into spinoglenoid notch (open arrow). Increased signal intensity in infraspinatus muscle (arrow) reflects denervation.

TERMINOLOGY

Abbreviations and Synonyms
- Spinoglenoid or suprascapular notch impingement

Definitions
- Suprascapular nerve: Motor nerve to supraspinatus and infraspinatus muscles (mm.)
- Impingement may occur at either spinoglenoid or suprascapular notch
- Spinoglenoid notch: At superior border of scapula, roofed by superior transverse ligament
- Suprascapular notch: Between neck and blade of scapula, roofed by spinoglenoid ligament

IMAGING FINDINGS

General Features
- Best diagnostic clue: Mass compressing nerve, and abnormal signal in innervated mm.
- Location
  - Occurs at suprascapular or spinoglenoid notch
    - Suprascapular notch: Entrapment affects both supraspinatus and infraspinatus mm.
    - Spinoglenoid notch: Entrapment affects infraspinatus mm. only

MR Findings
- T1WI
  - Low signal intensity mass or venous varicosities in suprascapular or spinoglenoid notch
  - Fatty atrophy in affected mm. if chronic
- T2WI
  - High signal intensity mass in suprascapular or spinoglenoid notch
  - Diffusely increased signal intensity (< fluid) in affected mm.
  - Posterosuperior labral tear
- STIR: Similar to T2WI
- T1 C+
  - May see rim enhancement around cyst
  - Venous varicosities, soft tissue masses enhance
- Venous varicosities
  - Serpentine, tubular structures, connect to draining vein

Other Modality Findings
- Electrodiagnosis standard in diagnosis

Imaging Recommendations
- Best imaging tool: MRI
- Protocol advice: Routine shoulder MRI, field of view to include spinoglenoid notch

DDx: Shoulder Girdle Weakness and Pain

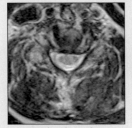

Radiculopathy

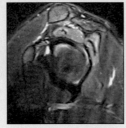

Parsonage-Turner

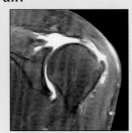

Rotator cuff tear

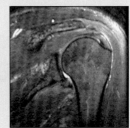

Tendinopathy

Key Facts

Imaging Findings
- Best diagnostic clue: Mass compressing nerve, and abnormal signal in innervated mm.
- Occurs at suprascapular or spinoglenoid notch

Top Differential Diagnoses
- Cervical radiculopathy
- Parsonage-Turner syndrome (brachial neuritis)
- Rotator cuff tear
- Rotator cuff tendinopathy

Pathology
- Paralabral cyst due to tear of posterosuperior glenoid labrum
- Venous varicosities
- Tumor compressing nerve

DIFFERENTIAL DIAGNOSIS

Cervical radiculopathy
- Disc protrusion, osteophytes

Parsonage-Turner syndrome (brachial neuritis)
- Increased signal in mm. on T2WI or STIR
- MM. atrophy on T1WI in chronic cases
- Muscles involved are variable

Rotator cuff tear
- Fluid signal in tendon defect
- MM. atrophy with chronic tear

Rotator cuff tendinopathy
- Increased signal < fluid in tendon on T2WI, STIR
- Abnormalities centered on tendon, not muscle belly

PATHOLOGY

General Features
- General path comments
  - Suprascapular nerve: C5 and C6 nerve roots
    - Through suprascapular notch
    - Innervates supraspinatus mm., extends deep to mm.
    - Through spinoglenoid notch
    - Innervates infraspinatus mm.
- Etiology
  - Paralabral cyst due to tear of posterosuperior glenoid labrum
  - Venous varicosities
  - Tumor compressing nerve
- Epidemiology: Overhead athletes

Gross Pathologic & Surgical Features
- Cyst often entered at arthroscopy via torn labrum
- Open surgery: Tense, slightly blue cyst visible
- Nerve: Normal, or may show attenuation or enlargement

Microscopic Features
- Cyst thin-walled; may be septated

CLINICAL ISSUES

Presentation
- Most common signs/symptoms: Weakness, pain

Demographics
- Age: Young or middle-aged patients
- Gender: M > F

Natural History & Prognosis
- Atrophy of mm. tends to progress without treatment
- Cysts may recur if labral tear not treated

Treatment
- Arthroscopic debridement of labral tear
- Open surgery for other masses

DIAGNOSTIC CHECKLIST

Image Interpretation Pearls
- Compare SI of rotator cuff mm. on sagittal T2WI

SELECTED REFERENCES

1. Carroll KW et al: Enlarged spinoglenoid notch veins causing suprascapular nerve compression. Skeletal Radiol. 32(2):72-7, 2003
2. Tung GA et al: MR imaging and MR arthrography of paraglenoid labral cysts. AJR Am J Roentgenol. 174(6):1707-15, 2000
3. Fabre T et al: Entrapment of the suprascapular nerve. J Bone Joint Surg Br. 81(3):414-9, 1999
4. Zehetgruber H et al: Suprascapular nerve entrapment. A meta-analysis. Int Orthop. 26(6):339-43, 2002;26(6):339-43.

IMAGE GALLERY

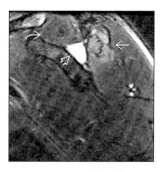 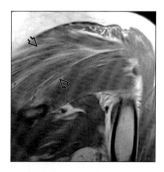

(Left) Sagittal T2WI MR shows cyst in spinoglenoid notch (open arrow) and denervation changes of infraspinatus muscle (arrow). Supraspinatus muscle (curved arrow) is normal signal intensity. *(Right)* Coronal T1WI MR shows infraspinatus muscle atrophy (arrows) due to longstanding impingement.

MEDIAN NERVE ENTRAPMENT

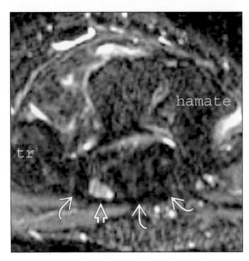 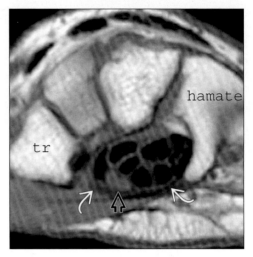

Axial STIR MR shows abnormal signal in median nerve (open arrow) due to infiltration of nerve by sarcoid. Flexor retinaculum (curved arrows) is normal in appearance. Tr = trapezium.

Axial T1WI MR shows mild enlargement of median nerve (open arrow) due to sarcoidosis. Flexor retinaculum (curved arrows) is normal. Tr = trapezium

TERMINOLOGY

Abbreviations and Synonyms
- Carpal tunnel syndrome: Entrapment at carpal tunnel
- Pronator syndrome: Entrapment at pronator teres

Definitions
- Carpal tunnel: Fibro-osseous tunnel at volar aspect of wrist
  - Contains median nerve and flexor tendons
- Tinel sign: Tingling along course of nerve when nerve tapped at point of entrapment

IMAGING FINDINGS

General Features
- Best diagnostic clue: Increased signal in nerve on STIR MRI
- Location: Elbow or wrist

MR Findings
- T1WI
  - Enlargement of nerve distal to region of entrapment
  - Focal flattening, rarely angular deformity of nerve
  - Increased anterior bowing of flexor retinaculum
    - Distance from hook of triquetrum to hook of hamate (TH)
    - Distance from this line to flexor retinaculum (PD = palmar displacement)
    - PD/TH < .15 in normals, .14-.26 in carpal tunnel syndrome
    - Ratio cumbersome, not highly accurate
- T2WI
  - Nerve high signal intensity, nerve fascicles indistinct
  - Increased signal intensity in innervated mm.
- STIR: Similar to T2WI
- T1 C+: Perineural enhancement
- Evaluate for mass causing compression on all sequences

Other Modality Findings
- Electrodiagnosis standard for diagnosis

Imaging Recommendations
- Best imaging tool: MRI
- Protocol advice
  - STIR sequences in long and short axis of nerve
  - T1WI or PDWI in axial plane for definition of anatomy

DIFFERENTIAL DIAGNOSIS

Cervical Radiculopathy
- Nerve impingement on MRI of cervical spine

DDx: Median nerve entrapment

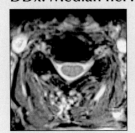 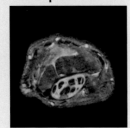 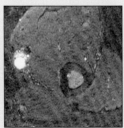 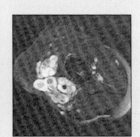

Radiculopathy   *Tenosynovitis*   *Schwannoma*   *Neurofibromatosis*

MEDIAN NERVE ENTRAPMENT

Key Facts

Terminology
- Carpal tunnel syndrome: Entrapment at carpal tunnel
- Pronator syndrome: Entrapment at pronator teres

Imaging Findings
- Best diagnostic clue: Increased signal in nerve on STIR MRI

Top Differential Diagnoses
- Cervical Radiculopathy
- Tenosynovitis
- Peripheral nerve sheath tumor

Clinical Issues
- Numbness, tingling along course of nerve
- Positive Tinel sign

Tenosynovitis
- Pain, muscle weakness
- May occur with or without nerve entrapment

Peripheral nerve sheath tumor
- Focal, globular enlargement of nerve

PATHOLOGY

General Features
- General path comments
  - Course of median nerve at elbow
    - Deep to bicipital aponeurosis, superficial to brachialis m.
    - Passes between ulnar and humeral heads of pronator teres m.
  - Course of median nerve at wrist
    - Superficial and radial aspect of carpal tunnel
- Etiology
  - Overuse
    - Carpal tunnel: Keyboarding, manual labor
    - Pronator: Athletes repeatedly pronating forearm
  - Arthritis
    - Rheumatoid arthritis, amyloid, gout, sarcoidosis
  - Tumors
    - Soft tissue tumor, ganglion cyst, osteochondroma
  - Fractures
    - Supracondylar humerus, distal radius
  - Anatomic variants
    - Muscle anomalies, small carpal tunnel
    - Supracondylar process of humerus

Gross Pathologic & Surgical Features
- Variable appearance of nerve: Normal, flattened or enlarged

Microscopic Features
- Perineural inflammation, +/- nerve ischemia

CLINICAL ISSUES

Presentation
- Most common signs/symptoms
  - Numbness, tingling along course of nerve
  - Positive Tinel sign
  - Tenderness at pronator region or carpal tunnel

Demographics
- Gender: Carpal tunnel: F:M = 3:1

Natural History & Prognosis
- Usually responds to conservative measures

Treatment
- Options, risks, complications
  - Surgery: Open or endoscopic
  - Complications: Reflex sympathetic dystrophy, median nerve injury, incomplete release
  - Conservative: Wrist splint in neutral position, steroid injection

DIAGNOSTIC CHECKLIST

Image Interpretation Pearls
- Nerve normally appears flattened at level of hook of hamate

SELECTED REFERENCES

1. Hochman MG et al: Nerves in a pinch: imaging of nerve compression syndromes. Radiol Clin North Am. 42(1):221-45, 2004
2. Witt JC et al: Neurologic disorders masquerading as carpal tunnel syndrome: 12 cases of failed carpal tunnel release. Mayo Clin Proc. 75(4):409-13, 2000
3. England JD: Entrapment neuropathies. Curr Opin Neurol. 12(5):597-602, 1999

IMAGE GALLERY

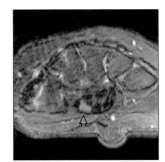 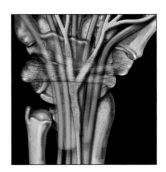

(Left) Axial T2WI MR shows persistent abnormal signal in median nerve (arrow) at level of proximal metacarpals following incomplete carpal tunnel release. *(Right)* Coronal graphic shows fibrous band of flexor retinaculum overlying median nerve (yellow). Nerve is edematous. Flexor tendons covered by tendon sheaths are shown deep to the median nerve.

COMMON PERONEAL NEUROPATHY

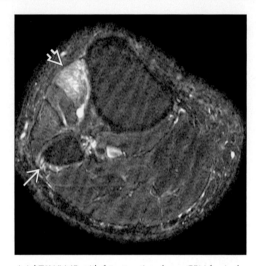

Axial T2WI MR with fat-saturation shows CPN fascicular enlargement, abnormal T2 hyperintensity (arrow) at fibular head & acute anterior compartment muscle denervation (open arrow).

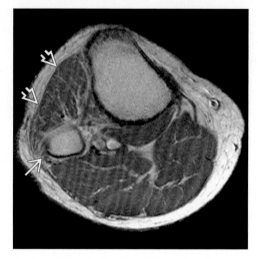

Axial T1WI MR reveals mild CPN fascicular enlargement (arrow) + anterior compartment muscle volume loss with fatty atrophy (open arrows) representing more chronic denervation change.

TERMINOLOGY

Abbreviations and Synonyms
- Synonyms: Common peroneal nerve (CPN) palsy, CPN entrapment

Definitions
- Common peroneal nerve entrapment at fibular head

IMAGING FINDINGS

General Features
- Best diagnostic clue: CPN enlargement +/- T2 hyperintensity, architectural distortion at fibular head in symptomatic patient
- Location: Knee (fibular head level)
- Morphology: Ranges mild CPN swelling +/- enlarged hyperintense fascicles (neuropraxic injury) → axonal injury, loss of internal architecture (axonotmesis) → complete transection (neurotmesis)

MR Findings
- T1WI: CPN enlargement +/- architectural distortion
- T2WI
  ○ CPN enlargement, abnormal T2 hyperintensity
  ○ Loss of internal architecture (more severe cases)
- STIR: Similar to fat-saturated T2WI
- T1 C+: +/- Mild enhancement of nerve, scar tissue

Other Modality Findings
- Nerve conduction velocity/EMG: Conduction block at fibular head, anterior compartment (tibial anterior, peroneus longus muscles) denervation

Imaging Recommendations
- Best imaging tool: High-resolution MR imaging (MR neurography)
- Protocol advice: Axial T1WI, fat-saturated T2WI, and STIR (T1 C+ MR if scar or neoplasm suspected) using surface or knee coil

DIFFERENTIAL DIAGNOSIS

Ganglion cyst
- Uncommon; variable location around knee
- +/- Synovial lining

Viral neuritis
- History, laboratory findings suggest diagnosis

Nerve sheath tumor
- Focal nerve enlargement, loss of fascicular architecture, tumoral enhancement
- Usually isolated, but search for NF1 stigmata
- Lacks soft tissue inflammatory changes seen in CPN entrapment

DDx: CPN Neuropathy

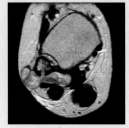

Ganglion Cyst

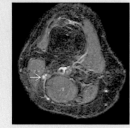

Viral Neuritis

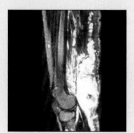

Neurofibrosarcoma

COMMON PERONEAL NEUROPATHY

Key Facts

Terminology
- Synonyms: Common peroneal nerve (CPN) palsy, CPN entrapment
- Common peroneal nerve entrapment at fibular head

Imaging Findings
- Best diagnostic clue: CPN enlargement +/- T2 hyperintensity, architectural distortion at fibular head in symptomatic patient

Top Differential Diagnoses
- Ganglion cyst
- Viral neuritis
- Nerve sheath tumor
- Direct acute CPN trauma

Diagnostic Checklist
- Focal CPN enlargement, abnormal T2 hyperintensity at fibular head diagnostic for CPN neuropathy

Direct acute CPN trauma
- Blunt or lacerating injury
- Rely on clinical history, exam findings

PATHOLOGY

General Features
- General path comments
  - Common peroneal nerve lies along fibular neck (floor of "fibular tunnel")
    - Tunnel entrance is rigid musculo-aponeurotic arch derived from soleus, peroneus longus muscles
- Etiology
  - Entrapment or sequelae of continued pressure on CPN at fibular head
  - Most commonly complication following orthopedic procedure around knee, less commonly acute direct nerve trauma, compression by traction splints, poor operative positioning, or following knee dislocation
- Epidemiology: Uncommon
- Associated abnormalities
  - Fibular osseous abnormalities
  - +/- Intraneural or extrinsic ganglion cyst

Gross Pathologic & Surgical Features
- Edematous/indurated CPN +/- thickened "fibular tunnel"

Microscopic Features
- Nerve edema +/- inflammatory cells, fibrous infiltration, fascicular atrophy/loss

CLINICAL ISSUES

Presentation
- Most common signs/symptoms: Foot drop, sensory abnormality along anterolateral leg
- Clinical profile: Foot drop +/- history of acute or chronic trauma to lateral knee

Demographics
- Age: Adults > > children, infants

Natural History & Prognosis
- Variable but frequently good recovery following conservative management
- Decompression in recalcitrant cases may produce improvement even after 6-12 months delay

Treatment
- Conservative: Physical therapy, rigid ankle-foot orthosis (AFO), avoidance of provocative maneuvers
- Surgical decompression if no improvement with conservative measures

DIAGNOSTIC CHECKLIST

Consider
- MR imaging is more sensitive for acute than chronic nerve injuries

Image Interpretation Pearls
- Focal CPN enlargement, abnormal T2 hyperintensity at fibular head diagnostic for CPN neuropathy

SELECTED REFERENCES

1. Agarwal M et al: Common peroneal nerve palsy after lateral unicompartmental knee arthroplasty. J Arthroplasty. 18(1):92-5, 2003
2. Ryan W et al: Relationship of the common peroneal nerve and its branches to the head and neck of the fibula. Clin Anat. 16(6):501-5, 2003
3. Thoma A et al: Decompression of the common peroneal nerve: experience with 20 consecutive cases. Plast Reconstr Surg. 107(5):1183-9, 2001
4. Yamazaki H et al: Peroneal nerve palsy caused by intraneural ganglion. Skeletal Radiol. 28(1):52-6, 1999

IMAGE GALLERY

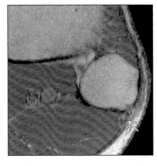 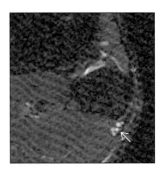

(Left) Axial T1WI MR shows isointense fascicular enlargement of left CPN at fibular head (arrow). (Right) Axial STIR MR confirms fascicular enlargement, abnormal T2 hyperintensity of left CPN at fibular head (arrow).

POSTERIOR TIBIAL NERVE ENTRAPMENT

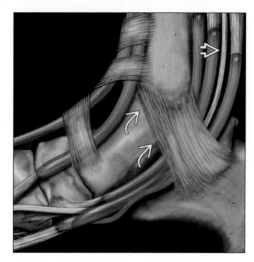

Sagittal graphic shows posterior tibial nerve (open arrow) coursing beneath flexor retinaculum (curved arrows) between flexor hallucis longus and flexor digitorum longus tendons.

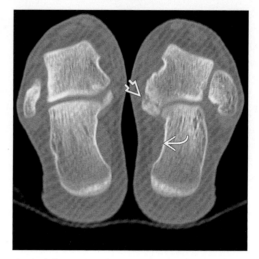

Coronal bone CT shows coalition variant with os sustentaculi (open arrow) narrowing tarsal tunnel. Note quadratus plantae atrophy (curved arrow) compared to normal contralateral side.

TERMINOLOGY

Abbreviations and Synonyms
- Synonym: Tarsal tunnel syndrome

Definitions
- Entrapment of posterior tibial nerve (n.) in the tarsal tunnel

IMAGING FINDINGS

General Features
- Best diagnostic clue: Space-occupying lesion in tarsal tunnel
- Location
  - Tarsal tunnel
    - Fibro-osseous tunnel beneath medial malleolus, inferior to sustentaculum tali
  - Anterior tarsal tunnel
    - Fascial continuation of constricting space along lateral and medial plantar nn.

MR Findings
- T1WI
  - Distinguishes between different etiologies
    - Mass, anomalous muscle, coalition
  - Fatty atrophy of intrinsic plantar mm.
- T2WI
  - Characterize mass if present
  - Edema in innervated mm.
- T1 C+: Differentiates cysts from enhancing soft tissue tumors

Other Modality Findings
- Electrodiagnosis (nerve conduction studies) standard for diagnosis

Imaging Recommendations
- Best imaging tool: MRI
- Protocol advice: Coronal, axial T2WI with fat-saturation

DIFFERENTIAL DIAGNOSIS

Plantar fasciitis
- Thickening, edema of plantar fascia evident on MRI

Calcaneus stress fracture
- Fracture line perpendicular to primary trabeculae of posterior process

Sciatica
- L5 or S1 disc herniation

Talocalcaneal coalition
- Bony, fibrous or cartilaginous bridge between sustentaculum tali and medial talus

DDx: Tibial Nerve Entrapment

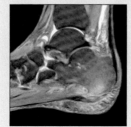

Plantar Fasciitis

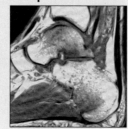

Stress Fracture

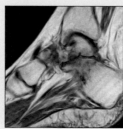

Coalition

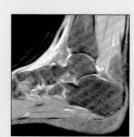

Rheumatoid

Key Facts

Terminology
- Synonym: Tarsal tunnel syndrome

Imaging Findings
- Distinguishes between different etiologies
- Fatty atrophy of intrinsic plantar mm.

Top Differential Diagnoses
- Plantar fasciitis

- Calcaneus stress fracture
- Sciatica
- Talocalcaneal coalition
- Peripheral neuropathy

Clinical Issues
- Vague heel pain, dysesthesias

Diagnostic Checklist
- Symptom vagueness ⇒ difficult clinical diagnosis

- Can lead to tarsal tunnel syndrome due to bony overgrowth

Peripheral neuropathy
- Burning foot pain, "stocking and glove" distribution
- Diabetic patients often have diffuse edema of plantar mm. on MRI

Inflammatory arthropathy (rheumatoid or seronegative)
- Subtalar joint involvement leads to heel pain, instability
- Tenosynovitis often involves multiple tendons
- Can lead to tarsal tunnel syndrome due to pannus

PATHOLOGY

General Features
- General path comments
  - Posterior tibial n. between flexor digitorum longus, flexor hallucis longus mm.
  - Innervates intrinsic plantar mm. of foot, also sensory
  - Passes through fibro-osseous tunnel in hindfoot
    - Beneath medial malleolus and sustentaculum tali
  - Divides into 3 branches
    - Medial plantar, lateral plantar, medial calcaneal
- Etiology
  - Overuse syndrome in runners
  - Space occupying lesion in tarsal tunnel (majority of patients)
    - Tumors: Nerve sheath, lipoma, rarely sarcoma
    - Non-neoplastic: Venous varicosities, tenosynovitis, ganglion cyst, accessory mm.
  - Fracture
  - Talocalcaneal coalition: Bony overgrowth can compress nerve
  - Valgus hindfoot: Stretches n.

Gross Pathologic & Surgical Features
- Nerve enlargement or flattening

CLINICAL ISSUES

Presentation
- Most common signs/symptoms
  - Vague heel pain, dysesthesias
  - Tinel sign: Tingling along course of nerve when nerve is tapped

Natural History & Prognosis
- Leads to mm. atrophy

Treatment
- Options, risks, complications
  - Conservative management of overuse syndrome
  - Flexor retinaculum surgical decompression
  - Resection of space-occupying lesions

DIAGNOSTIC CHECKLIST

Consider
- Symptom vagueness ⇒ difficult clinical diagnosis

SELECTED REFERENCES

1. Hochman MG et al: Nerves in a pinch: imaging of nerve compression syndromes. Radiol Clin North Am. 42(1):221-45, 2004
2. Kinoshita M et al: Tarsal tunnel syndrome associated with an accessory muscle. Foot Ankle Int. 24(2):132-6, 2003
3. Labib SA et al: Heel pain triad (HPT): the combination of plantar fasciitis, posterior tibial tendon dysfunction and tarsal tunnel syndrome. Foot Ankle Int. 23(3):212-20, 2002
4. Oh SJ et al: Entrapment neuropathies of the tibial (posterior tibial) nerve. Neurol Clin. 17(3):593-615, vii, 1999
5. Lau JT et al: Tarsal tunnel syndrome: a review of the literature. Foot Ankle Int. 20(3):201-9, 1999

IMAGE GALLERY

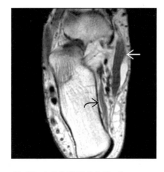 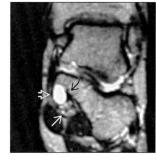

(Left) Axial T1WI MR shows anomalous flexor digitorum longus m. (arrow) compressing tarsal tunnel. Note atrophy of quadratus plantae (curved arrow). *(Right)* Coronal T2WI MR shows ganglion cyst (open arrow) in tarsal canal. Curved arrow shows flexor hallucis longus t.; straight arrow shows posterior tibial neurovascular bundle.

PART VII
Spine Post-Procedural Imaging

Post-Procedural Imaging and Complications　1

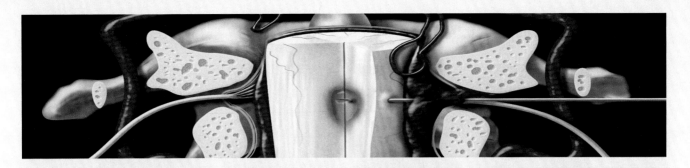

SECTION 1: Post-Procedural Imaging and Complications

MYELOGRAPHY COMPLICATIONS

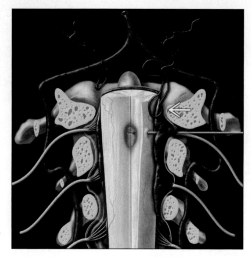

Coronal graphic shows complications of C1-2 puncture with cord injury from needle, + subarachnoid blood. Note close proximity to caudal loop of PICA (arrow).

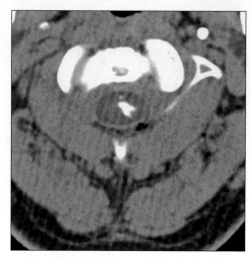

Axial CT following attempted myelogram shows focal contrast within cord substance + small amount of epidural gas.

TERMINOLOGY

Abbreviations and Synonyms
- Postdural puncture headache (PDPH)

Definitions
- Any unexpected sequela following myelography
  - Major complications: Cord injury, anaphylaxis, arachnoiditis, CSF leak, contrast reaction
  - Minor complications: PDPH, transient neurologic sequela, incorrect injection, contrast reaction
  - Delayed complications: Iatrogenic epidermoid

IMAGING FINDINGS

General Features
- Best diagnostic clue
  - Most common complications (e.g., headache) have no imaging findings
  - Incorrect injection: Epidural or mixed compartment
  - CSF leak: Radionuclide cisternography collection
  - Intracranial hydrocephalus: "Sagging" midbrain
  - Aseptic meningitis: Meningeal enhancement
  - Arachnoiditis: Clumped nerve roots, empty thecal sac, mild cauda equina enhancement
  - Cord injury: MRI cord contusion
  - Iatrogenic epidermoid: CSF intensity/density lesion

Radiographic Findings
- Myelography
  - Incorrect injection
    - Most often epidural injection
    - Contrast surrounding nerve root sleeves mimics sleeve filling during fluoroscopy → fools myelographer into believing they have good intradural injection
  - Lumbar approach
    - Neck extension should be minimized while obtaining radiographs for cervical myelogram
    - Replacing needle stylet before withdrawing helps to prevent headache
  - C1/2
    - Should be monitored with lateral fluoroscopy for accurate needle positioning & prevention of contrast medium injection into cord
    - Neck extension should be minimized

CT Findings
- CECT: Iatrogenic epidermoid: Nonenhancing hypodense lesion
- CT Myelography
  - Incorrect injection: Most often epidural
  - CSF leak: May reveal a small contrast collection at leakage site

---

DDx: Gamuts of Myelography Complication Mimics

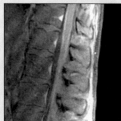

Infect. Arachnoiditis

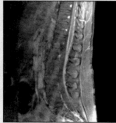

Carcinomatosis

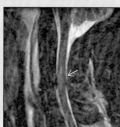

Traumatic Contusion

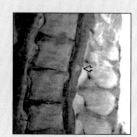

Myxo. Ependymoma

MYELOGRAPHY COMPLICATIONS

Key Facts

Terminology
- Any unexpected sequela following myelography
- Major complications: Cord injury, anaphylaxis, arachnoiditis, CSF leak, contrast reaction
- Minor complications: PDPH, transient neurologic sequela, incorrect injection, contrast reaction
- Delayed complications: Iatrogenic epidermoid

Imaging Findings
- Most common complications (e.g., headache) have no imaging findings
- CSF leak: Radionuclide cisternography collection
- Intracranial hydrocephalus: "Sagging" midbrain
- Aseptic meningitis: Meningeal enhancement
- Arachnoiditis: Clumped nerve roots, empty thecal sac, mild cauda equina enhancement

- Cord injury: MRI cord contusion
- Iatrogenic epidermoid: CSF intensity/density lesion
- Replacing needle stylet before withdrawing helps to prevent headache

Pathology
- Incidence of headache with 22 gauge atraumatic needle is 5% vs. 30% for 20 gauge bevelled needles

Clinical Issues
- Most common complication: Headache
- Usually begins within 3 days and lasts 3-5 days
- PDPH: Treatment for headache is supportive

MR Findings
- T1WI
  - CSF leak may lead to intracranial hypotension (best seen on sagittal technique)
    - Descent of brain, chiasm, brain stem with obliteration of basilar cisterns
    - Flattening of pons against the clivus
    - Secondary Chiari 1
    - May result in subdural hematoma → tearing of bridging veins occurs after "sagging" brain motion
  - Cord injury: Acutely isointense
  - Iatrogenic epidermoid: Well-defined intradural hyper-/isointense lesion to CSF
- T2WI
  - Cord injury: Acutely hyperintense
  - Iatrogenic epidermoid: Well-defined intradural hyper-/isointense lesion to CSF
- STIR: Cord injury: Acutely hyperintense
- T1 C+
  - CSF leak & intracranial hypotension
    - Diffuse, smooth meningeal enhancement
    - May involve both brain & spine
  - Aseptic meningitis: May see enhancement
  - Arachnoiditis → 3 patterns have been described
    - Smooth linear layer of enhancement outlining cord surface & nerve roots (most common)
    - Nodular pattern with discrete foci of enhancement along cord surface
    - Diffuse intradural enhancement completely filling the subarachnoid space (least common)
  - Iatrogenic epidermoid: Faint peripheral enhancement possible

Nuclear Medicine Findings
- CSF leak
  - Intrathecal Indium-111 DTPA radionuclide cisternography

Imaging Recommendations
- Best imaging tool
  - Incorrect injection: CT
  - CSF leak: Radionuclide cisternography followed by directed CT

- Intracranial hydrocephalus, aseptic meningitis, arachnoiditis, iatrogenic epidermoid: MRI C+
- Cord injury: MRI

DIFFERENTIAL DIAGNOSIS

Arachnoiditis
- Infection, inflammation, neoplastic, post-operative

Aseptic meningitis
- Infection, inflammation, neoplastic

Cord injury
- Traumatic

Iatrogenic epidermoid
- Congenital epidermoid, myxopapillary ependymoma

Intracranial hypotension
- Infection, inflammation, neoplastic

CSF leak
- Traumatic, post-operative, neoplastic

PATHOLOGY

General Features
- Etiology
  - PDPH
    - Most likely related to dural hole left after spinal needle has been withdrawn
    - Allows small CSF leak
  - Transient neurologic sequela: Neurotoxic effect
  - Cord injury
    - 2/3 due to cervical spine hyperextension & 1/3 after lateral C1-2 puncture
    - Contributing factors are a narrow canal diameter & severe cervical spondylosis
  - Iatrogenic epidermoid
    - Skin cells are implanted into spinal canal during lumbar puncture

MYELOGRAPHY COMPLICATIONS

- Majority are late complications of spinal puncture during the early neonatal period
- Have been discovered 2-23 yrs following apparent time of implantation
- Epidemiology
  - PDPH
    - Occurs in 36-58% of myelograms performed with 22-gauge Quincke needles
    - Incidence of headache with 22 gauge atraumatic needle is 5% vs. 30% for 20 gauge bevelled needles
    - Incidence with 24 gauge atraumatic needle is 1-2% but requires aspiration if CSF is needed
  - Arachnoiditis: Rare, dehydration increases incidence
  - Iatrogenic epidermoid
    - Epidermoid cysts are uncommon → 0.5-1% of all spinal tumors; acquired tumors account for ≈ 40%
    - Incidence significantly ↓ after nonstylet needles replaced by tight-fitting stylet needles
- Associated abnormalities
  - Subdural hematoma: Rare
  - Nerve rootlet avulsion: Rare

Microscopic Features

- CSF leak: Aseptic inflammatory reaction
- Iatrogenic epidermoid: Contains keratin, cholesterol crystals, desquamed epithelial cells

CLINICAL ISSUES

Presentation

- Most common signs/symptoms
  - Most common complication: Headache
    - Usually begins within 3 days and lasts 3-5 days
  - Nausea, vomiting, hearing loss, tinnitus, vertigo, dizziness, paresthesias
  - Seizures: Dehydration increases incidence
  - Visual disturbances such as diplopia or cortical blindness have been reported
  - Cranial nerve palsies are not uncommon
  - Transient neurologic sequela (e.g., expressive dysphasia); rare
  - Iatrogenic epidermoid: Progressive radicular & back pain, gait abnormalities, sphincter disturbances

Demographics

- Age: PDPH: More common in younger age patients
- Gender: PDPH: M:F = 1:2
- Body Habitus: Lower body mass index is a significant factor for PDPH in some series

Natural History & Prognosis

- PDPH
  - 72% resolve within 7 days, 87% in 6 mos
  - Decrease risk by using
    - Smaller gauge, atraumatic (blunt) needles
    - Paramedian approach
    - Parallel orientation of needle bevel to dural fibers
    - Replacing stylet before withdrawing
  - IV hydration, no removal of CSF, experience of myelographer, & inpatient status have been inconsistently associated with lower PDPH rates
  - When performed as an outpatient procedure does not have increased incidence of side effects or risk

Treatment

- Contrast reaction: Standard care
- PDPH: Treatment for headache is supportive
  - Non-narcotic analgesics, hydration, & time
  - Bed rest has been shown to be of no benefit
  - There is no clinical evidence that maintaining a supine position before/headache onset is effective
  - Epidural blood patch
    - Rarely necessary
    - Perform for PDPH persisting longer than one week
    - Place 15-30 cc of autologous blood within extradural space adjacent to puncture site
    - Very effective → produces remission in 89% of cases, and a further 8% relieved by a 2nd injection
- CSF leak
  - Large volume blood patch (60 cc) is often successful
  - Surgical closure of dural tear is option of last resort
- Iatrogenic epidermoid: Complete excision is usually possible and is curative

DIAGNOSTIC CHECKLIST

Consider

- Premyelography MRI screening recommended for patients with spinal canal stenosis, severe spondylosis, & myelopathy of any cause

SELECTED REFERENCES

1. Ziv ET et al: Iatrogenic intraspinal epidermoid tumor: two cases & review of the literature. Spine. 29(1):E15-8, 2004
2. Turnbull DK et al: Post-dural puncture headache: pathogenesis, prevention and treatment. Br J Anaesth. 91(5):718-29, 2003
3. Park JC et al: Iatrogenic spinal epidermoid tumor. A complication of spinal puncture in an adult. Clin Neurol Neurosurg. 105(4):281-5, 2003
4. Peterman SB: Postmyelography headache: a review. Radiology. 200(3):765-70, 1996
5. Nakakoshi T et al: Aseptic meningitis complicating iotrolan myelography. AJNR Am J Neuroradiol. 12(1):173, 1991
6. Robertson HJ et al: Cervical myelography: survey of modes of practice and major complications. Radiology. 174(1):79-83, 1990
7. Katoh Y et al: Complications of lateral C1-2 puncture myelography. Spine. 15(11):1085-7, 1990
8. Kostiner AI et al: Outpatient lumbar myelography with metrizamide. Radiology. 155(2):383-5, 1985
9. Sarno JB: Transient expressive (nonfluent) dysphasia after metrizamide myelography. AJNR Am J Neuroradiol. 6(6):945-7, 1985
10. Baker FJ et al: Aseptic meningitis complicating metrizamide myelography. AJNR Am J Neuroradiol. 3(6):662-3, 1982
11. Brodey PA et al: Nerve rootlet avulsion. A complication of myelography using the Chynn needle. Radiology. 125(3):734, 1977
12. Kennedy TF et al: Nerve rootlet avulsion as a complication of myelography with the Cualtico needle. Radiology. 119(2):389, 1976

IMAGE GALLERY

Typical

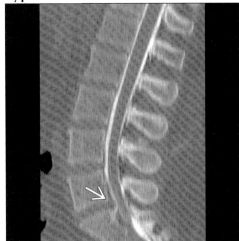
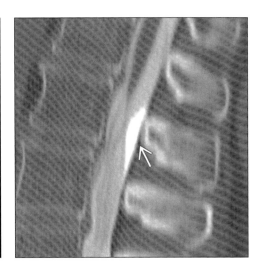

(Left) Sagittal CT myelography sagittal reformat reveals an incorrect epidural + subdural injection. Often the study is still diagnostic as pathology may efface the epidural contrast (arrow). *(Right)* Sagittal CT myelography reformat demonstrates a mixed compartment injection; normal intradural contrast is present as is a lentiform-shaped subdural collection (arrow).

Typical

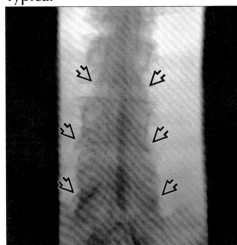
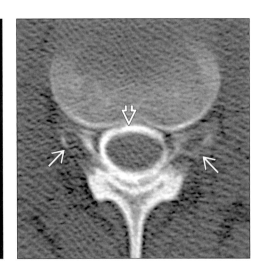

(Left) Fluoroscopy during myelography with an epidural injection can fool the myelographer as contrast surrounding nerve root sleeves (open arrows) can appear to be filling the sleeves. *(Right)* Axial CT myelography demonstrates contrast within the epidural space, surrounding (not filling) the nerve root sleeves (arrows), and subdural space (open arrow).

Typical

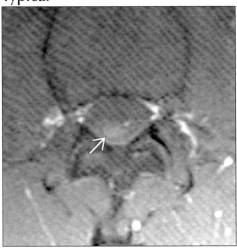
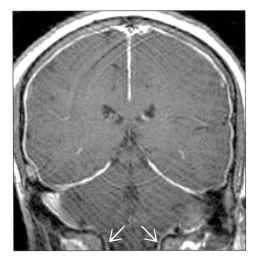

(Left) Axial T1WI MR shows an epidermoid as a well-defined mass lesion which is slightly hyperintense to CSF (arrow). It did not enhance (not shown). *(Right)* Coronal T1 C+ MR of intracranial hypotension due to CSF leak demonstrates diffuse, smooth, dural thickening & enhancement. Note this process extends into superior spinal canal (arrows).

VERTEBROPLASTY COMPLICATIONS

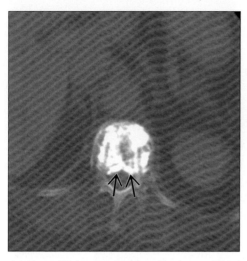

Axial bone CT shows cement in epidural space behind vertebral body of anterior spinal canal (arrows). Patient was asymptomatic after procedure.

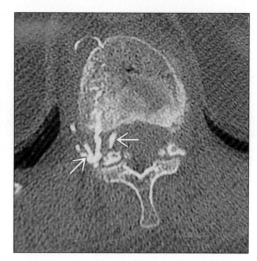

Axial bone CT shows cement in foramen (arrows). Slice above showed bulk of cement in vertebral body. Patient suffered pain and radiculopathy after procedure (Courtesy S. Dunnagan, MD).

TERMINOLOGY

Definitions
- Vertebroplasty: Placement of bone cement, typically polymethylmethacrylate, into compressed vertebral body (vb)
- Kyphoplasty: Same, but preceded by balloon inflation within vb to create cavity therein

IMAGING FINDINGS

General Features
- Best diagnostic clue
  - Extravasation of cement into spinal canal
    - Seen as cement beyond posterior vb border on fluoroscopy during procedure
  - Extravasation of cement into foramen
    - Cement in roof of foramen on oblique view
  - Extravasation of cement into vertebral plexus
    - Cement conforms to shape of vein, slowly flows towards central veins on fluoro
  - Pulmonary embolization of cement
    - Branching or globular hyperdense material in lung parenchyma on fluoro, x-ray, or CT
  - Vertebral Osteomyelitis
    - Rarefaction of vb on delayed x-rays, CT; high signal surrounding cement on T2WI, low on T1WI

- "Bounce back" fracture
  - New compression fracture of vb adjacent to treated level

Imaging Recommendations
- Best imaging tool
  - CT is best for defining cement extension beyond vb, into foramen, venous and pulmonary embolization
  - MR best for detecting osteomyelitis, early signs of "bounce back" fracture
- Protocol advice
  - Extravasation or embolization of cement - use post procedural plain films
    - Use CT if any question remains, or if symptoms present despite negative x-ray
    - Bone or wide soft tissue windows especially useful
    - Use of intrathecal dye can help prevent cement extravasation when visualization of vb borders suboptimal
  - Pre- and post-contrast MRI used for detecting osteomyelitis, "bounceback" fracture

DIFFERENTIAL DIAGNOSIS

Extravasation of cement into spinal canal
- Retropulsion of cement/bone fragment into canal

DDx: Complications of Vertebroplasty

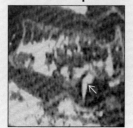

Foraminal Cement

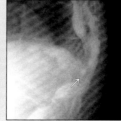

Cement In Canal

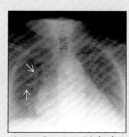

Lung Cement Emboli

VERTEBROPLASTY COMPLICATIONS

Key Facts

Imaging Findings

- Extravasation of cement into spinal canal
- Extravasation of cement into foramen
- Extravasation of cement into vertebral plexus
- Cement conforms to shape of vein, slowly flows towards central veins on fluoro
- Pulmonary embolization of cement
- Vertebral Osteomyelitis
- "Bounce back" fracture
- CT is best for defining cement extension beyond vb, into foramen, venous and pulmonary embolization
- MR best for detecting osteomyelitis, early signs of "bounce back" fracture
- Extravasation or embolization of cement - use post procedural plain films
- Bone or wide soft tissue windows especially useful

- Use of intrathecal dye can help prevent cement extravasation when visualization of vb borders suboptimal
- Pre- and post-contrast MRI used for detecting osteomyelitis, "bounceback" fracture

Clinical Issues

- Extravasation of cement into canal
- Most often asymptomatic

Diagnostic Checklist

- CT in any case of unexplained symptomatology following procedure

---

Extravasation of cement into foramen

- Bone spur or fragment in foramen

Extravasation of cement into perivertebral venous plexus

- Phlebolith

Pulmonary embolization of cement

- Calcified granuloma

Vertebral osteomyelitis

- Osteonecrosis

"Bounce back" fractures

- Progressive compression

PATHOLOGY

General Features

- Etiology
  - Extravasation or embolization of cement
    - Improper needle placement
    - Excessive force or rate of injection
    - Insufficient cement viscosity
    - Venous embolization common, as venous channels in vb communicate with perivertebral channels
    - Excessive volume of cement
    - Too many levels treated in one sitting
    - Underlying neoplasm
  - Vertebral osteomyelitis
    - Suboptimal sterile technique
    - Omission of prophylactic antibiotic
    - Immune compromise
  - "Bounce back" fractures
    - Seen in 10-15% of treated patients
    - Possibly due to creation of very hard focus ("hammer") within still osteoporotic spinal column
    - Cement extension into disc space may predispose
    - Sudden ambulation of previously bed ridden, still osteoporotic or compromised patient

- Obese patients more at risk as greater effect of gravity
- Not clear if true "complication", or natural history of process
- Epidemiology
  - Extravasation or venous embolization of cement
    - Most common complication
    - Seen in up to 20% of cases if looked for
  - Pulmonary embolization
    - Clinically significant embolization rare
    - Probably more common than recognized
    - Fat, displaced by cement placed in marrow, likely embolizes subclinically more often than cement
  - Osteomyelitis
    - Less than 1% incidence

Gross Pathologic & Surgical Features

- Extravasation, embolization of cement
  - Hardened cement beyond vb compromising canal, foramen or neural structures
    - Decompressive approach may reduce/resolve symptoms
  - Occlusion of vessel if embolization
- Osteomyelitis
  - Typical inflammatory changes, even liquefaction of bone surrounding cement
  - Treatment requires six weeks of intravenous antibiotics
    - In advanced cases may require vertebrectomy and fusion

CLINICAL ISSUES

Presentation

- Most common signs/symptoms
  - Extravasation of cement into canal
    - Most often asymptomatic
    - Back pain, radiculopathy most common symptoms
    - Myelopathy in severe cases
  - Extravasation into foramen
    - Severe radiculopathy immediately after procedure

VERTEBROPLASTY COMPLICATIONS

- ○ Embolization of cement into vein or lungs
  - Most often asymptomatic
  - Shortness of breath, chest pain in minority of pulmonary emboli
  - Compromised pulmonary function seen rarely
  - Cardiopulmonary collapse and death reported
  - Patients with advanced pulmonary compromise not good candidates for aggressive vertebroplasty
- ○ Osteomyelitis
  - Delayed onset of back pain
  - Elevated sedimentation rate, C-reactive protein, white cell count
  - Positive blood cultures
  - Positive aspirate or bone biopsy
- ○ "Bounce back" fractures
  - Delayed onset of new back pain

DIAGNOSTIC CHECKLIST

Consider
- CT in any case of unexplained symptomatology following procedure

SELECTED REFERENCES

1. Stricker K et al: Severe hypercapnia due to pulmonary embolism of polymethylmethacrylate during vertebroplasty. Anesth Analg. 98(4):1184-6, table of contents, 2004
2. Appel NB et al: Percutaneous vertebroplasty in patients with spinal canal compromise. AJR Am J Roentgenol. 182(4):947-51, 2004
3. Lin EP et al: Vertebroplasty: cement leakage into the disc increases the risk of new fracture of adjacent vertebral body. AJNR Am J Neuroradiol. 25(2):175-80, 2004
4. Brown DB et al: Treatment of chronic symptomatic vertebral compression fractures with percutaneous vertebroplasty. AJR Am J Roentgenol. 182(2):319-22, 2004
5. Tsai TT et al: Polymethylmethacrylate cement dislodgment following percutaneous vertebroplasty: a case report. Spine. 28(22):E457-60, 2003
6. Baroud G et al: Biomechanical explanation of adjacent fractures following vertebroplasty. Radiology. 229(2):606-7; author reply 607-8, 2003
7. Mathis JM: Percutaneous vertebroplasty: complication avoidance and technique optimization. AJNR Am J Neuroradiol. 24(8):1697-706, 2003
8. Childers JC Jr: Cardiovascular collapse and death during vertebroplasty. Radiology. 228(3):902; author reply 902-3, 2003
9. Kang JD et al: Cement augmentation of osteoporotic compression fractures and intraoperative navigation: summary statement. Spine. 28(15):S62-3, 2003
10. Gangi A et al: Percutaneous vertebroplasty: indications, technique, and results. Radiographics. 23(2):e10, 2003
11. Kelekis AD et al: Radicular pain after vertebroplasty: compression or irritation of the nerve root? Initial experience with the "cooling system". Spine. 28(14):E265-9, 2003
12. Mousavi P et al: Volumetric quantification of cement leakage following percutaneous vertebroplasty in metastatic and osteoporotic vertebrae. J Neurosurg. 99(1 Suppl):56-9, 2003
13. Koessler MJ et al: Fat and bone marrow embolism during percutaneous vertebroplasty. Anesth Analg. 97(1):293; author reply 294, 2003
14. Stallmeyer MJ et al: Optimizing patient selection in percutaneous vertebroplasty. J Vasc Interv Radiol. 14(6):683-96, 2003
15. Sarzier JS et al: Intrathecal injection of contrast medium to prevent polymethylmethacrylate leakage during percutaneous vertebroplasty. AJNR Am J Neuroradiol. 24(5):1001-2, 2003
16. Hodler J et al: Midterm outcome after vertebroplasty: predictive value of technical and patient-related factors. Radiology. 227(3):662-8, 2003
17. Yeom JS et al: Leakage of cement in percutaneous transpedicular vertebroplasty for painful osteoporotic compression fractures. J Bone Joint Surg Br. 85(1):83-9, 2003
18. Evans AJ et al: Vertebral compression fractures: pain reduction and improvement in functional mobility after percutaneous polymethylmethacrylate vertebroplasty retrospective report of 245 cases. Radiology. 226(2):366-72, 2003
19. Shapiro S et al: Surgical removal of epidural and intradural polymethylmethacrylate extravasation complicating percutaneous vertebroplasty for an osteoporotic lumbar compression fracture. Case report. J Neurosurg. 98(1 Suppl):90-2, 2003
20. Uppin AA et al: Occurrence of new vertebral body fracture after percutaneous vertebroplasty in patients with osteoporosis. Radiology. 226(1):119-24, 2003
21. Moreland DB et al: Vertebroplasty: techniques to avoid complications. Spine J. 1(1):66-71, 2001

IMAGE GALLERY

Typical

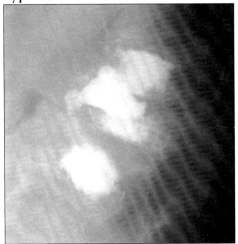
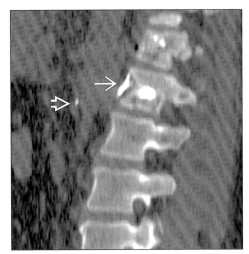

(Left) Lateral radiography shows large volume of cement beyond vertebral body in disc interspace and beyond, between two other vertebral bodies also treated which contain cement within their confines. *(Right)* Sagittal bone CT reformation shows cement in prevertebral vein (arrow), extending into renal vein (open arrow), the two foci were connected on contiguous slices. Patient was asymptomatic.

Typical

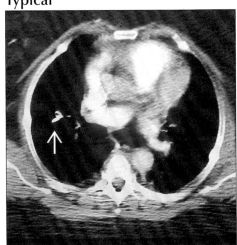
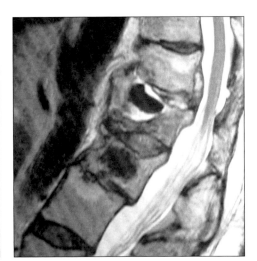

(Left) Axial CECT shows cement embolus bifurcating into tertiary branches of pulmonary artery (arrow) following vertebroplasty in asymptomatic patient. *(Right)* Sagittal T2WI MR shows high signal surrounding cement several weeks after vertebroplasty in patient on chronic steroid therapy. Aspiration showed staph. aureus infection (Courtesy S. Dunnagan, MD).

Typical

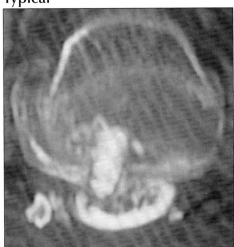
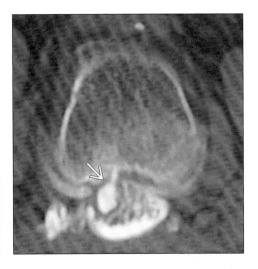

(Left) Axial bone CT shows column of cement extending into spinal canal, compressing contrast-filled thecal sac. *(Right)* Axial bone CT shows mushroom of cement (arrow) extravasating into thecal sac filled with contrast (Courtesy S. Dunnagan, MD).

CSF LEAKAGE SYNDROME

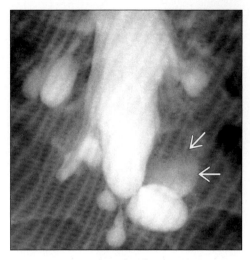

Anteroposterior myelography shows numerous nerve sleeve cysts, one of which leaks (amorphous contrast collection, arrows). Patient had SIH, with postural headaches and subdural effusion.

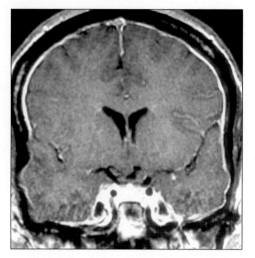

Coronal T1 C+ MR shows hyperemic, thickened dura, effacement of suprasellar cistern due to downward brain displacement in SIH patient with CSF leak from ruptured nerve sleeve cyst.

TERMINOLOGY

Abbreviations and Synonyms
- Spontaneous intracranial hypotension (SIH), intracranial hypotension (IH)
- Cerebrospinal fluid (CSF) hypovolemia
- Post-operative, iatrogenic, or post-traumatic CSF leak, pseudomeningocele

Definitions
- Symptomatic leakage of CSF

IMAGING FINDINGS

General Features
- Best diagnostic clue: Dural thickening and/or markedly enlarged epidural veins + CSF fluid collection
- Location
  - In spontaneous cases, dural thickening/engorgement most detectable in high cervical region
  - Fluid collections close to or remote from site of leakage
  - Can see intraspinal (epidural/subdural) hygromas

Radiographic Findings
- Myelography: Used to find site of occult CSF leak, relatively insensitive, unless combined with CT and/or Radionuclide cysternography

CT Findings
- NECT
  - Symmetric anterolateral epidural masses (dilated epidural veins)
  - +/- CSF collection (ventral sub/epidural or paraspinous)
  - +/- Arachnoid diverticula/meningocele(s)
  - Spinal hygromas within or beyond spinal canal
- CECT: May see "draped curtain" sign (intensely enhancing epidural veins)

MR Findings
- T1WI
  - Ventral/anterolateral fluid isointense with CSF, +/- "flow voids" in cervical spinal canal
  - Intra- or extraspinal fluid collections
- T2WI
  - Extra-axial fluid like CSF (may be hyperintense on PD)
  - +/- Arachnoid diverticula
- T1 C+
  - Enhancing, thickened ventral dura in cervical region
  - Intensely enhancing, greatly enlarged venous plexi

DDx: Postoperative Fluid Collections

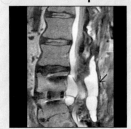

Phlegmon

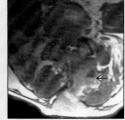

Hematoma

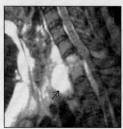

Abscess, Empyema

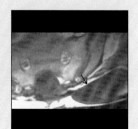

Pseudomeningocele

CSF LEAKAGE SYNDROME

Key Facts

Terminology
- Spontaneous intracranial hypotension (SIH), intracranial hypotension (IH)
- Post-operative, iatrogenic, or post-traumatic CSF leak, pseudomeningocele

Imaging Findings
- In spontaneous cases, dural thickening/engorgement most detectable in high cervical region
- Fluid collections close to or remote from site of leakage
- Can see intraspinal (epidural/subdural) hygromas
- Scan the brain first (look for cranial findings of SIH)
- Dural thickening, enhancement
- "Sagging midbrain"
- Tonsillar herniation
- Subdural hygroma
- Scan spine, search for actual leakage site only
- Use CT myelogram, isotope cisternography to search for sites of occult leakage
- Or to differentiate CSF leak from other causes of post-operative fluid collections

Top Differential Diagnoses
- Other causes of post-operative fluid collections
- Hematoma, phlegmon
- Empyema, abscess
- Pseudomeningocele

Diagnostic Checklist
- "Sagging" brain, posterior fossa with diffuse dural thickening in patient evaluated for headache should suggest CSF leak

Other Modality Findings
- Isotope cisternography
  - Rapid clearance ("washout") from CSF space
  - Early appearance of radionuclide in kidneys, bladder common
  - 60% demonstrate site of CSF leak
- Myelography/CT myelography
  - Arachnoid diverticula
  - May demonstrate CSF leak

Imaging Recommendations
- Scan the brain first (look for cranial findings of SIH)
  - Dural thickening, enhancement
  - "Sagging midbrain"
  - Tonsillar herniation
  - Subdural hygroma
  - Caution: Not all cases have all classic findings!
- Scan spine, search for actual leakage site only
  - If two technically adequate blood patches fail
  - Post-traumatic leak suspected
- Use CT myelogram, isotope cisternography to search for sites of occult leakage
  - Or to differentiate CSF leak from other causes of post-operative fluid collections

DIFFERENTIAL DIAGNOSIS

Other causes of post-operative fluid collections
- Hematoma, phlegmon
- Empyema, abscess
- Pseudomeningocele

Other causes of enlarged spinal venous plexi
- AVM
- Jugular vein or IVC thrombosis (collateral drainage)
- Venous engorgement above high grade spinal stenosis

Pachymeningopathies
- Infection
  - Epidural abscess
  - Rarely occurs in absence of bone, disc involvement
- Neoplasm (posterior cortex, pedicle often destroyed/infiltrated)
- Miscellaneous (e.g., sarcoid)

PATHOLOGY

General Features
- General path comments
  - Defect in dural sac
  - May be ruptured nerve sleeve or its diverticulum
- Genetics: 20% of spontaneous CSF leaks have minor skeletal features of Marfan syndrome
- Etiology
  - Reduced CSF pressure precipitated by
    - Surgery or trauma (including trivial fall)
    - Vigorous exercise, violent coughing
    - After lumbar puncture
    - Abnormal dura (e.g., Marfan syndrome)
    - Ruptured arachnoid diverticulum
    - Severe dehydration
- Epidemiology
  - M:F = 1:2 (spontaneous)
  - Peak age = 30-40 y
- Associated abnormalities
  - Subdural hematoma
  - Spina bifida
  - Marfan syndrome

Gross Pathologic & Surgical Features
- Fluid collection associated with dural defect

Microscopic Features
- Thick dura with fibrosis, numerous dilated thin-walled vessels
- No evidence for inflammation or neoplasia

CLINICAL ISSUES

Presentation
- Most common signs/symptoms
  - Postural headaches, unrelenting

CSF LEAKAGE SYNDROME

- ○ LP shows low CSF pressure +/- pleocytosis, increased protein
- ○ Other signs/symptoms
  - ▪ Cranial nerve palsies
  - ▪ Visual disturbance
  - ▪ Rare: Severe encephalopathy with disturbed consciousness, death
- • Clinical profile: Onset of postural headache after spinal surgery, or lumbar puncture

Natural History & Prognosis

- • 75% resolve spontaneously within 3 months (dural thickening, venous engorgement disappear; fluid collections resorbed)
- • 20-25% persistent leak, chronic headaches
- • Generally excellent
- • Rare: Coma, death from intracranial herniation

Treatment

- • Conservative Rx to restore CSF volume (fluid replacement, bed rest)
- • Other
  - ○ Autologous blood patch
  - ○ Epidural saline infusion
  - ○ Surgery if large dural tear, ruptured diverticulum or Tarlov cyst

DIAGNOSTIC CHECKLIST

Consider

- • Intracranial cisternography to look for congenital defects in middle fossa, or temporal bone

Image Interpretation Pearls

- • "Sagging" brain, posterior fossa with diffuse dural thickening in patient evaluated for headache should suggest CSF leak

SELECTED REFERENCES

1. Kelley GR et al: Sinking brain syndrome: craniotomy can precipitate brainstem herniation in CSF hypovolemia. Neurology. 62(1):157, 2004
2. Paolini S et al: Intraspinous postlaminectomy pseudomeningocele. Eur Spine J. 12(3):325-7, 2003
3. Luetmer PH et al: Dynamic CT myelography: a technique for localizing high-flow spinal cerebrospinal fluid leaks. AJNR Am J Neuroradiol. 24(8):1711-4, 2003
4. Rothrock JF: Low pressure headache and pseudosubdural hematomas. Headache. 43(9):1009, 2003
5. Eross EJ et al: Prolonged neurologic complication and MRI abnormalities consequent to intracranial hypotension. Headache. 43(4):415, 2003
6. Schievink WI et al: Recurrent spontaneous spinal cerebrospinal fluid leak associated with "nude nerve root" syndrome: case report. Neurosurgery. 53(5):1216-8; discussion 1218-9, 2003
7. Schievink WI et al: Recurrent spontaneous spinal cerebrospinal fluid leaks and intracranial hypotension: a prospective study. J Neurosurg. 99(5):840-2, 2003
8. Whiteley W et al: Spontaneous intracranial hypotension causing confusion and coma: a headache for the neurologist and the neurosurgeon. Br J Neurosurg. 17(5):456-8, 2003
9. Fujimaki H et al: Cerebrospinal fluid leak demonstrated by three-dimensional computed tomographic myelography in patients with spontaneous intracranial hypotension. Surg Neurol. 58(3-4):280-4; discussion 284-5, 2002
10. Black P: Cerebrospinal fluid leaks following spinal surgery: use of fat grafts for prevention and repair. Technical note. J Neurosurg. 96(2 Suppl):250-2, 2002
11. Chen CJ et al: Spinal MR findings in spontaneous intracranial hypotension. Neuroradiology. 44(12):996-1003, 2002
12. Schrijver I et al: Spontaneous spinal cerebrospinal fluid leaks and minor skeletal features of Marfan syndrome: a microfibrillopathy. J Neurosurg 96: 483-489, 2002
13. Yousry I et al: Cervical MR imaging in postural headache: MR signs and pathophysiological implications. AJNR 22(7):1239-50, 2001
14. Dillon WP: Spinal manifestations of intracranial hypotension. AJNR Am J Neuroradiol. 22(7):1233-4, 2001
15. Patel MR et al: CT-guided percutaneous fibrin glue therapy of cerebrospinal fluid leaks in the spine after surgery. AJR Am J Roentgenol. 175(2):443-6, 2000
16. O'Carroll CP et al: The syndrome of spontaneous intracranial hypotension. Cephalalgia. 19(2):80-7, 1999
17. Atkinson JL et al: Acquired Chiari I malformation secondary to spontaneous spinal cerebrospinal fluid leakage and chronic intracranial hypotension syndrome in seven cases. J Neurosurg. 88(2):237-42, 1998
18. Moayeri NN et al: Spinal dural enhancement on MRI associated with spontaneous intracranial hypotension. J Neurosrug 88: 912-8, 1998
19. Rabin BM et al: Spontaneous intracranial hypotension: Spinal MR findings. AJNR 19: 1034-9, 1998
20. Vakharia SB et al: Magnetic resonance imaging of cerebrospinal fluid leak and tamponade effect of blood patch in postdural puncture headache. Anesth Analg. 84(3):585-90, 1997
21. McCormack BM et al: Pseudomeningocele/CSF fistula in a patient with lumbar spinal implants treated with epidural blood patch and a brief course of closed subarachnoid drainage. A case report. Spine. 21(19):2273-6, 1996
22. Maycock NF et al: Post-laminectomy cerebrospinal fluid fistula treated with epidural blood patch. Spine. 19(19):2223-5, 1994
23. Lee KS et al: Postlaminectomy lumbar pseudomeningocele: report of four cases. Neurosurgery. 30(1):111-4, 1992
24. Waisman M et al: Postoperative cerebrospinal fluid leakage after lumbar spine operations. Conservative treatment. Spine. 16(1):52-3, 1991
25. Primeau M et al: Spinal cerebrospinal fluid leak demonstrated by radioisotopic cisternography. Clin Nucl Med. 13(10):701-3, 1988
26. Hanakita J et al: Spinal cord compression due to postoperative cervical pseudomeningocele. Neurosurgery. 17(2):317-9, 1985
27. Morris RE et al: Traumatic dural tears: CT diagnosis using metrizamide. Radiology. 152(2):443-6, 1984
28. Teplick JG et al: CT Identification of postlaminectomy pseudomeningocele. AJR Am J Roentgenol. 140(6):1203-6, 1983
29. Findler G et al: Continuous lumbar drainage of cerebrospinal fluid in neurosurgical patients. Surg Neurol. 8(6):455-7, 1977

IMAGE GALLERY

Typical

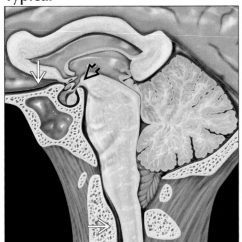

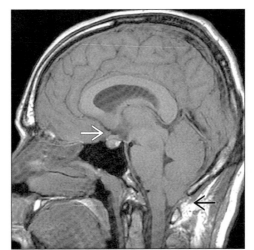

(Left) Sagittal graphic shows intracranial hypotension with dural venous engorgement (arrows), sagging midbrain, tonsil herniation, + inferiorly displaced hypothalamus (open arrows). (Right) Sagittal T1WI MR done for postural headaches (normal scan four months ago), shows sagging brain-obliteration of suprasellar cistern, descent of brain stem, tonsils (arrows). Occult CSF leak found.

Typical

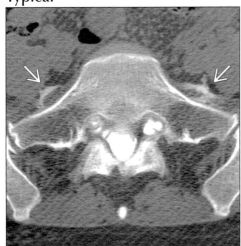

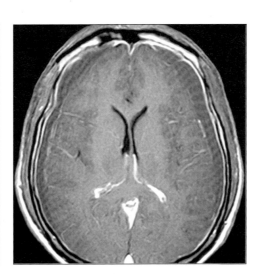

(Left) Axial bone CT myelogram shows nerve sleeve cysts in sacral foramina, leaking dye into pre-sacral space (arrows). Patient had low opening pressure, history of postural headaches, subdural effusions. (Right) Axial T1 C+ MR shows subdural effusions, small ventricles, dural hyperemia in patient with SIH.

Typical

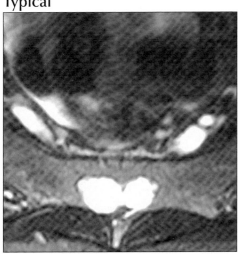

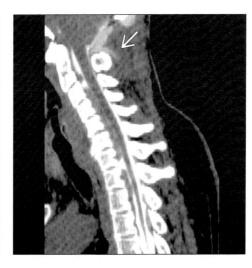

(Left) Axial T2WI MR shows sacral nerve sleeve cysts remodeling canal, loculated fluid in presacral space along the course of sacral roots consistent with CSF leak. (Right) Sagittal bone CT reformation with intrathecal dye shows CSF leak from suboccipital site of Chiari decompression (arrow). Note markedly hypertrophied veins anterior to the cervical cord.

HARDWARE FAILURE

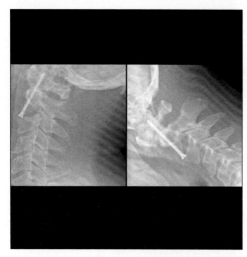

Lateral radiography flexion (left) and extension (right) views in patient with screw bridging type II odontoid fracture reveal motion between arch of C1 and the screw.

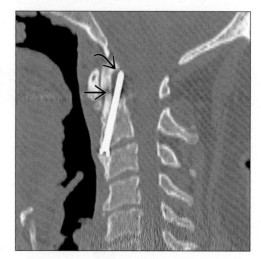

Axial bone CT with sagittal reformation in same patient confirms nonunion at the base of odontoid (arrow) with peri-implant lucency (curved arrow), compatible with hardware failure.

TERMINOLOGY

Abbreviations and Synonyms
- Implant or metal failure

Definitions
- Mechanical breakdown or malfunction of hardware

IMAGING FINDINGS

General Features
- Best diagnostic clue: Fractured or malpositioned metallic implant
- Location: Any spinal segment where instrumentations occur

Radiographic Findings
- Radiography
  - Cervical spine
    - Loose cannulated screw bridging type II odontoid fracture
    - Broken, extruded screw
    - Fractured, ventrally displaced plate
    - Dislodged allograft
    - Broken, detached posterior cervical wire
  - Thoracolumbar and lumbosacral spine
    - Broken sublaminar or subpars wire
    - Bent, loose, or fractured pedicle screw

- Disengaged hook
- Broken, dislodged rod
- Intervertebral cage/allograft migration
  - Pseudoarthrosis
    - Lucency between bone graft and adjacent vertebra
    - Sclerosis and rounding of unfused bones
  - Development or progression of vertebral malalignment
- Fluoroscopy
  - Pseudoarthrosis on flexion/extension views
    - 4 mm of translation or > 10° of angular motion between adjacent vertebrae
    - Up to 3 mm of translation considered normal

CT Findings
- Bone CT
  - Peri-implant lucency (suggests loosening)
  - Over-extension beyond posterior vertebral cortex by cervical bicortical screws
  - Medial cortex penetration by suboptimally placed lumbar pedicle screw
  - Occult osseous fractures
  - Osseous (non)union
    - Pseudoarthrosis

MR Findings
- MRI generally does not depict hardware location or integrity well

DDx: Types of Implant Failure

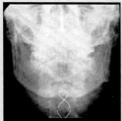

Broken Wire

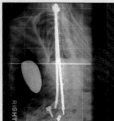

Dislodged Rods

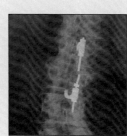

Fractured Rod

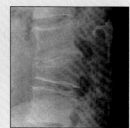

Fractured Rod

HARDWARE FAILURE

Key Facts

Terminology
- Implant or metal failure
- Mechanical breakdown or malfunction of hardware

Imaging Findings
- Best diagnostic clue: Fractured or malpositioned metallic implant
- Broken, extruded screw
- Fractured, ventrally displaced plate
- Bent, loose, or fractured pedicle screw
- Broken, dislodged rod
- Intervertebral cage/allograft migration
- Pseudoarthrosis on flexion/extension views
- 4 mm of translation or > 10° of angular motion between adjacent vertebrae
- Peri-implant lucency (suggests loosening)

- Plain films excellent in evaluating vertebral alignment, hardware integrity, fusion status
- MRI to identify soft tissue complications or spinal cord injury

Pathology
- 2-45% reoperation rate for implant failure

Clinical Issues
- Osseous fusion may be expected even if hardware fails

Diagnostic Checklist
- Important not only to evaluate hardware failure but also to look for complicating instability or osseous fracture

---

  - ○ Ineffective with extensive artifact from steel hardware
  - ○ Titanium hardware produces less artifact
- MRI useful for demonstrating impact on surrounding soft tissue and cord morphology

Nuclear Medicine Findings
- Bone Scan
  - ○ Increased uptake at fusion site suggests non-union
    - Nonspecific until one year after surgery

Other Modality Findings
- Anterior-posterior tomogram
  - ○ Lucency between sclerotic edges of bones suggests pseudoarthrosis

Imaging Recommendations
- Best imaging tool
  - ○ Plain films excellent in evaluating vertebral alignment, hardware integrity, fusion status
    - Cost-effective
    - Abnormalities frequently detected
    - Flexion extension views if hardware failure present
  - ○ CT evaluation if implant breakage suspected, but not definitive on radiography
    - Especially with complex constructs and/or in osteopenic patients
    - Sagittal and coronal reformation
  - ○ MRI to identify soft tissue complications or spinal cord injury
- Protocol advice
  - ○ MR techniques to minimize susceptibility artifact
    - Low magnetic field strength
    - Avoid gradient-echo sequences
    - Fast spin echo technique
    - Higher receiver bandwidths
    - Shorter TE
    - Smaller voxel size
    - Frequency encoding parallel to axis of hardware
  - ○ Increasing kilovolt peaks/milliamperes to reduce beam hardening on CT

DIFFERENTIAL DIAGNOSIS

None

PATHOLOGY

General Features
- General path comments
  - ○ Hardware intended to stabilize fusion construct while awaiting successful osseous fusion
    - All hardware eventually fails if fusion does not occur in timely fashion
    - Fusion rate improved with direct current electrical stimulation
    - Fusion occurs after 6-9 months, up to 18 months
  - ○ Fibrous union may provide satisfactory stability in absence of radiographic osseous fusion
    - Best confirmed with dynamic flexion extension views
- Genetics: No genetic predisposition
- Etiology
  - ○ Excessive stress loading on implant
    - Implant malpositioning at surgery
    - Gross spinal instability
    - Failed fusion with pseudoarthrosis
  - ○ Poor bone quality
    - Peri-implant bone resorption
    - Osteoporosis
    - Osteomyelitis
    - Residual or recurrent neoplasm
  - ○ Multi-segmental constructs
  - ○ Unconstrained cervical fusion plates: Orozco, Casper
    - Screw not locked to plate
    - Risk of screw extrusion
  - ○ Risks of pseudoarthrosis
    - Old age
    - Smoking
    - Obesity
    - Diabetes
    - Multiple spine surgeries
    - Multilevel fusions
    - ≥ Grade III anterolisthesis

HARDWARE FAILURE

- Epidemiology
  - 2-45% reoperation rate for implant failure
  - Hardware failure in scoliosis surgery
    - 31% with anterior approach
    - 1% with posterior approach
  - Unconstrained cervical fusion system
    - 22-46% failure rate vs. 18% in constrained system
  - Lumbar fusion with unconstrained pedicle screw system
    - 22% failure rate
    - 75% due to pseudoarthrosis
- Associated abnormalities
  - Pseudoarthrosis
  - Spinal instability
  - Osseous fractures
  - Dural laceration
  - Nerve injury

CLINICAL ISSUES

Presentation
- Most common signs/symptoms
  - May be incidental finding
  - Other signs/symptoms
    - Pain
    - Tenderness
    - Weakness
    - Paresthesia
    - Radiculopathy
- Clinical profile
  - Hardware failure in early post-operative period
    - Indication of continued gross spinal instability
  - Development or progression of neurologic symptoms
    - Osseous nonunion and/or hardware failure should be suspected

Demographics
- Age: Mostly adults
- Gender: No sex predilection

Natural History & Prognosis
- Osseous fusion may be expected even if hardware fails
  - Broken hardware need not be removed if spine clinically, radiographically stable
- Fibrous union without radiographic osseous fusion may be satisfactory
  - Best demonstrated on dynamic flexion extension views
- Repeat surgical fusion may be necessary
  - Especially if hardware failure occurs early

Treatment
- Conservative observation
- Surgical revision to prevent nonunion and instability

DIAGNOSTIC CHECKLIST

Consider
- Consulting references describing expected hardware appearance

Image Interpretation Pearls
- Important not only to evaluate hardware failure but also to look for complicating instability or osseous fracture
- Important to consider original indication for fusion in suspected implant failure
  - Failed fusion for trauma may indicate unsuspected ligamentous injury
  - Failed fusion for neoplasm may indicate tumor recurrence or progression

SELECTED REFERENCES

1. Singh SK et al: Occipitocervical reconstruction with the Ohio Medical Instruments Loop: results of a multicenter evaluation in 30 cases. J Neurosurg. 98(3 Suppl):239-46, 2003
2. Bagchi K et al: Hardware complications in scoliosis surgery. Pediatr Radiol. 32(7):465-75, 2002
3. Deckey JE et al: Loss of sagittal plane correction after removal of spinal implants. Spine. 25(19):2453-60, 2000
4. Glassman SD et al: The durability of small-diameter rods in lumbar spinal fusion. J Spinal Disord. 13(2):165-7, 2000
5. Apfelbaum RI et al: Direct anterior screw fixation for recent and remote odontoid fractures. J Neurosurg 93(2 Suppl): 227-36, 2000
6. Geiger F et al: Complications of scoliosis surgery in children with myelomeningocele. Eur Spine J. 8(1):22-6, 1999
7. Wetzel FT et al: Hardware failure in an unconstrained lumbar pedicle screw system. A 2-year follow-up study. Spine. 24(11):1138-43, 1999
8. Masferrer R et al: Efficacy of pedicle screw fixation in the treatment of spinal instability and failed back surgery: a 5-year review. J Neurosurg. 89(3):371-7, 1998
9. Lowery GL et al: The significance of hardware failure in anterior cervical plate fixation. Patients with 2- to 7-year follow-up. Spine. 15;23(2):181-6; discussion 186-7, 1998
10. Wellman BJ et al: Complications of posterior articular mass plate fixation of the subaxial cervical spine in 43 consecutive patients. Spine. 23(2):193-200, 1998
11. Shapiro SA et al: Spinal instrumentation with a low complication rate. Surg Neurol. 48(6):566-74, 1997
12. Paramore CG et al: Radiographic and clinical follow-up review of Caspar plates in 49 patients. J Neurosurg. 84(6):957-61, 1996
13. Blumenthal S et al: Complications of the Wiltse Pedicle Screw Fixation System. Spine. 18(13):1867-71, 1993
14. Slone RM et al: Spinal fixation. Part 3. Complications of spinal instrumentation. Radiographics. 13(4):797-816, 1993
15. Guidera KJ et al: Cotrel-Dubousset instrumentation. Results in 52 patients. Spine. 18(4):427-31, 1993
16. McLain RF et al: Early failure of short-segment pedicle instrumentation for thoracolumbar fractures. A preliminary report. J Bone Joint Surg Am. 75(2):162-7, 1993
17. Wilkinson RH et al: Radiographic evaluation of the spine after surgical correction of scoliosis. AJR Am J Roentgenol. 133(4):703-9, 1979

HARDWARE FAILURE

IMAGE GALLERY

Typical

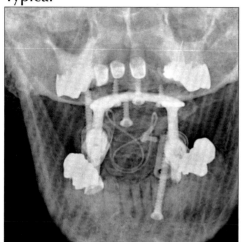 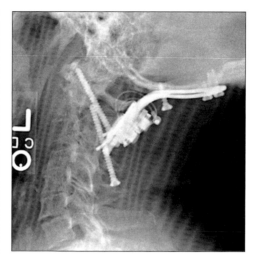

(Left) Anteroposterior radiography in a patient with C0-2 fusion shows asymmetric screw placement. *(Right)* Lateral radiography demonstrates dorsal extrusion of left transarticular screw from C1 and C2 lateral masses.

Typical

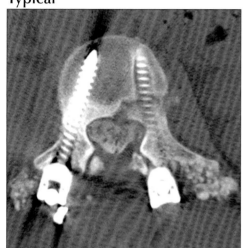 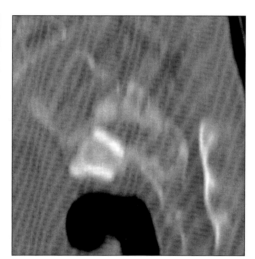

(Left) Axial bone CT through lumbar spine demonstrates subtle lucency medial to the left pedicle screw. A fracture is present at the base of left pedicle due to failed hardware. *(Right)* Axial bone CT with sagittal reformation through lumbosacral spine shows ventral extrusion of an intervertebral allograft at L5-S1.

Typical

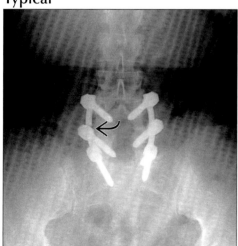 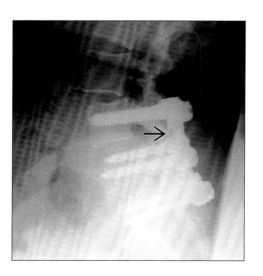

(Left) Anteroposterior radiography of lumbosacral spine in a patient with fusion from L4-S1 shows subtle discontinuity in the right rod (arrow). *(Right)* Lateral radiography confirms the rod fracture (arrow) with slight overlap of its ends.

ACCELERATED DEGENERATION

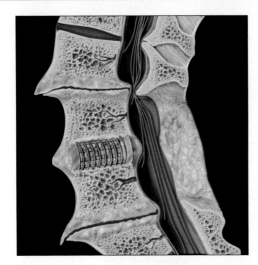

Sagittal graphic shows solid L4-5 interbody fusion and laminectomy. Severe disc degeneration at L3-4 with spondylolisthesis, loss of disc height, osteophytes and central stenosis.

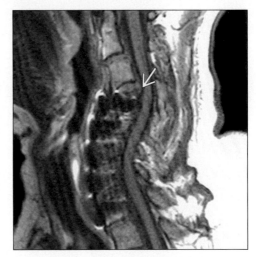

Sagittal T1WI MR shows patient post C4-T1 fusion with anterior plate/screws. There is herniation above fusion site at C3-4 (arrow) with impingement upon cord, and increased kyphosis.

TERMINOLOGY

Abbreviations and Synonyms
- Spinal "transitional" degenerative syndrome, accelerated segmental degeneration

Definitions
- Accelerated degeneration of disc space/facets at level(s) adjacent to surgical fusion

IMAGING FINDINGS

General Features
- Best diagnostic clue
  - Degenerative disc/facet changes directly above or below fusion
  - Also occurs adjacent to congenital segmentation anomalies
- Location: Degenerative disc/facet changes directly adjacent to fused vertebra
- Size: Varies from mild to severe disc degenerative change with deformity
- Morphology: Disc degenerative change related to disc, endplates, facets

Radiographic Findings
- Radiography

- Plain films show surgical change with adjacent segment degenerative changes
- Flexion/extension views for definition of instability
- Fluoroscopy: May show increased motion at degenerated level adjacent to fused segment
- Myelography
  - Nonspecific extradural disease (stenosis, herniation) at transitional level
  - May show myelographic block to contrast material with severe disease

CT Findings
- NECT
  - Findings of degenerative disc disease at transitional level
    - Loss of disc space height
    - Disc vacuum phenomenon
    - Bony endplate eburnation
    - Osteophyte
    - Facet degenerative arthropathy with foraminal stenosis
    - Anterolisthesis or retrolisthesis
    - Disc bulge, protrusion, extrusion
    - Central canal stenosis

MR Findings
- T1WI
  - Typical findings seen in degenerative disc and facet disease

DDx: T1 Hypointense Endplates

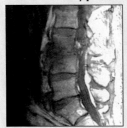

Infection

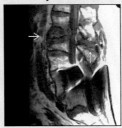

Pseudoarthosis

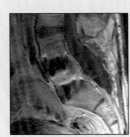

Metal Fusion Cages

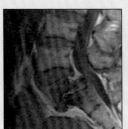

Instability

ACCELERATED DEGENERATION

Key Facts

Terminology
- Spinal "transitional" degenerative syndrome, accelerated segmental degeneration
- Accelerated degeneration of disc space/facets at level(s) adjacent to surgical fusion

Imaging Findings
- Also occurs adjacent to congenital segmentation anomalies

Pathology
- Produced by aberrant biophysical stresses from altered normal spinal motion
- Wolff law; living tissue responds to chronic changes in stresses & strains

- Increased mobility in these remaining mobile segments is hypothesized to cause accelerated degenerative pathologic changes
- Segmental motion above or below fusion increases
- Intradiscal pressure above or below fusion increases
- Lower lumbar fusions show more stress on adjacent levels than higher lumbar fusions

Clinical Issues
- May be asymptomatic
- Mechanical pain
- Radicular or myelopathic symptoms referable to level(s) above or below a surgical fusion
- Difficult to distinguish natural history of disc degeneration from accelerated degeneration following fusion

---

- Loss of disc space height
- Low signal foci within disc: Vacuum phenomena and/or calcification
- May show degenerative type I, II endplate changes
- Disc bulge, herniation
- Central and/or foraminal stenosis
- Facet degenerative arthropathy
- Malalignment
- T2WI
  - Typical findings seen in degenerative disc & facet disease
    - Loss of signal within intervertebral disc
    - Degenerative type I, II endplate changes
- STIR: High signal marrow edema with type I endplate changes at transitional level
- T1 C+
  - Adjacent vertebral body endplates may show marked enhancement with type I endplate changes
  - Linear enhancement within intervertebral disc due to degeneration
    - No endplate destruction

Nuclear Medicine Findings
- Bone Scan: Increased uptake related to disc degeneration
- PET
  - Hypometabolic as with degenerative disc disease
  - Hypermetabolic with disc space infection/osteomyelitis
  - PET accurate and specific to define infection from degenerative endplate changes

Imaging Recommendations
- Plain films most economical way to demonstrate presence of adjacent segment degenerative changes and to serially follow for progression
- MRI best identifies soft tissue abnormalities that are occult on plain film
  - Disc herniation, ligamentum flavum laxity, synovial proliferation

DIFFERENTIAL DIAGNOSIS

Disc space infection
- Low signal involving adjacent endplates similar to type I degenerative change
- Endplate destruction
- Hyperintense intervertebral disc on T2WI
- ± Paravertebral or epidural soft tissue phlegmon/abscess

Pseudoarthrosis
- Accelerated degenerative change may progress to pseudoarthrosis with abnormal motion, involvement of posterior elements/ligaments
- Abnormal horizontal signal extends through disc to posterior elements or interspinous ligament

Spondylolysis with spondylolisthesis
- Instability and abnormal biomechanics of fusion site may lead to stress fractures at transitional level
- Diagnosis rests with presence or absence of prior fusion, instrumentation, and level of listhesis

Normal post-operative changes
- Low signal from interbody fusion cages, with typical spatial mismapping of signal

PATHOLOGY

General Features
- General path comments
  - Not all patients at risk demonstrate accelerated degeneration
  - Pathological findings are typical of degenerative disc and facet disease
- Etiology
  - Produced by aberrant biophysical stresses from altered normal spinal motion
    - Wolff law; living tissue responds to chronic changes in stresses & strains
  - Solid fusion alters biomechanics at adjacent mobile levels

ACCELERATED DEGENERATION

- ○ Increased mobility in these remaining mobile segments is hypothesized to cause accelerated degenerative pathologic changes
  - Segmental motion above or below fusion increases
  - Intradiscal pressure above or below fusion increases
- ○ More common with multilevel fusion, but also seen following single level fusion
  - Lower lumbar fusions show more stress on adjacent levels than higher lumbar fusions
- • Epidemiology
  - ○ More common after surgical fusion than following decompression only
  - ○ Bertolotti syndrome refers to association of back pain with lumbosacral transitional vertebrae
    - Disc bulge/herniation 9x more common at interspace immediately above transitional vertebra than at any other level

Gross Pathologic & Surgical Features
- • Disc space height loss, disc bulge or herniation, central stenosis, facet osteoarthritic change

Microscopic Features
- • Disc dehydration, fissuring, anular disruption, disc protrusion or extrusion

Staging, Grading or Classification Criteria
- • Spondylolisthesis may be graded I-IV

CLINICAL ISSUES

Presentation
- • Most common signs/symptoms
  - ○ May be asymptomatic
  - ○ Mechanical pain
  - ○ Radicular or myelopathic symptoms referable to level(s) above or below a surgical fusion
  - ○ Herniation above site of fusion < 2%
- • Clinical profile: Prior surgical fusion, with new and progressing pain in different distribution than pre-operative pain

Demographics
- • Age: Adult
- • Gender: M = F

Natural History & Prognosis
- • Difficult to distinguish natural history of disc degeneration from accelerated degeneration following fusion
- • Progressively worsens
  - ○ Highly variable course
- • Decreased signal within adjacent discs on T2WI may occur as early as 12 months following fusion
- • Below scoliosis fusion chance of herniation up to 34%, chance of disc signal abnormality 50%

Treatment
- • Surgical decompression and fusion at adjacent symptomatic levels

DIAGNOSTIC CHECKLIST

Consider
- • Pseudoarthrosis if extensive signal abnormality involving anterior and posterior elements in a horizontal fashion

Image Interpretation Pearls
- • Presence of prior surgical fusion, instrumentation
- • Look for transitional lumbosacral vertebral body

SELECTED REFERENCES

1. Polikeit A et al: Factors influencing stresses in the lumbar spine after the insertion of intervertebral cages: finite element analysis. Eur Spine J. 12(4):413-20, 2003
2. Eck JC et al: Biomechanical study on the effect of cervical spine fusion on adjacent-level intradiscal pressure and segmental motion. Spine. 27(22):2431-4, 2002
3. Gertzbein SD et al: Disc herniation after lumbar fusion. Spine. 27(16):E373-6, 2002
4. Iseda T et al: Serial changes in signal intensities of the adjacent discs on T2-weighted sagittal images after surgical treatment of cervical spondylosis: anterior interbody fusion versus expansive laminoplasty. Acta Neurochir (Wien). 143(7):707-10, 2001
5. Miyakoshi N et al: Outcome of one-level posterior lumbar interbody fusion for spondylolisthesis and postoperative intervertebral disc degeneration adjacent to the fusion. Spine. 25(14):1837-42, 2000
6. Maiman DJ et al: Biomechanical effect of anterior cervical spine fusion on adjacent segments. Biomed Mater Eng. 9(1):27-38, 1999
7. Farcy JP: Review of surgical cases which have deteriorated over time. Bull Acad Natl Med 183(4): 775-82, 1999
8. Eck JC et al: Adjacent-segment degeneration after lumbar fusion: a review of clinical, biomechanical, and radiologic studies. Am J Orthop 28(6): 336-40, 1999
9. Hambly MF et al: The transition zone above a lumbosacral fusion. Spine. 23(16):1785-92, 1998
10. Balderston RA et al: Magnetic resonance imaging analysis of lumbar disc changes below scoliosis fusions. A prospective study. Spine. 23(1):54-8; discussion 59, 1998
11. Chow DH et al: Effects of short anterior lumbar interbody fusion on biomechanics of neighboring unfused segments. Spine. 21(5):549-55, 1996
12. Wu W et al: Degenerative changes following anterior cervical discectomy and fusion evaluated by fast spin-echo MR imaging. Acta Radiol 37(5): 614-7, 1996
13. Penta M et al: Magnetic resonance imaging assessment of disc degeneration 10 years after anterior lumbar interbody fusion. Spine. 20(6):743-7, 1995
14. Kim YE et al: Effect of disc degeneration at one level on the adjacent level in axial mode. Spine. 16(3):331-5, 1991
15. Dennis S et al: Comparison of disc space heights after anterior lumbar interbody fusion. Spine. 14(8):876-8, 1989
16. Elster AD: Bertolotti's syndrome revisited. Transitional vertebrae of the lumbar spine. Spine. 14(12):1373-7, 1989
17. Lee CK: Accelerated degeneration of the segment adjacent to a lumbar fusion. Spine. 13(3):375-7, 1988
18. Kurowski P et al: The relationship of degeneration of the intervertebral disc to mechanical loading conditions on lumbar vertebrae. Spine. 11(7):726-31, 1986
19. Lin PM et al: Posterior lumbar interbody fusion. Clin Orthop. (180):154-68, 1983

IMAGE GALLERY

Typical

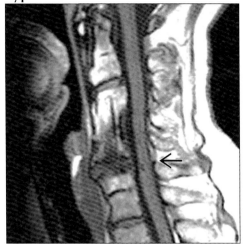 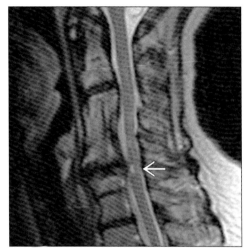

(Left) Sagittal T1WI MR shows patient post C3-5 fusion with graft. There is degeneration of C5-6 with central stenosis (arrow). Congenital fusion of C6-7 further increases biomechanical stress on C5-6. *(Right)* Sagittal T2WI MR shows patient post fusion of C3-5. Degeneration at C5-6 with central stenosis and narrowed subarachnoid space. Hyperintensity within cervical cord is due to myelomalacia (arrow).

Typical

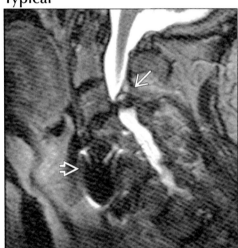 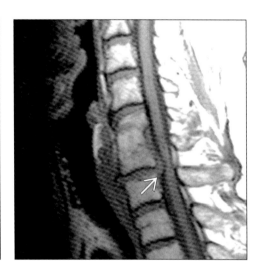

(Left) Sagittal T2WI MR shows patient post C4-7 fusion with anterior plating giving low signal artifact (open arrow). There is a large synovial cyst showing central hyperintensity at C3-4 level (arrow). *(Right)* Sagittal T1WI MR shows a solid fusion at C5-6 with normal fatty marrow signal. There is disc degeneration at C6-7 with decreased disc height, and large disc extrusion compressing cord (arrow).

Typical

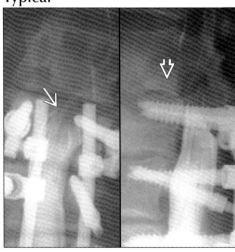 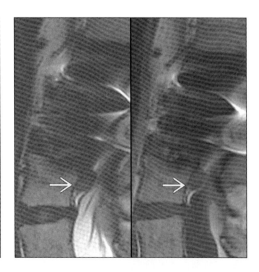

(Left) Anteroposterior myelography (L side) shows block to contrast at L1-2 (arrow) at upper margin of posterior fusion. Lateral view (R side) shows contrast block, & severe L1-2 degeneration (open arrow). *(Right)* Sagittal T2WI MR (L side), and T1WI C+ (R side) with lumbar pedicle screws giving artifact. There is peripheral enhancing disc extrusion (arrows) below fusion site with thecal sac compression.

POST-LAMINECTOMY SPONDYLOLISTHESIS

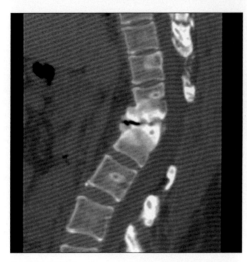

Sagittal NECT reformat shows increased kyphotic deformity, pseudoarthrosis at thoracolumbar junction following multilevel laminectomy for intramedullary ependymoma.

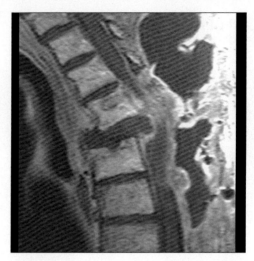

Sagittal T1WI MR shows upper thoracic body collapse, severe retrolisthesis with was progressive following multilevel laminectomy. There is a large post-operative pseudomeningocele.

TERMINOLOGY

Abbreviations and Synonyms
- Iatrogenic instability, postsurgical instability

Definitions
- Post-operative loss of spine motion segment stiffness, where applied force produces greater displacement than normal, with pain/deformity

IMAGING FINDINGS

General Features
- Best diagnostic clue: New post-operative deformity which increases with motion, and increases over time
- Location: Any spinal motion segment, most common involving cervical spine in children
- Size: Displacement may vary from few mm to width of vertebral body
- Morphology: Displacement of vertebral body with respect to adjacent body

Radiographic Findings
- Radiography
  - Various parameters used for degenerative instability by plain films
    - Dynamic slip > 3 mm in flexion/extension
    - Static slip of 4.5 mm or greater
    - Angulation > 10-15° suggests need for surgical intervention
- Fluoroscopy: Increased motion with flexion/extension or translation

CT Findings
- NECT: Nonspecific post-operative changes with malalignment

MR Findings
- T1WI: Anterolisthesis, retrolisthesis, lateral translation
- T2WI: Loss of disc signal, disc space height in adult with disc degeneration
- T1 C+: In adult, nonspecific enhancement of disc due to degenerative disc disease

Imaging Recommendations
- Best imaging tool: Flexion/extension plain films

DIFFERENTIAL DIAGNOSIS

Infection
- Endplate destruction, disc T2 hyperintensity

Tumor
- Enhancing soft tissue mass destroying vertebral body/posterior elements

DDx: Causes of Instability

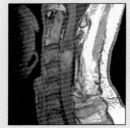

Tumor

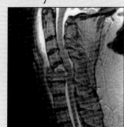

Infection

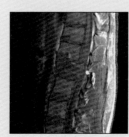

Trauma

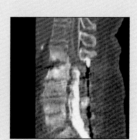

Disc Degeneration

Key Facts

Terminology
- Post-operative loss of spine motion segment stiffness, where applied force produces greater displacement than normal, with pain/deformity

Imaging Findings
- Best diagnostic clue: New post-operative deformity which increases with motion, and increases over time

Pathology
- Predisposing factors for post-operative instability
- Children > adults
- No preoperative lordosis in cervical spine
- Surgical disruption of facets
- C2 laminectomy ± increased risk
- More laminectomy levels ± increased risk

Degenerative instability
- Marked degenerative disc disease with intact endplates, no soft tissue mass

Isthmic spondylolisthesis
- Lysis involving pars interarticularis
- Progressive L5-S1 deformity in child (rarely unstable in adults)

Treatment
- Prophylactic fusion considered for patients at risk of post-operative kyphosis
  - Prevention of deformity easier than treatment
  - Facet fusion and lateral mass fixation of cervical spine
- Lower rate of cervical kyphotic deformity with laminoplasty compared to laminectomy

PATHOLOGY

General Features
- General path comments
  - Resection of ≥ 50% of both facets alters segmental stiffness
  - Plain films show new or worsening segmental motion
- Etiology
  - Post-operative alteration in spinal biomechanics
  - Postlaminectomy cervical kyphosis > 40% in children
  - Adult change in alignment > 20%, < 40% (but may not be clinically significant)
- Epidemiology
  - Predisposing factors for post-operative instability
    - Children > adults
    - No preoperative lordosis in cervical spine
    - Surgical disruption of facets
    - C2 laminectomy ± increased risk
    - More laminectomy levels ± increased risk

CLINICAL ISSUES

Presentation
- Most common signs/symptoms: Neck, back pain with later appearance of new neurologic symptoms
- Clinical profile: Early good operative result with progressive axial spine pain, new neurologic symptoms

Demographics
- Age: Children and adults
- Gender: No gender predilection

Natural History & Prognosis
- Generally progressive

SELECTED REFERENCES

1. Papagelopoulos PJ et al: Spinal column deformity and instability after lumbar or thoracolumbar laminectomy for intraspinal tumors in children and young adults. Spine. 22(4):442-51, 1997
2. Mullin BB et al: The effect of postlaminectomy spinal instability on the outcome of lumbar spinal stenosis patients. J Spinal Disord. 9(2):107-16, 1996
3. An HS et al: Spinal disorders at the cervicothoracic junction. Spine. 19(22):2557-64, 1994
4. Stromqvist B: Postlaminectomy problems with reference to spinal fusion. Acta Orthop Scand Suppl. 251:87-9, 1993
5. Butler JC et al: Postlaminectomy kyphosis. Causes and surgical management. Orthop Clin North Am. 23(3):505-11, 1992
6. Sano S et al: Unstable lumbar spine without hypermobility in postlaminectomy cases. Mechanism of symptoms and effect of spinal fusion with and without spinal instrumentation. Spine. 15(11):1190-7, 1990

IMAGE GALLERY

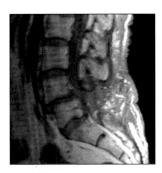 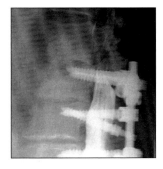

(Left) Sagittal T1WI MR shows spondylolisthesis of L4 on L5 following laminectomy, with disc degeneration. *(Right)* Sagittal myelography shows anterolisthesis of vertebral body at upper margin of lumbar fusion with accelerated disc degeneration.

PERIDURAL FIBROSIS

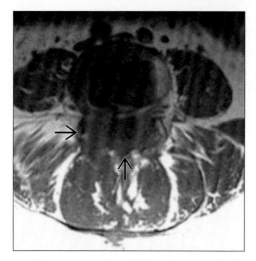

Axial T1WI MR in patient following posterior lumbar interbody fusion (PLIF) shows extensive low signal surrounding thecal sac (arrows). Artifact present in disc space from fusion cages.

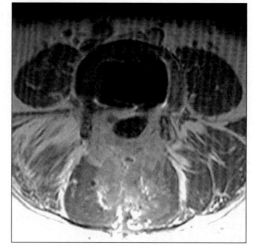

Axial T1 C+ MR in same patient following posterior lumbar interbody fusion (PLIF) shows diffuse enhancement of extensive epidural fibrosis with minimal thecal sac deformity.

TERMINOLOGY

Abbreviations and Synonyms
- Epidural fibrosis

Definitions
- Scar formation within epidural space after lumbar surgery
- Part of failed back surgery syndrome (FBSS)

IMAGING FINDINGS

General Features
- Best diagnostic clue: Infiltration of epidural/perineural fat by enhancing soft tissue density (intensity)
- Location: Epidural space at operative level
- Size: Few mm to 1-2 cm
- Morphology: Smooth marginated soft tissue, usually without mass effect

Radiographic Findings
- Radiography: Nonspecific post-operative changes
- Myelography: Nonspecific extradural defect on contrast column

CT Findings
- NECT: Nonspecific epidural soft tissue attenuation
- CECT
  - Epidural soft tissue density
    - Enhances after intravenous contrast

MR Findings
- T1WI
  - Peridural soft tissue intensity
    - Isointense on T1WI
    - Often surrounds nerve root
    - Occasionally can be mass-like
  - Combination of disc + scar may be present
  - Post-surgical changes in posterior elements
  - Can be associated with ipsilateral enlargement of exiting root sleeve (cicatrization)
- T2WI
  - Variable signal intensity on T2WI
  - Typically slightly increased in signal relative to disc herniation
- T1 C+
  - Immediate homogeneous post-contrast enhancement
    - Enhancement may persist for years after
    - Pre- and post-gadolinium enhanced MRI approximately 96% accurate in differentiating peridural fibrosis from disc herniation
  - Involved nerve root may show post-gadolinium enhancement

DDx: Epidural Disease

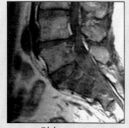

Phlegmon

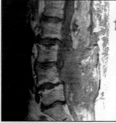

Postop Hemorrhage

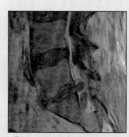

Recurrent Herniation

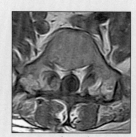

Arachnoiditis

PERIDURAL FIBROSIS

Key Facts

Terminology
- Scar formation within epidural space after lumbar surgery
- Part of failed back surgery syndrome (FBSS)

Top Differential Diagnoses
- Recurrent disc herniation
- Epidural abscess/phlegmon
- Pseudomeningocele
- Post-operative hemorrhage
- Arachnoiditis

Pathology
- Post-operative scarring is part of normal reparative mechanism
- May be asymptomatic; contribution to clinical symptoms controversial

- Extent of fibrosis possibly related to extent of surgical dissection
- Scar tissue compresses, irritates, puts abnormal traction on nerve roots
- Estimated 1 million spinal operations worldwide each year
- Peridural fibrosis implicated in 3-5% of cases as cause of FBSS

Clinical Issues
- Low back or radicular pain
- Numbness
- Weakness
- Worse reoperative success rates for only epidural fibrosis found at surgery, without disc herniation

Imaging Recommendations
- Fat suppression of T1WI (pre- and post-gadolinium) may increase sensitivity in detecting peridural fibrosis and differentiating fibrosis from disc

DIFFERENTIAL DIAGNOSIS

Recurrent disc herniation
- No central enhancement when imaged early after intravenous gadolinium
  - Peripheral enhancement common
- Delayed central enhancement if imaged after 30 minutes or later
  - Diffusion of contrast into disc

Epidural abscess/phlegmon
- May show homogeneous enhancement within epidural space
- Abscess shows peripheral enhancement
- Typical clinical and laboratory findings of infection (elevated sedimentation rate, C-reactive protein)

Pseudomeningocele
- CSF collection within dorsal soft tissues arising out of surgical bed

Post-operative hemorrhage
- Intermediate T1 signal if acute to subacute age
- Low T2 signal mass within epidural space at operative site
- Mass effect upon thecal sac/roots

Arachnoiditis
- Peripheral intradural clumping of roots in type II arachnoiditis may extend contiguous to epidural fibrosis
- May mimic epidural disease

PATHOLOGY

General Features
- General path comments
  - Post-operative scarring is part of normal reparative mechanism
  - May be asymptomatic; contribution to clinical symptoms controversial
  - Peridural fibrosis
    - Up to one-quarter of all FBSS cases
    - Most patients with some degree of fibrosis are asymptomatic
    - Whether a source of recurrent pain is still controversial
    - One prospective multicenter study (1996) shows that patients with extensive peridural fibrosis are 3.2 times more likely to have recurrent radicular pain than those with less extensive scarring
- Genetics: None
- Etiology
  - Extent of fibrosis possibly related to extent of surgical dissection
  - The degree of host inflammatory response also plays a role
  - Scar tissue compresses, irritates, puts abnormal traction on nerve roots
    - Blood supply compromised
    - Axoplasmic transport interrupted
- Epidemiology
  - Estimated 1 million spinal operations worldwide each year
    - 3/4 involve decompression of lumbar roots or cauda equina
    - Peridural fibrosis implicated in 3-5% of cases as cause of FBSS
- Associated abnormalities: Look for evidence of arachnoiditis

Gross Pathologic & Surgical Features
- Scar tissue surrounding thecal sac and exiting roots at operative level

PERIDURAL FIBROSIS

Microscopic Features

- Invasion of post-operative hematoma by dense fibrous tissue originating within deep surface of paravertebral musculature
- Fibrous tissue can extend to thecal sac, adhere to dura and roots

CLINICAL ISSUES

Presentation

- Most common signs/symptoms
  - Low back or radicular pain
  - Numbness
  - Weakness
  - 10% rate of recurrent back/radicular pain 6 months after discectomy
  - Causes of recurrent pain
    - Recurrent disc herniation
    - New herniation at another level
    - Peridural fibrosis
- Clinical profile: Adult with gradual onset low back pain following initially successful disc surgery

Demographics

- Age: Adult
- Gender: M = F

Natural History & Prognosis

- Chronic, indolent course of FBSS
- 30-35% success rate for repeat surgery (range 12-100%)
- Worse reoperative success rates for only epidural fibrosis found at surgery, without disc herniation
- 50-70% success rate for spinal cord stimulation

Treatment

- Symptomatic treatment with physical therapy, wide variety of pain medication
- Periradicular injection of corticosteroids and local anesthetics
- Spinal cord stimulation by implanted electrodes
- Surgical lysis of scar tissue rarely performed

DIAGNOSTIC CHECKLIST

Consider

- Identification of only epidural fibrosis in FBSS patient is contraindication to reoperation, yields poor reoperative result
- Best reoperative result in patients with herniation at new level
- Intermediate operative success results in patients with new herniation at previously operated level, better than scar only, worse than disc at non-operative level

Image Interpretation Pearls

- Classic imaging appearance: Enhancing epidural soft tissue surrounding the typically enlarged nerve root
- Primary function of imaging is to exclude recurrent disc herniation or other cause of FBSS (e.g., conus/filum tumor)

SELECTED REFERENCES

1. Gerszten PC et al: Low-dose radiotherapy for the inhibition of peridural fibrosis after reexploratory nerve root decompression for postlaminectomy syndrome. J Neurosurg. 99(3 Suppl):271-7, 2003
2. Van Goethem JW et al: Review article: MRI of the postoperative lumbar spine. Neuroradiology. 44(9):723-39, 2002
3. Anderson SR: A rationale for the treatment algorithm of failed back surgery syndrome. Curr Rev Pain. 4(5):395-406, 2000
4. Anderson VC et al: Failed back surgery syndrome. Curr Rev Pain. 4(2):105-11, 2000
5. Coskun E et al: Relationships between epidural fibrosis, pain, disability, and psychological factors after lumbar disc surgery. Eur Spine J. 9(3):218-23, 2000
6. Pearce JM: Aspects of the failed back syndrome: role of litigation. Spinal Cord. 38(2):63-70, 2000
7. Samy Abdou M et al: Epidural fibrosis and the failed back surgery syndrome: history and physical findings. Neurol Res. 21 Suppl 1:S5-8, 1999
8. Devulder J et al: Spinal cord stimulation: a valuable treatment for chronic failed back surgery patients. J Pain Symptom Manage. 13(5):296-301, 1997
9. Robertson JT: Role of peridural fibrosis in the failed back: a review. Eur Spine J. 5 Suppl 1:S2-6, 1996
10. Van Goethem JW et al: MRI after successful lumbar discectomy. Neuroradiology. 38 Suppl 1:S90-6, 1996
11. Fritsch EW et al: The failed back surgery syndrome: reasons, intraoperative findings, and long-term results: a report of 182 operative treatments. Spine. 21(5):626-33, 1996
12. Ross JS et al: Association between peridural scar and recurrent radicular pain after lumbar discectomy: Magnetic resonance evaluation. Neurosurgery 38: 855-61, 1996
13. Georgy BA et al: Fat-suppression contrast-enhanced MRI in the failed back surgery syndrome: a prospective study. Neuroradiology. 37(1):51-7, 1995
14. Kim SS et al: Revision surgery for failed back surgery syndrome. Spine. 17(8):957-60, 1992
15. North RB et al: Failed back surgery syndrome: 5-year follow-up in 102 patients undergoing repeated operation. Neurosurgery. 28(5):685-90; discussion 690-1, 1991
16. Ross JS et al: MR imaging of the postoperative lumbar spine: assessment with gadopentetate dimeglumine. AJR Am J Roentgenol. 155(4):867-72, 1990
17. Bundschuh CV et al: Distinguishing between scar and recurrent herniated disk in postoperative patients: value of contrast-enhanced CT and MR imaging. AJNR Am J Neuroradiol. 11(5):949-58, 1990
18. Ross JS et al: MR imaging of the postoperative lumbar spine: assessment with gadopentetate dimeglumine. AJNR Am J Neuroradiol. 11(4):771-6, 1990
19. Djukic S et al: Magnetic resonance imaging of the postoperative lumbar spine. Radiol Clin North Am. 28(2):341-60, 1990
20. Hueftle MG et al: Lumbar spine: postoperative MR imaging with Gd-DTPA. Radiology 167: 817-24, 1988

IMAGE GALLERY

Typical

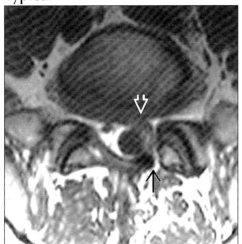
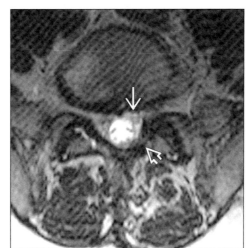

(Left) Axial T1WI MR shows small left hemilaminectomy site (arrow). Soft tissue signal surrounds the exiting left S1 root, without mass effect upon adjacent thecal sac (open arrow). *(Right)* Axial T2WI MR shows hemilaminectomy defect and absence of ligamentum flavum (open arrow). Epidural fibrosis surrounding left S1 root shows slight increased signal relative to adjacent disc (arrow).

Typical

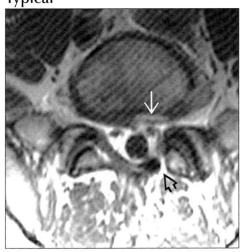
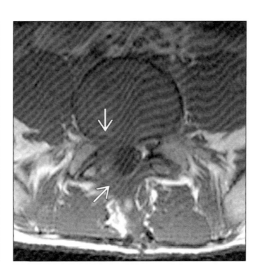

(Left) Axial T1 C+ MR shows left hemilaminectomy defect (open arrow). Small amount of epidural fibrosis surrounding left S1 root diffusely enhances, as does operative defect in posterior anulus (arrow). *(Right)* Axial T1WI MR shows right laminectomy defect, and extensive epidural fibrosis surrounding the right lateral and dorsal aspect of thecal sac, and exiting root (arrows).

Typical

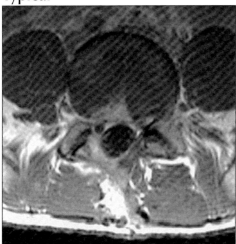
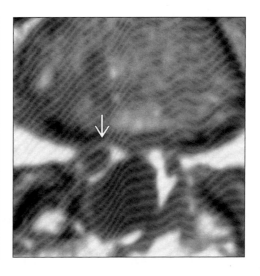

(Left) Axial T1 C+ MR shows right hemilaminectomy defect, and diffuse enhancement of epidural fibrosis surrounding the right lateral aspect of thecal sac. *(Right)* Axial T1 C+ MR shows right hemilaminectomy defect, and enlargement of exiting root sleeve on right, with peripheral enhancement due to scar cicatrization (arrow).

PSEUDOMENINGOCELE

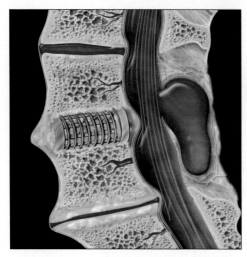

Sagittal graphic shows changes of L4-5 interbody fusion with cage. Large well-defined CSF collection extends into dorsal soft tissue from thecal sac, from site of operative dural tear.

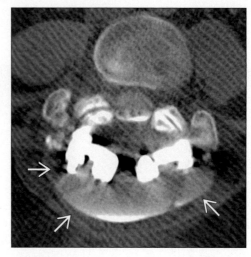

Axial CT post myelography shows contrast collection at laminectomy/fusion site in posterior soft tissues (arrows). There is incorporation of hardware into the collection.

TERMINOLOGY

Abbreviations and Synonyms
- Dural dehiscence, pseudocyst

Definitions
- Spinal cyst contiguous with thecal sac, not lined with meninges

IMAGING FINDINGS

General Features
- Best diagnostic clue: CSF filled spinal axis cyst with supportive post-operative or post-traumatic ancillary findings
- Location
  - Most common location is dorsal to thecal sac at lumbar laminectomy site
  - Rare reports of intraosseous location (lamina/spinous process)
- Size: 1 to > 10 cm
- Morphology: Round, lobulated CSF attenuation/signal collection

Radiographic Findings
- Radiography: Nonspecific post-operative changes, such as laminectomy defect
- Myelography

- Typical post-operative collection seen as round/lobulated contrast collection dorsal to thecal sac within subcutaneous tissues
  - +/- Ability to define precise point of communication with thecal sac
  - Note relationship to posterior fusion hardware; +/- incorporated into CSF collection
  - Note extension of contrast to skin surface
- Post-traumatic/post-surgical pseudomeningoceles usually devoid of neural elements
  - May see cord or nerve herniation into pseudomeningocele with severe dural laceration

CT Findings
- NECT
  - CSF density cyst adjacent to thecal sac
  - Post-operative pseudomeningocele cyst usually is oriented along operative approach
    - Dural connection is difficult to demonstrate without intrathecal contrast
  - Cervical root avulsions are anterolaterally oriented, contiguous with neural foramen, devoid of neural elements

MR Findings
- T1WI
  - CSF signal intensity cyst
    - Note relationship to posterior fusion hardware
    - +/- Incorporated into CSF collection

DDx: Posterior Soft Tissue Fluid Collections

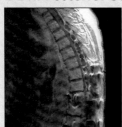
Epidural Abscess

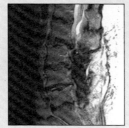
Hemorrhage

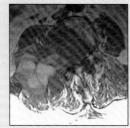
Osteosarcoma

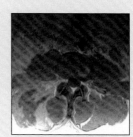
Rhabdomyolysis

PSEUDOMENINGOCELE

Key Facts

Terminology
- Dural dehiscence, pseudocyst
- Spinal cyst contiguous with thecal sac, not lined with meninges

Imaging Findings
- Best diagnostic clue: CSF filled spinal axis cyst with supportive post-operative or post-traumatic ancillary findings
- Most common location is dorsal to thecal sac at lumbar laminectomy site
- Fat-saturated T2WI best sequence to demonstrate pseudomeningocele and to localize dural communication
- Sagittal plane useful for diagnosis and to tailor thin section axial imaging for definitive localization

Top Differential Diagnoses
- Paraspinous abscess
- post-operative hematoma
- Soft tissue tumor
- Rhabdomyolysis

Pathology
- Epidemiology: 0.19 to 2% of patients undergoing lumbar laminectomies
- Reactive fibrous tissue forms cyst capsule

Clinical Issues
- Commonly asymptomatic
- Nonspecific back pain
- Occasionally extends superficially, palpable within subcutaneous tissues

---

- May be difficult to precisely define with presence of posterior fusion hardware/metal artifact
- T2WI: In post-operative cases, can frequently can identify thecal sac communication using axial and sagittal T2 weighted imaging
- DWI: CSF signal intensity lesion, with no restricted diffusion
- T1 C+
  - Does not enhance unless inflamed or infected; may see thin peripheral enhancement within 1 year of surgery
  - Spinal and intracranial dural thickening and enhancement in patients with symptomatic CSF hypotension

Ultrasonographic Findings
- Ultrasound - hypoechoic cyst; difficult to avoid bone shadow in adults

Other Modality Findings
- While radionuclide cisternography can show activity within pseudomeningoceles, generally CT/MR preferred for direct visualization

Imaging Recommendations
- Fat-saturated T2WI best sequence to demonstrate pseudomeningocele and to localize dural communication
- Sagittal plane useful for diagnosis and to tailor thin section axial imaging for definitive localization

DIFFERENTIAL DIAGNOSIS

Paraspinous abscess
- Clinical history of critical importance, with supportive lab values (sedimentation rate, C-reactive protein)
- May be indistinguishable from post-operative pseudomeningocele

post-operative hematoma
- Does not follow CSF signal on all pulse sequences
- T2* images show susceptibility artifact ("blooming")

Soft tissue tumor
- Cystic components of giant cell, aneurysmal bone cyst, osteosarcoma
- Easily distinguished from pseudomeningocele due to bone destruction, soft tissue component

Rhabdomyolysis
- Clinical/biochemical syndrome resulting from damage of integrity of skeletal muscle, with release of toxic muscle cell components into circulation
- Increased T2 signal within affected skeletal muscle group

True meningocele
- Lined with arachnoid
- Neurofibromatosis type 1, Marfan syndrome, homocystinuria, Ehlers-Danlos syndrome
- Does not have pertinent trauma or surgical history
- Often co-exists with dural dysplasia

Plexiform neurofibroma
- T2 hyperintense
  - Neurofibroma not as bright as CSF
- Avid contrast enhancement
- "Target sign" common

PATHOLOGY

General Features
- General path comments
  - CSF - containing cyst in contiguity with thecal sac
  - Not lined by meninges
  - Usually devoid of neural elements
  - In some cases neural elements may herniate into defect
- Genetics: None
- Etiology
  - Post-traumatic
    - Most commonly following cervical root avulsion
    - May also see with posterior element fractures + dural laceration
  - Post-surgical

PSEUDOMENINGOCELE

- ▪ Iatrogenic dural laceration with CSF leak
- ▪ May also see after dural graft following spinal tumor resection
- Epidemiology: 0.19 to 2% of patients undergoing lumbar laminectomies
- Associated abnormalities: May rarely show peripheral calcification/ossification

Gross Pathologic & Surgical Features

- CSF-containing collection

Microscopic Features

- No true meningeal covering
- Reactive fibrous tissue forms cyst capsule

CLINICAL ISSUES

Presentation

- Most common signs/symptoms
  - ○ Commonly asymptomatic
  - ○ Nonspecific back pain
  - ○ Headache if associated with CSF hypotension
  - ○ Occasionally extends superficially, palpable within subcutaneous tissues
  - ○ Meningitis/abscess if extends to/communicates with skin surface
- Clinical profile: Adult patient with palpable subcutaneous mass overlying lumbar laminectomy site

Demographics

- Age: Adult or children
- Gender: M = F

Natural History & Prognosis

- May be asymptomatic
- post-operative defects may close spontaneously if small, but can require treatment
- Cervical root avulsion with pseudomeningocele usually leaves permanent neurological deficits

Treatment

- Closure of underlying dural defect when possible
  - ○ Surgical repair for large defects
  - ○ Subarachnoid catheter drainage occasionally successful
  - ○ Blood patch may be effective for small defects

DIAGNOSTIC CHECKLIST

Consider

- Relationship of post-operative pseudomeningocele to patients pain difficult
- Causes of pain related to pseudomeningocele include
  - ○ Tension of cyst against nerve roots
  - ○ Entrapment of nerve roots
  - ○ Periradicular fibrosis

Image Interpretation Pearls

- Classic imaging appearance: CSF signal/density collection contiguous with thecal sac in correct clinical context

- May need to widen window on MR studies to visualize subcutaneous component due to surface coil signal inhomogeneity

SELECTED REFERENCES

1. Phillips CD et al: Depiction of a postoperative pseudomeningocele with digital subtraction myelography. AJNR Am J Neuroradiol. 23(2):337-8, 2002
2. Elbiaadi-Aziz N et al: Cerebrospinal fluid leak treated by aspiration and epidural blood patch under computed tomography guidance. Reg Anesth Pain Med. 26(4):363-7, 2001
3. Bosacco SJ et al: Evaluation and treatment of dural tears in lumbar spine surgery: a review. Clin Orthop 389: 238-47, 2001
4. Jinkins JR et al: The postsurgical lumbosacral spine. Magnetic resonance imaging evaluation following intervertebral disk surgery, surgical decompression, intervertebral bony fusion, and spinal instrumentation. Radiol clin North Am 39(1): 1-29, 2001
5. Ross JS: Magnetic resonance imaging of the postoperative spine. Semin Musculoskelet Radiol 4(3): 281-91, 2000
6. Stambough JL et al: Subarachnoid drainage of an established or chronic pseudomeningocele. J Spinal Disord. 13(1):39-41, 2000
7. Saunders RL et al: Four-level cervical corpectomy. Spine. 23(22):2455-61, 1998
8. McCormack BM et al: Pseudomeningocele/CSF fistula in a patient with lumbar spinal implants treated with epidural blood patch and a brief course of closed subarachnoid drainage. A case report. Spine. 21(19):2273-6, 1996
9. Hosono N et al: Postoperative cervical pseudomeningocele with herniation of the spinal cord. Spine. 20(19):2147-50, 1995
10. Aldrete JA et al: Postlaminectomy pseudomeningocele. An unsuspected cause of low back pain. Reg Anesth. 20(1):75-9, 1995
11. Shapiro SA et al: Closed continuous drainage of cerebrospinal fluid via a lumbar subarachnoid catheter for treatment or prevention of cranial/spinal cerebrospinal fluid fistula. Neurosurgery. 30(2):241-5, 1992
12. Lee KS et al: Postlaminectomy lumbar pseudomeningocele: report of four cases. Neurosurgery. 30(1):111-4, 1992
13. Murayama S et al: Magnetic resonance imaging of post-surgical pseudomeningocele. Comput Med Imaging Graph. 13(4):335-9, 1989
14. Tuvia J et al: Visualization of a pseudomeningocele on isotope cisternography. Clin Nucl Med. 13(12):889-91, 1988
15. Schumacher HW et al: Pseudomeningocele of the lumbar spine. Surg Neurol. 29(1):77-8, 1988
16. Teplick JG et al: CT Identification of postlaminectomy pseudomeningocele. AJR Am J Roentgenol. 140(6):1203-6, 1983
17. Helle TL et al: Postoperative cervical pseudomeningocele as a cause of delayed myelopathy. Neurosurgery. 9(3):314-6, 1981
18. Eismont FJ et al: Treatment of dural tears associated with spinal surgery. J Bone Joint Surg Am. 63(7):1132-6, 1981

IMAGE GALLERY

Typical

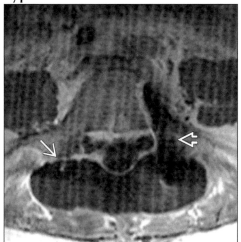
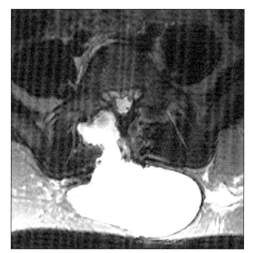

(Left) Axial T1WI MR shows ovoid CSF signal collection within dorsal soft tissues at prior laminectomy site (arrow). There is a left pedicle screw causing artifact (open arrow). (Right) Axial T2WI MR shows large hyperintense fluid collection within dorsal right hemilaminectomy site extending into subcutaneous tissues.

Typical

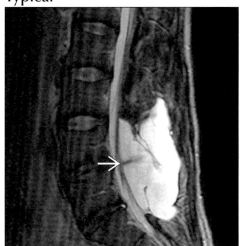
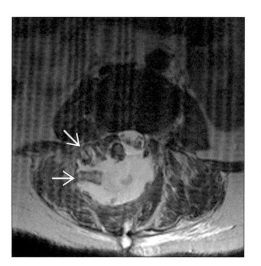

(Left) Sagittal T2WI MR shows hyperintense fluid collection at L4/ L5 levels. Focal low signal within collection is flow dephasing from CSF movement into collection at dural tear (arrow). (Right) Axial T2WI MR shows hyperintense fluid collection within dorsal soft tissues at laminectomy site. There are scattered pieces of bone graft material within the fluid collection (arrows).

Typical

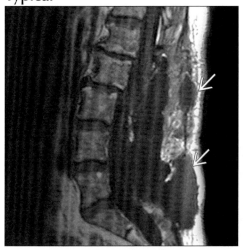
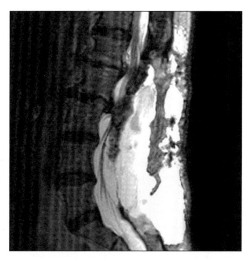

(Left) Sagittal T1WI MR shows large pseudomeningocele extending over the L2 to L5 levels with multiple loculations. Note the subcutaneous extension at several levels (arrows). (Right) Sagittal T2WI MR shows extensive hyperintense dorsal pseudomeningocele in this patient following multilevel lumbar laminectomy. There are multiple loculations and extension into subcutaneous tissues.

BONE GRAFT COMPLICATIONS

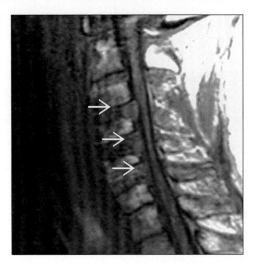

Sagittal T1WI MR shows interbody fusions spanning C3-4 through C5-6. Graft material is displaced posteriorly at all three levels abutting ventral cord with compression (arrows).

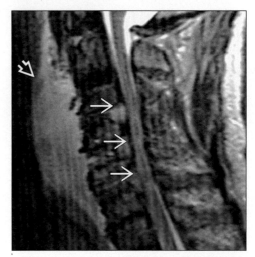

Sagittal T2WI MR shows 3 level interbody fusion. Three levels of grafts are placed posteriorly with effacement of thecal sac and cord (arrows). Note retropharyngeal hematoma (open arrow).

TERMINOLOGY

Abbreviations and Synonyms
- Synonyms: Graft migration, graft displacement, graft extrusion

Definitions
- Abnormal alignment, position, placement of graft or hardware ± associated neurologic deficit, instability, infection

IMAGING FINDINGS

General Features
- Best diagnostic clue: Abnormal position of graft material
- Location: Cervical > thoracic > lumbar
- Size: Variable depending upon graft construct (single level vs. multilevel strut)
- Morphology: Well-defined cortical graft material displaced with respect to interbody fusion site

Radiographic Findings
- Radiography: Essential for rapid intra-operative/post-operative evaluation of graft position
- Fluoroscopy: Not used acutely; useful for late nonfusion evaluation

- Myelography: Shows nonspecific extradural defect at level of dorsal graft migration

CT Findings
- NECT: MDCT with reformats shows graft position, endplate integrity, graft/vertebral body fractures

MR Findings
- T1WI
  - Variable appearance of graft material
    - Autogenous graft may show ↑ T1 signal with fatty marrow ⇒ ↓ signal (edema)
    - Allograft generally low signal
- T2WI: Variable appearance of graft material depending upon type (iliac crest, fibula), marrow state, and/or edema
- T2* GRE: Use for definition of graft cortical margins
- T1 C+: Little use in acute phase for graft malposition or epidural hemorrhage; mandatory if question of infection
- MRA: May be used for vertebral artery evaluation if question of surgical damage

Imaging Recommendations
- Best imaging tool: Plain films define graft position, ventral or dorsal migration, collapse
- Protocol advice: MRI: T1W, T2W, GRE axial + sagittal

DDx: Post-Operative Complications

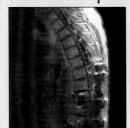

Abscess

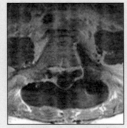

Pseudomeningocele

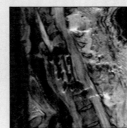

Cord Infarction

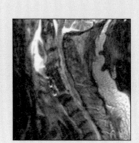

Epidural Hemorrhage

BONE GRAFT COMPLICATIONS

Key Facts

Terminology
- Synonyms: Graft migration, graft displacement, graft extrusion

Top Differential Diagnoses
- Abscess
- Hemorrhage
- Infarction
- Pseudoarthrosis

Pathology
- Graft migration occurs in 7% of cases after anterior cervical corpectomy
- 2 level corpectomy and fusion; 3 level (50%)
- Graft migration rate ↑ with more levels of fusion
- Graft migration rate ↑ with fusion ending at C7

DIFFERENTIAL DIAGNOSIS

Abscess
- Typical clinical and laboratory findings of infection (elevated sedimentation rate, C-reactive protein)

Hemorrhage
- Nonspecific T1 signal if acute ⇒ early subacute age (no increased signal)

Infarction
- Focal ↑ signal on T2WI in slightly expanded cord

Pseudoarthrosis
- Abnormal low T1 signal extending through disc, posterior elements and ligaments

PATHOLOGY

General Features
- General path comments
  - Graft migration rates vary widely depending on series, type
    - Graft migration occurs in 7% of cases after anterior cervical corpectomy
    - 2 level corpectomy and fusion; 3 level (50%)
  - Graft nonunion
    - Strut autograft 5-27%, allograft 40%
  - ↑ Nonunion rates in multilevel interbody grafting than corpectomy with strut grafting when ↑ vertebral levels involved
  - Similar fusion and complication rates for two level discectomy or single level corpectomy with plates
- Etiology
  - Graft migration rate ↑ with more levels of fusion
  - Graft migration rate ↑ with fusion ending at C7
  - ↑ Graft migration with strut graft compared to interbody graft

CLINICAL ISSUES

Presentation
- Most common signs/symptoms
  - May be asymptomatic, with only radiographic abnormality
  - New post-operative pain/focal deficit
  - Rare respiratory distress

Demographics
- Age: Adult
- Gender: M = F

Natural History & Prognosis
- ↑ Fusion rate after corpectomy/strut grafting (90%) than after multilevel discectomy/interbody graft (66%)
- Fusion less successful when anterior cervical arthrodesis is performed adjacent to prior fusion

Treatment
- May require reoperation for graft migration/extrusion/collapse

SELECTED REFERENCES

1. Wang JC et al: Graft migration or displacement after multilevel cervical corpectomy and strut grafting. Spine. 28(10):1016-21; discussion 1021-2, 2003
2. Hilibrand AS et al: Increased rate of arthrodesis with strut grafting after multilevel anterior cervical decompression. Spine. 27(2):146-51, 2002
3. Eleraky MA et al: Cervical corpectomy: report of 185 cases and review of the literature. J Neurosurg. 90(1 Suppl):35-41, 1999
4. Hilibrand AS et al: The success of anterior cervical arthrodesis adjacent to a previous fusion. Spine. 22(14):1574-9, 1997

IMAGE GALLERY

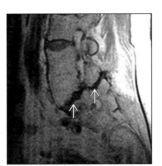 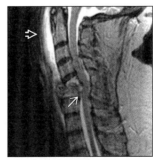

(Left) Sagittal T1WI MR shows pseudoarthrosis through L5-S1 level with linear low signal from disc level through posterior elements (arrows). Sold fusion at L4-5. *(Right)* Sagittal T2WI MR in patient with post-operative infection shows collapse of graft at C5-6 with kyphosis and subluxation (arrow), with cord compression. Note prevertebral edema (open arrow).

RECURRENT VERTEBRAL DISC HERNIATION

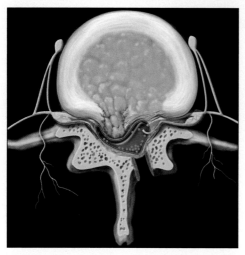

Axial graphic of lumbar spine shows left laminectomy defect. Large right central herniation is present compressing thecal sac & roots adjacent to site of prior discectomy.

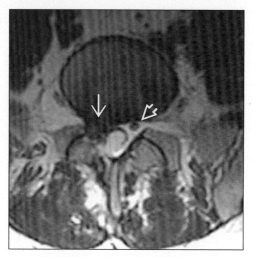

Axial T2WI MR shows right sided recurrent extrusion (arrow) as focal low signal mass displacing right S1 root & right lateral margin of thecal sac. Note normal left S1 root (open arrow).

TERMINOLOGY

Abbreviations and Synonyms
- Recurrent protrusion/extrusion
- Failed back surgery syndrome (FBSS)

Definitions
- Focal extension of disc material beyond endplate margins at previously operated intervertebral disc level

IMAGING FINDINGS

General Features
- Best diagnostic clue: Nonenhancing well-defined mass arising out of intervertebral disc
- Location: Primarily lumbar disc levels
- Size: Variable from few mm to > 10 mm
- Morphology
  - Round, smooth margined soft tissue
  - Protrusion
    - Protrusion is herniated disc with broad base at parent disc
    - Greatest diameter of protrusion in any plane < distance between edges of base in same plane
    - Focal: < 25% of disc circumference
  - Extrusion

- Extrusion is herniated disc with narrow or no base at parent disc
- Greatest diameter of extrusion in any plane > distance between edges of base in same plane
- Sequestered or free fragment: Extruded disc without contiguity to parent disc
- Migrated: Disc material displaced away from site of herniation, regardless of continuity to parent disc

Radiographic Findings
- Radiography: Plain film shows post-operative laminectomy site; not useful for disc herniation detection
- Myelography
  - Shows nonspecific extradural defect in contrast column centered at disc level
    - Root sleeves effaced or appear "cut off"
    - May fail to show L5-S1 herniation due to large epidural space

CT Findings
- NECT
  - Ventral epidural soft tissue density extending dorsally into spinal canal contiguous with disc
    - Changes of prior discectomy/laminectomy
- CECT

DDx: Epidural Masses

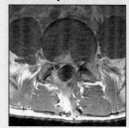

Peridural Fibrosus

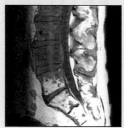

Tumor

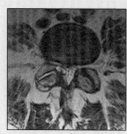

Synovial Cyst

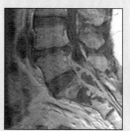

Abscess

Key Facts

Terminology
- Focal extension of disc material beyond endplate margins at previously operated intervertebral disc level

Imaging Findings
- Disc material shows no enhancement
- May enhance peripherally after intravenous contrast material due to granulation tissue or dilated epidural plexus
- Rare: Diffusely enhancement if associated with granulation tissue or if post-contrast imaging delayed
- Best imaging tool: Fat suppression of T1WI (pre-/post-gadolinium) may increase sensitivity in detecting peridural fibrosis, differentiating fibrosis from disc

Top Differential Diagnoses
- Peridural fibrosis
- Hemorrhage
- Abscess
- Osteophyte
- Synovial cyst/ganglion cyst
- Vertebral body/epidural tumor

Pathology
- Recurrent disc herniation implicated in FBSS in 7-12%

Diagnostic Checklist
- Immediate post-contrast MR 96-100% accurate detecting peridural fibrosis vs recurrent herniation

---

- ○ Herniation seen as soft tissue attenuation mass at disc level, +/- peripheral enhancement related to fibrosis or granulation tissue
- ○ Replaced by enhanced MR as primary diagnostic modality

MR Findings
- T1WI
  - ○ Isointense to parent disc
  - ○ May show low signal if calcified, or associated with vacuum phenomenon
- T2WI: Isointense to hyperintense
- T1 C+
  - ○ Disc material shows no enhancement
  - ○ May enhance peripherally after intravenous contrast material due to granulation tissue or dilated epidural plexus
  - ○ Rare: Diffusely enhancement if associated with granulation tissue or if post-contrast imaging delayed

Imaging Recommendations
- Best imaging tool: Fat suppression of T1WI (pre-/post-gadolinium) may increase sensitivity in detecting peridural fibrosis, differentiating fibrosis from disc
- Protocol advice: Sagittal, axial T1WI/T2WI; C+ sagittal, axial T1WI

DIFFERENTIAL DIAGNOSIS

Peridural fibrosis
- Immediate homogeneous post-contrast-enhancement
- Enhancement regardless the time elapsed since surgery
- Can be associated with ipsilateral enlargement of exiting root sleeve (cicatrization)

Hemorrhage
- Intermediate T1 signal if acute to subacute age
- Low T2 signal mass within epidural space at operative site

Abscess
- May show homogeneous enhancement within epidural space
- Abscess shows peripheral enhancement as do recurrent herniations
- Typical clinical/laboratory findings of infection (elevated sedimentation rate, C-reactive protein)

Osteophyte
- Sharp margins not arising directly from intervertebral disc level
- May show increased signal on T1WI due to fatty marrow content

Synovial cyst/ganglion cyst
- Extension of synovial cyst lateral to thecal sac may mimic ventral epidural process
- Central T2 hyperintensity, with peripheral enhancement

Vertebral body/epidural tumor
- Homogeneous enhancement
- Not arising out of intervertebral disc
- Irregular and infiltrative

PATHOLOGY

General Features
- General path comments
  - ○ Composed of combination of nucleus pulposus, fragmented anulus, cartilage, fragmented apophyseal bone
  - ○ Disc material may be intermixed with granulation tissue/fibrosis
- Etiology: Increased recurrent herniation with larger initial surgical anular defect
- Epidemiology
  - ○ Estimated 1 million spinal operations worldwide each year
  - ○ Recurrent disc herniation implicated in FBSS in 7-12%
- Associated abnormalities

RECURRENT VERTEBRAL DISC HERNIATION

○ Evidence of prior surgical intervention
  ▪ Fusion, peridural fibrosis, laminectomy defect, pseudomeningocele, arachnoiditis

Gross Pathologic & Surgical Features
- Nucleus pulposus
  ○ Gelatinous material with high water content, few collagen fibers
- Anulus fibrosus
  ○ Fibrocartilage, with collagen fibers in concentric lamellae

Microscopic Features
- Disc material surrounded by granulation tissue, capillaries, macrophages

Staging, Grading or Classification Criteria
- Three categories of post-operative disc/fibrosis
  ○ Recurrent herniation +/- peridural fibrosis
  ○ Herniation at new level
  ○ Peridural fibrosis only

CLINICAL ISSUES

Presentation
- Most common signs/symptoms
  ○ Low back pain or radiculopathy
  ○ Other signs/symptoms
    ▪ Weakness, numbness
- Clinical profile: Adult with new sudden onset low back pain/radiculopathy following initially successful disc surgery

Demographics
- Age: Adult
- Gender: M = F

Natural History & Prognosis
- FBSS complex, is multifactorial
- 7 year follow-up following microdiscectomy: 25% free of pain, 66% marked improvement, 9% had no improvement/worsening of pain
  ○ Of those that did not improve
  ○ 15% required changing profession following discectomy
  ○ 6% were incapacitated and unable to work
  ○ 14% were forced into early retirement

Treatment
- Conservative treatment
  ○ Exercise and physical conditioning
  ○ Nonsteroidal anti-inflammatory/opioid drugs
  ○ Epidural steroid injection
- 30-35% success rate for repeat surgery (range 12-100%)

DIAGNOSTIC CHECKLIST

Consider
- Best reoperative result in patients with herniation at new level away from operation site
- Intermediate operative success results in patients with new herniation at previously operated level, better than scar only, worse than disc at non-operative level

- Identification of only epidural fibrosis inFBSS patient is contraindication to reoperation, yields poor reoperative result

Image Interpretation Pearls
- Immediate post-contrast MR 96-100% accurate detecting peridural fibrosis vs recurrent herniation

SELECTED REFERENCES

1. Schofferman J et al: Failed back surgery: etiology and diagnostic evaluation. Spine J. 3(5):400-3, 2003
2. Carragee EJ et al: Clinical outcomes after lumbar discectomy for sciatica: the effects of fragment type and anular competence. J Bone Joint Surg Am. 85-A(1):102-8, 2003
3. Babar S et al: MRI of the post-discectomy lumbar spine. Clin Radiol. 57(11):969-81, 2002
4. Suk KS et al: Recurrent lumbar disc herniation: results of operative management. Spine. 26(6):672-6, 2001
5. Barrera MC et al: Post-operative lumbar spine: comparative study of TSE T2 and turbo-FLAIR sequences vs contrast-enhanced SE T1. Clin Radiol. 56(2):133-7, 2001
6. Ross JS: Magnetic resonance imaging of the postoperative spine. Semin Musculoskelet Radiol. 4(3):281-91, 2000
7. Loupasis GA et al: Seven- to 20-year outcome of lumbar discectomy. Spine. 24(22):2313-7, 1999
8. Spencer DL: The anatomical basis of sciatica secondary to herniated lumbar disc: a review. Neurol Res. 21 Suppl 1:S33-6, 1999
9. Bradley WG: Use of contrast in MR imaging of the lumbar spine. Magn Reson Imaging Clin N Am. 7(3):439-57, vii, 1999
10. Grane P: The postoperative lumbar spine. A radiological investigation of the lumbar spine after discectomy using MR imaging and CT. Acta Radiol Suppl. 414:1-23, 1998
11. Wilmink JT et al: MRI of the postoperative lumbar spine: triple-dose gadodiamide and fat suppression. Neuroradiology. 39(8):589-92, 1997
12. Bradley WG: Use of gadolinium chelates in MR imaging of the spine. J Magn Reson Imaging. 7(1):38-46, 1997
13. Fritsch EW et al: The failed back surgery syndrome: reasons, intraoperative findings, and long-term results: a report of 182 operative treatments. Spine. 21(5):626-33, 1996
14. Fiume D et al: Treatment of the failed back surgery syndrome due to lumbo-sacral epidural fibrosis. Acta Neurochir Suppl (Wien). 64:116-8, 1995
15. Djukic S et al: The lumbar spine: postoperative magnetic resonance imaging. Bildgebung. 59(3):136-46, 1992

RECURRENT VERTEBRAL DISC HERNIATION

IMAGE GALLERY

Typical

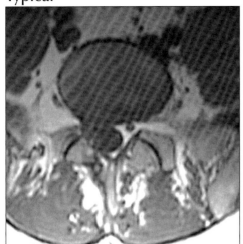 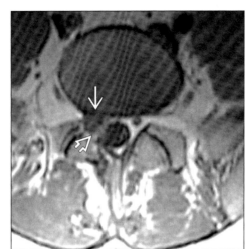

(Left) Axial T1WI MR shows right sided recurrent herniation as focal epidural mass of intermediate signal with compression of thecal sac. Exiting right S1 root is obscured by the herniation. *(Right)* Axial T1 C+ MR shows typical central lack of enhancement of herniation (arrow), with peripheral enhancement of granulation tissue (open arrow).

Typical

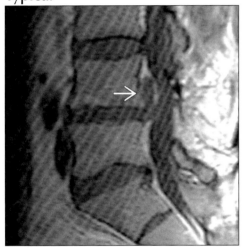 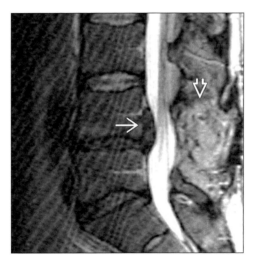

(Left) Sagittal T1 C+ MR shows recurrent disc extrusion as centrally nonenhancing mass with peripheral enhancing granulation tissue migrating superiorly from L4-5 level (arrow). *(Right)* Sagittal T2WI MR shows large recurrent extrusion (free fragment) migrating cephalad from L4-5 parent disc level (arrow). Note posterior laminectomy defect (open arrow).

Variant

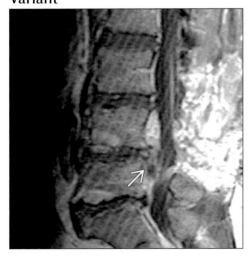 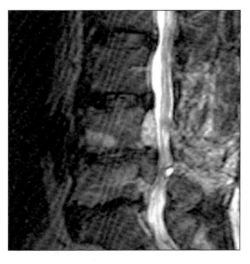

(Left) Sagittal T1 C+ MR shows recurrent nonenhancing herniation mixed with enhancing fibrosis at L4-5 (arrow). Severe multilevel disc degeneration is present with type II endplates. *(Right)* Sagittal T2WI MR shows large recurrent L4-5 extrusion effacing thecal sac, and migrating inferiorly behind L5 body.

POST-OPERATIVE INFECTION

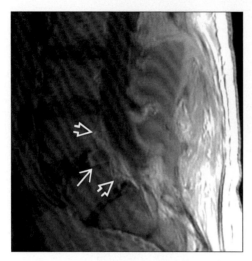

Sagittal T1 C+ MR demonstrates a large abscess posteriorly with an epidural component (open arrows) as well as disc enhancement (arrow).

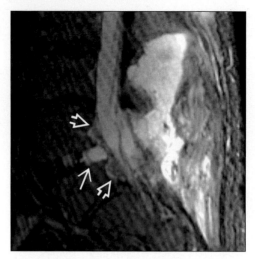

Sagittal STIR MR shows a large abscess posteriorly with an epidural component (open white arrows) as well as fluid signal in an adjacent disc (white arrow).

TERMINOLOGY

Definitions
- Infectious sequelae following operative procedures

IMAGING FINDINGS

General Features
- Best diagnostic clue: Unexpected abnormal MRI enhancement following spinal surgery
- Location
  ○ Begins at manipulated disc level as discitis
    ■ Less commonly at facets as facetitis
  ○ Spreads to adjacent local structures → "osteomyelitis-discitis"
  ○ Phlegmon/abscess may be paravertebral and/or epidural
- Size: Focal to widespread process
- Morphology: Epidural "curtain sign" = bilobed posterior bulging of an abscess (or other process) within epidural space to sides of septum/posterior longitudinal ligament complex

Radiographic Findings
- Radiography
  ○ Early: Insensitive
  ○ Later: Demineralization with end-plate lysis/erosion

- Chronic: Anterior wedging of affected vertebrae with fusion across disc space
    ■ May result in gibbus deformity
- Myelography
  ○ Abscess: Dye column defect from epidural abscess collection
  ○ Arachnoiditis: Nerve root clumping, adherence to thecal sac ("empty sac sign")

CT Findings
- CECT
  ○ Facetitis: May have associated facet/soft tissue enhancement
  ○ Phlegmon: Enhancing soft tissue collection without low density collection
  ○ Abscess: Hypodense collections within phlegmon
- Bone CT
  ○ Discitis: Adjacent endplate erosion
  ○ Facetitis: Osseous demineralization, ± erosion
- CT-Biopsy: Often needed to establish pathogen

MR Findings
- T1WI
  ○ Edema: Hypointense marrow
    ■ In children, normal marrow is relatively hypointense, thus T1WI often not helpful
  ○ Discitis: Disc hypointensity with loss of disc height; there may be complete obliteration of disc space
  ○ Facetitis: Relatively insensitive

DDx: Post-Operative Infection Mimics

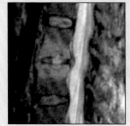
Hematogenous Discitis

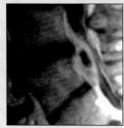
IVDA Epidural Abscess

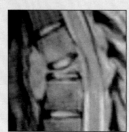
Tuberculosis

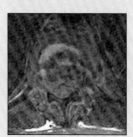
Renal Cell Carcinoma

POST-OPERATIVE INFECTION

Key Facts

Terminology
- Infectious sequelae following operative procedures

Imaging Findings
- Best diagnostic clue: Unexpected abnormal MRI enhancement following spinal surgery
- Begins at manipulated disc level as discitis
- Spreads to adjacent local structures → "osteomyelitis-discitis"
- Phlegmon/abscess may be paravertebral and/or epidural
- CT-Biopsy: Often needed to establish pathogen
- Best imaging tool: MRI C+; consider PET in presence of hardware susceptibility

Top Differential Diagnoses
- Hematogenous-seeded infection
- Local extension infection
- Neoplasm

Pathology
- Most common etiologic agent is Staph. aureus
- Overall uncommon; 0.2-3% spinal surgeries

Clinical Issues
- A variety of clinical symptoms are often found, but spontaneous drainage is most common
- Majority of patients have good long term outcomes, as high as 90%

Diagnostic Checklist
- Consider PET as an alternative to MRI
- Disc enhancement with fluid signal is discitis until proven otherwise

---

- ○ Phlegmon: Paravertebral soft tissue mass (intermediate signal intensity)
- ○ Abscess: Hypointense collections within phlegmon
- T2WI
  - ○ Edema: Hyperintense marrow
  - ○ Discitis: Disc hyperintensity or fluid intensity with loss of disc height
  - ○ Facetitis: Hyperintense facet fluid collection
  - ○ Phlegmon: Hyperintense paravertebral soft tissue
  - ○ Abscess: Hyperintense collections within phlegmon
  - ○ Arachnoiditis: Nerve root clumping, adherence to thecal sac ("empty sac sign")
- STIR: Best to visualize hyperintense marrow edema
- T1 C+
  - ○ Discitis: Disc enhancement
  - ○ Facetitis: Facet enhancement
  - ○ Phlegmon: Enhancing soft tissue
  - ○ Abscess: Fluid within enhancing phlegmon
  - ○ Osteomyelitis: Marrow enhancement
  - ○ Arachnoiditis: Nerve root clumping & enhancement
- Chronic MRI findings
  - ○ Anterior wedging of affected vertebrae with fusion across narrowed/abliterated disc space
  - ○ Normal marrow fat destroyed without restoration
- MRI may be non-diagnostic in the presence of hardware implanted during causative procedure

Ultrasonographic Findings
- Intra-operative: Hyperechoic epidural abscesses can be localized & decompression monitored

Nuclear Medicine Findings
- Bone Scan: Increased uptake, but limited value given uptake secondary to etiological procedure itself
- PET
  - ○ 18F-fluorodeoxyglucose (FDG) PET may become standard imaging technique
    - ↑ Glucose utilization of activated neutrophils & macrophages in inflammatory reactions
    - Not hindered by the presence of metallic implants
    - Provides rapid results (2 hours) & high-resolution images (4-5 mm)

- ○ Negative predictive value, sensitivity, specificity, & accuracy for diagnosing post-operative spine infection are 100%, 100%, 81%, & 86% respectively
- WBC Scan
  - ○ Often useless 2° to high uptake of labeled leukocytes in normal hematopoietically active bone marrow
- 99mTc-ciprofloxacin SPECT
  - ○ Sensitive for post-operative spine infections
  - ○ SPECT sensitivity much higher than planar imaging
  - ○ Specificity is limited, especially in recently operated patients (< 6 months)

Imaging Recommendations
- Best imaging tool: MRI C+; consider PET in presence of hardware susceptibility
- Protocol advice
  - ○ STIR best images marrow edema
  - ○ Fat suppressed techniques ↑ infection conspicuity

DIFFERENTIAL DIAGNOSIS

Hematogenous-seeded infection
- Most often bacterial (usually Staphylococcus aureus)
- IV drug abusers at higher risk
- Often single level or skips levels

Local extension infection
- Most often tuberculous (immunocompromised at ↑ risk)
- Often two or more contiguous levels
- May spare intervening disc

Neoplasm
- More often metastatic
- Two adjacent involved vertebral bodies typically spare intervening disc
- May have extensive epidural, paravertebral extension

PATHOLOGY

General Features
- Etiology

POST-OPERATIVE INFECTION

- ○ Most common etiologic agent is Staph. aureus
- ○ Three possible causes of a delayed infection
  - ▪ Intra-operative seeding
  - ▪ Metal fretting causing a sterile inflammatory response
  - ▪ Stimulating low-virulent organisms to fester with hematogenous seeding
- ○ Risk factors for spinal surgical site infection: Increasing age, post-operative incontinence, posterior approach, surgery for tumor resection, morbid obesity, increased blood loss, longer operative times, number of operated levels
- ○ Scoliosis surgery
  - ▪ Closure of thoracolumbar wounds after scoliosis surgery often difficult due to tautness & lack of usable tissue
  - ▪ Resulting dead space containing metallic fixation devices is predisposed to infection
- • Epidemiology
  - ○ Overall uncommon; 0.2-3% spinal surgeries
  - ○ Postprocedural discitis: Incidence ≈ 0.2%
  - ○ Scoliosis surgery: Post-operative infection due to lack of vascularized tissue & presence of metallic hardware near the wound is common

CLINICAL ISSUES

Presentation
- • Most common signs/symptoms
  - ○ A variety of clinical symptoms are often found, but spontaneous drainage is most common
  - ○ Symptoms & clinical findings are often nonspecific
  - ○ Practitioner must have a high index of suspicion in any patient presenting with ↑ back pain after an invasive spinal procedure
- • Clinical profile
  - ○ Abnormal erythrocyte sedimentation rate, C-reactive protein & blood cultures
  - ○ C-reactive protein is most sensitive clinical laboratory marker to assess presence of infection & effectiveness of treatment response
  - ○ Many patients have a fluctuant mass, localized drainage, or abscess
  - ○ Abscesses or drainage material is typically contiguous with instrumentation & fusion mass
- • Clinical setting & presentation are key in diagnosis
  - ○ 1-4 weeks following surgery patient develops back pain which may be severe
    - ▪ May radiate into abdomen, perineum, testes, legs
    - ▪ Accompanied by paravertebral muscle spasm
  - ○ Overlying signs of wound infection

Demographics
- • Age: Risk increases with age

Natural History & Prognosis
- • Majority of patients have good long term outcomes, as high as 90%

Treatment
- • Biopsy to establish pathogen
- • Effective treatment usually includes
  - ○ Removal of implants, irrigation, & debridement

- ○ Possible use of closed suction-irrigation system
- ○ Intravenous organism-specific antibiotic treatment & spinal immobilization
- • Prophylaxis
  - ○ One pre-operative administration of Cefotiam has been shown effective for ↓ rate of post-operative wound infections in lumbar disc surgery
    - ▪ Rate of infection 0.2 % after antibiotic administration vs. 2.8 % without prophylaxis
  - ○ Intraoperative antibiotic prophylaxis has been advocated by some
- • Scoliosis surgery
  - ○ Lower thoracic & thoracolumbar: Modified extended latissimus dorsi myocutaneous flap to close and supply blood to wounds
  - ○ Lumbosacral: Addition of gluteus maximus muscle flap to obtain covering caudal extent
  - ○ Allows for wound closure & drastically ↓ the risk of post-operative infection
  - ○ Effective for closure & increased blood supply to already infected wounds

DIAGNOSTIC CHECKLIST

Consider
- • Consider PET as an alternative to MRI

Image Interpretation Pearls
- • Disc enhancement with fluid signal is discitis until proven otherwise

SELECTED REFERENCES

1. De Winter F et al: 99mTc-ciprofloxacin planar and tomographic imaging for the diagnosis of infection in the postoperative spine: experience in 48 patients. Eur J Nucl Med Mol Imaging. 31(2):233-9, 2004
2. Brown MD et al: A randomized study of closed wound suction drainage for extensive lumbar spine surgery. Spine. 29(10):1066-8, 2004
3. Mitra A et al: Treatment of massive thoracolumbar wounds and vertebral osteomyelitis following scoliosis surgery. Plast Reconstr Surg. 113(1):206-13, 2004
4. Mastronardi L et al: Intraoperative antibiotic prophylaxis in clean spinal surgery: a retrospective analysis in a consecutive series of 973 cases. Surg Neurol. 61(2):129-35; discussion 135, 2004
5. Bavinzski G et al: Microsurgical management of postoperative disc space infection. Neurosurg Rev. 26(2):102-7, 2003
6. Olsen MA et al: Risk factors for surgical site infection in spinal surgery. J Neurosurg. 98(2 Suppl):149-55, 2003
7. De Winter F et al: 18-Fluorine fluorodeoxyglucose positron emission tomography for the diagnosis of infection in the postoperative spine. Spine. 28(12):1314-9, 2003
8. Carreon LY et al: Perioperative complications of posterior lumbar decompression and arthrodesis in older adults. J Bone Joint Surg Am. 85-A(11):2089-92, 2003
9. Schnoring M et al: Prophylactic antibiotics in lumbar disc surgery: analysis of 1,030 procedures. Zentralbl Neurochir. 64(1):24-9, 2003
10. Bose B: Delayed infection after instrumented spine surgery: case reports and review of the literature. Spine J. 3(5):394-9, 2003

POST-OPERATIVE INFECTION

IMAGE GALLERY

Typical

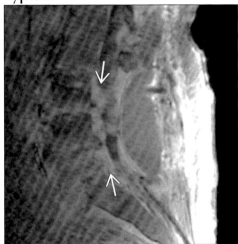
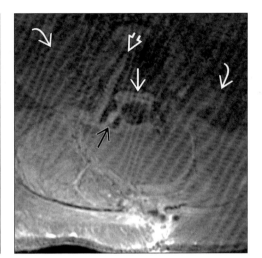

(Left) Sagittal fat-saturation T1 C+ MR demonstrates large abscess posteriorly with epidural component (arrows), L2 through S1 disc enhancement, & vertebral body enhancement (from osteomyelitis). *(Right)* Axial fat-saturation T1 C+ MR shows large abscess involving paraspinal tissues, epidural space (arrow), facet (black arrow), psoas muscles (curved arrows), & screw tract (open arrow).

Typical

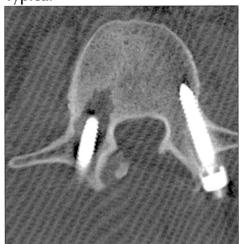
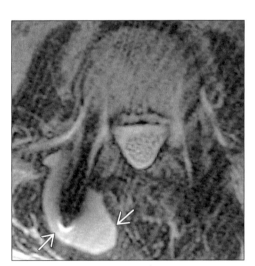

(Left) Axial bone CT reveals lucency around infected right screw prior to hardware removal. *(Right)* Axial T2WI MR demonstrates fluid collected (arrows) around infected right screw prior to hardware removal. Note FSE technique minimizes susceptibility yielding diagnostic scan.

Typical

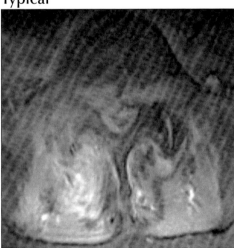
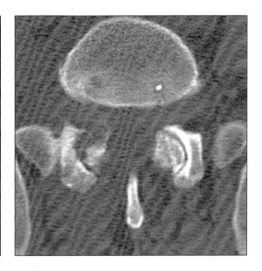

(Left) Axial fat-saturation T1 C+ MR reveals facetitis & widespread infection complicating right L5/S1 right facet injection in rheumatoid patient. *(Right)* Axial bone CT in same patient demonstrates erosions from facetitis complicating right L5/S1 right facet injection in rheumatoid patient.

POST-OPERATIVE SPINAL COMPLICATIONS

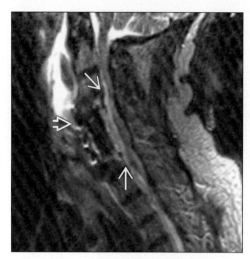

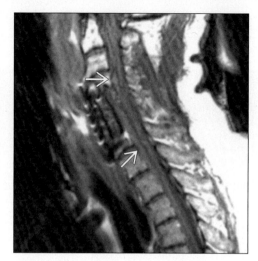

Sagittal T2WI MR shows C4-C7 strut graft placement + anterior plate for spondylosis (open arrow). Cord compression results from acute epidural hematoma (arrows) dorsal to operative site.

Sagittal T1WI MR shows strut graft placed from C4-C7 with anterior plate. Cord margin is indistinct from near isointense acute epidural hemorrhage (arrows).

TERMINOLOGY

Abbreviations and Synonyms
- Iatrogenic cord complication

Definitions
- Cord abnormality or neurologic deficit arising as direct or indirect result of prior surgery (including altered biomechanics)
- Multiple diverse etiologies
  - Hemorrhage with cord compression
    - Intramedullary
    - Subarachnoid/subdural
    - Epidural
    - Hemosiderosis (chronic sequelae)
  - Cord infarction
    - Aortic aneurysms repair with anterior spinal artery occlusion or embolization
    - Aortic or vertebral dissection following catheterization
    - Spinal vascular malformation repair/embolization
    - Direct operative cord trauma
    - Secondary to compression from hematoma
    - Hypoperfusion/cardiac tamponade
    - Rare: Hyperextension injury to cord from operative malpositioning of neck
    - Rare: Cord infarct associated with sitting position for posterior fossae/pineal tumor approach

- Spinal anesthesia related
  - Catheter-induced hematoma
  - Celiac plexus block (chemical toxicity)
  - Epidural catheter malposition with intracord injection of anesthetic
- Infection
  - Graft collapse with cord compression
  - Cord compression from abscess
  - Rare: Intramedullary abscess
- Instability
  - Altered biomechanics with accelerated degeneration
- Graft/hardware malposition
  - Graft extrusion/displacement with cord compression
  - Hardware (pedicle screw) malposition with cord/thecal sac compression
- Chronic: Radiation myelitis
- Chronic: Accelerated disc degeneration with herniation/stenosis

IMAGING FINDINGS

General Features
- Best diagnostic clue: New abnormality present post-operatively, outside usual scope of post-operative changes

DDx: Post-Operative Complications

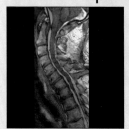

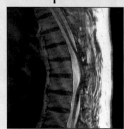

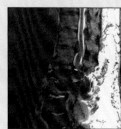

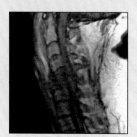

Subdural Hemorrhage

Tethered Cord

Disc Herniation

Infection

POST-OPERATIVE SPINAL COMPLICATIONS

Key Facts

Terminology

- Cord abnormality or neurologic deficit arising as direct or indirect result of prior surgery (including altered biomechanics)
- Multiple diverse etiologies
- Hemorrhage with cord compression
- Cord infarction
- Spinal anesthesia related
- Infection
- Graft/hardware malposition

Imaging Findings

- Hyperacute infarcts may show normal T1 signal
- "Snake eye" pattern of T2 central hyperintensity unfavorable prognostic factor for recovery of upper-extremity motor weakness

Pathology

- Epidemiology: Post-operative epidural hemorrhage associated with multilevel procedures + pre-operative coagulopathy

Clinical Issues

- Epidural post-operative hemorrhage acute symptoms within 24 hours of surgery
- New focal neurologic deficit
- Respiratory distress + flaccid quadriparesis/plegia
- Rare cases of more subacute post-operative hemorrhage 3-5 days after surgery
- Characterized with severe sharp pain with radiation to the extremities

---

- Location: Cervical, thoracic or lumbar spine
- Size
  - Variable depending upon etiology
    - Infarction: May involve several cord segments
    - Direct trauma: More focal abnormality
  - Hemorrhage extends over multiple segments
- Morphology
  - Variable depending upon etiology
    - Infarction: Fusiform cord enlargement in acute setting
  - Hemorrhage forms craniocaudal linear signal abnormality

Radiographic Findings

- Radiography: Defines hardware position
- Myelography
  - Secondary technique to MRI for post-operative complication imaging
    - Useful with MR contraindications (aneurysm clip, pacemakers)
    - May show nonspecific cord enlargement with infarct/extradural defect related to epidural hemorrhage

CT Findings

- NECT: MDCT show alignment, graft position, mass effect on thecal sac/cord

MR Findings

- T1WI
  - Infarct
    - Sight cord expansion, decreased signal
    - Hyperacute infarcts may show normal T1 signal
  - Hemorrhage
    - Isointense to hypointense in acute setting
    - Typical hyperintensity with subacute
- T2WI
  - Infarct
    - T2 hyperintensity in gray matter, gray matter with adjacent white matter, or entire cross sectional area of the cord
    - "Snake eye" pattern of T2 central hyperintensity unfavorable prognostic factor for recovery of upper-extremity motor weakness

- Hemorrhage
  - Isointense to markedly hypointense on T2WI in acute setting
- STIR
  - Infarct
    - Increased cord signal
- T2* GRE
  - Infarct
    - May show susceptibility effect from hemorrhage
  - Hemorrhage
    - Acute hemorrhage hypo- to isointense
- DWI
  - Infarct
    - Shows abnormal restricted diffusion (as in brain with infarct)
- T1 C+
  - Infarct
    - Generally does not acutely enhance
  - Enhanced studies limited usefulness in acute post-operative setting, although may increase conspicuity of post-operative fluid collections
  - Chronic myelomalacia may enhance, linear ⇒ focal

Imaging Recommendations

- Best imaging tool: MRI
- Protocol advice: T1W, T2W, GRE show intrinsic cord signal abnormality, cord deformity, epidural collections

DIFFERENTIAL DIAGNOSIS

Epidural hemorrhage

- Linear mass displacing low signal dura

Subdural hemorrhage

- Lobulated extramedullary signal abnormality, with well defined preserved dural peripheral margin

Disc herniation

- Focal abnormality arising out of parent disc

Graft extrusion/malposition

- Plain film/CT quick and accurate for graft position

POST-OPERATIVE SPINAL COMPLICATIONS

Abscess
- Subacute peripheral enhancing soft tissue mass, central nonenhancing fluid component

Subdural effusion
- Benign subdural CSF collection may extend into cervical spine following posterior fossa surgery
- May occur following lumbar puncture/surgery

Cord tethering
- Focal cord deformity with apposition of cord to dural surface at surgical site
- Cord displacement must be distinguished from mass effect from fluid collection

PATHOLOGY

General Features
- General path comments: Infarction: Soft pale, swollen cord tissue with increasingly distinct margin with more normal tissue over time
- Etiology: Post-operative complication
- Epidemiology: Post-operative epidural hemorrhage associated with multilevel procedures + pre-operative coagulopathy

Microscopic Features
- Acute infarction: Ischemic neurons with cytotoxic, vasogenic edema, swelling of endothelial cells + astrocytes

CLINICAL ISSUES

Presentation
- Most common signs/symptoms
  - Infarction
    - Anterior spinal syndrome presents with paralysis, loss of pain/temperature sensation, bladder/bowel dysfunction
    - Posterior spinal cord infarction characterized by loss of proprioception/vibration sense; paresis, and sphincter dysfunction
  - Epidural post-operative hemorrhage acute symptoms within 24 hours of surgery
    - New focal neurologic deficit
    - Respiratory distress + flaccid quadriparesis/plegia
  - Rare cases of more subacute post-operative hemorrhage 3-5 days after surgery
    - Characterized with severe sharp pain with radiation to the extremities
- Clinical profile: New neurologic deficit immediately following spinal surgery

Demographics
- Age: Child or adult
- Gender: M = F

Natural History & Prognosis
- Acute spinal cord ischemia syndrome has severe prognosis with permanent disabling sequelae
  - Substantial recovery < 20%

- Autonomic dysfunction, pain, paresthesia, and depression common sequelae and impede recovery

Treatment
- Immediate reoperation for decompression of hematoma, or graft malposition/compression
- Infarction without compression: Supportive care

DIAGNOSTIC CHECKLIST

Consider
- MR + CT for definition of soft tissue abnormality (hemorrhage, ischemia) plus bone/graft detail

Image Interpretation Pearls
- Hyperacute hemorrhage may show nonspecific T1WI + T2WI "fluid" signal, defined only by mass effect on neural structures

SELECTED REFERENCES

1. Uribe J et al: Delayed postoperative spinal epidural hematomas. Spine J. 3(2):125-9, 2003
2. Mizuno J et al: Clinicopathological study of "snake-eye appearance" in compressive myelopathy of the cervical spinal cord. J Neurosurg. 99(2 Suppl):162-8, 2003
3. Roberts DR et al: Hyperlordosis as a possible factor in the development of spinal cord infarction. Br J Anaesth. 90(6):797-800, 2003
4. Pelletier MP et al: Paraplegia after routine cardiac surgery: a rare complication. J Card Surg. 17(5):410-2, 2002
5. Kou J et al: Risk factors for spinal epidural hematoma after spinal surgery. Spine. 27(15):1670-3, 2002
6. Lin CC et al: Spinal cord infarction caused by cardiac tamponade. Am J Phys Med Rehabil. 81(1):68-71, 2002
7. Hong DK et al: Anterior spinal artery syndrome following total hip arthroplasty under epidural anaesthesia. Anaesth Intensive Care. 29(1):62-6, 2001
8. Bromage PR et al: Paraplegia following intracord injection during attempted epidural anesthesia under general anesthesia. Reg Anesth Pain Med. 23(1):104-7, 1998
9. Nitta H et al: Cervical spinal cord infarction after surgery for a pineal region choriocarcinoma in the sitting position: case report. Neurosurgery. 40(5):1082-5; discussion 1085-6, 1997
10. Singh U et al: Hypotensive infarction of the spinal cord. Paraplegia. 32(5):314-22, 1994
11. Waters RL et al: Recovery following ischemic myelopathy. J Trauma. 35(6):837-9, 1993
12. Yonenobu K et al: Neurologic complications of surgery for cervical compression myelopathy. Spine. 16(11):1277-82, 1991
13. Mawad ME et al: Spinal cord ischemia after resection of thoracoabdominal aortic aneurysms: MR findings in 24 patients. AJR Am J Roentgenol. 155(6):1303-7, 1990

POST-OPERATIVE SPINAL COMPLICATIONS

IMAGE GALLERY

Typical

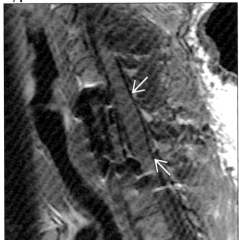 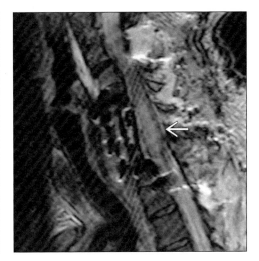

(Left) Sagittal T1WI MR shows multilevel corpectomy + strut graft placed for spondylosis. Cord shows fusiform enlargement with slight T1 hypointensity (arrows) from acute infarction. *(Right)* Sagittal T2WI MR shows anterior corpectomy + strut graft, posterior multilevel laminectomy. Cord shows fusiform enlargement and T2 hyperintensity (arrow) from acute infarction.

Typical

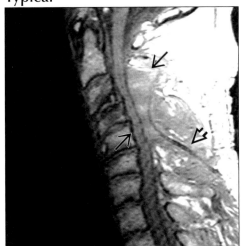 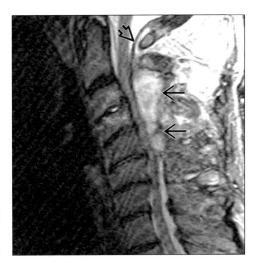

(Left) Sagittal T1WI MR shows multilevel laminectomy. Cord compressed from epidural hematoma (arrows), causing ventral cord deformity from disc/osteophytes. Note drainage catheter (open arrow). *(Right)* Sagittal T2WI MR shows laminectomy for spondylosis. Dorsal epidural hematoma (arrows) shows T2 hyperintensity compressing dorsal cord over multiple segments. Note distinct dural margin (open arrow).

Typical

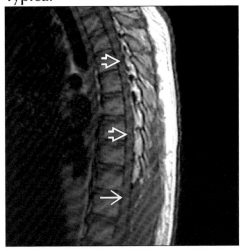 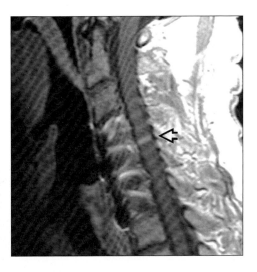

(Left) Sagittal T1WI MR shows laminectomy defect (arrow). Diffuse heterogeneous signal throughout dorsal thoracic spine from epidural hemorrhage and gas (open arrows), giving ventral cord displacement. *(Right)* Sagittal T1 C+ MR shows C4-C7 fusion + anterior plating with susceptibility artifact. Focal linear enhancement within cord at C5 level from myelomalacia (open arrow).

FAILED BACK SURGERY SYNDROME

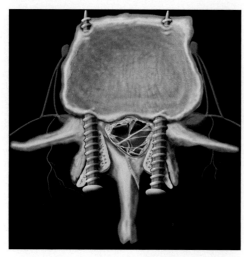

Axial graphic of lumbar spine shows post-operative change with bilateral pedicle screws and left laminectomy defect. There is clumping of nerve roots reflecting arachnoiditis.

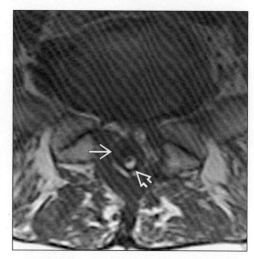

Axial T1WI MR shows laminectomy at L5-S1. There is peripheral clumping of roots in caudal thecal sac due to arachnoiditis (arrow), note droplet of T1 hyperintense Pantopaque (open arrow).

TERMINOLOGY

Abbreviations and Synonyms
- Abbreviation: Failed back surgery syndrome (FBSS)

Definitions
- Continued low back pain with or without radicular pain after lumber surgery

IMAGING FINDINGS

General Features
- Best diagnostic clue
  - Stenosis: "Trefoil" appearance of lumbar spinal canal on axial imaging
  - Instability: Deformity increases with motion, & increases over time
  - Recurrent herniation: Nonenhancing well-defined mass arising out of intervertebral disc
  - Fibrosis: Infiltration of epidural/perineural fat by enhancing soft tissue density (intensity)
  - Arachnoiditis: Clumping, adhesion of cauda equina nerve roots
- Location: Lumbar spine
- Size: Variable
- Morphology: Variable depending upon specific pathology

Radiographic Findings
- Radiography
  - Instability
    - Dynamic slip > 3 mm in flexion/extension
    - Static slip of 4.5 mm or greater
    - Angulation > 10-15° suggests need for surgical intervention
- Myelography
  - Stenosis: "Hourglass" constriction(s) at single or multiple levels
  - Herniation: Extradural defect at intervertebral disc level

CT Findings
- NECT: Herniation: Ventral epidural soft tissue density extending dorsally into spinal canal contiguous with disc

MR Findings
- T1WI
  - Stenosis: Trefoil appearance of spinal canal, thick ligamentum flavum
  - Instability: Anterolisthesis, retrolisthesis, lateral translation
  - Herniation: Isointense to parent disc ventral epidural mass
  - Fibrosis: Isointense on T1WI

DDx: Causes of Early Failed Surgery

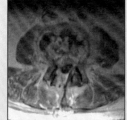

Infection

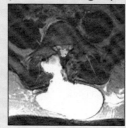

Pseudomeningocele

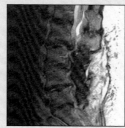

Hemorrhage

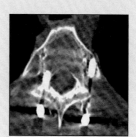

Hardware Malposition

FAILED BACK SURGERY SYNDROME

Key Facts

Terminology
- Abbreviation: Failed back surgery syndrome (FBSS)
- Continued low back pain with or without radicular pain after lumber surgery

Imaging Findings
- Stenosis: "Trefoil" appearance of lumbar spinal canal on axial imaging
- Instability: Deformity increases with motion, & increases over time
- Recurrent herniation: Nonenhancing well-defined mass arising out of intervertebral disc
- Fibrosis: Infiltration of epidural/perineural fat by enhancing soft tissue density (intensity)
- Arachnoiditis: Clumping, adhesion of cauda equina nerve roots

Pathology
- Multiple underlying etiologies for "late" failure
- Foraminal/central stenosis (20-60%)
- Pseudoarthrosis/instability (14%)
- Recurrent herniation (7-12%)
- Epidural fibrosis (5-25%)
- Arachnoiditis
- Some degree of FBSS found in 15% of operative patients

Clinical Issues
- Physiotherapy, back strengthening exercises
- Epidural steroids
- Surgery directed to specific pain generator: Recurrent herniation, foraminal stenosis, instability

---

  ○ Arachnoiditis: Peripheral or central clumping of cauda equina roots
- T2WI
  ○ Stenosis: Trefoil appearance of spinal canal, thick ligamentum flavum
  ○ Instability: Nonspecific loss of disc signal, disc space height
  ○ Herniation: Isointense to hyperintense ventral epidural lesion
  ○ Fibrosis: Typically slightly increased in signal relative to disc herniation
  ○ Arachnoiditis: Peripheral or central clumping of cauda equina
- T1 C+
  ○ Stenosis: Crowded ± enhancing nerve roots
  ○ Instability: Nonspecific enhancement of disc due to degenerative disc disease
  ○ Herniation: Disc material shows no enhancement, scar will enhance
  ○ Fibrosis: Immediate homogeneous post-contrast-enhancement
  ○ Arachnoiditis: Little or no enhancement of roots

Nuclear Medicine Findings
- Bone Scan: Nonspecific increased uptake with all degenerative disc disease
- PET
  ○ Hypometabolic with degenerative endplate changes
  ○ Hypermetabolic with disc space infection, vertebral osteomyelitis

Imaging Recommendations
- Best imaging tool
  ○ Flexion/extension plain films
  ○ MR defines degeneration, endplate changes, stenosis, fibrosis, herniation
- Protocol advice: Sagittal, axial T1WI and T2WI; C+ sagittal, axial T1WI

DIFFERENTIAL DIAGNOSIS

Infection
- Endplate destruction, disc T2 hyperintensity
- Abscess shows peripheral enhancement as do recurrent herniations
- Typical clinical and laboratory findings of infection (elevated sedimentation rate, C-reactive protein)

Tumor
- Enhancing soft tissue mass
- Not arising out of intervertebral disc
- Irregular and infiltrative

Hemorrhage
- Intermediate T1 signal if acute ⇒ subacute age

Pseudoarthrosis
- Abnormal low T1 signal extending through disc, posterior elements and ligaments

PATHOLOGY

General Features
- General path comments
  ○ Post-operative scarring is part of normal reparative mechanism
  ○ Herniation = combination of nucleus pulposus, fragmented anulus, cartilage, fragmented apophyseal bone
- Etiology
  ○ Multiple underlying etiologies for "late" failure
    ▪ Foraminal/central stenosis (20-60%)
    ▪ Pseudoarthrosis/instability (14%)
    ▪ Recurrent herniation (7-12%)
    ▪ Epidural fibrosis (5-25%)
    ▪ Arachnoiditis
  ○ Early surgical failure etiologies
    ▪ Post-operative hemorrhage with neural compression
    ▪ Disc space infection, vertebral osteomyelitis, meningitis

FAILED BACK SURGERY SYNDROME

■ Dural tear with pseudomeningocele
■ Hardware malposition
■ Wrong level surgery
○ Extent of fibrosis possibly related to the extent of surgical dissection
○ Increased recurrent herniation with larger initial surgical anular defect
○ Some degree of FBSS found in 15% of operative patients
• Epidemiology
○ Reintervention rates after lumbar discectomy range from 5-33%
○ Multiple revision: Rate of epidural fibrosis and instability increases to > 60%

Gross Pathologic & Surgical Features
• Multiple findings related to specific pathology such as fibrosis, nonunion, herniation, bony facet arthropathy

Microscopic Features
• Fibrous tissue can extend to vertebral canal, adhere to dura and roots
• Disc material surrounded by granulation tissue, capillaries, macrophages

Staging, Grading or Classification Criteria
• Best reoperative result in patients with herniation at new level away from operation site
• Intermediate operative success results in patients with new herniation at previously operated level
• Only fibrosis is contraindication to reoperation

CLINICAL ISSUES

Presentation
• Most common signs/symptoms
○ Continued low back pain or radiculopathy
○ Weakness, numbness
○ Other signs/symptoms
■ Patients may also be incapacitated by psychiatric, psychologic, social/vocational factors, which relate indirectly to back complaints
• Clinical profile: Continued back pain following lumbar discectomy

Demographics
• Age: Adult
• Gender: M = F

Natural History & Prognosis
• Better prognosis
○ Young female
○ History of good results from previous operations
○ Absence of epidural scar
○ Employment before surgery
○ Predominance of radicular (as opposed to axial) pain

Treatment
• Conservative measures
○ Physiotherapy, back strengthening exercises
○ Transcutaneous electrical nerve stimulation
○ Epidural steroids
• Spinal cord stimulators

• Surgery directed to specific pain generator: Recurrent herniation, foraminal stenosis, instability
○ 34% successful outcome (50% sustained relief of pain for 2 years and patient satisfaction with result)

DIAGNOSTIC CHECKLIST

Consider
• 30-35% success rate for repeat surgery (range 12-100%)

Image Interpretation Pearls
• Contrast-enhanced MR 96-100% accurate detecting peridural fibrosis vs. recurrent herniation

SELECTED REFERENCES

1. Schofferman J et al: Failed back surgery: etiology and diagnostic evaluation. Spine J. 3(5):400-3, 2003
2. Van Goethem JW et al: Review article: MRI of the postoperative lumbar spine. Neuroradiology. 44(9):723-39, 2002
3. Anderson VC et al: Failed back surgery syndrome. Curr Rev Pain. 4(2):105-11, 2000
4. Anderson SR: A rationale for the treatment algorithm of failed back surgery syndrome. Curr Rev Pain. 4(5):395-406, 2000
5. Coskun E et al: Relationships between epidural fibrosis, pain, disability, and psychological factors after lumbar disc surgery. Eur Spine J. 9(3):218-23, 2000
6. Anderson VC et al: A prospective study of long-term intrathecal morphine in the management of chronic nonmalignant pain. Neurosurgery. 44(2):289-300; discussion 300-1, 1999
7. Van Goethem JW et al: Imaging findings in patients with failed back surgery syndrome. J Belge Radiol. 80(2):81-4, 1997
8. Robertson JT: Role of peridural fibrosis in the failed back: a review. Eur Spine J. 5 Suppl 1:S2-6, 1996
9. Fritsch EW et al: The failed back surgery syndrome: reasons, intraoperative findings, and long-term results: a report of 182 operative treatments. Spine. 21(5):626-33, 1996
10. Georgy BA et al: Fat-suppression contrast-enhanced MRI in the failed back surgery syndrome: a prospective study. Neuroradiology. 37(1):51-7, 1995
11. Kim SS et al: Revision surgery for failed back surgery syndrome. Spine. 17(8):957-60, 1992
12. North RB et al: Failed back surgery syndrome: 5-year follow-up in 102 patients undergoing repeated operation. Neurosurgery. 28(5):685-90; discussion 690-1, 1991
13. Long DM: Failed back surgery syndrome. Neurosurg Clin N Am. 2(4):899-919, 1991
14. Ross JS et al: MR imaging of the postoperative lumbar spine: assessment with gadopentetate dimeglumine. AJNR Am J Neuroradiol. 11(4):771-6, 1990
15. Bundschuh CV et al: Distinguishing between scar and recurrent herniated disk in postoperative patients: value of contrast-enhanced CT and MR imaging. AJNR Am J Neuroradiol. 11(5):949-58, 1990

IMAGE GALLERY

Typical

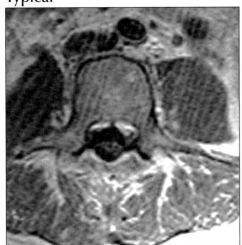
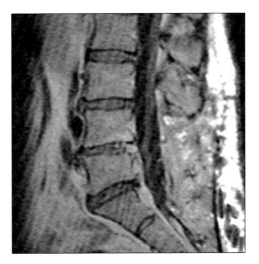

(Left) Axial T1 C+ MR shows abnormal central clumping of cauda equina at L3 level, reflecting arachnoiditis. There is no significant intradural enhancement. (Right) Sagittal T1 C+ MR shows central clumping of intrathecal roots into a central rope-like mass, simulating low lying cord. Note multilevel laminectomy defect, degenerative disc space enhancement.

Typical

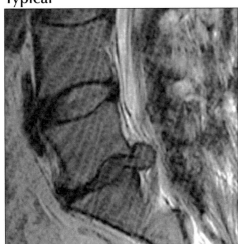
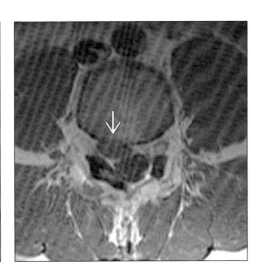

(Left) Sagittal T2WI MR shows large recurrent extrusion at L5-S1 level. There is disc degeneration at L5-S1 with loss of disc height and T2 signal. (Right) Axial T1 C+ MR shows large nonenhancing recurrent disc herniation (arrow) compressing anterior thecal sac in this patient status post laminectomy/discectomy.

Typical

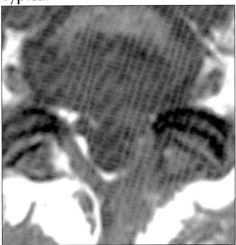
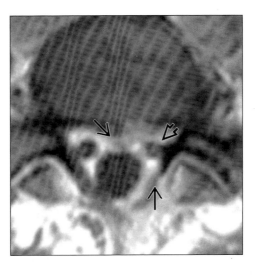

(Left) Axial T1WI MR shows homogeneous soft tissue surrounding ventral + left lateral aspect of thecal sac with minimal sac deformity from peridural fibrosis. (Right) Axial T1 C+ MR shows at L5-S1 diffuse enhancement ventral and lateral to thecal sac (arrows), surrounding exiting left S1 root (open arrow) from peridural fibrosis.

METAL ARTIFACT

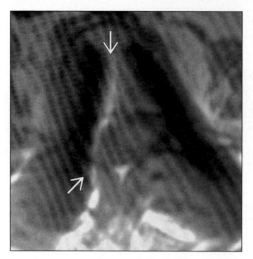

Axial T1WI MR shows metal artifact from bilateral pedicle screws. There is typical spatial mismapping with peripheral high signal (arrows). Frequency encoding direction is right to left.

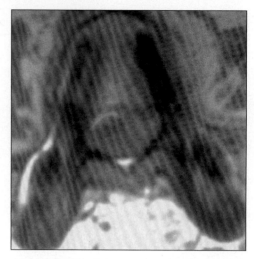

Axial T1WI MR shows metal artifact from pedicle screws. Frequency encode direction is oriented AP, minimizing artifact in transverse direction, and spreading artifact along AP direction.

TERMINOLOGY

Abbreviations and Synonyms
- CT: Beam hardening artifact
- MRI: Susceptibility artifact

Definitions
- Image degradation related to implanted metal
- Magnetic susceptibility
  - Phenomena where material becomes partially magnetized in presence of applied external magnetic field
  - Non ferromagnetic metals may produce local electrical currents induced by changing scanner magnetic field
  - Tissues with greatly different magnetic susceptibilities in uniform magnetic field ⇒
    - Difference of susceptibilities caused distortion in the magnetic field ⇒
    - Results in distortion on MR image
  - Magnetic susceptibility artifact consists of two independent but additive components
    - Geometric distortion + signal loss secondary to dephasing

IMAGING FINDINGS

General Features
- Best diagnostic clue
  - CT: Metal causes severe x-ray attenuation (missing data) in selected planes
    - Missing data or hollow projections cause classic "starburst" or streak artifacts during image reconstruction
    - Materials with lower x-ray attenuation coefficients produce less artifactual distortions
    - Plastic (best) < titanium << tantalum < stainless steel < cobalt chrome (worst)
    - Metal composition, mass, orientation + position of implant are important factors that determine magnitude of image artifact
  - Trade off must occur in choice of metal
    - Titanium wires exhibit least artifact on CT when compared to cobalt chrome or stainless steel but are more susceptible to failure
    - Titanium screws + cages produce fewer artifacts than tantalum but may not have desirable biologic properties
  - MRI: Potential safety and biologic considerations
    - Stainless steel is safe, but produces severe artifacts (especially with a low nickel content)
    - Titanium = tantalum implant artifact; much less relative to stainless steal

DDx: Causes of Low Signal

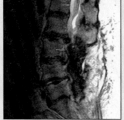

Epidural Hemorrhage

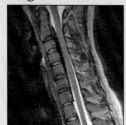

Intrathecal Gas

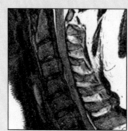

OPLL

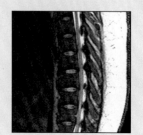

Ossif. Lig. Flavum

METAL ARTIFACT

Key Facts

Terminology
- Magnetic susceptibility
- Phenomena where material becomes partially magnetized in presence of applied external magnetic field
- Geometric distortion + signal loss secondary to dephasing

Imaging Findings
- CT: Metal causes severe x-ray attenuation (missing data) in selected planes
- Missing data or hollow projections cause classic "starburst" or streak artifacts during image reconstruction
- Materials with lower x-ray attenuation coefficients produce less artifactual distortions

- Plastic (best) < titanium << tantalum < stainless steel < cobalt chrome (worst)
- MRI general methods to minimize metal artifact
- Fast spin echo > conventional spin echo > gradient echo
- Larger field of view
- Higher readout bandwidth
- Smaller voxel size
- Appropriate geometric orientation of frequency encode direction
- Lower magnet field strength

Top Differential Diagnoses
- Bone/osteophyte
- Gas
- Hemorrhage
- Disc herniation

- ○ MRI general methods to minimize metal artifact
  - ■ Fast spin echo > conventional spin echo > gradient echo
  - ■ Larger field of view
  - ■ Higher readout bandwidth
  - ■ Smaller voxel size
  - ■ Appropriate geometric orientation of frequency encode direction
  - ■ Lower magnet field strength
- Location
  - ○ Intervertebral disc level related to fusion cages, anterior plates + screws, iatrogenic metal
  - ○ Pedicles related to pedicle screws
  - ○ Dorsal elements related to dorsal stabilization rods, interspinous process wiring
- Size: Variable
- Morphology: Central low signal, with indistinct margins, spatial mismapping of signal giving peripheral curvilinear high signal

Radiographic Findings
- Radiography: Visualize hardware malposition and alignment
- Myelography
  - ○ May be necessary if extensive hardware precludes adequate MR examination
  - ○ Fluoroscopic positioning will obtain most favorable projection with overlapping hardware

CT Findings
- NECT: Missing data from metal attenuation cause classic "starburst" or streak artifacts

MR Findings
- T1WI: Focal central signal loss with peripheral "halo" of ↑ signal related to spatial mismapping
- T2WI
  - ○ Focal central signal loss with peripheral "halo" of ↑ signal related to spatial mismapping
  - ○ Artifact minimized with FSE technique
- T2* GRE: Blooming of susceptibility artifact with gradient echo techniques, worse with increasing TE

Imaging Recommendations
- Best imaging tool: MRI best sequence choice: Fast spin echo > conventional spin echo > gradient echo
- Protocol advice
  - ○ CT: Thin-section, spiral imaging has improved quality compared to conventional discrete slices
  - ○ MRI: Optimum sequence should not contain gradient echos
    - ■ Preferably FSE technique
    - ■ FSE: Maintain short echo spacing (short echo train less critical)
    - ■ Single shot FSE sequences with half-Fourier (HASTE) useful
    - ■ Hybrid imaging sequences which use both gradient echo and spin echo components should not be used
    - ■ Frequency selective fat-saturation yields poor image quality with metal implants
    - ■ Orienting frequency encode direction along long axial of pedicle screws minimizes artifact (except in area just beyond tip of implant)

DIFFERENTIAL DIAGNOSIS

Bone/osteophyte
- Well defined low signal on all sequences; may show fatty marrow ↑ T1 signal

Gas
- No protons, no signal
- Iatrogenic epidural or subarachnoid gas
- Vacuum phenomena with degenerative disc disease

Hemorrhage
- Low signal deoxyhemoglobin

Disc herniation
- Dessication or calcification giving low signal
- Gas from adjacent vacuum phenomena

METAL ARTIFACT

PATHOLOGY

General Features
- General path comments: Post cervical discectomy/fusion, metallic susceptibility artifacts are produced by microscopic amounts of nickel, copper, and zinc
- Etiology: In anterior cervical discectomies, sufficient metals to produce artifacts are deposited only by contact of metal drill bits + suction tips
- Epidemiology: 5% of post-operative cervical discectomy cases have sufficient metal artifact to obscure thecal sac

CLINICAL ISSUES

Presentation
- Most common signs/symptoms: Typically asymptomatic, ancillary finding of surgical procedure

Demographics
- Age: Any age
- Gender: No gender predilection

DIAGNOSTIC CHECKLIST

Consider
- Following anterior cervical discectomy/fusion small amount of metal artifact is typical at fusion site
  - Contact between the drill burr and suction tip produced artifacts from metal flakes in soft tissues
- MRI pedicle screw artifact size correlates with reduction in ratio of FOV to number of pixels in frequency-encoding direction

Image Interpretation Pearls
- Minimize pedicle screw artifact by orienting frequency encode gradient parallel to screw long axis, using FSE technique
- Slice thickness 3-4 mm adequate, thinner sections yield little artifact reduction

SELECTED REFERENCES

1. Chang SD et al: MRI of spinal hardware: comparison of conventional T1-weighted sequence with a new metal artifact reduction sequence. Skeletal Radiol. 30(4):213-8, 2001
2. Viano AM et al: Improved MR imaging for patients with metallic implants. Magn Reson Imaging. 18(3):287-95, 2000
3. Henk CB et al: The postoperative spine. Top Magn Reson Imaging. 10(4):247-64, 1999
4. Rudisch A et al: Metallic artifacts in magnetic resonance imaging of patients with spinal fusion. A comparison of implant materials and imaging sequences. Spine. 23(6):692-9, 1998
5. Wang JC et al: A comparison of magnetic resonance and computed tomographic image quality after the implantation of tantalum and titanium spinal instrumentation. Spine. 23(15):1684-8, 1998
6. Taber KH et al: Pitfalls and artifacts encountered in clinical MR imaging of the spine. Radiographics. 18(6):1499-521, 1998
7. Frazzini VI et al: Internally stabilized spine: optimal choice of frequency-encoding gradient direction during MR imaging minimizes susceptibility artifact from titanium vertebral body screws. Radiology. 204(1):268-72, 1997
8. Doran SE et al: Internal fixation of the spine using a braided titanium cable: clinical results and postoperative magnetic resonance imaging. Neurosurgery. 38(3):493-6; discussion 496-7, 1996
9. Ortiz O et al: Postoperative magnetic resonance imaging with titanium implants of the thoracic and lumbar spine. Neurosurgery. 38(4):741-5, 1996
10. Petersilge CA et al: Optimizing imaging parameters for MR evaluation of the spine with titanium pedicle screws. AJR Am J Roentgenol. 166(5):1213-8, 1996
11. Shellock FG: MR imaging and cervical fixation devices: evaluation of ferromagnetism, heating, and artifacts at 1.5 Tesla. Magn Reson Imaging. 14(9):1093-8, 1996
12. Tominaga T et al: Magnetic resonance imaging of titanium anterior cervical spine plating systems. Neurosurgery. 36(5):951-5, 1995
13. Tartaglino LM et al: Metallic artifacts on MR images of the postoperative spine: reduction with fast spin-echo techniques. Radiology. 190(2):565-9, 1994
14. Vaccaro AR et al: Metallic spinal artifacts in magnetic resonance imaging. Spine. 19(11):1237-42, 1994
15. Yoshino MT et al: Metallic postoperative artifacts on cervical MR. AJNR Am J Neuroradiol. 14(3):747-9, 1993
16. Toro VE et al: MR artifacts after anterior cervical diskectomy and fusion: a cadaver study. J Comput Assist Tomogr. 17(5):696-9, 1993
17. Peterman SB et al: Magnetic resonance artifact in the postoperative cervical spine. A potential pitfall. Spine. 16(7):721-5, 1991

IMAGE GALLERY

Typical

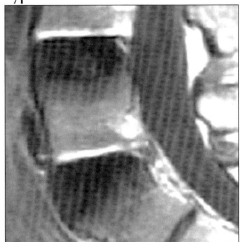

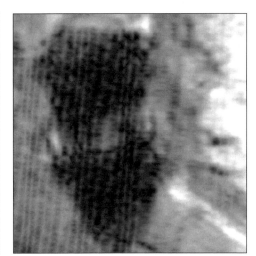

(Left) Sagittal T1WI MR shows metal artifact from L4-5, L5-S1 interbody fusion with cages. Artifact remains confined to vertebral body margins, allowing definition of epidural disease. *(Right)* Sagittal T2* GRE MR shows extensive metal susceptibility artifact in patient with L4-5, L5-S1 interbody fusion with cages.

Typical

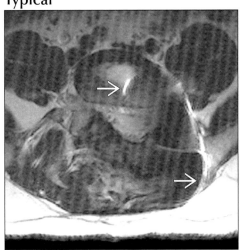

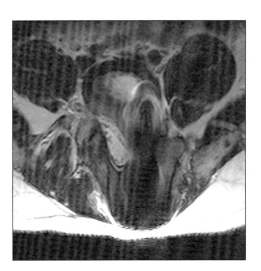

(Left) Axial T2WI MR shows susceptibility artifact from left pedicle screw with frequency encode direction oriented right-left. Note typical spatial mismapping with increase signal (arrows). *(Right)* Axial T2WI MR shows metal artifact from left pedicle screw. Frequency encode direction is oriented AP, stretching artifact along that direction, minimizing right-left direction artifact.

Typical

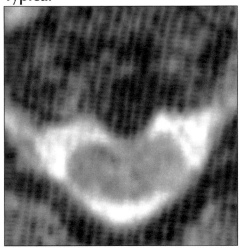

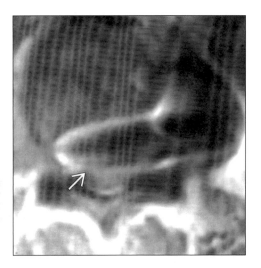

(Left) Axial T2* GRE MR shows focal low signal in anterior epidural region reflecting metal artifact from tiny metal shard, not visible on plain films or CT, mimicking osteophyte. *(Right)* Axial T1WI MR shows screw malposition. Linear metal artifact from vertebral body screw following thoracic fusion shows artifact is posterior within body, overlapping thecal sac and cord (arrow).

RADIATION MYELOPATHY

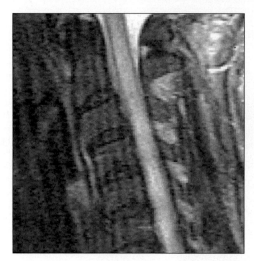

Sagittal T2WI MR shows diffusely enlarged hyperintense cervical cord in patient treated previously for nasopharyngeal cancer. T1 C+ MR showed focal enhancement.

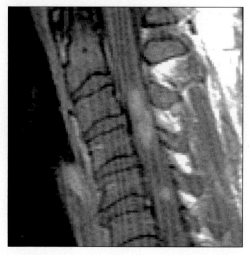

Sagittal T1 C+ MR in the same patient shows patchy enhancement within long segment of enlarged cord, low signal above, below. T2WI showed diffuse high signal throughout cord.

TERMINOLOGY

Abbreviations and Synonyms
- Chronic progressive radiation myelitis (CPRM)
- Delayed radiation myelopathy (DRM)
- Radiation necrosis

Definitions
- Damage of neural tissue in spinal cord following therapeutic radiation of intrinsic or nearby disease

IMAGING FINDINGS

General Features
- Best diagnostic clue: Cord swelling, intramedullary enhancement
- Location
  ○ Within radiation field
  ○ Mainly in white matter of lateral spinothalamic tracts, dorsal columns
- Size
  ○ Depends on dimension of radiation field
  ○ Clinical signs may reflect longer segment of damage than shown on MR
- Morphology
  ○ Spindle-shaped cord swelling with irregular, focal rind of enhancement

○ Focal cord atrophy in late stage

Radiographic Findings
- Myelography
  ○ Swollen cord
  ○ Atrophy in late stage

CT Findings
- CECT: May show enhancement within cord

MR Findings
- T1WI
  ○ Expanded cord, low signal intensity
  ○ Focal cord atrophy in late stage
- T2WI
  ○ Fusiform expansion of cord, with high signal intensity
  ○ Atrophic cord, with signal elevation in late stage
- STIR: Like T2WI
- T1 C+
  ○ Ring or irregular enhancement surrounded by edematous cord
  ○ Enhancing focus may be absent
  ○ Enhancing focus becomes site of focal atrophy in serial scans

Imaging Recommendations
- Best imaging tool: MRI with T1 C+
- Protocol advice: Fat-saturated T1 C+

DDx: Myelopathy

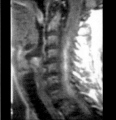

Transverse Myelitis

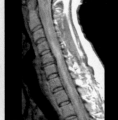

Multiple Sclerosis

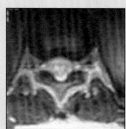

Cord Infarct

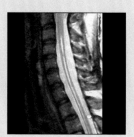

Syrinx

RADIATION MYELOPATHY

Key Facts

Terminology
- Chronic progressive radiation myelitis (CPRM)
- Delayed radiation myelopathy (DRM)
- Radiation necrosis

Imaging Findings
- Mainly in white matter of lateral spinothalamic tracts, dorsal columns
- Clinical signs may reflect longer segment of damage than shown on MR
- Spindle-shaped cord swelling with irregular, focal rind of enhancement
- Focal cord atrophy in late stage
- Ring or irregular enhancement surrounded by edematous cord
- Enhancing focus may be absent
- Enhancing focus becomes site of focal atrophy in serial scans

Top Differential Diagnoses
- Transverse myelitis
- Multiple sclerosis
- Astrocytoma

Pathology
- Radiation damage to cord
- Typically with doses over 50 Grey (Gy)
- Fractionation schedule - more than 2 Gy per treatment
- Demyelination in lateral, dorsal tracts
- Hyalinosis of intramedullary vessel walls
- Necrosis

DIFFERENTIAL DIAGNOSIS

Transverse myelitis
- More rapid onset of myelopathy
- Predisposing factors of infection, vaccination

Multiple sclerosis
- Multifocal
- Patchy high signal foci on T2WI
- Sensory symptoms at onset
- Waxing, waning signs and symptoms

Cord infarct
- Acute onset of paralysis
- Grey matter involvement predominates

Astrocytoma
- Very slow onset and progression

Syrinx
- More insidious onset
- Discrete cavity

PATHOLOGY

General Features
- General path comments: Swollen, boggy cord
- Etiology
  - Radiation damage to cord
  - Typically with doses over 50 Grey (Gy)
  - May see in cases below 50 Gy
  - Fractionation schedule - more than 2 Gy per treatment
  - Concurrent chemotherapy may be a predisposing factor, especially if intrathecal
- Epidemiology: Unusual complication

Gross Pathologic & Surgical Features
- Edematous, enlarged cord

Microscopic Features
- Demyelination in lateral, dorsal tracts
- Lipid ladened microphages
- Swollen astrocytes
- Endothelial damage
- Hyalinosis of intramedullary vessel walls
- Necrosis
- Local calcium deposits

CLINICAL ISSUES

Presentation
- Most common signs/symptoms
  - Progressive numbness and weakness
  - Other signs/symptoms
    - Sphincter dysfunction
- Clinical profile
  - Onset of weakness, numbness one month to several years following fractionated radiotherapy
  - Radiotherapy of lung or nasopharyngeal cancer; mantle lymphoma therapy especially with intrathecal methotrexate

Demographics
- Age: Any
- Gender: No predilection

Natural History & Prognosis
- Progressive, without significant improvement in most cases

Treatment
- Options, risks, complications: Hyperbaric oxygen helpful in some early cases

DIAGNOSTIC CHECKLIST

Consider
- Checking radiation field, fractionation schedule (especially if > 2 Gy per treatment)

Image Interpretation Pearls
- Late stage shows focal atrophy at sites of previous contrast enhancement

- Fatty replacement of marrow in vertebral bodies within treatment field
- Pathologic changes in cord not always visible on MRI

SELECTED REFERENCES

1. Warscotte L et al: Concurrent spinal cord and vertebral bone marrow radionecrosis 8 years after therapeutic irradiation. Neuroradiology. 44(3):245-8, 2002
2. Okada S et al: Pathology of radiation myelopathy. Neuropathology. 21(4):247-65, 2001
3. Maddison P et al: Clinical and MRI discordance in a case of delayed radiation myelopathy. J Neurol Neurosurg Psychiatry. 69(4):563-4, 2000
4. Maddison P et al: Clinical and MRI discordance in a case of delayed radiation myelopathy. J Neurol Neurosurg Psychiatry. 69(4):563-4, 2000
5. Macbeth F: Radiation myelitis and thoracic radiotherapy: evidence and anecdote. Clin Oncol (R Coll Radiol). 12(5):333-4, 2000
6. Calabro F et al: MRI of radiation myelitis: a report of a case treated with hyperbaric oxygen. Eur Radiol. 10(7):1079-84, 2000
7. Nieder C et al: Radiation myelopathy: new perspective on an old problem. Radiat Oncol Investig. 7(4):193-203, 1999
8. Rampling R et al: Radiation myelopathy. Curr Opin Neurol. 11(6):627-32, 1998
9. Alfonso ER et al: Radiation myelopathy in over-irradiated patients: MR imaging findings. Eur Radiol. 7(3):400-4, 1997
10. Koehler PJ et al: Delayed radiation myelopathy: serial MR-imaging and pathology. Clin Neurol Neurosurg. 98(2):197-201, 1996
11. Wong CS et al: Radiation myelopathy following single courses of radiotherapy and retreatment. Int J Radiat Oncol Biol Phys. 30(3):575-81, 1994
12. Hirota S et al: Chronological observation in early radiation myelopathy of the cervical spinal cord: gadolinium-enhanced MRI findings in two cases. Radiat Med. 11(4):154-9, 1993
13. Schultheiss TE et al: Invited review: permanent radiation myelopathy. Br J Radiol. 65(777):737-53, 1992
14. Dische S: Accelerated treatment and radiation myelitis. Radiother Oncol. 20(1):1-2, 1991
15. Jeremic B et al: Incidence of radiation myelitis of the cervical spinal cord at doses of 5500 cGy or greater. Cancer. 68(10):2138-41, 1991
16. Bloss JD et al: Radiation myelitis: a complication of concurrent cisplatin and 5-fluorouracil chemotherapy with extended field radiotherapy for carcinoma of the uterine cervix. Gynecol Oncol. 43(3):305-8, 1991
17. Magrini SM et al: Neurological damage in patients irradiated twice on the spinal cord: a morphologic and electrophysiological study. Radiother Oncol. 17(3):209-18, 1990
18. Marcus RB Jr et al: The incidence of myelitis after irradiation of the cervical spinal cord. Int J Radiat Oncol Biol Phys. 19(1):3-8, 1990
19. Dische S et al: Radiation myelitis and survival in the radiotherapy of lung cancer. Int J Radiat Oncol Biol Phys. 15(1):75-81, 1988
20. Goldwein JW: Radiation myelopathy: a review. Med Pediatr Oncol. 15(2):89-95, 1987
21. Hatlevoll R et al: Myelopathy following radiotherapy of bronchial carcinoma with large single fractions: a retrospective study. Int J Radiat Oncol Biol Phys. 9(1):41-4, 1983
22. Fitzgerald RH Jr et al: Chronic radiation myelitis. Radiology. 144(3):609-12, 1982
23. Worthington BS: Diffuse cord enlargement in radiation myelopathy. Clin Radiol. 30(1):117-9, 1979
24. Godwin-Austen RB et al: Observations on radiation myelopathy. Brain. 98(4):557-68, 1975
25. Burns RJ et al: Pathology of radiation myelopathy. J Neurol Neurosurg Psychiatry. 35(6):888-98, 1972

IMAGE GALLERY

Typical

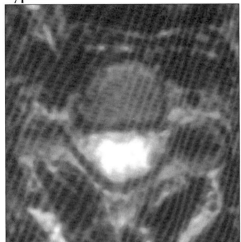 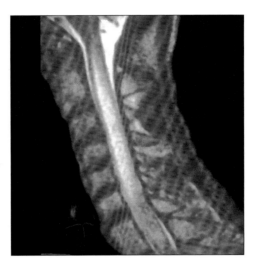

(Left) Axial T2WI MR shows obvious signal elevation in cord. Patient developed weakness and numbness several months after neck irradiation. *(Right)* Sagittal T2WI MR shows fusiform expansion and cord edema in patient after previous neck irradiation.

Typical

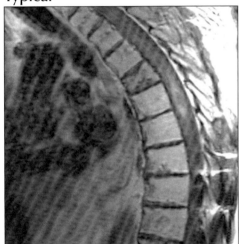 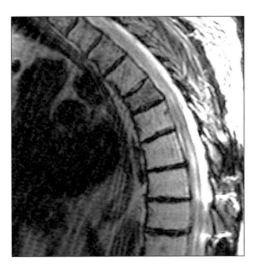

(Left) Sagittal T1 C+ MR shows spindle shaped enhancement in thoracic cord; fatty marrow replacement also noted in patient following previous radiation therapy for vertebral metastases. *(Right)* Sagittal T2WI MR shows increased signal within cord in patient previously treated for skeletal metastases.

Variant

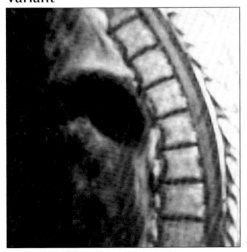 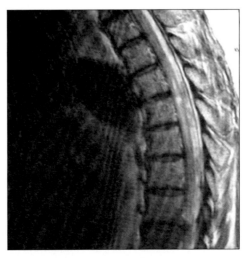

(Left) Sagittal T1WI MR shows focal low signal within atrophic cord. Patient was paraplegic several years after chest irradiation. Note fat signal in vertebral bodies. *(Right)* Sagittal T2WI MR shows atrophic cord, with signal elevation, in paraplegic patient several years after chest irradiation.

POST IRRADIATION VERTEBRAL MARROW

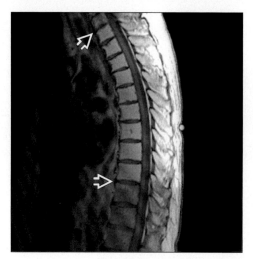

Sagittal T1WI MR shows homogeneous post irradiation fatty marrow in thoracic spine, with clear cranial and rostral demarcation (arrows), corresponding to radiotherapy portal.

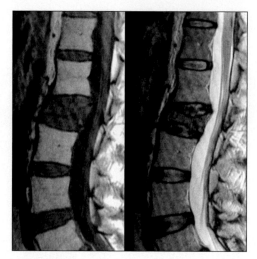

Sagittal T1WI MR (left) in a patient with previous lumbar irradiation shows diffuse hyperintense marrow, except in collapsed L2 vertebra. Fatty marrow is of intermediate SI on T2WI (right).

TERMINOLOGY

Definitions
- Transformation of vertebral marrow into fatty marrow after therapeutic irradiation

IMAGING FINDINGS

General Features
- Best diagnostic clue: Marrow signal intensity (SI) within radiotherapy portal similar to subcutaneous fat on T1WI
- Location: Corresponds to site of irradiation
- Size: Corresponds to extent of radiation field
- Morphology
  - Homogeneous marrow SI
    - Heterogeneity due to residual or recurrent marrow disease
  - Sharp demarcation between irradiated vs. untreated marrow

Radiographic Findings
- Radiography: Osteopenia, compression fractures may be present

CT Findings
- Bone CT
  - Compression fractures

MR Findings
- T1WI
  - Very high SI
  - Increased SI also in marrow outside radiation field
    - From scatter dose of radiation
- T2WI: Intermediate SI
- PD/Intermediate: Intermediate SI
- STIR
  - High SI in acute phase
  - Low SI thereafter
- T1 C+
  - Post-gadolinium enhancement in acute phase
    - Probably related to vascular congestion
  - No enhancement thereafter
    - Decreased vascularity and fibrosis
- First three weeks
  - No change or early marrow T1 hyperintensity
    - Hyperintensity suggestive of hemorrhage ± fatty replacement
  - Hyperintensity on STIR
    - Indicating marrow edema and necrosis
    - Peak incidence nine days after irradiation
    - Subsequent gradual decrease in SI
- Three to six weeks
  - Heterogeneous mottled pattern on T1WI
  - Increasing fat intensity within central vertebral marrow
    - Surrounding basivertebral vein

DDx: Hyperintense Marrow on T1WI

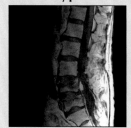

Fatty Marrow

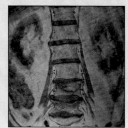

Fatty Marrow

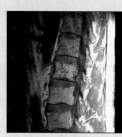

Hemangioma

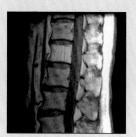

Hemangioma

Key Facts

Terminology
- Transformation of vertebral marrow into fatty marrow after therapeutic irradiation

Imaging Findings
- Best diagnostic clue: Marrow signal intensity (SI) within radiotherapy portal similar to subcutaneous fat on T1WI
- Homogeneous marrow SI
- Sharp demarcation between irradiated vs. untreated marrow
- T2WI: Intermediate SI
- Post-gadolinium enhancement in acute phase
- No enhancement thereafter
- Diffuse and homogenous hyperintensity on T1WI

- PET: Decreased marrow metabolic activity with FDG-18
- MRI is the modality of choice in marrow imaging

Top Differential Diagnoses
- Normal fatty marrow

Pathology
- Fatty marrow replaces cellular marrow and bone loss
- Marrow changes on MRI dependent on radiation dose, fractionation, and time elapsed after treatment

Clinical Issues
- Usually asymptomatic
- Return to normal marrow pattern on long term follow-up: > 10 yr

---

- After six weeks
  - Diffuse and homogenous hyperintensity on T1WI
  - Band pattern of peripheral intermediate SI
    - Surrounding central hyperintense marrow
    - May represent regenerating hematopoietic marrow
  - > 90% of treated marrow has this appearance

Nuclear Medicine Findings
- Bone Scan
  - Sharply delineated focal or diffuse diminished radio-tracer uptake
    - Loss of vascularity
- PET: Decreased marrow metabolic activity with FDG-18
- Tc-99m sulfur colloid scan
  - Sharply demarcated focal or diffuse photopenic region
    - Corresponds to radiation therapy portal

Other Modality Findings
- Dual energy CT study
  - Bone mass may be reduced

Imaging Recommendations
- Best imaging tool
  - MRI is the modality of choice in marrow imaging
    - T1WI most sensitive
- Protocol advice
  - STIR or FSE T2WI with fat-saturation to better assess recurrent or residual marrow disease
  - Pre- and post-gadolinium T1WI with fat-suppression also increases lesion conspicuity

DIFFERENTIAL DIAGNOSIS

Normal fatty marrow
- Age related
- Predominantly fat intensity
  - Some heterogeneity present
- No clear demarcation
- ± Compression fractures
- No abnormality on bone scan or PET

Vertebral hemangioma
- Well-circumscribed rounded lesion
- Typically hyperintense on T1WI and T2WI
  - Presence of fatty stroma
- Avid post-contrast-enhancement

PATHOLOGY

General Features
- General path comments: Fatty marrow replaces cellular marrow and bone loss
- Genetics: No genetic predisposition
- Etiology
  - Radiation destroys hematopoietic elements
    - Highly radiosensitive
  - Reduction of bone mass also occurs
  - Marrow changes on MRI dependent on radiation dose, fractionation, and time elapsed after treatment
    - No change in marrow SI with radiation dose of 1.25 Gy
    - At 50 Gy, persistent fat SI even after 9 years
    - Complete and irreversible eradication of cellular elements
    - Between 20-30 Gy, return to normal marrow pattern after long term follow-up: > 10 yr
    - Partial recovery between 2-9 years
    - Marrow reconversion in pediatric patients occurs 11-30 months after radiation treatment
    - Fatty marrow seen on MRI as early as 2 weeks after therapeutic irradiation
    - > 90% will show fatty marrow after 2 months
- Epidemiology: Expected finding on all post-radiotherapy patients
- Associated abnormalities
  - Osteonecrosis
    - Sharp border between normal and infarcted marrow
    - Hyperintense on STIR or T2WI with fat-saturation
    - Hypointense on T1WI
    - ± Enhance after intravenous gadolinium
    - ± Intravertebral fluid collection

POST IRRADIATION VERTEBRAL MARROW

- May see linear transverse intravertebral gas and sclerosis on radiography and CT
- No uptake on bone scan unless vertebral collapse
- May be difficult to distinguish from recurrent metastasis
- Biopsy indicated
○ Residual or recurrent metastases
  - Multifocal discrete lesions
  - Hypointense on T1WI surrounded by fatty marrow
  - Hyperintense on T2WI with fat-suppression or STIR
  - Treated lesions may not enhance
  - Paradural and paravertebral soft tissue extension
  - Pathologic fractures
○ Osteopenia
○ Compression fractures
○ Post radiation myelitis
  - Diffuse cord hyperintensity on T2WI within radiation treatment field
  - Mildly hypointense on T1WI
  - Cord enlargement
  - Irregular foci of enhancement suggestive of necrosis

Microscopic Features

- Based on rat model after single dose of irradiation at 20 Gy
- Initially decreased cellular elements and disrupted sinusoids
  ○ Associated edema and hemorrhage
- Early influx of cells to re-populate marrow
  ○ Concomitant increase in fatty marrow
- Subsequent depletion of cellularity and sinusoids
  ○ Fibrosis with further increase in fatty marrow
- Eventual regeneration of hematopoietic elements and sinusoids

CLINICAL ISSUES

Presentation

- Most common signs/symptoms
  ○ Usually asymptomatic
  ○ Other signs/symptoms
    - Pain
    - Myelopathy and radiculopathy from compression fracture or tumor infiltration
- Clinical profile
  ○ Development or worsening of pain and neurologic complaints
    - Indication of radiation necrosis, insufficiency fracture, or tumor recurrence or progression

Demographics

- Age: Children and adults
- Gender: Male and female equally affected
- Ethnicity: No racial predilection

Natural History & Prognosis

- Return to normal marrow pattern on long term follow-up: > 10 yr
- Dependent on underlying disease for which radiation therapy is employed

Treatment

- Supportive measures for compression fracture
- Surgical intervention if cord compromised or instability present

DIAGNOSTIC CHECKLIST

Consider

- T2WI with fat-suppression, STIR, and T1WI post-gadolinium with fat-suppression to evaluate residual or recurrent marrow disease

Image Interpretation Pearls

- Homogeneous fatty marrow sharply delineated from untreated vertebral marrow diagnostic of post irradiation change

SELECTED REFERENCES

1. Otake S et al: Radiation-induced changes in MR signal intensity and contrast enhancement of lumbosacral vertebrae: do changes occur only inside the radiation therapy field? Radiology. 222(1):179-83, 2002
2. Onu M et al: Early MR changes in vertebral bone marrow for patients following radiotherapy. Eur Radiol. 11(8):1463-9, 2001
3. Meyer MA et al: Reduced F-18 fluorodeoxyglucose uptake within marrow after external beam radiation. Clin Nucl Med. 25(4):279-80, 2000
4. Blomlie V et al: Female pelvic bone marrow: serial MR imaging before, during, and after radiation therapy. Radiology. 194(2):537-43, 1995
5. Cavenagh EC et al: Hematopoietic marrow regeneration in pediatric patients undergoing spinal irradiation: MR depiction. AJNR Am J Neuroradiol. 16(3):461-7, 1995
6. Steiner RM et al: Magnetic resonance imaging of diffuse bone marrow disease. Radiol Clin of North Am 31:383-409, 1993
7. Yankelevitz DF et al: Effect of radiation therapy on thoracic and lumbar bone marrow: evaluation with MR imaging. AJR Am J Roentgenol. 157(1):87-92, 1991
8. Stevens SK et al: Early and late bone-marrow changes after irradiation: MR evaluation. AJR Am J Roentgenol. 154(4):745-50, 1990
9. Naul LG et al: Avascular necrosis of the vertebral body: MR imaging. Radiology. 172(1):219-22, 1989
10. Casamassima F et al: Hematopoietic bone marrow recovery after radiation therapy: MRI evaluation. Blood. 73(6):1677-81, 1989
11. Rosenthal DI et al: Fatty replacement of spinal bone marrow due to radiation: demonstration by dual energy quantitative CT and MR imaging. J Comput Assist Tomogr. 13(3):463-5, 1989
12. Shih WJ et al: Thoracic vertebral photopenia may predict fatty changes of the corresponding bone marrow following irradiation. Radiat Med. 7(1):32-5, 1989
13. Ramsey RG et al: MR imaging of the spine after radiation therapy: easily recognizable effects. AJR Am J Roentgenol. 144(6):1131-5, 1985
14. Maldague BE et al: The intravertebral vacuum cleft: a sign of ischemic vertebral collapse. Radiology. 129(1):23-9, 1978

IMAGE GALLERY

Typical

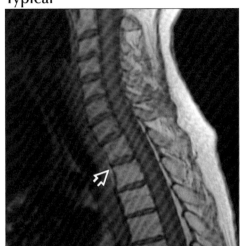 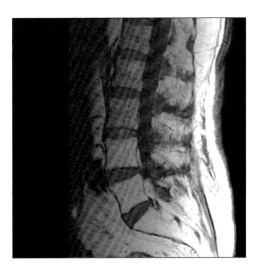

(Left) Sagittal T1WI MR demonstrates smooth marrow hyperintensity in thoracic vertebrae caudal to T1-2 (arrow), which is the upper boundary of radiotherapy field. *(Right)* Sagittal T1WI MR in another patient who received pelvic radiation shows fatty marrow replacement in L4 and L5 vertebrae and sacrum. Non-irradiated marrow in upper lumbar spine appears heterogeneous.

Typical

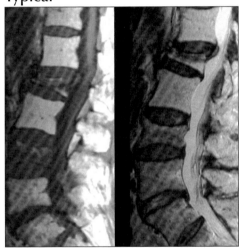 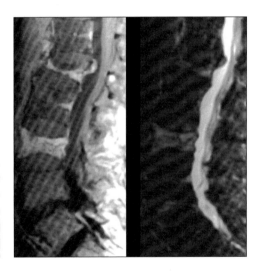

(Left) Sagittal T1WI MR (left) & T2WI (right) demonstrate post irradiation fatty marrow in lower thoracic & upper lumbar spine including L3. Benign compression fractures are present in L2 and L4 vertebrae. *(Right)* Sagittal T1 C+ MR with fat suppression (left) shows enhancing marrow in L2 & L4 vertebrae, which is hyperintense on STIR (right), compatible with marrow edema from acute benign fracture.

Typical

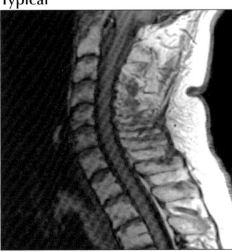 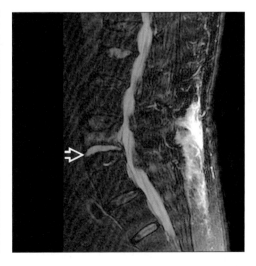

(Left) Sagittal T1WI MR of cervical spine in a patient with multiple myeloma and previous radiation therapy demonstrates scattered myelomatous deposits surrounded by hyperintense fatty marrow. *(Right)* Sagittal STIR MR shows vertebral osteonecrosis, which can be a complication of spinal radiation. Marrow edema, a fluid-filled cleft (arrow), and compression fracture are present in L4 vertebra.

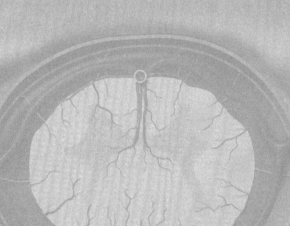

PART VIII

Potpourri

Gamuts ⬜1

VIII

1

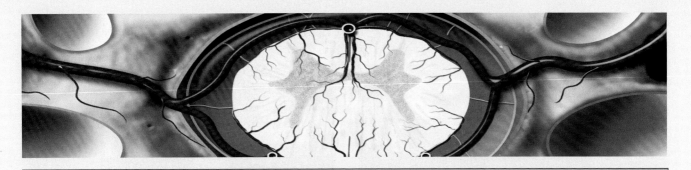

SECTION 1: Gamuts

SECONDARY ACUTE TRANSVERSE MYELITIS

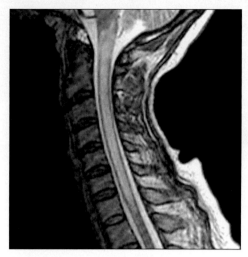

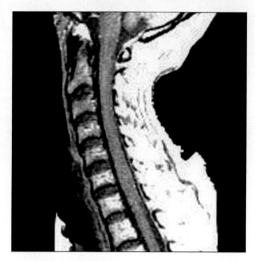

Sagittal T2WI MR in a patient with acute, progressive myelopathy shows diffuse homogeneous hyperintensity involving lower brain stem & entire cervical cord with slight cord swelling.

Sagittal T1 C+ MR in same patient does not demonstrate significant post-gadolinium enhancement. Findings are compatible with acute transverse myelitis.

TERMINOLOGY

Abbreviations and Synonyms
- Noncompressive myelopathy
- Acute transverse myelitis (ATM)

Definitions
- Inflammatory disorder of spinal cord associated with many etiologies

IMAGING FINDINGS

General Features
- Best diagnostic clue: Hyperintense lesion on T2WI with mild cord expansion without significant enhancement
- Location: Thoracic > cervical > conus medullaris
- Size: Segmental, multi-segmental, or holocord
- Morphology: Fairly well-defined signal abnormality

Radiographic Findings
- Myelography
  - Cord swelling
  - Cerebral spinal fluid flow may be impeded

CT Findings
- NECT: Mild cord enlargement
- CECT: Focal, diffuse, or heterogeneous enhancement

MR Findings
- T1WI
  - Normal
  - Focal or diffuse hypointensity
  - Mild hyperintensity due to petechial hemorrhage
- T2WI
  - Focal or diffuse hyperintensity
  - Swollen cord
- STIR: Hyperintense
- T1 C+
  - Variable enhancement
    - None
    - Focal, diffuse, heterogeneous
    - May be mass-like
    - Peripheral/meningeal
- Cord swelling and enhancement typically resolve
  - Corresponding to clinical improvement
- Cord atrophy may be present in later stage

Imaging Recommendations
- Best imaging tool
  - Sagittal and axial T1WI & T2WI MRI with gadolinium
    - 40% of clinical ATM with normal MRI findings

DDx: Intramedullary Hyperintense Lesions on T2WI

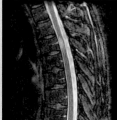

Multiple Sclerosis

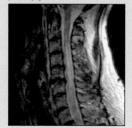

Idiopathic ATM

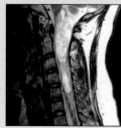

Astrocytoma

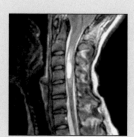

Syringohydromyelia

SECONDARY ACUTE TRANSVERSE MYELITIS

Key Facts

Terminology
- Noncompressive myelopathy
- Inflammatory disorder of spinal cord associated with many etiologies

Imaging Findings
- Best diagnostic clue: Hyperintense lesion on T2WI with mild cord expansion without significant enhancement
- Location: Thoracic > cervical > conus medullaris
- Size: Segmental, multi-segmental, or holocord
- Cord swelling
- Cerebral spinal fluid flow may be impeded
- Focal or diffuse hyperintensity
- Variable enhancement

Top Differential Diagnoses
- Multiple sclerosis (MS)
- Idiopathic ATM
- Acute disseminated encephalomyelitis (ADEM)
- Cord neoplasm
- Cord infarct

Pathology
- General path comments: Occlusive vasculitis, necrosis, gliosis, ± demyelination

Clinical Issues
- Sensory deficit
- Back ± radicular pain
- Paraplegia/quadriplegia
- Bladder and bowel urgency, frequency, and retention
- 30-50% with complete recovery after treatment

DIFFERENTIAL DIAGNOSIS

Multiple sclerosis (MS)
- May be difficult to distinguish from ATM by imaging alone
  - Lesion peripheral in location
  - Less than two vertebral segments in length
  - Less than half cross-sectional area of cord
  - Homogenous or ring enhancement in acute or subacute phase
- MS following ATM: 2-8%
- 90% with associated intracranial lesions
- Relapsing remitting clinical course

Idiopathic ATM
- Imaging features overlap with those in secondary ATM
  - Lesion centrally located
  - 3 to 4 segments in length
  - Occupying more than two thirds of cord's cross-sectional area
  - Variable enhancement
- Diagnosis of exclusion
  - 60% of ATM
- No associated intracranial lesions

Acute disseminated encephalomyelitis (ADEM)
- Indistinguishable from cord MS
- Thalamic involvement more common intracranially
- Younger age at presentation
- Constitutional symptoms
- Monophasic clinical course

Cord neoplasm
- Moderate cord expansion invariably present
- Diffuse or nodular contrast enhancement
- Extensive peri-tumoral edema
- Cystic ± hemorrhagic components
- More indolent clinical course

Cord infarct
- Ventral cord location
- Less mass effect initially
- Motor signs > sensory
- No enhancement in acute phase
- Immediate onset: Minutes, rather than hours, days

Neuromyelitis optica
- Devic disease
- Diffuse intramedullary hyperintensity on T2WI
- Cord swelling
- Bilateral retrobulbar optic neuritis preceding ATM
  - ATM as initial presentation in 20% of cases
- No clinical involvement beyond spinal cord and optic nerves

Vitamin B12 deficiency
- Mild cord enlargement
- Signal abnormality in dorsal ± lateral columns
  - Hypointense on T1WI and hyperintense on T2WI
- No enhancement
- Macrocytic anemia with decreased plasma B12 level

Syringohydromyelia
- Central cystic lesion
- Cerebral spinal fluid intensity on all pulse sequences
- No post-gadolinium enhancement
- Normal cord contour

PATHOLOGY

General Features
- General path comments: Occlusive vasculitis, necrosis, gliosis, ± demyelination
- Genetics: No genetic predilection
- Etiology
  - Collagen vascular disease
    - Autoimmune vasculitis
    - Systemic lupus erythematosus (SLE)
    - Antiphospholipid syndrome
    - Sjögren disease, scleroderma
    - Sarcoidosis
    - Mixed connective tissue disease
    - ATM may be the initial manifestation
  - Infectious: Typically viral

SECONDARY ACUTE TRANSVERSE MYELITIS

- Direct cord involvement ± autoimmune phenomenon
- Epstein-Barr virus, Cytomegalovirus
- Herpes zoster, varicella-zoster virus
- HIV, HTLV-1
- Enteroviruses
- Non-viral pathogens: Syphilis, Lyme disease, mycoplasma pneumoniae, schistosomiasis
  ○ Post-vaccination
    - Autoimmune response with small vessel vasculopathy
    - Polio, rubella, rabies, smallpox, influenza, hepatitis B vaccinations, etc.
  ○ Post irradiation
    - Dose of 45-50 Gy in daily 1.8-2 Gy fractions considered safe
    - Toxic radiation effect may be potentiated by concurrent chemotherapy
    - Symptoms develop 6-30 months after therapeutic irradiation
    - MRI may be normal even if symptoms present
  ○ Arterio-venous malformation (AVM)
    - Chronic ischemia/venous stasis
    - Course more indolent compared to other etiologies
  ○ Para-neoplastic syndrome
    - May be initial presentation of underlying neoplasm
    - Autoantibodies against proteins in spinal cord
    - Lung, breast, hepatocellular carcinoma, etc.
    - Lymphoma, leukemia, multiple myeloma
- Epidemiology: 4.6 new cases of transverse myelitis per million people per year in US
- Associated abnormalities
  ○ Optic neuritis in SLE
  ○ Fatty marrow in post irradiation
  ○ Abnormal surface vessels in cord AVM

Microscopic Features
- Necrosis of gray and white matter
- Destruction of neurons, axons, and myelin
- Astrocytic gliosis
- Perivascular lymphocytic infiltrate with vascular occlusion

CLINICAL ISSUES

Presentation
- Most common signs/symptoms
  ○ Sensory deficit
    - Loss of pain and temperature sensation
    - Well-defined upper level
    - Ascending paresthesia in bilateral upper/lower extremities
    - Band-like dysesthesia
  ○ Other signs/symptoms:
    - Back ± radicular pain
    - Paraplegia/quadriplegia
    - Bladder and bowel urgency, frequency, and retention
    - Hypotonia and hyporeflexia initially
    - Spasticity and hyperreflexia over time

- Clinical profile: Progression to severe neurologic deficits within days

Demographics
- Age
  ○ All ages can be effected
    - Peak incidence: 10-19 and 30-39 yo
- Gender
  ○ Female predominance in collagen vascular disease
  ○ Other etiologies without significant gender predilection

Natural History & Prognosis
- 30-50% with complete recovery after treatment

Treatment
- Collagen vascular disease
  ○ Corticosteroids
  ○ Immunosuppressive therapy
    - Cyclophosphamide, azathioprine, chlorambucil
  ○ Plasmapheresis
  ○ Intravenous immunoglobulin
- Infectious etiologies
  ○ Anti-viral, anti-bacterial medications
  ○ Corticosteroids
- Post irradiation myelitis
  ○ Hyperbaric oxygen treatment

DIAGNOSTIC CHECKLIST

Consider
- Brain MRI to exclude intracranial lesions associated with MS or ADEM

SELECTED REFERENCES
1. Harzheim M et al: Discriminatory features of acute transverse myelitis: a retrospective analysis of 45 patients. J Neurol Sci. 217(2):217-23, 2004
2. Sherer Y et al: Transverse myelitis in patients with antiphospholipid antibodies--the importance of early diagnosis and treatment. Clin Rheumatol. 21(3):207-10, 2002
3. Transverse Myelitis Consortium Working Group: Proposed diagnostic criteria and nosology of acute transverse myelitis. Neurology. 59(4):499-505, 2002
4. Goebels N et al: Extensive myelitis associated with Mycoplasma pneumoniae infection: magnetic resonance imaging and clinical long-term follow-up. J Neurol. 248(3):204-8, 2001
5. Scotti G et al: Diagnosis and differential diagnosis of acute transverse myelopathy. The role of neuroradiological investigations and review of the literature. Neurol Sci. 22 Suppl 2:S69-73, 2001
6. Kovacs B et al: Transverse myelopathy in systemic lupus erythematosus: an analysis of 14 cases and review of the literature. Ann Rheum Dis. 59(2):120-4, 2000
7. Tartaglino LM et al: MR imaging in a case of postvaccination myelitis. AJNR Am J Neuroradiol. 16(3):581-2, 1995
8. Austin SG et al: The role of magnetic resonance imaging in acute transverse myelitis. Can J Neurol Sci. 19(4):508-11, 1992

SECONDARY ACUTE TRANSVERSE MYELITIS

IMAGE GALLERY

Typical

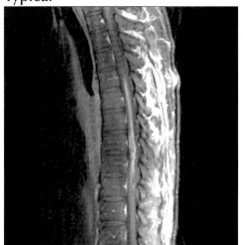 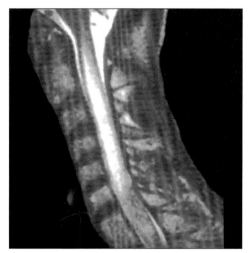

(Left) Sagittal T1 C+ MR with fat suppression in a patient with sarcoidosis & myelopathy demonstrates multisegmental thoracic intramedullary enhancement without significant mass effect. *(Right)* Sagittal T2WI MR in patient with history of head & neck cancer treated with radiotherapy demonstrates post irradiation ATM with diffuse hyperintensity + cord swelling from C2 to C6.

Typical

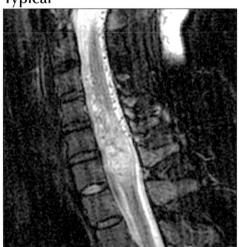 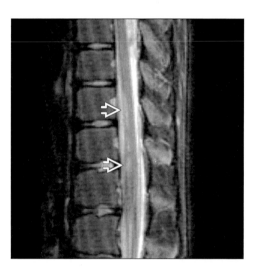

(Left) Sagittal STIR MR in patient with chronic cervical myelopathy shows fusiform hyperintense cord expansion from C4-C6 with multiple superficial flow voids, compatible with arterio-venous malformation. *(Right)* Sagittal T2WI MR with fat suppression in patient with rapid onset myelopathy after recent viral infection shows patchy hyperintensities (arrows) in ventral lower thoracic cord, consistent with ATM.

Typical

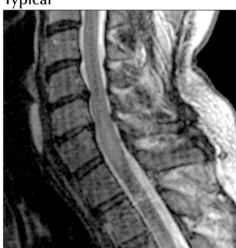 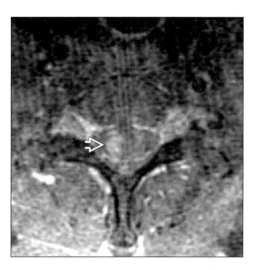

(Left) Sagittal T2WI MR in patient with HIV shows subtle hyperintensity from C5 to C6 & slight cord expansion. *(Right)* Axial T1 C+ MR with fat suppression in same patient shows right lateral cervical cord enhancement (arrow). A presumptive diagnosis of HIV associated ATM was made.

BACK PAIN IN CHILDREN

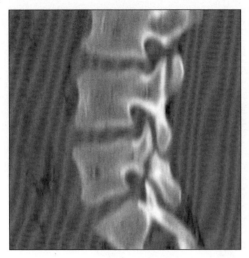

Sagittal reformation from an axial bone CT demonstrates L5 pars defect without anterolisthesis.

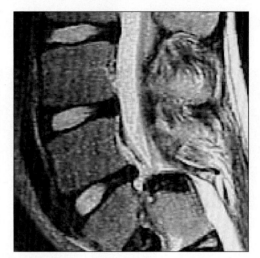

Sagittal T2WI MR shows grade 4 anterolisthesis of L5 on S1 secondary to bilateral L5 spondylolysis. There is severe central canal narrowing at superior endplate of S1.

TERMINOLOGY

Definitions
- Back pain in children & adolescents with or without underlying organic cause

IMAGING FINDINGS

General Features
- Best diagnostic clue: Imaging findings correspond to underlying etiology
- Location: Lumbar segment most common in nonspecific back pain

Imaging Recommendations
- Best imaging tool
  - Plain films and bone scan part of initial imaging work-up
  - MRI is the modality of choice if neurologic symptoms present
- Protocol advice
  - Start with plain films
    - AP, lateral, oblique, and odontoid views of cervical spine
    - AP, lateral thoracic spine
    - AP, lateral, & oblique lumbar spine with standing lateral spot film of L5-S1
    - If plain films positive, then thin-section CT
    - If negative, then bone scan
  - If bone scan positive, then thin-section CT
    - If negative, consider MRI
  - If MRI positive, also consider thin-section CT

DIFFERENTIAL DIAGNOSIS

Sports injuries
- Most common cause of back pain in children
- Muscle strain or ligamentous sprain
- History and clinical exam provide the diagnosis

Spondylolysis
- Defects in pars interarticularis
  - 5% in children
  - Most commonly identified cause of low back pain
- Pars defects result from chronic repetitive stress injury
- Discontinuity in neck of "Scotty dog" on oblique lumbar films

Spondylolisthesis
- Anterior translation of one vertebra with respect to another
- Usually at L5-S1 due to L5 spondylolysis
- 25% with associated disc degeneration

DDx: Vertebral Neoplasms Causing Back Pain in Children

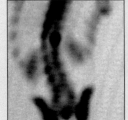

Osteoid Osteoma

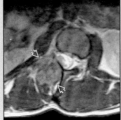

Osteoblastoma

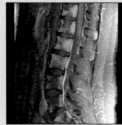

Leukemia

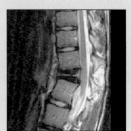

Eos. Granuloma

BACK PAIN IN CHILDREN

Key Facts

Terminology
- Back pain in children & adolescents with or without underlying organic cause

Imaging Findings
- Location: Lumbar segment most common in nonspecific back pain
- Plain films and bone scan part of initial imaging work-up
- MRI is the modality of choice if neurologic symptoms present

Top Differential Diagnoses
- Sports injuries
- Spondylolysis
- Spondylolisthesis
- Lumbar disc herniation

- Slipped vertebral ring apophysis
- Discitis and osteomyelitis
- Scheuermann disease
- Juvenile calcific discitis
- Idiopathic scoliosis
- Neoplasms
- Tethered cord
- Ankylosing spondylitis (AS)

Pathology
- General path comments: Up to 60% of back pain in children without underlying etiology
- Emotional, psychosocial, and conduct problems linked to development of low back pain without organic cause

Lumbar disc herniation
- 1% of surgically treated lumbar discs
- Etiology
  - Trauma
  - Congenital spinal anomalies: Transitional vertebrae, spina bifida occulta, congenital spinal stenosis
  - Familial predisposition: Up to 4-5x risk of disc herniation if + family history
- Correlates with low back pain in adolescence
  - Occurs after growth spurt
  - Increases linearly with age into adulthood
- 33% of 15 year olds in one series had degenerated discs
  - 89% in those with recurrent low back pain vs. 26% in asymptomatic individuals
- Disc height loss, desiccation, annular fissure, and disc herniation

Slipped vertebral ring apophysis
- Ring apophysis & adjacent disc displaced into spinal canal
  - Intraspinal bone fragment best seen on CT
- Rare, usually after heavy lifting
- Symptoms similar to disc herniation
  - L4-5 and L5-S1 most common
- Surgery indicated

Discitis and osteomyelitis
- Mean age for discitis 3 yo vs. 7.5 yo for osteomyelitis
- Lumbar spine most common in discitis vs. any spinal segment in osteomyelitis
- Staphylococcus aureus most common pathogen
- Hyperintense disc on T2WI
- Endplate erosive changes
- Subchondral marrow T2 hyperintensity and enhancement in adjacent vertebrae

Scheuermann disease
- 0.4-8% incidence
- Peak incidence: 13-17 yrs
- Probably caused by repetitive trauma in skeletally immature person
- ≥ 3 thoracic vertebrae with ≥ 5° of anterior wedging

- Endplate irregularities, disc space narrowing, limbus vertebrae

Juvenile calcific discitis
- Rare, idiopathic, and self-limiting
- Cervical spine most common
  - One or more discs with calcification
- Neck pain, fever, elevated erythrocyte sedimentation rate

Idiopathic scoliosis
- Most common of all scoliosis
- Typically in adolescents
- Pain due to worsening curvature ± degenerative facet and disc disease

Neoplasms
- Benign spinal tumors
  - Osteoid osteoma & osteoblastoma
    - Histologically identical, differing in size
    - Osteoid osteoma: Radiolucent nidus with surrounding sclerosis, < 1.5 cm
    - Osteoblastoma: Expansile lesion of neural arch, > 1.5 cm
    - Painful scoliosis
  - Eosinophilic granuloma
    - Abnormal histiocyte proliferation
    - 0.05-0.5 per 100,000 children per year
    - Vertebra plana
  - Aneurysmal bone cyst
    - 80% < 20 yo
    - Majority primary lesions
    - Expansile multiloculated neural arch mass with fluid-fluid levels
- Malignant spinal tumors
  - Enhancing soft tissue mass with variable paravertebral & intraspinal extension
  - Ewing sarcoma
    - Most common primary spinal malignant neoplasm
    - Mimics spinal infection clinically
  - Lymphoma, leukemia, and neuroblastoma metastases
- Cord glioma

○ 60% astrocytoma, 30% ependymoma in children
○ Astrocytoma more eccentric compared to ependymoma
○ Hemorrhage more common in ependymoma

Tethered cord
- Commonly discovered during growth spurts
- Neurologic symptoms invariably present
- Conus below inferior endplate of L2 with tethering mass or thick filum (> 2 mm)

Ankylosing spondylitis (AS)
- 10-20% of AS patients with onset of symptoms before 16 yrs
- Constitutional symptoms common at onset of disease
- Initial radiographs of spine + sacroiliac joints often normal in children

PATHOLOGY

General Features
- General path comments: Up to 60% of back pain in children without underlying etiology
- Genetics: Familial tendency in Scheuermann disease, idiopathic scoliosis, & disc herniation
- Etiology
  ○ Emotional, psychosocial, and conduct problems linked to development of low back pain without organic cause
    ▪ Preexisting somatic complaints also risk factor
  ○ Obesity may play a role in chronicity of symptoms
- Epidemiology
  ○ Prepubertal children: Rare
  ○ Adolescent children: Nonspecific low back pain
    ▪ Estimates of prevalence range between 8-57%, increasing with age
    ▪ Annual incidence between 12-22%, increasing with age
- Associated abnormalities
  ○ Pain without organic cause associated with
    ▪ Decreased lumbar extension with increased flexion
    ▪ Thoracic hyperkyphosis and lumbar hyperlordosis
    ▪ Decreased mobility at hips

CLINICAL ISSUES

Presentation
- Most common signs/symptoms
  ○ Nonspecific back pain
  ○ Other signs/symptoms
    ▪ Somatic complaints such as headaches and sore throat
- Clinical profile
  ○ Likelihood of serious underlying cause of back pain increased if following clinical signs present
    ▪ Prepubertal children, especially < 5 yo
    ▪ Functional disability
    ▪ Duration > 4 weeks
    ▪ Recurrent or worsening pain
    ▪ Fever, weight loss, malaise
    ▪ Postural change: Scoliosis ± kyphosis

- Decreased range of motion
- Neurologic symptoms
○ Imaging work-up indicated if above symptoms present

Demographics
- Gender
  ○ Slight male predominance
    ▪ Spondylolysis
    ▪ Slipped vertebral ring apophysis
    ▪ Scheuermann disease
    ▪ Osteoid osteoma, osteoblastoma
    ▪ Eosinophilic granuloma
    ▪ Ankylosis spondylitis
  ○ Female predominance in idiopathic scoliosis and nonspecific low back pain
- Ethnicity: No racial predilection

Natural History & Prognosis
- Back pain without underlying etiology
  ○ Self-limited
  ○ Small percentage with recurrent or continuous symptoms
  ○ Good prognosis
  ○ 8% with recurrent or continuous low back pain
  ○ 2-3% with symptoms continuing into early adulthood

Treatment
- Depends on underlying cause
- Conservative
  ○ Modification of activity
  ○ Limited bed rest
  ○ Analgesic medications
  ○ Back brace
  ○ Physical therapy

SELECTED REFERENCES

1. Watson KD et al: Low back pain in schoolchildren: the role of mechanical and psychosocial factors. Arch Dis Child. 88(1):12-7, 2003
2. Jones GT et al: Predictors of low back pain in British schoolchildren: a population-based prospective cohort study. Pediatrics. 111(4 Pt 1):822-8, 2003
3. Leboeuf-Yde C et al: Low back pain and lifestyle. Part II--Obesity. Information from a population-based sample of 29,424 twin subjects. Spine. 24(8):779-83; discussion 783-4, 1999
4. Salminen JJ et al: Recurrent low back pain and early disc degeneration in the young. Spine 24:1316-21, 1999
5. Leboeuf-Yde C et al: At what age does low back pain become a common problem? A study of 29,424 individuals aged 12-41 years. Spine 23:228-34, 1998
6. Hollingworth P: Back pain in children. Br J Rheumatol. 35(10):1022-8, 1996
7. Erkintalo MO et al: Development of degenerative changes in the lumbar intervertebral disk: Results of a prospective MR imaging study in adolescents with and without low-back pain. Radiology 196:529-33, 1995
8. Ventura N et al: Intervertebral disc calcification in childhood. Int Orthop. 19(5):291-4, 1995
9. Afshani E et al: Common causes of low back pain in children. Radiographics. 11(2):269-91, 1991

IMAGE GALLERY

Typical

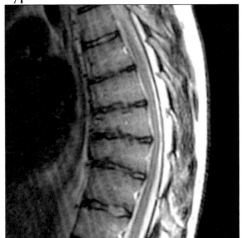 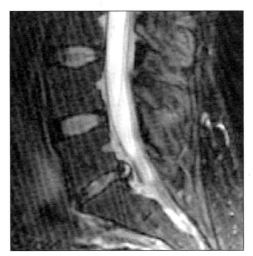

(Left) Sagittal T2WI MR in a patient with Scheuermann disease shows anterior wedging of three consecutive lower thoracic vertebrae. Disc space narrowing & endplate irregularities are also present. *(Right)* Sagittal STIR MR in teenager with low back pain shows disc height loss, annular fissure, and disc protrusion at L5-S1.

Typical

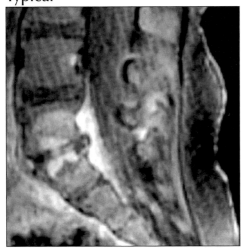 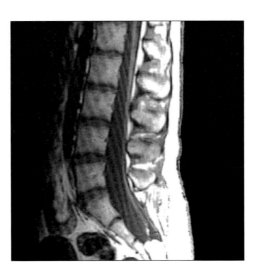

(Left) Sagittal T1 C+ MR with fat suppression in infant shows enhancing disc & endplates at L5-S1, with associated prevertebral, epidural enhancement, compatible with discitis, osteomyelitis. *(Right)* Sagittal T1WI MR in patient with worsening back pain and progressive neurologic symptoms demonstrates thickened filum terminale, tethered by intraspinal lipoma.

Typical

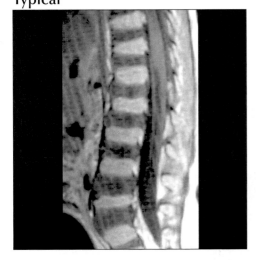 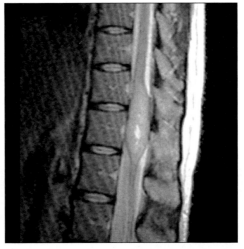

(Left) Sagittal T1 C+ MR in child with leukemia shows moderate compression of L5 vertebra with mild compression in upper lumbar & lower thoracic vertebrae, compatible with leukemic infiltration. *(Right)* Sagittal T2WI MR in child with back pain shows expansile mass involving the conus, with central cystic change. Cellular ependymoma was found at surgery.

KYPHOSIS

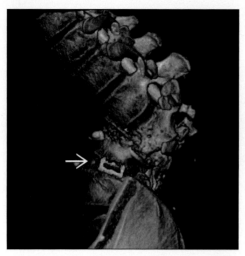

Sagittal 3D CT myelogram shows iatrogenic gibbus deformity due to infection above level of fusion. Arrow shows intact intervertebral cage below level of deformity.

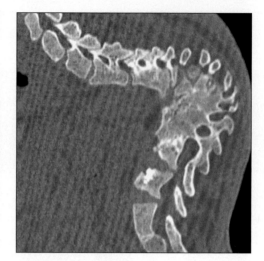

Sagittal bone CT reformation shows gibbus deformity and multiple vertebral fusions due to tuberculosis of the spine (Pott disease).

TERMINOLOGY

Definitions
- Increased apex dorsal curvature of spine in sagittal plane
- Gibbus deformity: Extreme, angular focal kyphosis

IMAGING FINDINGS

General Features
- Best diagnostic clue: Increased Cobb angle on lateral radiograph
- Location
  ○ Thoracic spine has normal kyphosis < 40°
  ○ Lumbar spine has normal lordosis 25-35°
  ○ Cervical spine has mild lordosis, large range of motion
- Morphology: Sagittal plane curvature changes gradually from cervical lordosis to thoracic kyphosis to lumbar lordosis

Radiographic Findings
- Radiography
  ○ Measure using method of Cobb
    ▪ Angle between superior and inferior endplates
    ▪ Interobserver variability 5-7°
  ○ Determining ends of curve
    ▪ Thoracic kyphosis normally measured from T3 to T12
    ▪ Fracture: Measure from 1 level above fracture to 1 level below
    ▪ Other deformity: Measure points of greatest inclination from horizontal
  ○ Determine flexibility of curve
    ▪ Lateral radiograph in full extension
    ▪ Decrease in kyphosis measured

CT Findings
- Bone CT
  ○ Kyphosis often underestimated because of supine position
  ○ Evaluate for underlying cause

MR Findings
- Evaluate for underlying cause

Imaging Recommendations
- Best imaging tool: CT scan
- Protocol advice: Sagittal, coronal reformations

DIFFERENTIAL DIAGNOSIS

Positional kyphosis
- Poor positioning of uncooperative patient

DDx: Causes of Kyphosis

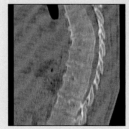

Scheuermann

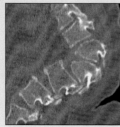

Achondroplasia

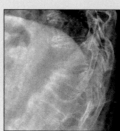

Insufficiency Fx

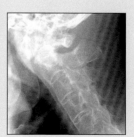

Ankylosing Spondylitis

KYPHOSIS

Key Facts

Terminology
- Increased apex dorsal curvature of spine in sagittal plane
- Gibbus deformity: Extreme, angular focal kyphosis

Imaging Findings
- Best diagnostic clue: Increased Cobb angle on lateral radiograph
- Thoracic spine has normal kyphosis < 40°

- Lumbar spine has normal lordosis 25-35°

Pathology
- Traumatic
- Congenital
- Developmental
- Infectious
- Neoplastic
- Iatrogenic
- Arthritis

PATHOLOGY

General Features
- General path comments
  - Infant spine has C-shaped curve in sagittal plane
  - Lumbar and cervical lordosis develop with erect posture
  - In adult, normal line of mechanical axis passes through C7, T1, L4
- Etiology
  - Traumatic
    - Compression, burst or Chance fracture
    - Ligamentous injury
    - Insufficiency fracture
  - Congenital
    - Failure of vertebral segmentation
    - Posterior hemivertebra
    - Syndromes: Including achondroplasia, Marfan, Ehlers Danlos, neurofibromatosis
    - Osteogenesis imperfecta
  - Developmental
    - Scheuermann disease
    - Postural (idiopathic) kyphosis
    - Neurogenic kyphosis
  - Infectious
    - Pyogenic
    - Tubercular (gibbus deformity)
    - Prevertebral abscess
  - Neoplastic
    - Primary or metastatic tumors
  - Iatrogenic
    - Post-surgical
    - Post-radiation in childhood
  - Arthritis
    - Ankylosing spondylitis (AS)
    - Crystals: Gout, CPPD, hemodialysis arthropathy

Staging, Grading or Classification Criteria
- Flexible vs. rigid
  - Determine with lateral radiographs in full extension

CLINICAL ISSUES

Demographics
- Age
  - Tumor: Any age; type of tumor varies with age
  - Child: Consider neurogenic, congenital causes
  - Adolescent or young adult: Consider Scheuermann, postural, post-traumatic
  - Older adult: Consider insufficiency fracture, post-traumatic

Natural History & Prognosis
- Premature degenerative disease, neurologic compromise

Treatment
- Options, risks, complications
  - Treatment of underlying entity
  - Brace vs. fusion

DIAGNOSTIC CHECKLIST

Consider
- Progressive kyphosis warrants CT scan

SELECTED REFERENCES

1. Keim HA et al: Spinal deformities. Scoliosis and kyphosis. Clin Symp. 41(4):3-32, 1989
2. Gutowski WT et al: Orthotic results in adolescent kyphosis. Spine. 13(5):485-9, 1988
3. Propst-Proctor SL et al: Radiographic determination of lordosis and kyphosis in normal and scoliotic children. J Pediatr Orthop. 3(3):344-6, 1983
4. Luque ER: The correction of postural curves of the spine. Spine. 7(3):270-5, 1982

IMAGE GALLERY

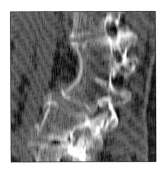 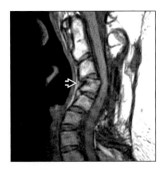

(Left) Sagittal bone CT reformation shows congenital kyphosis due to fusion of three vertebrae. This isolated, previously undiagnosed anomaly in 30 yo patient has led to premature DDD of lower lumbar spine. *(Right)* Sagittal T1WI MR shows iatrogenic kyphosis following wide cervical laminectomy. Anterolisthesis has developed at C3/4 and there is bone marrow edema of C4 (arrow) related to abnormal motion.

PERIPHERAL NEUROPATHY

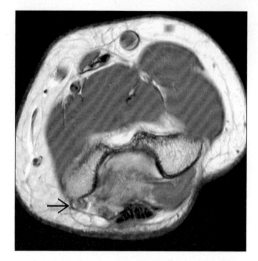

Axial PD/Intermediate MR of elbow shows enlarged ulnar n. (arrow) due to cubital tunnel syndrome, the second most common entrapment neuropathy in the upper extremity.

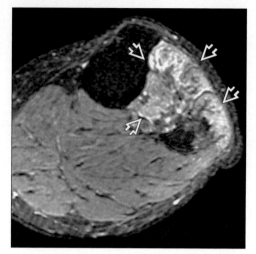

Axial STIR MR shows abnormal signal in the anterior muscles of the leg (arrows), which are innervated by the peroneal n. Images at level of knee showed tumor of peroneal n.

TERMINOLOGY

Definitions
- Primary disorder of one or more peripheral nerves (nn.)
- Mononeuropathy: Single nerve (n.) effected
- Multiple mononeuropathies: Multiple adjacent nn. effected
- Polyneuropathy: Effects multiple nn.; usually distal, symmetric involvement

IMAGING FINDINGS

General Features
- Best diagnostic clue: Abnormal T2 signal intensity in muscles innervated by effected nerve

Radiographic Findings
- Radiography
  - Charcot-Marie-tooth leads to characteristic pes cavus
  - Neuroarthropathy may develop

CT Findings
- NECT: Evaluate for mass involving n. or compressing n., muscle atrophy

MR Findings
- Evaluate for mass compressing or invading n.

- Denervation edema: High signal T2WI, STIR
- Fatty atrophy of (muscle) m. best seen on T1WI; occurs after denervation edema
- Nerve high signal T2WI, STIR, enhances with contrast

Imaging Recommendations
- Best imaging tool: MRI
- Protocol advice: Heavily T2 weighted and STIR sequences perpendicular to course of nerve

DIFFERENTIAL DIAGNOSIS

Radiculopathy
- Evaluate with MRI of spine

Myositis
- Diffusely increased signal on T2WI, may have focal abscess
- Muscle enlarged initially, atrophic later in course

Radiation
- Diffuse increase signal in muscle and surrounding soft tissues
- Conforms to geography of port, not distribution of n.

Post amputation or muscle detachment
- E.g., abnormal signal hamstrings after ACL graft harvest

DDx: Peripheral Neuropathy

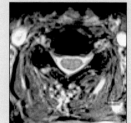

Radiculopathy

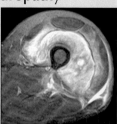

Myositis

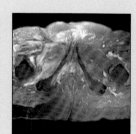

Radiation

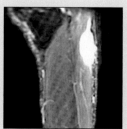

Nerve Sheath Tumor

PERIPHERAL NEUROPATHY

Key Facts

Terminology
- Primary disorder of one or more peripheral nerves (nn.)
- Mononeuropathy: Single nerve (n.) effected
- Multiple mononeuropathies: Multiple adjacent nn. effected
- Polyneuropathy: Effects multiple nn.; usually distal, symmetric involvement

Imaging Findings
- Best diagnostic clue: Abnormal T2 signal intensity in muscles innervated by effected nerve

Top Differential Diagnoses
- Radiculopathy
- Myositis

Muscular dystrophies
- Tend to involve proximal muscles more than distal

PATHOLOGY

General Features
- General path comments
  - Toxic peripheral neuropathies usually distal, "stocking and glove" distribution
  - Diabetes mellitus occasionally causes proximal neuropathy: "Diabetic amyotrophy"
  - Complex regional pain syndrome (formerly known as reflex sympathetic dystrophy) primarily effects autonomic nn.
  - Involvement of a single n. usually due to entrapment, trauma or tumor
  - Involvement of several adjacent nn. usually due to tumor or trauma
- Etiology
  - Nerve entrapment
    - Due to mass, arthritis (e.g., gout, rheumatoid arthritis) or fracture
  - Nerve injury
    - Laceration, electrical injury, radiation
  - Hereditary
    - Charcot-Marie-tooth syndrome effects peroneal n. primarily
    - Numerous hereditary motor, sensory and/or autonomic neuropathies
  - Neoplastic and paraneoplastic
  - Nerve ischemia
    - Vasculitis
    - Small vessel atherosclerosis (diabetes mellitus)
    - Thromboembolic disease
    - Arteriovenous shunt for hemodialysis
    - Following vascular surgery
  - Toxic/metabolic
    - Ethanol, uremia, hyperglycemia, drugs, vitamin B12 deficiency
  - Infectious, post-infectious/auto-immune
    - Guillain-Barre syndrome and chronic inflammatory demyelinating polyneuropathy
    - Parsonage-Turner syndrome
    - HIV, Lyme disease, leprosy, sarcoidosis
  - Complex regional pain syndrome

CLINICAL ISSUES

Presentation
- Most common signs/symptoms
  - Depend on whether motor, sensory or autonomic nn. most involved
  - Other signs/symptoms
    - Muscle wasting
    - Numbness, tingling, positive Tinel sign, loss of proprioception, pain

SELECTED REFERENCES
1. Rosai J: Surgical Pathology, vol 2. 9th ed. Edinburgh, Mosby .2629-2662, 2004
2. Crozier F et al: Magnetic resonance imaging in reflex sympathetic dystrophy syndrome of the foot. Joint Bone Spine. 70(6):503-8, 2003
3. Bus SA et al: Intrinsic muscle atrophy and toe deformity in the diabetic neuropathic foot: a magnetic resonance imaging study. Diabetes Care. 25(8):1444-50, 2002
4. Bendszus M et al: Sequential MR imaging of denervated muscle: experimental study. AJNR Am J Neuroradiol. 23(8):1427-31, 2002
5. Resnick D: Diagnosis of Bone and Joint disorders. vol 5. 3rd ed. Philadelphia, W.B. Saunders. 3383-3405, 1995

IMAGE GALLERY

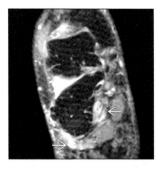 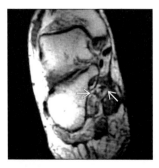

(Left) Coronal STIR MR shows abnormal signal intensity (arrows) in muscles innervated by lateral plantar n. Patient was status post failed tarsal tunnel surgery. (Right) Coronal T1WI MR shows severe muscle atrophy in distribution of lateral plantar n. following failed tarsal tunnel release. Scarring is evident in region of posterior tibial n. branches (arrows).

PATHOLOGIC VERTEBRAL FRACTURE

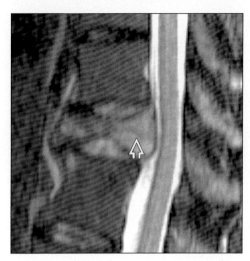

Sagittal STIR MR shows burst fracture of T11 due to breast cancer metastasis. Diffuse marrow infiltration is evident. Fracture line traverses vertebral body (arrow).

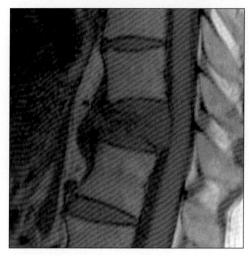

Sagittal T1WI MR shows pathologic T11 burst fracture due to metastasis. Uniform marrow replacement helps distinguish it from traumatic fracture.

TERMINOLOGY

Definitions
- Fracture occurring through bone weakened by tumor or infection

IMAGING FINDINGS

General Features
- Best diagnostic clue: Trabecular and/or cortical destruction
- Location
  - Vertebral body > neural arch
  - Isolated neural arch fractures seen in tumors of neural arch origin
    - Osteoblastoma, aneurysmal bone cyst, some sarcomas
  - Vertebral body + involvement of pedicles often viewed as sign of pathologic fracture
    - However, also seen in osteoporotic fractures
  - L5 compression fractures more likely to be pathologic (24%) than L1 (8%)
- Morphology
  - Rounded area of marrow replacement and trabecular destruction
  - May replace entire vertebral body marrow

  - Usually can be distinguished on MR from band-like signal abnormalities due to nonpathologic fracture
- Fracture may be compression or burst

Radiographic Findings
- Radiography
  - Often indistinguishable from benign fracture, especially in osteoporotic patients
  - Cortical destruction
  - Absent pedicle due to bone destruction
  - Focal osteopenia
  - Fracture less common in sclerotic metastases
  - Paraspinous mass not a reliable indicator
    - May be caused by tumor or hematoma

CT Findings
- Bone CT
  - Fracture line sclerotic, horizontal
    - Best seen on reformatted images
    - Compression or burst fracture
  - Highly sensitive in detecting underlying bone destruction
    - Rounded areas of trabecular destruction
    - Cortical breakthrough
    - Sagittal, coronal reformats help identify trabecular destruction
  - Detects additional areas of bone destruction in other vertebrae
  - More accurate than MRI in patients with myeloma

DDx: Pathologic Vertebral Fracture

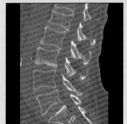
Osteoporosis

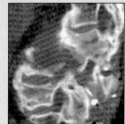
Neuoropathic

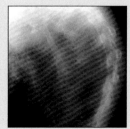
Idiopathic Kyphosis

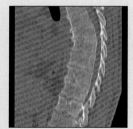
Scheuermann

PATHOLOGIC VERTEBRAL FRACTURE

Key Facts

Terminology
- Fracture occurring through bone weakened by tumor or infection

Imaging Findings
- Best diagnostic clue: Trabecular and/or cortical destruction
- Rounded area of marrow replacement and trabecular destruction
- May replace entire vertebral body marrow
- Usually can be distinguished on MR from band-like signal abnormalities due to nonpathologic fracture
- Fracture may be compression or burst
- Soft tissue paraspinous mass not a specific finding
- Can be mimicked by hematoma from nonpathologic fracture

- MR vs. CT scan still debatable as to best tool
- MR scan to evaluate rounded areas of tumor, pattern of enhancement
- CT scan to evaluate for trabecular, cortical destruction

Top Differential Diagnoses
- Osteoporotic compression fracture
- Neuropathic joint
- Idiopathic kyphosis
- Scheuermann disease
- Osteogenesis imperfecta

Pathology
- Epidemiology: Pathologic fracture may be presenting sign of tumor, especially breast carcinoma

---

- ○ Soft tissue paraspinous mass not a specific finding
  - ■ Can be mimicked by hematoma from nonpathologic fracture
- ○ Use to evaluate symptomatic patients after fracture fixation
  - ■ Artifact from most metallic fixators does not prevent diagnostic CT scan
  - ■ Thin sections, overlapping, multidetector helical CT needed

MR Findings
- T1WI
  - ○ Rounded or diffuse low signal intensity marrow replacement
  - ○ Very low signal intensity fracture line may or may not be visible
- T2WI
  - ○ Rounded or diffuse high signal intensity marrow replacement
  - ○ May be same signal intensity as fatty marrow
  - ○ Very low signal intensity fracture line
  - ○ Increase conspicuity of lesion by using fat-saturation sequences
- PD/Intermediate: Tumor may be indistinguishable from normal marrow
- STIR
  - ○ Rounded or diffuse high signal intensity marrow
    - ■ Corresponds to low signal area on T1WI
  - ○ Low signal may be seen in sclerotic metastases
  - ○ Very low signal intensity fracture line
- DWI
  - ○ Initially promising results with DWI not confirmed on subsequent studies
  - ○ No increase in accuracy compared to T1WI
- T1 C+
  - ○ Enhancement around fracture line and of underlying lesion
  - ○ Enhancement usually more rounded than in nonpathologic fracture
    - ■ Nonpathologic fractures enhance in band-like configuration
- Majority of cases can be distinguished from benign fracture by above criteria

- ○ Intraosseous hematoma can mimic tumor
- Pathologic fractures in myeloma often mimic osteoporotic compression fractures

Nuclear Medicine Findings
- Bone Scan
  - ○ Increased activity at fracture line
  - ○ Underlying lesion may show increased, normal or decreased uptake
- PET
  - ○ Fracture shows increased uptake with or without underlying lesion
  - ○ Accuracy improved by PET/CT

Imaging Recommendations
- Best imaging tool
  - ○ MR vs. CT scan still debatable as to best tool
    - ■ MR scan to evaluate rounded areas of tumor, pattern of enhancement
    - ■ CT scan to evaluate for trabecular, cortical destruction

DIFFERENTIAL DIAGNOSIS

Osteoporotic compression fracture
- Thinned trabeculae without focal destruction
- Cortical destruction is absent
- Often involves multiple levels
- Paraspinous hematoma mimics tumor mass

Neuropathic joint
- Fractures
- Bone debris
- Preserved bone density
- Subluxations of vertebral bodies
- Centered on discs and facet joints
- Soft tissue mass

Idiopathic kyphosis
- Mild wedging of several adjacent upper thoracic vertebrae
- Angular deformity endplates or anterior cortex absent

PATHOLOGIC VERTEBRAL FRACTURE

Scheuermann disease
- Schmorl nodes of at least 3 contiguous levels
- Wedging of at least 5 degrees at each of 3 contiguous levels

Osteogenesis imperfecta
- Mild forms may present in adulthood with vertebral fracture

PATHOLOGY

General Features
- General path comments
  - Risk of fracture from tumor depends on
    - Tumor type: Lytic tumor higher risk than blastic
    - Tumor volume
    - Pedicle involvement
    - Amount of cortical destruction, bowing of vertebral margins
    - Load on vertebra
- Etiology
  - Most common primary tumors
    - Malignant: Ewing sarcoma, lymphoma, leukemia
    - Benign: Hemangioma, Langerhans cell histiocytosis, fibrous dysplasia, unicameral bone cyst
    - Borderline: Giant cell tumor, chordoma
    - Vertebra plana manifestation of fracture
  - Most common metastatic tumors
    - Breast, lung, renal, gastrointestinal tumors
    - More common in lytic than blastic tumors
  - Osteomyelitis
    - Involvement of 2 adjacent vertebral bodies and intervening disc
    - Fracture may be extensive
  - Radiation
    - Bone sclerotic, fragmented
    - Sharp demarcation of abnormal bone in radiation field from normal bone outside it
  - Paget disease
    - Usually occurs in lytic phase
- Epidemiology: Pathologic fracture may be presenting sign of tumor, especially breast carcinoma

Gross Pathologic & Surgical Features
- Tumor or infection permeating bone

Microscopic Features
- Fracture callus can mimic tumors

CLINICAL ISSUES

Presentation
- Most common signs/symptoms
  - Back pain, greatest at night
  - Fracture with history of no trauma or minor trauma
  - Other signs/symptoms
    - Nerve or cord compression

Demographics
- Age: Usually in older patients

Natural History & Prognosis
- Pain improves with surgical stabilization or kyphoplasty/vertebroplasty

Treatment
- Options, risks, complications
  - Brace
  - Radiation
  - Kyphoplasty or vertebroplasty
  - Curettage + stabilization with bone graft or methylmethacrylate

DIAGNOSTIC CHECKLIST

Consider
- May be presenting sign of malignancy

SELECTED REFERENCES

1. Even-Sapir E et al: Assessment of malignant skeletal disease: initial experience with 18F-fluoride PET/CT and comparison between 18F-fluoride PET and 18F-fluoride PET/CT. J Nucl Med. 45(2):272-8, 2004
2. Roth SE et al: Metastatic burst fracture risk prediction using biomechanically based equations. Clin Orthop. (419):83-90, 2004
3. Fayad LM et al: Sacral fractures: a potential pitfall of FDG positron emission tomography. AJR Am J Roentgenol. 181(5):1239-43, 2003
4. Castillo M: Diffusion-weighted imaging of the spine: is it reliable? AJNR Am J Neuroradiol. 24(6):1251-3, 2003
5. Bertuna G et al: Marked osteoporosis and spontaneous vertebral fractures in children: don't forget, it could be leukemia. Med Pediatr Oncol. 41(5):450-1, 2003
6. Lieberman I et al: Vertebroplasty and kyphoplasty for osteolytic vertebral collapse. Clin Orthop. (415 Suppl):S176-86, 2003
7. Mahnken AH et al: Multidetector CT of the spine in multiple myeloma: comparison with MR imaging and radiography. AJR Am J Roentgenol. 178(6):1429-36, 2002
8. Castillo M et al: Diffusion-weighted MR imaging offers no advantage over routine noncontrast MR imaging in the detection of vertebral metastases. AJNR Am J Neuroradiol. 21(5):948-53, 2000
9. Lo LD et al: Are L5 fractures an indicator of metastasis? Skeletal Radiol. 29(8):454-8, 2000
10. Shih TT et al: Solitary vertebral collapse: distinction between benign and malignant causes using MR patterns. J Magn Reson Imaging. 9(5):635-42, 1999
11. Baur A et al: Diffusion-weighted MR imaging of bone marrow: differentiation of benign versus pathologic compression fractures. Radiology. 207(2):349-56, 1998
12. Lecouvet FE et al: Vertebral compression fractures in multiple myeloma. Part I. Distribution and appearance at MR imaging. Radiology. 204(1):195-9, 1997
13. Cuenod CA et al: Acute vertebral collapse due to osteoporosis or malignancy: appearance on unenhanced and gadolinium-enhanced MR images. Radiology. 199(2):541-9, 1996
14. Moulopoulos LA et al: MR prediction of benign and malignant vertebral compression fractures. J Magn Reson Imaging. 6(4):667-74, 1996
15. An HS et al: Can we distinguish between benign versus malignant compression fractures of the spine by magnetic resonance imaging? Spine. 20(16):1776-82, 1995

PATHOLOGIC VERTEBRAL FRACTURE

IMAGE GALLERY

Typical

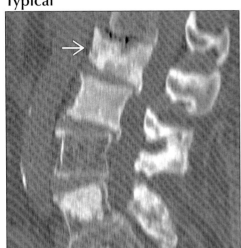 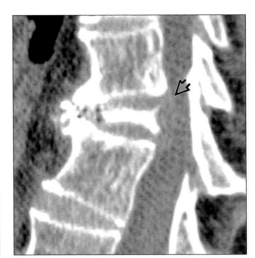

(Left) Sagittal bone CT shows prostate cancer metastases and pathologic fracture (arrow). Sclerotic metastases have lower rate of fracture than lytic ones, but are at increased risk compared to normal bone. *(Right)* Sagittal CT with soft tissue window shows vertebra plana from metastatic disease. Note tumor extension into spinal canal (arrow).

Typical

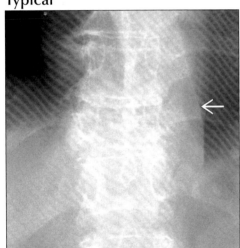 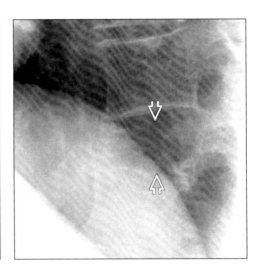

(Left) Anteroposterior radiography shows T11 fracture and large paraspinous mass (arrow) due to metastasis. Fracture not distinguishable on this view from osteoporotic compression fracture. *(Right)* Lateral radiography shows pathologic T11 fracture. Pathognomonic features on radiography for pathologic fracture are destruction of endplates (arrows) & focal lucency in vertebral body.

Variant

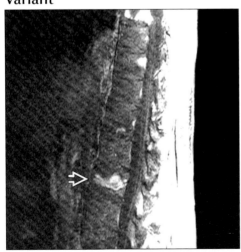 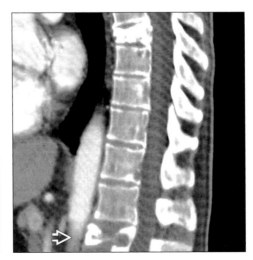

(Left) Sagittal T1 C+ MR shows L1 fracture (arrow) with band-like enhancement suggesting benign etiology. Enhancement of other lesions allowed diagnosis of malignancy. Patient with myeloma. *(Right)* Sagittal bone CT shows pathologic L1 fracture (arrow) due to myeloma. Trabecular destruction well seen adjacent to fracture. Multiple other lytic lesions visible, as well as T7 pathologic fracture.

DENSE VERTEBRAL BODY

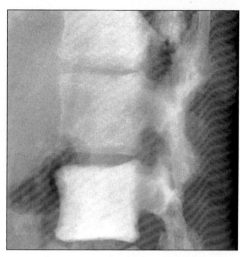

Lateral radiography shows "ivory vertebra" of L3 due to prostate metastasis. Less severe involvement seen at L1.

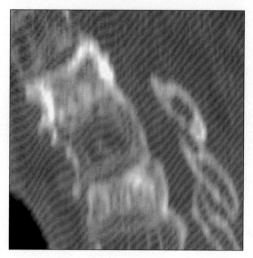

Sagittal bone CT shows sclerotic metastases with fractures and smudgy, amorphous increased density.

TERMINOLOGY

Abbreviations and Synonyms
- Osteosclerosis

Definitions
- Increased density of 1 or more vertebral bodies compared to normal patients

IMAGING FINDINGS

General Features
- Morphology
  - Several different appearances
    - Increased cortical and endplate thickness
    - Increased trabecular thickness
    - Amorphous increase in bone density
  - May involve 1 or multiple vertebrae
    - Diffuse involvement seen in systemic disease, widespread metastases

Radiographic Findings
- Radiography
  - Paget disease
    - Thickening of endplates and cortices: "Picture frame"
    - Thickened trabeculae: Corduroy vertebra
    - Enlarged vertebra
  - Blastic metastasis, lymphoma, osteosarcoma, sclerotic myeloma, myelofibrosis, radiation, fluorosis, hypervitaminosis A or D
    - Amorphous sclerosis
  - Infection
    - Amorphous sclerosis
    - Endplate erosions
  - Renal osteodystrophy
    - Thick, poorly defined bands of sclerosis at endplates: "Rugger jersey"
    - Poorly defined trabeculae
  - Osteopetrosis
    - Sharply demarcated bands of sclerosis at endplates
    - "Bone in bone" appearance
  - Sickle cell disease
    - Patchy sclerosis
    - H-shaped vertebrae
  - Healing fracture
    - Fracture deformity usually visible
    - Kümmell disease: Post-traumatic AVN
  - Discogenic sclerosis
    - Semicircular or band-like configuration
    - Centered at disk

CT Findings
- Bone CT
  - Features seen on radiographs more clearly identifiable

DDx: Dense Vertebral Body

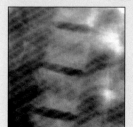
Osteopetrosis

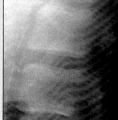
Renal OD

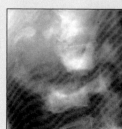
Neuropathic

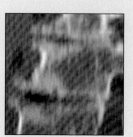
Discogenic

DENSE VERTEBRAL BODY

Key Facts

Terminology
- Osteosclerosis
- Increased density of 1 or more vertebral bodies compared to normal patients

Imaging Findings
- Best imaging tool: CT scan

Pathology
- Tumors and tumor-like conditions
- Systemic disorders
- Iatrogenic
- Infection
- Healing fracture
- Neuroarthropathy

- ○ Cortical breakthrough, paraspinous mass if present aids in differential diagnosis

MR Findings
- T1WI: Low signal intensity in bone marrow
- T2WI: Low to intermediate signal intensity in bone marrow
- STIR: Low to intermediate signal intensity in bone marrow
- Cortical breakthrough, paraspinous mass if present aids in differential diagnosis

Imaging Recommendations
- Best imaging tool: CT scan
- Protocol advice: Thin-section helical CT with sagittal and coronal reformations

DIFFERENTIAL DIAGNOSIS

Density in overlying soft tissues
- Usually clear on second projection

Technical factors
- Insufficient beam penetration in large patients

PATHOLOGY

General Features
- General path comments: Percutaneous biopsy difficult
- Etiology
  - ○ Tumors and tumor-like conditions
    - Blastic metastasis, lymphoma, osteosarcoma, sclerotic myeloma, Paget disease
    - Most common: Prostate, breast metastases
    - Treated lytic metastasis may become dense
    - Sclerotic myeloma usually in POEMS syndrome
    - POEMS: Polyneuropathy, organomegaly, endocrinopathy, M-spike, skin changes
  - ○ Systemic disorders
    - Sickle cell disease, osteopetrosis, renal osteodystrophy, myelofibrosis, fluorosis, hypervitaminosis A or D, mastocytosis
  - ○ Iatrogenic
    - Radiation
  - ○ Infection
  - ○ Healing fracture
  - ○ Neuroarthropathy

CLINICAL ISSUES

Presentation
- Most common signs/symptoms: Asymptomatic or back pain, neurologic symptoms

DIAGNOSTIC CHECKLIST

Consider
- First consideration in widespread sclerosis is metastatic disease

SELECTED REFERENCES

1. Multiple myeloma presenting with widespread osteosclerotic lesions: Joint Bone Spine. 71(1):79-83, 2004
2. Krishnan A et al: Primary bone lymphoma: radiographic-MR imaging correlation. Radiographics. 23(6):1371-83; discussion 1384-7, 2003
3. Jevtic V: Imaging of renal osteodystrophy. Eur J Radiol. 46(2):85-95, 2003
4. Thrall JH et al: Skeletal metastases. Radiol Clin North Am. 25(6):1155-70, 1987
5. Burgener FA et al: Differential diagnosis in Conventional Radiology. New York, Georg Thieme Verlag.11-24, 1985
6. Galasko CS: Mechanisms of lytic and blastic metastatic disease of bone. Clin Orthop. (169):20-7, 1982

IMAGE GALLERY

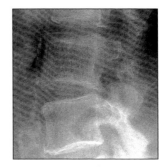 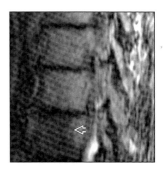

(Left) Lateral radiography shows Paget disease of L3 with enlargement of the vertebra, thickened endplates, and thickened trabeculae. Pedicles are also involved. (Right) Sagittal STIR MR shows very low signal intensity of blastic metastasis (arrow). Metastasis was also low signal intensity on T1WI. Despite lack of visible edema, metastasis was active and painful.

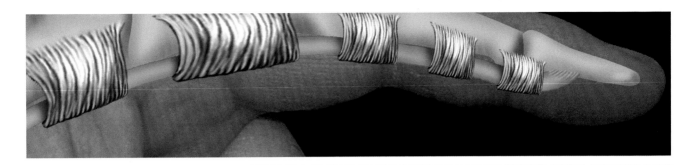

INDEX

INDEX

INDEX

INDEX

INDEX

INDEX

INDEX

L

INDEX

i

xvii

INDEX

INDEX

INDEX

INDEX

INDEX

i

xxix

INDEX

INDEX

i

xxxi